BM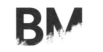

KT-528-420

FROM LIBRARY

WITHDRAWN

BRITISH MEDICAL ASSOCIATION

0970088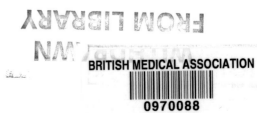

Berek & Hacker's Gynecologic Oncology

Sixth Edition

Jonathan S. Berek, MD, MMS

Laurie Kraus Lacob Professor
Director, Stanford Women's Cancer Center
Stanford Cancer Institute
Chair, Department of Obstetrics and Gynecology
Stanford University School of Medicine
Stanford, California

Neville F. Hacker, AM, MD

Professor of Gynaecologic Oncology
Conjoint, University of New South Wales
Director, Gynaecologic Cancer Centre
Royal Hospital for Women
Sydney, Australia

Illustrations and design by
Deborah Berek, MA
Tim Hengst, CMI, FAMI

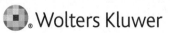 Wolters Kluwer

Philadelphia • Baltimore • New York • London
Buenos Aires • Hong Kong • Sydney • Tokyo

WITHDRAWN FROM LIBRARY

Acquisitions Editor: Jamie M. Elfrank
Product Development Editor: Ashley Fischer
Editorial Assistant: Brian Convery
Production Project Manager: Bridgett Dougherty
Design Coordinator: Stephen Druding
Illustration Coordinator: Jennifer Clements
Manufacturing Coordinator: Beth Welsh
Marketing Manager: Stephanie Kindlick
Prepress Vendor: Aptara, Inc.

6th edition

Copyright © 2015 Wolters Kluwer

Copyright © 2010 Wolters Kluwer Health/Lippincott Williams & Wilkins. Copyright © 2005 by Lippincott Williams & Wilkins. All rights reserved. This book is protected by copyright. No part of this book may be reproduced or transmitted in any form or by any means, including as photocopies or scanned-in or other electronic copies, or utilized by any information storage and retrieval system without written permission from the copyright owner, except for brief quotations embodied in critical articles and reviews. Materials appearing in this book prepared by individuals as part of their official duties as U.S. government employees are not covered by the above-mentioned copyright. To request permission, please contact Wolters Kluwer at Two Commerce Square, 2001 Market Street, Philadelphia, PA 19103, via email at permissions@lww.com, or via our website at lww.com (products and services).

9 8 7 6 5 4 3 2 1

Printed in China

Library of Congress Cataloging-in-Publication Data

Berek & Hacker's gynecologic oncology / [edited by] Jonathan S. Berek, Neville F. Hacker ; illustrations and design by Tim Hengst, George Barile, Deborah Berek. – 6th edition.
     p. ; cm.
  Berek and Hacker's gynecologic oncology
  Gynecologic oncology
  Includes bibliographical references and index.
  ISBN 978-1-4511-9007-6 (alk. paper)
  I. Berek, Jonathan S., editor. II. Hacker, Neville F., editor. III. Title: Berek and Hacker's gynecologic oncology. IV. Title: Gynecologic oncology.
  [DNLM: 1. Genital Neoplasms, Female. 2. Genitalia, Female–physiopathology. WP 145]
  RC280.G5
  616.99'465–dc23

2014032705

This work is provided "as is," and the publisher disclaims any and all warranties, express or implied, including any warranties as to accuracy, comprehensiveness, or currency of the content of this work.

This work is no substitute for individual patient assessment based upon healthcare professionals' examination of each patient and consideration of, among other things, age, weight, gender, current or prior medical conditions, medication history, laboratory data and other factors unique to the patient. The publisher does not provide medical advice or guidance and this work is merely a reference tool. Healthcare professionals, and not the publisher, are solely responsible for the use of this work including all medical judgments and for any resulting diagnosis and treatments.

Given continuous, rapid advances in medical science and health information, independent professional verification of medical diagnoses, indications, appropriate pharmaceutical selections and dosages, and treatment options should be made and healthcare professionals should consult a variety of sources. When prescribing medication, healthcare professionals are advised to consult the product information sheet (the manufacturer's package insert) accompanying each drug to verify, among other things, conditions of use, warnings and side effects and identify any changes in dosage schedule or contradictions, particularly if the medication to be administered is new, infrequently used or has a narrow therapeutic range. To the maximum extent permitted under applicable law, no responsibility is assumed by the publisher for any injury and/or damage to persons or property, as a matter of products liability, negligence law or otherwise, or from any reference to or use by any person of this work.

LWW.com

CCS1014

To Deborah and Estelle, and to our patients, from whom we are always learning, and who continue to inspire us with their courage.

Contributors

Spencer R. Adams, MD

Assistant Clinical Professor
Department of Internal Medicine
UCLA David Geffen School of Medicine
Internal Medicine Hospitalist
Director of Perioperative Medical Services
Los Angeles, California

Frédéric Amant, MD, PhD

Head, Scientific Section of Gynecological Oncology
Catholic University of Leuven
Staff Member, Gynecological Oncology
University Hospitals of Leuven
Leuven, Belgium

Barbara L. Andersen, PhD

Professor
Department of Psychology
James Cancer Hospital
Solove Research Institute
The Ohio State University
Columbus, Ohio

Walter F. Baile, MD

Professor
Department of Behavioral Science and Psychiatry
Psychiatrist and Director
Program for Interpersonal Communication and
Relationship Enhancement
MD Anderson Cancer Center
University of Texas
Houston, Texas

Andrew Berchuck, MD

Professor and Director
Department of Obstetrics and Gynecology
Division of Gynecologic Oncology
Duke University School of Medicine
Durham, North Carolina

Ross S. Berkowitz, MD

William H. Baker Professor of Gynecology
Department of Obstetrics, Gynecology and
Reproductive Biology
Harvard Medical School
Director of Gynecologic Oncology
Co-Director, New England Trophoblastic Disease Center
Brigham and Women's Hospital
Dana Farber Cancer Institute
Boston, Massachusetts

Michael J. Campion, MD

Director of Preinvasive Disease
Gynaecological Cancer Centre
Royal Hospital for Women
Sydney, Australia

Karen Canfell, DPhil

Associate Professor
Lowry Cancer Research Centre
Prince of Wales Clinical School
University of New South Wales
Sydney, Australia

David Cibula, MD, PhD

Professor
First Faculty of Medicine
Charles University
Chair, Gynecologic Oncology Centre
General University Hospital in Prague
Prague, Czech Republic

Daniel W. Cramer, MD

Professor
Department of Obstetrics, Gynecology and
Reproductive Biology
Harvard Medical School
Brigham and Women's Hospital
Boston, Massachusetts

Catherine M. Dang, MD

Associate Director
Wasserman Breast Cancer Risk Reduction Program
Department of Surgery
Cedars-Sinai Medical Center
Los Angeles, California

Oliver Dorigo, MD, PhD

Associate Professor and Director
Division of Gynecologic Oncology
Director, Mary Lake Polan
Gynecologic Oncology Research Laboratory
Department of Obstetrics and Gynecology
Stanford University School of Medicine
Director, Gynecologic Cancer Care Program
Stanford Women's Cancer Center
Stanford Cancer Institute
Stanford, California

Patricia J. Eifel, MD

Professor
Department of Radiation Oncology
MD Anderson Cancer Center
University of Texas
Houston, Texas

Patricia Eshaghian, MD

Assistant Clinical Professor of Medicine
Division of Pulmonary and Critical Care Medicine
UCLA David Geffen School of Medicine
Santa Monica, California

Michael L. Friedlander, MBChB, PhD

Conjoint Professor of Medicine
University of New South Wales
Director of Medical Oncology
The Prince of Wales Hospital
Consultant Medical Oncologist
Royal Hospital for Women
Sydney, Australia

Stéphanie Gaillard, MD, PhD

Assistant Professor
Division of Medical Oncology
Duke Cancer Institute
Durham, North Carolina

Alexandra Gentry-Mararaj, PhD

Senior Research Associate
Department of Women's Cancer
EGA Institute for Women's Health
University College London
England, United Kingdom

Arnando E. Giuliano, MD

Clinical Professor of Surgery
UCLA David Geffen School of Medicine
Executive Vice Chair
Department of Surgery
Cedars-Sinai Medical Center
Los Angeles, California

Donald P. Goldstein, MD

Professor
Department of Obstetrics, Gynecology and
Reproductive Biology
Harvard Medical School
Co-Director, New England Trophoblastic Disease Center
Brigham and Women's Cancer Center
Boston, Massachusetts

Walter H. Gotlieb, MD, PhD

Professor
Department of Oncology
Department of Obstetrics and Gynecology
McGill University
Director of Gynecology
Segal Cancer Center
Jewish General Hospital
Montreal, Canada

Kenneth D. Hatch, MD

Professor
Department of Obstetrics and Gynecology
University of Arizona School of Medicine
University Medical Center
Tucson, Arizona

Michael R. Hendrickson, MD

Professor Emeritus
Department of Pathology
Stanford University School of Medicine
Director of Surgical Pathology
Stanford Health Care
Stanford, California

Ian Jacobs, MBBS, MD

Vice Chancellor
University of New South Wales
Sydney, Australia

Amer Karam, MD

Associate Clinical Professor
Associate Director and Director of Outreach
Division of Gynecologic Oncology
Department of Obstetrics and Gynecology
Stanford University School of Medicine
Stanford Women's Cancer Center
Stanford, California

Reza Khorsan, MD

Assistant Professor of Medicine
Department of Medicine
UCLA David Geffen School of Medicine
Los Angeles, California
Nephrologist, Department of Medicine
Santa Monica-UCLA Medical Center
Santa Monica, California

Christina S. Kong, MD

Associate Professor
Department of Pathology
Stanford University School of Medicine
Director of Cytopathology
Stanford Health Care
Stanford, California

Roger M. Lee, MD

Assistant Clinical Professor
Department of Internal Medicine
UCLA David Geffen School of Medicine
Los Angeles, California
Santa Monica-UCLA Medical Center
Santa Monica, California

J. Norelle Lickiss, MD

Clinical Professor
University of Sydney
Consultant Emeritus
Royal Prince Alfred Hospital, Camperdam &
Royal Hospital for Women
New South Wales, Australia

Teri A. Longacre, MD

Professor
Department of Pathology
Stanford University School of Medicine
Associate Director of Surgical Pathology
Stanford Health Care
Stanford, California

Paul M. Maggio, MD

Assistant Professor
Department of Surgery
Stanford University School of Medicine
Co-director, Critical Care Medicine
Stanford Health Care
Stanford, California

Maurie Markman, MD

Clinical Professor of Medicine
Drexel University College of Medicine
President of Medicine and Science
Cancer Treatment Centers of America
Philadelphia, Pennsylvania

G. Larry Maxwell, MD

Professor of Obstetrics and Gynecology
Virginia Commonwealth University School of Medicine
Chair, Department of Obstetrics and Gynecology
Inova Fairfax Hospital
Falls Church, Virginia

Usha Menon, MD

Head, Department of Gynaecological Oncology
Gynaecological Cancer Research Centre
Institute for Women's Health
Consultant Gynaecologist
University College London
England, United Kingdom

Roseanne Moses, MMed, MBBS

Senior Staff Specialist
Palliative Medicine
Gynaecological Cancer Centre
Royal Hospital For Women
New South Wales, Australia

Jennifer A. M. Philip, PhD, MMed, MBBS

Associate Professor
Center for Palliative Care
University of Melbourne
Deputy Director, Palliative Medicine
St. Vincent's Hospital
Melbourne, Australia

Joshua Z. Press, MD, MSc

Gynecologic Oncologist
Pacific Gynecology Specialists
Division of Oncology and Pelvic Surgery
Seattle, Washington

Norman W. Rizk, MD

Berthod and Bell N. Guggenhime Professor in Medicine
Senior Associate Dean for Clinical Affairs
Stanford University School of Medicine
Chief Medical Officer
Stanford Health Care
Stanford University School of Medicine
Stanford, California

Samuel A. Skootsky, MD

Chief Medical Officer
UCLA Faculty Practice Group and Medical Group
Professor of Medicine
UCLA David Geffen School of Medicine
Los Angeles, California

M. Iain Smith, MD

Assistant Clinical Professor
Department of Medicine
UCLA David Geffen School of Medicine
Los Angeles, California

Anil K. Sood, MD

Professor
Department of Gynecologic Oncology
MD Anderson Cancer Center
Houston, Texas

Kathryn L. Terry, ScD

Assistant Professor
Obstetrics, Gynecology, and Reproductive Biology
Harvard Medical School
Associate Epidemiologist
Brigham and Women's Hospital
Boston, Massachusetts

Laszlo Ungar, MD

Professor
Department of Obstetrics and Gynecology
Albert Szentgyorgyi Medical University
Head, Metropolitan Gynecological Service
St. Stephen and Jahn Ferenc Hospitals
Budapest, Hungary

Jan B. Vermorken, MD, PhD

Emeritus Professor of Medical Sciences
Antwerp University
Antwerp, Belgium
Consultant in Medical Oncology
Antwerp University Hospital
Edegem, Belgium

Kristen C. Williams, MA

Department of Psychology
James Cancer Hospital
Solove Research Institute
The Ohio State University
Columbus, Ohio

Foreword to the First Edition

Close to the beginning of this century, William Osler observed, "The practice of medicine is an art, based on science." That brief characterization of our profession rings true, even as we approach the next century in the midst of brilliant, accelerating scientific discovery.

Some aspects of the art—including compassion and the basic skills of history taking and physical examination—are, or should be, common to all physicians and remain largely unchanged by a century of research. In other ways, the "art," which can also be translated as "craft" from the original Greek work "techne," has been greatly enlarged and diversified by science and technology. Thus, the special skills required by a gynecologic oncologist derive not only from experience and practice, but also from the proliferation of knowledge in many branches of science. Indeed, it is mainly the developments of science in obstetrics and gynecology—and in some other disciplines— that have evolved the clinical subspecialty of gynecologic oncology.

The art and the science are connected not only by ancestry, however. Their relationship continues to be an interdependent one. One of the ever-expanding glories of medicine is that what is learned in the laboratory can enhance learning at the bedside and what is learned from experience with patients helps to shape and direct scientific inquiry.

Doctors who remain lifelong students are exhilarated by these interconnections and make the best teachers of clinical medicine. It is in the scholarly tradition that Jonathan S. Berek and Neville F. Hacker, with contributions from distinguished colleagues in their own discipline and in fields that bear upon it, have brought together the salient information required to develop the acumen and skills that enable clinicians to understand and to care for women suffering from tumors.

Practical Gynecologic Oncology reflects the indivisibility of art and science in medicine. The two editors—one in Los Angeles and one in Sydney—worked and studied together for 7 years in the same hospital and laboratories and remain mutually helpful intellectual allies on opposite shores of the Pacific Ocean.

Sherman M. Mellinkoff, MD
Dean Emeritus
Professor of Medicine
UCLA David Geffen School of Medicine
Los Angeles, California

Preface

The discipline of gynecologic oncology has changed since its inception as a subspecialty of Obstetrics and Gynecology in the United States in 1973. In its early years, the gynecologic oncologist was seen as the physician who was able to deal with virtually all of the surgical needs of a woman with a gynecologic malignancy, and usually all of the chemotherapeutic needs as well. With significant advances in all fields of surgery and the establishment of medical oncology as a legitimate subspecialty of medicine, the role of the gynecologic oncologist has evolved into that of the leader of a large multidisciplinary team. The team includes not only a variety of medical specialists, but also oncology nurses and paramedical personnel, including psychologists, social workers, physiotherapists, and dietitians.

The surgical management of advanced ovarian cancer has become more radical, with increasing emphasis on the need to resect all macroscopic metastatic disease. This has necessitated collaboration with hepatobiliary and even thoracic surgeons in selected cases. On the other hand, a more conservative approach to the lymph nodes has been advocated by some for vulvar, cervical, and endometrial cancer, and these concepts are addressed in this new edition.

All chapters have been extensively revised and updated, but special mention should be made of the contributions of new authors. Robotic surgery is being more widely practiced, and a new chapter, written by Joshua Press and Walter Gottlieb from Canada, leading exponents of this technique, has been devoted to this topic. David Cibula, an internationally acknowledged surgeon from Prague, and Amer Karam from Stanford contributed to the chapter on surgical techniques.

The changing concepts of the biology of cervical cancer precursors, the more widespread introduction of the vaccine against the human papilloma—virus (HPV), and the recent modifications to the screening guidelines for cervical cancer are addressed by Michael Campion and a new co-author, Karen Canfell, an acknowledged international authority on cancer screening. The chapter on Cancer in Pregnancy has been rewritten by Frederic Amant from Belgium and Laszlo Ungar from Budapest, who have extensively studied this topic.

The multidisciplinary approach to gynecologic cancer has been acknowledged by the inclusion as co-authors of Patricia Eifel, a radiation oncologist from the M–D Anderson Hospital in Houston, on the chapters on vulvar and vaginal cancer, Jan Vermorken, a medical oncologist from Antwerp on the chapter on cervical cancer, and Michael Friedlander, a medical oncologist from Sydney, on the chapters on uterine, ovarian, and germ cell tumors. Dr. Friedlander, who has been the consultant medical oncologist at the Royal Hospital for Women for the past 25 years, has also extensively revised the chapter on chemotherapy.

The first four editions of our book were titled *Practical Gynecologic Oncology*. In recognition of its sustained utility, Lippincott Williams & Wilkins renamed the fifth edition *Berek & Hacker's Gynecologic Oncology*, and we have retained that title for this sixth edition. Since the fourth edition, our book has been officially translated into Chinese and Spanish, an acknowledgment of its international appeal.

This edition preserves the basic format and style of the previous editions, being divided into four sections: general principles, disease sites, medical and surgical topics, and quality of life. As with previous editions, where level I evidence is not available, we have interjected our personal biases, but have tried to justify our position with adequate reference to the available literature.

We are most grateful to Tim Hengst for his outstanding illustrations and drawings, and to Deborah Berek for her valuable assistance with design and editing. We thank Estelle Hacker for her assistance with the manuscript. We gratefully acknowledge Kerry Garcia for her assistance at Stanford. We appreciate the important contribution of the Lippincott Williams & Wilkins staff, especially Rebecca Gaertner, Ashley Fisher, Bridgett Dougherty, and Indu Jawwad. Finally, we extend special thanks to Charley Mitchell who has been supportive of our book since its inception.

At Stanford, we acknowledge the generosity of our benefactors, especially Laurie Kraus Lacob, Nicole Kidman, Keith Urban, Garth Brooks, Trisha Yearwood, and the Under One Umbrella Committee on behalf of the Stanford Women's Cancer Center; and the support of our colleagues—Dean Emeritus Philip Pizzo, Stanford University School of Medicine; Beverly Mitchell, Director, Stanford Cancer Institute; Amir Rubin, CEO, Stanford Health Care; and Sri Seshadri,

Vice President, Stanford Health Care. In Sydney, we acknowledge the support of our multidisciplinary team at the Gynecological Cancer Center of the Royal Hospital for Women. All are committed to excellence in patient-centered care, and all are constantly striving to improve outcomes for gynecologic cancer patients. At both institutions, the enduring support of our benefactors has been critical to our gynecologic oncology research and clinical programs.

Our book is written primarily for gynecologic oncologists, fellows undertaking training in gynecologic oncology and consultant gynecologists as well as medical oncologists and radiation oncologists whose practices involve a significant component of gynecologic cancer care.

We offer this book to those who strive to improve the care of women with gynecologic malignancies.

Jonathan S. Berek

Neville F. Hacker

Contents

Section I
General Principles

Section II
Disease Sites

GENERAL
PRINCIPLES

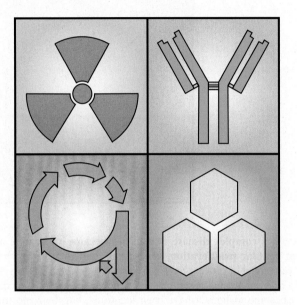

1 Biology and Genetics

Stéphanie Gaillard
G. Larry Maxwell
Anil K. Sood
Andrew Berchuck

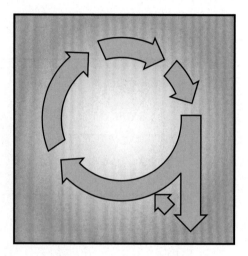

Cancer is a complex disease that arises because of genetic and epigenetic alterations that disrupt cellular proliferation, senescence, and death (Fig. 1.1). The alterations that underlie the development of cancers have a diverse etiology, and the loss of DNA repair mechanisms often plays a role in allowing mutations to accumulate. Specific molecular changes that cause a normal cell to become malignant have been identified, but their spectrum varies considerably between cancer types.

The malignant phenotype is characterized by the ability to invade surrounding tissues and metastasize. The development of a cancer elicits a considerable molecular response in the local microenvironment that is characterized by recruitment of stromal elements such as new blood vessels and by an active immunologic response. These secondary events play a critical role in the evolution and progression of cancers. Although the molecular pathogenesis of gynecologic cancers has been only partially elucidated, advances in the understanding of these diseases are providing the opportunity for improvements in diagnosis, treatment, and prevention.

The initial sections of this chapter will outline what is known regarding the basic molecular mechanisms involved in the development of cancers and the evolution of the malignant phenotype. The molecular alterations characteristic of gynecologic cancers will be outlined in the later sections.

Growth Regulation

Proliferation

The number of cells in normal tissues is tightly regulated by a balance between cellular proliferation and death. The final common pathway for cell division involves distinct molecular switches that control cell cycle progression from G_1 to the S phase of DNA synthesis. These include the retinoblastoma (*Rb*) and E2F proteins and their various regulatory cyclins, cyclin-dependent kinases (cdks), and cdk inhibitors. Likewise, the events that facilitate progression from G_2 to mitosis and cell division are regulated by other cyclins and cdks (Fig. 1.2).

In some tissues—such as the bone marrow, epidermis and gastrointestinal tract—the life span of mature cells is relatively short, and high rates of proliferation by progenitor cells are required to

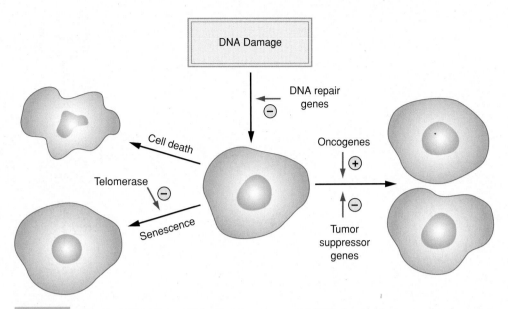

Figure 1.1 Role of proliferation, cell death, senescence, and DNA damage in cancer development.

maintain the population. In other tissues—such as liver, muscle, and brain—cells are long lived, and proliferation rarely occurs. **Complex molecular mechanisms have evolved to closely regulate proliferation.** These involve a finely tuned balance between stimulatory and inhibitory growth signals.

Dysregulation of cellular proliferation is one of the main hallmarks of cancer. There may be increased activity of genes involved in stimulating proliferation (oncogenes) or loss of growth inhibitory (tumor suppressor) genes or both. In the past, it was thought that cancer might arise solely because of more rapid proliferation or a higher fraction of proliferating cells. Although increased proliferation is a characteristic of many cancers and is an appealing therapeutic target (1), the fraction of cancer cells actively dividing, and the time required to transit the cell cycle, is not strikingly different between many cancers and corresponding normal cells of the same lineage. Altered regulation of proliferation is only one of several factors that contribute to malignant transformation. Ultimately, the relative balance of growth stimulatory factors and inhibitory factors is shifted in malignancy to promote unregulated cellular proliferation.

Cell Death

In addition to being driven by increased proliferation, growth of a cancer may be attributable to cellular resistance to death. **At least three distinct types of cell death pathways have been characterized, including apoptosis, necrosis, and autophagy** (2). **All three pathways may be ongoing simultaneously within a tumor** and methods that distinguish between them are far from perfect.

Apoptosis

The term *apoptosis* is derived from Greek, and alludes to a process akin to leaves dying and falling off a tree. **Apoptosis is an active, energy-dependent process that involves cleavage of the DNA by endonucleases and proteins by proteases called *caspases*.** Morphologically, apoptosis is characterized by condensation of chromatin, nuclear and cytoplasmic blebbing, and cellular shrinkage. The molecular events that affect apoptosis in response to various stimuli are complex and have been only partially elucidated (3), but several reliable markers of apoptosis have been discovered including annexin V, caspase-3 activation, and DNA fragmentation (4).

External stimuli such as tumor necrosis factor, tumor necrosis factor-related apoptosis-inducing ligand, fatty acid synthase (Fas), and other death ligands that interact with cell surface receptors can induce activation of caspases, and lead to apoptosis via an extrinsic pathway (Fig. 1.3). The intrinsic pathway is activated in response to a wide range of stresses including DNA damage and deprivation of growth factors. **The intrinsic apoptosis pathway is regulated by a complex interaction**

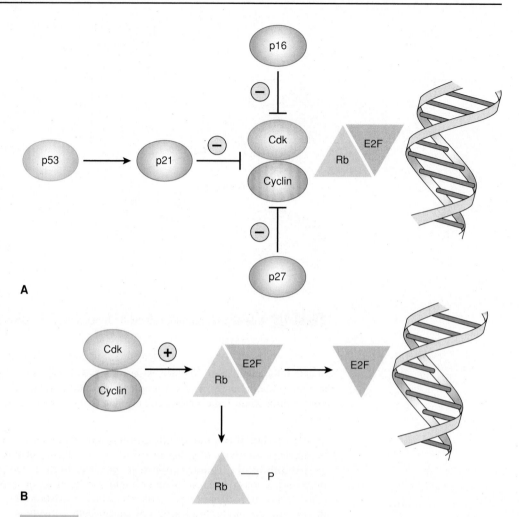

Figure 1.2 Regulation of cell cycle arrest in G₁ by cyclin-dependent kinase (cdk) inhibitors. **A:** Cell cycle arrest. **B:** Cell cycle progression.

of proapoptotic and antiapoptotic proteins in the mitochondrial membrane that affect its permeability. Proteins that increase permeability allow the release of cytochrome c, which activates the apoptosome complex leading to the activation of caspases leading to apoptosis. Conversely, proteins that stabilize mitochondrial membranes inhibit apoptosis. The first major insight that led to the understanding of the intrinsic apoptotic pathway was the finding that an activating translocation of the *bcl-2* gene in B-cell lymphomas resulted in essentially a complete inhibition of apoptosis (5). Subsequent studies have demonstrated that the antiapoptotic effect of *bcl-2* is attributable to stabilization of the mitochondrial membrane. Additional genes related to *bcl-2* (such as *BAD, BCL-XL,* and others) block apoptosis by inhibiting membrane permeability. Other genes in the *BCL* family (such as *BAX, BAK,* and others) increase membrane permeability and are proapoptotic. **An increased understanding of the complex system of molecular checks and balances involved in regulation of apoptosis provides opportunities for targeted cancer therapies;** several strategies are under development (6).

In addition to restraining the number of cells in a population, apoptosis serves an important role in preventing malignant transformation by allowing the elimination of cells that have undergone genetic damage. Following exposure of cells to mutagenic stimuli, including radiation and carcinogenic drugs, the cell cycle is arrested so that DNA damage may be repaired. If DNA repair is not sufficient, apoptosis occurs so that damaged cells do not survive. This serves as an anticancer surveillance mechanism by which mutated cells are eliminated before they become fully transformed. In this regard, **the *TP53* tumor suppressor gene is a critical regulator of cell cycle arrest and apoptosis in response to DNA damage, and the frequency of *TP53* mutations in human cancers reflects its critical role in preventing tumorigenesis.**

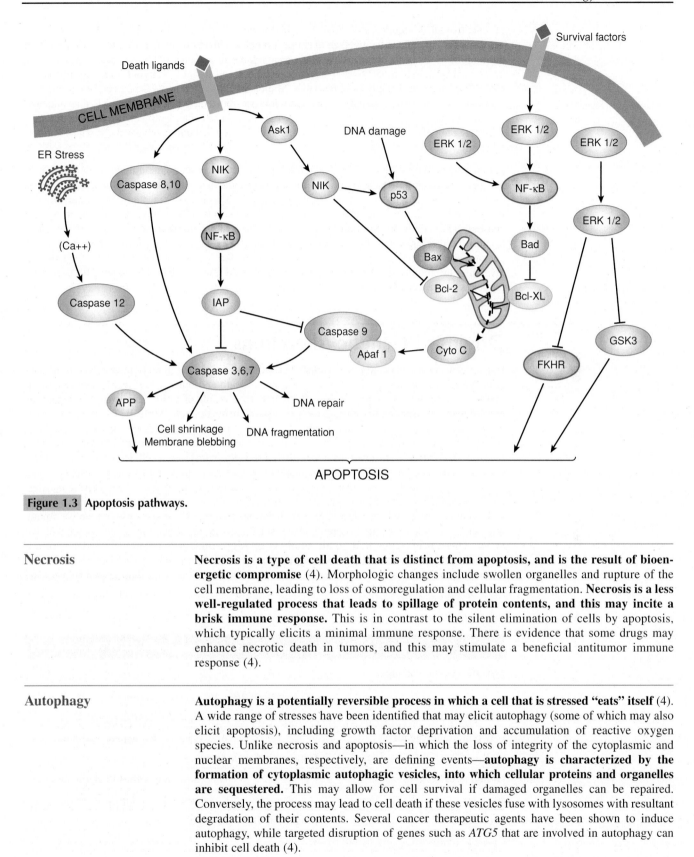

Figure 1.3 Apoptosis pathways.

Necrosis	Necrosis is a type of cell death that is distinct from apoptosis, and is the result of bioenergetic compromise (4). Morphologic changes include swollen organelles and rupture of the cell membrane, leading to loss of osmoregulation and cellular fragmentation. **Necrosis is a less well-regulated process that leads to spillage of protein contents, and this may incite a brisk immune response.** This is in contrast to the silent elimination of cells by apoptosis, which typically elicits a minimal immune response. There is evidence that some drugs may enhance necrotic death in tumors, and this may stimulate a beneficial antitumor immune response (4).
Autophagy	**Autophagy is a potentially reversible process in which a cell that is stressed "eats" itself** (4). A wide range of stresses have been identified that may elicit autophagy (some of which may also elicit apoptosis), including growth factor deprivation and accumulation of reactive oxygen species. Unlike necrosis and apoptosis—in which the loss of integrity of the cytoplasmic and nuclear membranes, respectively, are defining events—**autophagy is characterized by the formation of cytoplasmic autophagic vesicles, into which cellular proteins and organelles are sequestered.** This may allow for cell survival if damaged organelles can be repaired. Conversely, the process may lead to cell death if these vesicles fuse with lysosomes with resultant degradation of their contents. Several cancer therapeutic agents have been shown to induce autophagy, while targeted disruption of genes such as *ATG5* that are involved in autophagy can inhibit cell death (4).
Cellular Senescence	**Normal cells are capable of undergoing division only a finite number of times before becoming senescent. Cellular senescence is regulated** by a biologic clock related to progressive shortening

of repetitive DNA sequences (TTAGGG) called **telomeres** that cap the ends of each chromosome. Telomeres are thought to be involved in chromosomal stabilization and in preventing recombination during mitosis. At birth, chromosomes have long telomeric sequences (150,000 bases) that become progressively shorter by 50 to 200 bases each time a cell divides. **Telomeric shortening is the molecular clock that triggers senescence.** Malignant cells often avoid senescence by turning on expression of telomerase activity to prevent telomeric shortening (7). Telomerase is a ribonucleoprotein complex, and both the protein and RNA subunits have been identified. The RNA component serves as a template for telomeric extension, and the protein subunit catalyzes the synthesis of new telomeric repeats.

Telomerase activity is detectable in a high fraction of many cancers, including ovarian (8), cervical (9,10), and endometrial (11). It has been suggested that detection of telomerase might be useful for early diagnosis of cancer, but the lack of specificity is a significant issue. In this regard, endometrium is one of the normal adult tissues in which telomerase expression is most common (12). Perhaps this relates to the need for a large number of lifetime cell divisions because of the rapid growth and shedding of this tissue each month during the reproductive years. Therapeutic approaches to inhibiting telomerase are under development, focusing on reversing the immortalized state of cancer cells to make them susceptible once again to normal replicative senescence (7).

Origins of Genetic Alterations

Human cancers arise because of a series of genetic and epigenetic alterations that lead to disruption of normal mechanisms that govern cell growth, death and senescence (13,14). **Genetic damage may be inherited or may arise after birth as a result of either exposure to exogenous carcinogens or endogenous mutagenic processes within the cell** (Table 1.1). The incidence of most cancers increases with aging because the longer one is alive, the higher the likelihood that a cell will acquire sufficient damage to become fully transformed. **It is thought that at least three to six critical "driver" alterations are required to fully transform a cell.** However, most cancer cells are genetically unstable, with an average of 30 to 100 acquired mutations per cancer. Some of these may be simply "passenger" mutations that occur as a result of generalized genetic instability. Although not involved in malignant transformation, these may contribute to evolution of the malignant phenotype with respect to growth, invasion, metastasis, and response to therapy, among other characteristics. Genetic instability also results in evolution of heterogeneous clones within a tumor. **There is evidence that small numbers of progenitor cells (stem cells) exist within a tumor and have the capacity to regenerate tumors.** The stem cell theory suggests that these dormant or quiescent stem cells may be more resistant to therapy, and thus responsible for the development of recurrent disease (15).

Table 1.1 Origins of Genetic Damage in Human Cancers	
Type of Genetic Damage	*Examples*
Hereditary	
High-penetrance genes	BRCA1, BRCA2, MLH1, MSH2
Low-penetrance genes	APC I1307 K in colorectal cancer
Exogenous Carcinogens	
Ultraviolet radiation	TP53 and other genes in skin cancer
Tobacco	K-ras and TP53 in lung cancer
Endogenous DNA Damage	
Cytosine methylation and deamination	TP53 in ovarian and other cancers
Hydrolysis	Various genes
Spontaneous errors in DNA synthesis	Various genes
Oxidative stress with free radical damage	Various genes

Inherited Cancer Susceptibility

Although most cancers arise sporadically in the population because of acquired genetic damage, inherited mutations in cancer susceptibility genes are responsible for some cases. Families with these mutations exhibit a high incidence of specific types of cancers. The age of cancer onset is younger in these families and it is not unusual for some individuals to be affected with multiple primary cancers.

The most common forms of hereditary cancer syndromes predispose to breast/ovarian (*BRCA1*, *BRCA2*) and colon/endometrial (Lynch syndrome genes such as *MSH2* and *MLH1*) cancers (Table 1.2). Examples of other hereditary cancer syndromes are outlined in Table 1.2. Beyond this list of known hereditary cancer syndromes, additional high penetrance genes have been discovered that are mutated infrequently but confer dramatically increased cancer risks. For example, in addition to BRCA1–2, germline mutations in a number of other genes in the homologous recombination (HR) DNA repair pathway confer susceptibility to breast/ovarian cancer (e.g., *RAD51 C/D*, *BRIP1*, *PALB2*). **This is leading to the development of hereditary cancer genetic test panels that will likely replace testing for individual genes.**

Tumor suppressor genes have been implicated most frequently in hereditary cancer syndromes, and many of these are DNA repair genes such as BRCA1–2 and the Lynch syndrome genes. In only a few instances are germline mutations in oncogenes responsible for hereditary cancers (Table 1.2). Although affected individuals carry the germline alteration in every cell of

Table 1.2 Hereditary Cancer Syndromes		
Syndrome	*Genes*	*Predominant Cancers*
Cancer Types in Which Hereditary Syndromes Are Common		
Hereditary breast/ovarian cancer	*BRCA1[a], BRCA2[a]*	Breast, ovary
Hereditary colorectal cancer	*MSH2[a], MLH1[a], PMS1[a], PMS2[a], MSH6[a]*	Colon, endometrium, other GI tract, ovary
Familial adenomatous polyposis	*APC*	Colonic polyps and brain cancers
Familial melanoma	*CMM1, CMM2, CDK4, CDKN2 (p16)*	Melanoma
Rare Hereditary Cancer Syndromes		
Li–Fraumeni syndrome	*TP53[a]*	Sarcomas, leukemias, breast, brain, and others
Wilms tumor	*WT1*	Kidney
von Hippel–Lindau	*VHL*	Kidney and others
Neurofibromatosis	*NF1, NF2*	Neurofibromas, GIST
Retinoblastoma	*Rb*	Retinoblastoma, sarcomas
Multiple-endocrine neoplasia 1	*MEN1*	Thyroid, adrenal, pancreas, pituitary, parathyroid
Multiple-endocrine neoplasia 2	*ret[b]*	Thyroid, adrenal, parathyroid
Hereditary papillary renal cancer	*met[b]*	Papillary kidney
Cowden	*PTEN*	Hamartomatous tumors, breast cancer, variety of other cancers
Hereditary GIST	*cKIT[b]*	Gastric and small bowel GIST, GI paragangliomas
Ataxia telangiectasia	*ATM[a]*	Lymphoma, acute leukemia
Xeroderma pigmentosum	*XPA-G[a], POLH[a]*	Cutaneous basal cell and squamous cell carcinomas
Fanconi anemia	*FANCA-N[a]*	Leukemia, squamous cell carcinomas
Nijmegen breakage	*NBS1[a]*	Lymphoma
Peutz–Jeghers syndrome	*STK11*	GI cancers, ovarian granulosa cell tumors

[a]DNA repair genes.

[b]Oncogenes.

GI, gastrointestinal; GIST, gastrointestinal stromal tumor.

their bodies, paradoxically, cancer susceptibility genes are characterized by a limited repertoire of cancers. There is no relationship between expression patterns of these genes in various organs and the development of specific types of cancers. For example, *BRCA1* expression is high in the testis, but men who inherit mutations in this gene are not predisposed to develop testicular cancer. **The penetrance of cancer susceptibility genes is incomplete because not all individuals who inherit a mutation develop cancer.** The emergence of cancers in carriers depends on the occurrence of additional genetic alterations.

The familial cancer syndromes described above result from rare mutations that occur in less than 1% of the population. Low-penetrance common genetic polymorphisms may also affect cancer susceptibility, albeit less dramatically (16). There are more than 10 million polymorphic genetic loci in the human genome, and many of these polymorphisms are common in the population. **Although genetic polymorphisms do not increase risk sufficiently to produce familial cancer clustering, they could account for a significant fraction of cancers currently classified as sporadic,** because of their relatively high prevalence. For example, 6% of Ashkenazi Jews carry the less common allele of a polymorphism in codon 1,307 of the *APC* gene that changes a single amino acid in the protein, and this increases the risk of colorectal cancer by about 50% (17). The recent development of genomic technologies that can assess hundreds of thousands of polymorphisms simultaneously in large numbers of individuals is fueling the search for additional genetic susceptibility polymorphisms (16). It is estimated that dozens to a few hundred of these likely exist for each cancer type. A more complete understanding of the genetic factors that affect cancer susceptibility could facilitate implementation of screening and preventive approaches in subsets of the population at increased risk.

Acquired Genetic Damage

The etiology of acquired genetic damage in cancers also has been elucidated to some extent. For example, a strong causal link exists between cigarette smoke and cancers of the aerodigestive tract and between ultraviolet radiation and skin cancer. **For many common forms of cancer** (colon, breast, endometrium, ovary), **a strong association with specific carcinogens does not exist.** It is thought that the genetic alterations responsible for these cancers arise mainly because of endogenous mutagenic processes such as methylation, deamination, and hydrolysis of DNA. Furthermore, spontaneous errors in DNA synthesis may occur during the process of DNA replication associated with normal proliferation. Finally, free radicals generated in response to inflammation and other cellular damage may cause DNA damage. These endogenous processes produce many mutations each day in every cell in the body. **While the multiple cellular mechanisms for DNA damage surveillance and repair are highly effective, some mutations may elude them.** The efficiency of these DNA damage-response systems varies between individuals because of genetic and other factors and may affect susceptibility to cancer.

Epigenetic Changes

Epigenetics changes are heritable changes that do not result from alterations in DNA sequence (14). Methylation of cytosine residues that reside next to guanine residues is the primary mechanism of epigenetic regulation, and this process is regulated by a family of DNA methyltransferases. **Most cancers have globally reduced DNA methylation, which may contribute to genomic instability.** Conversely, selective hypermethylation of cytosines in the promoter regions of tumor suppressor genes may lead to their inactivation and contribute to carcinogenesis.

There is a family of **imprinted genes** in which either the maternal or paternal copy is normally completely silenced because of methylation. Loss of imprinting in genes that stimulate proliferation, such as *insulin-like growth factor 2 (IGF2),* may provide an oncogenic stimulus further disrupting the balance between proliferation and cell death. **Acetylation and methylation of the histone proteins that coat DNA represent another level of epigenetic regulation** that is altered in cancer. While the underlying cause of these epigenetic alterations remains poorly understood, they represent appealing therapeutic targets. Histone deacetylase inhibitors and hypomethylating agents can reactivate the expression of genes silenced by acetylation and methylation, respectively, and are used for the treatment of some hematologic malignancies, such as myelodysplastic syndromes and lymphomas.

Oncogenes

Alterations in genes that stimulate cellular growth (oncogenes) can cause malignant transformation (13). Oncogenes can be activated via several mechanisms. Amplification of some oncogenes results in multiple copies of a gene with resultant overexpression of the corresponding protein. *HER2-neu* amplification in a subset of breast cancers is an example of a tumor driven by amplification of a single gene that can be therapeutically targeted using an anti-HER2 antibody, **trastuzumab.** Other oncogenes, such as **KIT** in gastrointestinal stromal tumors (GIST), may become overactive when affected by point mutations at codons that change a single amino acid leading to gain of function. Finally, oncogenes may be translocated from one chromosomal location to another and then come under the influence of promoter sequences that cause overexpression of the gene. This latter mechanism frequently occurs in leukemias and lymphomas (e.g., the BCR-ABL translocation in chronic myelogenous leukemia), but is relatively uncommon in gynecologic and other solid tumors. For tumorigenesis driven by activation of individual oncogenes, targeting the oncogene can be a useful therapeutic approach.

In cell culture systems, **many genes that are involved in normal growth regulatory pathways can elicit transformation when altered to overactive forms via amplification, mutation, or translocation.** On this basis, a large number of genes have been classified as oncogenes. Studies in human cancers have suggested that the actual spectrum of genes altered in the development of human cancers is more limited. A number of genes that elicit transformation when activated *in vitro* have not been documented to undergo alterations in human cancers. In this section, the various classes of oncogenes will be summarized and particular attention paid to those that are altered in gynecologic cancers.

Cell Membrane Oncogenes—Peptide Growth Factors and Their Receptors	**Peptide growth factors in the extracellular space–such as those of the epidermal growth factor (EGF), platelet-derived growth factor (PDGF), and fibroblast growth factor (FGF) families—stimulate a cascade of molecular events that leads to proliferation by binding to cell membrane receptors.** Growth factors are involved in normal cellular processes such as development, stromal–epithelial communication, tissue regeneration, and wound healing. Unlike endocrine hormones, which are secreted into the blood stream and act in distant target organs, peptide growth factors typically act in the local environment where they have been secreted.

Aberrant proliferative signaling through these peptide growth factor pathways can occur through a number of mechanisms: (1) Increased or inappropriate autocrine production of growth factors, (2) increased paracrine production of growth factors by tumor stromal environment, (3) increased responsiveness of receptors to growth factor ligands or ligand independent activation of the receptor, and (4) constitutive activation of components downstream of the receptor. Autocrine growth stimulation may be a key strategy by which cancer cell proliferation becomes autonomous. In this model, it is postulated that cancers secrete stimulatory growth factors that interact with receptors on the same cell. Although peptide growth factors provide a growth stimulatory signal, **there is little evidence to suggest that overproduction of growth factors is a precipitating event in the development of most cancers.** Increased expression of peptide growth factors likely serves to promote rather than initiate malignant transformation.

Cell membrane receptors that bind peptide growth factors are composed of an extracellular ligand-binding domain, a membrane spanning region, and a cytoplasmic tyrosine kinase domain (18). Binding of a growth factor to the extracellular domain results in aggregation and conformational shifts in the receptor and activation of the inner tyrosine kinase (Fig. 1.4). This kinase phosphorylates tyrosine residues on both the growth factor receptor itself (**autophosphorylation**) and on molecular targets in the cell interior, leading to activation of secondary signals.

Growth of some cancers is driven by overexpression of receptor tyrosine kinases. Therapeutic strategies that target receptor tyrosine kinases have been an active area of investigation. **Trastuzumab** is a monoclonal antibody that **blocks the HER-2/*neu* receptor** and it is widely used in the treatment of breast and gastric cancers that overexpress this tyrosine kinase (19). **Cetuximab** is a monoclonal antibody that targets the epidermal growth factor receptor (EGFR), whereas **gefitinib is a direct inhibitor of the EGFR tyrosine kinase** (20). Both are used in the treatment of EGFR-expressing nonsmall cell lung cancers. **Lapatinib** is a dual EGFR/HER-2 kinase inhibitor approved for treatment of HER-2 overexpressing breast cancers. **Imatinib antagonizes the activity of the BCR-ABL, c-kit, and PDGF receptor tyrosine kinases** and has proven effective in treatment of chronic myelogenous leukemias and gastrointestinal stromal tumors.

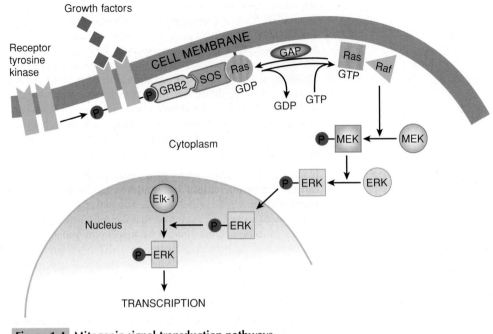

Figure 1.4 Mitogenic signal transduction pathways.

WNT Pathway

β-catenin (*CTNNB1*) is involved along with cadherins in cell-cell adhesion junctions and may play a role in inhibition of excessive growth when cells come in contact with each other (Fig. 1.5). β-catenin may be translocated to the nucleus and play a role in regulating transcription of genes involved in embryonic development, cell differentiation and cell polarity. β-catenin activity is regulated by the WNT pathway (21,22). The WNT family of genes encodes secreted peptides that interact with Frizzled family cell surface receptors. Frizzled activates the intracellular Dishevelled protein, resulting in an increase in the amount of β-catenin translocated to the nucleus. Dishevelled accomplishes this by inhibiting a complex of proteins that includes axin, GSK-3β, and APC that normally promote proteolytic degradation of β-catenin. This allows β-catenin to enter the nucleus and interact with TCF/LEF family transcription factors to promote gene expression.

Genes encoding WNT signaling inhibitors are often downregulated during carcinogenesis and driver mutations in several of these genes (*APC, Axin, GSK-3β, β-catenin*) occur frequently in human cancers, including endometrial cancers. Germline mutations in the APC gene are responsible for familial adenomatous polyposis of the colon.

Intracellular Oncogenes

Following the interaction of peptide growth factors and their receptors, secondary molecular signals are generated to transmit the growth stimulus to the nucleus. This function is served by a multitude of complex and overlapping signal transduction pathways that occur in the inner cell membrane and cytoplasm. Many of these signals involve phosphorylation of proteins by enzymes known as **nonreceptor kinases** (23). **These kinases transfer a phosphate group from ATP to specific amino acid residues of target proteins. The kinases that are involved in growth regulation include those that phosphorylate tyrosine residues on proteins, and others that are specific for serine or threonine residues such as *AKT*** (24). In addition, phosphatidylinositol (PIK) 3-kinases are a class of growth regulatory lipid kinases that phosphorylate inositol in the cell membrane (25). **The activity of kinases is regulated by phosphatases, such as *PTEN*, which act in opposition to the kinases by removing phosphates from the target proteins** (Fig. 1.6).

Guanosine-triphosphate–binding proteins (G proteins) represent another class of molecules involved in transmission of growth signals. They are located on the inner aspect of the cell membrane and have intrinsic GTPase activity that catalyzes the exchange of guanine-triphosphate (GTP) for guanine-diphosphate (GDP). In their active GTP-bound form, G proteins interact with kinases that are involved in relaying the mitogenic signal, such as those of the MAP kinase family. Conversely, hydrolysis of GTP to GDP, which is stimulated by GTPase-activating proteins (GAPs), leads to inactivation of G proteins.

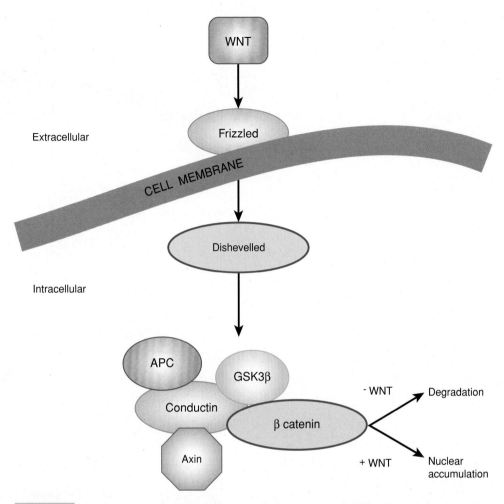

Figure 1.5 **Wingless (WNT) Beta-catenin signaling.** WNT extracellular ligands bind Frizzled receptors and regulate the phosphorylation status of axin. Axin functions as part of the destruction complex that regulates the stability of Beta-catenin, a transcriptional regulator. (Redrawn from **Berchuck A, Levine DA, Farley JH, et al.** Molecular pathogenesis of gynecologic cancers. In: Barakat RR, ed. *Principles and Practice of Gynecologic Oncology.* Lippincott Williams and Wilkins; 2013.)

The *ras* family of G proteins is among the most frequently mutated oncogenes in human cancers (e.g., gastrointestinal and endometrial cancers). Activation of *ras* genes usually involves point mutations in codons 12, 13, or 61 that result in constitutively activated molecules (26). Therapeutic approaches to interfering with *ras* signaling are being developed. The most successful approach involves inhibition of BRAF, a kinase that interacts with *ras* proteins in activating the MAP kinase pathway. *BRAF* mutations occur in many cancers that lack *ras* mutations, such as melanoma, where a mutation resulting in the substitution of glutamic acid for valine at amino acid 600 (V600E) is common. *Vemurafenib,* an inhibitor of the kinase domain of mutant *BRAF,* improves survival of melanoma patients whose tumors carry a *BRAF* mutation; however, the tumors ultimately develop resistance to the *BRAF* inhibitor by developing other mechanisms to activate growth pathways and circumvent BRAF inhibition (27).

Nuclear Oncogenes

If proliferation is to occur in response to signals generated in the cell membrane and cytoplasm, these events must lead to activation of nuclear transcription factors and other genetic products responsible for stimulating DNA replication and cell division. **Expression of several genes that encode nuclear proteins increases dramatically within minutes of treatment of cells with peptide growth factors.** When induced, the products of these genes bind to specific DNA regulatory elements and induce transcription of genes involved in DNA synthesis and cell division. Examples include the *fos* and *jun* oncogenes, which dimerize to form the activator protein 1 (AP1) transcription complex. When inappropriately overexpressed, these transcription factors can act as

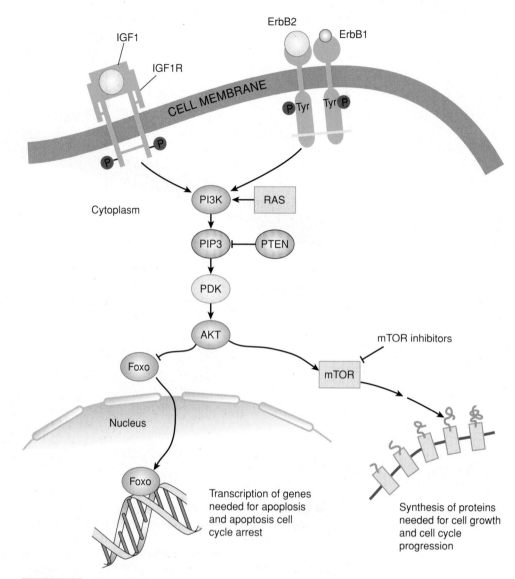

Figure 1.6 **The phosphatidylinositol 3-kinase (PI3 K) pathway is activated by RAS and by a number of growth factor receptors,** here exemplified by IGFIR and the RebB1/ErbB2 heterodimer. Activated PI3K generates phosphatidylinositol-3,4,5-triphophate (PIP3), which activates phosphoinositide-dependent kinse-1 (PDK). In turn, PDK phosphorylates AKT. PTEN is an endogenous inhibitor of AKT activation. Phosphorylated AKT tranduces multiple downstream signals, including activation of the mTOR and inhibition of the FOXO family of transcription factors. mTOR activation promotes the synthesis of proteins required for cell growth and cell cycle progression. (Redrawn from **Berchuck A, Levine DA, Farley JH, et al.** Molecular pathogenesis of gynecologic cancers. In: Barakat RR, ed. *Principles and Practice of Gynecologic Oncology.* Lippincott Williams and Wilkins; 2013.)

oncogenes. Among the nuclear transcription factors involved in stimulating proliferation, **amplification or overexpression of members of the *myc* family has most often been implicated in the development of human cancers.** Many of the nuclear regulatory genes such as *myc* that control proliferation also affect the threshold for apoptosis. Genes that positively regulate cell cycle progression may be amplified and/or overexpressed in some cancers leading to unrestrained proliferation (e.g., cyclin D1, cyclin E1). Finally, as discussed previously, genes encoding nuclear proteins that inhibit apoptosis (e.g., *bcl-2*) can act as oncogenes when altered to constitutively active forms.

Tumor Suppressor Genes

Loss of tumor suppressor gene function plays a role in the development of most cancers. This usually involves a two-step process in which both copies of a tumor suppressor gene are inactivated.

In most cases, there is mutation of one copy of a tumor suppressor gene and loss of the other copy caused by deletion of a segment of the chromosome where the gene resides. Some tumor suppressor genes may be inactivated because of methylation of the promoter region of the gene (14). The promoter is an area proximal to the coding sequence that regulates whether the gene is transcribed from DNA to RNA. When the promoter is methylated, it is resistant to activation and the gene is essentially silenced despite remaining structurally intact.

This two-hit paradigm is relevant to both hereditary cancer syndromes, in which one mutation is inherited and the second acquired, and sporadic cancers, in which the two hits are acquired. Tumor suppressor gene products are found throughout the cell, reflecting their diverse functions. With the recognition that inactivation of tumor suppressor genes is a defining feature of cancers, genetic therapeutic strategies have been developed that aim to deliver functional copies of these genes lost to cancer cells.

Nuclear Tumor Suppressor Genes

The retinoblastoma gene was the first tumor suppressor gene discovered (Table 1.2) (28). **The *Rb* gene plays a key role in the regulation of cell cycle progression** (Fig. 1.2). In the G_1 phase of the cell cycle, *Rb* protein binds to the E2F transcription factor and prevents it from activating transcription of other genes involved in cell cycle progression. G_1 arrest is maintained by cdk inhibitors that prevent phosphorylation of *Rb*, such as *p16, p21,* and *p27* (29). When *Rb* is phosphorylated by cyclin–cdk complexes, E2F is released and stimulates entry into the DNA synthesis phase of the cell cycle. Other cyclins and cdks are involved in progression from G_2 to mitosis. **Mutations in the *Rb* gene have been noted primarily in retinoblastomas and sarcomas,** but may occur rarely in other types of cancers. By maintaining G_1 arrest, the cdk inhibitors *p16, p21, p27,* and others act as tumor suppressor genes. Loss of *p16* tumor suppressor function as a result of genomic deletion or promoter methylation occurs in some cancers, including familial melanomas. Likewise, loss of *p21* and *p27* has been noted in some cancers.

Mutation of the *TP53* tumor suppressor gene is the most frequent genetic event described in human cancers (Fig. 1.7) (30,31). The *TP53* gene encodes a 393 amino acid protein that plays a central role in the regulation of both proliferation and apoptosis. In normal cells, p53 protein resides in the nucleus and exerts its tumor suppressor activity by binding to transcriptional regulatory elements of genes, such as the cdk inhibitor *p21,* that act to arrest cells in G_1. The *MDM2* gene product degrades p53 protein when appropriate, whereas p14ARF downregulates *MDM2* when upregulation of p53 is needed to initiate cell cycle arrest.

Many cancers have missense mutations in one copy of the *TP53* gene that result in substitution of a single amino acid in exons 5 through 8, which encode the DNA binding domains. Although these **mutant *TP53* genes encode full-length proteins, they are unable to bind to DNA and regulate transcription of other genes.** Mutation of one copy of the *TP53* gene often is accompanied by deletion of the other copy, leaving the cancer cell with only mutant p53 protein. If the cancer cell retains one normal copy of the *TP53* gene, mutant p53 protein can complex with wild-type p53 protein and prevent it from oligimerizing and interacting with DNA. Because inactivation of both *TP53* alleles is not required for loss of p53 function, mutant p53 is said to act in a "dominant negative" fashion. Although normal cells have low levels of p53 protein because it is rapidly degraded, missense mutations encode protein products that are resistant to degradation. The resultant overaccumulation of mutant p53 protein in the nucleus can be detected immunohistochemically. A smaller fraction of cancers have mutations in the *TP53* gene that encode truncated protein products. In these cases, loss of the other allele occurs as the second event as is seen with other tumor suppressor genes.

Beyond simply inhibiting proliferation, normal p53 is thought to play a role in preventing cancer by stimulating apoptosis of cells that have undergone excessive genetic damage. In this regard, p53 has been described as the "guardian of the genome" because it delays entry into S phase until the genome has been cleansed of mutations. If DNA repair is inadequate, then p53 may initiate apoptosis, thereby eliminating cells with genetic damage. Likewise, other genes that repair damage to the DNA nucleotide sequence or strand breakage sometimes are classified as tumor suppressors. These other genes will be discussed in the next sections in the context of hereditary gynecologic cancer syndromes.

Extranuclear Tumor Suppressor Genes

Although many tumor suppressor genes—including *TP53, Rb,* and *p16*—encode nuclear proteins, **some extranuclear tumor suppressors have been identified.** Theoretically, any protein that normally is involved in inhibition of proliferation has the potential to act as a tumor suppressor. In this regard, appealing candidates include phosphatases such as *PTEN* that normally

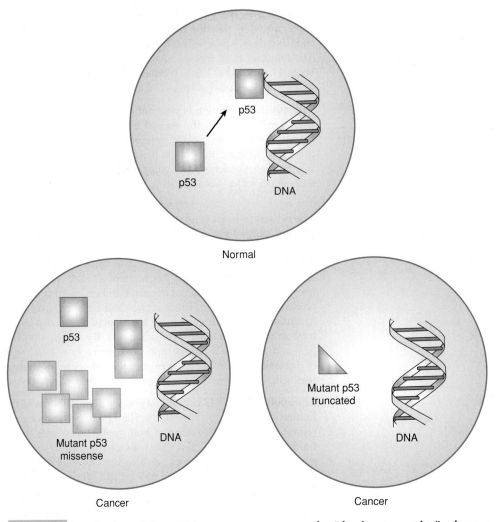

Normal

Cancer

Cancer

Figure 1.7 Inactivation of the *p53* tumor suppressor gene by "dominant negative" missense mutation or by truncation mutation and deletion.

oppose the action of the tyrosine kinases by dephosphorylating tyrosine residues. In addition to its phosphatase activity, *PTEN* is homologous to the cytoskeleton proteins tensin and axin. It has been postulated that *PTEN* might act to inhibit invasion and metastasis through modulation of the cytoskeleton. The *APC* tumor suppressor gene encodes a cytoplasmic protein involved in the WNT signaling pathway that regulates both cellular proliferation and adhesion (see section on Adhesion). **Inactivation of *APC* leads to malignant transformation and inherited mutations in this gene are responsible for familial adenomatous polyposis syndrome.**

The transforming growth factor-beta (TGF-β) family of peptide growth factors inhibits proliferation of normal epithelial cells and serves as a tumor suppressive pathway (22). It is thought that TGF-β causes G_1 arrest by inducing expression of cdk inhibitors such as *p27*. Three closely related forms of TGF-β that are encoded by separate genes (TGF-β1, TGF-β2, and TGF-β3) have been discovered. TGF-β is secreted from cells in an inactive form bound to a portion of its precursor molecule from which it must be cleaved to release biologically active TGF-β. Active TGF-β interacts with type I and type II cell surface TGF-β receptors and initiates serine or threonine kinase activity. **Prominent intracellular targets include a class of molecules called Smads that translocate to the nucleus and act as transcriptional regulators.**

MicroRNA

In addition to primary dysregulation of oncogenes and tumor suppressor genes, altered expression of microRNAs that regulate the expression of these genes occurs in many cancers. **MicroRNA genes consist of a single RNA strand of approximately 21 to 23 nucleotides that does not encode proteins. They bind to messenger RNAs that contain complementary sequences and can block protein translation** (32). MicroRNAs can function as either tumor suppressors or oncogenes and the disruption of normal microRNA function can occur through genetic changes (e.g., mutation, amplification), epigenetic silencing, or dysregulation by transcription factors. Approaches are being developed to target microRNAs involved in tumorigenesis.

Invasion and Metastasis

Metastasis is a process by which cancer cells spread from the primary tumor to distant sites (33). Cancer metastasis can proceed only if a series of sequential steps are completed, including proliferation, angiogenesis, invasion, embolisation or circulation, transportation, adherence in organs, adherence to vessel wall, and extravasation (Fig. 1.8).

Most types of cancer have an organ-specific pattern of metastasis. The propensity of various types of cancer to form metastases in specific organs was first proposed by Paget, who hypothesized that these patterns resulted from the "dependence of the seed (cancer cell) on the soil (the metastatic site)" (34). This hypothesis was suggested by the nonrandom pattern of metastasis. Paget concluded that metastases formed only when the seed and soil were compatible. **It is now appreciated at a molecular level that metastasis is dependent on a balance between stimulating factors from both the tumor and host cells *versus* inhibitory signals.** To produce metastasis, the balance must be weighted toward the stimulatory signals.

Cancer progression is a product of an evolving crosstalk between different cell types within the tumor and its surrounding supporting tissue, the tumor stroma (35). The tumor stroma contains a specific extracellular matrix as well as cellular components such as fibroblasts, immune and inflammatory cells, and blood vessel cells. The interactive signaling between tumor and stroma contributes to the formation of a complex multicellular organ. The organ microenvironment can markedly change the gene-expression patterns of cancer cells and therefore their behavior and growth potential (35). Recent studies regarding chemokines and their receptors provide important clues regarding why some cancers metastasize to specific organs. For example, **breast cancer cells frequently express chemokine receptors CXCR4 and CCR7 at high levels. The specific ligands for these receptors, CXCL12 and CCL 21, are found at high levels in lymph nodes, lung, liver, and bone marrow, which are common sites for breast cancer metastasis.**

Angiogenesis

All cells require oxygen and other nutrients for survival and growth, and cells must reside within 100 μm of a capillary in order to receive oxygen (36). Therefore, growth of new vessels, termed *angiogenesis,* is required for sustained malignant growth beyond approximately 1 mm in diameter (Fig. 1.9). **Angiogenesis occurs as a result of a shift in balance toward proangiogenic factors within the tumor microenvironment** along with down regulation of antiangiogenic influences. **One of the primary mediators of angiogenesis is vascular endothelial growth factor A (VEGF-A)** (37), which increases vascular permeability, stimulates endothelial cell proliferation and migration, and promotes endothelial cell survival (38). **Other mediators of angiogenesis include tumor-derived factors and host stromal factors including interleukin-8, alpha v-beta 3 integrin, the tyrosine kinase receptor EphA2, and matrix metalloproteinases** (39). From a translational perspective, patient-specific tumor microenvironmental characteristics may influence the response to antiangiogenic therapy (40). Therapeutic strategies to target angiogenesis include VEGF-A neutralizing antibodies (*Bevacizumab*) and multikinase inhibitors that target the VEGF-receptors along with other kinases. *Bevacizumab* is widely used in the treatment of metastatic colorectal cancer, advanced nonsmall cell lung cancer, glioblastoma, and metastatic renal cell carcinoma. *Sorafenib* and *pazopanib* are two examples of multikinase inhibitors that are approved for the treatment of metastatic renal cell carcinoma. There has been much enthusiasm for these drugs in the treatment of ovarian cancer; however, their benefit appears limited to improving time to progression with no overall survival benefit.

Invasion

Invasion through the basement membrane is a critical first step in metastasis and the primary feature that defines malignancy. Invasion requires the interplay between cancer cells and a permissive underlying stroma (41). Invasion of malignant cells through the basement membrane and endothelial cell migration for angiogenesis require degradation of the extracellular matrix. **This process is facilitated by a group of enzymes called matrix metalloproteinases (MMPs),** which are a family of zinc-dependent endopeptidases that digest collagen and other extracellular matrix components. They also stimulate proliferation and induce release of VEGF. **Ovarian tumors overexpress MMP-2 and MMP-9, and this increased expression correlates with aggressive clinical features** (42).

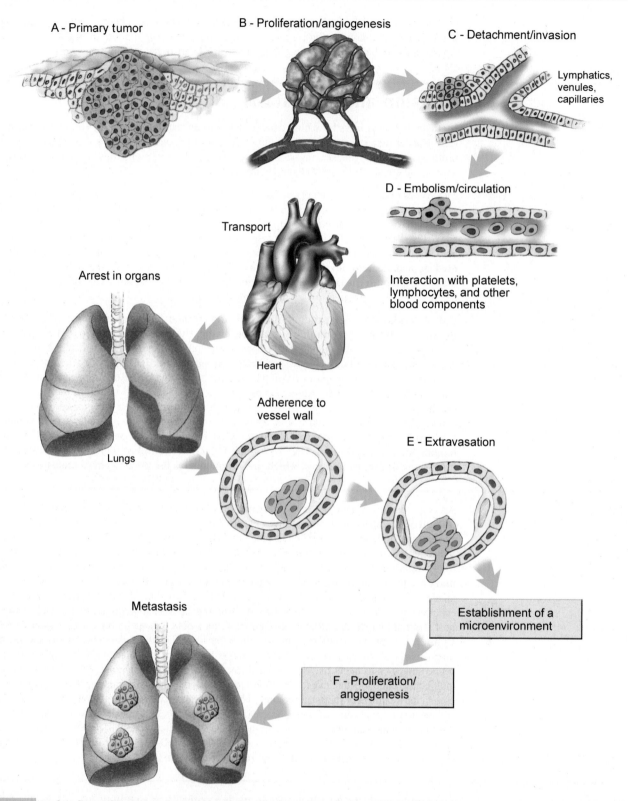

A - Primary tumor

B - Proliferation/angiogenesis

C - Detachment/invasion

Lymphatics, venules, capillaries

D - Embolism/circulation

Transport

Interaction with platelets, lymphocytes, and other blood components

Arrest in organs

Heart

Lungs

Adherence to vessel wall

E - Extravasation

Establishment of a microenvironment

Metastasis

F - Proliferation/ angiogenesis

Figure 1.8 Molecular pathways involved in invasion and metastasis. (Redrawn from **Fidler IJ.** The pathogenesis of cancer metastasis: The "seed and soil" hypothesis revisited. *Nat Rev Cancer.* 2003;3:453–458.)

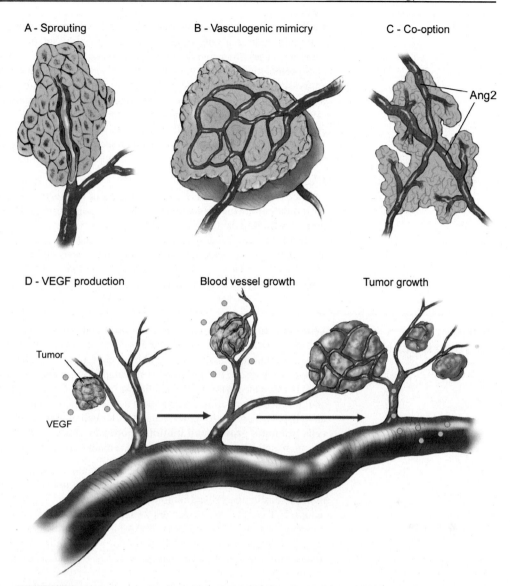

Figure 1.9 **Mechanism of tumor neovascularization. A:** Endothelial sprouting results from luminal endothelial cells migrating through the vessel basement membrane into underlying extracellular matrix, which is the dominant process for vessel growth. **B:** Aggressive tumor cells can form microvascular channels in a process termed "vasculogenic mimicry." **C:** Tumors may co-opt pre-existing host tissue vasculature. **D:** A shift in the balance favoring the release of pro-angiogenic factors (e.g., VEGF) leads to endothelial activation, blood vessel growth, and tumor expansion. (Redrawn from **Spannuth WA, Sood AK, Coleman RL.** Angiogenesis as a strategic target for ovarian cancer therapy. *Nat Clin Pract Oncol.* 2008;5:194–204.)

Adhesion

Tumor cell adhesion to the extracellular matrix within tissues greatly influences the ability of a malignant cell to invade and metastasize (43). Given the shedding nature of ovarian cancer, adhesion molecules such as focal adhesion kinase, integrins, and E-cadherin have been evaluated for their role in peritoneal metastasis (44). The proteins of the extracellular matrix consist of type I and IV collagens, laminins, heparin sulfate proteoglycan, fibronectin, and other noncollagenous glycoproteins (45). Cell adhesion to these proteins is mediated in part by a group of heterodimeric transmembrane proteins called *integrins,* which are composed of a noncovalently associated α and β subunit that define the integrin–ligand specificity (46). Approximately 18 β subunits and eight α subunits have been identified, and at least 24 receptor combinations exist (47). The intracellular domains of integrins interact with cytoskeletal components and are actively involved in generating intracellular signals.

17

Cadherins **are another group of cell–cell adhesion molecules that are involved in development and maintenance of solid tissues.** E-cadherins are the subgroup predominantly found in epithelial cells (48). These transmembrane proteins mediate cell–cell adhesion: Cadherins on neighboring cells preferentially bind to the same types of cadherins on adjacent cells. **E-cadherin is uniformly expressed in ovarian cancer, in low–malignant-potential tumors, in benign neoplasms, and—notably—in inclusion cysts of normal ovaries, but not in the normal surface epithelium** (49). Cadherin dysfunction is associated with loss of cell–cell cohesion, altered cellular motility, and increased invasiveness and metastatic potential. Changes in the composition of the cadherin–catenin complex, phosphorylation of components in the complex and alterations in the interactions with the actin cytoskeleton have all been suggested as playing a role in regulating adhesion.

E-cadherin mutations occur only rarely (50), but cadherin expression may be downregulated in the absence of mutations. **The cytoplasmic tails of cadherins exist as a macromolecular complex with β-catenin, which is involved in the WNT signaling pathways that regulate both adhesion and growth.** Regulation of β-*catenin* activity also depends on the *APC* gene product and others in the WNT pathway. Mutations in the *APC* gene that abrogate its ability to inhibit β-*catenin* activity are common in the hereditary adenomatous polyposis coli syndrome and sporadic colon cancers (51). Likewise, mutations in the β-*catenin* gene that result in constitutively activated molecules have been observed in some cancers, including endometrial cancers (52).

Tumor Microenvironment

Within the tumor microenvironment, other cell types also play a critical role in tumor growth and progression. For example, certain types of inflammatory cells, including macrophages and mast cells and their associated cytokines, confer an unfavorable prognosis and increased tumor growth. Conversely, the presence of an adaptive immune response characterized by cytotoxic T cells is associated with improved clinical outcome. Cancer cells may evade immune recognition and destruction by various means, such as Fas ligand production to induce lymphocytic apoptosis and HLA-G secretion to inhibit natural-killer cell activity (53). **Cytokine production by cancer cells promotes growth and inhibits apoptosis.** However, the mechanistic relationships between the microenvironment and tumor growth remain only partially understood.

Immune checkpoints, crucial for maintaining immune self-tolerance and preventing auto-immune diseases, can be exploited by tumors to allow them to avoid immune surveillance (54). There are multiple costimulatory and inhibitory interactions that regulate T cell responses. Among them, cytotoxic T-lymphocyte-associated antigen 4 (CTLA4) is expressed exclusively on T cells and downregulates T cell activation. CTLA4-blocking antibodies, such as *ipilimumab,* increase T-cell proliferation and activation, leading to improved anti-tumor responses. *Ipilimumab* is used in the treatment of malignant melanoma and is under evaluation for the treatment of multiple cancers.

Energy Metabolism

Cancer cells uptake increased amounts of glucose to satisfy their metabolic demands (55). Normal tissues generate energy using mitochondrial oxidative phosphorylation and switch to breaking down glucose only to derive energy in the absence of oxygen, which leads to the accumulation of lactate. In contrast, **glycolysis of glucose to lactate occurs in cancers even in the presence of oxygen, a phenomenon called "aerobic glycolysis."** This is referred to as the Warburg effect, in honor of its discoverer (56). Because cancers often outgrow their blood supply and become hypoxic, the ability to survive using aerobic glycolysis instead of oxidative phosphorylation may be selected for during malignant transformation. Aerobic glycolysis may serve the increased metabolic requirement for carbon atoms to produce the macromolecules needed to build new cancer cells. If glucose is completely broken down to carbon dioxide via the citric acid cycle, these carbon building blocks are lost.

The hypoxia-inducible transcription factor-1α (HIF-1α) plays an important role in the cellular response to decreased oxygen in the local environment. When oxygen is absent, HIF-1α accumulates and promotes transcription of pro-angiogenesis genes as well as those involved in glucose transport and glycolysis. HIF-1α accumulation may be a consequence of loss of the VHL tumor suppressor gene, providing a link between the loss of a tumor suppressor and the altered metabolic phenotype of malignant cells. **Another link between glucose metabolism and cancer is the finding that isocitrate dehydrogenase (IDH), an enzyme involved in glycolysis, is frequently mutated in glioblastomas.** The common amino acid changing *IDH* mutations result in increased production of 2-hydroxyglutarate, which accumulates to high levels and plays a role in the development of these cancers.

Differences in metabolism between normal and malignant cells represent an appealing therapeutic target. In this regard, **there is a suggestion that the diabetic drug metformin may have efficacy in the treatment and prevention of cancer.** This appears to be independent of blood glucose level and the exact mechanism is unclear.

DNA Repair

Loss of DNA repair activity increases the likelihood of mutations being fixed in the genome and this is a hallmark of many cancers. Thousands of mutations occur in humans on a daily basis (57). Cells in many organs such as the skin, gastrointestinal tract, and respiratory tract that are exposed most directly to the environment constantly undergo renewal with shedding of differentiated cells that may contain mutations. **Mammalian cells have highly evolved and complex DNA repair systems to maintain the integrity of the genome. A series of cell cycle checkpoints exist that allow the opportunity to pause for successful DNA repair,** or alternatively for cell death if repair cannot be accomplished. DNA damage checkpoints occur at the boundaries between G1/S and G2/M and during S phase and mitotic spindle assembly. These checkpoints serve to protect against genetic damage that can lead to malignant transformation being fixed in the genome.

There are several repair mechanisms that operate on specific types of DNA damage during these checkpoints (55,56,58,59). **Mismatch repair (MMR) excises nucleotides that are incorrectly paired with the correct nucleotide on the opposite DNA strand.** Inherited mutations in MMR genes are responsible for Lynch syndrome. The nucleotide excision repair (NER) and base excision repair (BER) pathways respond to damage caused by DNA damaging agents. Mutations in the *POLE* gene have been found in a subset of endometrial cancers with the highest mutation rates. **HR is a process that provides high-fidelity repair of complex DNA damage** such as DNA cross-links, double-strand breaks, single-strand DNA gaps, and DNA interstrand cross-links. **Inherited mutations in BRCA1–2 and other genes in the HR pathway cause familial breast/ovarian cancer susceptibility.**

Gynecologic Malignancies

Gynecologic cancers vary with respect to grade, histology, stage, response to treatment, and survival. This clinical heterogeneity is attributable to differences in underlying molecular pathogenesis. Some cancers arise in a setting of inherited mutations in cancer susceptibility genes, but most occur sporadically in the absence of a strong hereditary predisposition. **The spectrum of genes that are mutated varies between cancer types.** For each type of cancer, there are a few genes that are frequently mutated, while a wider spectrum are altered in a small fraction of cases (13).

There is significant variety with respect to the spectrum of genetic changes within a given type of cancer. Cancers with a similar microscopic appearance may differ greatly at the molecular level. In some instances, molecular features may be predictive of clinical phenotypes such as stage, histologic type, and survival. With a more complete understanding of the clinical implications of various genetic alterations in gynecologic cancers, **the molecular profile may prove valuable in predicting clinical behavior and response to treatment.**

Endometrial Cancer

Epidemiologic and clinical studies of endometrial cancer have suggested that there are two distinct types of endometrial cancer (60). **Type I cases are associated with unopposed estrogen stimulation and often develop in a background of endometrial hyperplasia.** Obesity is the most common cause of unopposed estrogen and is part of a metabolic syndrome that includes insulin resistance and overexpression of insulin-like growth factors that may play a role in carcinogenesis. **Type I cancers are well differentiated, endometrioid, early stage lesions, and have a favorable outcome. In contrast, type II cancers are poorly differentiated, often nonendometrioid (serous, clear cell), and are more virulent.** Some may arise from serous carcinoma in situ of the endometrium. They often present at an advanced stage and survival is relatively poor. In practice, not all cancers can be neatly characterized as either pure type I or II lesions either clinically or based on their underlying genetic mutations (Table 1.3).

Similar to other human cancers, **endometrial cancers are believed to arise because of a series of genetic alterations that result in progression from normal to precancer to invasive cancer.** Unopposed estrogenic stimulation may contribute to the development of endometrial cancer

Table 1.3 Characteristics of Type 1 versus Type 2 Endometrial Cancers		
Clinical Features	*Type 1*	*Type 2*
BMI	Obese	Normal
Etiology	Unopposed estrogen	Sporadic
Precursor	Endometrial hyperplasia	Serous in situ carcinoma
Histology	Endometrioid	Serous or clear cell
Grade	1, 2	2, 3
Stage	I, II	III, IV
Survival	Favorable	Poor
Molecular Features		
Ploidy	Diploid	Aneuploid
Microsatellite instability	40%	Rare
Tumor Suppressor Genes		
TP53 mutation	15%	90%
FWXW7 mutation	10%	30%
PP2R1A mutation	Rare	25%
ARID1A mutation	40%	10%
PTEN mutation	80%	Rare
MLH1 methylation	35%	Rare
CTCF mutation	25%	Rare
POLE mutation	10%	Rare
Oncogenes		
CTNNB1 (β-catenin) mutation	40%	Rare
PIK3CA mutation	55%	40%
PIC3R1 mutation	40%	Rare
KRAS mutation	25%	Rare
HER-2/neu amplification	Rare	30%
FGFR2 mutation	15%	10%
MYC amplification	Rare	25%

Mutation frequencies obtained from TCGA data, which are available to the cancer research community through the TCGA Data Portal (http://tcga-data.nci.nih.gov/tcga).

through its mitogenic effect on the endometrium. **A higher rate of proliferation in response to estrogens may lead to an increased frequency of spontaneous mutations.** In addition, when genetic damage occurs, regardless of the cause, the presence of estrogens may facilitate clonal expansion. Estrogens may act as "complete carcinogens" that not only promote carcinogenesis by stimulating proliferation but also act as initiating agents by virtue of their carcinogenic metabolites. In contrast, **progestins oppose the action of estrogens by downregulating estrogen receptor levels, decreasing proliferation, and increasing apoptosis. A small minority of endometrial cancers occur in women with a strong hereditary predisposition because of germline mutations in DNA repair genes causing Lynch syndrome.**

Hereditary Endometrial Cancer

Approximately 3% of endometrial cancers arise because of inherited mutations in DNA repair genes in the context of Lynch syndrome, which typically manifests as familial clustering of early onset colon cancer (61,62). Endometrial cancer is the most common extracolonic malignancy in women with Lynch syndrome. **The risk of a woman developing endometrial cancer has ranged from 20% to 60%** in various reports (63–65) and in some studies this exceeds the risk of colon cancer. In addition, **the risk of ovarian cancer is increased to approximately 5% to 12%.** Patients with Lynch syndrome also have a modestly increased risk of stomach, small bowel, hepatobiliary, pancreatic, and genitourinary cancers.

The identification of the DNA mismatch repair genes responsible for Lynch syndrome has facilitated the development of genetic testing (66). **Most Lynch syndrome cases result from alterations in *MSH2* and *MLH1*, although *MSH6*, *MSH3*, *PMS1*, and *PMS2* have been implicated in a small number of these cancers** (67). Loss of mismatch repair leads to a "mutator phenotype" in which genetic mutations accumulate throughout the genome, particularly in repetitive DNA sequences called **microsatellites.** Examples of microsatellite sequences include mono-, di-, and trinucleotide repeats (AAAA, CACACACA, and CAGCAGCAGCAG). **The propensity to accumulate mutations in microsatellite sequences is referred to as *microsatellite instability* (MSI).** Some microsatellite sequences are in noncoding areas of the genome, whereas others are within genes. It is thought that the accumulation of mutations in microsatellite sequences of tumor suppressor genes may inactivate them and accelerate the process of malignant transformation.

The Amsterdam and Bethesda criteria have been developed to provide clinical guidelines for the diagnosis of Lynch syndrome. These criteria are inexact, and **analysis of cancers for microsatellite instability has been proposed as a genetic screening test for Lynch syndrome. Among families with germline mutations in mismatch repair genes, MSI is seen in greater than 90% of colon cancers and approximately 75% of endometrial cancers** (68,69). However, MSI is found in 20% to 25% of endometrial **cancers** (70) and 15% to 20% of colorectal cancers overall (71), and most of these cases are attributable to silencing of the *MLH1* gene because of promoter methylation rather than germline mutation (72,73).

Another screening approach for Lynch syndrome is immunohistochemical staining of tumors to determine where there has been a loss of MSH2 or MLH1 protein (74). In cancers with MSI or loss of expression of one of the mismatch repair proteins, these genes can be sequenced to identify the disease-causing mutations, most of which cause truncated protein products. **Mutational analysis of the responsible genes remains the gold standard for diagnosis of Lynch syndrome** (66). Although it has been suggested that it may be cost-effective to do these tests on all endometrial cancers (75), this approach has not been widely adopted.

Lynch syndrome-related cancers are distinguished by their onset typically at least 10 years earlier than sporadic cases. The average age of women with sporadic endometrial cancers is in the early 60s, whereas cancers that arise in association with Lynch syndrome are often diagnosed before the menopause (average age in the 40s) (63,76,77). **The clinical features of Lynch syndrome-associated endometrial cancers are similar to those of most sporadic cases** (well differentiated, endometrioid, early stage) and survival is approximately 90% (76,78).

The mean age of onset of ovarian cancer in Lynch syndrome families is in the early 40s, and the clinical features of these cancers generally are more favorable than sporadic cases (79). They are usually early stage, well or moderately differentiated and approximately 20% occur in the setting of synchronous endometrial cancers. However, **analysis of groups of patients with synchronous cancers of the ovary and endometrium has revealed that few of these exhibit microsatellite instability and most probably are not attributable to Lynch syndrome** (80).

The optimal strategy for prevention of Lynch syndrome-associated mortality is unclear. Screening and surgical prophylaxis are both employed for colonic and extracolonic malignancies. Surveillance and prophylactic surgery should be considered early (between ages 25 and 35), generally 10 years before the earliest onset of cancer in other relatives who have had a Lynch syndrome-related malignancy (77). **Transvaginal ultrasound is used as a screening test for endometrial and ovarian cancer, but there is no strong evidence that this decreases mortality from these cancers** (81). There is no evidence that CA125 or other blood markers facilitate early detection of endometrial cancer, but CA125 can be justified as a means of screening for Lynch syndrome-associated ovarian cancer in view of the increased incidence. **Endometrial biopsy may be the only screening test with sufficient sensitivity,** and it has been suggested that this should be employed periodically beginning around age 30 to 35. No data have been published demonstrating that this approach is superior with respect to decreasing mortality compared to simply performing biopsies in response to abnormal uterine bleeding (see Chapter 9).

One study demonstrated that there were no cases of endometrial cancer in 61 Lynch syndrome carriers who underwent prophylactic hysterectomy, compared to 69 of 210 (33%) who did not undergo surgery (82). Survival of women with Lynch syndrome-associated endometrial cancers is approximately 90%, so prophylactic hysterectomy may not appreciably decrease mortality.

Some women in Lynch syndrome families elect to undergo prophylactic colectomy, either via laparoscopy or laparotomy. **This provides an opportunity to remove the uterus as well, and concomitant prophylactic salpingo-oophorectomy should be strongly considered in view of the increased risk of ovarian cancer.** At least an endometrial biopsy should be performed before prophylactic hysterectomy to exclude endometrial cancer. Estrogen-replacement therapy following oophorectomy is not contraindicated, and postmenopausal estrogen-replacement therapy in the general population substantially decreases colon cancer risk (83).

Sporadic Endometrial Cancer

Several approaches have been undertaken to evaluate the spectrum of genetic changes involved in the pathogenesis of sporadic endometrial cancers. **Cytogenetic studies have described gross chromosomal alterations in endometrial cancers, including changes in the number of copies of specific chromosomes** (84). Comparative genomic hybridization (CGH) studies have demonstrated areas of chromosomal loss and gain in both endometrial cancers and atypical hyperplasias (85,86). The most common sites of chromosomal gain are 1q, 8q, 10p, and 10q (87–89). Chromosomal losses are frequently observed using CGH and in loss of heterozygosity (LOH) studies (90). A correlation has been noted between higher numbers of chromosomal alterations on CGH and more virulent clinical features (91). The overall number of chromosomal alterations detected using CGH is lower in endometrial cancers relative to other cancer types.

Ploidy analysis measures total nuclear DNA content. **Approximately 80% of endometrial cancers have a normal diploid DNA content as measured by ploidy analysis.** Aneuploidy occurs in 20% and is associated with advanced stage, poor grade, nonendometrioid histology, and poor survival (92). The frequency of aneuploidy (20%) is relatively low in endometrial cancers relative to ovarian cancers (80%).

The Cancer Genome Atlas (TCGA) Project

The National Institutes of Health has directed the TCGA project to perform an integrated genomic and proteomic analysis of more than 20 types of cancer. The data generated by the TCGA are available to the cancer research community through the TCGA Data Portal (http://tcga-data.nci.nih.gov/tcga) (93). The analyses include evaluation of mRNA and microRNA expression, exome sequencing of the entire coding regions, along with evaluation of copy number alternations and methylation events.

Ovarian and endometrial cancers were among the first cancer types evaluated. In the endometrial carcinoma project, tumor samples were collected from 373 patients, consisting primarily of endometrioid histology (82.3%) with fewer serous (14.2%) or mixed histology (3.5%) cases (93). The frequency of alterations in various genes found by TCGA is shown in Table 1.3. **Based on the integrated analysis, four broad categories of endometrial cancers were identified:**

1. **Microsatelite instability cancers:** One third of cancers were characterized by microsatellite instability. These consisted predominantly of type I endometrioid tumors exhibiting mutation rates 10-fold higher than microsatellite stable tumors, few copy number alternations, and frequent *KRAS* mutations.

2. **Microsatellite stable cancers, low copy-number alteration endometrioid cancers:** These exhibited a high frequency of mutations in β-catenin (*CTNNB1*), a protein involved in cell–cell adhesion and WNT signaling pathway.

3. **Microsatellite stable cancers, high copy-number alteration cancers:** These had frequent *TP53* mutations, and comprised the serous cases and some grade 3 endometrioid tumors. This group shared similar molecular features with high-grade serous ovarian carcinomas and basal-like breast cancers.

4. **Ultrahigh mutation rate cancers:** These are a very small subgroup, characterized by an ultrahigh mutation rate (100-fold or greater than the mutation rate seen in low-mutation tumors), but without significant microsatellite instability. This group is characterized by hotspot mutations in *POLE*, a catalytic subunit of DNA polymerase epsilon involved in nuclear DNA replication and repair. Mutations in *POLE* have also been associated with an ultramutation phenomenon in other cancers, particularly colorectal cancers (94).

Tumor Suppressor Genes

Inactivation of the *TP53* tumor suppressor gene is among the most frequent genetic events in endometrial cancers (29). **Overexpression of mutant p53 protein occurs in approximately 20% of endometrial adenocarcinomas and is associated with several known poor prognostic factors, including advanced stage, high-grade, and nonendometrioid histology** (95–97). Overexpression occurs in about 10% of stages I and II cancers and 40% of stages III and IV (95). In some of these studies, *p53* overexpression has been associated with worse survival even after controlling for stage and histology (98). In studies of serous endometrial carcinomas, *TP53* mutation and p53 protein overexpression have been observed in the vast majority of cases, as well as in its putative dysplastic glandular precursor lesion (99,100). Although little is known regarding molecular alterations in uterine sarcomas, overexpression of mutant *p53* occurs in a majority of mixed mesodermal sarcomas of the uterus (74%) and in some leiomyosarcomas (101,102).

Mutations in the *PTEN* tumor suppressor gene occur in a very high fraction of endometrial cancers (103,104). Most of these mutations are deletions, insertions, and nonsense mutations that lead to truncated protein products, whereas only about 15% are missense mutations that change a single amino acid in the critical phosphatase domain. The *PTEN* gene encodes a phosphatase that opposes the activity of cellular kinases. For example, loss of *PTEN* in endometrial cancers is associated with increased activity of the PI3 kinase, with resultant phosphorylation of its downstream substrate Akt (105). **Mutations in the *PTEN* gene are associated with endometrioid histology, early stage and favorable clinical behavior** (106). ***PTEN* mutations have been observed in 20% of endometrial hyperplasias,** suggesting this is an early event in the development of some endometrioid type I endometrial cancers (107). Loss of *PTEN* may even occur in normal appearing endometrial glands, and it has been proposed that this may represent the earliest event in endometrial carcinogenesis (108,109).

Endometrial cancer is the second most common malignancy observed in women with Lynch syndrome. Cancers that arise in women with Lynch syndrome are characterized by mutations in multiple microsatellite repeat sequences throughout the genome. **Microsatellite instability is also apparent in approximately 20% of sporadic endometrial cancers** (110,111). Endometrial cancers that exhibit microsatellite instability tend to be type I cancers. **Loss of mismatch repair in these cases usually results from silencing of the *MLH1* gene by promoter methylation** (72,73). Methylation of the *MLH1* promoter has been noted in endometrial hyperplasias (111,112) and normal endometrium adjacent to cancers, suggesting this is an early event in the development of some of these cancers (113). Global changes in methylation resulting in decreased expression of a number of tumor suppressor and DNA repair genes may be a characteristic of some endometrial cancers, particularly type I cases (114). Loss of DNA mismatch repair may accelerate the process of malignant transformation by facilitating accumulation of mutations in microsatellite sequences present in genes involved in malignant transformation. Several other tumor suppressor genes may play a role in the development of some endometrial cancers (Table 1.3).

Oncogenes

Alterations in oncogenes have been demonstrated in endometrial cancers (Table 1.3). Increased expression of the HER-2/*neu* receptor tyrosine kinase was described many years ago (115,116) and was associated with advanced stage and poor outcome. **HER-2/*neu* overexpression is more prevalent in patients with serous endometrial cancers** (117,118). **Therapies that target HER-2/*neu* such as *trastuzumab* (anti-HER-2/*neu* antibody) may have a role in the treatment of serous endometrial carcinomas,** although levels of HER-2/*neu* overexpression in endometrial cancers are much less striking than in breast cancers. While initial studies of single-agent *trastuzumab* in endometrial cancer were disappointing, a large percentage of tumors in the trial did not show HER-2/*neu* amplification (119). Clinical trials of *trastuzumab* in combination with chemotherapy for the treatment of uterine papillary serous carcinomas are ongoing.

The *ras* oncogenes undergo point mutations in codons 12, 13, or 61 that result in constitutively activated molecules in many types of cancers. Codon 12 of K-*ras* was found to be mutated many years ago in approximately 10% of U.S. cases and 20% of Japanese cases (120–122). These mutations typically occur in type I endometrial cancers. K-*ras* mutations have been identified in some endometrial hyperplasias (121,123), which suggests that this may be a relatively early event in the development of some type I cancers.

As noted previously, the *PTEN* tumor suppressor gene, which normally acts to restrain *PI3K* activity, is frequently inactivated in type I endometrial cancers. Conversely, **activating mutations in** the catalytic subunit of *PI3 K* (*PIK3CA*) have been described in several types of cancers. In one study, *PIK3CA* mutations were seen in 36% of endometrial cancers, and 24% of cases had mutations in both *PTEN* and *PIK3CA* (124), suggesting an additive effect of two mutations in the same pathway. In addition, the TCGA study found a high frequency of mutations in the *PIK3R1* gene that encodes a PIK3 regulatory subunit.

Both inactivation of *PTEN* or unrestrained *PIK3* can lead to activation of AKT, which in turn leads to upregulation of the mammalian target of *rapamycin* (mTOR), a key regulator of apoptosis and cellular growth. Clinical trials with the mTOR inhibitors, temsirolimus, everolimus, and ridaforolimus, have shown promising single agent activity in the treatment of type I endometrial cancer (125–128). Studies evaluating combinations of these agents with hormonal therapies, other targeted therapies, or chemotherapy are underway.

Alterations in the WNT pathway involving E-cadherin, *APC*, and β-*catenin* (*CTNNB1* gene) have been noted in some endometrial cancers. E-cadherin is a transmembrane glycoprotein involved in cell–cell adhesion, and decreased expression in cancer cells is associated with increased invasiveness and metastatic potential. E-cadherin mutations occur only rarely in endometrial cancers (50), but cadherin expression may be downregulated in the absence of mutations and low E-cadherin expression has been found to be an independent poor prognostic factor in stage IV and recurrent endometrial cancers. The cytoplasmic tail of E-cadherin exists as a macromolecular complex with the β-*catenin* and *APC* gene products, which link it to the cytoskeleton.

Germline *APC* mutations are responsible for the adenomatous polyposis coli syndrome and somatic mutations are common in sporadic colon cancers, but *APC* mutations have not been described in endometrial cancers (51,129). The *APC* gene may be inactivated in some endometrial cancers because of promoter methylation. It has been shown that missense mutations in exon 3 of β-*catenin* lead to the same end result—namely, abrogation of the ability of *APC* to induce β-*catenin* degradation—which results in abnormal transcriptional activity. **Mutation of β-*catenin* was found in 40% of type I endometrial cancers in the TCGA study.**

Activating mutations have been observed in the fibroblast growth factor receptor 2 (*FGFR2*) gene in approximately 10% of endometrial cancers (130) and in early stage cancers have been associated with worse disease-free and overall survival (131). *FGFR2* mutations were found almost exclusively in endometrioid cancers (131). Several FGFR inhibitors are being evaluated for the treatment of recurrent endometrial cancer in early phase clinical trials.

Among nuclear transcription factors involved in stimulating proliferation, amplification of members of the *myc* family has most often been implicated in the development of human cancers. Several **studies have suggested that *myc* may be amplified in a fraction of endometrial cancers** (132), **and this has been found in about 25% of type II cases.**

Ovarian Cancer

Approximately 10% of ovarian cancers arise in women who carry germline mutations in cancer susceptibility genes—predominantly BRCA1 or BRCA2 (133). The vast majority of ovarian cancers are sporadic, and they arise because of acquired genetic damage. The causes of acquired genetic alterations remain uncertain, but exogenous carcinogens have not been strongly implicated. Cellular proliferation and oxidative stress with free radical formation with associated inflammation at the time of ovulation or in association with endometriosis or infection may also contribute to accumulation of DNA damage. Regardless of the mechanisms involved, **reproductive events that decrease lifetime ovulatory cycles (e.g., pregnancy and birth control pills) are protective against ovarian cancer** (134).

The protective effect of these factors is greater in magnitude than one would predict based on the extent that ovulation is interrupted. **Five years of oral contraceptive use reduces the risk of developing ovarian cancer by 50%, while decreasing the total years of ovulation by less than 20%.** The progestagenic milieu of pregnancy and the pill may protect against ovarian cancer by increasing apoptosis of ovarian epithelial cells, thereby cleansing the ovary of cells that have acquired genetic damage (135). The action of other reproductive hormones such as estrogens, androgens, and gonadotropins also may contribute to the development of ovarian cancers.

Epithelial ovarian cancers are heterogeneous with respect to behavior (borderline versus invasive) and histologic type (serous, mucinous, endometrioid, clear cell). Although the strongest epidemiologic risk factors generally affect risk of all disease subsets, differences have been

Table 1.4 Clinical and Molecular Characteristics of Histologic Types of Ovarian Cancers

Endometrioid and clear cell cancers	Associated with endometriosis
	Usually early stage and favorable survival
	Frequent mutations in *PTEN, PIK3CA, CTNNB1* (β-catenin), *ARID1A, PPP2R1A*
Mucinous ovarian cancers	Usually early stage
	Frequent mutations in K-*ras*
Low-grade serous ovarian cancer (borderline, well differentiated)	Favorable survival
	Frequent mutations in K-*ras* and *BRAF*
High-grade serous ovarian cancer	Most common ovarian cancer histology in *BRCA1* and *BRCA2* mutation carriers
	Usually advanced stage and poor survival
	Frequent mutations in *TP53, BRCA1,* and *BRCA2* Homologous recombination pathway inactivation
	Genomic instability

observed with respect to etiology and molecular alterations (Table 1.4). It has been proposed that ovarian tumors can be classified as low-grade or high-grade based on histology, clinical behavior, and molecular phenotypes (136). Low-grade tumors are genetically stable and are characterized by mutations in a number of genes, including *K-ras, BRAF, PTEN,* and β-*catenin.* High-grade cancers, predominantly serous, have a high level of genetic instability and are characterized by mutation of *TP53.*

There is strong evidence to suggest that all epithelial ovarian cancers have an extraovarian origin (137). High-grade serous cancers of the ovary, fallopian tube, and peritoneum are likely to be derived from epithelial cells of the tubal fimbriae (138). In this regard, most early serous cancers discovered in *BRCA1–2* carriers undergoing prophylactic surgery have been found to originate in the fallopian tube fimbria and are associated with preinvasive serous tubal in situ carcinomas (STICs) that overexpress mutant *TP53.* **In contrast, most endometrioid and clear cell cancers are thought to develop in deposits of endometriosis on the ovary or other pelvic structures.** The origin of mucinous ovarian cancers is less clear and some may originate from mucinous borderline tumors, while others may represent metastases from gastrointestinal cancers. It has been postulated that some mucinous and Brenner tumors arise from embryonic nests near the ovary (137).

Elucidation of the molecular basis for the clinical heterogeneity of ovarian cancer has the potential to facilitate future improvements in diagnosis, treatment, and prevention. **Using next generation sequencing techniques, mutations that present in ovarian cancers can be detected in liquid PAP smears,** potentially paving the way for a new approach to screening and early detection (139).

Hereditary Ovarian Cancer

Inherited mutations in *BRCA1* and *BRCA2* strongly predispose women to breast and ovarian cancer. Inherited mutations in the DNA mismatch repair genes involved in Lynch syndrome are responsible for about 1% of ovarian cancer cases. **About two-thirds of hereditary ovarian cancers are caused by *BRCA1* mutations and one-third by *BRCA2* mutations.** Hereditary cases account for about 10% of all invasive epithelial ovarian cancers and 20% of high-grade serous cases. **The lifetime risk of ovarian cancer increases from a baseline of 1.5% to about 15–25% in *BRCA2* carriers and 25–40% in *BRCA1* carriers (140–145).**

***BRCA1* and *BRCA2* mutations are rare and carried by fewer than 1 in 500 individuals in most populations (144–146). Most *BRCA1–2* mutations involve deletions or insertions encoding truncated protein products that are clearly dysfunctional.** Less frequently, disease causing point mutations may occur that alter a single amino acid, but most of these missense variants represent innocent polymorphisms (147). **The clinical significance of missense mutations can**

sometimes be elucidated by determining whether they track with cancer in other family members. The search for *BRCA1–2* genetic alterations may also involve sequencing of introns that lie between the coding exons. Intronic mutations may affect RNA splicing and can result in deletion of adjacent exons. In addition, genomic rearrangements may occur that inactivate *BRCA1* or 2, and identification of such alterations requires molecular testing beyond sequencing.

The *BRCA1* and *BRCA2* gene products complex with Rad51 and other proteins involved in repair of double-stranded DNA breaks by HR (148,149). *BRCA1* and *BRCA2* have been classified as tumor suppressor genes because the nonmutated copy is invariably deleted in breast and ovarian cancers that arise in women who inherit a mutant gene. **There are other genes that cooperate with *BRCA1–2* in repair of double-stranded DNA cross-links and breaks by HR. Inherited mutations in several of these genes are associated with high penetrance ovarian cancer predisposition, including *RAD51C* (150), *RAD51D* (151), *PALB2* (152), and *BRIP1* (153).** Women with a strong personal and family history of ovarian and breast cancer who are not found to have *BRCA1–2* mutations can be tested for mutations in the genes noted above. In the near future, it is likely that gene panels will replace testing that examines only *BRCA1–2* (154–165).

Sporadic Ovarian Cancer

High-grade Serous Cancers

High-grade serous ovarian cancer was the second cancer analyzed by the Cancer Genome Atlas (TCGA) project (166). **This comprehensive genomic analysis confirmed that these cancers were characterized by a high degree of genetic instability, with many copy number alterations, as well as inactivation of *TP53*, *BRCA1–2*, and other genes in the homologous DNA repair pathway** (Table 1.4).

DNA Copy Number Alterations

High-grade serous ovarian cancers are characterized by extensive genetic instability. Initially, gains and losses of various segments of the genome were demonstrated using karyotyping, and later at a finer level using CGH (167). Likewise, loss of heterozygosity, indicative of deletion of specific genetic loci, was demonstrated to occur at a high frequency on many chromosomal arms (168). It has been possible using next-generation sequencing to characterize chromosomal rearrangements at the level of the actual base sequence, which has facilitated analysis of their functional significance (169). TCGA examined DNA copy number alterations in 489 cases using a variety of high resolution platforms (166). There were eight chromosomal regions with recurrent gains and 22 with losses. There were 63 recurrent focal amplifications that encoded eight or fewer genes. **The most common focal amplifications included *CCNE1* (cyclin E), *MYC*, and *MECOM*, each of which was amplified in more than 20% of cancers.**

Amplification of *MYC* has been reported to occur in some ovarian cancers (170) as has amplification and overexpression of *CCNE1* (171,172). In studies of advanced ovarian cancers, high cyclin E expression has been associated with poor outcome (171,173). Alterations of the PI3K pathway are frequent in ovarian cancer, and it has been previously reported that the *AKT2* (174) and PIK3CA genes were amplified in some cases (175). Several PI3K-AKT pathway inhibitors have shown efficacy in preclinical models of ovarian cancer, and are under development in early phase clinical trials (176–179).

TCGA found 50 focal deletions in patients with high-grade serous cancers and the known tumor suppressor genes *PTEN*, *RB*, and *NF1* were deleted, albeit only in a small fraction of cases (166). RB and NF1 were targeted by mutations, consistent with the two-hit paradigm of tumor suppressor gene inactivation. Although mutations in the RB tumor suppressor gene are not a common feature of ovarian cancers, evidence suggests that inactivation of RB greatly enhances tumor formation in the presence of TP53 mutations (180). A large number of other candidate genes are in regions that are recurrently amplified or deleted in high-grade serous ovarian cancers. Considerable effort will be required to elucidate which of these represent driver events.

About 30% of breast cancers express increased levels of the HER-2/neu oncogene (181), usually caused by gene amplification. Overexpression of HER-2/neu in breast cancer has been associated with poor survival. **Expression of HER-2/neu is increased in a fraction of ovarian cancers, and overexpression has been associated with poor survival in some studies** (181,182). However, ovarian cancers with HER-2/neu overexpression rarely have high-level gene amplification. Anti-HER-2/neu antibody therapy (*trastuzumab*) has demonstrated great efficacy in breast cancer and often is administered with chemotherapy in the context of both adjuvant therapy and treatment of metastatic disease (183). The use of this drug is restricted to patients whose cancers have been shown to overexpress HER-2/neu based on immunohistochemical analysis of protein levels and/or FISH analysis of gene amplification in paraffin tumor tissue blocks.

A study performed by the Gynecologic Oncology Group found that only 11% of ovarian cancers exhibited significant HER-2/neu overexpression (184). The response rate to single-agent *trastuzumab* therapy was disappointingly low (7%), but there may be some benefit using it in regimens that include cytotoxics or other biologic agents. A phase 2 study of *trastuzumab, carboplatin,* and *paclitaxel* in patients with recurrent ovarian cancer that overexpressed Her2/neu identified overexpression/amplification in only 6.4% of the 320 cases screened (185). Only seven patients were eligible to receive treatment on study; of these, there was one complete response, two serologic complete responses, three with stable disease, and one with progression. **The number of patients enrolled was too small to determine whether the addition of *trastuzumab* increased efficacy.**

The cdk inhibitors act as tumor suppressors by virtue of their inhibition of cell cycle progression from G1 to S phase. Expression of several cdk inhibitors appears to be decreased in some ovarian cancers. *CDKN2A* (p16) undergoes homozygous deletions in about 15% of ovarian cancers (186). There is evidence to suggest that *CDKN2A* (187) and *CDKN2B* (p15) (188) may be inactivated via transcriptional silencing caused by promoter methylation, rather than by mutation and/or deletion. Likewise, decreased expression of the p21/*WAF1* cdk inhibitor has been noted in a significant fraction of ovarian cancers despite the absence of inactivating mutations (189). Loss of p27 (*CDKN1B*) also may occur, and correlates with poor survival in some studies (190). Aberrant expression of p27 in the cytoplasm may be most associated with poor outcome (191).

Mutations

TCGA performed sequencing of the coding regions and splice sites of about 18,500 genes in DNA isolated from 316 high-grade serous ovarian cancers (166). **Although several genes were identified that were mutated at low frequencies, *TP53*, *BRCA1*, and *BRCA2* were confirmed to be the most frequently mutated genes in high-grade ovarian cancers.**

TCGA confirmed that mutation of the *TP53* tumor suppressor gene is the most frequent genetic event in high-grade serous ovarian cancers (192,193). This is an early event that is found in tubal serous carcinoma *in situ* (138). **About two-thirds of high-grade serous ovarian cancers have TP53 missense mutations in the DNA binding regions of exons 5 through 8 of the gene** that result in p53 protein overexpression caused by increased stability of the protein. Codons 175, 248, and 273 are mutational hot spots. These missense mutants act as dominant negative transforming genes because of their loss of transcriptional activity (Fig. 1.7). Loss of the other copy of the *TP53* gene is not required. Most *TP53* missense mutations are transitions rather than transversions or microdeletions (194), which suggests that they occur spontaneously, rather than as a result of exogenous carcinogens. **Most high-grade serous ovarian cancers that do not overexpress p53 protein have *TP53* mutations that result in truncated protein products** (192,195). These are usually accompanied by loss of the other copy of the gene, consistent with the classic two-hit model of tumor suppressor gene inactivation. **TCGA found *TP53* mutations in 303 of 316 samples,** suggesting that this is essentially a requisite event in the development of high-grade serous cancers.

***BRCA1* and *BRCA2* germline mutations were found in 9% and 8% of high-grade serous cases respectively in the TCGA study and somatic mutations occurred in an additional 3%** (166). Silencing of *BRCA1* caused by promoter methylation was observed in 11% of cases as has been previously described (196). Defective HR repair of double-stranded DNA damage resulting from loss of *BRCA1–2* was predicted in 31% of high-grade serous ovarian cancers. Other genes in the HR pathway are inactivated in some cancers and the HR pathway may be compromised in about half of the cases. **Patients with *BRCA1* or *BRCA2* mutations have increased sensitivity to platinum chemotherapy and favorable survival relative to sporadic cases** (197,198). Conversely, the emergence of platinum resistance in these cancers may occur as a result of "back mutations" in which the normal *BRCA1* or *BRCA2* sequence is restored (199).

Cancers with defects in the double-stranded DNA HR repair pathway caused by mutations in *BRCA1–2* or other genes can be targeted effectively by inducing a second hit in the form of inhibition of the single stranded DNA repair pathway. In the TCGA study, about half the high-grade serous ovarian cancers had defects in genes in the HR pathway. This concept of synthetic—the combination of two genetic alterations, which on their own are nonlethal, but together result in a lethal phenotype—has led to interest in inhibitors of enzymes such as poly-ADP ribose polymerase (PARP) that are involved in single stranded base excision repair (200). Inhibition of PARP leads to the persistence of DNA lesions normally repaired by HR and makes HR-deficient cells more likely to undergo apoptosis, which can be further enhanced by chemotherapy-induced DNA injury (201). While normal cells can repair the damage and survive, the BRCA-deficient cells cannot activate the HR system and therefore die (202). **PARP inhibitors have demonstrated promising results in ongoing trials in ovarian cancer, both when combined with cytotoxic chemotherapy and as a single agent in the maintenance setting** (203).

Six other genes were found to be significantly mutated by TCGA, including RB, NF1, FAT3, CSMD3, GABRA6, and CDK12, but none was mutated in more than 6% of cancers (166). RB and NF1 are known tumor suppressor genes, while CDK12 has been implicated in regulation of RNA splicing. GABRA6 and FAT3 both appeared as significantly mutated but did not seem to be expressed in high-grade serous ovarian cancer or fallopian tube tissue, so it is less likely that mutation of these genes has a significant role in high-grade serous ovarian cancer. A number of other known oncogenic mutations were found in KRAS, NRAS, PIK3CA, and BRAF, but at frequencies less than 1%, although these mutations have been shown to have transforming activity and probably represent important drivers of some cancers.

Gene Expression

Microarray chips that contain sequences complementary to thousands of genes have been created that allow global assessment of the level of expression of each gene. Many genes have been identified that appear to be up- or downregulated in the process of malignant transformation (204). In addition, microarrays have demonstrated patterns of gene expression that distinguish between histologic types (205), borderline versus invasive cases (206), and between early and advanced stage disease (207). Molecular signatures have been identified that are predictive of response to therapy (208) and survival (208,209).

In the TCGA ovarian cancer project, a 193 gene expression signature predictive of survival was developed and validated in several other existing data sets (166). **The TCGA identified four gene expression subtypes of high-grade serous ovarian cancer (166). These were named mesenchymal, immunoreactive, differentiated, and proliferative based on the genes that characterized each subtype.** Although the subtypes were independently validated in several other microarray data sets, they are not strongly predictive of response or outcome. Alterations in gene expression may be attributable to methylation of their promoters. The TCGA found 168 epigenetically altered genes compared to normal fallopian tube epithelium. Pathway analysis showed that the RB and PI3K/RAS pathways were frequently abnormally expressed. Further validation of genomic signatures is needed, but genomic approaches hold the potential to guide selection of therapy in the future. **Patients identified as having a "poor prognosis" molecular profile might be the best candidates for investigational trials of new therapies.**

Borderline and Invasive Low-grade Serous Ovarian Cancers

Similar to high-grade serous cancers, it is thought that borderline and low-grade serous cancers likely arise from cells that originated in the fallopian tube epithelium. However, **the underlying genetic alterations in borderline and low-grade tumors are different from those of high-grade cancers** (Table 1.4), suggesting that they are distinct entities, rather than a single disease with varying degrees of differentiation.

Activating mutations in codons 12 and 13 of the *KRAS* oncogene are common in borderline serous ovarian tumors, occurring in about 25% to 50% of cases (210). **In addition, activating mutations in codon 600 of *BRAF* (V600E), which is a downstream effector of *KRAS*, occur in about 20% of serous borderline tumors** (211). Mutations in these two genes are mutually exclusive and result in constitutive activation of the MAP kinase pathway. Mutations in *KRAS* and *BRAF* have been noted in cystadenoma epithelium adjacent to serous borderline tumors, suggesting that this is an early event in their development (212). Likewise, mutations in *BRAF* and *KRAS* occur in some low-grade serous ovarian cancers (137), but these mutations are rarely seen in high-grade serous ovarian cancers. In one study, 35% of patients with serous borderline or low-grade serous ovarian cancers had evidence of a *BRAF* V600E mutation, and the presence of the mutation was associated with early stage disease and improved prognosis (213). Because metastatic low-grade serous and borderline cancers are generally resistant to *platinum/taxane* therapy, the MAP kinase pathway downstream of *KRAS/BRAF* represents an appealing target for ongoing clinical trials (214).

Overexpression of p53 protein is rare in stage I serous borderline tumors and well-differentiated serous cancers, but occurs in a minority of advanced stage borderline cases (215,216). In a study of advanced serous borderline tumors, p53 overexpression was associated with a sixfold higher risk of death (215). In some cases, invasive low-grade serous cancers may arise following an earlier diagnosis of borderline tumor. It has been shown that *TP53* mutational status was not concordant between the original borderline tumor and the subsequent invasive cancer (217). This suggests that the invasive cancer either arises independently or as a clonal outgrowth within the original tumor.

Endometrioid and Clear Cell Ovarian Cancers

About 20% of epithelial ovarian cancers have endometrioid or clear cell histology and these are thought to arise in pelvic endometriosis, usually on the ovary. **Clear cell cancers and low-grade endometrioid cancers have a lower level of genetic instability than high-grade serous cases. The most common alterations in clear cell cancers are mutations of the *ARID1A* tumor suppressor gene, which is involved in chromatin remodeling; this occurs in about 50% of cases** (218,219). *ARID1A* mutations have been observed in the tumor and contiguous atypical endometriosis, but not in distant endometriotic lesions. This suggests that *ARID1A* mutations are an early event in the development of these cancers. The PI3K pathway is frequently altered in clear cell cancers; activating mutations of *PIK3CA* occur in about 50% of cases and deletion of the *PTEN* tumor suppressor in about 20% (220). *PPP2R1A* encodes the α-isoform of the scaffolding subunit of the serine/threonine protein phosphatase 2A (PP2A) holoenzyme. This putative tumor suppressor complex is involved in growth and survival pathways. Missense mutations in this gene have been noted in about 5% of clear cell carcinomas (218).

Mutations of these same genes occur in endometrioid cancers (Table 1.4): **ARID1A (30%), PIK3CA (20%), PTEN (20%), PPP2R1A (10%)** (221,222). In addition, about 30% of endometrioid cancers have mutations in the *CTNNB1* gene that encodes β-catenin, a nuclear transcription factor involved in the WNT pathway. These mutations occur in exon 3 at or adjacent to the serine/threonine phosphorylation sites and stabilize the protein product, leading to nuclear overexpression and increased transcriptional activity. In some endometrioid ovarian cancers with abnormal nuclear accumulation of β-catenin that lack mutations in this gene, the *APC, AXIN1,* or *AXIN2* genes that regulate β-catenin activity are mutated (223). This suggests that in addition to the mutations that are present in clear cell cancers, endometrioid cancers frequently have alterations in the WNT signaling pathway (Table 1.4). Inactivation of the WNT and the PIK3/PTEN pathways in mouse models leads to the development of endometriosis and endometrioid cancers (224,225).

Some high-grade endometrioid ovarian cancers have molecular features similar to high-grade serous ovarian cancers, including genetic instability and *TP53* mutations. This suggests that these cases may sometimes be misclassified by pathologists based on light microscopy.

Synchronous Endometrioid Ovarian and Endometrial Cancers

As noted above, about 20% of endometrioid ovarian cancers have *PTEN* mutations (222). Synchronous endometrioid cancers are sometimes encountered in the endometrium and ovary that are indistinguishable microscopically. In some of these cases, identical *PTEN* mutations have been identified, suggesting that the ovarian tumor represents a metastasis from the endometrium (226). In other cases, the *PTEN* mutation seen in the endometrial cancer has not been found in the ovarian tumor, suggesting that these represent two distinct primary cancers. **Mutational analysis of PTEN, CTNNB1, and other genes frequently mutated in endometrioid cancers is helpful when a mutation is present in both cancers or in one cancer and absent in the other, but this approach may often be uninformative.** It has been reported that mitochondrial DNA mutations are fairly common in endometrial cancers (227) and mitochondrial DNA sequencing has been proposed as an alternative method of determining whether synchronous endometrioid cancers of the ovary and endometrium represent separate primary cancers.

Mucinous Ovarian Cancer

Similar to mucinous colorectal cancers, mucinous ovarian cancers frequently have *KRAS* mutations (137). These mutations occur in 50% to 75% of mucinous ovarian cancers and are missense changes in the hotspot codons. Identical *KRAS* mutations have been found in mucinous carcinomas and adjacent mucinous cystadenomas and borderline tumors, suggesting that the latter lesions represent premalignant precursors (137). Amplification of HER-2/*neu* has also been described in a subset of mucinous ovarian cancers (137).

Stromal Ovarian Tumors

The genetic alterations driving stromal tumors of the ovary were unknown until it became possible to screen the entire genome using next-generation sequencing. **Essentially all adult granulosa tumors have been found to have a missense mutation in codon 134 of *FOXL2*,** a gene encoding a transcription factor known to be critical for granulosa cell development (228). This mutation was also found in about 20% of thecomas and in 10% of juvenile granulosa cell tumors, but not in other types of sex cord stromal tumors. In addition, *DICER1* mutations in the RNase IIIb domain have been found in about 30% of nonepithelial ovarian tumors, predominantly in Sertoli–Leydig cell tumors (60%) (229). These mutations were restricted to codons encoding metal-binding sites within the RNase IIIb catalytic centers, which are critical for microRNA interaction and cleavage.

Cervical Cancer

Etiology

Although the incidence of cervical cancer has fallen by over 80% in developed countries as a result of the widespread implementation of cervical screening, in developing areas of the world it is still the most common cancer in women. **Unlike most other types of human cancers that occur because of mutations in oncogenes and tumor suppressors, cervical cancers arise as a consequence of viral inactivation of the *TP53* and *RB* tumor suppressors by the HPV E6 and E7 oncoproteins, respectively** (Fig. 1.10) (230). Almost all cervical cancers are caused by sexually transmitted human papilloma virus (HPV) infection, as are many vaginal and vulvar cancers (231). Only a small minority of women who are infected with HPV develop invasive cervical cancer. This suggests that other genetic or environmental factors are involved in cervical carcinogenesis. For example, individuals who are immunosuppressed because of either HIV infection (232) or immunosuppressive drugs are more likely to develop dysplasia and invasive cervical cancer following HPV infection. Vaccination against specific oncogenic HPV subtypes has reduced the incidence of high-grade cervical intraepithelial neoplasia in young women who were not previously infected with HPV-16 or HPV-18 (233) (see Chapter 7 for a complete discussion).

The E6 and E7 oncoproteins are the main transforming genes of oncogenic strains of HPV (230). **The HPV E7 protein acts primarily by binding to and inactivating the *Rb* tumor suppressor gene product.** E7 contains two domains, one of which mediates binding to *Rb* while the other serves as a substrate for casein kinase II (CKII) phosphorylation, enhancing binding of E7 to proteins controlling cell growth (234). Variations in oncogenic potential between HPV subtypes may be related to differences in the binding efficacy of E7 to *Rb*. High-risk HPV types contain E7 oncoproteins that bind Rb with more affinity than E7 from low-risk types.

The E6 proteins of oncogenic HPV subtypes bind to and inactivate the *TP53* tumor suppressor gene product (234–236). There is a correlation between oncogenicity of various HPV strains

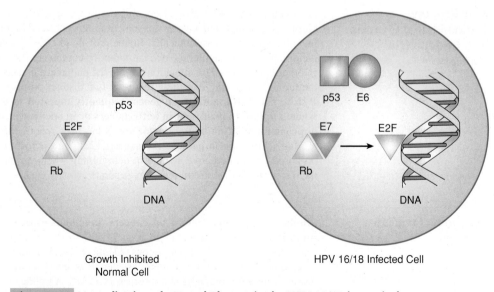

Growth Inhibited
Normal Cell

HPV 16/18 Infected Cell

Figure 1.10 Neutralization of p53 and Rb proteins by HPV 16/18 in cervical cancer.

and the ability of their E6 oncoproteins to inactivate p53. Inactivation of Rb and p53 by E6 and E7 circumvents the need for mutational inactivation of these key growth regulatory genes. In some studies, the levels of E6 and E7 in invasive cervical cancers have been found to predict outcome, whereas HPV viral load has not (237). There is evidence that HPV E6/E7 may interact directly with other genes such as telomerase that enhance growth and inhibit apoptosis.

HPV-negative cervical cancers are uncommon but have been reported to exhibit overexpression of mutant p53 protein (238). This suggests that **inactivation of the TP53 tumor suppressor gene either by HPV E6 or by mutation is a requisite event in cervical carcinogenesis.** Finally, the cdk inhibitor p16 is strikingly upregulated in most cervical dysplasias and cancers (239). **P16 detection may represent a useful adjunct to improve the positive predictive value of high-risk HPV testing for detection of cervical dysplasia** (see Chapter 7 for a full discussion of the clinical aspects of HPV).

Secondary Genomic Changes

HPV associated cervical carcinogenesis with inactivation of the *TP53* tumor suppressor gene leads to genomic instability that results in secondary genetic alterations that play a role in the development and phenotype of these cancers. Over time this ongoing instability leads to significant intratumoral heterogeneity as genetic damage continues to accumulate.

Most cervical cancers are aneuploid and CGH studies have shown that areas of DNA copy number gain or loss are common. A strikingly consistent finding is the high frequency of gains on chromosome 3q in both squamous cancers (240,241) and adenocarcinomas (242). Other chromosomes that exhibit frequent gains include 1q and 11q. The most common areas of chromosomal loss include chromosomes 3p, 2q, and 13q (243). Abnormalities seen in invasive cancers using CGH have been identified in high-grade dysplasias, suggesting that these are early and perhaps requisite events in cervical carcinogenesis (241,244,245).

Alterations in genetic dosage caused by chromosomal gains or losses have the potential to lead to changes in expression of genes involved in regulation of processes central to malignant transformation such as growth, differentiation, and apoptosis. Cervical carcinogenesis is also accompanied by changes in DNA methylation that affect genetic expression. Some changes in genetic dosage likely represent collateral damage and have no effect on development and evolution of the malignant phenotype, but it is likely that over time, there is selection for clones that exhibit enhanced growth and invasive potential. It is possible that genetic instability may enhance the emergence of resistance to radiation and chemotherapy.

A recent study examined genetic dosage in locally advanced cervical cancers using microarrays (243). Alterations were frequent and there were 14 regions with recurrent gains and 14 with recurrent losses. The most common alterations were gains on 1q, 3q, 5p, 20q, and Xq and losses on 2q, 3p, 4p, 11q, and 13q, each involving 44% to 76% of the patients. Four genes on 3p (*RYBP, GBE1*) and 13q (*FAM48A, MED4*) correlated with outcome at both the genetic dosage and expression level and were validated in the independent cohort. **Despite circumstantial evidence provided by studies such as this, with the exception of the fragile histidine triad (*FHIT*) gene on chromosome 3p14, it has been difficult to prove that genomic gains and losses result in alterations in specific oncogenes or tumor suppressor genes that are directly involved in tumor development.**

The *FHIT* gene is frequently deleted in many different cancers, including cervical cancer (246–248). Decreased expression of this putative tumor suppressor gene is an early event in some cervical cancers (248,249). In one study, FHIT protein expression was markedly reduced or absent in 71% of invasive cancers, 52% of HSILs associated with invasive cancer, and 21% of HSILs without associated invasive cancer (248). In addition, reduced expression was associated with a poor prognosis in advanced cervical cancers (250).

The role of several oncogenes has been examined in cervical carcinomas including most prominently the RAS and MYC genes. Mutant RAS genes are capable of cooperating with HPV in transforming cells *in vitro*. There is some evidence that mutations in either *KRAS* or *HRAS* may play a role in a subset of cervical cancers (238,251,252). *MYC* amplification and overexpression may be an early event in the development of some cervical cancers (253). Overexpression of *MYC* has been demonstrated in one-third of early invasive carcinomas and some CIN 3 lesions. In some studies, amplification has correlated with a poor prognosis in early stage cases (254).

Gene silencing due to promoter hypermethylation also may play a role in cervical carcinogenesis (255,256). In this regard, expression of the *RASSF1A* gene on chromosome 3p21 is frequently lost in cervical cancers, particularly adenocarcinomas (257,258). The function of this gene is not completely understood, but is thought to be involved in ras-mediated signal transduction pathways. Hypermethylation of tumor suppressor genes and genes associated with programmed cell death (apoptosis) have also been described in cervical cancers (255).

Gestational Trophoblastic Neoplasia

The genetic alterations that underlie gestational trophoblastic disease have been elucidated to a great extent. **The most prominent feature of these tumors is an imbalance of parental chromosomes.** In partial moles, this involves an extra haploid copy of one set of paternal chromosomes (XXY, XXX, or XYY). Complete moles generally are characterized by two pairs of one paternal haploid set of chromosomes (XX) and an absence of maternal chromosomes, while a minority is (XY) as a result of dispermy. Although the risk of repeated molar pregnancy is only about 1%, women who have had two molar pregnancies have about a 25% risk of developing another mole. **Mutations in the *NLRP7* gene have been found to be responsible for a recurrent form of molar pregnancy, and women with these mutations have an impaired inflammatory response** (259).

There is little convincing evidence that damage to specific tumor suppressor genes or oncogenes contributes to the development of sporadic gestational trophoblastic disease. However, **the presence of two identical copies of each chromosome in most complete moles could facilitate transformation caused by increased or decreased expression of imprinted genes involved in growth regulatory pathways. In addition, inactivation of a tumor suppressor gene on a paternal chromosome that might not normally be manifest because of the presence of a wild-type allele on the maternal chromosome could become significant in cells with two copies of the same haploid paternal genome.**

Microarray studies have identified several genes that are differentially expressed compared to normal villi, particularly genes associated with cellular apoptosis, immune suppression, and cell invasion (260,261). One study, in which genomic techniques were used to compare genetic expression between moles that spontaneously regressed and those that subsequently developed metastatic GTN, identified 16 differentially expressed transcripts (261). Downregulation of ferritin light polypeptide (*FTL*) and insulin-like growth factor binding protein 1 (*IGFBP1*) were confirmed in cases that subsequently developed GTN compared with those that regressed. Studies have suggested that changes in expression of genes involved in apoptosis, such as greater expression of the antiapoptotic gene *Mcl-1*, may be involved in progression of a molar pregnancy to invasive cancer (262). In addition, c-myc, mTOR, MAPK, and EGFR pathway alterations have been identified in gestational trophoblastic neoplasias, suggesting that inhibition of these pathways may be beneficial for patients who develop recurrent disease after primary treatment or are refractory to chemotherapy (263).

References

1. **Schwartz GK, Shah MA.** Targeting the cell cycle: A new approach to cancer therapy. *J Clin Oncol.* 2005;23:9408–9421.
2. **Benz EJ Jr, Nathan DG, Amaravadi RK, et al.** Targeting the cell death-survival equation. *Clin Cancer Res.* 2007;13:7250–7253.
3. **Danial NN.** BCL-2 family proteins: Critical checkpoints of apoptotic cell death. *Clin Cancer Res.* 2007;13:7254–7263.
4. **Amaravadi RK, Thompson CB.** The roles of therapy-induced autophagy and necrosis in cancer treatment. *Clin Cancer Res.* 2007; 13:7271–7279.
5. **Chao DT, Korsmeyer SJ.** BCL-2 family: Regulators of cell death. *Annu Rev Immunol.* 1998;16:395–419.
6. **Verdine GL, Walensky LD.** The challenge of drugging undruggable targets in cancer: Lessons learned from targeting BCL-2 family members. *Clin Cancer Res.* 2007;13:7264–7270.
7. **Shay JW, Keith WN.** Targeting telomerase for cancer therapeutics. *Br J Cancer.* 2008;98:677–683.
8. **Kyo S, Takakura M, Tanaka M, et al.** Quantitative differences in telomerase activity among malignant, premalignant, and benign ovarian lesions. *Clin Cancer Res.* 1998;4:399–405.
9. **Takakura M, Kyo S, Kanaya T, et al.** Expression of human telomerase subunits and correlation with telomerase activity in cervical cancer. *Cancer Res.* 1998;58:1558–1561.
10. **Kyo S, Takakura M, Tanaka M, et al.** Telomerase activity in cervical cancer is quantitatively distinct from that in its precursor lesions. *Int J Cancer.* 1998;79:66–70.
11. **Brien TP, Kallakury BV, Lowry CV, et al.** Telomerase activity in benign endometrium and endometrial carcinoma. *Cancer Res.* 1997; 57:2760–2764.
12. **Kyo S, Takakura M, Kohama T, et al.** Telomerase activity in human endometrium. *Cancer Res.* 1997;57:610–614.
13. **Vogelstein B, Papadopoulos N, Velculescu VE, et al.** Cancer genome landscapes. *Science.* 2013;339:1546–1558.
14. **Esteller M.** Epigenetics in cancer. *N Engl J Med.* 2008;358:1148–1159.
15. **Wicha MS, Liu S, Dontu G.** Cancer stem cells: An old idea–a paradigm shift. *Cancer Res.* 2006;66:1883–1890.
16. **Bolton KL, Ganda C, Berchuck A, et al.** Role of common genetic variants in ovarian cancer susceptibility and outcome: Progress to date from the Ovarian Cancer Association Consortium (OCAC). *J Intern Med.* 2012;271:366–378.
17. **Gryfe R, Di Nicola N, Lal G, et al.** Inherited colorectal polyposis and cancer risk of the APC I1307 K polymorphism. *Am J Hum Genet.* 1999;64:378–384.

18. **Bublil EM, Yarden Y.** The EGF receptor family: Spearheading a merger of signaling and therapeutics. *Curr Opin Cell Biol.* 2007; 19:124–134.

19. **Shepard HM, Jin P, Slamon DJ, et al.** Herceptin. *Handb Exp Pharmacol.* 2008;181:183–219.

20. **Kumar A, Petri ET, Halmos B, et al.** Structure and clinical relevance of the epidermal growth factor receptor in human cancer. *J Clin Oncol.* 2008;26:1742–1751.

21. **Cantley LC, Carpenter CL, Hahn WC, et al.** Cell signaling. In: DeVita VT, Lawrence TS, Rosenberg SA, eds. *DeVita, Hellman, and Rosenberg's Cancer: Priniciples & Practice of Oncology.* 9th ed. Philadelphia, PA: Lippincott Williams & Wilkins; 2011:57–67.

22. **Elliott RL, Blobe GC.** Role of transforming growth factor Beta in human cancer. *J Clin Oncol.* 2005;23:2078–2093.

23. **Schwartzberg PL.** The many faces of Src: Multiple functions of a prototypical tyrosine kinase. *Oncogene.* 1998;17:1463–1468.

24. **Tokunaga E, Oki E, Egashira A, et al.** Deregulation of the Akt pathway in human cancer. *Curr Cancer Drug Targets.* 2008;8:27–36.

25. **Courtney KD, Corcoran RB, Engelman JA.** The PI3 K pathway as drug target in human cancer. *J Clin Oncol.* 2010;28:1075–1083.

26. **Prior IA, Lewis PD, Mattos C.** A comprehensive survey of Ras mutations in cancer. *Cancer Res.* 2012;72:2457–2467.

27. **Salama AK, Flaherty KT.** BRAF in melanoma: Current strategies and future directions. *Clin Cancer Res.* 2013;19:4326–4334.

28. **Leiderman YI, Kiss S, Mukai S.** Molecular genetics of RB1—The retinoblastoma gene. *Semin Ophthalmol.* 2007;22:247–254.

29. **Shapiro GI.** Cyclin-dependent kinase pathways as targets for cancer treatment. *J Clin Oncol.* 2006;24:1770–1783.

30. **Berchuck A, Kohler MF, Marks JR, et al.** The p53 tumor suppressor gene frequently is altered in gynecologic cancers. *Am J Obstet Gynecol.* 1994;170:246–252.

31. **Edlund K, Larsson O, Ameur A, et al.** Data-driven unbiased curation of the TP53 tumor suppressor gene mutation database and validation by ultradeep sequencing of human tumors. *Proc Natl Acad Sci U S A.* 2012;109:9551–9556.

32. **Croce CM.** Causes and consequences of microRNA dysregulation in cancer. *Nat Rev Genet.* 2009;10:704–714.

33. **Fidler IJ.** The pathogenesis of cancer metastasis: The "seed and soil" hypothesis revisited. *Nat Rev Cancer.* 2003;3:453–458.

34. **Paget S.** The distribution of secondary growths in cancer of the breast. 1889. *Cancer Metastasis Rev.* 1989;8:98–101.

35. **Mueller MM, Fusenig NE.** Friends or foes—Bipolar effects of the tumour stroma in cancer. *Nat Rev Cancer.* 2004;4:839–849.

36. **Folkman J.** Angiogenesis in cancer, vascular, rheumatoid and other disease. *Nat Med.* 1995;1:27–31.

37. **Frumovitz M, Sood AK.** Vascular endothelial growth factor (VEGF) pathway as a therapeutic target in gynecologic malignancies. *Gynecol Oncol.* 2007;104:768–778.

38. **Senger DR, Galli SJ, Dvorak AM, et al.** Tumor cells secrete a vascular permeability factor that promotes accumulation of ascites fluid. *Science.* 1983;219:983–985.

39. **Spannuth WA, Sood AK, Coleman RL.** Angiogenesis as a strategic target for ovarian cancer therapy. *Nat Clin Pract Oncol.* 2008;5: 194–204.

40. **Jung YD, Ahmad SA, Akagi Y, et al.** Role of the tumor microenvironment in mediating response to anti-angiogenic therapy. *Cancer Metastasis Rev.* 2000;19:147–157.

41. **Liotta LA, Kohn EC.** The microenvironment of the tumour-host interface. *Nature.* 2001;411:375–379.

42. **Kamat AA, Fletcher M, Gruman LM, et al.** The clinical relevance of stromal matrix metalloproteinase expression in ovarian cancer. *Clin Cancer Res.* 2006;12:1707–1714.

43. **Boudreau N, Bissell MJ.** Extracellular matrix signaling: Integration of form and function in normal and malignant cells. *Curr Opin Cell Biol.* 1998;10:640–646.

44. **Hood JD, Cheresh DA.** Role of integrins in cell invasion and migration. *Nat Rev Cancer.* 2002;2:91–100.

45. **Hay E.** *Biology of the Extracellular Matrix.* New York: Plenum Press; 1991.

46. **Hynes RO.** Integrins: Versatility, modulation, and signaling in cell adhesion. *Cell.* 1992;69:11–25.

47. **Morgan MR, Humphries MJ, Bass MD.** Synergistic control of cell adhesion by integrins and syndecans. *Nat Rev Mol Cell Biol.* 2007; 8:957–969.

48. **Hirohashi S.** Inactivation of the E-cadherin-mediated cell adhesion system in human cancers. *Am J Pathol.* 1998;153:333–339.

49. **Sundfeldt K, Piontkewitz Y, Ivarsson K, et al.** E-cadherin expression in human epithelial ovarian cancer and normal ovary. *Int J Cancer.* 1997;74:275–280.

50. **Risinger JI, Berchuck A, Kohler MF, et al.** Mutations of the E-cadherin gene in human gynecologic cancers. *Nat Genet.* 1994;7: 98–102.

51. **O'Sullivan MJ, McCarthy TV, Doyle CT.** Familial adenomatous polyposis: From bedside to benchside. *Am J Clin Pathol.* 1998;109: 521–526.

52. **Fukuchi T, Sakamoto M, Tsuda H, et al.** Beta-catenin mutation in carcinoma of the uterine endometrium. *Cancer Res.* 1998;58:3526–3528.

53. **Paul P, Rouas-Freiss N, Khalil-Daher I, et al.** HLA-G expression in melanoma: A way for tumor cells to escape from immunosurveillance. *Proc Natl Acad Sci U S A.* 1998;95:4510–4515.

54. **Pardoll DM.** The blockade of immune checkpoints in cancer immunotherapy. *Nat Rev Cancer.* 2012;12:252–264.

55. **Vander Heiden MG.** Cancer metabolism. In: DeVita VT, Lawrence DK, Rosenberg SA, eds. *DeVita, Hellman, and Rosenberg's Cancer: Principles & Practice of Oncology.* 9th ed. Philadelphia, PA: Lippincott Williams and Wilkins; 2011:91–100.

56. **Hirschhaeuser F, Sattler UG, Mueller-Klieser W.** Lactate: A metabolic key player in cancer. *Cancer Res.* 2011;71:6921–6925.

57. **Jackson SP, Bartek J.** The DNA-damage response in human biology and disease. *Nature.* 2009;461:1071–1078.

58. **Gordon DJ, Barbie DA, D'Andrea AD, et al.** Mechanisms of genomic instability. In: DeVita VT, Lawrence DK, Rosenberg SA, eds. *DeVita, Hellman, and Rosenberg's Cancer: Principles & Practice of Oncology.* 9th ed. Philadelphia, PA: Lippincott Williams and Wilkins; 2011:23–40.

59. **Jalal S, Earley JN, Turchi JJ.** DNA repair: From genome maintenance to biomarker and therapeutic target. *Clin Cancer Res.* 2011; 17:6973–6984.

60. **Deligdisch L, Holinka CF.** Endometrial carcinoma: Two diseases? *Cancer Detect Prev.* 1987;10:237–246.

61. **Lynch HT, Lynch J.** Lynch syndrome: Genetics, natural history, genetic counseling, and prevention. *J Clin Oncol.* 2000;18:19S–31S.

62. **Annie Yu HJ, Lin KM, Ota DM, et al.** Hereditary nonpolyposis colorectal cancer: Preventive management. *Cancer Treat Rev.* 2003;29:461–470.

63. **Watson P, Vasen HF, Mecklin JP, et al.** The risk of endometrial cancer in hereditary nonpolyposis colorectal cancer. *Am J Med.* 1994;96:516–520.

64. **Dunlop MG, Farrington SM, Carothers AD, et al.** Cancer risk associated with germline DNA mismatch repair gene mutations. *Hum Mol Genet.* 1997;6:105–110.

65. **Aarnio M, Mecklin JP, Aaltonen LA, et al.** Life-time risk of different cancers in hereditary non-polyposis colorectal cancer (HNPCC) syndrome. *Int J Cancer.* 1995;64:430–433.

66. **Giardiello FM, Bresinger JD, Peterson GM.** American Gastroenterological Association technical review: Hereditary colorectal cancer and genetic tesing. *Gastroenterology.* 2001;121:198–213.

67. **Wijnen J, de Leeuw W, Vasen H, et al.** Familial endometrial cancer in female carriers of MSH6 germline mutations. *Nat Genet.* 1999;23: 142–144.

68. **Peltomaki P, Lothe RA, Aaltonen LA, et al.** Microsatellite instability is associated with tumors that characterize the hereditary non-polyposis colorectal carcinoma syndrome. *Cancer Res.* 1993; 53:5853–5855.

69. **Aaltonen LA, Peltomaki P, Leach FS, et al.** Clues to the pathogenesis of familial colorectal cancer. *Science.* 1993;260:812–816.

70. **Kowalski LD, Mutch DG, Herzog TJ, et al.** Mutational analysis of MLH1 and MSH2 in 25 prospectively- acquired RER +endometrial cancers. *Genes Chromosomes Cancer.* 1997;18:219–227.

71. **Thibodeau SN, French AJ, Roche PC, et al.** Altered expression of hMSH2 and hMLH1 in tumors with microsatellite instability and genetic alterations in mismatch repair genes. *Cancer Res.* 1996;56: 4836–4840.

72. **Simpkins SB, Bocker T, Swisher EM, et al.** MLH1 promoter methylation and gene silencing is the primary cause of microsatellite instability in sporadic endometrial cancers. *Hum Mol Genet.* 1999; 8:661–666.

73. Salvesen HB, MacDonald N, Ryan A, et al. Methylation of hMLH1 in a population-based series of endometrial carcinomas. *Clin Cancer Res.* 2000;6:3607–3613.

74. Hampel H, Frankel W, Panescu J, et al. Screening for Lynch syndrome (hereditary nonpolyposis colorectal cancer) among endometrial cancer patients. *Cancer Res.* 2006;66:7810–7817.

75. Resnick K, Straughn JM Jr, Backes F, et al. Lynch syndrome screening strategies among newly diagnosed endometrial cancer patients. *Obstet Gynecol.* 2009;114:530–536.

76. Vasen HF, Watson P, Mecklin JP, et al. The epidemiology of endometrial cancer in hereditary nonpolyposis colorectal cancer. *Anticancer Res.* 1994;14:1675–1678.

77. Brown GJ, John DJ, Macrae FA, et al. Cancer risk in young women at risk of hereditary nonpolyposis colorectal cancer: Implications for gynecologic surveillance. *Gynecol Oncol.* 2001;80:346–349.

78. Boks DE, Trujillo AP, Voogd AC, et al. Survival analysis of endometrial carcinoma associated with hereditary nonpolyposis colorectal cancer. *Int J Cancer.* 2002;102:198–200.

79. Watson P, Butzow R, Lynch HT, et al. The clinical features of ovarian cancer in hereditary nonpolyposis colorectal cancer. *Gynecol Oncol.* 2001;82:223–228.

80. Shannon C, Kirk J, Barnetson R, et al. Incidence of microsatellite instability in synchronous tumors of the ovary and endometrium. *Clin Cancer Res.* 2003;9:1387–1392.

81. Dove-Edwin I, Boks D, Goff S, et al. The outcome of endometrial carcinoma surveillance by ultrasound scan in women at risk of hereditary nonpolyposis colorectal carcinoma and familial colorectal carcinoma. *Cancer.* 2002;94:1708–1712.

82. Schmeler KM, Lynch HT, Chen LM, et al. Prophylactic surgery to reduce the risk of gynecologic cancers in the Lynch syndrome. *N Engl J Med.* 2006;354:261–269.

83. Rossouw JE, Anderson GL, Prentice RL, et al. Writing Group for the Women's Health Initiative Investigators. Risks and benefits of estrogen plus progestin in healthy postmenopausal women: Principal results from the women's health initiative randomized controlled trial. *JAMA.* 2003;288:321–333.

84. Shah NK, Currie JL, Rosenshein N, et al. Cytogenetic and FISH analysis of endometrial carcinoma. *Cancer Genet Cytogenet.* 1994;73:142–146.

85. Baloglu H, Cannizzaro LA, Jones J, et al. Atypical endometrial hyperplasia shares genomic abnormalities with endometrioid carcinoma by comparative genomic hybridization. *Hum Pathol.* 2001;32:615–622.

86. Kiechle M, Hinrichs M, Jacobsen A, et al. Genetic imbalances in precursor lesions of endometrial cancer detected by comparative genomic hybridization. *Am J Pathol.* 2000;156:1827–1833.

87. Suzuki A, Fukushige S, Nagase S, et al. Frequent gains on chromosome arms 1q and/or 8q in human endometrial cancer. *Hum Genet.* 1997;100:629–636.

88. Sonoda G, du Manoir S, Godwin AK, et al. Detection of DNA gains and losses in primary endometrial carcinomas by comparative genomic hybridization. *Genes Chromosomes Cancer.* 1997;18:115–125.

89. Hirasawa A, Aoki D, Inoue J, et al. Unfavorable prognostic factors associated with high frequency of microsatellite instability and comparative genomic hybridization analysis in endometrial cancer. *Clin Cancer Res.* 2003;9:5675–5682.

90. Risinger JI, Maxwell GL, Chandramouli GV, et al. Microarray analysis reveals distinct gene expression profiles among different histologic types of endometrial cancer. *Cancer Res.* 2003;63:6–11.

91. Suehiro Y, Umayahara K, Ogata H, et al. Genetic aberrations detected by comparative genomic hybridization predict outcome in patients with endometrioid carcinoma. *Genes Chromosomes Cancer.* 2000;29:75–82.

92. Lukes AS, Kohler MF, Pieper CF, et al. Multivariable analysis of DNA ploidy, p53, and HER-2/neu as prognostic factors in endometrial cancer. *Cancer.* 1994;73:2380–2385.

93. The Cancer Genome Atlas Research Network. Integrated genomic analysis of endometrial cancer. *Nature.* 2013;497:67–73.

94. Briggs S, Tomlinson I. Germline and somatic polymerase epsilon and delta mutations define a new class of hypermutated colorectal and endometrial cancers. *J Pathol.* 2013;230:148–153.

95. Kohler MF, Berchuck A, Davidoff AM, et al. Overexpression and mutation of p53 in endometrial carcinoma. *Cancer Res.* 1992;52:1622–1627.

96. Hachisuga T, Fukuda K, Uchiyama M, et al. Immunohistochemical study of p53 expression in endometrial carcinomas: Correlation with markers of proliferating cells and clinicopathologic features. *Int J Gynecol Cancer.* 1993;3:363–368.

97. Ito K, Watanabe K, Nasim S, et al. Prognostic significance of p53 overexpression in endometrial cancer. *Cancer Res.* 1994;54:4667–4670.

98. Kohler MF, Carney P, Dodge R, et al. p53 overexpression in advanced-stage endometrial adenocarcinoma. *Am J Obstet Gynecol.* 1996;175:1246–1252.

99. Tashiro H, Isacson C, Levine R, et al. p53 gene mutations are common in uterine serous carcinoma and occur early in their pathogenesis. *Am J Pathol.* 1997;150:177–185.

100. Jia L, Liu Y, Yi X, et al. Endometrial glandular dysplasia with frequent p53 gene mutation: A genetic evidence supporting its precancer nature for endometrial serous carcinoma. *Clin Cancer Res.* 2008;14:2263–2269.

101. Liu FS, Kohler MF, Marks JR, et al. Mutation and overexpression of the p53 tumor suppressor gene frequently occurs in uterine and ovarian sarcomas. *Obstet Gynecol.* 1994;83:118–124.

102. Hall KL, Teneriello MG, Taylor RR, et al. Analysis of Ki-ras, p53, and MDM2 genes in uterine leiomyomas and leiomyosarcomas. *Gynecol Oncol.* 1997;65:330–335.

103. Risinger JI, Hayes AK, Berchuck A, et al. PTEN/MMAC1 mutations in endometrial cancers. *Cancer Res.* 1997;57:4736–4738.

104. Tashiro H, Blazes MS, Wu R, et al. Mutations in PTEN are frequent in endometrial carcinoma but rare in other common gynecologic malignancies. *Cancer Res.* 1997;57:3935–3940.

105. Kanamori Y, Kigawa J, Itamochi H, et al. Correlation between loss of PTEN expression and Akt phosphorylation in endometrial carcinoma. *Clin Cancer Res.* 2001;7:892–895.

106. Risinger JI, Hayes K, Maxwell GL, et al. PTEN mutation in endometrial cancers is associated with favorable clinical and pathologic characteristics. *Clin Cancer Res.* 1998;4:3005–3010.

107. Milner J, Ponder B, Hughes-Davies L, et al. Transcriptional activation functions in BRCA2. *Nature.* 1997;386:772–773.

108. Mutter GL, Ince TA, Baak JP, et al. Molecular identification of latent precancers in histologically normal endometrium. *Cancer Res.* 2001;61:4311–4314.

109. Mutter GL, Lin MC, Fitzgerald JT, et al. Altered PTEN expression as a diagnostic marker for the earliest endometrial precancers. *J Natl Cancer Inst.* 2000;92:924–930.

110. Risinger JI, Berchuck A, Kohler MF, et al. Genetic instability of microsatellites in endometrial carcinoma. *Cancer Res.* 1993;53:5100–5103.

111. Faquin WC, Fitzgerald JT, Lin MC, et al. Sporadic microsatellite instability is specific to neoplastic and preneoplastic endometrial tissues. *Am J Clin Pathol.* 2000;113:576–582.

112. Esteller M, Catasus L, Matias-Guiu X, et al. hMLH1 promoter hypermethylation is an early event in human endometrial tumorigenesis. *Am J Pathol.* 1999;155:1767–1772.

113. Kanaya T, Kyo S, Maida Y, et al. Frequent hypermethylation of MLH1 promoter in normal endometrium of patients with endometrial cancers. *Oncogene.* 2003;22:2352–2360.

114. Risinger JI, Maxwell GL, Berchuck A, et al. Promoter hypermethylation as an epigenetic component in Type I and Type II endometrial cancers. *Ann N Y Acad Sci.* 2003;983:208–212.

115. Berchuck A, Rodriguez G, Kinney RB, et al. Overexpression of HER-2/neu in endometrial cancer is associated with advanced stage disease. *Am J Obstet Gynecol.* 1991;164:t-21.

116. Lu KH, Bell DA, Welch WR, et al. Evidence for the multifocal origin of bilateral and advanced human serous borderline ovarian tumors. *Cancer Res.* 1998;58:2328–2330.

117. Santin AD, Bellone S, Van SS, et al. Determination of HER2/neu status in uterine serous papillary carcinoma: Comparative analysis of immunohistochemistry and fluorescence in situ hybridization. *Gynecol Oncol.* 2005;98:24–30.

118. Morrison C, Zanagnolo V, Ramirez N, et al. HER-2 is an independent prognostic factor in endometrial cancer: Association with outcome in a large cohort of surgically staged patients. *J Clin Oncol.* 2006;24:2376–2385.

119. **Fleming GF, Sill MW, Darcy KM, et al.** Phase II trial of trastuzumab in women with advanced or recurrent, HER2-positive endometrial carcinoma: A Gynecologic Oncology Group study. *Gynecol Oncol.* 2010;116:15–20.

120. **Ignar-Trowbridge D, Risinger JI, Dent GA, et al.** Mutations of the Ki-*ras* oncogene in endometrial carcinoma. *Am J Obstet Gynecol.* 1992;167:227–232.

121. **Duggan BD, Felix JC, Muderspach LI, et al.** Early mutational activation of the c-Ki-ras oncogene in endometrial carcinoma. *Cancer Res.* 1994;54:1604–1607.

122. **Fujimoto I, Shimizu Y, Hirai Y, et al.** Studies on *ras* oncogene activation in endometrial carcinoma. *Gynecol Oncol.* 1993;48:196–202.

123. **Mutter GL, Wada H, Faquin WC, et al.** K-ras mutations appear in the premalignant phase of both microsatellite stable and unstable endometrial carcinogenesis. *Mol Pathol.* 1999;52:257–262.

124. **Oda K, Stokoe D, Taketani Y, et al.** High frequency of coexistent mutations of PIK3CA and PTEN genes in endometrial carcinoma. *Cancer Res.* 2005;65:10669–10673.

125. **Oza AM, Elit L, Tsao MS, et al.** Phase II study of temsirolimus in women with recurrent or metastatic endometrial cancer: A trial of the NCIC Clinical Trials Group. *J Clin Oncol.* 2011;29:3278–3285.

126. **Ray-Coquard I, Favier L, Weber B, et al.** Everolimus as second- or third-line treatment of advanced endometrial cancer: ENDORAD, a phase II trial of GINECO. *Br J Cancer.* 2013;108:1771–1777.

127. **Colombo N, McMeekin DS, Schwartz PE, et al.** Ridaforolimus as a single agent in advanced endometrial cancer: Results of a single-arm, phase 2 trial. *Br J Cancer.* 2013;108:1021–1026.

128. **Slomovitz BM, Burke TW, Eifel P, et al.** Uterine papillary serious carcinoma (UPSC): A single institution review of 129 cases. *Gynecol Oncol.* 2010;91:463–469.

129. **Moreno-Bueno G, Hardisson D, Sanchez C, et al.** Abnormalities of the APC/beta-catenin pathway in endometrial cancer. *Oncogene.* 2002;21:7981–7990.

130. **Byron SA, Gartside M, Powell MA, et al.** FGFR2 point mutations in 466 endometrioid endometrial tumors: Relationship with MSI, KRAS, PIK3CA, CTNNB1 mutations and clinicopathological features. *PLoS ONE.* 2012;7:e30801.

131. **Pollock PM, Gartside MG, Dejeza LC, et al.** Frequent activating FGFR2 mutations in endometrial carcinomas parallel germline mutations associated with craniosynostosis and skeletal dysplasia syndromes. *Oncogene.* 2007;26:7158–7162.

132. **Konopka B, Janiec-Jankowska A, Paszko Z, et al.** The coexistence of ERBB2, INT2, and CMYC oncogene amplifications and PTEN gene mutations in endometrial carcinoma. *J Cancer Res Clin Oncol.* 2013;130:114–121.

133. **Walsh T, Casadei S, Lee MK, et al.** Mutations in 12 genes for inherited ovarian, fallopian tube, and peritoneal carcinoma identified by massively parallel sequencing. *Proc Natl Acad Sci U S A.* 2011;108:18032–18037.

134. **Whittemore AS, Harris R, Itnyre J.** Characteristics relating to ovarian cancer risk. Collaborative analysis of twelve US case-control studies: IV. The pathogenesis of epithelial ovarian cancer. *Am J Epidemiol.* 1992;136:1212–1220.

135. **Rodriguez GC, Walmer DK, Cline M, et al.** Effect of progestin on the ovarian epithelium of macaques: Cancer prevention through apoptosis? *J Soc Gynecol Investig.* 1998;5:271–276.

136. **Kurman RJ, Shih I.** Pathogenesis of ovarian cancer: Lessons from morphology and molecular biology and their clinical implications. *Int J Gynecol Pathol.* 2008;27:151–160.

137. **Kurman RJ, Shih I.** Molecular pathogenesis and extraovarian origin of epithelial ovarian cancer–shifting the paradigm. *Hum Pathol.* 2011;42:918–931.

138. **Mehra K, Mehrad M, Ning G, et al.** STICS, SCOUTs and p53 signatures; a new language for pelvic serous carcinogenesis. *Front Biosci (Elite Ed).* 2011;3:625–634.

139. **Kinde I, Bettegowda C, Wang Y, et al.** Evaluation of DNA from the Papanicolaou test to detect ovarian and endometrial cancers. *Sci Transl Med.* 2013;5:167ra4.

140. **Whittemore AS, Gong G, Itnyre J.** Prevalence and contribution of BRCA1 mutations in breast cancer and ovarian cancer: Results from three U.S. population-based case- control studies of ovarian cancer. *Am J Hum Genet.* 1997;60:496–504.

141. **Struewing JP, Hartge P, Wacholder S, et al.** The risk of cancer associated with specific mutations of BRCA1 and BRCA2 among Ashkenazi Jews. *N Engl J Med.* 1997;336:1401–1408.

142. **Risch HA, McLaughlin JR, Cole DE, et al.** Prevalence and penetrance of germline BRCA1 and BRCA2 mutations in a population series of 649 women with ovarian cancer. *Am J Hum Genet.* 2001;68:700–710.

143. **Antoniou A, Pharoah PD, Narod S, et al.** Average risks of breast and ovarian cancer associated with BRCA1 or BRCA2 mutations detected in case Series unselected for family history: A combined analysis of 22 studies. *Am J Hum Genet.* 2003;72:1117–1130.

144. **Szabo CI, King MC.** Invited editorial: Population genetics of BRCA1 and BRCA2. *Am J Hum Genet.* 1997;60:1013–1020.

145. **Struewing JP, Abeliovich D, Peretz T, et al.** The carrier frequency of the BRCA1 185delAG mutation is approximately 1 percent in Ashkenazi Jewish individuals. *Nat Genet.* 1995;11:198–200.

146. **Schrader KA, Hurlburt J, Kalloger SE, et al.** Germline BRCA1 and BRCA2 mutations in ovarian cancer: Utility of a histology-based referral strategy. *Obstet Gynecol.* 2012;120:235–240.

147. **Deffenbaugh AM, Frank TS, Hoffman M, et al.** Characterization of common BRCA1 and BRCA2 variants. *Genet Test.* 2002;6:119–121.

148. **Powell SN, Kachnic LA.** Roles of BRCA1 and BRCA2 in homologous recombination, DNA replication fidelity and the cellular response to ionizing radiation. *Oncogene.* 2003;22:5784–5791.

149. **Jasin M.** Homologous repair of DNA damage and tumorigenesis: The BRCA connection. *Oncogene.* 2002;21:8981–8993.

150. **Meindl A, Hellebrand H, Wiek C, et al.** Germline mutations in breast and ovarian cancer pedigrees establish RAD51 C as a human cancer susceptibility gene. *Nat Genet.* 2010;42:410–414.

151. **Loveday C, Turnbull C, Ramsay E, et al.** Germline mutations in RAD51D confer susceptibility to ovarian cancer. *Nat Genet.* 2011;43:879–882.

152. **Dansonka-Mieszkowska A, Kluska A, Moes J, et al.** A novel germline PALB2 deletion in Polish breast and ovarian cancer patients. *BMC Med Genet.* 2010;11:20.

153. **Rafnar T, Gudbjartsson DF, Sulem P, et al.** Mutations in BRIP1 confer high risk of ovarian cancer. *Nat Genet.* 2011;43:1104–1107.

154. **King MC, Marks JH, Mandell JB.** Breast and ovarian cancer risks due to inherited mutations in BRCA1 and BRCA2. *Science.* 2003;302:643–646.

155. **Kauff ND, Satagopan JM, Robson ME, et al.** Risk-reducing salpingo-oophorectomy in women with a BRCA1 or BRCA2 mutation. *N Engl J Med.* 2002;346:1609–1615.

156. **Rebbeck TR, Lynch HT, Neuhausen SL, et al.** Prophylactic oophorectomy in carriers of BRCA1 or BRCA2 mutations. *N Engl J Med.* 2002;346:1616–1622.

157. **Finch A, Beiner M, Lubinski J, et al.** Salpingo-oophorectomy and the risk of ovarian, fallopian tube, and peritoneal cancers in women with a BRCA1 or BRCA2 Mutation. *JAMA.* 2006;296:185–192.

158. **Stratton JF, Gayther SA, Russell P, et al.** Contribution of BRCA1 mutations to ovarian cancer. *N Engl J Med.* 1997;336:1125–1130.

159. **Callahan MJ, Crum CP, Medeiros F, et al.** Primary fallopian tube malignancies in BRCA-positive women undergoing surgery for ovarian cancer risk reduction. *J Clin Oncol.* 2007;25:3985–3990.

160. **Medeiros F, Muto MG, Lee Y, et al.** The tubal fimbria is a preferred site for early adenocarcinoma in women with familial ovarian cancer syndrome. *Am J Surg Pathol.* 2006;30:230–236.

161. **Shaw PA, Rouzbahman M, Pizer ES, et al.** Candidate serous cancer precursors in fallopian tube epithelium of BRCA1/2 mutation carriers. *Mod Pathol.* 2009;22:1133–1138.

162. **Lu KH, Garber JE, Cramer DW, et al.** Occult ovarian tumors in women with BRCA1 or BRCA2 mutations undergoing prophylactic oophorectomy. *J Clin Oncol.* 2000;18:2728–2732.

163. **Colgan TJ, Murphy J, Cole DE, et al.** Occult carcinoma in prophylactic oophorectomy specimens: Prevalence and association with BRCA germline mutation status. *Am J Surg Pathol.* 2001;25:1283–1289.

164. **Piver MS, Jishi MF, Tsukada Y, et al.** Primary peritoneal carcinoma after prophylactic oophorectomy in women with a family history of ovarian cancer. A report of the Gilda Radner Familial Ovarian Cancer Registry. *Cancer.* 1993;71:2751–2755.

165. **Struewing JP, Watson P, Easton DF, et al.** Prophylactic oophorectomy in inherited breast/ovarian cancer families. *Monogr Natl Cancer Inst.* 1995;17:33–35.

166. **The Cancer Genome Atlas Research Network.** Integrated genomic analyses of ovarian carcinoma. *Nature.* 2011;474:609–615.

167. **Kallioniemi A, Kallioniemi OP, Sudar D, et al.** Comparative genomic hybridization for molecular cytogenetic analysis of solid tumors. *Science.* 1992;258:818–821.

168. **Cliby W, Ritland S, Hartmann L, et al.** Human epithelial ovarian cancer allelotype. *Cancer Res.* 1993;53:2393–2398.

169. **McBride DJ, Etemadmoghadam D, Cooke SL, et al.** Tandem duplication of chromosomal segments is common in ovarian and breast cancer genomes. *J Pathol.* 2012;227:446–455.

170. **Tashiro H, Niyazaki K, Okamura H, et al.** c-*myc* overexpression in human primary ovarian tumors: Its relevance to tumor progression. *Int J Cancer.* 1992;50:828–833.

171. **Farley J, Smith LM, Darcy KM, et al.** Cyclin E expression is a significant predictor of survival in advanced, suboptimally debulked ovarian epithelial cancers: A Gynecologic Oncology Group study. *Cancer Res.* 2003;63:1235–1241.

172. **Etemadmoghadam D, George J, Cowin PA, et al.** Amplicon-dependent CCNE1 expression is critical for clonogenic survival after cisplatin treatment and is correlated with 20q11 gain in ovarian cancer. *PLoS One.* 2010;5:e15498.

173. **Rosen DG, Yang G, Deavers MT, et al.** Cyclin E expression is correlated with tumor progression and predicts a poor prognosis in patients with ovarian carcinoma. *Cancer.* 2006;106:1925–1932.

174. **Bellacosa A, de Feo D, Godwin AK, et al.** Molecular alterations of the AKT2 oncogene in ovarian and breast carcinomas. *Int J Cancer.* 1995;64:280–285.

175. **Shayesteh L, Lu Y, Kuo WL, et al.** PIK3CA is implicated as an oncogene in ovarian cancer. *Nat Genet.* 1999;21:99–102.

176. **Santiskulvong C, Konecny GE, Fekete M, et al.** Dual targeting of phosphoinositide 3-kinase and mammalian target of rapamycin using NVP-BEZ235 as a novel therapeutic approach in human ovarian carcinoma. *Clin Cancer Res.* 2011;17:2373–2384.

177. **Wallin JJ, Guan J, Prior WW, et al.** Nuclear phospho-Akt increase predicts synergy of PI3 K inhibition and doxorubicin in breast and ovarian cancer. *Sci Transl Med.* 2010;2:48ra66.

178. **Hirai H, Sootome H, Nakatsuru Y, et al.** MK-2206, an allosteric Akt inhibitor, enhances antitumor efficacy by standard chemotherapeutic agents or molecular targeted drugs in vitro and in vivo. *Mol Cancer Therapy.* 2010;9:1956–1967.

179. **Mabuchi S, Altomare DA, Cheung M, et al.** RAD001 inhibits human ovarian cancer cell proliferation, enhances cisplatin-induced apoptosis, and prolongs survival in an ovarian cancer model. *Clin Cancer Res.* 2007;13:4261–4270.

180. **Flesken-Nikitin A, Choi KC, Eng JP, et al.** Induction of carcinogenesis by concurrent inactivation of p53 and Rb1 in the mouse ovarian surface epithelium. *Cancer Res.* 2003;63:3459–3463.

181. **Slamon DJ, Godolphin W, Jones LA, et al.** Studies of HER-2/*neu* proto-oncogene in human breast and ovarian cancer. *Science.* 1989;244:707–712.

182. **Berchuck A, Kamel A, Whitaker R, et al.** Overexpression of HER-2/*neu* is associated with poor survival in advanced epithelial ovarian cancer. *Cancer Res.* 1990;50:4087–4091.

183. **Slamon D, Eiermann W, Robert N, et al.** Adjuvant trastuzumab in HER2-positive breast cancer. *N Engl J Med.* 2011;365:1273–1283.

184. **Bookman MA, Darcy KM, Clarke-Pearson D, et al.** Evaluation of monoclonal humanized anti-HER2 antibody, trastuzumab, in patients with recurrent or refractory ovarian or primary peritoneal carcinoma with overexpression of HER2: A phase II trial of the Gynecologic Oncology Group. *J Clin Oncol.* 2003;21:283–290.

185. **Ray-Coquard I, Guastalla JP, Allouache D, et al.** HER2 Overexpression/amplification and trastuzumab treatment in advanced ovarian cancer: A GINECO phase II study. *Clin Ovarian Cancer.* 2008;1:54–59.

186. **Schultz DC, Vanderveer L, Buetow KH, et al.** Characterization of chromosome 9 in human ovarian neoplasia identifies frequent genetic imbalance on 9q and rare alterations involving 9p, including CDKN2. *Cancer Res.* 1995;55:2150–2157.

187. **McCluskey LL, Chen C, Delgadillo E, et al.** Differences in p16 gene methylation and expression in benign and malignant ovarian tumors. *Gynecol Oncol.* 1999;72:87–92.

188. **Liu Z, Wang LE, Wang L, et al.** Methylation and messenger RNA expression of p15INK4b but not p16INK4 a are independent risk factors for ovarian cancer. *Clin Cancer Res.* 2005;11:4968–4976.

189. **Levesque MA, Katsaros D, Massobrio M, et al.** Evidence for a dose-response effect between p53 (but not p21WAF1/Cip1) protein concentrations, survival, and responsiveness in patients with epithelial ovarian cancer treated with platinum-based chemotherapy. *Clin Cancer Res.* 2000;6:3260–3270.

190. **Korkolopoulou P, Vassilopoulos I, Konstantinidou AE, et al.** The combined evaluation of p27Kip1 and Ki-67 expression provides independent information on overall survival of ovarian carcinoma patients. *Gynecol Oncol.* 2002;85:404–414.

191. **Rosen DG, Yang G, Cai KQ, et al.** Subcellular localization of p27kip1 expression predicts poor prognosis in human ovarian cancer. *Clin Cancer Res.* 2005;11:632–637.

192. **Casey G, Lopez ME, Ramos JC, et al.** DNA sequence analysis of exons 2 through 11 and immunohistochemical staining are required to detect all known p53 alterations in human malignancies. *Oncogene.* 1996;13:1971–1981.

193. **Marks JR, Davidoff AM, Kerns B, et al.** Overexpression and mutation of p53 in epithelial ovarian cancer. *Cancer Res.* 1991;51:2979–2984.

194. **Kohler MF, Marks JR, Wiseman RW, et al.** Spectrum of mutation and frequency of allelic deletion of the p53 gene in ovarian cancer. *J Natl Cancer Inst.* 1993;85:1513–1519.

195. **Havrilesky L, Hamdan H, Darcy K, et al.** Relationship between p53 mutation, p53 overexpression and survival in advanced ovarian cancers treated on Gynecologic Oncology Group studies #114 and #132. *J Clin Oncol.* 2003;21:3814–3825.

196. **Baldwin RL, Nemeth E, Tran H, et al.** BRCA1 promoter region hypermethylation in ovarian carcinoma: A population-based study. *Cancer Res.* 2000;60:5329–5333.

197. **Rubin SC, Benjamin I, Behbakht K, et al.** Clinical and pathological features of ovarian cancer in women with germ-line mutations of BRCA1. *N Engl J Med.* 1996;335:1413–1416.

198. **Bolton KL, Chenevix-Trench G, Goh C, et al.** Association between BRCA1 and BRCA2 mutations and survival in women with invasive epithelial ovarian cancer. *JAMA.* 2012;307:382–390.

199. **Norquist B, Wurz KA, Pennil CC, et al.** Secondary somatic mutations restoring BRCA1/2 predict chemotherapy resistance in hereditary ovarian carcinomas. *J Clin Oncol.* 2011;29:3008–3015.

200. **Annunziata CM, O'Shaughnessy J.** Poly (ADP-ribose) polymerase as a novel therapeutic target in cancer. *Clin Cancer Res.* 2010;16:4517–4526.

201. **Farmer H, McCabe N, Lord CJ, et al.** Targeting the DNA repair defect in BRCA mutant cells as a therapeutic strategy. *Nature.* 2005;434:917–921.

202. **Banerjee S, Kaye SB, Ashworth A.** Making the best of PARP inhibitors in ovarian cancer. *Nat Rev Clin Oncol.* 2010;7:508–519.

203. **Ledermann J, Harter P, Gourley C, et al.** Olaparib maintenance therapy in platinum-sensitive relapsed ovarian cancer. *N Engl J Med.* 2012;366:1382–1392.

204. **Welsh JB, Zarrinkar PP, Sapinoso LM, et al.** Analysis of gene expression profiles in normal and neoplastic ovarian tissue samples identifies candidate molecular markers of epithelial ovarian cancer. *Proc Natl Acad Sci U S A.* 2001;98:1176–1181.

205. **Schwartz DR, Kardia SL, Shedden KA, et al.** Gene expression in ovarian cancer reflects both morphology and biological behavior, distinguishing clear cell from other poor- prognosis ovarian carcinomas. *Cancer Res.* 2002;62:4722–4729.

206. **Bonome T, Lee JY, Park DC, et al.** Expression profiling of serous low malignant potential, low-grade, and high-grade tumors of the ovary. *Cancer Res.* 2005;65:10602–10612.

207. **Shridhar V, Lee J, Pandita A, et al.** Genetic analysis of early- versus late-stage ovarian tumors. *Cancer Res.* 2001;61:5895–5904.

208. **Spentzos D, Levine DA, Kolia S, et al.** Unique gene expression profile based on pathologic response in epithelial ovarian cancer. *J Clin Oncol.* 2005;23:7911–7918.

209. **Berchuck A, Iversen ES, Luo J, et al.** Microarray analysis of early stage serous ovarian cancers shows profiles predictive of favorable outcome. *Clin Cancer Res.* 2009;15:2448–2455.

210. **Mok SCH, Bell DA, Knapp RC, et al.** Mutation of K-*ras* protooncogene in human ovarian epithelial tumors of borderline malignancy. *Cancer Res.* 1993;53:1489–1492.

211. **Singer G, Oldt R III, Cohen Y, et al.** Mutations in BRAF and KRAS characterize the development of low-grade ovarian serous carcinoma. *J Natl Cancer Inst.* 2003;95:484–486.

212. **Ho CL, Kurman RJ, Dehari R, et al.** Mutations of BRAF and KRAS precede the development of ovarian serous borderline tumors. *Cancer Res.* 2004;64:6915–6918.

213. **Grisham RN, Iyer G, Garg K, et al.** BRAF mutation is associated with early stage disease and improved outcome in patients with low-grade serous ovarian cancer. *Cancer.* 2013;119:548–554.

214. **Diaz-Padilla I, Malpica AL, Minig L, et al.** Ovarian low-grade serous carcinoma: A comprehensive update. *Gynecol Oncol.* 2012;126:279–285.

215. **Gershenson DM, Deavers M, Diaz S, et al.** Prognostic significance of p53 expression in advanced-stage ovarian serous borderline tumors. *Clin Cancer Res.* 1999;5:4053–4058.

216. **Berchuck A, Kohler MF, Hopkins MP, et al.** Overexpression of p53 is not a feature of benign and early-stage borderline epithelial ovarian tumors. *Gynecol Oncol.* 1994;52:232–236.

217. **Ortiz BH, Ailawadi M, Colitti C, et al.** Second primary or recurrence? Comparative patterns of p53 and K-ras mutations suggest that serous borderline ovarian tumors and subsequent serous carcinomas are unrelated tumors. *Cancer Res.* 2001; 61:7264–7267.

218. **Jones S, Wang TL, Shih I, et al.** Frequent mutations of chromatin remodeling gene ARID1 A in ovarian clear cell carcinoma. *Science.* 2010;330:228–231.

219. **Wiegand KC, Shah SP, Al-Agha OM, et al.** ARID1 A mutations in endometriosis-associated ovarian carcinomas. *N Engl J Med.* 2010; 363:1532–1543.

220. **Anglesio MS, Carey MS, Kobel M, et al.** Clear cell carcinoma of the ovary: A report from the first Ovarian Clear Cell Symposium, June 24th, 2010. *Gynecol Oncol.* 2011;121:407–415.

221. **McConechy MK, Anglesio MS, Kalloger SE, et al.** Subtype-specific mutation of PPP2R1 A in endometrial and ovarian carcinomas. *J Pathol.* 2011;223:567–573.

222. **Obata K, Morland SJ, Watson RH, et al.** Frequent PTEN/MMAC mutations in endometrioid but not serous or mucinous epithelial ovarian tumors. *Cancer Res.* 1998;58:2095–2097.

223. **Wu R, Zhai Y, Fearon ER, et al.** Diverse mechanisms of beta-catenin deregulation in ovarian endometrioid adenocarcinomas. *Cancer Res.* 2001;61:8247–8255.

224. **Wu R, Hendrix-Lucas N, Kuick R, et al.** Mouse model of human ovarian endometrioid adenocarcinoma based on somatic defects in the Wnt/beta-catenin and PI3 K/Pten signaling pathways. *Cancer Cell.* 2007;11:321–333.

225. **Dinulescu DM, Ince TA, Quade BJ, et al.** Role of K-ras and Pten in the development of mouse models of endometriosis and endometrioid ovarian cancer. *Nat Med.* 2005;11:63–70.

226. **Lin WM, Forgacs E, Warshal DP, et al.** Loss of heterozygosity and mutational analysis of the PTEN/MMAC1 gene in synchronous endometrial and ovarian carcinomas. *Clin Cancer Res.* 1998;4:2577–2583.

227. **Guerra F, Kurelac I, Magini P, et al.** Mitochondrial DNA genotyping reveals synchronous nature of simultaneously detected endometrial and ovarian cancers. *Gynecol Oncol.* 2011;122:457–458.

228. **Shah SP, Kobel M, Senz J, et al.** Mutation of FOXL2 in granulosa-cell tumors of the ovary. *N Engl J Med.* 2009;360:2719–2729.

229. **Heravi-Moussavi A, Anglesio MS, Cheng SW, et al.** Recurrent somatic DICER1 mutations in nonepithelial ovarian cancers. *N Engl J Med.* 2012;366:234–242.

230. **Scheffner M, Werness BA, Huibregtse JM, et al.** The E6 oncoprotein encoded by human papillomavirus types 16 and 18 promotes the degradation of p53. *Cell.* 1990;63:1129–1136.

231. **Munoz N, Bosch FX, de Sanjose S, et al.** Epidemiologic classification of human papillomavirus types associated with cervical cancer. *N Engl J Med.* 2003;348:518–527.

232. **Sun XW, Kuhn L, Ellerbrock TV, et al.** Human papillomavirus infection in women infected with the human immunodeficiency virus. *N Engl J Med.* 1997;337:1343–1349.

233. **The Future II Study Group.** Quadrivalent vaccine against human papillomavirus to prevent high-grade cervical lesions. *N Engl J Med.* 2013;356:1915–1927.

234. **Massimi P, Pim D, Storey A, et al.** HPV-16 E7 and adenovirus E1 a complex formation with TATA box binding protein is enhanced by casein kinase II phosphorylation. *Oncogene.* 1996;12:2325–2330.

235. **Scheffner M, Munger K, Byrne JC, et al.** The state of the p53 and retinoblastoma gene in human cervical carcinoma cell lines. *Proc Natl Acad Sci U S A.* 1991;88:5523–5527.

236. **Werness BA, Levine AJ, Howley PM.** Association of human papillomavirus types 16 and 18 E6 proteins with p53. *Science.* 1990;248: 76–79.

237. **de Boer MA, Jordanova ES, Kenter GG, et al.** High human papillomavirus oncogene mRNA expression and not viral DNA load is associated with poor prognosis in cervical cancer patients. *Clin Cancer Res.* 2007;13:132–138.

238. **Parker MF, Arroyo GF, Geradts J, et al.** Molecular characterization of adenocarcinoma of the cervix. *Gynecol Oncol.* 1997;64:242–251.

239. **Wang SS, Trunk M, Schiffman M, et al.** Validation of p16INK4 a as a marker of oncogenic human papillomavirus infection in cervical biopsies from a population-based cohort in Costa Rica. *Cancer Epidemiol Biomarkers Prev.* 2004;13:1355–1360.

240. **Narayan G, Pulido HA, Koul S, et al.** Genetic analysis identifies putative tumor suppressor sites at 2q35-q36.1 and 2q36.3-q37.1 involved in cervical cancer progression. *Oncogene.* 2003;22:3489–3499.

241. **Umayahara K, Numa F, Suehiro Y, et al.** Comparative genomic hybridization detects genetic alterations during early stages of cervical cancer progression. *Genes Chromosomes Cancer.* 2002;33:98–102.

242. **Yang YC, Shyong WY, Chang MS, et al.** Frequent gain of copy number on the long arm of chromosome 3 in human cervical adenocarcinoma. *Cancer Genet Cytogenet.* 2001;131:48–53.

243. **Lando M, Holden M, Bergersen LC, et al.** Gene dosage, expression, and ontology analysis identifies driver genes in the carcinogenesis and chemoradioresistance of cervical cancer. *PLoS Genet.* 2009; 5:e1000719.

244. **Lin WM, Michalopulos EA, Dhurander N, et al.** Allelic loss and microsatellite alterations of chromosome 3p14.2 are more frequent in recurrent cervical dysplasias. *Clin Cancer Res.* 2000;6:1410–1414.

245. **Kirchhoff M, Rose H, Petersen BL, et al.** Comparative genomic hybridization reveals a recurrent pattern of chromosomal aberrations in severe dysplasia/carcinoma in situ of the cervix and in advanced-stage cervical carcinoma. *Genes Chromosomes Cancer.* 1999;24:144–150.

246. **Birrer MJ, Hendricks D, Farley J, et al.** Abnormal Fhit expression in malignant and premalignant lesions of the cervix. *Cancer Res.* 1999;59:5270–5274.

247. **Huang LW, Chao SL, Chen TJ.** Reduced Fhit expression in cervical carcinoma: Correlation with tumor progression and poor prognosis. *Gynecol Oncol.* 2003;90:331–337.

248. **Connolly DC, Greenspan DL, Wu R, et al.** Loss of fhit expression in invasive cervical carcinomas and intraepithelial lesions associated with invasive disease. *Clin Cancer Res.* 2000;6:3505–3510.

249. **Liu FS, Hsieh YT, Chen JT, et al.** FHIT (fragile histidine triad) gene analysis in cervical intraepithelial neoplasia. *Gynecol Oncol.* 2001;82:283–290.

250. **Krivak TC, McBroom JW, Seidman J, et al.** Abnormal fragile histidine triad (FHIT) expression in advanced cervical carcinoma: A poor prognostic factor. *Cancer Res.* 2001;61:4382–4385.

251. **Riou G, Barrois M, Sheng ZM, et al.** Somatic deletions and mutations of c-Ha-*ras* gene in human cervical cancers. *Oncogene.* 1988;3:329–333.

252. **Van Le L, Stoerker J, Rinehart CA, et al.** H-*ras* condon 12 mutation in cervical dysplasia. *Gynecol Oncol.* 1993;49:181–184.

253. **Riou G, Le MG, Favre M, et al.** Human papillomavirus-negative status and c-*myc* gene overexpression: Independent prognostic indicators of distant metastasis for early-stage invasive cervical cancers. *J Natl Cancer Inst.* 1992;84:1525–1526.

254. **Bourhis J, Le MG, Barrois M, et al.** Prognostic value of c-myc proto-oncogene overexpression in early invasive carcinoma of the cervix. *J Clin Oncol.* 1990;8:1789–1796.

255. **Dong SM, Kim HS, Rha SH, et al.** Promoter hypermethylation of multiple genes in carcinoma of the uterine cervix. *Clin Cancer Res.* 2001;7:1982–1986.

256. **Virmani AK, Muller C, Rathi A, et al.** Aberrant methylation during cervical carcinogenesis. *Clin Cancer Res.* 2001;7:584–589.

257. **Wong YF, Selvanayagam ZE, Wei N, et al.** Expression genomics of cervical cancer: Molecular classification and prediction of radiotherapy response by DNA microarray. *Clin Cancer Res.* 2003;9:5486–5492.

258. **Kuzmin I, Liu L, Dammann R, et al.** Inactivation of RAS association domain family 1A gene in cervical carcinomas and the role of human papillomavirus infection. *Cancer Res.* 2003;63:1888–1893.

259. **Deveault C, Qian JH, Chebaro W, et al.** NLRP7 mutations in women with diploid androgenetic and triploid moles: A proposed mechanism for mole formation. *Hum Mol Genet.* 2009;18:888–897.

260. **Kim SJ, Lee SY, Lee C, et al.** Differential expression profiling of genes in a complete hydatidiform mole using cDNA microarray analysis. *Gynecol Oncol.* 2006;103:654–660.

261. **Feng HC, Tsao SW, Ngan HY, et al.** Differential expression of insulin-like growth factor binding protein 1 and ferritin light polypeptide in gestational trophoblastic neoplasia: Combined cDNA suppression subtractive hybridization and microarray study. *Cancer.* 2005;104:2409–2416.

262. **Fong PY, Xue WC, Ngan HY, et al.** Mcl-1 expression in gestational trophoblastic disease correlates with clinical outcome: A differential expression study. *Cancer.* 2005;103:268–276.

263. **Shih I.** Gestational trophoblastic neoplasia—Pathogenesis and potential therapeutic targets. *Lancet Oncol.* 2013;8:642–650.

Note: Portions of this chapter have previously appeared in Principles and Practice of Gynecologic Oncology, 6th ed./editor, Richard R. Barakat. Lippincott Williams & Wilkins, 2013, with permission of the publisher.

2 Biologic, Targeted, and Immune Therapy

Oliver Dorigo
Jonathan S. Berek

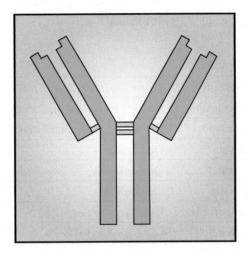

Cancer is caused by a series of events that include the accumulation of successive molecular lesions and alterations in the tumor microenvironment (1). Molecular lesions include overexpression, amplification, or mutations of oncogenes; deletion of tumor suppressor genes; and the inappropriate expression of growth factors and their cellular receptors. In addition to these molecular changes, the formation of new blood vessels (angiogenesis) and the lack of effective host antitumor immune responses create a microenvironment that supports the growth of cancer (2). Our improved understanding of these mechanisms presents an opportunity for the development of novel therapeutic approaches (3). This chapter provides an overview of biologic, targeted, and immunotherapeutic strategies for gynecologic cancers.

Biologic and Targeted Therapies

The growth of cancer cells is crucially dependent on oncogenic signal transduction pathways. Extracellular signals are transmitted to the cancer cell via transmembrane receptors. Activation of the **epidermal growth factor receptors (EGFRs, HER2, HER3, and HER4),** for example, stimulates a cascade of intracellular proteins that ultimately lead to changes in gene expression. **Novel therapeutics are targeted to modulate these signal transduction pathways by blocking the extracellular transmembrane receptors or interfering with intracellular proteins such as tyrosine kinases further downstream. This novel therapeutic approach is also termed** *molecular targeting* (4). It is accomplished by either monoclonal antibodies that bind to transmembrane receptors and serum proteins such as **vascular endothelial growth factor (VEGF)** or chemical, small-molecule inhibitors that prevent activation of signal transduction proteins. **Targeting the signaling cascade inhibits the proliferation of cancer cells, induces apoptosis, and blocks metastasis. The specificity of these molecules is based on the assumption that cancer cells are overexpressing various proteins in the signal transduction pathways, therefore presenting a preferred target compared to normal cells.** Conceptually, this should result in more cancer cell–specific therapy and less clinical side effects because of sparing of normal tissue (5). At this time, a large variety of molecular-targeting strategies are being tested for efficacy in clinical trials (Table 2.1).

Table 2.1 Targeted Cancer Therapies

Targeted Pathway	Drug	Chemistry	Main Molecular Targets
Angiogenesis	Bevacizumab	Humanized monoclonal antibody	VEGF-A
	VEGF-Trap	Fusion protein	VEGF-A (B, C, D, E)
	Cediranib	Quinazoline	VEGFR-1, VEGFR-2, VEGFR-3
	Pazopanib	Indazolylpyrimidine	VEGFR-1, VEGFR-2, VEGFR-3, PDGFR-α/β, c-kit
	Trebananib	Peptide–Fc fusion protein (peptibody)	Angiopoietin 1 and 2
	Nintedanib	Indolinone	VEGFR-1, VEGFR-2, and VEGFR-3, PDGFR-α/β, FGFR-1, FGFR-2, FGFR-3, members of the v-src sarcoma viral oncogene homolog (Src) family, and Flt-3
Epidermal growth factor receptors	Trastuzumab	Humanized monoclonal antibody	HER2
	Pertuzumab	Humanized monoclonal antibody	HER2
	Cetuximab	Chimerized monoclonal antibody	EGFR
	Gefitinib	Quinazoline	EGFR ATP-binding domain
	Erlotinib	Quinazoline	EGFR ATP-binding domain
	Lapatinib	Quinazoline	EGFR, HER2, ERK1 and 2, Akt
Tyrosine kinases	Temsirolimus	Rapamycin analog	mTOR
Multiple kinases	Sorafenib	Carboxamide derivative	raf, c-kit, VEGFR-2, 3, FLT-3, PDGFR-β
	Sunitinib	Carboxamide derivative	PDGFR, VEGFR-1, 2, 3, c-kit, FLT-3
PARP	Niraparib	Carboxamide derivative	PARP
	Olaparib	Phthalazinone derivative	
	Rucaparib	Indole derivative	
	Veliparib	Carboxamide derivative	

VEGF, vascular endothelial growth factor; VEGFR, vascular endothelial growth factor receptor; PDGFR, platelet-derived endothelial cell growth factor receptor; HER2, human epidermal growth factor; EGFR, epidermal growth factor receptor; mTOR, mammalian target of rapamycin; FLT3, fms-like tyrosine kinase 3; raf, raf oncogene; PARP, Poly(ADP-ribose) polymerase.

Angiogenesis

The formation of new blood vessels (neoangiogenesis) is a normal process during embryonic development, tissue remodeling, and wound healing (6). Malignant tumors are able to induce angiogenesis by secreting paracrine factors that promote the formation of new blood vessels. **Angiogenesis is a complex process that is influenced by various pro- and antiangiogenic factors, including VEGF, interleukin 8, platelet-derived endothelial cell growth factor, and angiopoietins. Overexpression of these angiogenic factors leads to neovascularization and increased supply of nutrients and oxygen to the tumor.**

Three main therapeutic strategies that target angiogenesis are currently being explored for the treatment of cancer patients (7). One group of agents targets VEGF (e.g., *bevacizumab*, *VEGF-Trap*), the second group prevents VEGF from binding to its receptor (*pertuzumab*), and the third group of agents inhibits tyrosine kinase activation and downstream signaling in the angiogenesis signaling cascade (*vatalanib*, *sunitinib*) (8).

Vascular Endothelial Growth Factor

VEGF is overexpressed in gynecologic malignancies, therefore presenting an excellent target for therapy (9). Inhibition of VEGF-induced angiogenic signaling decreases tumor microvascular density and causes death of solid tumors in various preclinical models. Several agents are now available for clinical use; all target the VEGF signaling pathway. The most widely used agent at this time is *bevacizumab*, a humanized, recombinant monoclonal antibody that binds to all isoforms of VEGF-A (12). *Bevacizumab* has been approved for the treatment of colorectal carcinoma based on improved overall survival in combination with chemotherapy in patients with metastatic disease, single agent therapy in glioblastoma with progressive disease, first-line treatment in combination with *carboplatin* and *paclitaxel* for lung cancer, and in combination with *interferon alpha* for metastatic renal cell carcinoma (10,11).

In ovarian carcinoma, various clinical trials have demonstrated the efficacy of *bevacizumab* treatment (see Chapter 11 for more discussion). The initial studies by the Gynecologic Oncology Group included 62 patients treated with single agent *bevacizumab* 15 mg/kg intravenously every 21 days (13). Thirteen patients (21%) showed clinical responses with two complete and eleven partial responses. The median response duration was 10 months, and 25 patients (41.3%) survived progression free for at least 6 months. In a second trial, *bevacizumab* treatment of 44 patients with recurrent, platinum-resistant ovarian carcinoma resulted in partial responses in seven patients (15.9%) and stable disease in 27 (61.4%) (14). Median progression-free survival (PFS) was 4.4 months with a median survival of 10.7 months.

Based on these promising data, Phase III first-line clinical trials of *bevacizumab* were conducted. The GOG-0218 and ICON7 studies assessed the efficacy of *bevacizumab* added to *carboplatin* and *paclitaxel* followed by maintenance therapy in patients with epithelial ovarian cancer (15,16). **Significant improvements were demonstrated in progression-free survival in both studies with concurrent and maintenance *bevacizumab* treatment. In addition, an overall survival benefit of almost 8 months** (28.8 vs. 36.6 months; HR, 0.64; 95% confidence interval [CI], 0.48 to 0.85; $p < 0.002$) **was found for the subgroup of patients with high-risk disease when treated with *bevacizumab*. This high-risk group was defined as having FIGO stage IV or stage III disease with suboptimal tumor debulking.** *Bevacizumab* did not show an overall survival benefit when the entire cohort was analyzed.

***Bevacizumab* has likewise demonstrated efficacy in recurrent ovarian cancer,** both in the so-called AURELIA and OCEANS studies (17,18). In the AURELIA trial, patients with platinum-resistant disease were treated with *bevacizumab* in combination with chemotherapy (either *topotecan, pegylated liposomal doxorubicin,* or weekly *paclitaxel*). A statistically significant improvement in PFS (3.4 vs. 6.7 months; HR, 0.48; $p < 0.001$) was found in patients treated with the combination. In the OCEANS study, *bevacizumab* in combination with *carboplatin* and *gemcitabine* followed by maintenance therapy in platinum-sensitive patients resulted in a significant improvement in PFS compared to chemotherapy alone (8.4 vs. 12.4 months; HR, 0.48; $p < 0.0001$). Neither the OCEANS nor AURELIA trial showed a benefit in overall survival, but both demonstrated the efficacy of *bevacizumab* even in platinum-resistant disease.

A recent trial conducted by the GOG has demonstrated the efficacy of *bevacizumab* in combination with *cisplatin* and *paclitaxel* or *cisplatin* with *topotecan* in locally advanced and metastatic cervical cancer. The median PFS in the *bevacizumab* group was 8.2 months, compared with 5.9 months in the chemotherapy alone group. In addition, the median overall survival (OS) for patients who received *cisplatin* plus *paclitaxel* was 14.3 months, significantly less than the 17.5 months for the *bevacizumab* group ($p = 0.0348$). Similarly, the median OS for those who received *topotecan* plus *paclitaxel* was 12.7 months, compared with 16.2 months with *bevacizumab* ($p = 0.0896$).

***Bevacizumab*-related side effects include venous and arterial thrombosis, hemorrhage, nephrotic syndrome with proteinuria, hypertension, rare leukoencephalopathy, and bowel perforation** (20–24). There are no predictors of response to *bevacizumab* at this time, but prospective clinical trials are currently investigating the utility of novel imaging technologies to monitor the clinical response.

Other antiangiogenic strategies are being pursued in clinical trials. Angiopoietin 1 and 2 have been identified as important mediators of angiogenesis in ovarian cancer via their binding to the Tie2 receptor. *Trebananib* (AMG386) is a peptide–Fc fusion protein that blocks the interactions between angiopoetin-1 and angiopoetin-2, which are expressed on vascular endothelial cells with the Tie2 receptor (19). This results in blocking of VEGF stimulation and vascular maturation. The ongoing first-line (TRINOVA-3) and recurrent (TRINOVA-1 and 2) ovarian cancer clinical trials combine *trebananib* with chemotherapy, and also use it as maintenance.

***VEGF-Trap* (AVE 0005)** is a recombinant fusion protein that consists of the extracellular domain of VEGF receptors VEGFR1 and VEGFR2 fused to the FC portion of immunoglobulin G1 (25). VEGF is inactivated by binding to the ligand-binding domain of this fusion protein followed by destruction of this complex via immune system–mediated mechanisms. **Small-molecule tyrosine kinase inhibitors that target the VEGF pathway include *pazopanib, vatalanib,* and *sunitinib*. *Pazopanib* is a multitarget tyrosine kinase inhibitor which is directed against VEGFR1,**

VEGFR2, VEGFR3, platelet-derived growth factor receptor (PDGFR), and c-kit (3). Similarly, *vatalanib* (PTK787) targets multiple VEGF-receptor tyrosine kinases. *Sunitinib* (SU11248) inhibits PDGR, VEGFR, c-kit, and SLT3, and has shown promising results in renal cell cancer and gastrointestinal stromal tumors. Trials in gynecologic malignancies are ongoing.

Epidermal Growth Factor Receptor

The epidermal growth factor receptor pathway plays an important role in regulation of growth and differentiation of epithelial cells through regulation of cell division, migration, adhesion, differentiation, and apoptosis (26). **The epidermal growth factor receptor family consists of four members including EGFR (HER1), HER2, HER3, and HER4** (27). **EGFR overexpression has been reported in 35–70% of patients with epithelial ovarian cancer** (28,29). **In endometrial cancer, EGFR is overexpressed in 43–67% of tumors, and is associated with a shortened disease-free and overall survival** (30–32). In addition, amplification of the HER2 gene is commonly found in endometrial carcinoma. Overexpression of the HER2 receptor is more prevalent in nonendometrial cancer and is associated with an aggressive form of the disease. In uterine serous carcinomas, HER2 gene amplification can be demonstrated in as many as 42% of cases (33).

Various agents directed against epidermal growth factor receptors are available (34). *Trastuzumab* is a humanized monoclonal antibody that binds to the extracellular domain of HER2 (35). Blockade of HER2 affects various molecules that ultimately decrease cell proliferation. *Pertuzumab* is another humanized monoclonal antibody that binds to a different epitope of HER2 compared to *trastuzumab*. Binding to HER2 prevents dimerization of the receptor, which is required for its function (36). *Cetuximab* is a chimeric monoclonal antibody that binds to EGFR, thereby preventing dimerization and activation (37). *Gefitinib* is a small-molecule tyrosine kinase inhibitor of EGFR that prevents phosphorylation of the receptor by binding to the intracellular ATP-binding domain of the receptor (38). *Erlotinib* is a small-molecule tyrosine kinase inhibitor of EGRF that prevents phosphorylation of the intracellular domain of the EGFR receptor. *Lapatinib* (GW572016) inhibits both EGFR and HER2 (Fig. 2.1).

Inhibition of EGFR signaling is accomplished by using either monoclonal antibodies against the extracellular receptor or small-molecule inhibitors against the intracellular kinase domain. Both strategies result in inhibition of phosphorylation or receptor activation.

Erlotinib is a potent reversible inhibitor of EGFR tyrosine kinase that blocks receptor autophosphorylation and has been used for the treatment of ovarian carcinoma. In one study, 34 patients were treated with single agent *erlotinib* (150 mg/day orally) for as long as 48 weeks (39). Two patients showed a partial response lasting 8 and 17 weeks. Fifteen patients (44%) had stable

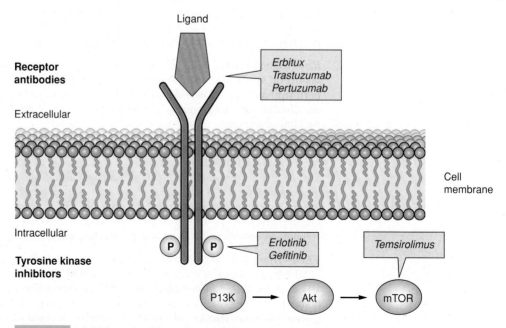

Figure 2.1 Inhibition of epidermal growth factor receptor signaling.

disease, and 17 patients (50%) progressed under treatment. The side effects of *erlotinib* were mainly confined to tissues with strong expression of EGFR: skin rashes and diarrhea were observed in 68% and 38% of patients, respectively.

Erlotinib has been used in combination with *docetaxel* and *carboplatin* as first-line treatment after surgical cytoreduction in patients with ovarian, fallopian tube, and peritoneal cancers (40). In this study, 23 evaluable patients showed five complete and seven partial responses. The treatment was well tolerated; main side effects were neutropenia and skin rashes. The study demonstrated the feasibility and tolerability of *erlotinib* in conjunction with chemotherapy.

Cetuximab (C225, *Erbitux*) is a chimerized monoclonal antibody against EGFR. Treatment of patients with primary ovarian or peritoneal cancer using *cetuximab* has shown only modest activity in screened patients with EGFR-positive tumors. *Cetuximab* in combination with *carboplatin* resulted in three complete (10.7%) and six partial (21.4%) responses in 28 patients with recurrent ovarian cancer (41). Twenty-six of these 28 patients (92.8%) had EGFR-positive tumors. **The combination of *paclitaxel*, *carboplatin*, and *cetuximab* for first-line chemotherapy of stage III ovarian cancer patients resulted in progression-free survival of 14.4 months and was therefore not significantly prolonged compared to historical data** (42).

Gefitinib (ZD1839 *Iressa*) is a low–molecular-weight quinazoline derivative that inhibits the activation of EGFR tyrosine kinase via competitive binding of the ATP-binding domain of the receptor. In a Gynecologic Oncology Group clinical trial, 27 patients with recurrent or persistent epithelial ovarian cancer were treated with 500-mg *gefitinib* daily (43). Four patients (14.8%) survived progression free for more than 6 months, with one objective response (3.6%). Commonly observed toxicity included skin rash and diarrhea. Interestingly, EGFR expression was associated with longer progression-free survival and possibly longer survival. The patient with the only objective antitumor response had a tumor with a mutation in the catalytic domain of the tumor's EGFR (2235dEL15). This patient received 29 cycles of *gefitinib* and had a progression-free survival of approximately 27 months.

In a separate trial, 24 patients with recurrent epithelial ovarian cancer were treated with *gefitinib* 500 mg daily (44). All tumor samples had detectable levels of EGFR and PGFR. Of 16 patients who completed more than two cycles of therapy, no complete or partial responses were observed. However, analysis of clinical samples showed that *gefitinib* inhibited phosphorylation of EGFR, thereby providing a conceptual proof of targeted therapy.

Treatment of patients with recurrent ovarian cancer using the combination of *gefitinib*, *carboplatin*, and *paxitaxel* has resulted in an overall response rate of 63% (45). Interestingly, antitumor responses were observed in 35% of patients with platinum-resistant disease compared to 73% of patients with platinum-sensitive disease. Based on these preliminary data, none of the 18 patients treated showed EGFR receptor mutations.

Gefitinib has also been used in combination with *tamoxifen*. In 56 patients with primary ovarian or fallopian tube cancer, treatment with *tamoxifen* (40 mg/day) and *gefitinib* (500 mg/day) did not result in objective antitumor responses, but 16 patients had stable disease (46). In squamous and adenocarcinoma of the cervix, *gefitinib* (500 mg/day) treatment resulted in disease stabilization in 6 of 28 patients (20%) but no clinical responses (47). The median duration of stable disease was 111.5 days, with a median overall survival of 107 days.

Lapatinib is a small-molecule inhibitor of both the HER2 and EGFR tyrosine kinase receptor. The rationale for using *lapatinib* in endometrial carcinoma is supported mainly by studies in human cancer cell lines. Its efficacy in endometrial cancer is being investigated currently in clinical trials (33).

HER2/*neu*

The HER2/*neu* receptor is activated by homo- or heterodimerization, resulting in tyrosine phosphorylation and subsequent activation of various downstream signals that among other functions control cellular proliferation, migration, and invasion. *Trastuzumab* is a recombinant, humanized IgG1 monoclonal antibody that is specific for the extracellular domain of HER2/*neu*. **Binding of the antibody to HER2/*neu* prevents activation of the receptor with a subsequent increase of apoptosis in vitro and in vivo, impaired DNA damage repair, and inhibition of tumor neovascularization** (35). Preclinical models have suggested that the therapeutic activity may also depend on innate immune effector cells that mediate antibody-dependent cellular cytotoxicity (ADCC). In addition, *trastuzumab* influences the adaptive immune response and augments antigen processing and presentation (48). In breast cancer, the addition of *trastuzumab* to adjuvant chemotherapy for patients with HER2/*neu*-positive tumors significantly decreases the hazard ratio for recurrence and subsequently improves survival (49).

The HER2/*neu* oncogene is overexpressed in several gynecologic malignancies, including 20% to 30% of ovarian cancers (50). The largest clinical trial evaluating HER2/*neu* as a target in ovarian or peritoneal carcinoma was conducted by the Gynecologic Oncology Group (51). **Of 837 tumor samples screened for HER2/*neu* expression, 95 patients (11.4%) were found to have tumors with HER/*neu* overexpression.** Forty-one patients with HER2/*neu*-positive tumors received *trastuzumab* weekly. Single agent treatment resulted in one complete (2.4%) and two partial (4.9%) responses, with a median duration of response of 8 weeks (range: 2 to 104 weeks). The authors concluded that **single agent *trastuzumab* in recurrent ovarian cancer was of limited value because of the low frequency of HER2/*neu*** overexpression and the low rate of clinical antitumor response.

HER2/*neu* overexpression is infrequent in cervical cancer. In one study, only one of 35 (2.9%) cervical carcinomas showed strong expression of HER2/*neu* (52). In uterine serous carcinoma, 12 of 68 tumors (18%) showed HER2/*neu* overexpression; this was associated with a worse overall prognosis (53). In a separate study, 5 of 19 specimens (26%) stained strongly for HER2/*neu* protein receptor (54).

Mitogen-activated Protein Kinase Pathways

The mitogen-activated protein (MAP) kinase cascades are activated by various cofactors, inflammatory cytokines, and stress (55). The signaling cascades include various molecules, including RAS, MEK1/2, ERK1/2, and p38 MAPK. Various molecules have been developed that target this pathway but are mostly still under investigation. *Sorafenib* is among the first of the agents with clinically proven efficacy. *Sorafenib* is a competitive inhibitor of *raf* that has been approved for treatment of renal cell carcinoma and hepatocellular carcinoma (56). Besides targeting *raf, sorafenib* also inhibits VEGFR2 and VEGFR3, FT3, c-kit, and PDGFR-β.

Targeting the MAPKinase pathway has been a particular focus of clinical studies in low-grade serous ovarian carcinomas. The latter are characterized by younger age at presentation, indolent growth pattern, and poor response to systemic therapy (57). **Up to one-third of low-grade serous ovarian carcinomas have been found to have a mutation in either BRAF or KRAS, and hence activated MAPKinase pathway signaling** (58). A phase II trial of the MEK1/2 inhibitor *selumetinib* (AZD6244) in 52 patients with recurrent low-grade serous ovarian carcinoma showed an overall response rate of 15.4%, stable disease in 65% of patients, and a PFS of 11 months (59). The 6% BRAF, 41% KRAS, and 15% NRAS mutations did not correlate with response to therapy.

PARP Inhibitors

The enzyme poly (adenosine diphosphate-ribose) polymerase (PARP) and the BRCA proteins are involved in DNA repair as induced by cytotoxic agents like platinum chemotherapy or radiation. The recent development of PARP inhibitors has allowed the therapeutic targeting of DNA repair pathways and exploited the concept of synthetic lethality. In essence, in a synthetic lethal pair, targeting of one gene product or protein (PARP) while the other gene is defective (*BRCA* mutation) selectively kills tumor cells while sparing normal cells (60). It has therefore been hypothesized that patients harboring mutations in *BRCA1–2* would be highly susceptible to treatment with PARP inhibitors. Several clinical trials have documented proof of this mechanism, including a large phase I study of the PARP inhibitor *olaparib* in women with *BRCA1* or *BRCA2* germline mutations (61,62). In a randomized phase II trial, patients with platinum-sensitive recurrent ovarian cancer who achieved a response to platinum-based chemotherapy were treated with maintenance *olaparib* (63). Among the 265 women, 22.8% had *BRCA* mutations, while 13.2% were wild type and 64% unknown. Treatment with *olaparib* at a dose of 400 mg twice daily resulted in a significantly longer median PFS compared to a placebo (median: 8.4 months vs. 4.8 months; HR = 0.35; 95% CI 0.25 to 0.49). Similarly, a randomized phase II trial of *paclitaxel–carboplatin* with or without *olaparib* followed by *olaparib* or placebo maintenance showed a significant prolongation of the median PFS in the experimental arm (median: 12.2 months vs. 9.6 months; HR = 0.51; 95% CI 0.34 to 0.77) (64). PARP inhibitors are currently being extensively studied in various clinical trials and include *olaparib, niraparib, BMN-673, rucaparib,* and *veliparib.* **The efficacy of PARP inhibitors might not be restricted to patients with mutated *BRCA*, but may also be seen in tumors with functional defects in other DNA repair pathway proteins.**

The PI3-kinase/Akt/mTOR Pathway

The phosphoinositide3-kinase (PI3-kinase)/Akt/mammalian target of rapamycin (mTOR) pathway is a major oncogenic signaling pathway in various cancers (65). Activation of this pathway can be demonstrated in more than 80% of endometrial cancers, 50% to 70% of epithelial ovarian cancers, and approximately 50% of cervical cancers (66–68). Activation of PI3-kinase by various growth factors such as platelet-derived growth factor (PDGF) or insulin growth factor results in phosphorylation and therefore activation of the central oncogenic protein Akt. Activated Akt is released from the membrane and elicits downstream effects, mainly by phosphorylating signal transduction proteins such as *BAD,* FKHR, Caspase 9, and the mTOR. Activation of these downstream signals leads to an increase in cellular proliferation, invasiveness, drug resistance, and neoangiogenesis. The *PTEN* gene (phosphatase and tensin homolog deleted on chromosome 10) is a tumor suppressor gene that is located on chromosome 10q23 and encodes a dual-specificity phosphatase for both lipid and protein substrates (69). *PTEN* decreases the activation of Akt in the *PTEN*/PI3-kinase/Akt pathway.

Several inhibitors of PI3-kinase/Akt/mTOR signaling are currently in clinical trials (70,71). *Rapamycin* or *rapamycin* analogs, for example, block the activity of mTOR, a protein complex responsible for increasing protein synthesis and cellular proliferation (72). Several mTOR inhibitors, including RAD001 and CCI779, and specific PI3-kinase inhibitors are currently under development in preclinical models and clinical trials. PI3-kinase/Akt/mTOR inhibitors have been used in endometrial cancer with limited benefit (73). However, the results from clinical trials using mTOR inhibitors in renal cell carcinomas and glioblastomas are encouraging (74).

Inhibitors of the PI3K pathway signaling might have greater antitumor effects in combination with other targeting strategies, including PARP inhibition or targeting VEGF, based on the following rationale: **PI3K inhibition is associated with the loss of homologous recombinant repair capability resulting in sensitization to PARP inhibitors.** PARP inhibitors can increase VEGFR2 phosphorylation and the subsequent activation of endothelial cell survival pathways that can be blocked with antiangiogenic therapies.

Immunotherapy

Failure of functional immunity contributes to the genesis of virus-associated cancers, such as those caused by human papillomavirus (HPV) or Epstein–Barr virus. Although many effective induced antitumor immune responses have been described, **the relative role of natural antitumor immune responses in the detection and destruction of cancer cells,** at least as was envisioned originally when the concept of immune surveillance was first defined (76), **is still unclear.** Some researchers have suggested that immune responses are mainly involved in protection from virus-associated cancers, but not from other forms of cancer (77).

Cancer is a common disease, and overt immune deficiency certainly is not necessary for its development. However, recent studies have shown that many cancers, including those that are not known to have a viral etiology, are seen with increased frequency in patients who have dysfunctional immunity. In a meta-analysis of cancer incidence in populations known to be immune deficient (e.g., organ transplant recipients, patients with HIV infection), Grulich et al. (78) found an increased incidence of several common cancers, suggesting that impaired immunity may contribute to the development of cancer.

Components of the Immune System Involved in Antitumor Responses

Various types of human immune responses can target tumor cells. Immune responses can be categorized as humoral or cellular, a distinction based on the observation in experimental systems that some immune responses could be transferred by serum (humoral) and others by cells (cellular). In general, humoral responses refer to antibody responses; antibodies are antigen-reactive, soluble, bifunctional molecules composed of specific antigen-binding sites associated with a constant region that directs the biologic activities of the antibody molecule, such as binding to effector cells or complement activation (Fig. 2.2). Cellular immune responses generally refer to cytotoxic responses mediated directly by activated immune cells, rather than by the production of antibodies (Fig. 2.3).

Nearly all immune responses involve both humoral and cellular components and require the coordinated activities of populations of lymphocytes operating in concert with each other

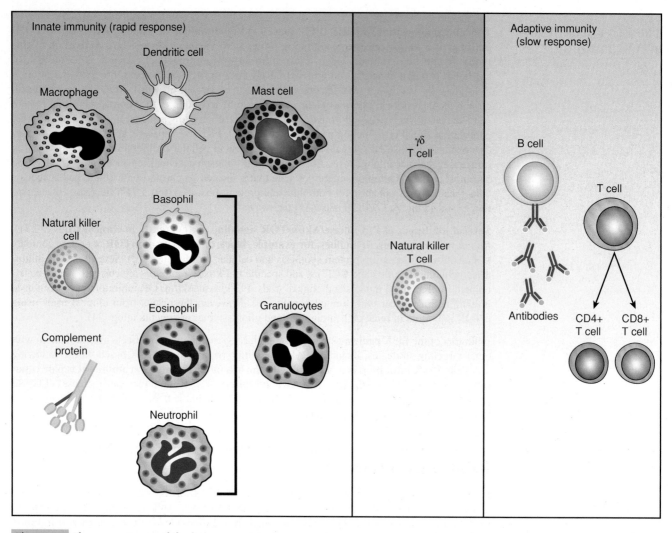

Figure 2.2 The components of the immune system.

and with antigen-presenting cells. These activities result in various effector functions such as antibody production, cytokine secretion, and the stimulation and expansion of cytotoxic T cells. Cellular interactions involved in immune responses include direct cell–cell contact as well as cellular interactions mediated by the secretion of, and response to, cytokines. The latter are biologic messenger molecules that play important roles in the genesis, amplification, and effector functions of immune responses.

T lymphocytes play a pivotal role by acting as helper cells in the generation of humoral and cellular immune responses and by acting as effector cells in cellular responses. Cytotoxic T cells are effector T cells that can directly interact with, and kill, target cells by the release of cytotoxic molecules and the induction of target cell apoptosis. T lymphocyte precursors mature into functional T lymphocytes in the thymus, where they learn to recognize antigen in the context of the major histocompatibility complex (MHC) molecules of the individual. Most T lymphocytes with the capability of responding to self-antigens are removed during thymic development. T lymphocytes are distinguished from other types of lymphocytes by their biologic activities and by the expression of distinctive cell surface molecules, including the T cell antigen receptor and the CD3 molecular complex. T lymphocytes recognize specific antigens by interactions that involve the T cell antigen receptor (Fig. 2.2) (79).

There are two major subsets of T lymphocytes: T helper/inducer cells, which express the CD4 cell surface marker; and T suppressor/cytotoxic cells, which express the CD8 marker. CD4 T lymphocytes can provide help to B lymphocytes, resulting in antibody production, and also can act as helper cells for other T lymphocytes. Much of the helper activity of T lymphocytes is mediated by the production of cytokines. CD4 T cells have been further

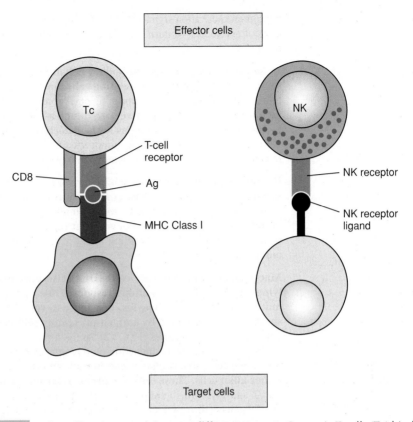

Figure 2.3 **Cell-mediated cytotoxicity: two different types:** 1. Cytotoxic T cells (Tc) bind to their target by recognizing specific antigens (Ag) in the context of major histocompatibility complex (MHC) determinants. 2. Natural killer (NK) cells recognize target cells in an unspecific manner via NK receptor ligands.

subdivided into TH1 (cellular immunity/proinflammatory) and TH2 (antibody response–promoting) subsets, based on the patterns of cytokine production and the biologic properties of these cells. Recent studies have identified a subset of T cells that inhibit autoreactive cells, perhaps acting to prevent autoimmune responses (80). This subset of T cells has been called *regulatory T (Treg) cells.* Other recently described T cell subsets include TH17 cells, which are important in driving responses to bacteria and fungi (81,82).

The CD8 T lymphocyte subset includes cells that are cytotoxic and can directly kill target cells. A major biologic role of such cytotoxic T lymphocytes is the lysis of virus-infected cells. Cytotoxic T lymphocytes can directly mediate the lysis of tumor cells. **Effector T cells also can contribute to antitumor immune responses by producing cytokines,** such as tumor necrosis factor (TNF), that induce tumor cell lysis and can enhance other antitumor cell effector responses.

Both CD4 and CD8 T cells respond to antigen only when it is presented in the context of major histocompatibility complex (MHC) molecules on antigen-presenting cells, target cells, or both. The T cell receptor on CD4 T cells is restricted to responding to antigen plus MHC class II molecules; the receptor on CD8 T cells is restricted to responding to antigen plus MHC class I molecules. In addition, both T cell subsets require a second simultaneous costimulatory signal for optimal stimulation, in the absence of which the T cells may be induced to enter a state of unresponsiveness or even apoptosis. **Therefore, provision of effective costimulatory signals is necessary for the induction of effective antitumor responses by activated T cells.**

In ovarian cancer, the presence of tumor-infiltrating lymphocytes (TILs) correlates both with progression-free and overall survival (83,84). In particular CD8-positive TILs are prognostic markers, since their presence correlates with survival across all stages of disease and all histologic types. In contrast, the presence of immunosuppressive Treg cells (classified as CD4+/CD25+/FoxP3+ T cells), in ovarian cancers has been associated with decreased survival (85,86).

B lymphocytes are the cells that produce and secrete antibodies, which are antigen-binding molecules (Fig. 2.2). B lymphocytes develop from pre-B cells tand, after exposure to antigen and appropriate activation signals, differentiate to become plasma cells—cells that produce large quantities of antibodies. Mature B lymphocytes use cell-surface immunoglobulin molecules as antigen receptors.

In addition to producing antibodies, B lymphocytes play another important role: they can serve as efficient antigen-presenting cells for T lymphocytes. Although the production of antitumor antibodies does not appear to play a central role in host antitumor immune responses, **monoclonal antibodies reactive with tumor-associated antigens have proven to be very useful in antitumor therapy, as well as in the detection of tumors or of tumor-associated molecules.** Unfortunately, no truly unique tumor-specific antigens have been identified, and most tumor-related antigens are also expressed to some extent on nonmalignant tissues.

Because some monoclonal antibodies are of murine and not human origin, the host's immune system can recognize and respond to murine monoclonal antibodies. This has led to the development of "humanized" monoclonal antibodies (genetically engineered monoclonal antibodies composed of human constant regions with specific antigen-reactive murine variable regions), with the aim of avoiding many of the problems associated with the administration of murine monoclonal antibodies.

Macrophages and dendritic cells (DCs) also play key roles in the generation of adaptive, lymphocyte-mediated immune responses by acting as antigen-presenting cells. Helper/ inducer (CD4) T lymphocytes, bearing a T cell receptor of appropriate antigen and self-specificity, are activated by antigen-presenting cells that display processed antigen combined with self-MHC molecules (Fig. 2.2). Antigen-presenting cells also provide costimulatory signals that are important for the induction of T lymphocyte activation. In addition to serving as antigen-presenting cells, **macrophages can ingest and kill microorganisms, and act as cytotoxic antitumor killer cells. These cells also produce various cytokines,** including IL-1, IL-6, chemokines, IL-10, and TNF, which are involved in many immune responses. These monocyte-produced cytokines can have direct effects on tumor cell growth and development, both as growth-inducing and growth-inhibiting factors.

Natural killer (NK) cells are cells that have large granular lymphocytic morphology, do not express the CD3 T cell receptor complex, and do not respond to specific antigens. NK cells can lyse target cells, including tumor cells, unrestricted by the expression of antigen or self-MHC molecules on the target cell. Therefore, NK cells are effector cells in an innate (nonantigen-restricted) immune response, and may play a vital role in immune responses to tumor cells. The cells that can affect ADCC are NK-like cells.

Cytokines are soluble mediator molecules that induce, enhance, or affect immune responses. Cytokines are produced by various types of cells and play critical roles not only in immune responses, but also in biologic responses outside of the immune response, such as hematopoiesis or the acute phase response. T helper 1 (TH1) and TH2 cells, which control the nature of an immune response by secreting characteristic and mutually antagonistic sets of cytokines (9–11), are defined by the cytokines they produce. TH1 clones produce IL-2 and IFN-γ, whereas TH2 clones produce IL-4, IL-5, IL-6, and IL-10. TH1 cytokines promote cell-mediated and inflammatory responses, whereas TH2 cytokines enhance antibody production. Most immune responses involve both TH1 and TH2 components.

Research has identified CD4-positive T cells that participate in the maintenance of immunologic self-tolerance by actively suppressing the activation and expansion of self-reactive lymphocytes. These cells are called Treg cells. Treg cells are characterized by the expression of CD25 (the IL-2 receptor chain) and the transcription factor FoxP3 (87,88). Treg cell activity is thought to be important in preventing the development of autoimmune diseases. Removal of Treg also may enhance immune responses against infectious agents or cancer. Although much remains to be learned about the role of Treg activity in antitumor immunity, it is clear that such cells may play a role in modulating host responses to cancer.

Therapeutic Strategies

There has been great interest in developing effective biologic and immunologic therapies for gynecologic malignancies. For example, patients with small-volume or microscopic residual peritoneal ovarian cancer are attractive candidates for peritoneal immune or biologic therapy (89,90). Also, many patients with advanced disease are immunocompromised, suggesting a role for immune-enhancing therapeutic approaches. Advances in molecular biology, biotechnology, immunology, and cytokine biology have resulted in the availability of many new, promising immunotherapeutic approaches for gynecologic cancers.

The state of the art in immunotherapy for ovarian cancer and other gynecologic malignancies has been discussed in detail in several recent reviews (91–94), and the reader is referred to these publications for more detailed information. Examples of the current use of immunotherapy in clinical trials are provided below.

Cancer Vaccines

Cancers may develop or progress because immune cells are not given a strong enough signal to become activated and destroy the tumor cells. In some cases, cancers are able to downregulate immune responses. For example, cytokines or other molecules produced by tumor cells, such as IL-10 (132), are able to inhibit antitumor immune responses. It may be possible to counter this lack of antitumor immune responsiveness by enhancing antigen presenting cell (APC) activity, providing tumor-associated antigens in a manner that can better induce the generation of antitumor effector T cells (tumor vaccine therapy), or both.

Cervical Cancer

The greatest success story involving the enhancement of immunity to combat gynecologic cancer is the development of vaccines against human papilloma virus (HPV), which are highly effective for the prevention of cervical dysplasia and cancer (94). In addition, dysplastic and cancerous cervical epithelial cells infected with HPV, an oncogenic virus, also present an attractive target for immune enhancement-based therapeutic strategies, including the development of therapeutic vaccines for HPV.

HPV—specifically, HPV subtypes 16, 18, 31, and 45—has been implicated as the major etiologic agent in cervical cancer. HPV-infected dysplastic and cancerous cervical epithelial cells consistently retain and express two of the viral genes, *E6* and *E7,* that respectively interact with, and disrupt, the function of the *p53* and retinoblastoma tumor suppressor gene products. **Factors other than infection with HPV, such as cellular immune function, play an important role in determining whether the infection of cervical epithelial cells regresses or progresses to cancer.** This has led to the development of prophylactic and therapeutic vaccines to HPV as well as treatment approaches based on the enhancement of host immune function.

HPV vaccines have been shown to have an exceptional level of efficacy (75), **clearly reducing the incidence of both HPV-16 and HPV-18 infections, and HPV-16 and HPV-18–related cervical intraepithelial neoplasia.** The HPV vaccines *Gardasil* and *Cervarix* use HPV-like particles as immunogens to generate neutralizing antibodies for HPV. HPV-based therapeutic cancer vaccines may ultimately be effective for the control of cervical cancer (94).

HPV *E6* and *E7* are attractive antigens for use in therapeutic vaccines because these HPV-encoded proteins are involved in cellular transformation, and therefore are consistently expressed in HPV-positive tumor cells. Candidate therapeutic HPV vaccines include DNA vaccines, with recent research aimed at enhancing the potency and delivery of such vaccines (94,134–136). Clinical trials with such DNA-based vaccines are currently being planned (94).

Ovarian Cancer

Therapeutic vaccines for ovarian cancer have been developed and studied in various clinical trials. A thorough overview of the rationale and design of potential vaccines can be found in recent review papers (91,92). At this time, tumor vaccine approaches include (i) vaccination with defined tumor-associated antigens, or DNA vaccines that encode for tumor-associated antigens; and (ii) vaccination with whole tumor cell preparations, with and without the coadministration of antigen-presenting cells such as dendritic cells (DCs).

Peptide vaccines are designed to stimulate antitumor immune responses against various target antigens that are expressed on ovarian cancer, such as NY-ESO-1, p53, WT-1, HER-2, and VEGF (133). These vaccines are generally well tolerated and can generate measurable, sustained immune responses (95). Peptide vaccines are frequently administered with adjuvants, such as Montanide or **granulocyte–macrophage colony-stimulating factor** (GM-CSF) to enhance immune responses in vivo.

One of the candidate antigen for vaccine development is NY-ESO-1 which is a highly immunogenic cancer-testis antigen. It is expressed in up to 40% of ovarian cancers (96). Two recent clinical trials have shown the ability of an NY-ESO-1 peptide vaccine with *Montanide* ISA51 as adjuvant to induce both antigen-specific CD4+ and CD8+ T cell responses in patients with minimal residual ovarian cancer (97). The second trial used HLA-A*0201-restricted NY-ESO-1b peptide vaccination with *Montanide* in patients with ovarian cancer in complete clinical remission after first-line treatment (98). Three of four patients with NY-ESO-1-positive tumors and four of five patients with NY-ESO-1-negative tumors showed T cell immunity. Three patients with NY-ESO-1-negative tumors remained in complete clinical remission. Another trial used intradermally injected recombinant vaccinia and fowlpox viruses expressing NY-ESO-1 in 19 women with NY-ESO-1 expressing ovarian cancers in complete remission after primary therapy (50). About 50% of patients showed NY-ESO-1-specific immune responses, resulting in a mean disease-free interval of 19.9 months (99).

Other vaccination strategies have used p53 peptides as the immunogenic antigen, since the vast majority of serous cancers in particular overexpress p53 (100–102). In general, p53 vaccination trials have resulted in the successful generation of p53-specific immune responses, and the vaccines have been well tolerated. Clinical responses have been demonstrated in up to 20% of patients, but these responses have not necessarily correlated with vaccine-mediated antip53 immunity.

Various multipeptide vaccines have been studied in ovarian cancer patients. One of these vaccines combines peptides from various antigens, including the adenomatous polyposis coli, ubiquitin-conjugating enzyme E2, BAP31, replication protein A, Abl-binding protein 3c, cyclin I, topoisomerase IIα, integrin β eight subunit precursor, cell division control protein 2 (CDC2), TACE/ADAM17, g-catenin, and EDDR1, administered along with *Montanide* ISA-51 and GM-CSF. This vaccine generated peptide-specific T cell responses in patients with breast and ovarian cancer without evidence of disease, but 50% of patients with ovarian cancer recurred during the observation period (103).

Recombinant vaccinia and fowlpox viruses have been used to express CEA and MUC1 as well as the T cell costimulatory molecules B7.1, ICAM-1, and LFA-3. The vaccine showed efficacy in one of the three ovarian cancer patients treated in a pilot study that enrolled patients with MUC1-positive cancers (104).

In addition to using specific tumor-associated antigen, whole tumor antigen vaccines can potentially provide a wider range of tumor antigens. These vaccines can be created using autologous tumor lysates or tumor-derived RNA, and are in general administered with adjuvants like GM-CSF, Montanide ISA-51, or toll-like receptor agonists. **Patients may have a better clinical response to whole tumor antigen vaccination** (105,106).

Dendritic cells are highly effective antigen-presenting cells, and play a central role in the induction of both CD4 and CD8 T cell responses. DCs can be pulsed with tumor antigen peptides, or bioengineered to express tumor antigens, allowing them to be used in experimental therapies that aim to enhance antitumor immunity. Exposure of T cells to DCs pulsed with ovarian cancer–derived antigenic preparations has resulted in the generation of cytolytic effector T cells that are capable of killing autologous tumor cells in vitro (137–139).

In a phase I clinical trial, Hernando et al. (140) showed that patients with advanced gynecologic malignancies could be effectively vaccinated with DCs pulsed with a nontumor test antigen, keyhole limpet hemocyanin (KLH), and autologous tumor antigens. Lymphoproliferative responses to KLH and to tumor lysate stimulation were noted. The treatment was safe, well tolerated, immunologically active, and generally devoid of significant adverse effects.

Given the exceptional ability of DCs to serve as potent antigen-presenting cells in the induction of T cell responses, an attractive approach would be to combine tumor vaccines with *ex vivo*–generated DC preparations. DCs can be generated *ex vivo* from peripheral blood mononuclear cells, using various strategies (91,141–144). Such *ex vivo*–generated DCs can be pulsed with tumor antigens or vaccines, or with DNA- or RNA-encoding tumor antigens before administration, and have resulted in the induction of antitumor responses in preclinical studies (91,145–147).

Several major challenges need to be overcome for the successful development of effective DC-based therapies for ovarian cancer: (i) **The identification of tumor-associated or tumor-specific antigens,** (ii) **the development of means to induce optimal DC maturation after antigen uptake,** (iii) **the development of schemes for generation of DCs that maintain optimal antigen-presenting cell activity** and do not produce immunosuppressive factors, and (iv) **the development of *ex vivo* expansion techniques that provide sufficient numbers of DCs** for effective immunotherapy (91,148–150). As more is learned about the immunogenicity of current tumor-associated antigens, novel cancer-associated antigens are identified, and the techniques of DC activation and antigen expression are better developed, **DC-based immunotherapy may provide a therapeutic alternative for the treatment of these cancers.**

Monoclonal Antibodies and Antibody-based Immunotherapy

Monoclonal antibodies have played an important role in both the development of immunotherapeutic agents and tumor markers. Monoclonal antibodies also have been used for radioimmunodetection (107,108) **and are being used for treatment.** Monoclonal antibodies can potentially induce antitumor responses in various ways: (i) By complement activation and subsequent tumor cell lysis; (ii) by directly inducing antiproliferative effects, perhaps by interaction with tumor cell surface signaling molecules; (iii) by enhancing the activity of phagocytic cells, which can interact with immune complexes containing monoclonal antibodies; and (iv) by mediating ADCC via interactions of the Fc portion of monoclonal antibodies with Fc receptors on cells that mediate ADCC (109). In addition, monoclonal antibodies can be labeled with either radioactive particles or antitumor drugs and used to focus these agents onto tumor cells (110).

Some monoclonal antibody-based drugs are currently approved for the treatment of cancer. FDA-approved monoclonal antibody-based anticancer drugs include **bevacizumab** (*Avastin*) for the treatment of colon and lung cancer, **cetuximab** (*Erbitux*) for the treatment of colon and head and neck cancer, **gemtuzumab** (*Mylotarg*) for the treatment of acute myelogenous leukemia, **rituximab** (*Rituxan*) for the treatment of nonHodgkin lymphoma, and **trastuzumab** (*Herceptin*) for the treatment of breast cancer.

Various antigens have been found to be expressed by ovarian cancers and are being explored as therapeutic targets (111). **In general, these antigens can be classified as specific tumor-associated antigens or universal tumor antigens.** Examples of ovarian tumor-associated antigens include CA125, the folate receptor, MUC1, mesothelin, and NY-ESO-1. Survivin and hTERT are universal tumor antigens, etc., since they are expressed on a variety of tumors, and not on most normal human cells.

Several clinical trials have utilized monoclonal antibodies directed against ovarian cancer antigens, including CA125, folate receptor, MUC1 antigen, and tumor-associated glycoprotein 72 (93). Evidence that CA125 can act as a tumor antigen and stimulate humoral and cellular immune responses has been derived from various in vitro studies and clinical trials. *Oregovomab* (B43.13) **is a murine monoclonal antibody to CA125 that has been used for the treatment of ovarian cancer.** The antibody binds to circulating CA125, resulting in the formation of immune complexes (antibody–antigen complexes). These immune complexes are recognized as foreign, mainly because of the murine component. They are taken up by antigen-presenting cells, allowing the processing of the autologous CA125 antigen, ultimately leading to induction of CA125-specific antibodies, helper T cells, and cytolytic T cells.

In 2004, Berek et al. reported on the use of *oregovomab* **for maintenance therapy in patients with ovarian cancer after first-line treatment.** A subgroup of patients with favorable prognostic factors had a significantly longer time to relapse compared to patients in the placebo group (112). This subgroup was studied in a subsequent trial and oregovomab maintenance therapy failed to show a survival benefit (113,114). *Oregovomab* **is currently being studied in combination with** *carboplatin* **and** *paclitaxel,* **and might provide immune adjuvant properties in this setting, as suggested by recent clinical observations** (115).

Another antibody network–based strategy has employed anti-idiotypic vaccines in patients with relapsed ovarian cancer. ACA125 is a murine anti-idiotypic antibody that mimics an antigenic epitope on CA125 (92,93,116,117). Therefore, antibodies generated to ACA125 have the potential to react with antigenic epitopes on CA125, with ACA125 serving as an anti-idiotypic vaccine that would enhance immune responses to CA125 (92). Treatment with ACA125 has resulted in both humoral and cellular responses, and those patients who had detectable anti-ACA125 responses showed a longer mean survival time (118,119).

Abagovomab is an anti-idiotypic antibody that mimics the CA125 antigen. The initial results of *abagovomab* treatment in patients with ovarian cancer have been reported by Sabbatini et al. (120) and have shown that all patients developed an anti-idiotypic antibody response (Ab3). In addition, the generation of T cell immunity to CA125 was demonstrated in five patients. While patients had measurable serum CA125 levels in both trials, neither trial analyzed CA125 expression in tumor tissue. A large international, multicenter trial is investigating the effect of *abagovomab* as consolidation treatment in patients with ovarian cancer. **Preliminary data from the trial does not show a clinical benefit of abagovomab as consolidation therapy.**

Adoptive Immunotherapy

Adoptive immunotherapy involves the *ex vivo* expansion of antitumor immune cells followed by the administration of such effector cells. It has provided another immune system–based approach for antitumor therapy (91,92,121–124). **Adoptive immunotherapy, involving the infusion of large numbers of autologous *ex vivo*–activated immune effector cells, has been shown to produce tumor regression in various animal and human tumors** (122), and it has produced the best results to date in tumor immunotherapy (91). This approach can provide large numbers of tumor-specific T cells with the capacity to specifically kill tumor cells, and can potentially lead to the complete elimination of residual tumor cells (91).

Early approaches used peripheral blood mononuclear cells exposed to IL-2 *ex vivo* to lead to the generation of lymphokine-activated killer (LAK) cells that are cytotoxic for a variety of tumor cells (125,126). Although experimental treatment of human subjects with LAK cells and IL-2 yielded some responses, considerable toxicity was seen (89,121–124,126–130), and **adoptive immunotherapy with LAK cells does not appear to be a practical option for the treatment of ovarian cancer.**

The use of immunotherapy based on *ex vivo*–stimulated tumor-infiltrating lymphocytes or tumor-associated lymphocytes from ascites, with or without added IL-2, also has been examined in ovarian cancer (91,124,129,130). It is clear that optimization of such adoptive immunotherapies is needed in terms of the cell source, the forms of stimulation, the methods for *ex vivo* expansion, and the cytokines that are given during such treatment (91). Potentially important refinements of these approaches include the use of DCs as antigen-presenting cells (APCs) to stimulate T cells, the provision of effective costimulatory signals to the responding T cells by *APC*, host conditioning with immunosuppressive chemotherapy before the adoptive transfer of cells (91,131), and the genetic modification of T cells to express tumor-specific antigens like NY-ESO-1.

Cytokine Therapy: Modulation of Host Immunity

Most early experimental biologic therapies for metastatic ovarian cancer involved biologic response modifiers such as *Corynebacterium parvum* (a heat-killed, gram-negative anaerobic bacillus), *bacillus Calmette–Guérin* (BCG), or modifications of these agents (152–155). Intraperitoneal (IP) treatment with *C. parvum* induced a profound local reaction, including peritoneal fibrosis, and its toxicity precluded more widespread testing.

Malignancies that tend predominantly to grow in the peritoneal cavity, such as ovarian cancer, have been treated in many experimental trials with IP administered drugs, most frequently with cytotoxic chemotherapeutic agents (156). **IP biologic response modifier therapy, immunotherapy with cytokines, and gene therapy have been proposed.** These approaches have the additional advantage of potentially inducing the activation of regional immune effector mechanisms in the peritoneal cavity (90). This might be particularly true for cytokine-based treatment strategies or for adoptive immunotherapies, because activated immune effector cells may require direct contact with the malignant target cells for most effective antitumor activity.

Various cytokines have been tested in clinical trials, to date producing mixed results (91). **This includes trials of IFN-α and IFN-γ, TNF-α, and IL-2.** IP IL-2 therapy was studied in women with platinum-resistant or refractory ovarian cancer in a phase I/II trial (157,158). Among 35 assessable patients, there were 6 complete responses and 3 partial responses, for an overall response rate of 25.7% (9 of 35) with a median survival of 2.1 years.

Treatment with IP IFN-α combined with *cisplatin* or *carboplatin* has resulted in pathologic complete and long-term remission in 14 of 27 patients in two trials for recurrent or refractory ovarian cancer (159,160). Treatment of patients with refractory ovarian cancer with intravenous recombinant human IL-12, a TH1-inducing cytokine, has resulted in disease stabilization in about half of the treated patients (161).

IP treatment with IL-12 in patients with carcinomatosis from mesotheliomas, Müllerian, or gastrointestinal carcinomas has shown disease stabilization in 2 of 12 treated patients (162). In a phase II trial, treatment with subcutaneously administered IL-2 and oral *retinoic acid* was reported to improve survival in 44 patients who had ovarian cancer responding to chemotherapy (163).

GM-CSF stimulates the proliferation and differentiation of granulocytes and monocytes, and has demonstrated antitumor efficacy in patients with recurrent Müllerian malignancies. In one clinical trial that included 72 patients, GM-CSF treatment resulted in one complete response and 20 patients had stable disease (164). GM-CSF in combination with *interferon gamma 1b* (IFN-γ 1b) and *carboplatin* in women with recurrent, platinum-sensitive ovarian cancer (165). Of 54 patients evaluable for response, 9 (17%) had a complete response, 21 (39%) had a partial response, and 24 (44%) had progressive disease. The overall response rate was 56%. With a median follow-up of 6.4 months, the PFS was 6 months.

The identification of T cell subpopulations that have potent immunoregulatory properties, such as Treg and TH17 cells, has provided new opportunities for the design of host immune system–modulating therapies with the aim of enhancing immune responses to cancer. Treg cells are immunoinhibitory, and can inhibit the induction of cytotoxic T cells, and may thereby inhibit host antitumor immune responses. Increased levels of Treg cells in ascites, blood, and tumor have been seen in patients with advanced ovarian cancer (166). These Treg cells can inhibit antitumor immunity and promote tumor cell growth in ovarian cancer (85). Therefore, blocking the action of these Treg cells is an important target in the development of new immunotherapeutic approaches.

Studies aimed at blocking Treg activity in patients with cancer have been initiated using monoclonal antibodies targeting CD25, a cell-surface molecule commonly expressed on these cells. To date, these studies have not resulted in enhanced anticancer immune responses (167), and more refined approaches to targeting Treg need to be developed.

TH17 cells are another recently identified Treg cell subpopulation, characterized by the secretion of IL-17. They have the ability to modulate Treg activity (81,82,168). The role of TH17 cells in cancer has not been clearly defined. An animal study reported that provision of IL-2 in the tumor microenvironment was associated with decreased TH17 activity and increased Treg activity (168). Although much more work needs to be done to define the role of TH17 cells in downregulating Treg activity, and perhaps in enhancing antitumor responses, future experimental treatment strategies aimed at enhancing TH17 activity may be of value in enhancing antitumor immune responses.

References

1. **Hanahan D, Weinberg RA.** The hallmarks of cancer. *Cell.* 2000; 100:57–70.
2. **Collinson FJ, Hall GD, Perren TJ, et al.** Development of antiangiogenic agents for ovarian cancer. *Expert Rev Anticancer Ther.* 2008;8:21–32.
3. **Ashouri S, Garcia AA.** Current status of signal transduction modulators in the treatment of gynecologic malignancies. *Curr Treat Options Oncol.* 2007;8:383–392.
4. **Markman M.** The promise and perils of "targeted therapy" of advanced ovarian cancer. *Oncology.* 2008;74:1–6.
5. **Murdoch D, Sager J.** Will targeted therapy hold its promise? An evidence-based review. *Curr Opin Oncol.* 2008;20:104–111.
6. **Goede V, Schmidt T, Kimmina S, et al.** Analysis of blood vessel maturation processes during cyclic ovarian angiogenesis. *Lab Invest.* 1998;78:1385–1394.
7. **Martin L, Schilder R.** Novel approaches in advancing the treatment of epithelial ovarian cancer: The role of angiogenesis inhibition. *J Clin Oncol.* 2007;25:2894–2901.
8. **Grothey A, Ellis LM.** Targeting angiogenesis driven by vascular endothelial growth factors using antibody-based therapies. *Cancer J.* 2008;14:170–177.
9. **Alvarez AA, Krigman HR, Whitaker RS, et al.** The prognostic significance of angiogenesis in epithelial ovarian carcinoma. *Clin Cancer Res.* 1999;5:587–591.
10. **Cohen MH, Gootenberg J, Keegan P, et al.** FDA drug approval summary: Bevacizumab plus FOLFOX4 as second-line treatment of colorectal cancer. *Oncologist.* 2007;12:356–361.
11. **Hurwitz H, Fehrenbacher L, Novotny W, et al.** Bevacizumab plus irinotecan, fluorouracil, and leucovorin for metastatic colorectal cancer. *N Engl J Med.* 2004;350:2335–2342.
12. http://www.cancer.gov/cancertopics/druginfo/fda-bevacizumab
13. **Burger RA, Sill MW, Monk BJ, et al.** Phase II trial of bevacizumab in persistent or recurrent epithelial ovarian cancer or primary peritoneal cancer: A Gynecologic Oncology Group Study. *J Clin Oncol.* 2007;25:5165–5171.
14. **Cannistra SA, Matulonis UA, Penson RT, et al.** Phase II study of bevacizumab in patients with platinum-resistant ovarian cancer or peritoneal serous cancer. *J Clin Oncol.* 2007;25:5180–5186.
15. **Burger RA, Brady MF, Bookman MA, et al.** Incorporation of bevacizumab in the primary treatment of ovarian cancer. *N Engl J Med.* 2011;365:2473–2483.
16. **Perren TJ, Swart AM, Pfisterer J, et al.** A phase 3 trial of bevacizumab in ovarian cancer. *N Engl J Med.* 2011;365:2484–2496.
17. **Aghajanian C, Blank SV, Goff BA, et al.** OCEANS: A randomized, double-blind, placebo-controlled phase III trial of chemotherapy with or without bevacizumab in patients with platinum-sensitive recurrent epithelial ovarian, primary peritoneal, or fallopian tube cancer. *J Clin Oncol.* 2012;30:2039–2045.
18. **Pujade-Lauraine E, Hilpert F, Weber B, et al.** AURELIA: A randomized phase III trial evaluating bevacizumab (BEV) plus chemotherapy (CT) for platinum (PT)-resistant recurrent ovarian cancer (OC). *J Clin Oncol.* 2012;30(18 Suppl):LBA5002.
19. **Karlan BY, Oza AM, Richardson GE, et al.** Randomized, double-blind, placebo-controlled phase II study of AMG 386 combined with weekly paclitaxel in patients with recurrent ovarian cancer. *J Clin Oncol.* 2012;30:362–371.
20. **Garcia AA, Hirte H, Fleming G, et al.** Phase II clinical trial of bevacizumab and low-dose metronomic oral cyclophosphamide in recurrent ovarian cancer: A trial of the California, Chicago, and Princess Margaret Hospital phase II consortia. *J Clin Oncol.* 2008;26: 76–82.
21. **Cohn DE, Valmadre S, Resnick KE, et al.** Bevacizumab and weekly taxane chemotherapy demonstrates activity in refractory ovarian cancer. *Gynecol Oncol.* 2006;102:134–139.
22. **Wright JD, Secord AA, Numnum TM, et al.** A multi-institutional evaluation of factors predictive of toxicity and efficacy of bevacizumab for recurrent ovarian cancer. *Int J Gynecol Cancer.* 2008;18:400–406.
23. **Badgwell BD, Camp ER, Feig B, et al.** Management of bevacizumab-associated bowel perforation: A case series and review of the literature. *Ann Oncol.* 2008;19:577–582.
24. **Auranen A, Grénman S.** Radiation therapy and biological compounds for consolidation therapy in advanced ovarian cancer. *Int J Gynecol Cancer.* 2008;18(Suppl 1):44–46.
25. **Lu C, Thaker PH, Lin YG, et al.** Impact of vessel maturation on antiangiogenic therapy in ovarian cancer. *Am J Obstet Gynecol.* 2008; 198:477.e1–e9; discussion 477.e9–10.

26. **Kumar A, Petri ET, Halmos B, et al.** Structure and clinical relevance of the epidermal growth factor receptor in human cancer. *J Clin Oncol.* 2008;26:1742–1751.

27. **Wieduwilt MJ, Moasser MM.** The epidermal growth factor receptor family: Biology driving targeted therapeutics. *Cell Mol Life Sci.* 2008;65:1566–1584.

28. **Psyrri A, Kassar M, Yu Z, et al.** Effect of epidermal growth factor receptor expression level on survival in patients with epithelial ovarian cancer. *Clin Cancer Res.* 2005;11:8637–8643.

29. **de Graeff P, Crijns AP, Ten Hoor KA, et al.** The ErbB signalling pathway: Protein expression and prognostic value in epithelial ovarian cancer. *Br J Cancer.* 2008;99:341–349.

30. **Khalifa MA, Abdoh AA, Mannel RS, et al.** Prognostic utility of epidermal growth factor receptor overexpression in endometrial adenocarcinoma. *Cancer.* 1994;73:370–376.

31. **Scambia G, Benedetti Panici P, Ferrandina G, et al.** Significance of epidermal growth factor receptor expression in primary human endometrial cancer. *Int J Cancer.* 1994;56:26–30.

32. **Wang D, Konishi I, Koshiyama M, et al.** Expression of c-erbB-2 protein and epidermal growth receptor in endometrial carcinomas. Correlation with clinicopathologic and sex steroid receptor status. *Cancer.* 1993;72:2628–2637.

33. **Konecny GE, Venkatesan N, Yang G, et al.** Activity of lapatinib, a novel HER2 and EGFR dual kinase inhibitor in human endometrial cancer cells. *Br J Cancer.* 2008;98:1076–1084.

34. **Vaidya AP, Parnes AD, Seiden MV.** Rationale and clinical experience with epidermal growth factor receptor inhibitors in gynecologic malignancies. *Curr Treat Options Oncol.* 2005;6:103–114.

35. **Hudis CA.** Trastuzumab—mechanism of action and use in clinical practice. *N Engl J Med.* 2007;357:39–51.

36. **Attard G, Kitzen J, Blagden SP, et al.** A phase Ib study of pertuzumab, a recombinant humanised antibody to HER2, and docetaxel in patients with advanced solid tumours. *Br J Cancer.* 2007;97:1338–1343.

37. **Galizia G, Lieto E, De Vita F, et al.** Cetuximab, a chimeric human mouse anti-epidermal growth factor receptor monoclonal antibody, in the treatment of human colorectal cancer. *Oncogene.* 2007;26:3654–3660.

38. **Wang S, Guo P, Wang X, et al.** Preclinical pharmacokinetic/pharmacodynamic models of gefitinib and the design of equivalent dosing regimens in EGFR wild-type and mutant tumor models. *Mol Cancer Ther.* 2008;7:407–417.

39. **Gordon AN, Finkler N, Edwards RP, et al.** Efficacy and safety of erlotinib HCl, an epidermal growth factor receptor (HER1/EGFR) tyrosine kinase inhibitor, in patients with advanced ovarian carcinoma: Results from a phase II multicenter study. *Int J Gynecol Cancer.* 2005;15:785–792.

40. **Vasey PA, Gore M, Wilson R, et al.** A phase Ib trial of docetaxel, carboplatin, and erlotinib in ovarian, fallopian tube, and primary peritoneal cancers. *Br J Cancer.* 2008;98:1774–1780.

41. **Secord AA, Blessing JA, Armstrong DK, et al.** Phase II trial of cetuximab and carboplatin in relapsed platinum-sensitive ovarian cancer and evaluation of epidermal growth factor receptor expression: A Gynecologic Oncology Group study. *Gynecol Oncol.* 2008;108:493–499.

42. **Konner J, Schilder RJ, DeRosa FA, et al.** A phase II study of cetuximab/paclitaxel/carboplatin for the initial treatment of advanced-stage ovarian, primary peritoneal, or fallopian tube cancer. *Gynecol Oncol.* 2008;110:140–145.

43. **Schilder RJ, Sill MW, Chen X, et al.** Phase II study of gefitinib in patients with relapsed or persistent ovarian or primary peritoneal carcinoma and evaluation of epidermal growth factor receptor mutations and immunohistochemical expression: A Gynecologic Oncology Group Study. *Clin Cancer Res.* 2005;11:5539–5548.

44. **Posadas EM, Liel MS, Kwitkowski V, et al.** A phase II and pharmacodynamic study of gefitinib in patients with refractory or recurrent epithelial ovarian cancer. *Cancer.* 2007;109:1323–1330.

45. **Lacroix L, Pautier P, Duvillard P, et al.** Response of ovarian carcinomas to gefitinib-carboplatin-paclitaxel combination is not associated with EGFR kinase domain somatic mutations. *Int J Cancer.* 2006;118:1068–1069.

46. **Wagner U, du Bois A, Pfisterer J, et al.** Gefitinib in combination with tamoxifen in patients with ovarian cancer refractory or resistant to platinum-taxane based therapy—a phase II trial of the AGO Ovarian Cancer Study Group (AGO-OVAR 2.6). *Gynecol Oncol.* 2007;105:132–137.

47. **Goncalves A, Fabbro M, Lhomme C, et al.** A phase II trial to evaluate gefitinib as second- or third-line treatment in patients with recurring locoregionally advanced or metastatic cervical cancer. *Gynecol Oncol.* 2008;108:42–46.

48. **Reich O, Liegl B, Tamussino K, et al.** p185HER2 overexpression and HER2 oncogene amplification in recurrent vulvar Paget's disease. *Mod Pathol.* 2005;18:354–357.

49. **De Laurentiis M, Cancello G, Zinno L, et al.** Targeting HER2 as a therapeutic strategy for breast cancer: A paradigmatic shift of drug development in oncology. *Ann Oncol.* 2005;16(suppl 4):iv7–13.

50. **Tuefferd M, Couturier J, Penault-Llorca F, et al.** HER2 status in ovarian carcinomas: A multicenter GINECO study of 320 patients. *PLoS ONE.* 2007;2:e1138.

51. **Bookman MA, Darcy KM, Clarke-Pearson D, et al.** Evaluation of monoclonal humanized anti-HER2 antibody, trastuzumab, in patients with recurrent or refractory ovarian or primary peritoneal carcinoma with overexpression of HER2: A phase II trial of the Gynecologic Oncology Group. *J Clin Oncol.* 2003;21:283–290.

52. **Chavez-Blanco A, Perez-Sanchez V, Gonzalez-Fierro A, et al.** HER2 expression in cervical cancer as a potential therapeutic target. *BMC Cancer.* 2004;4:59.

53. **Slomovitz BM, Broaddus RR, Burke TW, et al.** Her-2/*neu* overexpression and amplification in uterine papillary serous carcinoma. *J Clin Oncol.* 2004;22:3126–3132.

54. **Villella JA, Cohen S, Smith DH, et al.** HER-2/*neu* overexpression in uterine papillary serous cancers and its possible therapeutic implications. *Int J Gynecol Cancer.* 2006;16:1897–1902.

55. **McCubrey JA, Milella M, Tafuri A, et al.** Targeting the *Raf*/MEK/ERK pathway with small-molecule inhibitors. *Curr Opin Investig Drugs.* 2008;9:614–630.

56. **Adnane L, Trail PA, Taylor I, et al.** Sorafenib (BAY 43–9006, Nexavar), a dual-action inhibitor that targets *RAF*/MEK/ERK pathway in tumor cells and tyrosine kinases VEGFR/PDGFR in tumor vasculature. *Methods Enzymol.* 2006;407:597–612.

57. **Diaz-Padilla I, Malpica AL, Minig L, et al.** Ovarian low-grade serous carcinoma: A comprehensive update. *Gynecol Oncol.* 2012;126:279–285.

58. **Singer G, Oldt R III, Cohen Y, et al.** Mutations in BRAF and KRAS characterize the development of low-grade ovarian serous carcinoma. *J Natl Cancer Inst.* 2003;95:484–486.

59. **Farley J, Brady WE, Vathipadiekal V, et al.** Selumetinib in women with recurrent low-grade serous carcinoma of the ovary or peritoneum: An open-label, single-arm, phase 2 study. *Lancet Oncol.* 2013;14:134–140.

60. **Ashworth A.** A synthetic lethal therapeutic approach: Poly(ADP) ribose polymerase inhibitors for the treatment of cancers deficient in DNA double-strand break repair. *J Clin Oncol.* 2008;26:3785–3790.

61. **Fong PC, Boss DS, Yap TA, et al.** Inhibition of poly(ADP-ribose) polymerase in tumors from BRCA mutation carriers. *N Engl J Med.* 2009;361(2):123–134.

62. **Audeh MW, Carmichael J, Penson RT, et al.** Oral poly(ADP-ribose) polymerase inhibitor olaparib in patients with BRCA1 or BRCA2 mutations and recurrent ovarian cancer: A proof-of-concept trial. *Lancet.* 2010;376:245–251.

63. **Ledermann J, Harter P, Gourley C, et al.** Olaparib maintenance therapy in platinum-sensitive relapsed ovarian cancer. *N Engl J Med.* 2012;366(15):1382–1392.

64. **Oza AM, Cibula D, Oaknin A, et al.** Olaparib plus paclitaxel and carboplatin (P/C) followed by olaparib maintenance treatment in patients (pts) with platinum-sensitive recurrent serous ovarian cancer (PSR SOC): A randomized, open-label phase II study [abstract]. *J Clin Oncol.* 2012;30(Suppl):a5001.

65. **Jiang BH, Liu LZ.** PI3 K/*PTEN* signaling in tumorigenesis and angiogenesis. *Biochem Biophys Acta.* 2008;1784:150–158.

66. **Mutter GL, Lin MC, Fitzgerald JT, et al.** Altered *PTEN* expression as a diagnostic marker for the earliest endometrial precancers. *J Natl Cancer Inst.* 2000;92:924–930.

67. **Cully M, You H, Levine AJ, et al.** Beyond *PTEN* mutations: The PI3 K pathway as an integrator of multiple inputs during tumorigenesis. *Nat Rev Cancer.* 2006;6:184–192.

68. Castellvi J, Garcia A, Rojo F, et al. Phosphorylated 4E binding protein 1: A hallmark of cell signaling that correlates with survival in ovarian cancer. *Cancer.* 2006;107:1801–1811.

69. Salmena L, Carracedo A, Pandolfi PP. Tenets of *PTEN* tumor suppression. *Cell.* 2008;133:403–414.

70. LoPiccolo J, Blumenthal GM, Bernstein WB, et al. Targeting the PI3 K/Akt/mTOR pathway: Effective combinations and clinical considerations. *Drug Resist Updat.* 2008;11:32–50.

71. Marone R, Cmiljanovic V, Giese B, et al. Targeting phosphoinositide 3-kinase: Moving towards therapy. *Biochim Biophys Acta.* 2008;1784:159–185.

72. Wullschleger S, Loewith R, Hall MN. TOR signaling in growth and metabolism. *Cell.* 2006;124:471–484.

73. Gadducci A, Tana R, Cosio S, et al. Molecular target therapies in endometrial cancer: From the basic research to the clinic. *Gynecol Endocrinol.* 2008;24:239–249.

74. Motzer RJ, Escudier B, Oudard S, et al. Efficacy of everolimus in advanced renal cell carcinoma: A double-blind, randomised, placebo-controlled phase III trial. *Lancet.* 2008;372:449–456.

75. FUTURE II Study Group. Quadrivalent vaccine against human papillomavirus to prevent high-grade cervical lesions. *N Engl J Med.* 2007;356:1915–1927.

76. Burnet FM. The concept of immunological surveillance. *Prog Exp Tumor Res.* 1970;13:1–27.

77. Klein G, Klein E. Surveillance against tumors—is it mainly immunological? *Immunol Lett.* 2005;100:29–33.

78. Grulich AE, van Leeuwen MT, Falster MO, et al. Incidence of cancers in people with HIV/AIDS compared with immunosuppressed transplant recipients: A meta-analysis. *Lancet.* 2007; 370:59–67.

79. Owen M. T-cell receptors and MHC molecules. In: Roitt I, Borstoff J, Male D, eds. *Immunology.* 5th ed. St. Louis, MO: Mosby-Year Book; 1998.

80. Zou W. Regulatory T cells, tumour immunity and immunotherapy. *Nat Rev Immunol.* 2006;6:295–307.

81. Bettelli E, Carrier Y, Gao W, et al. Reciprocal developmental pathways for the generation of pathogenic effector TH17 and regulatory T cells. *Nature.* 2006;441:235–238.

82. Bronte V. TH17 and cancer: Friends or foes? *Blood.* 2008;112:214.

83. Zhang L, Conejo-Garcia JR, Katsaros D, et al. Intratumoral T cells, recurrence, and survival in epithelial ovarian cancer. *N Engl J Med.* 2003;348:203–213.

84. Hwang WT, Adams SF, Tahirovic E, et al. Prognostic significance of tumor-infiltrating T cells in ovarian cancer: A meta-analysis. *Gynecol Oncol.* 2012;124:192–198.

85. Curiel TJ, Coukos G, Zou L, et al. Specific recruitment of regulatory T cells in ovarian carcinoma fosters immune privilege and predicts reduced survival. *Nat Med.* 2004;10:942–949.

86. Sato E, Olson SH, Ahn J, et al. Intraepithelial CD8+ tumor-infiltrating lymphocytes and a high CD8+/regulatory T cell ratio are associated with favorable prognosis in ovarian cancer. *Proc Natl Acad Sci U S A.* 2005;102:18538–18543.

87. Sakaguchi S, Sakaguchi N, Shimizu J, et al. Immunologic tolerance maintained by CD25+ CD4+ regulatory T cells: Their common role in controlling autoimmunity, tumor immunity, and transplantation tolerance. *Immunol Rev.* 2001;182:18–32.

88. Shevach EM. CD4+ CD25+ suppressor T cells: More questions than answers. *Nat Rev Immunol.* 2002;2:389–400.

89. Bookman MA, Bast RC Jr. The immunobiology and immunotherapy of ovarian cancer. *Semin Oncol.* 1991;18:270–291.

90. Bookman MA. Biological therapy of ovarian cancer: Current directions. *Semin Oncol.* 1998;25:381–396.

91. Mantia-Smaldone GM, Corr B, Chu CS. Immunotherapy in ovarian cancer. *Hum Vaccin Immunother.* 2012;8(9):1179–1191. doi:10.4161/hv.20738. Review.

92. Motz GT, Coukos G. Deciphering and reversing tumor immune suppression. *Immunity.* 2013;39(1):61–73.

93. Charbonneau B, Goode EL, Kalli KR, et al. The immune system in the pathogenesis of ovarian cancer. *Crit Rev Immunol.* 2013;33(2):137–164. Review.

94. Hopkins TG, Wood N. Female human papillomavirus (HPV) vaccination: Global uptake and the impact of attitudes. *Vaccine.* 2013;31(13):1673–1679.

95. Liu B, Nash J, Runowicz C, et al. Ovarian cancer immunotherapy: Opportunities, progresses and challenges. *J Hematol Oncol.* 2010;3:7. PMID:20146807.

96. Odunsi K, Jungbluth AA, Stockert E, et al. NY-ESO-1 and LAGE-1 cancer-testis antigens are potential targets for immunotherapy in epithelial ovarian cancer. *Cancer Res.* 2003;63:6076–6083.

97. Odunsi K, Qian F, Matsuzaki J, et al. Vaccination with an NY-ESO-1 peptide of HLA class I/II specificities induces integrated humoral and T cell responses in ovarian cancer. *Proc Natl Acad Sci U S A.* 2007;104:12837–12842.

98. Diefenbach CS, Gnjatic S, Sabbatini P, et al. Safety and immunogenicity study of NY-ESO-1b peptide and montanide ISA-51 vaccination of patients with epithelial ovarian cancer in high-risk first remission. *Clin Cancer Res.* 2008;14:2740–2748.

99. Odunsi KRK, Lele S. Diversified prime and boost vaccination using recombinant vaccinia and fowlpox expressing NY-ESO-1 efficiently induces anti-body, CD4+ and CD8+ anti tumor immune responses in patients with ovarian cancer. *Proceedings of the 38th Society of Gynecologic Oncologists,* San Diego, CA, USA. Abstract 200.

100. Rahma OE, Ashtar E, Czystowska M, et al. A Gynecologic Oncology Group phase II trial of two p53 peptide vaccine approaches: Subcutaneous injection and intravenous pulsed dendritic cells in high recurrence risk ovarian cancer patients. *Cancer Immunol Immunother.* 2012;61:373–384.

101. Leffers N, Lambeck AJ, Gooden MJ, et al. Immunization with a P53 synthetic long peptide vaccine induces P53-specific immune responses in ovarian cancer patients, a phase II trial. *Int J Cancer.* 2009;125:2104–2113.

102. Leffers N, Vermeij R, Hoogeboom BN, et al. Long-term clinical and immunological effects of p53-SLP® vaccine in patients with ovarian cancer. *Int J Cancer.* 2012;130:105–112.

103. Morse MA, Secord AA, Blackwell K, et al. MHC class I-presented tumor antigens identified in ovarian cancer by immunoproteomic analysis are targets for T-cell responses against breast and ovarian cancer. *Clin Cancer Res.* 2011;17:3408–3419.

104. Gulley JL, Arlen PM, Tsang KY, et al. Pilot study of vaccination with recombinant CEA-MUC-1-TRICOM poxviral-based vaccines in patients with metastatic carcinoma. *Clin Cancer Res.* 2008;14:3060–3069.

105. Chiang CL, Kandalaft LE, Coukos G. Adjuvants for enhancing the immunogenicity of whole tumor cell vaccines. *Int Rev Immunol.* 2011;30:150–182.

106. Buckanovich RJ, Facciabene A, Kim S, et al. Endothelin B receptor mediates the endothelial barrier to T cell homing to tumors and disables immune therapy. *Nat Med.* 2008;14:28–36.

107. Epenetos AA, Shepherd J, Britton KE, et al. 123I radioiodinated antibody imaging of occult ovarian cancer. *Cancer.* 1985;55:984–987.

108. Epenetos AA, Hooker G, Krausz T, et al. Antibody-guided irradiation of malignant ascites in ovarian cancer: A new therapeutic method possessing specificity against cancer cells. *Obstet Gynecol.* 1986;68:71S–74S.

109. Berek JS, Martinez-Maza O, Montz FJ. The immune system and gynecologic cancer. In: Coppelson MT, Morrow CP, eds. *Gynecologic Oncology.* Edinburgh: Churchill-Livingstone; 1992:119–151.

110. Ortiz-Sanchez E, Helguera G, Daniels TR, et al. Antibody-cytokine fusion proteins: Applications in cancer therapy. *Expert Opin Biol Ther.* 2008;8:609–632.

111. Kandalaft LE, Powell DJ Jr, Singh N, et al. Immunotherapy for ovarian cancer: What's next? *J Clin Oncol.* 2011;29:925–933.

112. Berek JS, Taylor PT, Gordon A, et al. Randomized, placebo-controlled study of oregovomab for consolidation of clinical remission in patients with advanced ovarian cancer. *J Clin Oncol.* 2004; 22:3507–3516.

113. Berek JS, Taylor PT, Nicodemus CF. CA125 velocity at relapse is a highly significant predictor of survival post relapse: Results of a 5-year follow-up survey to a randomized placebo-controlled study of maintenance oregovomab immunotherapy in advanced ovarian cancer. *J Immunother.* 2008;31:207–214.

114. Berek J, Taylor P, McGuire W, et al. Oregovomab maintenance monoimmunotherapy does not improve outcomes in advanced ovarian cancer. *J Clin Oncol.* 2009;27:418–425.

115. **Nicodemus CF, Chu C, Collins Y, et al.** The immune adjuvant properties of front-line carboplatin-paclitaxel: A randomized phase 2 study of alternative schedules of intravenous oregovomab chemoimmunotherapy in advanced ovarian cancer. *J Immunother.* 2009;32:54–65.

116. **Schlebusch H, Wagner U, Grunn U, et al.** A monoclonal anti-idiotypic antibody ACA125 mimicking the tumor-associated antigen CA125 for immunotherapy of ovarian cancer. *Hybridoma.* 1995;14:167–174.

117. **Wagner U.** Antitumor antibodies for immunotherapy of ovarian carcinomas. *Hybridoma.* 1993;12:521–528.

118. **Reinartz S, Köhler S, Schlebusch H, et al.** Vaccination of patients with advanced ovarian carcinoma with the anti-idiotype ACA125: Immunological response and survival (phase Ib/II). *Clin Cancer Res.* 2004;10:1580–1587.

119. **Wagner U, Köhler S, Reinartz S, et al.** Immunological consolidation of ovarian carcinoma recurrences with monoclonal anti-idiotype antibody ACA125: Immune responses and survival in palliative treatment. *Clin Cancer Res.* 2001;7:1154–1162. Commentary by **Foon K, Bhattacharya-Chatterjee M**. Are solid tumor anti-idiotype vaccines ready for prime time? *Clin Cancer Res.* 2001;7:1112–1115.

120. **Sabbatini P, Dupont J, Aghajanian C, et al.** Phase I study of abagovomab in patients with epithelial ovarian, fallopian tube, or primary peritoneal cancer. *Clin Cancer Res.* 2006;12:5503–5510.

121. **Rosenberg SA.** Immunotherapy of cancer by systemic administration of lymphoid cells plus interleukin-2. *J Biol Response Mod.* 1984; 3:501–511.

122. **Rosenberg SA, Lotze MT.** Cancer immunotherapy using interleukin-2 and interleukin-2-activated lymphocytes. *Annu Rev Immunol.* 1986; 4:681–709.

123. **Rosenberg SA, Lotze MT, Muul LM, et al.** Observations on the systemic administration of autologous lymphokine-activated killer cells and recombinant interleukin-2 to patients with metastatic cancer. *N Engl J Med.* 1985;313:1485–1492.

124. **Lotzova E.** Role of human circulating and tumor-infiltrating lymphocytes in cancer defense and treatment. *Nat Immun Cell Growth Regul.* 1990;9:253–264.

125. **Urba WJ, Clark JW, Steis RG, et al.** Intraperitoneal lymphokine-activated killer cell/interleukin-2 therapy in patients with intra-abdominal cancer: Immunologic considerations. *J Natl Cancer Inst.* 1989;81:602–611.

126. **Steis RG, Urba WJ, VanderMolen LA, et al.** Intraperitoneal lymphokine-activated killer-cell and interleukin-2 therapy for malignancies limited to the peritoneal cavity. *J Clin Oncol.* 1990;8:1618–1629.

127. **Berek JS, Lichtenstein AK, Knox RM, et al.** Synergistic effects of combination sequential immunotherapies in a murine ovarian cancer model. *Cancer Res.* 1985;45:4215–4218.

128. **West WH, Tauer KW, Yannelli JR, et al.** Constant-infusion recombinant interleukin-2 in adoptive immunotherapy of advanced cancer. *N Engl J Med.* 1987;316:898–905.

129. **Topalian SL, Solomon D, Avis FP, et al.** Immunotherapy of patients with advanced cancer using tumor-infiltrating lymphocytes and recombinant interleukin-2: A pilot study. *J Clin Oncol.* 1988;6:839–853.

130. **Aoki Y, Takakuwa K, Kodama S, et al.** Use of adoptive transfer of tumor-infiltrating lymphocytes alone or in combination with cisplatin-containing chemotherapy in patients with epithelial ovarian cancer. *Cancer Res.* 1991;51:1934–1939.

131. **Dudley ME, Wunderlich JR, Yang JC, et al.** Adoptive cell transfer therapy following nonmyeloablative but lymphodepleting chemotherapy for the treatment of patients with refractory metastatic melanoma. *J Clin Oncol.* 2005;23:2346–2357.

132. **Gotlieb WH, Abrams JS, Watson JM, et al.** Presence of interleukin 10 (IL-10) in the ascites of patients with ovarian and other intra-abdominal cancers. *Cytokine.* 1992;4:385–390.

133. **Disis ML, Schiffman K, Guthrie K, et al.** Effect of dose on immune response in patients vaccinated with an HER-2/*neu* intracellular domain protein–based vaccine. *J Clin Oncol.* 2004;22:1916–1925.

134. **Brulet JM, Maudoux F, Thomas S, et al.** DNA vaccine encoding endosome-targeted human papillomavirus type 16 E7 protein generates CD4+ T cell-dependent protection. *Eur J Immunol.* 2007;37:376–384.

135. **Wu TC, Guarnieri FG, Staveley-O'Carroll KF, et al.** Engineering an intracellular pathway for major histocompatibility complex class II presentation of antigens. *Proc Natl Acad Sci U S A.* 1995;92:11671–11675.

136. **Ji H, Wang TL, Chen CH, et al.** Targeting human papillomavirus type 16 E7 to the endosomal/lysosomal compartment enhances the antitumor immunity of DNA vaccines against murine human papillomavirus type 16 E7-expressing tumors. *Hum Gene Ther.* 1999; 10:2727–2740.

137. **Santin AD, Hermonat PL, Ravaggi A, et al.** *In vitro* induction of tumor-specific human lymphocyte antigen class I-restricted CD8 cytotoxic T lymphocytes by ovarian tumor antigen-pulsed autologous dendritic cells from patients with advanced ovarian cancer. *Am J Obstet Gynecol.* 2000;183:601–609.

138. **Santin AD, Hermonat PL, Ravaggi A, et al.** Development, characterization and distribution of adoptively transferred peripheral blood lymphocytes primed by human papillomavirus 18 E7–pulsed autologous dendritic cells in a patient with metastatic adenocarcinoma of the uterine cervix. *Eur J Gynaecol Oncol.* 2000;21:17–23.

139. **Zhao X, Wei YQ, Peng ZL.** Induction of T cell responses against autologous ovarian tumors with whole tumor cell lysate-pulsed dendritic cells. *Immunol Invest.* 2001;30:33–45.

140. **Hernando JJ, Park TW, Kubler K, et al.** Vaccination with autologous tumour antigen-pulsed dendritic cells in advanced gynaecological malignancies: Clinical and immunological evaluation of a phase I trial. *Cancer Immunol Immunother.* 2002;51:45–52.

141. **Inaba K, Turley S, Yamaide F, et al.** Efficient presentation of phagocytosed cellular fragments on the major histocompatibility complex class II products of dendritic cells. *J Exp Med.* 1998;188: 2163–2173.

142. **Mackensen A, Herbst B, Chen JL, et al.** Phase I study in melanoma patients of a vaccine with peptide-pulsed dendritic cells generated *in vitro* from CD34(+) hematopoietic progenitor cells. *Int J Cancer.* 2000;86:385–392.

143. **Thurner B, Roder C, Dieckmann D, et al.** Generation of large numbers of fully mature and stable dendritic cells from leukapheresis products for clinical application. *J Immunol Methods.* 1999;223:1–15.

144. **Thurner B, Haendle I, Roder C, et al.** Vaccination with mage-3A1 peptide-pulsed mature, monocyte-derived dendritic cells expands specific cytotoxic T cells and induces regression of some metastases in advanced stage IV melanoma. *J Exp Med.* 1999;190: 1669–1678.

145. **Finn OJ.** Cancer vaccines: Between the idea and the reality. *Nat Rev Immunol.* 2003;3:630–641.

146. **Paul S, Acres B, Limacher JM, et al.** Cancer vaccines: Challenges and outlook in the field. *IDrugs.* 2007;10:324–328.

147. **Tabi Z, Man S.** Challenges for cancer vaccine development. *Adv Drug Deliv Rev.* 2006;58:902–915.

148. **Cannon MJ, O'Brien TJ, Underwood LJ, et al.** Novel target antigens for dendritic cell-based immunotherapy against ovarian cancer. *Exp Rev Anticancer Ther.* 2002;2:97–105.

149. **McIlroy D, Gregoire M.** Optimizing dendritic cell-based anticancer immunotherapy: Maturation state does have clinical impact. *Cancer Immunol Immunother.* 2003;52:583–591.

150. **McIlroy D, Tanguy-Royer S, Le Meur N, et al.** Profiling dendritic cell maturation with dedicated microarrays. *J Leukoc Biol.* 2005;78: 794–803.

151. **Berek JS, Knapp RC, Hacker NF, et al.** Intraperitoneal immunotherapy of epithelial ovarian carcinoma with *Corynebacterium parvum. Am J Obstet Gynecol.* 1985;152:1003–1010.

152. **Lichtenstein A, Berek J, Bast R, et al.** Activation of peritoneal lymphocyte cytotoxicity in patients with ovarian cancer by intraperitoneal treatment with *Corynebacterium parvum. J Biol Response Mod.* 1984;3:371–378.

153. **Bast RC Jr, Berek JS, Obrist R, et al.** Intraperitoneal immunotherapy of human ovarian carcinoma with *Corynebacterium parvum. Cancer Res.* 1983;43:1395–1401.

154. **Mantovani A, Sessa C, Peri G, et al.** Intraperitoneal administration of *Corynebacterium parvum* in patients with ascitic ovarian tumors resistant to chemotherapy: Effects on cytotoxicity of tumor-associated macrophages and NK cells. *Int J Cancer.* 1981;27:437–446.

155. **Gusdon JP Jr, Homesley HD, Jobson VW, et al.** Treatment of advanced ovarian malignancy with chemoimmunotherapy using autologous tumor and *Corynebacterium parvum. Obstet Gynecol.* 1983; 62:728–735.

156. **Howell SB, Kirmani S, Lucas WE, et al.** A phase II trial of intraperitoneal cisplatin and etoposide for primary treatment of ovarian epithelial cancer. *J Clin Oncol.* 1990;8:137–145.

157. **Edwards RP, Gooding W, Lembersky BC, et al.** Comparison of toxicity and survival following intraperitoneal recombinant interleukin-2 for persistent ovarian cancer after platinum: Twenty-four-hour versus 7-day infusion. *J Clin Oncol.* 1997;15:3399–3407.

158. **Vlad AM, Budiu RA, Lenzner DE, et al.** A phase II trial of intraperitoneal interleukin-2 in patients with platinum-resistant or platinum-refractory ovarian cancer. *Cancer Immunol Immunother.* 2010;59:293–301.

159. **Nardi M, Cognetti F, Pollera CF, et al.** Intraperitoneal recombinant alpha-2-interferon alternating with cisplatin as salvage therapy for minimal residual-disease ovarian cancer: A phase II study. *J Clin Oncol.* 1990;8:1036–1041.

160. **Repetto L, Chiara S, Guido T, et al.** Intraperitoneal chemotherapy with carboplatin and interferon alpha in the treatment of relapsed ovarian cancer: A pilot study. *Anticancer Res.* 1991;11:1641–1643.

161. **Hurteau JA, Blessing JA, DeCesare SL, et al.** Evaluation of recombinant human interleukin-12 in patients with recurrent or refractory ovarian cancer: A Gynecologic Oncology Group study. *Gynecol Oncol.* 2001;82:7–10.

162. **Lenzi R, Rosenblum M, Verschraegen C, et al.** Phase I study of intraperitoneal recombinant human interleukin 12 in patients with Müllerian carcinoma, gastrointestinal primary malignancies, and mesothelioma. *Clin Cancer Res.* 2002;8:3686–3695.

163. **Recchia F, Saggio G, Cesta A, et al.** Interleukin-2 and 13-cis retinoic acid as maintenance therapy in advanced ovarian cancer. *Int J Oncol.* 2005;27:1039–1046.

164. **Roche MR, Rudd PJ, Krasner CN, et al.** Phase II trial of GM-CSF in women with asymptomatic recurrent müllerian tumors. *Gynecol Oncol.* 2010;116:168–172.

165. **Schmeler KM, Vadhan-Raj S, Ramirez PT, et al.** A phase II study of GM-CSF and rIFN-gamma1b plus carboplatin for the treatment of recurrent, platinum-sensitive ovarian, fallopian tube and primary peritoneal cancer. *Gynecol Oncol.* 2009;113:210–215.

166. **Woo EY, Chu CS, Goletz TJ, et al.** Regulatory CD4(+)CD25(+) T cells in tumors from patients with early-stage non-small cell lung cancer and late-stage ovarian cancer. *Cancer Res.* 2001;61:4766–4772.

167. **Powell DJ Jr, Felipe-Silva A, Merino MJ, et al.** Administration of a CD25-directed immunotoxin, LMB-2, to patients with metastatic melanoma induces a selective partial reduction in regulatory T cells *in vivo. J Immunol.* 2007;179:4919–4928.

168. **Kryczek I, Wei S, Zou L, et al.** Cutting edge: TH17 and regulatory T cell dynamics and the regulation by IL-2 in the tumor microenvironment. *J Immunol.* 2007;178:6730–6733.

3 Chemotherapy

Michael L. Friedlander
Maurie Markman

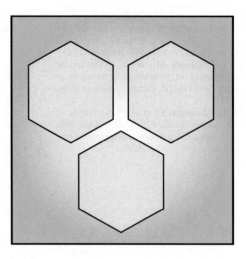

General Principles

Tumor Growth and Chemotherapy

There are a wide variety of chemotherapeutic agents and a growing number of targeted agents available to treat women with gynecologic cancers. The selection of a treatment regimen should be based on the results of randomized phase III trials, but this may not be possible, particularly when treating patients with uncommon cancers.

Treatment recommendations and choice of drugs are determined by the known efficacy and potential toxicities of chemotherapeutic agents and the clinical context, that is, first-line treatment or treatment for recurrent disease after one or more lines of prior therapy. Most antineoplastic agents have a relatively narrow therapeutic index, and treatment decisions are based on multiple factors, including age, performance status, medical comorbidities, organ function, tumor type, previous chemotherapy, objectives of therapy, and the predicted likelihood of benefit, which should be communicated clearly to the patient and her family (Table 3.1).

It is important to consider the natural history and biology of the cancer being treated. For example, low-grade serous cancers or granulosa cell tumors are typically indolent and slow growing, in contrast to undifferentiated sarcomas, which are rapidly progressive. This may influence decisions regarding initiation of treatment, particularly when chemotherapy is administered with palliative intent. It may be appropriate to withhold or delay chemotherapy in asymptomatic patients with relatively indolent metastatic disease.

It is a fundamental principle that chemotherapy should be administered only to patients in whom the diagnosis of cancer has been confirmed with a biopsy. Cytology may provide acceptable confirmation, depending on the clinical context, for example, in a patient with a large volume of ascites, multiple peritoneal nodules, an adnexal mass, and an elevated CA125 titer, it would be acceptable to give neoadjuvant chemotherapy if the cytology was consistent with a primary ovarian cancer.

All chemotherapeutic agents have potential side effects and potential benefits. It is important to ascertain whether the patient has measurable disease or elevated tumor markers before commencing treatment, particularly in patients with metastatic disease, so that response can be assessed. The extent of previous therapy and the patient's age, general health, and other relevant medical problems (e.g., neuropathy from long-standing diabetes or prior chemotherapy with taxanes)

58

Table 3.1 Issues When Considering Cancer Chemotherapy

1. Natural History of the Malignancy

    a. Diagnosis of a malignancy made by biopsy or cytology

    b. Rate of disease progression

    c. Extent of disease spread

2. Patient Factors

    a. Age, general health, medical comorbidities, performance status

    b. Extent of previous treatment

    c. Availability of facilities to evaluate, monitor, and treat potential drug toxicities

    d. The emotional, social, and financial situation of the patient

3. Likelihood of Achieving a Clinical Benefit

    a. Cancers in which chemotherapy is curative (e.g., ovarian germ cell tumors and gestational trophoblastic tumors)

    b. Cancers in which chemotherapy has demonstrated improvement in survival (e.g., epithelial ovarian cancer)

    c. Cancers that respond to treatment but in which improved survival has not been clearly demonstrated (e.g., metastatic leiomyosarcoma)

    d. Cancers with marginal or no response to chemotherapy (e.g., platinum refractory ovarian cancer)

should all be taken into consideration when deciding on the choice of treatment. The patient's emotional, social, and financial status must be respected as part of the considerations. It is essential to clearly communicate the aims and objectives of therapy, that is, cure or palliation, the likelihood of benefit, and the side effects of treatment, so the patient can make an informed decision regarding chemotherapy.

Gynecologic cancers can be grouped into the following three categories, based on the likelihood of chemotherapeutic response and treatment benefit:

1. **Highly chemosensitive tumors**—treatment administered with curative intent. This group includes ovarian germ cell tumors and gestational trophoblastic tumors, where chemotherapy is curative for most patients. Toxicity is acceptable if the probability of cure is high, but every effort should be made to limit toxicity and reduce side effects without compromising the chance of cure by inappropriate dose reductions or prolonged delay between cycles.

2. **Chemosensitive, but cure is uncommon.** This group includes advanced high-grade serous epithelial ovarian cancer, where response rates range from 70% to 90%. Chemotherapy increases progression-free and overall survival in patients with advanced ovarian cancer, but the majority of patients will relapse and die of disease.

3. **Response to chemotherapy is relatively low.** This group includes uterine leiomyosarcomas and platinum-resistant ovarian cancers, and the impact of treatment on overall survival is unclear. In this setting, it is important to consider the patient's performance status, other medical comorbidities, extent of disease, rate of progression, and symptoms when discussing the relative risks and benefits of cytotoxic drug therapy.

Differential Sensitivity

Most cancer chemotherapeutic agents target DNA in malignant and normal cells. **DNA damage results in cancer cell death and is responsible for many of the benefits and side effects of therapy** (1). Most combinations of chemotherapy are administered using doses that are close to, or at, the maximum tolerated dose (MTD), based on the concept that a combination of drugs with nonoverlapping mechanisms of action administered at full dose may prevent or delay the emergence of drug-resistant tumor cells, and result in greater cell kill. **The therapeutic window between antitumor effect and normal tissue toxicity may be narrow, because there are many similarities between normal cells and malignant cells,** particularly those normal cell populations in which constant cell proliferation is common (e.g., bone marrow, gastrointestinal epithelium, and hair follicles). As a result, the differential effect of antineoplastic drugs on tumors compared with normal tissues is quantitative rather than qualitative. **Some degree of injury to normal tissue occurs with all chemotherapeutic agents** (1). The normal tissue toxicity produced by most chemotherapeutic agents commonly correlates with the intrinsic rate of cellular proliferation in the target tissue, which explains why blood count suppression, mucosal injury, and alopecia are common with many chemotherapeutic regimens.

Therapeutic Index

For any chemotherapeutic agent, the net effect on the patient is referred to as the drug's *therapeutic index* **(i.e., a ratio of the doses at which therapeutic effect and toxicity occur).** The mechanism of action does not distinguish between normal cells and proliferating cancer cells, so there is a narrow therapeutic window between antitumor effect and toxicity (1). Cancer chemotherapy requires a balance of therapeutic effect and toxicity to optimize the therapeutic index, which may be influenced by pharmacologic and biologic factors, including pharmacogenomics in an individual patient.

Biologic Factors Influencing Treatment

Cell Kinetic Concepts

The growth capacity of normal and malignant cells is closely regulated by a complex process of signaling and inhibitory pathways. The increased or selective cytotoxicity of chemotherapy in chemosensitive cancers was previously thought to result from the differential rates of proliferation in normal and malignant cells. It was believed that cancer cells simply grew faster than normal cells, which caused their sensitivity to chemotherapy. This is not the case for most solid tumors, and the efficacy of chemotherapy cannot be explained by this reductionist theory (1). Cancers are characterized by continuous dysregulated cellular proliferation, greater sensitivity to cytotoxic chemotherapy than normal cells, limited ability to repair DNA damage, and cell death through apoptosis (2). For example, **ovarian cancers that occur in patients with germline BRCA mutations appear to be much more sensitive to platinum-based chemotherapeutic agents, because of the deficiency in homologous recombination repair, nonhomologous endjoining, and an inability to repair DNA double-strand breaks (DSBs), rather than because of more rapid proliferation.**

Patterns of Normal Growth

All normal tissues have the capacity for cellular division and growth. There are three general types of normal tissue growth: static, expanding, and renewing.

1. The **static** population comprises relatively well-differentiated cells that, after initial proliferative activity in the embryonic and neonatal period, rarely undergo cell division. Typical examples are striated muscle and neurons.

2. The **expanding** population of cells is characterized by the capacity to proliferate under special stimuli (e.g., tissue injury). Under those circumstances, the normally quiescent tissue (e.g., liver or kidney) undergoes a surge of proliferation with regrowth.

3. The **renewing** population of cells is constantly in a proliferative state. There is constant cell division, a high degree of cell turnover, and constant cell loss. This occurs in bone marrow, epidermis, and gastrointestinal mucosa.

Normal tissues with a static pattern of growth are rarely seriously injured by drug therapy, whereas renewing cell populations such as bone marrow, gastrointestinal mucosa, and spermatozoa are commonly injured, which explains many of the side effects of chemotherapy.

Cancer Cell Growth

Tumor cell growth represents a disruption in the normal cellular brake mechanisms, resulting in continued proliferation and eventual death of the host. It is not the rate of cellular proliferation per se, but the failure of the regulated balance between cell loss and cell proliferation that differentiates malignant cells from normal cells.

Gompertzian Growth

The characteristics of cancer growth have been assessed by multiple studies in animals and more limited studies in humans. When tumors are extremely small, growth follows an exponential pattern that later seems to slow. In 1825, Gompertz proposed that tumors grow in a sigmoidal pattern, with the fastest growth occurring when tumors are about one-third of their maximum size, with growth slowing as tumors get larger. Experimental models suggest that this observation is the result of decreased cell production, rather than increased cell loss in larger tumors. Put simply, Gompertzian growth means that as a tumor mass increases in size, the time required to double the tumor's volume also increases. This suggests that small tumors and micrometastases should be more sensitive to chemotherapy (3).

Doubling Time

The doubling time of a human tumor is the time it takes for the mass to double its size. There is considerable variation in doubling times of human tumors. For example, germ cell tumors and some lymphomas have relatively fast doubling times (20 to 40 days), whereas adenocarcinomas and squamous cell carcinomas have relatively slow doubling times (50 to 150 days). In general, metastases have faster doubling times than primary tumors.

If it is assumed that **exponential growth occurs early in a tumor's history and that a tumor starts from a single malignant stem cell,** then:

1. A 1-mm mass will have undergone approximately 20 tumor doublings
2. A 5-mm mass (a size that might be first visualized on a radiograph) will have undergone 27 doublings
3. A 1-cm mass will have undergone 30 doublings

When a 1-cm tumor is diagnosed, it is commonly assumed that the tumor was detected early. In reality, it probably has undergone 30 doublings and been present for approximately 60% of its life span (4).

Unfortunately, our current diagnostic methods detect tumors only relatively late in their growth, and metastases may have occurred long before there is obvious evidence of the primary lesion. The second implication of tumor kinetics is that, in late stages of tumor growth, very few doublings in tumor mass have a dramatic impact on the size of the tumor. After a tumor becomes palpable (1 cm in diameter), only three more doublings are necessary to produce a large tumor mass (8 cm in diameter) (4,5).

Cell Cycle

The cell cycle is controlled by a complex system with multiple overlapping checkpoints that regulate progression through the cell cycle (6). Loss of normal cell cycle control and disabled checkpoints are a hallmark of cancer, with somatic events that promote entry and progression through the cell cycle. Cyclins and their associated cyclin-dependent kinases (CDKs) are the key drivers of the cell cycle, and specific transitions in the cell cycle are controlled by specific CDKs (6,7).

Cell cycle progression is controlled by successive changes in cyclin–CDK activity. Several checkpoints can stall the cell cycle in response to genotoxic insults. To minimize the possibility of errors, checkpoints exist at four different points in the cell cycle, G_1/S, intra-S, G_2/M, and at metaphase to anaphase. The TP53-dependent G_1/S checkpoint blocks initiation of DNA replication. The intra-S phase checkpoint is initiated by ATR-CHK1 to stabilize stalled replication forks and block replication. The G_2/M checkpoint inhibits mitotic entry, and the spindle assembly checkpoint inhibits anaphase until there is bipolar attachment of chromosomes to microtubules of the mitotic spindle (6,7). **The complex cell cycle and its controls are simplified by the classic cell cycle model shown in Figure 3.1.**

1. **G_1 phase (postmitotic phase).** Cyclin D–CDK4/6 promotes entry into the cell cycle at the restriction point, and is the initial driver of the G_1 phase. This is a period of variable duration when enzymes necessary for DNA and RNA synthesis and other proteins occur in preparation for cell division.
2. **S phase (DNA synthetic phase)** is the period in which new DNA replication occurs. Cyclin E–CDK 2 activity increases during late G_1 and peaks in S phase, and cyclin A–CDK2 complexes are active in S and G_2 phases.
3. **G_2 phase (postsynthetic phase)** is the period during which the cell has a diploid number of chromosomes and twice the DNA content of the normal cell. The cell remains in this phase for a relatively short time before it reenters the mitotic phase. Cyclin B–CDK1 is essential for G_2–M transition and mitosis. PLK and Aurora A are critical for

61

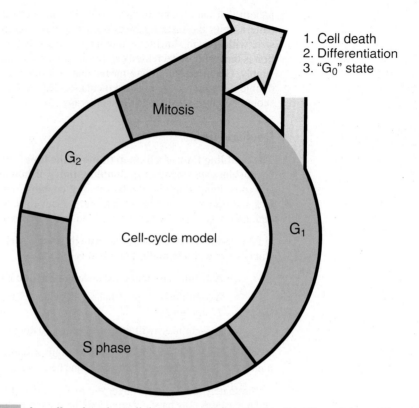

1. Cell death
2. Differentiation
3. "G_0" state

Figure 3.1 **The cell cycle.** After cell division, a cell can *(1)* die, *(2)* differentiate, or *(3)* enter resting (G_0) phase. Cells in the latter two phases can reenter the cycle at G_1.

centrosome maturation, formation of the mitotic spindle, and also play a role in chromosomal segregation and cytokinesis.

4. **M phase (mitotic phase)** of the cell cycle is the phase of cell division.

5. **G_0 phase (the resting phase)** is the time during which cells are quiescent and do not divide. Cells may move in and out of the G_0 phase.

The generation time is the duration of the cycle from M phase to M phase. Variation occurs in all phases of the cell cycle, but the variation is greatest during the G_1 period. The two gap phases serve as more than time delays to allow cell growth. They also provide time for the cell to monitor the internal and external environment, to ensure that conditions are suitable and preparations are complete before the cell commits itself to the S phase and mitosis. The G_1 phase can vary greatly depending on external conditions and extracellular signals. If extracellular conditions are unfavorable, cells delay progress through G_1 and may enter a resting state known as G_0, in which they can remain for long periods before resuming proliferation (8).

These cell cycle events have important implications for cancer therapy. **Tumors consist of pools of proliferating and nonproliferating or quiescent cells. Dividing cancer cells that are actively traversing the cell cycle are more sensitive to chemotherapeutic agents. Cells in a resting state (G_0) are relatively insensitive to chemotherapeutic agents. These may include cancer stem cells and a hypoxic cell population, which are relatively drug resistant (9).**

Cell Kinetics

In cell kinetic studies performed on human tumors, the duration of the S phase (DNA synthesis phase) is relatively similar for most human tumors and is about 8 hours while the M phase is about 1 hour. In mammalian cells, the length of the G_2 phase is about 2 hours. The length of the G_1 phase is highly variable and can range from about 6 hours to several days or longer (10). The length of the cell cycle in human tumors varies from slightly more than half a day to perhaps 5 days. With cell cycle times in the range of 24 hours and doubling times in the range of 10 to 1,000 days, it is clear that only a small proportion of tumor cells are in active cell division at any one time.

Table 3.2 Cell Cycle Specificity of Chemotherapeutic Agents

Classification	Examples
Cell cycle–specific, proliferation dependent	Hydroxyurea, cytosine arabinoside
Cell cycle–specific, less proliferation dependent	5-fluorouracil, methotrexate
Cell cycle–nonspecific, proliferation dependent	Cyclophosphamide, actinomycin D, carboplatin, cisplatin
Cell cycle–nonspecific, less proliferation dependent	Paclitaxel, topotecan

Two major factors that affect the rate at which tumors grow are the growth fraction and the rate of cell loss from the population due to terminal differentiation or cell death. **The growth fraction is the number of cells in the tumor mass that are actively dividing.** There is a marked variation in the growth fraction of tumors in humans. In the past, it was thought that human tumors contained billions of cells, all growing slowly. In actuality, there is a small fraction of cells in a tumor mass that is rapidly proliferating, while the remainder, including a stem cell component, are out of the cell cycle and quiescent. **Cancer "stem cells" are a small population of the tumor mass. They appear to be relatively chemoresistant, and are thought to be responsible for the high rate of recurrence of many solid tumors.** For example, studies have shown an enriched population of cancer stem cells and stem cell pathway mediators in recurrent ovarian cancers, suggesting that these cells contribute to the development of recurrence (11,12). Several developmental pathways, including Notch, Wnt, Hedgehog, and TNF beta, have been shown to be crucial for the regulation and maintenance of ovarian cancer stem cells, and they are potentially amenable to targeted therapies (13).

Cell Cycle–Specific versus Cell Cycle–Nonspecific Drugs

Antineoplastic agents have complex mechanisms of action and induce damage to cells in a wide variety of ways. They may have different sites of action in the cell cycle, and their activity is a function of the proliferative capacity of the tumor being treated. Chemotherapeutic agents can be divided into two main classes based on their site of action in the cell cycle: Cell cycle–nonspecific and cell cycle–specific, although this is an oversimplification of how chemotherapy works (Table 3.2).

Cell Cycle–Nonspecific **Cell cycle–nonspecific agents kill in all phases of the cell cycle and have limited dependency on proliferative activity.** They have a linear dose response and are active on cells in either a dividing or resting state. They include alkylating agents, antitumor antibiotics, and hormonal therapies.

Cell Cycle–Specific **Cell cycle–specific agents act only at particular phases of the cell cycle,** and include antimetabolites that are S-phase specific, vinca alkaloids and taxanes that are M-phase dependent, and *Bleomycin* and *Topotecan* that are G_2-phase dependent. Between these two broad classifications, there is a spectrum of drugs with variable degrees of cell cycle and proliferation dependence (Table 3.3).

Table 3.3 Site of Action in the Cell Cycle

Portion of Cell Cycle	Drugs
G_1	Actinomycin D
Early S	Hydroxyurea, cytosine arabinoside, 5-fluorouracil, methotrexate
Late S	Doxorubicin
G_2	Bleomycin, etoposide, teniposide, carboplatin, cisplatin, topotecan
M	Paclitaxel, vincristine, vinblastine

Log Kill Hypothesis

From knowledge of basic cellular kinetics, concepts of chemotherapy have emerged that have proven useful in the design of chemotherapeutic combination regimens (2). In experimental tumor systems in mouse models, survival is inversely proportional to the number of cells implanted, or to the size of the tumor at the time treatment is initiated (14). **Treatment immediately after tumor implantation, or when the tumor is subclinical in size, results in a higher chance of cure than if the tumor is clinically obvious and large** (14). Skipper's cell kill hypothesis, published over 60 years ago, suggested that if tumors were treated at the level of micrometastases rather than larger volume tumors, it was more likely that the treatment would be effective. This is supported by the results of adjuvant chemotherapy in many solid tumors.

Skipper used a murine leukemic model to define the concept of logarithmic cancer cell growth and specific log cell kill with chemotherapy (14). They suggested that **chemotherapeutic agents work by first-order kinetics; that is, they kill a constant fraction of cells rather than a constant number of cells.** This concept has had important implications for the development of chemotherapeutic regimens and adjuvant chemotherapeutic trials. For instance, a single exposure of tumor cells to an antineoplastic drug might be capable of producing 2- to 5-logs of cell kill. With typical body tumor burdens of 10^{12} cells (1 kg), a single dose of chemotherapy is unlikely to be curative. This explains the need for intermittent courses of chemotherapy to achieve the magnitude of cell kill necessary to produce tumor regression and cure. It also provides a rationale for multiple-drug or combination chemotherapy.

The cure rate in mouse models is significantly improved if only micrometastases are present, that is, 10^1 to 10^4 cells, which are too small for clinical detection (14). This is the basis for using adjuvant chemotherapy in apparently localized cancers, when subclinical metastases are likely to be present in many patients.

Drug Resistance and Tumor Cell Heterogeneity

Chemotherapeutic agents often are active when initially used, but tumors commonly develop resistance to chemotherapy (15). Many patients have an initial response and then develop a recurrence that is no longer responsive to the drugs that were previously effective. It is unclear why some cancers, such as germ cell tumors and gestational trophoblastic tumors, are usually cured with chemotherapy, even at an advanced stage, while the majority of solid tumors, such as high-grade serous ovarian cancers, ultimately develop drug resistance (16).

It has been postulated that cancers that are curable with chemotherapy have an increased intrinsic sensitivity to induction of apoptosis by a DNA damaging agent, and have wild-type TP53 (16). Malignant cells with intact function of p53 recognize recombination checkpoints that activate apoptosis in the presence of DNA strand breaks caused by chemotherapy. The majority of germ cell tumors retain intact apoptotic pathways, including the expression of wild-type p53, and these patients respond very well to platinum-based chemotherapy. In contrast, germ cell tumors with p53 mutations are frequently resistant to chemotherapy (17). Similarly, gestational choriocarcinomas express high levels of wild-type p53, have a high BAX: Bcl2 ratio, and high levels of apoptosis (16).

There is a lot of evidence to support the key role of apoptotic pathways in causing cell death in response to chemotherapy, and signaling pathways activated by p53 appear to be very important. Many solid tumors, such as high-grade serous ovarian cancer, are characterized by TP53 mutations, which may explain why recurrence is so common after initial response to chemotherapy (18). There are many possible mechanisms for drug resistance related to the instability of the cancer cell genome, which is characterized by gene amplifications and deletions, rearrangements, and multiple mutations. There is often epigenetic silencing of genes and many cellular mechanisms involved in drug resistance (2,15,18). Resistant tumor cells may display increased deactivation or decreased activation of drugs, allow increased drug efflux, or resist normal drug uptake (15,17–19).

Theories for Overcoming Drug Resistance

It has been suggested that spontaneous mutation to a drug-resistant phenotype occurs in rapidly growing malignant tumors, and this is called the somatic mutation theory (20). The theory suggests that most mammalian tumor cells start with intrinsic sensitivity to antineoplastic drugs, but develop spontaneous resistance at variable rates. This concept—**the Goldie–Coldman hypothesis**—was applied to the growth of malignant tumors and has important clinical implications (20). A fundamental assumption of this hypothesis is that mutations conferring resistance to chemotherapy occur in 10^3 to 10^6 cells, which are substantially below the level of clinical detection.

Goldie and Coldman (20) developed a mathematical model that relates curability to the initial appearance of singly or doubly resistant cells. Assuming a natural mutation rate, the model predicts a variation in size of the resistant fraction in tumors of the same size and type, depending on the mutation rate and the point at which the first mutation develops. Given these assumptions, **the proportion of resistant cells in any untreated tumor is likely to be small, and the initial response to treatment would not be influenced by the number of resistant cells.** In clinical practice, this means that a complete remission could be obtained even if resistant cells were present. The failure to cure such a patient, however, would be directly dependent on the presence of resistant cells.

This model of spontaneous drug resistance implies that (20):

1. Tumors are curable with chemotherapy if no permanently resistant cells are present and if chemotherapy begins before resistance develops.

2. If only one antineoplastic agent is used, then the probability of cure diminishes rapidly with the development of a single resistant line.

3. Minimizing the emergence of drug-resistant clones requires multiple effective drugs that are used as early as possible in the course of the patient's disease.

4. The rate of spontaneous mutation to resistance occurs at approximately the natural frequency of 1 in 10,000 to 1 in 1,000,000 cell divisions.

This model predicts that alternating cycles of treatment should be superior to the sequential use of particular agents, because sequential use of antineoplastic drugs would allow for the development and regrowth of a doubly resistant line. The intrinsic frequency of spontaneous mutation to drug resistance is likely to be influenced by the etiologic factors responsible for tumor development. Lung or bladder cancers, for instance, result from exposure to multiple carcinogenic chemicals and may have a higher spontaneous mutation rate than is seen in other tumors. Under these circumstances, numerous drug-resistant clones may be present before the tumors are clinically evident. This is an attractive theory that could explain the inability of antineoplastic therapy to cure a number of common malignancies (20), but it has not been confirmed in clinical trials using alternating noncross–resistant chemotherapeutic regimens to treat many solid tumors, including breast and ovarian cancer (21–23).

An alternative hypothesis, developed by Norton and Simon, focuses on the Gompertzian growth rates exhibited by malignant tumors (24,25). This mathematical model suggests that the efficacy of treatment for tumors exhibiting sensitivity to particular chemotherapeutic agents will be enhanced if single agents, or combination regimens, are delivered at their optimal dose levels in a so-called dose-dense manner, rather than as alternating regimens.

The fundamental difference between these two models is that in the **Goldie–Coldman model,** the individual drugs are given in sequence at their optimal levels to produce a cytotoxic effect, whereas in the **Norton–Simon model,** which focuses on the rapid administration of as many active agents as possible, dose levels of individual drugs will frequently need to be modified because of overlapping toxic effects (e.g., bone marrow suppression).

Randomized trials in breast cancer and ovarian cancer provided evidence in support of the Norton–Simon hypothesis (26,27). High-risk gestational trophoblastic tumors are very chemosensitive, and treatment with EMA-CO every 6 to 7 days is an example of a dose-dense regimen that is highly effective (see Chapter 15).

These models have been useful in progressing clinical trials, developing combination chemotherapeutic regimens, and the timing of adjuvant chemotherapy (28). The simplicity of the models is challenged by the biologic complexity of cancer, and the many nonkinetic reasons why chemotherapy may not work.

Drug Resistance

Resistance to chemotherapy continues to be a major problem in cancer treatment, and can be broadly classified into primary or acquired (15). Primary resistance is a common feature of a number of cancers, such as metastatic uterine leiomyosarcoma and clear cell ovarian cancer. Acquired resistance occurs after an initial response to chemotherapy.

The vast majority of patients with advanced solid tumors will eventually develop acquired resistance, and there are many potential explanations and mechanisms for this (2,11,12,15). Both primary and acquired resistance may be caused by alterations in drug metabolism, including changes in drug uptake, efflux, and detoxification. Enhanced efflux is caused by increased expression of P Glycoprotein and Multidrug Resistance associated Protein1 (MRP1). P Glyco-protein transports a number of hydrophobic agents, such as *doxorubicin, paclitaxel,* and vinca alkaloids, while MRP-1 transports topoisomerase inhibitors and anthracyclines (19).

Many other mechanisms of resistance to chemotherapy and targeted agents have been described, including modification of drug targets, dysregulation of apoptotic pathways, and enhanced DNA repair (15). Drug-resistant subpopulations may be present before starting chemotherapy, and may be selected out over time. These subpopulations may be made up of cancer stem cells, often quiescent and not cycling, which are intrinsically resistant to chemotherapy (12,13).

Dose Intensity, Dose-Dense, and High-Dose Chemotherapy

Studies in human solid tumors in vitro frequently demonstrate steep dose–response curves, suggesting the importance of administering the maximum tolerated dose, particularly in the first-line setting, or when the aim of treatment is cure or prolongation of survival (29).

Dose intensity (DI) is a measure of the amount of drug delivered per unit of time, generally expressed as $mg/m^2/wk$ (30).

Relative dose intensity (RDI) is the ratio of the delivered dose of a single drug (or of several drugs in a combination chemotherapeutic regimen) to the planned dose of the drug.

In very chemosensitive tumors, such as lymphoma and germ cell tumors, there is a steep dose–response curve. Relatively small increases in the dose of chemotherapy will have a substantial effect on the number of tumor cells killed.

Although retrospective data suggest that dose intensity may be important in ovarian cancer, several prospective randomized trials in epithelial ovarian cancer have failed to demonstrate an improved outcome either by increasing the dose of *cisplatin* or *carboplatin* per cycle or by extending the duration of treatment beyond six cycles in the first-line setting (31–33). Randomized studies of high-dose chemotherapy (with bone marrow or peripheral progenitor stem cell support) for advanced ovarian cancer also have failed to demonstrate superior survival compared to standard dose regimens (34,35).

Although evidence does not suggest that dose-intensive approaches improve outcome, there is a minimum dose below which response rates and survival will be compromised. In general, the goal should be to maintain dose intensity consistent with an acceptable toxicity in each patient. The severity of neutropenia can frequently be reduced through the administration of a bone marrow stimulatory agent (e.g., granulocyte colony stimulating factor [GCSF]). These drugs can be given prophylactically with certain chemotherapeutic regimens that commonly cause grade 3 or 4 myelosuppression and a high risk of febrile neutropenia.

Mathematical modeling of the growth of tumor cells supports the concept of dose intensification by increasing the frequency of chemotherapy administration: the so-called dose-dense chemotherapy. There is evidence that dose-dense chemotherapy with weekly *paclitaxel* is more effective than standard 3 weekly dosing in ovarian cancer. The Japanese GOG reported the results of a randomized trial comparing *carboplatin* and *paclitaxel* administered every 3 weeks at standard dose with the same dose of *carboplatin* (AUC = 6) every 3 weeks and *paclitaxel* given weekly (80 mg/M^2) in the experimental arm (27). There was a significantly longer progression-free and overall survival in the experimental arm. This study was repeated in the United States (GOG 252) and in the United Kingdom (ICON 8) to see whether the findings could be replicated in a Caucasian population. It is possible that the benefit may be due to pharmacogenomic variations in Japanese women. The results of these two studies are eagerly awaited.

Pharmacologic Factors Influencing Treatment

Pharmacologically, it is useful to describe effective chemotherapy as concentration over time of the active agent or its metabolite at the primary site of antitumor action. Although it is not possible to determine exact pericellular pharmacokinetics, substantial information on important pharmacokinetic factors is available (36).

$$\text{Drug effect} = \text{drug concentration} \times \text{duration of exposure (C} \times \text{T)}$$

Because direct measurements often are not possible, considerable focus is given to plasma concentration $\times$ time (C $\times$ T) analyses. Many factors influence this pharmacokinetic result, including route of administration and drug absorption, transportation, distribution, biotransformation, inactivation, excretion, and interactions with other drugs.

Route of Administration and Absorption

Traditionally, drugs have been given orally, intravenously, or intramuscularly. Over the past decade, considerable attention has been given to the regional administration of chemotherapeutic agents, particularly in ovarian cancer (37–41). The intraperitoneal approach is based on the finding that the peritoneal clearance of the agent is slower than its plasma clearance and, as a result, an increased concentration of the drug in the peritoneal cavity can be maintained, while plasma concentrations are low.

Studies of a wide variety of chemotherapeutic agents have demonstrated a differential concentration of 30- to 1,000-fold, depending on the molecular weight, charge, and lipid solubility of the drug. Clinical trials in ovarian cancer were performed with IP *cisplatin, carboplatin, and paclitaxel* combinations (37–41).

Several randomized trials have revealed that the intraperitoneal administration of *cisplatin* as primary therapy for small volume advanced ovarian cancer (largest tumor nodule within the peritoneal cavity ≤1 cm in maximal diameter) resulted in an improvement in progression-free survival, and an overall survival comparable to intravenous administration, but with increased toxicity (38–40). There is ongoing research with intraperitoneal therapy to develop less toxic regimens (41).

Drug Distribution

Antineoplastic agents usually produce their antitumor effect by interacting with intracellular target molecules. It is critically important that a drug or active metabolite reach the cancer cell in sufficient concentration to have a lethal effect. After absorption, drugs may be bound to serum albumin or other blood components. Their ability to penetrate various body compartments, vascular spaces, and extracellular sites is highly influenced by plasma protein binding, relative ionization at physiologic pH, molecular size, and lipid solubility (36).

Sanctuary Sites

Unique circumstances may produce sanctuary sites, which are areas where the tumor is inaccessible to anticancer drugs and the drug concentration over time is insufficient for cell kill. Examples of such sanctuary sites include the cerebrospinal fluid and areas of large tumor masses with central tumor necrosis and a low oxygen tension.

Cell Penetration

Some drugs enter the target cell by simple diffusion; in other instances, cellular penetration is an active process. As an example, many of the alkylating agents depend on a carrier transport system for cellular penetration. For large macromolecules, it may be necessary for pinocytosis to accomplish cellular entry.

Drug Metabolism

Many antineoplastic agents are active as intact molecules, while others require metabolism to an active form (42). Many of the antimetabolites require phosphorylation for cell entry. The alkylating agent *cyclophosphamide* requires absorption and liver metabolism to be activated. Attention to these unique metabolic requirements is needed for appropriate drug selection. For example, if direct installation of an alkylating agent is required, an agent that is active as an intact drug should be selected (e.g., *Thiotepa*), rather than *cyclophosphamide,* because the latter drug requires hepatic biotransformation. Initial activation is important, as is the rate of metabolic degradation of the active drug or metabolite in determining antitumor activity. As an example, one mechanism of drug resistance in ovarian cancer is increased metabolism of alkylating agents because of increased intracellular enzymes (e.g., glutathione-S-transferase) (42).

Excretion

Most chemotherapeutic agents are excreted through the kidney or liver. Overall, kidney or liver function is critical to normal drug excretion, so it is necessary to modify the dosage of certain agents if either of these organs is functionally impaired.

Certain drugs (e.g., *vincristine, doxorubicin, paclitaxel*) are excreted primarily through the liver, and others (e.g., *methotrexate*) are excreted almost entirely by the kidney. Extreme care should be

Table 3.4 Drug Interactions in Cancer Chemotherapy

Effect	Caused by	Interaction	Resulting in	Bioavailable Drug
↓ Renal function/excretion	nephrotoxic antibiotics	*methotrexate; cisplatin*	↓ Excretion	↑
↓ Hepatic metabolism/biliary excretion	*vincristine*	*doxorubicin*	↓ Excretion	↑
↓ Displacement from albumin or plasma proteins	sulfonamides; salicylates	*methotrexate; cisplatin*	↓ Binding	↑
↓ Intestinal absorption	*neomycin*	*methotrexate*	↓ Absorption	↓
↓ Direct chemical interaction	*mannitol*	*cisplatin*	↑ Excretion	↓
↓ Direct effect on metabolism	phenobarbitol *methotrexate* *5-fluorouracil*	cyclophosphamide *5-fluorouracil* *methotrexate*	↑ Metabolism ↑ Activation ↓ Metabolism	↑

taken with appropriate dose reduction in patients with impaired renal function. Most experimental protocols and cooperative group trials contain formulas for dose modification, or dose omission, for specific organ impairments (43).

Drug Interactions

There are multiple opportunities for clinically important drug interactions to occur during cancer treatment (44,45). These interactions may increase or decrease the antitumor activity of an agent, or they may increase or modify its toxicity. Types of drug interaction of potential importance include those listed in Table 3.4.

Important drug interactions with antineoplastic drugs include the following:

1. The alkylating agents are highly reactive compounds and may produce direct chemical or physical inactivation when multiple drugs are mixed.

2. Intestinal absorption of certain oral chemotherapeutic agents is altered by antibiotics that suppress bowel flora (e.g., reduced absorption of oral *methotrexate*), resulting in its decreased circulating level.

3. Drugs such as *cisplatin* or *methotrexate* bind to albumin or plasma proteins and may be displaced from that binding by drugs that bind to similar sites, such as *aspirin* or *sulfa*, thereby increasing the circulating level of bioavailable *cisplatin* or *methotrexate*.

4. Alterations in drug activation may occur, as when *methotrexate* increases *5-fluorouracil* activation; conversely, a drug interaction may antagonize an antitumor effect, as when *5-fluorouracil* impairs the antifolate action of *methotrexate*.

5. Nephrotoxic antibiotics frequently alter *methotrexate* excretion, and may also increase the renal toxicity of *cisplatin*.

Principles of Combination Chemotherapy

There is a solid theoretic basis for combination chemotherapy founded on cellular kinetics, drug metabolism, drug resistance, and tumor heterogeneity (46). Combination chemotherapy is the standard approach to the management of many adult solid tumors, including breast cancer and gynecologic malignancies, particularly when given as adjuvant or first-line therapy, where the aim is to achieve a high response rate and durable remission. There is no evidence that outcomes are improved with combination chemotherapy compared to single agents when the aim of treatment is palliation (e.g., platinum-resistant ovarian cancer or metastatic breast cancer).

Combination Chemotherapy

Combination chemotherapeutic regimens typically include active chemotherapeutic agents that act in different phases of the tumor cell cycle. General principles for the development of successful combinations are shown in Table 3.5. The use of multiple drugs is more likely to reduce

Table 3.5 Important Factors in the Design of Drug Combinations

1. The drugs used must be active as single agents against the particular tumor.

2. The drugs should have different mechanisms of action to minimize emergence of drug resistance.

3. The combination of drugs should have additive or preferably synergistic effects.

4. The drugs chosen should have a different spectrum of toxicity so that they can be used for maximum cell kill at (or near) full doses.

5. The drugs chosen should be administered intermittently so that cell kill is enhanced and prolonged myelosuppression is minimized.

the tumor volume than the use of a single chemotherapeutic agent, and should theoretically decrease the likelihood of developing drug resistance (46). For instance, if a cell cycle–nonspecific agent is administered, producing a 2-log cell kill in a tumor mass with 10^9 cells, and no further therapy is given, a minor tumor response will occur, followed by tumor regrowth, and there will be no impact on survival. If a cell cycle–specific agent produces a similar degree of cell kill, only those cells coming into cell cycle will be affected by the agent. The use of combinations of cell cycle–specific and cell cycle–nonspecific agents can enhance log kill in tumors. Combining drugs may achieve sufficient log kill to produce a cure or prolonged remission.

This does not necessarily mean that three or four drugs are better than two drugs in advanced cancers where cure is unlikely. This was illustrated by the GOG 182 study, which included more than 4,000 women with advanced ovarian cancer. The study demonstrated that *carboplatin* and *paclitaxel* had the same median progression-free and overall survival as triplet or alternating doublet combinations, which included agents such as *liposomal doxorubicin, gemcitabine,* or *topotecan* (47).

Although the probability of the emergence of drug-resistant cells in any given population is reduced if two or more agents with different mechanisms of action are used in a tightly sequenced treatment scheme, the majority of advanced cancers ultimately develop drug resistance (47).

Drug Interaction

Drug interactions may be additive, synergistic, or antagonistic. Combinations that result in higher response rates than those achieved with either drug alone are said to be synergistic. Additive therapies have response rates equivalent to the sum of both agents acting singly. Some antitumor agents may antagonize the effect of each other, producing a lesser therapeutic effect than when used singly (48). For example, *5-fluorouracil* prevents the antifolate action of *methotrexate* when used before *methotrexate* administration.

The principles allowing the development of successful combinations are shown in Table 3.5. Although these cannot be used in every regimen and overlapping toxicities are common, these concepts are the central feature of most of the regimens being used in cancer treatment.

Clinical Benefit

When a treatment regimen has been selected, it is necessary to have a standardized method to evaluate the response and to determine whether there has been a clinical benefit. The terms *complete* response, *partial* response, stable disease, and progressive disease are generally accepted.

Complete Response **is the complete disappearance of all objective evidence of tumor, and the resolution of all signs and symptoms referable to the tumor. Complete response is often associated with significant prolongation in progression-free survival, but is not synonymous with cure in patients with most advanced solid cancers.**

Partial Response **is defined as a 30% reduction in the sum of the diameters of all target measurable lesions. Partial responses may be associated with improved well-being, symptom benefit for the patient, and delayed progression time.**

RECIST Criteria

The Response Evaluation Criteria in Solid Tumors (RECIST) is used in all clinical trials. The criteria were modified in 2009, and RECIST1.1 is used in clinical trials (Table 3.6) (49).

Table 3.6 RECIST 1.1 Definitions of Response	
Complete response (CR)	Disappearance of all target lesions
Partial response (PR)	At least a 30% decrease in the sum of the longest diameter (LD) of target lesions, taking as reference the baseline sum LD
Progressive disease (PD)	At least a 20% increase in the sum of the LD of target lesions, taking as reference the smallest sum LD recorded since the treatment started or the appearance of one or more new lesions
Stable disease (SD)	Neither sufficient shrinkage to qualify for PR nor sufficient increase to qualify for PD, taking as reference the smallest sum LD since the treatment started

Baseline documentation of "target" and "nontarget" lesions before treatment in clinical trials is essential. All measurable lesions up to a maximum of two lesions per organ and five lesions in total, representative of all involved organs, should be identified as target lesions and recorded and measured at baseline. Target lesions should be selected on the basis of their size (lesions with the longest diameter [LD]) and their suitability for accurate repeated measurements by radiologic imaging with CT scans or MRI.

A sum of the LD for all target lesions should be calculated and reported as the baseline sum LD, and should be used as the reference to characterize the objective response. All other lesions (or sites of disease) should be identified as nontarget lesions and recorded at baseline. Measurements of these lesions are not required, but the presence or absence of each should be noted throughout follow-up.

Dose Adjustment

Patients vary in their tolerance to chemotherapy, and tailoring the treatment is necessary, particularly when treatment is administered with palliative intent. All clinical trial protocols stipulate dose modification and dose reductions based on toxicities, particularly grade 3 or 4 toxicities. It is beyond the scope of this chapter to detail the dose modifications, but all cancer centers have protocols and guidelines to ensure safe administration of treatment (43).

Carboplatin Dose Calculation

Carboplatin-based chemotherapy remains the mainstay of treatment for many patients with gynecologic malignancies, and it is important to have a good understanding of how *carboplatin* dose is calculated (50,51). It is cleared renally, and severe marrow toxicity may occur in some patients with impaired renal function; hence, the dose is based on renal function. Typically, the *carboplatin* dose is calculated using an estimated creatinine clearance or GFR, which is derived from formulas that use the patient's creatinine, age, and weight. The **Cockcroft–Gault equation** is most commonly used, but the **Jellife formula,** which does not use the patient's weight, is also used.

The Calvert formula is used to calculate the *carboplatin* dose, for example, total *carboplatin* dose (mg) = target AUC × (GFR + 25) (51). The target AUC is commonly 4 to 5 mg/mL for previously treated patients and 5 to 6 mg/mL for those previously untreated.

The switch to the isotope dilution mass spectrometry (IDMS) method to measure serum creatinine has resulted in creatinine values that are 10% to 20% lower than older non-IDMS values. In patients with a relatively low serum creatinine, the IDMS method will result in a lower creatinine and an overestimation of creatinine clearance, with a potentially higher calculated *carboplatin* dose. In view of this, **NCI/CTEP has recommended that the GFR used in the Calvert formula should not exceed 125 mL/min, and that the maximum *carboplatin* dose based on the AUC should be capped. For example, if the target AUC is 6, the dose should not exceed 900 mg; for AUC 5, it should not exceed 750 mg, and for AUC 4, it should not exceed 600 mg** (52).

The Cockcroft–Gault equation is unreliable in patients who are obese, cachectic, or have an abnormally low serum creatinine. Ideally these patients should have an EDTA clearance to more accurately measure GFR, but if this is not possible, guidelines are available from the GOG (53).

Drug Toxicity

Antineoplastic drugs have many potential side effects with predictable and at times unpredictable toxicities. In almost all instances, chemotherapeutic agents are used in doses that produce some degree of toxicity to normal tissues.

Severe debility, advanced age, poor nutritional status, or impaired organ function can result in severe side effects of chemotherapy. Idiosyncratic drug reactions can have severe and unexpected consequences. As a result, careful monitoring of patients receiving cancer chemotherapy is a major responsibility of the treating physician.

Hematologic Toxicity

The proliferating cells of the erythroid, myeloid, and megakaryocytic series of the bone marrow are highly susceptible to damage by many of the commonly used antineoplastic agents. Granulocytopenia and thrombocytopenia are predictable side effects of most of the commonly used antitumor agents, and are seen with all effective regimens of combination chemotherapy. The severity and duration of these side effects are variable, and depend on the drugs, the dose, the schedule, and the patient's previous exposure to radiation or chemotherapy.

In general, acute granulocytopenia occurs 6 to 12 days after administration of most myelosuppressive chemotherapeutic agents, and recovery occurs within 21 days; platelet suppression occurs 4 to 5 days later, with recovery after white cell count recovery. Several agents are unique in producing delayed bone marrow suppression, among them *mitomycin C* and the nitrosoureas. Marrow suppression from these drugs commonly occurs at 28 to 42 days, with recovery 40 to 60 days after treatment.

Granulocytopenia

Patients with an absolute granulocyte count of less than 500/mm^3 for 5 days or longer are at high risk of febrile neutropenia, which can be rapidly fatal. The widespread use of empiric, broad-spectrum antibiotics in febrile granulocytopenic patients with cancer significantly decreases the likelihood of life-threatening toxicity (54), and the importance of quickly initiating such antibiotics in the presence of fever in a granulocytopenic patient cannot be overemphasized.

Granulocytopenic patients should have their temperature checked every 4 hours, and must be examined frequently for evidence of infection. The availability of hematopoietic growth factors has enabled physicians to reduce the duration of granulocytopenia in certain patients. The use of granulocyte stimulating factor (GCSF) for high-risk patients with established febrile neutropenia is controversial. Trials and meta-analyses have suggested that therapeutic GCSF use is associated with a 1 day (statistically significant) reduction in length of stay and time to neutrophil recovery, but has no effect on mortality. **The most recent guidelines of the Infectious Diseases Society of America continue to recommend against therapeutic GCSF for all patients with febrile neutropenia, given the cost and adverse effects of the drugs** (54).

Before the initiation of antibiotics in a febrile granulocytopenic patient, cultures of possible sites of infection (e.g., blood, urine, sputum, recent surgical wound, indwelling intravenous delivery device) should be obtained. A detailed physical examination (including the throat, perianal region, and skin) should be performed, looking for a specific site of infection, which may influence the choice of antibiotic therapy (e.g., vancomycin in patients with central lines or indwelling venous access devices).

There are published guidelines for the selection of patients with febrile neutropenia for outpatient management. Selection should begin with a validated risk index (e.g., Multinational Association for Supportive Care in Cancer [MASCC] score). Patients with MASCC scores ≥21, and without other risk factors, may be considered for outpatient treatment. The guidelines advise that febrile neutropenic patients should receive initial doses of empirical antibacterial therapy within an hour of triage, and should either be monitored for at least 4 hours to determine suitability for outpatient management or be admitted to the hospital. An oral fluoroquinolone plus amoxicillin/clavulanate (or clindamycin if penicillin allergic) is recommended as empiric therapy, unless fluoroquinolone prophylaxis had been used before the fever developed (55).

Thrombocytopenia

Patients with sustained thrombocytopenia, who have platelet counts below 10,000/mm^3 are at risk of spontaneous hemorrhage, particularly gastrointestinal or intracranial, and platelet transfusions significantly reduce the risk. For patients who are critically ill with fever, sepsis, or coagulopathy, the platelet count should be maintained above 20×10^9/L. Patients with

platelet counts exceeding 50,000/mm³ do not usually experience severe bleeding. Transfusion at this level is only indicated if the patient is actively bleeding or about to undergo an urgent surgical procedure.

A post-transfusion platelet count performed 1 hour after platelet administration should show an appropriate incremental increase. If no platelet increase occurs, it is likely that there has been previous sensitization to random donor platelets, and the patient may require single-donor human leukocyte antigen-matched platelets for future transfusions.

Gastrointestinal Toxicity

Mucositis caused by a direct effect on the rapidly dividing epithelial mucosal cells is common, and concomitant granulocytopenia may allow the injured mucosa to become infected and serve as a portal of entry for bacteria and fungi into the bloodstream. Impaired cellular immunity because of underlying disease or corticosteroid therapy can contribute to extensive infection of the gastrointestinal tract (56). Other side effects related to the gastrointestinal tract include impaired intestinal motility, resulting from the autonomic neuropathic effect of vinca alkaloids (*vincristine* and *vinblastine*), and nausea and vomiting, induced by many anticancer drugs (57).

Upper Gastrointestinal

The onset of mucositis is frequently 3 to 5 days earlier than that of myelosuppression. Lesions of the mouth and pharynx are difficult to distinguish from candidiasis and herpes simplex infection. Esophagitis resulting from direct drug toxicity can be confused with radiation esophagitis or infections with bacteria, fungi, or herpes simplex because they all produce dysphagia and retrosternal burning pain. Mild oral candidiasis (thrush) responds to several oral agents. More intensive therapy will be required for esophageal or severe oral candidiasis or herpes simplex infections. Symptomatic management of painful upper gastrointestinal inflammation includes warm saline mouth rinses and topical anesthetics such as viscous lidocaine. Intravenous fluids may be indicated, and hyperalimentation may rarely be required (56).

Lower Gastrointestinal

Mucositis in the lower gastrointestinal tract is invariably associated with diarrhea. Serious complications include bowel perforation, hemorrhage, and necrotizing enterocolitis.

Necrotizing enterocolitis includes a spectrum of severe diarrheal illnesses that can be fatal in a granulocytopenic patient. Broad-spectrum antibiotic therapy may predispose the patient to necrotizing enterocolitis, as may cytotoxic chemotherapy, which can interfere with the integrity of the bowel wall. This condition is more common in patients receiving intensive chemotherapy (e.g., patients with leukemia), but it can also occur with treatment of gynecologic malignancies. The most commonly involved organism is *Pseudomonas aeruginosa*. Symptoms of necrotizing enterocolitis include watery or bloody diarrhea, abdominal pain, sore throat, nausea, vomiting, and fever. Physical examination usually reveals abdominal tenderness and distention. The performance of an abdominal or pelvic computed tomographic scan or ultrasound will be helpful in the evaluation of this constellation of signs and symptoms. Treatment includes the administration of broad-spectrum antibiotics with specific activity against aerobic gram-negative organisms and anaerobes. Nasogastric decompression, intravenous fluids, and bowel rest may be required. In the neutropenic patient, recovery of normal blood counts is essential for improvement of the condition. Surgical intervention is occasionally necessary.

Immunosuppression

Most anticancer drugs are capable of producing suppression of cellular and, to a lesser extent, humoral immunity. The magnitude and duration of the immunosuppression vary with the dose and schedule of drug administration, and are inadequately characterized for most chemotherapeutic agents. **Most of the acute immunosuppressive side effects do not persist after the completion of drug treatment.** Laboratory studies suggest a decrease in host defenses during treatment associated with a rebound to complete or nearly complete restoration 2 to 3 days after treatment is completed. This short-term immunosuppressive effect has led to increased use of intermittent chemotherapy regimens to allow immunologic recovery. Individuals with cancer who undergo certain cytotoxic or immunosuppressive therapies and have hepatitis B virus (HBV) infection or prior exposure to HBV may be at elevated risk of liver failure from HBV reactivation (58). HBV screening requires clinical judgment, but should be considered in patients who may be at potential risk. When evidence for chronic HBV infection is found, antiviral therapy before and throughout the course of chemotherapy may be considered to reduce the risk of HBV reactivation.

Dermatologic Reactions

Several important drug toxicities involve skin reactions. Skin necrosis and sloughing may result from extravasation of certain irritating chemotherapeutic agents, such as *doxorubicin, actinomycin D, mitomycin C, vinblastine, vincristine,* and *nitrogen mustard.* The extent of necrosis depends on the quantity of drug extravasated and can vary from local erythema to chronic ulcerative necrosis (59). All cancer centers have guidelines and protocols in place to deal with extravasation incidents, and the approach is dependent on the agent. Long-term monitoring of the affected area is required, and surgical debridement and full-thickness skin grafting may be necessary in selected patients.

Alopecia is a very common side effect of many chemotherapeutic agents and may have significant emotional consequences for patients. Agents commonly associated with severe hair loss include the anthracycline antibiotics, taxanes such as *paclitaxel or docetaxel,* and alkylating agents such as *cyclophosphamide.* Most commonly used drug combinations produce variable degrees of alopecia. Alopecia is reversible, and regrowth usually begins several weeks after treatment is completed. Attempts to minimize alopecia by using a variety of methods such a scalp cooling have been tried with varying degrees of success (60).

Generalized allergic skin reactions can occur with chemotherapeutic agents and can sometimes be severe. Other skin reactions occasionally seen with chemotherapeutic agents include increased skin pigmentation (*bleomycin*), photosensitivity reactions, transverse banding or nail loss, folliculitis (*actinomycin D, methotrexate*), and radiation recall reactions (*doxorubicin*).

Liposomal doxorubicin can produce a painful dermatologic syndrome characterized by desquamation of the skin, most often involving **the hands and feet** (61). Blistering, focal or disseminated, may be observed.

Hepatic Toxicity

Modest elevations in aminotransferase, alkaline phosphatase, and bilirubin levels are frequently seen with many anticancer agents, but they usually resolve quickly (62). More severe reactions may occur, and long-term administration of *methotrexate* can induce hepatic fibrosis that can progress to cirrhosis. The cirrhosis and drug-induced hepatitis should be managed by withdrawal of the toxic agent, with the same supportive measures that are used for hepatitis or cirrhosis of any cause. Pre-existing liver disease or exposure to other hepatotoxins may increase the risk.

Pulmonary Complications

Respiratory compromise resulting from lung metastases, pulmonary emboli, radiation pneumonitis, and pneumonia may be significant complications associated with an underlying malignancy, but direct pulmonary toxicity from commonly used anticancer drugs is sometimes seen (63).

Interstitial Pneumonitis

Interstitial pneumonitis with pulmonary fibrosis is the usual pattern of lung damage associated with cytotoxic drugs. Likely agents include *bleomycin,* alkylating agents, *gemcitabine,* and the nitrosoureas. The physical and chest radiologic findings are not easily distinguishable from those of interstitial pneumonitis resulting from infectious agents or lymphangitic spread of cancer.

Management of drug-induced interstitial pneumonitis includes discontinuation of the suspected agent and supportive care. Steroids may be of symptomatic benefit in some patients.

Cardiac Toxicity

Cardiac toxicity is seen with several important cancer chemotherapeutic agents. Although the myocardium consists of largely nondividing cells, drugs of the anthracycline antibiotic class—specifically, *doxorubicin* and *daunomycin*—can cause severe cardiomyopathy (64).

The risk of cardiac toxicity increases with the total cumulative dose of *doxorubicin*. For this reason, a cumulative dose of 450 to 500 mg/m^2 of ideal body surface area is now widely used as the maximum tolerable dose of *doxorubicin.* With careful and frequent monitoring of left ventricular function by means of ejection fraction studies, therapy can be continued to higher doses if no satisfactory alternative exists. Occasionally, anthracyclines and *paclitaxel* can cause acute arrhythmias that are not related to total drug dose. Anthracycline cardiac toxicity is potentiated by radiation.

The medical management of cardiomyopathy induced by anthracyclines is supportive but usually unsatisfactory. Use of radionuclide cardiac scintigraphy to allow early detection of cardiac compromise before the clinical manifestations of congestive heart failure appear is important. Discontinuation of the drug at the first indication of decreasing left ventricular function minimizes the risk of cardiovascular decompensation (64).

Rarely, *cyclophosphamide* produced cardiotoxicity, particularly in the massive doses used in conjunction with bone marrow transplantation. With conventional doses of *cyclophosphamide,* this complication is unlikely. *Busulfan* and *mitomycin C* may cause endocardial fibrosis and myocardial fibrosis, respectively. Rarely, *5-fluorouracil* may cause symptoms of angina pectoris due to coronary artery spasm.

Cardiac toxicity is an important side effect of *trastuzumab,* a targeted therapy (HER2 receptor) commonly used in the management of patients with HER2 positive breast cancer, especially when the agent is delivered with *doxorubicin* (65).

A common toxicity of the antiangiogenic agent *bevacizumab* is the development of hypertension (66). In a patient with pre-existing cardiac abnormalities, this has the potential to cause deterioration of heart function. This concern is likely to increase as use of this class of agent becomes more standard in the clinical management of gynecologic malignancies.

Genitourinary Toxicity

In patients with cancer, chronic azotemia or acute renal failure may be produced by fluid depletion, infection, tumor infiltration of the kidney, ureteric obstruction by tumor, radiation damage, and tumor lysis syndrome (67,68).

Drugs that cause kidney damage include the following:

1. *Cisplatin,* which produces renal tubular toxicity associated with azotemia and calcium and magnesium wasting (69)
2. *Methotrexate,* which can precipitate in the renal tubules, causing oliguric renal failure. *Methotrexate* toxicity can be prevented by maintenance of a high urine volume and alkalinization of the urine
3. *Nitrosoureas,* which cause a chronic interstitial nephritis with chronic renal failure
4. *Mitomycin C,* which causes a systemic microangiopathic hemolysis and acute renal failure

Metabolites of *cyclophosphamide* are irritants to the bladder mucosa and rarely cause a chronic hemorrhagic cystitis, particularly during high-dose or prolonged treatment. Vigorous hydration and diuresis can reduce the risk of this complication.

N-acetylcysteine or ***mesna*** (*sodium mercaptoethanesulfonate*) was used in conjunction with very high doses of *cyclophosphamide* or *ifosfamide* to prevent bladder toxicity by inactivating the toxic metabolite (*acrolein*). Persistent hemorrhagic cystitis that does not respond to conservative management may be treated with epsilon-aminocaproic acid.

Neurotoxicity

Many antineoplastic drugs are associated with some central or peripheral neurotoxicity. These neurologic side effects usually are mild, but occasionally may be severe (70,71).

Vinca Alkaloids

The vinca alkaloids (***vincristine, vinblastine,*** and ***vindesine***) are commonly associated with peripheral motor, sensory, and autonomic neuropathies, which are the major side effects of *vincristine.* Toxicity first appears as loss of deep tendon reflexes with distal paresthesiae. Cranial nerves can be affected, and the autonomic neuropathy can appear as adynamic ileus, urinary bladder atony with retention, or postural hypotension. All of these neurologic toxicities from the vinca alkaloids may be slowly reversible after cessation of the drug.

Cisplatin

Cisplatin produces ototoxicity, peripheral neuropathy, and, rarely, retrobulbar neuritis and blindness. High doses of *cisplatin* are particularly likely to produce a progressive and somewhat delayed peripheral neuropathy. This defect is characterized by sensory impairment and loss of proprioception, whereas motor strength usually is preserved. Progression of this neuropathy 1 to 2 months after cessation of high-dose *cisplatin* has been reported (72,73).

Paclitaxel

Paclitaxel is associated with the development of a peripheral sensory neuropathy. The incidence and severity of symptoms relate to the peak levels of the agent reached in the plasma (74). The combination of *paclitaxel* and *cisplatin* (or *carboplatin*) has the potential to be more neurotoxic than either agent used alone.

Other Drugs

Rarely, *5-fluorouracil* can be associated with an acute cerebellar toxicity, apparently related to its metabolism to fluorocitrate, a neurotoxic metabolite of the parent compound. *Hexamethylmelamine* has also been reported to produce peripheral neuropathy and encephalopathy (75).

Vascular and Hypersensitivity Reactions	Occasionally, severe hypersensitivity reactions in the form of anaphylaxis develop with chemotherapeutic agents (76). In rare cases, this has been associated with *cyclophosphamide, doxorubicin, cisplatin,* intravenous *melphalan,* and high-dose *methotrexate. Bleomycin* administration may be associated with marked fever reactions or anaphylaxis. The same reactions have been reported with *procarbazine, etoposide,* and *teniposide.*

Hypersensitivity reactions are sometimes seen with *paclitaxel,* and are believed to result from hypersensitivity to the *cremophor* vehicle. They can be ameliorated with the use of *dexamethasone, diphenhydramine,* and *cimetidine* before *paclitaxel* is administered.

Carboplatin and **cisplatin** may be associated with a significant risk of hypersensitivity reactions in patients who have been treated with more than six courses of a platinum agent (77).

Second Malignancies	**Many antineoplastic agents are mutagenic and teratogenic.** The potential for these agents to induce second malignancies appears to vary with the class of agent (78). Alkylating agents (especially *melphalan*), *procarbazine,* and the nitrosoureas seem to be the major offenders. Prolonged use of *etoposide* has been associated with the development of leukemia.

The cumulative 7-year risk of acute nonlymphocytic leukemia developing in patients treated primarily with oral *melphalan* for ovarian cancer has been reported to be as high as 9.6% in patients receiving therapy for more than 1 year (79). Although *cisplatin* has been associated with the development of acute leukemia, the risk is lower than with the alkylating agents (80).

Evidence from long-term studies of Hodgkin disease suggests a major risk with combined chemotherapy and radiation therapy (81,82). In such patients, there is a risk of acute leukemia and an increasd incidence of solid tumors, seen particularly within the radiation fields. The long-term follow-up of women cured of choriocarcinoma, primarily with antimetabolite therapy, has revealed no increased risk of a second malignancy.

Radiation alone appears to produce a relatively low risk of late leukemia, as do chemotherapeutic regimens alone, particularly those without alkylating agents or *procarbazine.* Combination chemotherapy (including *cisplatin*-based treatment of ovarian cancer) and limited-field radiation therapy only slightly increase the risk.

Patients at increased risk include those who have received the following:

1. Extensive radiation therapy plus combination chemotherapy
2. Prolonged alkylating agent therapy (longer than 1 year)
3. High doses of certain drugs such as *etoposide*

Gonadal Dysfunction	**Many cancer chemotherapeutic agents have profound and lasting effects on testicular and ovarian function.** Chemotherapeutic agents, particularly alkylating agents, can cause azoospermia and amenorrhea. Secondary sexual characteristics related to hormonal function are usually less disturbed. Prolonged intensive combination chemotherapy commonly produces azoospermia in men, and recovery is uncommon.

The onset of amenorrhea and ovarian failure is accompanied by an elevation of the serum follicle-stimulating hormone (FSH) and luteinizing hormone (LH) levels, and a decrease in the serum estradiol level.

When short-term intensive chemotherapy is used, particularly with antimetabolites, vinca alkaloids, or antitumor antibiotics, injury to the reproductive system is less common. For example, men treated for testicular cancer, children with acute leukemia, and women cured of gestational tropho-blastic disease or ovarian germ cell malignancies usually recover reproductive capacity after therapy (83–86).

Chemotherapy in Pregnancy

The risk of congenital abnormalities from chemotherapeutic agents is highest during the first trimester, especially when antimetabolites (e.g., *cytosine arabinoside* or *methotrexate*) and alkylating agents are used (87). Chemotherapy administered during the second or third trimesters usually is not associated with an increased risk of fetal abnormalities, although the number of patients studied is relatively small (see Chapter 17).

Antineoplastic Drugs

Alkylating Agents

This class of antineoplastic agent acts primarily by chemically interacting with DNA. These drugs form extremely unstable alkyl groups that react with nucleophilic (electron-rich) sites on many important organic compounds such as nucleic acids, proteins, and amino acids. These interactions produce the primary cytotoxic effects.

Mechanism

Alkylating agents commonly bind to the N-7 position of guanine and to other key DNA sites. In doing so, they interfere with accurate base pairing, crosslink DNA, and produce single- and double-stranded breaks. This results in the inhibition of DNA, RNA, and protein synthesis.

Because some effects of alkylating agents are similar to those of irradiation, these drugs are often called **radiomimetic**. Most of the effective alkylating agents are bifunctional or polyfunctional, and have two or more potentially unstable alkyl groups per molecule. These bifunctional alkylating agents allow cross-linkage of DNA that results in cellular disruption.

Because all alkylating agents have similar mechanisms of action, there tends to be cross-resistance to other agents of the same class.

Drugs

There are many alkylating agents; those most commonly used include *cyclophosphamide, melphalan, chlorambucil,* and *ifosfamide.* In addition to the more common alkylating agents, several antineoplastic agents of different types are usually classified as alkylating-like agents and include the nitrosoureas, *DTIC (dacarbazine),* and the platinum analogs *cisplatin* and *carboplatin.*

Cisplatin and *carboplatin* are considered to be cell cycle–nonspecific bifunctional alkylating agents. As opposed to classical alkylating agents, they bind to DNA to cause intrastrand cross-links and adducts that change the conformation of DNA and affect DNA replication. Although they are considered to be cell cycle–nonspecific, they are believed to cause G_2 cell cycle arrest and apoptotic cell death.

The characteristics of the commonly used alkylating agents are listed in Table 3.7, and the alkylating-like agents are listed in Table 3.8.

Antitumor Antibiotics

The antitumor antibiotics are antineoplastic drugs that were isolated as natural products from fungi found in the soil. These natural products usually have extremely complex and different chemical structures, although they function by forming complexes with DNA.

Mechanism

The interaction between these drugs and DNA often involves intercalation, that is, the compound is inserted between DNA base pairs. A second mechanism thought to be important in their antitumor action is the formation of free radicals capable of damaging DNA, RNA, and vital proteins. Other effects include metal ion chelation and alteration of tumor cell membranes. This class of antineoplastic agents is thought to be *cell cycle–nonspecific.*

Drugs

Major drugs in this family include actinomycin D, bleomycin, mitomycin C, and the anthracycline antibiotics doxorubicin and liposomal doxorubicin.

Table 3.7 Alkylating Agents Used for Gynecologic Cancer

Drug	Route of Administration	Common Toxicities	Diseases Treated
Cyclophosphamide (Cytoxan)	PO, IV	Myelosuppression, cystitis ± bladder fibrosis, alopecia, hepatitis, amenorrhea, azoospermia	Breast, ovarian cancer, soft tissue sarcomas
Chlorambucil (Leukeran)	PO	Myelosuppression, nausea, dermatitis, hepatotoxicity	Ovarian cancer
Melphalan (Alkeran, L-PAM)	PO	Myelosuppression, nausea and vomiting (rare), second malignancies	Ovarian, breast cancer
Triethylenethiophosphoramide	IV	Myelosuppression, nausea and vomiting, headaches, fever (rare)	Ovarian, breast cancer
Ifosphamide (Ifex)	IV	Myelosuppression, bladder toxicity, central nervous system dysfunction, renal toxicity	Cervical, ovarian cancer

Anthracyclines

Anthracyclines are antibiotics isolated from the fungi *Streptomyces*. These pigmented compounds have an anthraquinone nucleus attached to an amino sugar and have multiple mechanisms of action. Because of the planar structure of the anthraquinone moiety, these agents act as intercalators in the DNA double helix. They chelate divalent cations and are avid calcium binders. They cause single-stranded DNA breaks, inhibit DNA repair, and actively generate free radicals that are capable of producing DNA damage. Anthracyclines are capable of reacting directly with cell membranes, disrupting membrane structure, and altering membrane function.

Bleomycin

Bleomycin was **isolated from the *Streptomyces* fungus.** Its structure contains a DNA-binding fragment and an ion-binding unit. It appears to produce its antitumor action by producing single- and double-stranded breaks in DNA, mainly at sites of guanine bases. The drug is primarily excreted in the urine, and increased toxicity may be seen in patients with impaired renal function.

Mitomycin C

Mitomycin C is another antibiotic that was **isolated from the *Streptomyces* fungus.** It is activated *in vivo* into an alkylating agent that can bind DNA, producing crosslinks and inhibiting DNA synthesis. It has a quinone moiety that can generate free radical reactions similar to those seen with

Table 3.8 Alkylating-like Agents Used for Gynecologic Cancer

Drug	Route of Administration	Common Toxicities	Diseases Treated
Cisplatin	IV	Nephrotoxicity, tinnitus and hearing loss, nausea and vomiting, myelosuppression, peripheral neuropathy	Ovarian and germ cell carcinomas, cervical, endometrial cancer
Carboplatin	IV	Less neuropathy, ototoxicity, and nephrotoxicity than cisplatin; more hematopoietic toxicity, especially thrombocytopenia, than cisplatin	Ovarian carcinomas, endometrial and cervical cancer
Dacarbazine (DTIC)	IV	Myelosuppression, nausea and vomiting, flu-like syndrome, hepatotoxicity	Uterine sarcomas, soft tissue sarcomas

Drug	Route of Administration	Common Toxicities	Diseases Treated
Actinomycin D (dactinomycin, Cosmegen)	IV	Nausea and vomiting, skin necrosis, mucosal ulceration, myelosuppression	Germ cell ovarian tumors, choriocarcinoma, soft tissue sarcoma
Bleomycin (Blenoxane)	IV, IM	Fever, dermatologic reactions, pulmonary toxicity, anaphylactic reactions	Germ cell ovarian tumors
Doxorubicin (Adriamycin)	IV	Myelosuppression, alopecia, cardiotoxicity, local vesicant, nausea and vomiting, mucosal ulcerations	Ovarian, breast, endometrial cancer
Liposomal doxorubicin (Doxil, Caelyx)	IV	Palmar–plantar erythrodysesthesia, myelosuppression, stomatitis	Ovarian and endometrial cancers

Table 3.9 Antitumor Antibiotics Used for Gynecologic Cancer

IV, intravenous; IM, intramuscular.

the anthracycline antibiotics. It is administered intravenously and is degraded primarily by metabolism. Renal clearance is not a major mechanism of excretion.

Some of the important characteristics of the antitumor antibiotics are listed in Table 3.9.

Antimetabolites

The antimetabolite agents interact with vital intracellular enzymes, leading to their inactivation, or to the production of fraudulent products incapable of normal intracellular function. Their structures resemble analogs of normal purines and pyrimidines, or they resemble normal substances that are vital for cellular function. Some antimetabolites are active as intact drugs, and others require biotransformation to active agents.

Mechanism

Although many of these agents act at different sites in biosynthetic pathways, they appear to exert their antitumor activity by disrupting functions crucial to the viability of the cell. These effects are usually more disruptive to actively proliferating cells; thus, the antimetabolites are classed in general as **cell cycle–specific** agents.

Drugs

Although hundreds of antimetabolites have been investigated, only a few are commonly used. They include the following:

1. The folate antagonist *methotrexate*, which inhibits the enzyme dihydrofolate reductase
2. The purine antagonists *6-mercaptopurine* and *6-thioguanine*
3. The pyrimidine antagonists *5-fluorouracil (5-FU)* and *cytosine arabinoside*
4. The ribonucleotide reductase inhibitor *hydroxyurea*
5. The nucleoside analog *gemcitabine*

In most instances, the antimetabolites are used in combinations because of their cell cycle specificity and their capacity for complementary inhibition. Antimetabolites commonly used in the treatment of gynecologic malignancies are summarized in Table 3.10.

Plant Alkaloids

The most commonly used plant alkaloids are the vinca alkaloids, natural products derived from the common periwinkle plant (*Vinca rosea*), although the *epipodophyllotoxins* and *paclitaxel* are used frequently in gynecologic malignancies (Table 3.11). Like most natural products, these compounds are large and complex molecules, but *vincristine* and *vinblastine* differ only by a single methyl group on one side chain.

Table 3.10 Antimetabolites Used for Gynecologic Cancer

Drug	Route of Administration	Common Toxicities	Diseases Treated
5-Fluorouracil (fluorouracil, 5-FU)	IV	Myelosuppression, nausea and vomiting, anorexia, alopecia	Breast, cervical cancer
Methotrexate (MTX, amethopterin)	PO, IV, IT	Mucosal ulceration, myelosuppression, hepatotoxicity, allergic pneumonitis; with intrathecal: meningeal irritation	Choriocarcinoma, breast cancer
Gemcitabine (Gemzar)	IV	Myelosuppression, fever	Ovarian, breast cancer, leiomyosarcoma

IV, intravenous; PO, oral; IT, intrathecal.

Vincristine and *vinblastine* act primarily by binding to vital intracellular microtubular proteins, particularly tubulin. Tubulin binding produces inhibition of microtubular assembly, destruction of the mitotic spindle, and arrest in mitosis. This class of antineoplastic agent is believed to be cell cycle–specific. At high concentrations, these drugs have effects on nucleic acid and protein synthesis.

Paclitaxel has a unique mechanism of action. It binds preferentially to microtubules and results in their polymerization and stabilization. *Paclitaxel*-treated cells contain large numbers of microtubules, free and in bundles that result in disruption of microtubular function and, ultimately, cell death. Renal clearance is only 5%.

Vinblastine has been used primarily in the treatment of ovarian germ cell tumors, but is now rarely used to treat any gynecologic cancer. Its primary toxicity is myelosuppression. In contrast, *vincristine* causes little myelosuppression. Its primary dose-limiting toxicity is peripheral neuropathy. *Vincristine* was used in the treatment of cervical carcinoma, but is rarely used today.

A second family of plant alkaloids has been documented to have significant antitumor properties. Members of this family, known as the *epipodophyllotoxins*, are extracts from the mandrake plant. Although the primary plant extracts have tubulin-binding properties similar to those of the vinca alkaloids, the active derivative, *etoposide*, does not seem to function either by inhibiting mitotic

Table 3.11 Plant Alkaloids

Drug	Route of Administration	Common Toxicities	Diseases Treated
Vincristine (Oncovin)	IV	Neurotoxicity, myelosuppression, cranial nerve palsies, gastrointestinal	Ovarian germ cell, sarcomas, cervical cancer
Vinblastine (Velban)	IV	Myelosuppression, alopecia, nausea and vomiting, neurotoxicity	Ovarian germ cell
Epipodophyllotoxin (etoposide, VP-16)	IV/PO	Myelosuppression, alopecia	Ovarian germ cell, choriocarcinoma Ovarian cancer
Paclitaxel (Taxol)	IV	Myelosuppression, alopecia, allergic reactions, cardiac arrhythmias	Ovarian, breast cancer
Vinorelbine (Navelbine)	IV	Myelosuppression, constipation, peripheral neuropathy	Ovarian, breast cancer
Docetaxel (Taxotere)	IV	Myelosuppression, alopecia, hypersensitivity reactions, peripheral edema	Breast, ovarian cancer

IV, intravenous; PO, oral.

Table 3.12 Topoisomerase 1 Inhibitors			
Drug	Route of Administration	Common Toxicity	Disease Treated
Topetecan (Hycamtin)	IV	Myelosuppression	Ovarian cancer
Irinotecan (Camptosar)	IV	Myelosuppression, diarrhea	Cervical, ovarian cancer

spindle formation or by tubulin binding. Rather, the drug appears to function by causing single-stranded DNA breaks. Unlike many of the other compounds that act primarily by DNA interactions, the agent appears to be cell cycle specific and schedule dependent. The dose-limiting toxicity is myelosuppression. Other toxicities include an infusion rate-limited hypotension, nausea, vomiting, anorexia, and alopecia. *Etoposide* is used to treat ovarian germ cell tumor and choriocarcinomas.

Paclitaxel is a complex agent in the class of drugs known as *taxanes*. Its major toxicity includes bone marrow suppression, alopecia, myalgias, arthralgias, and hypersensitivity reactions (87). The most common dose-limiting toxicity is granulocytopenia, although with certain schedules, the limiting toxicity is peripheral sensory neuropathy. The drug is active in cancers of the ovary, endometrium, cervix, and breast.

A second taxane, *docetaxel,* is active in cancers of the ovary, endometrium, and breast (87). The dose-limiting toxicity of *docetaxel* is bone marrow suppression, principally neutropenia. Hypersensitivity reactions are occasionally observed.

Topoisomerase 1 and 2 Inhibitors

Topoisomerase 1 and 2 inhibitors include *irinotecan* and *topotecan* (Table 3.12). Before replication, topoisomerases introduce temporary breaks in the DNA strands to allow the DNA to unwind. Inhibition of topoisomerases stabilizes the topoisomerase–DNA complex and causes the arrest of DNA replication forks and double-stranded DNA breaks.

Topotecan, the first topoisomerase 1 inhibitor approved for clinical use in the United States, is active in platinum-refractory ovarian cancer and cervical cancer. Its major toxicity is bone marrow suppression. The drug was developed for administration on a 5-day schedule, but is frequently given weekly for convenience.

Irinotecan, a second topoisomerase 1 inhibitor, has demonstrated activity in ovarian and cervical cancers, but is rarely used (88). Its major side effects are bone marrow suppression and diarrhea.

Targeted Therapies

There is increasing use of targeted therapies in gynecologic oncology, and they will play an increasingly important role in the future. Some of the targets and the targeted therapies are briefly reviewed below (Table 3.13).

Angiogenesis

The formation of new blood vessels from the pre-existing vasculature, is a critical component of cancer growth and metastasis (89). The vascular endothelium growth factor (VEGF) family

Table 3.13 Anti-angiogenesis Agents			
Drug	Route of Administration	Common Toxicities	Disease Treated
Bevacizumab (Avastin)	IV	Hypertension, proteinuria, bowel perforation	Breast, ovarian, and cervical cancer
VEGF Trap (Afilbercept)	IV	Hypertension, proteinuria, fatigue	Colon cancer

and its receptors (VEGFR) are among the major pathways involved in tumor angiogenesis. The VEGF family consists of seven structurally related glycoproteins—VEGF-A, VEGF-B, VEGF-C, VEGF-D, VEGF-E, and placental growth factors 1 and 2 (90). The major mediator of tumor angiogenesis is VEGF-A, which is upregulated in tumors by a variety of environmental factors including hypoxia-inducible transcription factors, low pH, inflammatory cytokines, and a variety of growth factors. The VEGF ligands bind to three structurally similar receptors—VEGFR1, VEGRF2, and VEGFR3. VEGF-A binds with the receptors VEGFR1 and VEGFR2, which are found mainly on vascular endothelial cells. After ligand binding to the VEGFRs, each tyrosine kinase activates the intracellular signaling cascade, including the mitogen-activated protein kinase (MAPK) and phosphatidylinositol 3, 4, 5-kinase (PI3 K)/Akt pathways. Subsequently, proangiogenic effects, such as stimulation of endothelial progenitor cell mobilization from the bone marrow, promotion of endothelial cell proliferation, migration, survival, and differentiation are activated (90).

VEGF increases vascular permeability and vasodilation, and is thought to play an important role in the formation of ascites. Overexpression of VEGF is observed in many solid tumors, including ovarian cancer, and is associated with an increased risk of metastatic disease and a poor prognosis. The VEGF signaling pathways are promising targets to treat ovarian and other gynecologic cancers (90,91).

Bevacizumab (Avastin)

This is a recombinant, humanized monoclonal IgG1 antibody that targets VEGF-A, and binds to and neutralizes biologically active forms of VEGF-A. This results in suppression of tumor growth, and appears to inhibit metastatic pathways. Bevacizumab improves the structure and function of tumor vessels, leading to decreased interstitial fluid pressure, increased tumor oxygenation, and improved penetration of drugs, potentially making tumors more sensitive to chemotherapy. Bevacizumab is administered intravenously every 3 weeks, either in conjunction with chemotherapy or alone as a maintenance therapy. There are many potential side effects of bevacizumab, including hypertension, thromboembolism, bleeding, impaired wound healing, proteinuria, and an increased risk of bowel perforation (91,92).

VEGF Trap (Aflibercept)

This is a fusion protein that combines the Fc region of IgG1 with domain two of VEGFR1 and domain three of VEGFR2. It acts as a decoy receptor, binding with high affinity to the VEGF-A ligand and thus preventing VEGFR1 and VEGFR2 binding and subsequent stimulation. It has strong binding affinity for PIGF. It is being investigated in clinical trials in ovarian cancer. It has similar side effects to bevacizumab (93).

Tyrosine Kinase Inhibitors (pazopanib, cediranib, sunitinib)	Tyrosine kinase inhibitors are potent small-molecule inhibitors of several tyrosine kinases, including VEGFR-1, VEGFR-2, VEGFR-3, c-kit and PDGF, and are being actively investigated in ovarian cancers (94).
Targeting DNA Repair—Polyadenosine Diphosphate-Ribose Polymerase Inhibitors	An increased understanding of DNA repair pathways led to the development of drugs designed specifically to target DNA repair. Targeting the base excision repair pathway with polyadenosine diphosphate-ribose polymerase (PARP) inhibitors is very promising in ovarian cancer, particularly in patients with the *BRCA*-associated subtype (95). Synthetic lethality describes a process by which defects in two different genes or pathways together result in cell death, but independently do not affect cell viability. The concept of synthetic lethality explains the selective and targeted effect of PARP inhibitors in cells with dysfunction in the Homologous Repair (HR) pathway.

Loss of function of BRCA1 or BRCA2 results in exquisite sensitivity to inhibition of PARP1, resulting from accumulation of unrepaired single-strand DNA breaks in proliferating cells. This leads to the collapse of replication forks, and consequently to double-strand breaks (DSBs). These DSBs are not repaired in BRCA1 or BRCA2 tumor cells, which are deficient in Homologous Repair, and this causes genetic instability and cell death.

The synthetic lethal interactions between PARP1 inhibitors and homozygous BRCA1 or BRCA2 tumors have been confirmed *in vitro,* and in phase I and II clinical trials in women with recurrent ovarian cancer (96,97). **PARP inhibitors are likely to play an increasingly important role in** |

the management of ovarian cancer patients with BRCA mutations, and at least 50% of sporadic high-grade serous cancers have dysfunction of the HR DNA repair pathway, and also may be sensitive to PARP1 inhibition (98).

References

1. **Mitchison T.** The proliferation rate paradox in antimitotic chemotherapy. *Mol Biol Cell.* 2012;23:1–6.

2. **Crawford S.** Is it time for a new paradigm for systemic cancer treatment? Lessons from a century of cancer chemotherapy. *Front Pharmacol.* 2013;4:68.

3. **Norton L.** Kinetic concepts in the systemic drug therapy of breast cancer. *Semin Oncol.* 1999;26(suppl 2):11–20.

4. **Talmadge JE.** Clonal selection of metastasis within the life history of a tumor. *Cancer Res.* 2007;67:11471–11475.

5. **Norton L.** Theoretical concepts and the emerging role of taxanes in adjuvant therapy. *Oncologist.* 2001;6(suppl 3):30–35.

6. **Kastan MB, Bartek J.** Cell cycle checkpoints and cancer. *Nature.* 2004;432:316–323.

7. **Aarts M, Linardopoulos S, Turner NC.** Tumour selective targeting of cell cycle kinases for cancer treatment. *Curr Opin Pharmacol.* 2013;13:529–535.

8. **Alberts B, Johnson A, Lewis J, et al.** An overview of the cell cycle. In: *Molecular Biology of the Cell.* 4th ed. New York, NY: Garland Science; 2002.

9. **Jordan C, Guzman ML, Noble M.** Cancer stem cells. *NEJM.* 2006; 355(12):1253–1261.

10. **Andreeff M, Goodrich DW, Pardee AB.** Cell proliferation, differentiation, and apoptosis. In: **Bast RC Jr, Kufe DW, Pollock RE, et al. eds.** *Holland-Frei Cancer Medicine.* 5th ed. Hamilton, ON: BC Decker; 2000. Chapter 2.

11. **Steg AD, Bevis KS, Katre AA, et al.** Stem cell pathways contribute to clinical chemoresistance in ovarian cancer. *Clin Cancer Res.* 2012; 18(3):869–881.

12. **Latifi A, Luwor RB, Bilandzic M, et al.** Isolation and characterization of tumor cells from the ascites of ovarian cancer patients: Molecular phenotype of chemoresistant ovarian tumors. *PLoS One.* 2012;7(10):e46858.

13. **Kwon MJ, Shin YK.** Regulation of ovarian cancer stem cells or tumor-initiating cells. *Int J Mol Sci.* 2013;14(4):6624–6648.

14. **Skipper HE, Schabel FM Jr, Mullett LB.** Implications of biochemical, cytokinetic, pharmacologic, and toxicologic relationships in the design of optimal therapeutic schedules. *Cancer Chemother Rep.* 1950;54:431–450.

15. **Zahreddine H, Borden K.** Mechanisms and insights into drug resistance in cancer. *Front Pharmacol.* 2013;4:28.

16. **Savage P, Stebbing J, Bower M, et al.** Why does cytotoxic chemotherapy cure only some cancers? *Nat Clin Pract Oncol.* 2009; 6(1):43–52.

17. **Houldsworth J, Xiao H, Murty VV, et al.** Human male germ cell tumor resistance to cisplatin is linked to TP53 gene mutation. *Oncogene.* 1998;16(18):2345–2349.

18. **Ali AY, Farrand L, Kim JY, et al.** Molecular determinants of ovarian cancer chemoresistance: New insights into an old conundrum. *Ann N Y Acad Sci.* 2012;1271:58–67.

19. **Ling V.** Drug resistance and membrane alteration in mutants of mammalian cells. *Can J Genet Cytol.* 1975;17:503–515.

20. **Goldie JH, Coldman AJ.** A mathematical model for relating the drug sensitivity of tumors to their spontaneous mutation rate. *Cancer Treat Rep.* 1979;63:1727–1733.

21. **De Placido S, Perrone F, Carlomagno C, et al.** CMF vs alternating CMF/EV in the adjuvant treatment of operable breast cancer. A single centre randomised clinical trial (Naples GUN-3 study). *Br J Cancer.* 1995;71(6):1283–1287.

22. **Boccardo F, Rubagotti A, Amoroso D, et al.** Lack of effectiveness of adjuvant alternating chemotherapy in node-positive, estrogen-receptor-negative premenopausal breast cancer patients: Results of a multicentric Italian study. The Breast Cancer Adjuvant Chemo-Hormone Therapy Cooperative Group (GROCTA). *Cancer Invest.* 1997;15(6): 505–512.

23. **Lund B, Hansen M, Hansen HH, et al.** A randomized study of sequential versus alternating combination chemotherapy in advanced ovarian carcinoma. *Ann Oncol.* 1990;1(2):134–140.

24. **Norton L, Simon R.** Predicting the course of Gompertzian growth. *Nature.* 1976;264:542–544.

25. **Norton L, Simon R.** The Norton–Simon hypothesis revisited. *Cancer Treat Rep.* 1986;70:163–169.

26. **Lemos Duarte I, da Silveira Nogueira Lima JP, Passos Lima CS, et al.** Dose-dense chemotherapy versus conventional chemotherapy for early breast cancer: A systematic review with meta-analysis. *Breast.* 2012;21(3):343–349.

27. **Katsumata N, Yasuda M, Takahashi F, et al.** Dose-dense paclitaxel once a week in combination with carboplatin every 3 weeks for advanced ovarian cancer: A phase 3, open-label, randomized controlled trial. *Lancet.* 2009;374(9698):1331–1338.

28. **Comen E, Morris PG, Norton L.** Translating mathematical modelling of tumor growth patterns into novel therapeutic approaches for breast cancer. *J Mammary Gland Biol Neoplasia.* 2012;17(3–4): 241–249.

29. **Skipper HE.** Criteria associated with destruction of leukemia and solid tumor cells in animals. *Cancer Res.* 1967;27:2636–2645.

30. **Hryniuk W, Levine MN.** Analysis of dose intensity for adjuvant chemotherapy trials in stage II breast cancer. *J Clin Oncol.* 1986;4: 1162–1170.

31. **Hakes TB, Chalas E, Hoskins WJ, et al.** Randomized prospective trial of 5 versus 10 cycles of cyclophosphamide, doxorubicin, and cisplatin in advanced ovarian carcinoma. *Gynecol Oncol.* 1992;45: 284–289.

32. **McGuire WP, Hoskins WJ, Brady MS, et al.** Assessment of dose-intensive therapy in suboptimally debulked ovarian cancer: A Gynecologic Oncology Group study. *J Clin Oncol.* 1995;13:1589–1599.

33. **Gore M, Mainwaring P, A'Hern R, et al.** Randomized trial of dose-intensity with single-agent carboplatin in patients with epithelial ovarian cancer. *J Clin Oncol.* 1998;16:2426–2434.

34. **Mobus V, Wandt H, Frickhofen N, et al.** Phase III trial of high-dose sequential chemotherapy with peripheral blood stem cell support compared with standard dose chemotherapy for first-line treatment of advanced ovarian cancer: Intergroup trial of the AGO-Ovar-AIO and EBMT. *J Clin Oncol.* 2007;25:4187–4193.

35. **Grenman S, Wiklund T, Jalkanen J, et al.** A randomized phase III study comparing high-dose chemotherapy to conventionally dosed chemotherapy for stage III ovarian cancer: The Finnish Ovarian Cancer (FINOVA) study. *Eur J Cancer.* 2006;42:2196–2199.

36. *Drug Absorption, Distribution and Elimination; Pharmacokinetics.* Columbia University. Available online at: http://www.columbia.edu/itc/gsas/g9600/2004/GrazianoReadings/Drugabs.pdf

37. **Markman M.** Intraperitoneal antineoplastic drug delivery: Rationale and results. *Lancet Oncol.* 2003;4:277–283.

38. **Alberts DS, Liu PY, Hannigan EV, et al.** Intraperitoneal cisplatin plus intravenous cyclophosphamide versus intravenous cisplatin plus intravenous cyclophosphamide for stage III ovarian cancer. *N Engl J Med.* 1996;335:1950–1955.

39. **Markman M, Bundy BN, Alberts DS, et al.** Phase III trial of standard-dose intravenous cisplatin plus paclitaxel versus moderately high-dose carboplatin followed by intravenous paclitaxel and intraperitoneal cisplatin in small-volume stage III ovarian carcinoma: An intergroup study of the Gynecologic Oncology Group, Southwestern Oncology Group, and Eastern Cooperative Oncology Group. *J Clin Oncol.* 2001;19:1001–1007.

40. **Armstrong DK, Bundy B, Wenzel L, et al.** Intraperitoneal cisplatin and paclitaxel in ovarian cancer. *N Engl J Med.* 2006;354:34–43.

41. **Markman M, Walker JL.** Intraperitoneal chemotherapy of ovarian cancer: A review, with a focus on practical aspects of treatment. *J Clin Oncol.* 2006;24:988–994.

42. **Riddick DS, Lee C, Ramji S, et al.** Cancer chemotherapy and drug metabolism. *Drug Metab Dispos.* 2005;33(8):1083–1096.

43. **Canal P, Chatelut E, Guichard S.** Practical treatment guide for dose individualisation in cancer chemotherapy. *Drugs.* 1998;56(6):1019–1038.

44. **Beijnen JH, Schellens JH.** Drug interactions in oncology. *Lancet Oncol.* 2004;5(8):489–496.

45. **Blower P, de Wit R, Goodin S, et al.** Drug-drug interactions in oncology: Why are they important and can they be minimized? *Crit Rev Oncol Hematol.* 2005;55(2):117–142.

46. **Frei E III, Eder JP.** Principles of dose, schedule, and combination therapy. In: **Kufe DW, Pollock RE, Weichselbaum RR, et al., eds.** *Holland-Frei Cancer Medicine.* 6th ed. Hamilton, ON: BC Decker; 2003. Chapter 44.

47. **Bookman MA, Brady MF, McGuire WP, et al.** Evaluation of new platinum-based treatment regimens in advanced-stage ovarian cancer: A Phase III Trial of the Gynecologic Cancer Intergroup. *J Clin Oncol.* 2009;27(9):1419–1425.

48. **Mayer LD, Janoff AS.** Optimizing combination chemotherapy by controlling drug ratios.*Mol Interv.* 2007;7(4):216–223.

49. **Eisenhauer EA, Therasse P, Bogaerts J, et al.** New response evaluation criteria in solid tumours: Revised RECIST guideline (version 1.1). *Eur J Cancer.* 2009;45(2):228–247.

50. **Collins IM, Roberts-Thomson R, Faulkner D, et al.** Carboplatin dosing in ovarian cancer: Problems and pitfalls. *Int J Gynecol Cancer.* 2011;21(7):1213–1218.

51. **Calvert AH, Newell DR, Gumbrell LA, et al.** Carboplatin dosage: Prospective evaluation of a simple formula based on renal function. *J Clin Oncol.* 1989;7:1748–1756.

52. http://ctep.cancer.gov/content/docs/carboplatin_information letter.pdf

53. https://gogmember.gog.org

54. **Freifeld AG, Bow EJ, Sepkowitz KA, et al.** Clinical practice guideline for the use of antimicrobial agents in neutropenic patients with cancer: 2010 update by the Infectious Diseases Society of America. *Clin Infect Dis.* 2011;52:e56–e93.

55. **Flowers CR, Seidenfeld J, Bow EJ, et al.** Antimicrobial prophylaxis and outpatient management of fever and neutropenia in adults treated for malignancy: American Society of Clinical Oncology clinical practice guideline. *J Clin Oncol.* 2013; 31(6):794–810.

56. **Bensinger W, Schubert M, Ang KK, et al.** NCCN Task Force Report. prevention and management of mucositis in cancer care. *J Natl Compr Canc Netw.* 2008;6(suppl 1):S1–S21.

57. **Schnell FM.** Chemotherapy-induced nausea and vomiting: The importance of acute antiemetic control. *Oncologist.* 2003;8(2):187–198.

58. **Artz AS, Somerfield MR, Feld JJ, et al.** American Society of Clinical Oncology provisional clinical opinion: Chronic hepatitis B virus infection screening in patients receiving cytotoxic chemotherapy for treatment of malignant diseases. *J Clin Oncol.* 2010;28(19):3199–3202.

59. **de Wit M, Ortner P, Lipp HP, et al.** Management of cytotoxic extravasation—ASORS expert opinion for diagnosis, prevention and treatment *Onkologie.* 2013;36(3):127–135.

60. **Komen MM, Smorenburg CH, van den Hurk CJ, et al.** Factors influencing the effectiveness of scalp cooling in the prevention of chemotherapy-induced alopecia. *Oncologist.* 2013;18(7):885–891.

61. **Muggia FM, Hainsworth JD, Jeffers S, et al.** Phase II study of liposomal doxorubicin in refractory ovarian cancer: Antitumor activity and toxicity modification by liposomal encapsulation. *J Clin Oncol.* 1997;15:987–993.

62. **King PD, Perry MC.** Hepatotoxicity of chemotherapy. *Oncologist.* 2001;6(2):162–176

63. **Limper AH.** Chemotherapy-induced lung disease. *Clin Chest Med.* 2004;25:53–64.

64. **Bovelli D, Platanioitis G, Roila F, On behalf of the ESMO Guidelines.** Cardiotoxicity of chemotherapeutic agents and radiotherapy-related heart disease: ESMO Clinical Practice Guidelines. *Ann Oncol.* 2010;21(suppl 5):v277–v282.

65. **Perez EA, Rodeheffer R.** Clinical cardiac tolerability of trastuzumab. *J Clin Oncol.* 2004;22:322–329.

66. **Burger RA, Sill MW, Monk BJ, et al.** Phase II trial of bevicizumab in persistent or recurrent epithelial ovarian cancer or primary peritoneal cancer: A Gynecologic Oncology Group study. *J Clin Oncol.* 2007;25:5165–5171.

67. **Lameire N, Kruse V, Rottey S.** Nephrotoxicity of anticancer drugs—An underestimated problem? *Acta Clin Belg.* 2011;66(5):337–345.

68. **Perazella MA, Moeckel GW.** Nephrotoxicity from chemotherapeutic agents: Clinical manifestations, pathobiology, and prevention/therapy Semin Nephrol. 2010;30(6):570–581.

69. **Xin Y, Kessarin P, Neil K, et al.** Cisplatin nephrotoxicity: A review. *Am J Med Sci.* 2007;334(2):116–124.

70. **Park SB, Krishnan AV, Lin CS, et al.** Mechanisms underlying chemotherapy-induced neurotoxicity and the potential for neuroprotective strategies. *Curr Med Chem.* 2008;15(29):3081–3094.

71. **Argyriou AA, Koltzenburg M, Polychronopoulos P, et al.** Peripheral nerve damage associated with administration of taxanes in patients with cancer. *Crit Rev Oncol Hematol.* 2008;66(3):218–228.

72. **Roelofs RI, Hrushesky W, Rogin J, et al.** Peripheral sensory neuropathy and cisplatin chemotherapy. *Neurology.* 1984;34(7):934–938.

73. **Amptoulach S, Tsavaris N.** Neurotoxicity caused by the treatment with platinum analogues. *Chemother Res Pract.* 2011; 2011:843019.

74. **Connelly E, Markman M, Kennedy A, et al.** Paclitaxel delivered as a 3-hr infusion with cisplatin in patients with gynecologic cancers: Unexpected incidence of neurotoxicity. *Gynecol Oncol.* 1996;62:166–168.

75. **Hansen LA, Hughes TE.** Altretamine. *DICP.* 1991;25(2):146–152.

76. **Joerger M.** Prevention and handling of acute allergic and infusion reactions in oncology. *Ann Oncol.* 2012;23 (suppl 10):313–319.

77. **Markman M, Kennedy A, Webster K, et al.** Clinical features of hypersensitivity reactions to carboplatin. *J Clin Oncol.* 1999;17:1141–1145.

78. **Van Leeuwen FE, Travis LB.** Second cancers. In: **DeVita VT Jr, Hellman S, Rosenberg SA, eds.** *Cancer: Principles and Practice of Oncology.* 7th ed. Philadelphia, PA: Lippincott–Raven Publishers, 2005:2575–2601.

79. **Greene MH, Boice JD Jr, Greer BE, et al.** Acute nonlymphocytic leukemia after therapy with alkylating agents for ovarian cancer: A study of five randomized clinical trials.*N Engl J Med.* 1982;307:1416–1421.

80. **Travis LB, Holowaty EJ, Bergfeldt K, et al.** Risk of leukemia after platinum-based chemotherapy for ovarian cancer. *N Engl J Med.* 1999;340:351–357.

81. **Wood M, Vogel V, Ng A, et al.** Second malignant neoplasms: Assessment and strategies for risk reduction. *J Clin Oncol.* 2012;30(30):3734–3745.

82. **Travis LB.** Therapy-associated solid tumors. *Acta Oncol.* 2002;41:323–333.

83. **Bower M, Newlands ES, Holden L, et al.** EMA/CO for high-risk gestational trophoblastic tumors: Results from a cohort of 272 patients. *J Clin Oncol.* 1997;15:2636–2643.

84. **Brewer M, Gershenson DM, Herzog CE, et al.** Outcome and reproductive function after chemotherapy for ovarian dysgerminoma. *J Clin Oncol.* 1999;17:2670–2675.

85. **Tangir J, Zelterman D, Ma W, et al.** Reproductive function after conservative surgery and chemotherapy for malignant germ cell tumors of the ovary. *Obstet Gynecol.* 2003;101:251–257.

86. **Amant F, Han SN, Gziri MM, et al.** Chemotherapy during pregnancy. *Curr Opin Oncol.* 2012;24(5):580–586.

87. **Gelmon K.** The taxoids: Paclitaxel and docetaxel. *Lancet.* 1994; 344:1267–1272.

88. **Pizzolato JF, Saltz LB.** The camptothecins. *Lancet.* 2003;361:2235–2242.

89. **Kieran MW, Kalluri R, Cho YJ.** The VEGF pathway in cancer and disease: Responses, resistance, and the path forward. *Cold Spring Harb Perspect Med.* 2012;2(12):a006593.

90. **Itamochi H.** Targeted therapies in epithelial ovarian cancer: Molecular mechanisms of action. *World J Biol Chem.* 2010;1(7):209–220.

91. **Garcia A, Singh H.** Bevacizumab and ovarian cancer. *Ther Adv Med Oncol.* 2013;5(2):133–141.

92. **Stone RL, Sood AK, Coleman RL.** Collateral damage: Toxic effects of targeted antiangiogenic therapies in ovarian cancer. *Lancet Oncol.* 2010;(5):465–475.

93. **Moroney JW, Sood AK, Coleman RL.** Aflibercept in epithelial ovarian carcinoma. *Future Oncol.* 2009;5(5):591–600.

94. **Smolle E, Tauche Vr, Pichler M, et al.** Targeting signaling pathways in epithelial ovarian cancer. *Int J Mol Sci.* 2013;14(5):9536–9555.

95. **Curtin NJ, Szabo C.** Therapeutic applications of PARP inhibitors: Anticancer therapy and beyond. *Mol Aspects Med.* 2013;34(6): 1217–1256.

96. **Fong PC, Yap TA, Boss DS, et al.** Poly (ADP)-ribose polymerase inhibition: Frequent durable responses in BRCA carrier ovarian cancer correlating with platinum-free interval. *J Clin Oncol.* 2010;28: 2512–2519.

97. **Audeh MW, Carmichael J, Penson RT, et al.** Oral poly(ADP-ribose) polymerase inhibitor olaparib in patients with BRCA1 or BRCA2 mutations and recurrent ovarian cancer: A proof-of-concept trial. *Lancet.* 2010;376:245–251.

98. **Rigakos G, Razis E.** BRCAness: Finding the Achilles heel in ovarian cancer. *Oncologist.* 2012;17(7):956–962.

4 Radiation Therapy

Patricia J. Eifel

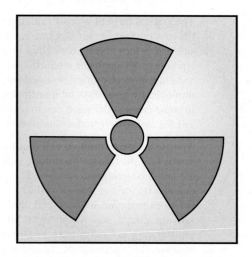

Radiation therapy plays a major role in the treatment of patients with gynecologic malignancies. For women with cervical cancer, radiation therapy is the primary treatment for patients with advanced disease (1,2), yields cure rates equal to those seen after radical surgery for patients with early tumors (3–5), and reduces the risk of local recurrence after surgery for patients with high-risk features (6,7). For women with endometrial cancer, radiation therapy reduces the risk of local recurrence after hysterectomy for patients with high-risk features (8–11) and is a potentially curative primary treatment for patients with recurrent disease and for those who are unfit for primary surgery (12–15). Radiation therapy is an effective treatment for selected patients with ovarian cancer (16,17) and is the primary curative treatment for most patients with invasive vaginal cancer (18,19). It has an expanding role in the management of carcinomas of the vulva (20–22).

Computer technology and information systems have transformed many aspects of radiation therapy practice in the past two decades, making possible three-dimensional treatment planning based on computed tomography (CT) and magnetic resonance imaging (MRI), optimized inverse planning, computer-controlled treatment delivery, and remote afterloading brachytherapy. These techniques enable radiation oncologists to restrict radiation-dose distributions to specified target volumes, thereby delivering the maximal dose to the tumor while sparing normal tissues as much as possible. However, the planning and delivery of these advanced techniques are labor-intensive, costly, and potentially more prone to error than the planning and delivery of traditional, generally simpler techniques.

Radiation biologists and clinicians continue to advance our understanding of the molecular mechanisms involved in radiation-induced cell death, the nature of drug–radiation interactions, and the importance of radiation dose, the time over which the dose is given, and the dose per fraction. **In 1999 and 2000, the results of randomized clinical trials demonstrated a significant improvement in pelvic disease control and survival when concurrent chemotherapy was added to radiation therapy for patients with locally advanced cervical cancer** (20–22). These results led to one of the most significant changes in the standard treatment of gynecologic cancers in decades.

In this chapter, the basic principles of radiation therapy, radiation biology, and radiation physics are reviewed, and an overview of the indications for, and techniques of, radiation therapy in the treatment of gynecologic malignancies is presented.

Radiation Biology

Radiation Damage and Repair

Cell death can be defined as the loss of clonogenic capacity (i.e., the ability of the cell to reproduce). Most cell death caused by ionizing radiation is mitotic cell death. Ionizing radiation may also cause programmed cell death (apoptosis).

The critical target for most radiation-induced cell death is the DNA within the cell's nucleus. Photons or charged particles interact with intracellular water to produce highly reactive free radicals that in turn interact with DNA to produce strand breaks that interfere with the cell's ability to reproduce. Although this interaction may cause a cell's "reproductive death," the cell may continue to be metabolically alive for some time. **Radiation-induced damage may not be expressed morphologically until days or months later when the cell attempts to divide (mitotic cell death).** In some cases, a damaged cell may undergo a limited number of divisions before it dies, having lost the ability to reproduce indefinitely.

Apoptosis (programmed cell death) may play an important role in radiation-induced cell death (23). In contrast to mitotic cell death, apoptosis may occur before cell division or after the cell has completed mitosis. The plasma membrane and nuclear DNA may both be important targets for this type of cell death. Apoptosis appears to be a particularly important mechanism of radiation-induced cell death in certain postmitotic normal tissues, including human salivary glands and lymphocytes. Radiation-induced apoptosis has been observed in some proliferating normal tissues and tumors. Biologists are actively studying the pathways that regulate the expression of radiation-induced apoptosis, in the hope that they can be exploited to improve local tumor control.

Cell Survival Curves

The effects of ionizing radiation on the survival of mammalian cell populations in vitro are typically expressed graphically as dose–response or *"cell survival"* curves (24). The surviving fraction of cells is plotted (on an exponential scale) against the dose of radiation (on a linear scale). **Experimental data using single doses of sparsely ionizing radiation (e.g., x-rays, gamma rays, electrons, or protons) typically produce cell survival curves with two components** (Fig. 4.1): **A shoulder region and an exponential region.**

Several mathematical models, based on different hypothetical mechanisms of cell killing, have been devised to describe radiation dose–response relationships. These include the following:

1. **The multitarget model (also referred to as the N-D_0 model).**
2. **The linear-quadratic model (also referred to as the α/β model).**

The multitarget model (Fig. 4.1A) is described by the expression $\log_e N = D_q/D_0$, where N and D_q measure the width of the shoulder and D_0 is the slope of the final exponential portion of the survival curve. This model derives from the classic target theory, which holds that each cell contains multiple sensitive targets, all of which must be hit to kill the cell. The presence of a shoulder region is believed to reflect accumulation of **sublethal injury** in some of the irradiated cells (24,25). Although the multitarget model accurately describes the exponential portion of the dose–response curve, it is a poor fit to experimental data in the shoulder region. In particular, it fails to predict the approximately linear slope (D_1) of the initial portion of the shoulder (Fig. 4.1B).

The linear-quadratic model describes the dose–response relationship according to the equation $S = exp - (\alpha D + \beta D^2)$, where S is the surviving fraction, D is the dose of radiation, and α and β are constants (Fig. 4.1B). This model presupposes two components of cell death: one that is proportional to the dose (αD) and one that is proportional to the square of the dose (βD^2). The dose at which the linear and quadratic components are equal is α/β (Fig. 4.1A). This model fits experimental data particularly well for the first few logs of cell death, which are most relevant to fractionated and low-dose-rate (LDR) irradiation, but it is continuously bending on a log-linear plot. This bend is inconsistent with experimental data that demonstrate a straight line on a log-linear plot for the distal portion of the cell survival curve. For this reason, the linear-quadratic model may not accurately predict the effect of treatment schedules that involve very large doses per radiation fraction.

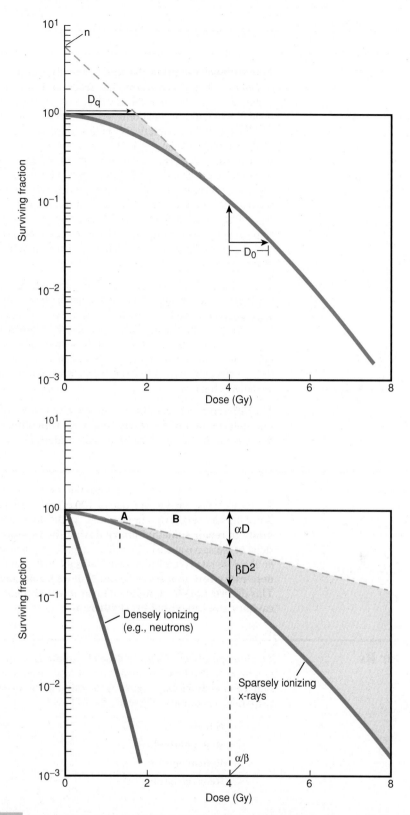

Figure 4.1 Parameters commonly used to characterize the relationship between radiation dose and cell survival in mammalian culture. In the multitarget, or $N\text{-}D_0$, model **(A)**, N is the extrapolation number, N and D_q measure the width of the shoulder, and D_0 represents the slope of the final exponential portion of the survival curve. The multitarget model provides an accurate description of experimental data in the exponential portion of the survival curve. The linear-quadratic model **(B)** more accurately describes the shape of the initial shoulder portion of the curve. Because the shoulder has more influence on fractionated radiation therapy, the linear-quadratic model is more often used to predict the results of fractionated clinical radiation therapy. (Modified from **Hall EJ**. *Radiobiology for the Radiologist*. 5th ed. Philadelphia, PA: Lippincott Williams & Wilkins; 2000, with permission.)

Fractionation

Conventional radiation therapy is usually given in a fractionated course with daily doses of 180 to 200 cGy (centiGray) per fraction. Hypothetical cell survival curves for normal tissue and tumor cells illustrate the advantage of fractionation (Fig. 4.2). When a dose of radiation is divided into multiple smaller doses separated by an interval sufficient to allow maximum repair of sublethal injury, a relatively shallow dose–response curve is achieved, reflecting a repetition of the shoulder of the single-dose cell survival curve. The slope of the fractionated-dose cell survival curve depends on the character of the shoulder (N and D_q). The sparing effect of fractionation is greatest for cells with a response to radiation characterized by a relatively broad shoulder, reflecting the cells' greater ability to accumulate and repair sublethal damage during the interfraction interval. Many normal tissues and some poorly responsive tumors exhibit this type of response to fractionated irradiation in vivo and in vitro. In contrast, most tumors and some acutely responding normal tissues (e.g., bone marrow and intestinal crypt cells) have a dose–response curve with a relatively narrow shoulder, implying relatively little sparing effect of fractionation.

The biologic effects of various fractionation schemes can be estimated and compared using the linear-quadratic formula. For a total radiation dose d divided in n well-separated fractions, the biologic effect is given by $E = n (\alpha d + \beta d^2)$. Some rearrangement of the equation gives: $E/\alpha = nd \times (1 + d/(\alpha/\beta))$. The quantity E/$\alpha$ is termed the **biologically effective dose** (BED) and is the value used to compare various fractionation schedules. The value of α/β provides an estimate of the fractionation sensitivity of a tissue. Tissues that are greatly spared by fractionation (most normal tissues) generally have a low α/β value, while tumors and acutely responding tissues tend to have a relatively high value.

The difference between the *fractionation sensitivity* of tumors and normal tissues is an important determinant of the *therapeutic ratio* (the difference between tumor control and normal tissue complications) of fractionated irradiation.

Dose-rate Effect

So far, this discussion of cell survival curves and fractionation has referred to radiation given in acute exposures—that is, at a rate of 100 cGy per minute or greater. At these dose rates, the shoulder of the survival curve is pronounced. **As the dose rate is decreased, cells have a greater opportunity to repair sublethal injury during the exposure. This is called the *dose-rate effect.*** The slope of the survival curve becomes increasingly shallow and the shoulder less apparent (Fig. 4.3) until a dose rate is reached at which all sublethal injury is repaired. **In experimental systems, the dose-rate effect appears to be much more pronounced for normal cells than for tumor cells. This differential effect implies a favorable therapeutic ratio that is exploited with LDR intracavitary and interstitial brachytherapy.**

The Four Rs

The biologic effect of a given dose of radiation is influenced by the dose, fraction size, interfraction interval, and time over which the dose is given. **Four factors, classically referred to as "the four Rs of radiobiology," govern the influence of dose, time, and fractionation on the cellular response to radiation.** These are the following:

1. **Repair**
2. **Repopulation**
3. **Redistribution**
4. **Reoxygenation**

Repair

Because fractionated irradiation permits greater recovery of sublethal injury during treatment, a higher total dose of radiation is required to achieve a given biologic effect when the total dose is divided into smaller fractions. The broader the shoulder of the survival curve, the greater the increase in dose required to achieve the same level of cell death as achieved by a single dose. Two-dose experiments with varying interfraction intervals have indicated that a space of at least 4 hours, and probably more than 6 hours, is necessary to complete repair of accumulated sublethal injury. Clinical studies tend to confirm these findings; for this reason, altered-fractionation protocols usually require a minimum interval of 4 to 6 hours between treatments.

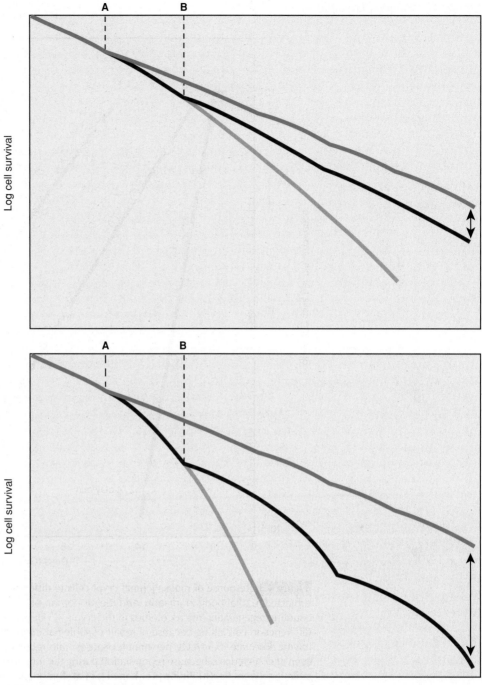

Figure 4.2 Relationship between radiation dose and surviving fraction of cells treated in vitro with radiation delivered in a single dose or in fractions. **Top:** Most tumors and acutely responding normal tissues. **Bottom:** Late-responding normal tissues. For most tumors and acutely responding normal tissues, the cellular response to single doses of radiation is described by a curve with a relatively shallow initial shoulder (**Top,** *yellow line*). Cellular survival curves for late-responding normal tissues (**Bottom,** *yellow line*) have a more pronounced shoulder, suggesting that these cells have a greater capacity to accumulate and repair sublethal radiation injury. When the total dose of radiation is delivered in several smaller fractions (Dose A [*dose/fraction*] = *blue line,* or a larger fraction Dose B [*dose/fraction*] = *red line*), the response to each fraction is similar and the overall radiation survival curve reflects multiple repetitions of the initial portion of the single-dose survival curve. Note that the total dose required to kill a specific proportion of the cells decreases as the dose per fraction increases (*red line*). Arrows indicate the differential effects of relatively large versus small fractions of radiation. The greater differential effects of fractionated irradiation on normal tissues (**Bottom**) than on tumor (**Top**) reflect the greater capacity of late-responding normal tissues to accumulate and repair sublethal radiation injury. (From **Karcher KH, Kogelnik HD, Reinartz G, eds**. *Progress in Radio-Oncology II*. New York, NY: Raven Press; 1982:287–296.)

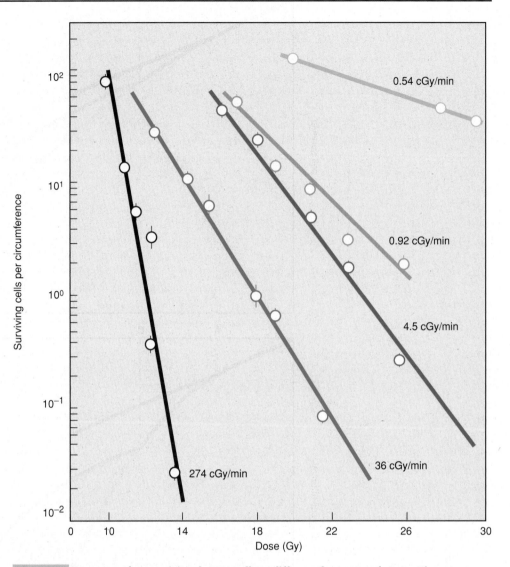

Figure 4.3 **Response of mouse jejunal crypt cells to different dose rates of γ rays.** The mice were subjected to total body irradiation, and the proportion of surviving crypt cells was determined by counting regenerating microcolonies in the crypts 3.5 days after irradiation. There was a dramatic difference in cell killing because of repair of sublethal injury at low dose rates. In this system, the lowest dose rate (0.54 cGy per minute) causes little reduction in the number of surviving cells even after high doses because repopulation during the long exposure balances the cell killing from radiation. (From **Fu KK, Phillips TL, Kane LJ, et al.** Tumor and normal tissue response to irradiation in vivo: Variation with decreasing dose rates. *Radiology.* 1975;114:709–716, with permission.)

Repopulation

Repopulation **refers to the cell proliferation that occurs during the delivery of radiation.** The magnitude of the effect of repopulation on the dose required to produce a given level of cell death depends on the doubling time of the cells involved. For cells with a relatively short doubling time, a significant increase in dose may be required to compensate for a protraction in the delivery time. This phenomenon may be of considerable practical importance. The speed of repopulation of normal tissues that manifest radiation injury soon after exposure (skin, mucosal surfaces, etc.) limits contraction of a course of fractionated irradiation. Unnecessary protraction probably reduces the effectiveness of a dose of radiation by permitting time for repopulation of malignant clonogens during treatment (26,27). **Cytotoxic treatments—including chemotherapy, radiation therapy, and possibly surgical resection—may trigger an increase in the proliferation rate of surviving clonogens.** This *accelerated repopulation* **may increase the detrimental effect of treatment delays and may influence the effectiveness of sequential multimodality treatments** (28,29).

Redistribution

Studies of synchronized cell populations show significant differences in the radiosensitivity of cells in different phases of the cell cycle (30). Cells are usually most sensitive to radiation in the late G_2 phase and during mitosis and are most resistant in the mid- to late S and early G_1 phases. When asynchronous dividing cells receive a fractionated dose of radiation, the first fraction tends to synchronize the cells by killing off those in sensitive phases of the cell cycle. Cells remaining in the S phase begin to progress to a more sensitive phase of the cell cycle during the interval before the next fraction is given. This redistribution of cells to a more sensitive phase of the cell cycle tends to increase the overall cell death achieved from a fractionated dose of ionizing radiation, particularly if the cells have a relatively short cell cycle time.

Reoxygenation

The sensitivity of fully oxygenated cells to sparsely ionizing radiation is approximately three times that of cells irradiated under anoxic conditions. This makes oxygen the most effective known radiation sensitizer. The molecular interactions responsible for the oxygen effect are not completely understood, but it is believed that oxygen stabilizes the reactive free radicals produced by the ionizing events. The ratio between the dose needed to achieve a given level of cell death under oxygenated versus hypoxic conditions is referred to as the oxygen enhancement ratio (Fig. 4.4).

Most normal tissues are fully oxygenated, but significant hypoxia occurs in at least some solid tumors, rendering the tumor cells relatively resistant to the effects of radiation. **The clinical**

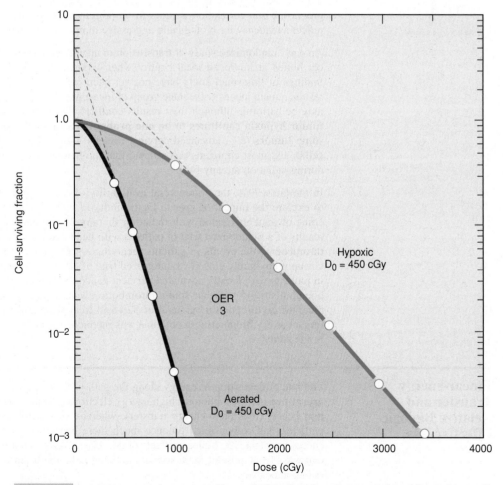

Figure 4.4 Survival curves for mammalian cells irradiated under aerated and hypoxic conditions. The dose required to produce a given level of damage is approximately three times greater under hypoxic or anoxic conditions than under fully oxygenated conditions. The ratio of doses is the oxygen enhancement ratio (OER). Sometimes the shoulder also is reduced under hypoxic conditions. (Modified from **Hall EJ**. *Radiobiology for the Radiologist*. 5th ed. Philadelphia, PA: Lippincott Williams & Wilkins; 2000, with permission.)

importance of tumor hypoxia is uncertain, because hypoxic cells initially tend to become better oxygenated during a course of fractionated irradiation (31). This phenomenon, called **reoxygenation,** tends to increase the response of tumors to a dose of fractionated radiation.

Treatment Strategies for Overcoming Radioresistance of Hypoxic Cells

Many treatment strategies have been explored to overcome the relative radioresistance of hypoxic cells in human solid tumors (32–37). These include the following:

1. Hyperbaric oxygen or carbogen breathing
2. Red cell transfusion or use of growth factors
3. Pharmacologic agents that act as hypoxic cell sensitizers (e.g., misonidazole) or that selectively kill potentially radioresistant hypoxic cells (e.g., tirapazamine)
4. High-linear-energy-transfer radiation

None of these approaches have clearly demonstrated an improvement in outcome; however, many of the relevant studies were severely compromised by technical or logistical problems.

Numerous retrospective studies have found a correlation between the minimum hemoglobin level during treatment and outcome, but all of them were compromised by possible confounding risk factors (38–40). Even with multivariate analysis, investigators have been unable to sort out whether anemic patients have poorer responses to radiation because of their low hemoglobin levels or have low hemoglobin levels because poorly responsive tumors are more likely to bleed. Studies of intratumoral oxygen tension have suggested that patients with hypoxic tumors tend to have a poor prognosis; this correlation appears to be present in surgically treated patients, and may in part reflect a tendency for biologically aggressive tumors to be hypoxic (41).

An early randomized study of transfusion in anemic patients with locally advanced cervical cancer hinted at improved local control when oxygen-carrying capacity was increased (41). The findings of this small study have not yet been confirmed in a larger prospective trial, and the results remain inconclusive. One group of investigators (42) suggested that allogeneic transfusion may be harmful, although their results conflict with those of most other studies. Nevertheless, **tumor hypoxia continues to be one probable cause of the failure of irradiation to control some tumors** (e.g., advanced cervical cancers with a significant population of hypoxic tumor cells), and most clinicians recommend that the hemoglobin level be maintained above 10 g/dL during radiation therapy (43).

In the late 1990s, the commercial availability of recombinant *erythropoietin* led investigators to explore the impact of growth factor–induced increases in the hemoglobin level on the outcome of patients treated with radiation therapy. Initial enthusiasm was tempered by negative results of a randomized trial in patients with head and neck cancer and by reports of increased thromboembolic events in patients receiving *erythropoietin* (44). The Gynecologic Oncology Group prematurely closed a randomized trial of chemoradiation with or without *erythropoietin* in patients with locally advanced cervical cancer because of concerns about the risk of thromboembolism (45). In that study, thrombotic events occurred in 11 of 57 patients (19%) who received erythropoietin versus 4 of 52 (8%) treated with chemoradiation alone ($p = NS$); the impact of erythropoietin on outcome was inconclusive because of the small number of patients in the study.

Linear-energy Transfer and Relative Biologic Effectiveness

The rate of deposition of energy along the path of the radiation beam is referred to as its *linear-energy transfer* (46). Photons, high-energy electrons, and protons produce sparsely ionizing radiation beams (low-linear-energy transfer), whereas larger atomic particles (e.g., neutrons, alpha particles, and carbon ions) produce much more densely ionizing radiation beams (high-linear-energy transfer). The biologic effects of densely ionizing radiation beams differ in several important ways from those of more sparsely ionizing radiation beams. With high-linear-energy-transfer radiation beams:

1. There is little or no repairable injury and therefore no shoulder on the tumor cell survival curve.
2. The magnitude of cell death from a given dose is greater, increasing the terminal slope of the survival curve.
3. The oxygen enhancement ratio is diminished.

The unit of **relative biologic effectiveness** is used to compare the effects of different radiation beams. Relative biologic effectiveness is defined as the ratio between a test radiation dose and the dose of 250-kV x-rays needed to produce a specific biologic effect. The relative biologic effectiveness may differ somewhat according to the tissue and biologic end point being studied.

In practice, few facilities exist for the production of high-linear-energy-transfer beams, and their use has had no major impact on the results of treatment for gynecologic malignancies.

Hyperthermia

Temperature is another factor that can modify the effect of ionizing radiation (24). Supraphysiologic temperatures alone can be toxic to cells because heat is preferentially toxic to cells in a low-pH environment (frequent in areas of hypoxia) and to cells in the relatively radioresistant S phase of the cell cycle. **Temperatures in the range of 42°C to 43°C sensitize cells to radiation by reducing the shoulder and increasing the slope of the cell survival curve.** Because of the different vascular supplies of tumors and normal tissues, hyperthermia may produce greater temperature elevations in tumors, increasing the possible therapeutic advantage when heat is combined with irradiation. Biologists and clinicians tried to find ways to exploit this effect for many years but were hampered by technologic limitations on the ability to selectively heat deep-seated tumors (47). A trial from Amsterdam (48) reported that survival was improved when hyperthermia was used with irradiation in patients with locally advanced cervical cancer. The patients in this study received relatively low doses of radiation, did not receive concurrent chemotherapy, and had poorer than expected pelvic disease control in the control arm, but the findings suggest that the approach may deserve further study.

Interactions between Radiation and Drugs

Drugs and radiation interact in a number of ways to modify cellular responses. Steel and Peckham (49) categorized these interactions into four groups: Spatial cooperation (independent action), additivity, supra-additivity, and subadditivity.

Spatial Cooperation— Independent Action

Spatial cooperation is the situation in which drugs and radiation act independently with different targets and mechanisms of action so that the total effect of the combination is equal to that of each agent separately. For example, a site that is protected from chemotherapy (e.g., the brain) may be treated with radiation to prevent recurrence. Alternatively, a drug may be used to destroy microscopic distant disease, while radiation is used to sterilize local tumor.

Additivity

Additivity is the situation in which two agents act on the same target to cause damage that is equal to the sum of their individual toxic effects.

Supra-additivity

When there is supra-additivity, a drug potentiates the effect of radiation, causing a greater response than would be expected from simple additivity.

Subadditivity

With subadditivity, the amount of cell death that results from the use of the two agents is less than that expected from simple additivity (the amount may still be greater than expected from either treatment alone).

Clinically, it is difficult to determine which mode of interaction occurs when two agents are used concurrently. When a greater response is observed than would be expected from radiation alone, the interaction is often described as synergistic, but may be only additive or even subadditive.

Therapeutic Ratio

Ionizing radiation interacts with all the tissues in its path, not exclusively tumor tissue. Radiation can be considered an effective cancer treatment only if there is a differential biologic effect on tumor and normal tissues. **The difference between tumor control and normal tissue complications is referred to as the therapeutic gain or therapeutic ratio.**

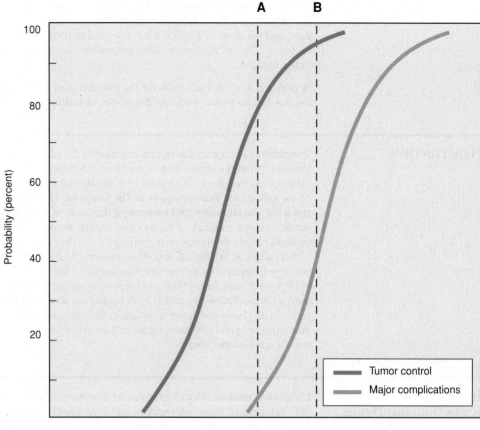

Figure 4.5 **Theoretical sigmoid dose–response curves for tumor control and severe complications.** The therapeutic ratio is related to the distance between the two curves. Dose A controls tumor in 80% of cases with a 5% incidence of complications (blue curve). Dose B yields a 10–15% increase in the tumor control probability but a much greater risk of complications, narrowing the therapeutic ratio (orange curve).

In general, the relationship between the probability of tumor cure or the probability of normal tissue injury and the dose of radiation can be described by a sigmoid curve (Fig. 4.5). At relatively low radiation doses, there is an insufficient amount of cell death to produce any likelihood of tumor cure. As the dose is increased, a threshold is reached at which some cures begin to be observed. For most tumor systems, the likelihood of cure rises rapidly as the radiation dose is increased beyond this threshold and then reaches a plateau. The shape and slope of the dose–response curve vary according to the tumor type and size (50,51).

A similar sigmoid relationship is seen when the likelihood of complications is plotted against the radiation dose. If the sigmoid curve for normal tissue complications is to the right of the sigmoid curve for tumor control, then treatment with doses that fall between the two curves may achieve tumor control without causing complications. **The difference between these curves represents the therapeutic ratio.** The primary goal of radiation research efforts is to improve the therapeutic ratio by increasing the separation between these dose–response curves, maximizing the probability of complication-free tumor control.

Effects of Radiation on Normal Tissues

The extent of radiation damage to normal tissues depends on a number of factors, including the radiation dose, the organ, the volume of tissue irradiated, and the division rate of the irradiated cells. **Tissues that have rapid cell turnover (i.e., tissues whose functional activity requires constant cell renewal) tend to manifest radiation injury soon after exposure,** often during a fractionated course of radiation therapy. **Examples of acutely responding tissues include most epithelia (e.g., skin, hair, gastrointestinal mucosa, bone marrow, and reproductive tissues).** In contrast, **tissues that have slower cell turnover (i.e., tissues whose functional activity does not require constant cell renewal) tend to manifest radiation injury months or years after exposure to radiation. Examples of late-responding tissues are the connective tissues, muscle, and neural tissues.**

In some normal tissues, cell death may occur through the mechanism of apoptosis. Although apoptosis is not the primary mechanism of damage in most normal tissue injury, it is important in the response of lymphocytes, salivary gland cells, and a small proportion of intestinal crypt cells (23).

Acute Reactions

Acute reactions to pelvic irradiation, such as diarrhea, are usually associated with mucosal denudation, which in turn stimulates an increase in cell proliferation (52). This regenerative response is usually sufficient to prevent serious side effects with weekly doses of 900 to 1,000 cGy given in five fractions. This empirically derived schedule is the most commonly used for clinical radiation therapy. If treatment is accelerated to deliver the dose over much shorter periods, then the regenerative capacity of the epithelium may be overwhelmed and the acute reaction so severe that a break in treatment is needed to allow for epithelial regeneration. The severity of acute reactions depends on the volume of the normal tissues irradiated and the specific nature of the tissues.

Late Reactions

The pathogenesis of late radiation complications (i.e., those that occur months to years after radiation therapy) differs from that of acute reactions and is still incompletely understood. **It is hypothesized that late effects of radiation result from the following:**

1. Damage to vascular stroma that causes an epithelial proliferation with decreased blood supply and subsequent fibrosis.
2. Damage to slowly or infrequently proliferating parenchymal stem cells that eventually results in loss of tissue or organ function (52).

The likelihood of developing serious late effects from radiation depends on many factors, including, but not limited to, the dose of radiation, the radiation dose per fraction, the volume of tissue irradiated, the radiation dose-rate, patient characteristics, other treatments (such as surgery or chemotherapy), and the end point being measured.

Because late-responding tissues are not proliferating rapidly, the duration of a course of radiation treatment does not alter their tolerance. Late-responding normal tissues tend to be quite sensitive to changes in the dose per fraction so that **for a given dose of radiation administered over a given period, the risk of late effects will be greater with larger fractions.** This fractionation effect is responsible for the advantage of altered fractionation schedules in clinical settings in which late normal tissue reactions are severely dose limiting (Fig. 4.2) (53–55). **This fractionation effect has important implications for treatments such as high-dose-rate (HDR) brachytherapy, intensity-modulated radiation therapy (IMRT), and stereotactic body radiation therapy (SBRT)** where a portion of the target (and possibly adjacent normal tissues) frequently receives doses of more than 2 Gy per fraction.

Some tissues—such as the liver, kidney, and lung—consist of functional subunits that are arranged more or less in parallel; these tissues can tolerate a high dose of radiation given to a small portion of the organ without serious late effects, but tend to be relatively sensitive to moderate whole-organ doses. Other organs, such as bowel or ureter, are organized in a serial fashion—delivery of a damaging dose to even a small portion of the organ can cause total organ failure. For all of the reasons discussed previously, normal tissue tolerances cannot be described in terms of simple dose limits. **Some generalizations can be made about the tolerance of individual tissues** (doses refer to external radiation given in daily fractions of 1.8 to 2 Gy or with LDR brachytherapy).

Uterus   **The uterus and cervix are typically described as resistant to radiation;** however, what is really meant by this is that the uterus can be treated to very high doses (more than 100 Gy in some cases) without the patient developing serious complications in adjacent critical structures (e.g., bowel and bladder). The uterus probably cannot sustain pregnancy after such doses. **Even moderate doses of 40 to 50 Gy probably cause enough smooth muscle atrophy to prohibit successful term pregnancy,** but this is rarely tested. Women who have received 20 to 30 Gy or more to the uterus during the perimenarchal period have become pregnant, but have tended to have spontaneous second trimester abortions, probably because of underdevelopment of the uterus. Patches of endometrium frequently continue to function after doses of 50 Gy or more.

Ovary   **The radiation dose required to cause ovarian failure is highly dependent on the patient's age.** Perimenarchal girls may continue to menstruate and can become pregnant after receiving as much as 30 Gy to the ovaries; however, they usually experience premature menopause 10 to 20 years later. **Most adult women have ovarian failure after 20 Gy;** as little as 5 to 10 Gy can induce menopause in older premenopausal women.

Vagina   **The radiation tolerance of the vagina depends on the region** (upper, middle, lower, anterior, posterior, or lateral), length of vagina treated and radiation dose, fraction size, dose rate, hormonal support, and other factors. **Small portions of the surface of the lateral apical vagina can be treated to a very high dose (≥140 Gy) without causing major complications in adjacent structures.** However, these high doses cause atrophy and shortening of the apical vagina. The vaginal tolerance dose is less if treatment includes more than the apical vagina, or if the dose includes the posterior, or distal, vagina. Even moderate doses (40 to 50 Gy) may decrease the elasticity of the vagina, although it is sometimes difficult to distinguish the direct effects of radiation from those of tumor, altered hormonal environment, aging, and other factors.

Small Intestine   The risk of small intestinal side effects is highly dependent on the radiation dose and volume irradiated and on the patient's history. **In the absence of complicating factors, the entire small intestine can tolerate doses up to 30 Gy without major late effects.** Smaller volumes can tolerate 45 to 50 Gy with a low risk of complications; the risk of chronic diarrhea and bowel obstruction increases rapidly with doses greater than 50 to 60 Gy and approaches 100% if a significant volume of small bowel receives 70 Gy or more. The risk of bowel obstruction is significantly increased in patients who have a history of major transperitoneal surgery, pelvic infection, or heavy smoking (56).

Rectum   **In most cases, the entire rectum can tolerate 45 to 50 Gy with a low risk of major sequelae.** Small portions of the anterior rectal wall can tolerate doses of at least 70 to 75 Gy. The risk of serious late effects (severe bleeding, obstruction, or fistula) increases steeply as the volume of rectum treated to high dose is increased.

Bladder   **The entire bladder can be treated to 45 to 50 Gy with a very low rate of serious morbidity.** This dose may have subtle effects on bladder contractility, particularly in patients who have undergone radical hysterectomy. Small portions of the bladder can tolerate doses of 80 Gy or more with a low risk of major morbidity (severe bleeding, contracture, or fistula). The dose–response relationship is poorly defined in this range, because traditional methods of bladder dose estimation have used reference points that systematically underestimated the maximum dose. Newer CT- and MRI-based treatment planning methods yield more accurate estimates that should provide the basis for a better understanding of bladder tolerance doses in the future.

Ureter   **Surgically undisturbed ureters appear to tolerate 85 to 90 Gy** of combined external beam radiation and LDR intracavitary treatment with a low risk of stricture.

Kidney   **Most patients can tolerate as much as 18 to 22 Gy to both kidneys** with very little risk of long-term damage. Higher doses cause permanent damage to renal parenchyma. If the patient has normal renal function, 50% or more of the renal parenchyma can be treated to a high dose without causing renal failure; however, renal hypertension may occur if an entire kidney is obliterated with radiation. Underlying renal disease or concurrent use of chemotherapy can decrease renal tolerance.

Liver   **In most cases, the liver can tolerate as much as 30 Gy** (at 1.5 Gy per fraction) to the entire organ, although this dose will cause transient elevation of alkaline phosphatase levels and can cause dysfunction in a small proportion of patients. Higher doses cause serious damage to liver parenchyma but can be tolerated if delivered to only a portion of the liver. Tolerance is highly dependent on underlying hepatic function and can be markedly decreased with concurrent delivery of some chemotherapeutic agents and during periods of hepatocyte regeneration (e.g., after partial hepatectomy).

Spinal Cord and Nerves   Transverse myelitis and paralysis can occur in a small proportion of patients who receive doses as low as 50 Gy to the spinal cord, and the risk increases rapidly as the dose approaches 60 Gy at 2 Gy per fraction. **Peripheral nerves, including the cauda equina, are** rarely affected after 50 Gy and **usually tolerate doses as high as 60 Gy without serious sequelae.**

Bone   **As little as 10 to 15 Gy of radiation causes transient depletion of bone marrow elements.** With doses of more than 30 to 40 Gy, permanent damage is done to supporting elements, and bone marrow within the irradiated area will not repopulate normally. This damage can be seen as fatty replacement of the marrow cavity on MRI. The risk of fracture after radiation therapy depends on the bone irradiated, the volume of bone in the high-dose region, bone density, concomitant steroid use, and other factors.

Symptomatic fracture is rare after treatment with 40 to 45 Gy of pelvic radiation. However, routine MRI sometimes detects small, usually asymptomatic, insufficiency fractures of the pelvis after this dose (57). Hip fracture may be seen after doses as low as 40 Gy to the entire femoral head and neck, and the risk probably increases rapidly as the dose approaches 60 Gy.

Treatment Strategies to Exploit Differences between Tumor and Normal Tissue in the Response to Fractionated Radiation Therapy

A variety of altered fractionation schemes have been devised to exploit the different sensitivities of tumor and normal tissues to fractionation and the possible effects of tumor cell repopulation. These include **hyperfractionation,** in which the dose per fraction is reduced, the number of fractions and total dose are increased, and the overall treatment time is relatively unchanged; **accelerated fractionation,** in which the dose per fraction is unchanged, the overall treatment duration is reduced, and the total dose is unchanged or decreased; and **hypofractionation,** in which the dose per fraction is increased, the number of fractions and total dose are reduced, and the overall treatment time is decreased.

With **hyperfractionation,** treatment is usually given two or more times daily with at least 4 to 6 hours between fractions to allow repair of sublethal injury. This scheme should permit delivery of a higher dose of radiation without increasing the risk of late complications or the overall duration of treatment. Hyperfractionation schemes may have an advantage if the increased dose delivered per day does not cause unacceptable acute effects and if patients are willing to accept the added inconvenience of two or three treatments daily.

Accelerated fractionation schemes do not reduce the risk of late effects and tend to increase the acute effects of treatment, but may be advantageous because treatment is completed over a shorter time, reducing tumor cell repopulation during treatment (55). Such schemes are likely to be of limited value in the management of gynecologic malignancies, because acute side effects tend to limit the rate of treatment delivery.

Hypofractionation schedules are usually avoided when treatment is likely to cure the patient, because the α/β of late-responding normal tissues is less than the α/β of most tumors, meaning that large fractions have a therapeutic disadvantage. Malignant melanoma, which appears to have a relatively low α/β, may be a rare exception to this pattern. Hypofractionated schedules are frequently used for palliative treatment because they are convenient and produce rapid symptom relief. However, the necessary reduction in dose reduces the likelihood of complete eradication of tumor within the treatment field. Hypofractionation may be particularly beneficial if the tumor target is some distance from critical structures and if the radiation treatment plan is characterized by a steep dose gradient such that the target receives a relatively high dose per fraction, while normal tissue structures receive no more than approximately 2 Gy per fraction. Under ideal circumstances, HDR brachytherapy plans and some highly conformal external beam plans achieve this favorable geometry.

SBRT, sometimes referred to as stereotactic radiosurgery, is an extreme form of hypofractionation in which a small number of large doses of radiation (usually five or fewer) are used to ablate tumor. Because there is very little sublethal injury with these schedules, tight geometrical conformality is needed to obtain a favorable balance between tumor control and normal tissue preservation. For this reason, great care must be taken to avoid exposing vulnerable normal tissues to the target dose.

Treatment is usually delivered using highly conformal treatment plans with precise patient positioning and immobilization. These techniques are particularly useful for treatment of tumors surrounded by normal tissues that have a parallel structure (e.g., lung or liver) because ablation of a small volume of these normal tissues has little effect on the overall organ function. SBRT may be more dangerous in situations where tumor is very close to serially structured organs, which can be seriously compromised if even a small portion of the organ is severely damaged (e.g., bowel, ureter, or bladder).

For this reason, **SBRT should be used with extreme caution in the pelvis,** where tumors are typically surrounded by vulnerable structures and where very tightly conforming treatment plans may lead to undertreatment of a portion of the tumor.

Combinations of Surgery and Radiation Therapy

Because surgery and radiation therapy are both effective treatments, clinicians have tried to improve locoregional control or reduce treatment morbidity by combining the two modalities. **Theoretically, surgery may remove bulky tumor that may be difficult to control with tolerable doses of radiation, and radiation may sterilize microscopic disease at the periphery of the surgical bed.** The two modalities are combined in a number of ways:

1. Preoperative irradiation
2. Diagnostic surgery (surgical staging) followed by definitive irradiation
3. Intraoperative irradiation
4. Surgical resection followed by postoperative irradiation
5. Combinations of these approaches

Preoperative Irradiation

Preoperative irradiation is sometimes used to sterilize possible microscopic disease at the margins of a planned operative site. This is potentially most useful when the surgeon anticipates close margins adjacent to a critical structure (e.g., the urethra or anus in a patient with locally advanced vulvar cancer).

In patients with uterine cancer, preoperative irradiation has largely been abandoned in favor of postoperative irradiation, which can be planned when information from the surgical specimen is available and which avoids unnecessarily treating patients with very-early-stage disease. Preoperative irradiation is sometimes used to treat patients with stage II endometrial cancer that grossly involves the cervix, and is used in some patients with bulky cervical cancers. This is because the dose deliverable to paravaginal tissues is much greater when the uterus is still in place to hold an intrauterine applicator than after surgery, when only an intravaginal applicator can be used.

Some studies suggested that lower doses of radiation may be required to sterilize microscopic disease in a tumor bed undisturbed by surgery because an intact vascular supply is better able to deliver oxygen. Because the risk of operative complications is increased after high-dose radiation therapy, doses given when surgical resection is anticipated are usually lower than doses given when a tumor is irradiated definitively. **The greatest risk of preoperative radiation therapy is that if the tumor remains unresectable, the effectiveness of additional irradiation will be markedly decreased by the long interval between treatments.**

Intraoperative Irradiation

In some cases, intraoperative irradiation can be delivered with a permanent implant (using ^{125}I or ^{198}Au), with afterloading catheters in the operative bed (using ^{192}Ir), or with a special electron beam or orthovoltage unit in the operating room. These approaches deliver radiation directly to the site of maximum risk when the target can be visualized directly and normal tissues nearest the treatment area can be removed from the radiation field. **Removal of normal tissues from the treatment field is an important physical advantage of intraoperative external beam techniques** that may counterbalance the biologic disadvantage to any normal tissues remaining in the field when an entire dose is delivered in a single large fraction.

Postoperative Irradiation

Postoperative irradiation improves locoregional control and survival in several settings important to gynecologic oncologists. **In vulvar cancer,** postoperative pelvic and groin irradiation reduces the risk of groin recurrence and improves the survival rate of patients with multiple positive inguinal nodes (55). **In endometrial cancer,** postoperative pelvic irradiation reduces the incidence of pelvic recurrence in patients with high-risk disease (8,9,11). **In cervical cancer,** postoperative pelvic irradiation reduces the incidence of pelvic recurrence in patients with lymph node involvement and in those with high-risk features in the primary tumor (6,7).

Combination Approaches

Combined surgery and radiation therapy is optimized when the treatment plan exploits the complementary advantages of the two treatments. This requires close cooperation between specialists at the time of the patient's initial evaluation. Because the morbidity of combined therapy is often greater than that of single-modality therapy, combined treatment should usually be limited to situations in which a combined approach is likely to improve survival, permit organ preservation, or significantly reduce the risk of local recurrence compared with the expected results from treatment with either modality alone (58).

Physical Principles

Ionizing Radiations Used in Therapy

Ionizing radiations lie on the high-energy portion of the electromagnetic spectrum and are characterized by their ability to excite, or ionize, atoms in an absorbing material. **The decay of radioactive nuclei can produce several types of radiation, including uncharged gamma (γ) rays, negatively charged beta (β) rays (electrons), positively charged alpha (α) particles (helium ions), and neutrons.** The resulting ionizing radiations are exploited therapeutically in brachytherapy treatments (using ^{226}Ra, ^{137}Cs, ^{186}Ir, and other isotopes) or to produce teletherapy beams (e.g., ^{60}Co). The average energy of the photons produced by the decay of radioactive cobalt is 1.2 million eV (MeV).

Most external beam therapy is delivered via linear accelerators that produce photon beams (x-rays) by bombarding a target such as tungsten with accelerated electrons. Varying the energy of the accelerated electrons produces therapeutic x-rays of different energies. X-rays and γ-rays are both composed of photons and differ only in that x-rays are produced by extranuclear forces and γ-rays are produced by intranuclear forces.

Interactions of Radiation with Matter

X-rays and γ-rays

Photons interact with matter by means of three distinct mechanisms: The photoelectric effect, Compton scatter, and pair production.

The photoelectric effect is most important at energies used for diagnostic purposes. Absorption by the photoelectric effect is proportional to Z^3, where Z is the atomic number of the absorbing material. This effect is responsible for the increased absorption of bone that provides contrast between bone and soft tissue with diagnostic x-ray beams of 250 kV or less. However, the increased bone absorption, high skin dose, and poor penetration with such beams make them unsuitable for most modern therapeutic applications. Superficial kilovoltage radiation beams, delivered using a transvaginal cone, are occasionally used for patients with large bleeding exophytic tumors to achieve hemostasis before definitive treatment (59).

Modern therapeutic beams of 1 to 20 megavolts (MV) produce photons that interact with tissues primarily by Compton scatter. In this process, incident photons interact with loosely bound outer-shell electrons, ejecting them from the atom. Both the photon and the electron go on to interact with other atoms, causing additional ionizations. Compton-scatter absorption is independent of Z, but varies according to the density of the absorbing material. This accounts for the poor contrast of radiation portal verification films.

Photons that are absorbed by Compton scatter produce an increasing number of scattered electrons and ionizations as they penetrate beneath the surface of an absorbing material. This creates a buildup region just below the surface that is responsible for the **skin-sparing** characteristic of modern high-energy therapy beams (Fig. 4.6). **The maximum dose from a megavoltage beam is reached at 0.5 to 3 cm below the skin surface, depending on the photon energy.** At greater depths, the dose decreases at a fairly constant rate that is related to the beam energy. The greater skin-sparing effects and penetration of beams with energies of 15 MV or greater make such beams particularly useful for pelvic treatment.

Pair production absorption is related to Z^2. In soft tissue, this type of absorption begins to dominate only at photon energies of more than approximately 30 MeV, so pair production is of limited importance in the current radiation therapy planning.

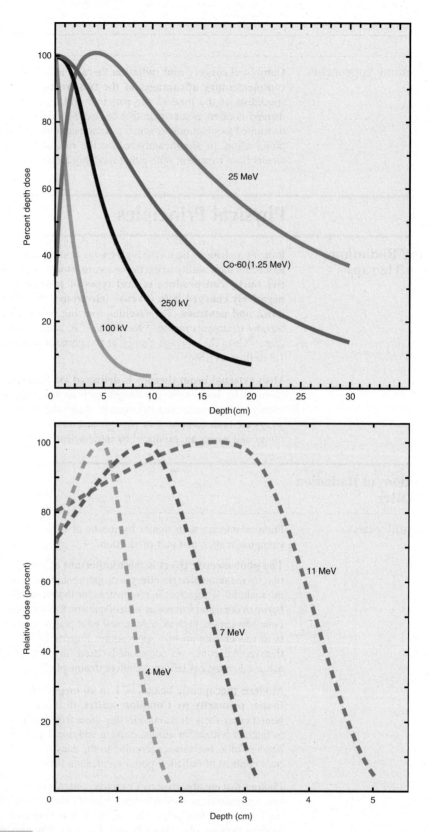

Figure 4.6 **Depth dose curves for selected x-ray and γ-ray beams (top).** As the energy increases, the depth of maximum dose (D_{max} or D_{100}) increases. For kilovoltage beams, the dose is maximum at the skin surface. With appositionally directed megavoltage beams (e.g., ^{60}Co or 25-MeV photon beams), the maximum dose is reached at a depth beyond the skin surface, producing skin sparing. High-energy beams also penetrate more deeply, making them more useful for treatment of deep-seated pelvic tumors. **Depth dose curves for electron beam fields of selected energies (bottom).** The depth of maximum dose increases with increasing energy. At depths just below the maximum, the dose falls off rapidly, sparing deeper tissues.

Electrons and Other Particles

Several types of particle beams are used in radiation therapy: Electron beams, proton beams, and neutron beams.

Electrons are very light particles. When they interact with matter, they tend to lose most of their energy in a single interaction. The dose from an electron beam is relatively homogeneous up to a depth that is related to the beam's energy (Fig. 4.6). Beyond this depth, the dose decreases very rapidly to nearly zero. Electrons are used to treat relatively superficial targets without delivering a significant dose to underlying tissues. The approximate depth (in centimeters) at which the rapid falloff in dose occurs can be estimated by dividing the electron energy by 3.

Protons are positively charged particles that are much heavier than electrons. Protons scatter minimally as they interact with matter, deposit increasing amounts of energy as they slow down, and then stop at a depth related to their initial energy. This results in rapid deposition of most of their energy at depth (called the **Bragg peak**), with a steep falloff in dose to near zero shortly after the peak. Modulating the energy can spread this peak out. **The absence of an exit dose makes proton beams ideal for conformal therapy, and interest in their use has increased as the cost of producing proton generators has become somewhat more reasonable.**

The physics support, quality assurance, and clinical requirements needed to safely treat patients with protons are complex, highly specialized, and time-consuming. In some difficult clinical situations, protons clearly provide at least a theoretical dosimetric advantage over photons, but there are as yet no randomized comparisons. Because the depth of penetration of protons is highly dependent on the density of intervening tissue, the presence of variable gas-filled structures (e.g., bowel) in the midpelvis may limit applications in gynecologic radiation oncology.

Neutrons are neutral particles that tend to deposit most of their energy in a single intranuclear event. For this reason, there is little or no repairable injury and therefore no shoulder on the tumor cell survival curve. The falloff of a neutron dose is similar to that of a photon beam of 4 to 6 MV, but the high relative biologic effectiveness of densely ionizing neutron beams is of interest to clinical investigators. **Clinical studies of neutron treatments in cervical cancer patients have been plagued by high complication rates** (60), and neutrons are rarely if ever used to treat gynecologic tumors today.

Measurement of Absorbed Dose

Absorbed dose is a measure of the energy deposited by the radiation source in the target material. The unit currently used to measure radiation dose is the Gray (Gy), where 1 Gy is equal to 1 J/kg of absorbing material. Before the early 1980s, absorbed doses of radiation were measured in radians (rads), where 1 rad = 1 cGy and 1 Gy = 100 rad.

The rate of decay of a sample of radioactive material (such as radium or cesium) is referred to as the activity of the sample and is measured in curies (Ci), where $1\ Ci = 3.7 \times 10^{10}$ disintegrations per second and $1\ mCi = 10^{-3}\ Ci$.

Safe delivery of radiation depends on precise calibration of radiation source activities and machine output. These are measured using sensitive ionization chambers in *phantoms* that simulate tissue density. Periodic calibrations of equipment and sources are a vital part of quality assurance in any radiation oncology department.

Inverse Square Law

The dose of radiation from a source to any point in space varies according to the inverse of the square of the distance from the source to the point (61). This relationship is particularly important for brachytherapy applications, because it results in a rapid falloff of dose as distance from an intracavitary or interstitial source is increased.

Radiation Techniques

Radiation therapy is delivered in three ways:

1. **Teletherapy:** X-rays are delivered from a source at a distance from the body (external beam therapy).

2. **Brachytherapy:** Radiation sources are placed within or adjacent to a target volume (intracavitary or interstitial therapy).

3. **Radioactive solutions:** Solutions that contain isotopes (e.g., radioactive colloidal gold or 32P) are introduced into a cavity (e.g., the peritoneum) to treat the walls of the cavity.

Teletherapy

Several terms are commonly used to describe the dose distributions produced by external beam irradiation of tissues.

Percentage depth dose is the change in dose with depth along the central axis of a radiation beam (Fig. 4.6).

D_{max} is the maximum dose delivered to the treated tissue. With a single appositional photon beam, the D_{max} is located at a distance below the tissue surface that increases with the energy of the photon beam (Fig. 4.6).

Source to skin distance is the distance between the source of x-rays (e.g., a cobalt source or the target in a linear accelerator) and the skin surface.

Isocenter is a point within the patient that remains a fixed distance from the radiation source as the treatment source (gantry) is rotated around the patient (Fig. 4.7).

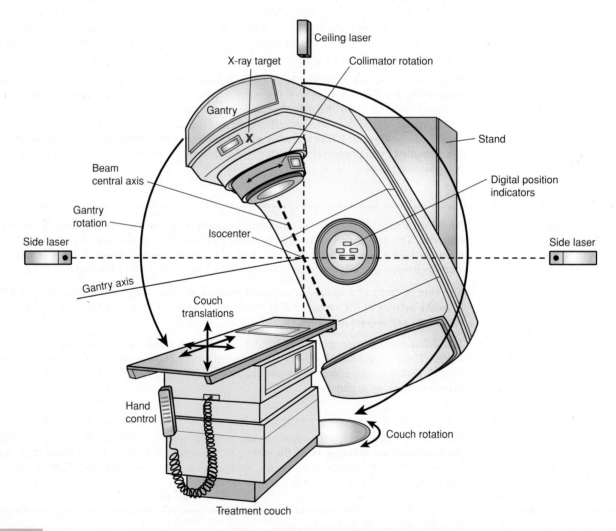

Figure 4.7 Diagram of a therapeutic linear accelerator. Patients are positioned on the treatment couch with a system of lasers that are aligned precisely with the center of the radiation beam. Collimators in the treatment head, located on a rotating gantry, define the size and rotation of the radiation field. The treatment couch can also be rotated around the central axis of the radiation beam. Beam-modifying devices such as shielding blocks and wedges can be attached to a tray beneath the collimator (not shown). (From **Karzmark CJ, Nunan CS, Tanabe E**. *Medical Electron Accelerators*. New York, NY: McGraw-Hill; 1993, with permission.)

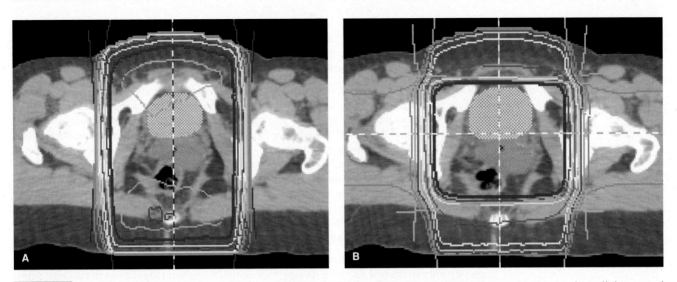

Figure 4.8 **Isodose distribution for external beam irradiation of the pelvis using an 18-MV beam. A:** A pair of parallel opposed anterior and posterior fields. **B:** Anterior, posterior, and two lateral fields (four-field box technique). The heavy red isodose line represents the region of tissue treated to ≥45 Gy.

Source to axis distance is the distance from the source of x-rays to the isocenter.

Isodose curve is a line or surface that connects points of equal radiation dose (Fig. 4.8).

Many factors influence the dose distribution in tissue from a single external beam of photons. These include the following:

1. **The energy of the beam** (determined by its voltage). Higher-energy photon beams are more penetrating than lower-energy beams. In other words, the dose of radiation delivered to deep tissues relative to more superficial tissues is greater with higher-energy beams. Higher-energy beams have a larger **buildup region** than lower-energy beams; this results in a relative sparing of the skin surface, facilitating irradiation of deep tissues (Fig. 4.6).

2. **The distance from the source to the patient.** As the source to skin distance increases, the percentage depth dose increases.

3. **The size of the radiation field.** The percentage depth dose increases with increasing field size because of the increasing contribution of internal scatter to the radiation dose. This effect is greatest with relatively low-energy radiation beams.

4. **The patient's contour and the angle of the beam's incidence.**

5. **The density of tissues in the target volume** (particularly air versus soft tissue).

6. **A variety of beam-shaping devices placed between the radiation source and the patient** that alter the shape or distribution of the radiation dose.

Modern linear accelerators permit many variations in these factors (Fig. 4.7). A rotational gantry permits *isocentric* beam arrangements that maintain a fixed distance between the beam's source and a point within the patient. This facilitates accurate patient setup and treatment planning.

Most radiation therapy treatment plans combine two or more beams to create a dose distribution designed to accomplish three aims: (i) to maximize the dose of radiation delivered to the target; (ii) to produce a relatively homogeneous dose within the volume of interest to minimize hot or cold spots that would increase the risks of complications or recurrence, respectively; and (iii) **to minimize the dose delivered to uninvolved tissues,** taking into account the different tolerances of various normal tissues.

The treatment plan must include the primary target volume (gross tumor or tumor bed), any areas at risk for microscopic spread of disease, and a margin of tissue to account for uncertainties in the location of the target, reproducibility of the setup, and organ motion. The overall plan is often designed to deliver different doses to areas of greater or lesser risk (e.g., gross vs. microscopic residual disease) by boosting areas at greater risk with smaller treatment fields after initial delivery of treatment to a relatively large volume. Two opposing beams (e.g., anterior–posterior and poste-rior–anterior) usually produce a relatively homogeneous distribution of dose within the intervening tissue with some sparing of the skin surface. In many cases, **multiple fields are used to "focus" the high-dose region to conform more closely to a deep target volume** (Fig. 4.8).

Modern technology has made it possible to use computers to optimize the beam arrangements that are required in treatment plans that incorporate many fields and beam-shaping devices. These conformal treatment plans may provide a very tight distribution of dose around the target volume. The simplest form of conformal therapy uses fairly conventional beam arrangements, but exploits modern CT-based treatment-planning techniques to more accurately define the target volume and to design blocks that conform closely to that volume. CT reconstructions permit more accurate shaping of fields that enter the patient from oblique angles. Multileaf collimators have computer-controlled leaves that can form irregularly shaped fields, replacing hand-loaded beam-shaping devices. Because the therapist no longer needs to enter the room to replace blocks on each field, it is possible to treat patients with more fields and more complex beam arrangements in a single treatment visit of acceptable duration.

Attention has focused on Intensity Modulated Radiation Therapy (IMRT) (Fig. 4.9). This form of highly conformal radiation therapy uses complex computer algorithms to optimize deliv-ery of radiation from multiple beam angles. The physician must carefully contour target volumes and all critical normal tissue structures on each slice of a CT scan that is obtained while the patient is in the treatment position. The minimum and maximum acceptable doses of radiation to be deliv-ered to each area are specified. Inverse planning techniques (based on the physician's designation of targets and avoidance structures rather than specific radiation fields) are used to design an opti-mized plan, which usually includes multiple irregularly shaped fields from each of several (usually six to nine) beam angles. In other cases, treatment may be delivered in a sequence of slices as the patient moves past a rotating source (tomotherapy) or in a continuous arc as the gantry rotates around the patient (volumetric modulated arc therapy). **In all cases, the leaves of multileaf col-limators enter the field or retract dynamically during treatment to deliver the desired amount of radiation to tissues within the target.** Very tightly conforming radiation distributions can be obtained with this approach. However, the time required to plan treatments is lengthened, and the duration of daily treatments may also be lengthened.

Quality assurance is very demanding for IMRT because the fields are less readily visualized than static radiation fields. **In the past 5 years, the use of IMRT and other highly conformal radia-tion techniques has increased exponentially.** In many cases, **these techniques can be used to reduce the dose delivered to normal tissues** during a course of radiation therapy. The opportuni-ties for error have increased; unlike traditional treatments that were based on relatively simple,

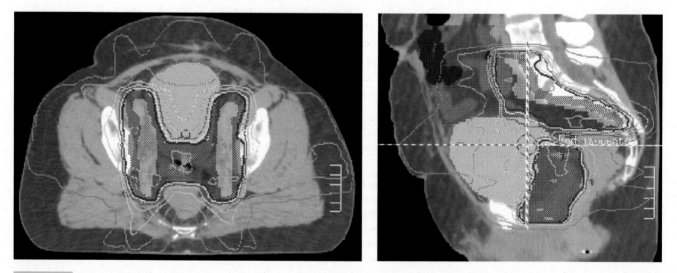

Figure 4.9 **Dose distribution obtained using intensity-modulated radiation therapy (IMRT) to treat the pelvic lymph nodes after hysterectomy.** In this case, each of seven fields was modulated to obtain a distribution that covered the iliac and presacral lymph nodes while sparing bowel in the central pelvis from high dose. A somewhat larger volume receives low-dose radiation than with standard techniques, and the very tight dose distribution requires an accurate understanding of anatomy, tissues at risk, and internal organ motion.

empirically tested field shapes and distributions, **IMRT plans are entirely dependent on the clinician's understanding of the target volume and tissues at risk.** If the clinician misses or fails to correctly designate tissues at risk for disease, the computerized inverse planning process will tend to result in exclusion of areas of possible tumor involvement or overtreatment of critical structures. **Because the dose of radiation falls off rapidly outside the designated target volume, IMRT plans require a high degree of confidence in the distribution of disease, a clear understanding of internal organ motion, and meticulous patient immobilization. Because there are as yet no level-1 data confirming the benefit of IMRT in treatment of gynecologic neoplasms,** payers may consider the treatment experimental and decline payment.

Brachytherapy

Brachytherapy is a highly specialized form of treatment that is particularly critical to the successful management of vaginal and cervical cancers. Surveys indicate that patients who are treated for cervical cancer in small, nonacademic radiation oncology facilities are less likely to receive brachytherapy and are more likely to have unacceptably prolonged treatment courses than are patients treated in large academic centers (62). **Gynecologic oncologists who are counseling newly diagnosed patients should always ascertain the level of specialized experience and adequacy of resources before referring patients who may require brachytherapy to a radiation oncologist.**

Intracavitary Treatment

Any treatment that involves placement of radioactive sources within an existing body cavity is termed *intracavitary* **treatment.** The most common gynecologic applications of intracavitary therapy involve placement of intrauterine or intravaginal applicators that are subsequently loaded with encapsulated radioactive sources (e.g., ^{137}Cs or ^{192}Ir) (Table 4.1). Applicator systems vary in their appearance and configuration, but those used for radical treatment of cervical or uterine cancer tend to have several features in common. These applicators usually consist of a hollow tube, or **tandem,** and some form of intravaginal receptacle for additional sources. The greatest variation between systems is in the vaginal applicators, which differ in their shape, the orientation of sources, and the presence or absence of shielding (63,64). One applicator that is commonly used to treat intact carcinomas of the cervix is the Fletcher–Suit–Delclos system. Important characteristics of this system are the arrangement of vaginal sources perpendicular to the tandem, and the presence of internal shielding that reduces the dose to the rectum from the vaginal sources by as much as 25%. The Fletcher–Williamson applicator (Fig. 4.10) is similar to the Fletcher–Suit–Delclos applicator but is adapted for use with a stepping source of ^{192}Ir (65). **The vaginal ring applicator is commonly used with HDR systems** and has geometry similar to that of the unshielded Delclos miniovoids used with Fletcher-type applicator systems. Other applicator systems, such as the Delclos dome cylinder, were designed specifically for treatment of the vaginal apex after hysterectomy (66).

Figure 4.11 illustrates a typical pear-shaped isodose distribution produced by a line of intrauterine sources and Fletcher–Suit–Delclos vaginal colpostats loaded with ^{137}Cs. **Intracavitary brachytherapy is useful in the treatment of cervical cancer because it allows a very high dose of radiation to be delivered to a small volume surrounding the applicator** (i.e., the cervix and paracervical

Table 4.1 Isotopes Used in Gynecologic Oncology

Element	Isotope	Half-life	Eγ (MeV)	Eβ (MeV)
Phosphorus	^{32}P	14.3 d	None	1.7 (max)
Iodine	^{125}I	60.2 d	0.028_{avg}	None
	^{131}I	8.06 d	0.08–0.63	0.61 (max)
Cesium	^{137}Cs	30 yrs	0.662	0.514, 1.17
Iridium	^{192}Ir	74 d	0.32–0.61	0.24, 0.67
Gold	^{198}Au	2.7 d	0.41–1.1	0.96 (max)
Radium	^{226}Ra	1,620 yrs	0.19–0.6	3.26 (max)
Cobalt	^{60}Co	5.26 yrs	1.17–1.33	0.313 (max)

Eγ, gamma-ray energy; Eβ, beta-ray energy; MeV, million electron volts.

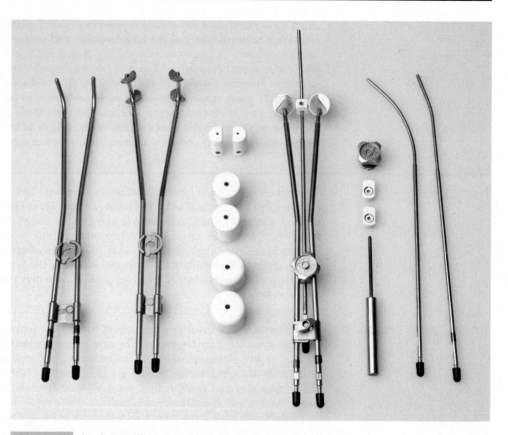

Figure 4.10 Fletcher–Williamson type applicators used for high-dose-rate and pulsed-dose-rate intracavitary applications. Note the tungsten shields located in the inferior-medial position anteriorly and posteriorly in the small (2 cm) ovoid inserts.

tissues) without excessive treatment of normal tissues that are more distant from the sources. Because of the rapid change in dose over short distances, accurate positioning of the intracavitary applicator and sources is very important. Packing or retraction of the bladder and rectum can significantly reduce the dose to portions of these organs by distancing them from the vaginal sources.

To minimize the exposure of medical personnel to radiation, most modern applicator systems are loaded with radioactive sources after adequate positioning is confirmed with anterior–posterior and lateral x-rays of the pelvis. In most cases, remote afterloading devices are used to automatically retract sources from the applicator to a lead-lined safe when someone enters the patient's room, further reducing the radiation exposure to visitors and medical personnel.

Dose Rate

Historically, most brachytherapy has been delivered at a low dose rate, most commonly 40 to 60 cGy per hour. These dose rates take maximum advantage of the dose-rate effect described above, differentially sparing late-responding normal tissues as compared with acutely responding tissues and tumor cells. The dose of LDR intracavitary therapy needed to radically treat cervical cancer is usually delivered in 72 to 96 hours during one or two hospital admissions. Although some investigators have tried to reduce the duration of these treatments by doubling the dose rate (from 40 cGy per hour to 80 cGy per hour), the limited clinical data on this approach suggest that doubling the dose rate results in a less favorable therapeutic ratio (67).

In the past 25 years, the advent of computer-controlled remote afterloading has made it possible to deliver brachytherapy treatments at high dose rates (in minutes rather than hours). HDR treatment may offer practical advantages for the patient because it is typically performed on an outpatient basis, although more applications are usually required. With this technique, a single very high activity source of ^{192}Ir is remotely inserted into the intracavitary applicator. According to the treatment plan, during each treatment the source is advanced in individual "steps" to deliver radiation throughout the treatment volume. Because of the high activity of the source (usually about 10 Ci), treatment must be delivered in a heavily shielded room, and strict safety and quality assurance standards must be met.

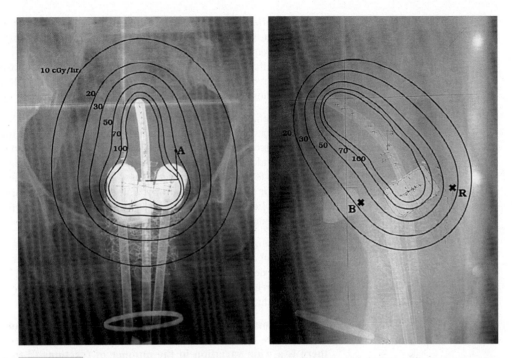

Figure 4.11 Posterior–anterior and lateral views of a Fletcher–Suit–Delclos applicator system loaded with ^{137}Cs sources for treatment of invasive cervical cancer. Units on the isodose contours are cGy per hour. Point A *(A)*, bladder *(B)*, and rectal *(R)* reference points are indicated on the figure. (From **Eifel PJ, Berek JS, Thigpen JT**. Cancer of the cervix, vagina, and vulva. In: **DeVita V, Hellman S, Rosenberg S, eds.** *Cancer: Principles and Practice of Oncology.* Philadelphia, PA: JB Lippincott Co.; 2001;1526–1556, with permission).

HDR therapy has gained steadily in popularity over the past 20 years, particularly for intracavitary gynecologic applications. This is partly because of the practical advantages for physicians who center most of their practice in an outpatient setting, but another factor has been the recent interruption in the supply of cesium sources suitable for LDR gynecologic brachytherapy. Some clinicians remain reluctant to change to HDR therapy because of the **theoretical radiobiologic disadvantages of large-fraction irradiation and the absence of well-controlled randomized clinical trials comparing HDR and LDR regimens** (68). Other practical considerations have led most US radiation oncologists to move to HDR brachytherapy.

An alternative to HDR therapy that is commonly used in Europe but has only recently been introduced in the United States is pulsed-dose-rate (PDR) brachytherapy. With this approach, treatment is given in intermittent pulses, using a single stepping source of ^{192}Ir, which is similar to, but lower in activity than, the source used for HDR brachytherapy. If treatment is delivered in hourly pulses of 40 to 50 cGy, the tissue sparing should be nearly identical to that achieved with LDR brachytherapy.

PDR holds several advantages over true LDR brachytherapy. The sources are readily obtainable, patients are able to receive nursing care and have visitors as they wish during the intervals between pulses, and the stepping source method permits somewhat more flexibility in treatment planning. The equipment can be used for either interstitial or intracavitary brachytherapy, and because the applicators are identical to those used for HDR brachytherapy, clinicians who choose to have both options available to their patients require only one set of applicators.

The total brachytherapy dose to point A must be reduced to convert from LDR to HDR regimens. The appropriate dose and dose per fraction are based on calculations of the estimated biologically effective dose (BED) for tumor and normal tissues. BED is derived from the linear-quadratic formula described earlier in this chapter and is equal to the total nominal dose (nd) times the relative effectiveness: **BED = (nd) × (1 + d/[α/β])**, where d is the dose per fraction. For example, assuming α/β values of 10 and 3 for tumor and for normal tissues, respectively, a fractionation scheme in which a total dose of 30 Gy is given in five fractions of 6 Gy each would result in:

$$\text{Tumor BED} = (30) \times (1 + 6/10) = 48 \text{ Gy}_{10}$$

$$\text{Normal tissue BED} = (30) \times (1 + 6/3) = 90 \text{ Gy}_3$$

Clinicians often express these doses in the more familiar terms of the equivalent dose at 2 Gy per fraction, which is equal to BED/(1 + 2/[α/β]). Using this calculation, the above example would yield equivalent doses of 40 and 54 Gy, respectively, for tumor and normal tissues. In other words, the effect on normal tissues is about 35% greater than would be expected from the same tumor-effective dose given at 2 Gy per fraction or with LDR brachytherapy (which, at 40 to 45 cGy per hour, has an effect similar to that of a dose divided in 2-Gy fractions).

This differential effect would make HDR unacceptable if the normal tissues received the same dose as tumor. With good applicator positioning, effective packing of the bladder and rectum, and optimal source positioning, the total dose and dose per fraction delivered to normal tissues are usually considerably lower than those delivered to tumor, making it possible to achieve a ratio of tumor effect to normal tissue effect that is similar to what is achieved with LDR. **If the tumor is very large or the vaginal anatomy is unfavorable, the nominal doses to tumor and normal tissues may be similar;** in these cases, patients may be more effectively treated with LDR, PDR, or a larger than usual number of HDR fractions (68–71).

It is important that dose fractionation schemes used for HDR therapy be designed to produce tumor control and complication rates approximately equivalent to those seen with LDR therapy. The optimal dose per fraction for HDR therapy is unknown and is probably patient specific but, in general, increasing the number of fractions and concomitantly decreasing the dose per fraction appear to reduce the rate of moderate and severe complications (72,73).

The most common HDR regimen used for the treatment of cervical cancer in the United States is five fractions of 5.5 to 6 Gy each to point A after 45 Gy to the pelvis, although there is a wide variation in the number of fractions (2 to 13) and the dose per fraction (3 to 9 Gy) (62,73).

During the past 5 to 10 years, clinicians have begun to more effectively integrate sophisticated imaging into the brachytherapy planning process. Most radiation therapy simulators are now based on CT rather than fluoroscopic or plain images. Many facilities use intraoperative ultrasonography to confirm correct positioning of applicators, and increasingly MRI is being used to delineate target volumes and critical structures (Fig. 4.12).

The extent to which these resources are exploited in brachytherapy planning varies between facilities. At a minimum, ultrasonography, CT, or MRI can be used to rule out uterine perforations, which, if undetected, can lead to life-threatening complications. Clinicians are increasingly exploring the use of true three-dimensional image-guided brachytherapy planning based on CT or MRI of the pelvis with the applicators in place. Tumor volumes and critical structures are contoured as is done with modern external beam radiation therapy planning. The application of these methods in brachytherapy is complex because of the heterogeneous distribution of radiation doses around the brachytherapy sources. Although the transition to image-guided brachytherapy needs to be implemented with caution, there is reason to hope that the greater understanding of anatomical relationships obtained with image-based planning will improve future disease control rates and decrease the complication rates (74,75).

Interstitial Implants

Interstitial brachytherapy refers to the placement of radioactive sources within tissues. Various sources of radiation—such as ^{192}Ir, ^{198}Au, ^{103}Pd, and ^{125}I—may be obtained as radioactive wires or seeds. ^{192}Ir may be obtained as separate sources that are usually distributed at regular intervals (usually 1 cm) in Teflon tubes or as wires with activity specified in terms of the mCi per centimeters. Sources may be positioned in the tumor or tumor bed in a variety of ways:

1. **Permanent seed implants (usually ^{125}I, ^{103}Pd, or ^{198}Au)** can be inserted using a specialized seed inserter. These implants are most commonly used to treat prostate cancer but are sometimes used to treat pelvic or aortic lymph nodes, particularly in the case of nodal recurrence after irradiation.

2. **Temporary Teflon catheter implants** can be placed intraoperatively and subsequently loaded with radioactive sources (usually ^{192}Ir). These are sometimes used to treat tumor beds (76).

3. **Temporary transperineal template-guided interstitial needle implants** can be placed using a Lucite template with regularly spaced holes and a central obturator that can hold a tandem or additional needles. Needles are afterloaded, usually with ^{192}Ir. These implants are used to treat vaginal and some cervical tumors (77–79). In some cases,

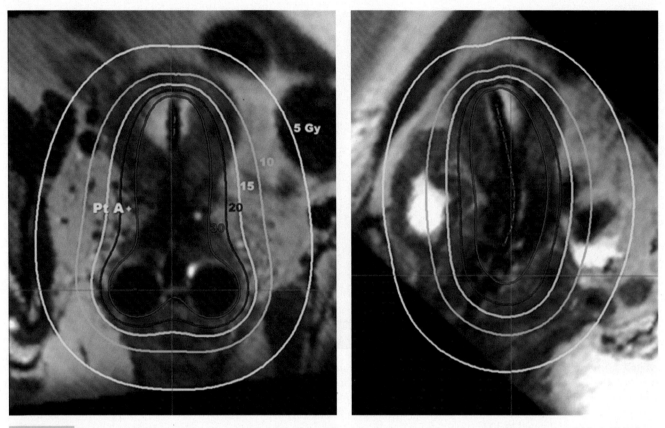

Figure 4.12 Reconstructed coronal and sagittal MRI views through the approximate center of the uterus with a Fletcher–Williamson applicator in place. Numbers represent the total doses delivered during a 48-hour pulsed-dose-rate treatment. Note the high dose delivered to the central cervical tumor and the rapid fall-off of dose close to the sources. Although lateral structures receive a much lower dose of radiation, the obturator nodal region (visible at the edge of the coronal view) received approximately 5 Gy from this first of two planned implants. This dose must be considered in planning boosts that may be required for any involved nodes in this region.

particularly for treatment of apical vaginal lesions, guidance by laparoscopy or laparotomy may facilitate needle placement (80).

4. **Temporary transperineal implants can be placed freehand,** an approach that may allow better control of needle placement in selected cases. Freehand implants are particularly useful for treating urethral and vaginal tumors (Fig. 4.13) (18,81).

Most gynecologic interstitial implants are temporary LDR implants. Although HDR techniques may be used for some interstitial treatments, the very close proximity of bladder, rectum, and other hollow viscera makes it particularly difficult to achieve adequate doses to tumors involving the vagina, urethra, or vulva without exposing critical structures to unacceptably high fractional doses. Like intracavitary therapy, interstitial therapy delivers a relatively high dose of radiation to a small volume, sparing the surrounding normal tissues. However, **the risk to normal tissues adjacent to the tumor or in the tumor bed may still be significant, particularly if the needle placement is inaccurate.**

Some investigators have advocated the use of template-guided interstitial brachytherapy to treat difficult cases of locally advanced cervical cancer (Fig. 4.14) (82,83). The ability to place sources in the lateral parametrium with this technique suggests a theoretical advantage over intracavitary treatment for patients with pelvic sidewall involvement. Some investigators have claimed high local control rates with this approach (82,83). Survival rates are not clearly superior to those achieved with combined external beam and intracavitary therapy, and the risk of major complications may be greater (78,79).

The radiation oncology community remains polarized as to the appropriateness of interstitial therapy for patients with intact cervical carcinomas and as yet no randomized trials have been conducted to compare the therapeutic ratio of conventional intracavitary irradiation with that of interstitial treatment. Interstitial implants may be used for a variety of other

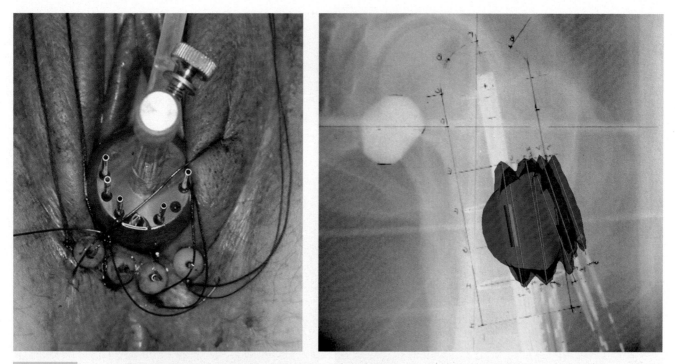

Figure 4.13 Interstitial implant for a stage II distal vaginal cancer. Needles are individually inserted transperineally; a finger is placed in the vagina while the needles are inserted to monitor the position of each needle relative to the tumor and mucosal surface. **Left:** A Lucite cylinder in the vagina displaces uninvolved vagina from the needles and has channels for additional sources at the periphery of the cylinder. **Right:** Postoperative radiographs show placement of the needles with a superimposed dose cloud that encloses the volume treated to 30 Gy.

gynecologic indications, including vaginal cancer, vaginal recurrence of cervical or endometrial cancer, and urethral cancer.

Intraperitoneal Radioisotopes

Intraperitoneal radioisotopes have been used to treat epithelial ovarian cancer in an effort to address the transperitoneal spread of the disease (84). Radioactive chromic phosphate (^{32}P) has largely replaced colloidal gold (^{198}Au) for peritoneal treatment. The longer half-life (14.3 days), pure β decay, and higher mean energy (0.698 MeV) of ^{32}P yield slightly longer exposures, fewer radiation protection problems, and deeper tissue penetration than what is observed with ^{198}Au.

If a radioisotope is evenly distributed within the peritoneum, it is theoretically possible to irradiate the entire peritoneal surface. However, the pattern of energy deposition within the abdomen and the dose delivered beneath the peritoneal surfaces depend on many factors, including the physical characteristics of the isotope used, the energies of its decay products, and the distribution of the isotope within the peritoneal cavity. **In practice, isotope is seldom distributed uniformly to the peritoneal and omental surfaces** (85). Postsurgical adhesions may limit the free flow of fluid, and this nonuniform distribution may result in underdosage of some peritoneal sites and overdosage of some normal tissues. This may result in unacceptable complications, particularly if intraperitoneal isotope therapy and external beam irradiation are combined (86). Although randomized studies have demonstrated similar survival rates for patients with early ovarian cancer treated with ^{32}P or single-agent chemotherapy, the role of intraperitoneal treatment has not been clearly established (87), and this approach is rarely used today.

Clinical Uses of Radiation

Cervical Cancer

Although specific radiation-therapy techniques may vary, the curative treatment of cervical cancer usually includes a combination of external pelvic irradiation and brachytherapy,

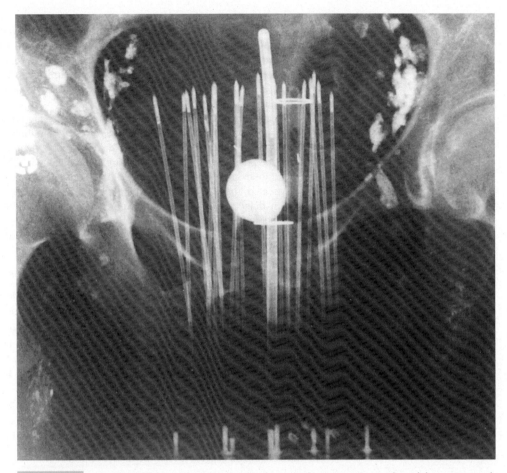

Figure 4.14 Interstitial implant for an advanced cervical cancer. (Reproduced from Dr. Mark Schray, Division of Radiation Oncology, Mayo Clinic, with permission.)

often with concurrent chemotherapy. The goal of radiation therapy is to eliminate cancer in the cervix, paracervical tissues, and regional lymph nodes (63). All of these regions can be encompassed in a pelvic radiation field. The dose that can be delivered to the pelvis is limited by the tolerance of intrapelvic normal tissues, most importantly the rectosigmoid, bladder, and small bowel. Because the bulkiest tumor is usually in the cervix, this region typically requires higher doses than the rest of the pelvis to achieve locoregional control. It is usually possible to deliver these high doses with intracavitary therapy.

Patients with International Federation of Gynecology and Obstetrics (FIGO) stage IA1 disease and some patients with stage IA2 disease can be treated with intracavitary irradiation alone. Patients with higher stage cancers have a sufficiently high risk of metastasis to the pelvic lymph nodes to justify a course of external beam irradiation to sterilize possible microscopic regional disease. For most patients with locally advanced cervical cancers, an initial course of treatment is given with external beam irradiation and concurrent chemotherapy. Four to five weeks (40 to 45 Gy) of chemoradiation usually decreases endocervical disease and shrinks exophytic tumor, facilitating optimal intracavitary therapy. The dose to the central tumor is supplemented with one or two LDR intracavitary treatments or with a variable number of HDR treatments. If the initial tumor volume is small or there is an excellent tumor response to external beam irradiation and concurrent chemotherapy, brachytherapy may be given earlier in the patient's treatment. Because the number of brachytherapy treatments is greater with HDR therapy than with LDR therapy, practitioners who use the HDR approach often begin brachytherapy before external beam therapy is completed, if the initial tumor response has been adequate. The balance between external beam and intracavitary therapy may vary somewhat according to the tumor extent (63). Several studies have suggested that intracavitary therapy is critically important to successful treatment, even for patients with very bulky stage IIIB tumors (1,88).

External Beam Irradiation

Typical external beam fields are designed to include the primary tumor, paracervical tissues, and iliac and presacral lymph nodes, all with 1.5- to 2-cm margins. If the common iliac or aortic nodes are involved, the treatment fields are usually extended to include at least the lower para-aortic region. Every effort should be made to minimize the high-dose treatment volume while adequately encompassing the tumor and its regional lymph nodes. Using four beams (anterior, posterior, and right and left lateral) rather than an opposed pair of anterior and posterior beams (Fig. 4.8) can reduce the volume of tissue irradiated to a high dose. Great care must be taken not to shield the primary tumor, uterosacral disease, or external iliac nodes when lateral fields are used (89,90). For some patients with locally advanced tumors, the amount of tissue spared with lateral fields may be relatively small after these areas are included. The additional bone marrow treated with lateral fields may be a consideration if chemotherapy is part of the treatment plan. When the pelvis is treated after hysterectomy, four or more fields usually produce a more favorable dose distribution than two opposed fields. Some clinicians advocated the use of highly conformal radiation-therapy techniques such as IMRT to treat the whole pelvis (91). When these highly conformal techniques are used, particular care must be taken to adequately cover the target volume and account for tumor response and internal organ motion.

The borders of the typical anterior–posterior and posterior–anterior pelvic fields are as follows:

1. **Inferior**—at the midpubis or 3 to 4 cm below the most distal disease in the cervix or vagina (usually demonstrated using a radiopaque vaginal marker).

2. **Superior**—at the L4–L5 interface or at the bifurcation of the aorta so that the common iliac nodes are encompassed. For patients with very small tumors that are at minimal risk for extensive nodal spread, the upper border may be placed at the L5–S1 interface. For patients who have lymph node involvement, the field may be extended to include para-aortic nodes.

3. **Lateral**—1.5 to 2 cm lateral to the pelvic lymph nodes as contoured on a CT scan, or at least 1 cm lateral to the margins of the bony pelvis. Appropriate shielding along the common iliac nodes decreases the amount of sigmoid and small bowel in the field.

The borders of the typical lateral fields are as follows:

1. **Inferior and superior**—same as the borders described above for anterior–posterior and posterior–anterior pelvic fields.

2. **Anterior**—1.5 to 2 cm anterior to the iliac nodes. Inferiorly, the field usually splits the pubis to achieve adequate coverage of the distal obturator/hypogastric nodes. In most cases, the field should be designed to include the entire uterus, taking into account possible intratreatment motion.

3. **Posterior**—1.5 to 2 cm posterior to the iliac nodes. This usually places the posterior border at the posterior margin of S1–S3. Caudad to S3, the field must be designed to encompass the cervix and vagina, again taking into account possible intratreatment motion.

For patients who have grossly enlarged lymph nodes, extensive paracervical disease, or other disease that is inadequately covered by brachytherapy, additional treatment may be given using reduced external beam fields. These are called "boosts." These boosts must be carefully planned, taking into consideration the estimated dose delivered to these regions from brachytherapy.

Intracavitary Brachytherapy for Cervical Cancer

The total doses of radiation to the central tumor and regional nodes are tailored according to the amount of disease in those sites (74,75,92). A number of methods have been used to prescribe and specify the doses delivered with intracavitary therapy. **Most radiation oncologists specify treatment using some variation of the Manchester system, which uses two primary reference points** (Fig. 4.11):

1. **Point A**—a point 2 cm lateral and 2 cm superior to the external cervical os in the plane of the implant.

2. **Point B**—a point 3 cm lateral to point A.

Although the doses from intracavitary and external beam radiation therapy may not be biologically equivalent (particularly with HDR therapy), these doses are frequently summed to determine the total doses to points A and B. **The total dose to point A (from external beam and LDR** intracavitary therapy) believed to be adequate to achieve central disease control is usually between 75 Gy (for small stage IB1 cancers) and 90 Gy (for bulky or locally advanced disease). The prescribed dose to point B is 45 to 65 Gy, depending on the extent of parametrial and sidewall disease.

Prescription and treatment planning cannot be limited to specification of the dose to these reference points. Other factors that should be considered include the following:

1. The position and length of the intrauterine tandem, which influence the loading of the tandem.
2. The type and position of vaginal applicators, which influence the loading of the vaginal applicators.
3. The quality of the vaginal packing.
4. The size of the central tumor before and after external beam treatment.
5. The vaginal surface dose (usually limited to 120 to 140 cGy).
6. The proximity of the system to the bladder and rectum.
7. The dose rate (or fraction size).

A number of methods and reference doses have been described to estimate the maximum dose to the bladder and rectum on the basis of orthogonal reference films of the implants. **The most common method for specifying normal tissue doses is to calculate the doses to reference points defined by the International Commission on Radiation Units and Measurements** (Fig. 4.11) (93). Using this method, the bladder reference point is placed at the posterior edge of a Foley bulb filled with 7 cc of contrast material; the rectal point is located 5 mm posterior to the vaginal applicator or packing (whichever is most posterior) at the level of the vaginal sources. Three-dimensional reconstructions of intracavitary placements suggest that most methods that use orthogonal x-rays to estimate the dose to normal structures tend to underestimate the true maximum dose (94).

Image-guided techniques permit much more precise estimates of the doses to critical structures. A variety of methods have been proposed for reporting critical structure doses using advanced imaging. The method that has been most actively studied involves estimating the minimum dose to the most irradiated 2-cc volume ($D_{2\,cc}$) of rectum, bladder, and sigmoid (95). Estimates of critical structure doses, particularly bladder doses, tend to be much higher with this method than with traditional reference points, suggesting that these tissues may tolerate higher doses than was once believed. However, clinicians are still learning how to use these estimates in decision making.

Some centers that use LDR brachytherapy document the total milligram-Radium-equivalent hours (mgRaEq-hr) of each intracavitary system. This number, obtained by multiplying the mgRaEq of cesium or radium in the system by the number of hours the radioactive sources are left in place, cannot be used as the sole measure of any treatment, but is sometimes used to limit the total integral dose to the pelvis. The doses to points at a substantial distance from the system are roughly proportional to the total mgRaEq-hr because as the distance increases, the dose rate approaches that from a single point source of similar activity. In general, after 40 to 45 Gy of external beam irradiation, the total mgRaEq-hr (from intracavitary radiation therapy given at 40 to 60 cGy/hr) should not exceed 6,000 to 6,500 mgRaEq-hr. **An alternative measure is the reference air kerma, defined as the total dose delivered at 1 meter from the center of the activity and measured in μGy m²;** this unit serves the same purpose as mgRaEq-hr but can be used with isotopes other than radium or cesium.

There is a growing movement toward the use of image-guided brachytherapy, with treatment planning based on CT or MRI images obtained with the implant in place (Fig. 4.12) (74,75). Ideally, image-guided brachytherapy would include true three-dimensional imaging and calculations of the distribution of dose to tumor and normal tissues with accompanying dose limits derived from clinically derived dose-effect data. There are very few clinical data derived from patients treated with image-guided brachytherapy; logistical problems create significant impediments to true image-guided brachytherapy.

Results of Treatment

Radiation therapy is extremely effective in the treatment of stage IB1 cervical cancer, producing central and pelvic disease control rates of greater than 98% and greater than 95%, respectively, and disease-specific survival rates of approximately 90% (2,4). Pelvic control rates decrease as tumor size and FIGO stage increase, although large single institution experiences report 5-year pelvic control rates of 60–70% and 5-year disease-specific survival rates of 40–50% even for bulky stage IIIB cancers treated with radiation alone, before routine use of concurrent chemotherapy (1,2). That such large tumors can be controlled even half the time with radiation therapy alone reflects the remarkable effectiveness of carefully planned combinations of external beam and intracavitary radiation therapy.

During the past decade, studies have demonstrated a significant improvement in pelvic disease control and survival when *cisplatin*-**containing chemotherapy has been delivered concurrently with radiation for patients with locoregionally advanced cervical cancer** (96–100). Several of the regimens tested in these studies have included *5-fluorouracil*. This drug is known to be a potent radiation sensitizer, which is particularly effective in the treatment of gastrointestinal malignancies, but its contribution to chemoradiation in patients with carcinoma of the cervix is uncertain. Other randomized trials have suggested that *mitomycin C* (101,102), *epirubicin* (103), and *gemcitabine* (104) may improve outcomes when they are delivered concurrently with radiation to patients with locally advanced cervical cancer.

Adjuvant Pelvic Radiation Therapy after Radical Hysterectomy

For patients with stage IB and IIA cervical cancer treated with radical hysterectomy and pelvic lymphadenectomy, lymph node involvement is probably the strongest predictor of local recurrence and death. Retrospective studies from the late 1980s reported that patients with nodal involvement had survival rates of only 50–60% of those with negative nodes (105,106). With modern postoperative chemoradiation, these results have improved (99,107), but lymph node involvement is still associated with an increased rate of distant metastasis. Parametrial involvement and involvement of surgical margins also predict a high rate of pelvic recurrence and are considered to be indications for postoperative irradiation.

In 2000, the Southwest Oncology Group published results of a study comparing postoperative radiation with combined chemoradiation in patients who had positive lymph nodes, parametrium, or surgical margins; the study demonstrated a 50% reduction in the risk of recurrence when *cisplatin* and *fluorouracil* were added to pelvic irradiation (99).

For patients with negative nodes but high-risk primary tumor features (i.e., tumor size >4 cm, deep stromal invasion, or vascular space involvement), studies of postoperative irradiation have demonstrated a significant reduction in the risk of recurrence (7,107).

The drawback of adjuvant pelvic radiation therapy is a somewhat greater risk of major complications than with surgery alone or radiation alone (5,7,107).

Recurrent Cervical Cancer

Patients who have an isolated pelvic recurrence after radical hysterectomy can sometimes be treated successfully with aggressive radiation therapy. The prognosis is best for patients with an isolated central recurrence that is not fixed to the pelvic wall and does not involve pelvic nodes. These patients have 5-year survival rates as high as 60–70% (108). For patients whose tumor involves the pelvic wall or lymph nodes, most reported 5-year survival rates have been between 20% and 30% following treatment with radiation alone (109–111). Some groups have reported encouraging results with combined chemoradiation (109). It probably is reasonable to extrapolate from randomized trials that demonstrate improved survival with concurrent chemoradiation for locally advanced cervical cancer to justify a similar approach in patients with pelvic recurrences, although reports have so far been largely anecdotal (110,112).

Some patients who have an isolated locoregional recurrence outside the prior pelvic radiation field can be cured with definitive radiation therapy. IMRT is particularly useful in the treatment of these complex cases.

Complications

Late complications of radical irradiation for cervical cancer occur in 5–15% of patients and are related to the dose per fraction, the total dose administered, and the volume irradiated (110). Patient factors such as a history of pelvic infection, heavy smoking, previous abdominal surgery, and diabetes mellitus may increase the risk of complications (56,111). The positioning of the intracavitary system may influence the risk of complications. Late effects may be seen in the bladder (hematuria, fibrosis and contraction, or fistulas) and in the rectosigmoid or terminal ileum (bleeding, stricture, obstruction, or perforation). Agglutination of the apex of the vagina is common. Severe vaginal shortening is less common and is probably correlated with the patient's age, menopausal status and sexual activity, and with the initial extent of disease (112,113). Our understanding of the factors influencing sexual dysfunction in patients treated for cervical cancer is incomplete. Most gastrointestinal complications occur within 30 months of radiation therapy, although late effects may occur many years after treatment (113).

In the United States, **late complications of radiation therapy (occurring more than 90 days after treatment) are usually scored according to the Radiation Therapy Oncology Group/ European Organization for Research and Treatment of Cancer Late Radiation Morbidity Scheme,** which is part of the National Cancer Institute's system for reporting of adverse events (Table 4.2). With today's multimodality treatments, several factors may contribute to adverse events. In Europe, many groups use the Franco-Italian Glossary, a scoring system that incorporates early and late surgical and radiation-related side effects (114).

Palliation

Radiation therapy plays an important role in the palliation of metastatic cervical cancer. Short courses of palliative irradiation, such as 2,000 cGy in five fractions or 3,000 cGy in 10 fractions, usually will alleviate symptoms related to bony metastases or para-aortic nodal disease. Such treatment may relieve symptoms related to pressure from enlarging mediastinal or supraclavicular nodal disease.

Endometrial Cancer

The role of radiation therapy in the treatment of endometrial carcinoma is a subject of considerable controversy and is discussed in greater detail in Chapter 10. **Indications for radiation therapy in the treatment of endometrial cancer are as follows:**

1. **Adjuvant treatment to prevent locoregional recurrence** after hysterectomy and bilateral salpingo-oophorectomy.

2. **Preoperative treatment for patients with very extensive cervical stromal involvement.**

3. **Curative treatment for some patients with medical problems that preclude surgery** and for occasional patients with stage III disease involving the vagina.

4. **Curative treatment for patients with isolated vaginal or pelvic recurrence,** usually using a combination of external beam and intracavitary or interstitial radiation therapy.

5. **Palliative treatment of massive pelvic or metastatic disease.**

In the past, disease confined to the uterus was often treated with preoperative intracavitary radiation therapy. An intracavitary line source was placed in the uterus, or the uterus was packed with multiple radium (Heyman's) capsules or cesium (Simon's) capsules (115). Preoperative irradiation reduced the risk of vaginal apex recurrence, but was never proven to improve survival, although no randomized studies were ever done to compare preoperative and postoperative irradiation (116,117). **Because tailored postoperative irradiation appears to achieve similar pelvic control rates and avoids unnecessary overtreatment of patients whose hysterectomy findings predict a negligible risk of recurrence, preoperative irradiation has been abandoned for most patients** (116,118,119).

Most patients with stage I endometrial cancer have minimally invasive grade 1 to 2 tumors, which rarely recur after hysterectomy alone, and usually need no additional treatment. The use of adjuvant pelvic radiation therapy is usually confined to patients with multiple high-risk features, particularly those with deeply invasive lesions or other high-risk findings at surgery (e.g., lymph node involvement or cervical stromal involvement) (9,116,118,119).

Adjuvant pelvic radiation therapy reduces the risk of pelvic recurrence, but was never proven to improve survival. In 2004, the Gynecologic Oncology Group reported results of a randomized trial addressing this question in patients with intermediate-risk FIGO stage I cancers (9). This study demonstrated a reduction in the overall risk of pelvic (particularly vaginal) recurrence without a significant difference in overall survival for patients who received postoperative pelvic radiation therapy. However, using subset analysis, the authors identified a subset of patients with high-intermediate-risk disease who may benefit from adjuvant radiation therapy. In another randomized trial, Creutzberg et al. (11) found that postoperative radiation therapy reduced the risk of pelvic recurrence but had no significant impact on survival. Both of these trials included a large number of patients who had relatively favorable findings (grade 1 disease or <50% invasion); **neither trial included a sufficient number of patients who had grade 3 tumors or deep myometrial invasion**

Table 4.2 RTOG and EORTC Late Radiation Morbidity Scoring Scheme[a]

Adverse Event[b]	Grade				
	0	**1**	**2**	**3**	**4**
Bladder	No change from baseline	Slight epithelial atrophy; minor telangiectasia (microscopic hematuria)	Moderate frequency; generalized telangiectasia; intermittent macroscopic hematuria	Severe frequency and dysuria; severe generalized telangiectasia (often with petechiae); frequent hematuria; reduction in bladder capacity (<150 mL)	Necrosis; contracted bladder (capacity <100 mL), severe hemorrhagic cystitis, fistula
Bone	No change from baseline	Asymptomatic; reduced bone density	Moderate pain or tenderness; irregular bone sclerosis	Severe pain or tenderness; dense bone sclerosis	Necrosis; spontaneous fracture
Joint	No change from baseline	Mild joint stiffness; slight limitation of movement	Moderate stiffness; intermittent or moderate joint pain; moderate limitation of movement	Severe joint stiffness; pain with severe limitation of movement	Necrosis; complete fixation
Kidney	No change from baseline	Transient albuminuria; no hypertension; mild impairment of renal function; urea 25–35 mg%; creatinine 1.5–2 mg%; creatinine clearance >75%	Persistent moderate albuminuria (2+); mild hypertension; no related anemia; moderate impairment of renal function; urea. >36–60 mg%; creatinine clearance >50–74%	Severe albuminuria; severe hypertension; persistent anemia (<10 g%; severe renal failure; urea >60 mg%; creatinine clearance <50%)	Malignant hypertension; uremic coma; urea >100 mg%
Liver	No change from baseline	Mild lassitude; nausea; dyspepsia; slightly abnormal liver function	Moderate symptoms; some abnormal liver function tests; serum albumin normal	Disabling hepatic insufficiency; liver function tests grossly abnormal; low albumin; edema or ascites	Necrosis; hepatic coma or encephalopathy
Vagina	No change from baseline	Partial stenosis or shortening but less than complete occlusion	Complete occlusion; telangiectasis with frequent bleeding	Radionecrotic ulcer	Fistula to bladder, bowel, or peritoneal cavity
Small, large intestine	No change from baseline	Mild diarrhea; mild cramping; bowel movement ≥5 × daily; slight rectal discharge or bleeding	Moderate diarrhea and colic; bowel movement >5 × daily; excessive rectal mucus or intermittent bleeding	Obstruction or bleeding, requiring surgery	Necrosis; perforation fistula
Spinal cord	No change from baseline	Mild Lhermitte's syndrome	Severe Lhermitte's syndrome	Objective neurologic findings at or below cord level treatment	Mono-, para-, quadriplegia
Subcutaneous tissue	No change from baseline	Slight induration (fibrosis) and loss of subcutaneous fat	Moderate fibrosis but asymptomatic; slight field contracture; <10% linear reduction	Severe induration and loss of subcutaneous tissue; field contracture; >10% linear reduction	Necrosis

[a]Used for adverse events occurring more than 90 days after radiation therapy.

[b]Includes sites most pertinent to treatment of gynecologic malignancies.

RTOG, Radiation Therapy Oncology Group; EORTC, European Organization for Research and Treatment of Cancer.

to rule out clinically important differences in these subgroups. In a subsequent trial, Nout et al. (120) reported no significant difference in survival for patients treated with adjuvant pelvic irradiation or vaginal cuff irradiation; although this study was intended to include relatively high intermediate risk cancers, subsequent pathology review suggested that the patients in this trial had a much lower risk of recurrence than those in the Gynecologic Oncology Group high-intermediate-risk group (9).

Uterine serous cancers are associated with a particularly poor prognosis and tend to spread intraperitoneally in a manner similar to that seen with ovarian cancers. Whole abdominal irradiation may be a valuable treatment for some such patients who have minimal residual disease after hysterectomy (121,122), although many groups favor the use of adjuvant chemotherapy, with or without local radiation therapy, for this group of patients.

For patients with endometrial cancer, the potential benefit of adjuvant treatment must be balanced against the risk of complications for each patient (123). Extensive staging lymphadenectomy appears to increase the risk of serious bowel complications after radiation therapy (124,125).

Ovarian Cancer

In the 1980s, several independent investigators demonstrated that whole abdominal and pelvic irradiation was potentially curative for certain subsets of patients with epithelial ovarian cancer (126–128). Survival rates were strongly correlated with the initial disease stage and volume of residual disease. Although these results were encouraging, the subsequent development of increasingly successful chemotherapeutic treatments consigned radiation therapy for ovarian cancer to a largely palliative role.

One major limitation of the use of whole abdominal irradiation in the treatment of müllerian carcinomas is the radiosensitivity of normal tissues in the upper abdomen (e.g., kidney, liver, bowel, and spinal cord), which prevents delivery of more than approximately 22 to 30 Gy to the whole abdomen. This dose is inadequate to control areas of gross or even extensive microscopic disease.

Several investigators have evaluated the use of whole abdominal irradiation after chemotherapy. A retrospective analysis of the Toronto data suggested an improved outcome for high-risk patients treated with sequential chemotherapy and whole abdominal irradiation when compared with historical controls treated with radiation alone (129). However, three randomized studies comparing chemotherapy alone with multimodality treatment (130–132) reported disappointing results. Some patients with minimal residual disease may benefit, but **in general the data do not support routine use of sequential chemotherapy and abdominopelvic irradiation.** Poor tolerance after extensive chemotherapy and the possible induction of accelerated repopulation of resistant clonogens during treatment are among the reasons suggested for the failure of this approach in most studies (126,133,134).

Occasionally, patients who have localized recurrences may experience prolonged disease-free survival after localized radical radiation therapy. Patients who have initially platinum-sensitive disease and who have isolated recurrences in the pelvis or lymph nodes tend to be good candidates for second-line radiation therapy (17). Patients with clear cell carcinoma appear to have particularly favorable outcomes after second-line radiation therapy, although long-term disease-free intervals have also been observed in patients with other histologic types (17).

Radiation therapy may be helpful in the palliation of pain, bleeding, or other symptoms of ovarian cancer.

Vulvar Cancer

The role of radiation therapy in the treatment of vulvar cancer has expanded dramatically during the past 25 years. Improved radiation-therapy equipment and techniques have reduced the toxicity that discouraged early attempts to treat the vulva with radiation, and prospective studies have increased interest in this modality. In particular, a landmark randomized study published by Homesley et al. (21) in 1986 demonstrated a marked improvement in survival when patients with positive lymph nodes were treated with pelvic and inguinal irradiation after vulvectomy and lymphadenectomy. The role of radiation for treatment of vulvar cancer is explored in more detail in Chapter 13.

In brief, **the possible benefits of radiation therapy in the treatment of vulvar cancer** include (i) reduced risk of regional recurrence and improved survival in patients with **inguinal node metastases** (21); (ii) reduced risk of vulvar recurrence in patients with **positive surgical margins, multiple local recurrences,** or other high-risk features (135,136); and (iii) **avoidance of exenterative surgery in patients whose disease involves the anus or urethra** (137). Radiation therapy may be an alternative to inguinal lymphadenectomy in selected patients with clinically negative groins (22,138).

Several reports have emphasized the critical importance of careful radiation-therapy technique in treating patients with vulvar cancer (22,138,139). A number of approaches have been developed to decrease the dose to the femoral heads from groin irradiation. In most cases, adequate coverage of the volume at risk is readily achieved without risking serious femoral morbidity. This can only be accomplished with detailed CT-based treatment planning.

In general, the total dose of radiation should be tailored to the amount of residual disease, with doses of approximately 45 to 50 Gy for microscopic disease and 60 Gy or higher for positive margins, extracapsular nodal extension, or macroscopic residual disease.

When necessary, the dose to portions of the vulva at high risk for recurrence can be "boosted" with an *en face* electron field. This approach minimizes the amount of tissue exposed to high doses and thereby reduces acute skin reactions. **Carefully designed IMRT may be useful in selected cases.** The techniques required for effective vulvar IMRT are complex, requiring a detailed understanding of the three-dimensional anatomy of this region and specialized treatment planning techniques. **Bolus may be needed to increase the dose to superficial tissues in the "build-up region" of photon and low-energy electron beams. Treatment interruptions should be minimized** to avoid possible tumor proliferation during breaks in radiation therapy.

The use of concurrent "sensitizing" chemotherapy (e.g., continuous-infusion *fluorouracil* or *cisplatin*) to improve control rates has been explored in a number of uncontrolled studies (140–146). The encouraging response rates and long-term control of gross disease reported in these trials and the successful use of chemoradiation in cervical and anal cancer are bound to increase interest in this approach.

Acute moist desquamation of the skin of the inguinal creases and vulva is expected. Symptoms may be reduced with careful local care, sitz baths, avoidance of tight clothing, and immediate treatment of superimposed fungal or bacterial infections. Superinfection with *Candida* species is particularly frequent during treatment. **Late complications may include lymphedema, particularly after radical groin dissection. Atrophy, telangiectasia, and fibrosis of the skin or subcutaneous tissues can occur** and may be related to the daily fraction size and total dose, tissue destruction from tumor, and the extent of local surgery.

Vaginal Cancer

Although small apical vaginal lesions can sometimes be resected, the intimate relationship of the vagina to the bladder and rectum usually makes it impossible to perform curative surgical resection of vaginal lesions without sacrificing those organs. For this reason, **most patients who have invasive vaginal cancers are treated with radiation therapy, which achieves cure rates that are, stage for stage, similar to those achieved with radiation therapy for patients with cervical cancer** (18,19,147). Treatment usually consists of a combination of external beam irradiation and brachytherapy. Interstitial or intracavitary techniques may be used, depending on the size and site of the primary lesion and its response to external beam therapy (Fig. 4.13). Because the dose gradient from intracavitary therapy is very steep, interstitial techniques are usually used to treat tumors that are more than 3 to 5 mm thick. Tumors that are very advanced, diffuse, or fixed, or that extensively involve the rectovaginal septum, may be boosted to a high dose using conformal external beam therapy or IMRT. The vaginal apex can move 2 to 3 cm with bladder filling and emptying; this internal organ motion should be carefully considered during treatment planning.

Concurrent chemoradiation may have a role in the treatment of vaginal cancers, although there are no randomized trials. Many clinicians believe that similarities in histology and behavior between cervical and vaginal cancer justify the use of similar regimens to treat locally advanced vaginal cancers. Because vaginal cancer is very rare and the radiation-therapy techniques used to treat this disease are specialized, patients with vaginal cancer may benefit from referral to centers with relatively large gynecologic radiation oncology practices.

References

1. **Logsdon MD, Eifel PJ.** FIGO stage IIIB squamous cell carcinoma of the uterine cervix: An analysis of prognostic factors emphasizing the balance between external beam and intracavitary radiation therapy. *Int J Radiat Oncol Biol Phys.* 1999;43:763–775.

2. **Stehman F, Perez C, Kurman R, et al.** Uterine cervix. In: **Hoskins W, Perez C, Young R,** eds. *Principles and Practice of Gynecologic Oncology.* Philadelphia, PA: Lippincott; 2000:591–662.

3. **Eifel PJ.** Radiotherapy versus radical surgery for gynecologic neoplasms: Carcinomas of the cervix and vulva. *Front Radiat Ther Oncol.* 1993;27:130–142.

4. **Eifel PJ, Morris M, Wharton JT, et al.** The influence of tumor size and morphology on the outcome of patients with FIGO stage IB squamous cell carcinoma of the uterine cervix. *Int J Radiat Oncol Biol Phys.* 1994;29:9–16.

5. **Landoni F, Maneo A, Colombo A, et al.** Randomised study of radical surgery versus radiotherapy for stage Ib–IIa cervical cancer. *Lancet.* 1997;350:535–540.

6. **Morrow CP.** Is pelvic radiation beneficial in the postoperative management of Stage Ib squamous cell carcinoma of the cervix with pelvic node metastases treated by radical hysterectomy and pelvic lymphadenectomy? *Gynecol Oncol.* 1980;10:105–110.

7. **Sedlis A, Bundy BN, Rotman MZ, et al.** A randomized trial of pelvic radiation therapy versus no further therapy in selected patients with stage IB carcinoma of the cervix after radical hysterectomy and pelvic lymphadenectomy: A Gynecologic Oncology Group study. *Gynecol Oncol.* 1999;73:177–183.

8. **Aalders J, Abeler V, Kolstad P, et al.** Postoperative external irradiation and prognostic parameters in Stage I endometrial carcinoma. *Obstet Gynecol.* 1980;56:419–427.

9. **Keys HM, Roberts JA, Brunetto VL, et al.** A phase III trial of surgery with or without adjunctive external pelvic radiation therapy in intermediate risk endometrial adenocarcinoma: A Gynecologic Oncology Group study. *Gynecol Oncol.* 2004;92:744–751.

10. **Creutzberg CL, van Putten WL, Warlam-Rodenhuis CC, et al.** Outcome of high-risk stage IC, grade 3, compared with stage I endometrial carcinoma patients: The Postoperative Radiation Therapy in Endometrial Carcinoma Trial. *J Clin Oncol.* 2004;22:1234–1241.

11. **Creutzberg CL, van Putten WL, Koper PC, et al.** Surgery and postoperative radiotherapy versus surgery alone for patients with stage-1 endometrial carcinoma: Multicentre randomised trial. PORTEC Study Group. Post Operative Radiation Therapy in Endometrial Carcinoma. *Lancet.* 2000;355:1404–1411.

12. **Grigsby PW, Perez CA.** Radiotherapy alone for medically inoperable carcinoma of the cervix: Stage IA and carcinoma in situ. *Int J Radiat Oncol Biol Phys.* 1991;21:375–378.

13. **Kupelian PA, Eifel PJ, Tornos C, et al.** Treatment of endometrial carcinoma with radiation therapy alone. *Int J Radiat Oncol Biol Phys.* 1993;27:817–824.

14. **Jhingran A, Burke TW, Eifel PJ.** Definitive radiotherapy for patients with isolated vaginal recurrence of endometrial carcinoma after hysterectomy. *Int J Radiat Oncol Biol Phys.* 2003;56:1366–1372.

15. **Shirvani SM, Klopp AH, Likhacheva A, et al.** Intensity modulated radiation therapy for definitive treatment of paraortic relapse in patients with endometrial cancer. *Pract Radiat Oncol.* 2013;3:e21–e28.

16. **Dembo AJ.** Radiotherapeutic management of ovarian cancer. *Semin Oncol.* 1984;11:238–250.

17. **Brown AP, Jhingran A, Klopp AH, et al.** Involved-field radiation therapy for locoregionally recurrent ovarian cancer. *Gynecol Oncol.* 2013;130:300–305.

18. **Frank SJ, Jhingran A, Levenback C, et al.** Definitive treatment of vaginal cancer with radiation therapy. *Int J Radiat Oncol Biol Phys.* 2003;57:S194.

19. **Kirkbride P, Fyles A, Rawlings GA, et al.** Carcinoma of the vagina—Experience at the Princess Margaret Hospital (1974–1989). *Gynecol Oncol.* 1995;56:435–443.

20. **Boronow RC.** Combined therapy as an alternative to exenteration for locally advanced vulvo-vaginal cancer: Rationale and results. *Cancer.* 1982;49:1085–1091.

21. **Homesley HD, Bundy BN, Sedlis A, et al.** Radiation therapy versus pelvic node resection for carcinoma of the vulva with positive groin nodes. *Obstet Gynecol.* 1986;68:733–740.

22. **Katz A, Eifel PJ, Jhingran A, et al.** The role of radiation therapy in preventing regional recurrences of invasive squamous cell carcinoma of the vulva. *Int J Radiat Oncol Biol Phys.* 2003;57:409–418.

23. **Dewey WC, Ling CC, Meyn RE.** Radiation-induced apoptosis: Relevance to radiotherapy. *Int J Radiat Oncol Biol Phys.* 1995;33:781–796.

24. **Hall EJ, Giaccia AJ.** *Radiobiology for the Radiologist.* 7th ed. Philadelphia, PA: Lippincott Williams & Wilkins; 2011.

25. **Elkind MM, Sutton H.** Radiation response of mammalian cells grown in culture: 1. Repair of x-ray damage in surviving Chinese hamster cells. *Radiat Res.* 1960;13:556–593.

26. **Fyles A, Keane TJ, Barton M, et al.** The effect of treatment duration in the local control of cervix cancer. *Radiother Oncol.* 1992;25:273–279.

27. **Lanciano RM, Pajak TF, Martz K, et al.** The influence of treatment time on outcome for squamous cell cancer of the uterine cervix treated with radiation: A Patterns-of-Care Study. *Int J Radiat Oncol Biol Phys.* 1993;25:391–397.

28. **Parsons JT, Bova FJ, Million RR.** A re-evaluation of split-course technique for squamous cell carcinoma of the head and neck. *Int J Radiat Oncol Biol Phys.* 1980;6:1645–1652.

29. **Tannock IF, Browman G.** Lack of evidence for a role of chemotherapy in the routine management of locally advanced head and neck cancer. *J Clin Oncol.* 1986;4:1121–1126.

30. **Terasima R, Tolmach LJ.** X-ray sensitivity and DNA synthesis in synchronous populations of HeLa cells. *Science.* 1963;140:490–492.

31. **Kallman RF.** The phenomenon of reoxygenation and its implications for fractionated radiotherapy. *Radiology.* 1972;105:135–142.

32. **Dische S, Anderson PJ, Sealy R, et al.** Carcinoma of the cervix—Anaemia, radiotherapy and hyperbaric oxygen. *Br J Radiol.* 1983;56:251–255.

33. **Sundfør K, Trope C, Suo Z, et al.** Normobaric oxygen treatment during radiotherapy for carcinoma of the uterine cervix. Results from a prospective controlled randomized trial. *Radiother Oncol.* 1999;50:157–165.

34. **Leibel S, Bauer M, Wasserman T, et al.** Radiotherapy with or without misonidazole for patients with stage IIIB or IVA squamous cell carcinoma of the uterine cervix: Preliminary report of a Radiation Therapy Oncology Group randomized trial. *Int J Radiat Oncol Biol Phys.* 1987;13:541–549.

35. **Overgaard J, Bentzen SM, Kolstad P, et al.** Misonidazole combined with radiotherapy in the treatment of carcinoma of the uterine cervix. *Int J Radiat Oncol Biol Phys.* 1989;16:1069–1072.

36. **Thomas G.** The effect of hemoglobin level on radiotherapy outcomes: The Canadian experience. *Semin Oncol.* 2001;28:60–65.

37. **Reddy SB, Williamson SK.** Tirapazamine: A novel agent targeting hypoxic tumor cells. *Expert Opin Investig Drugs.* 2009;18:77–87.

38. **Girinski T, Pejovic-Lenfant M, Bourhis J, et al.** Prognostic value of hemoglobin concentrations and blood transfusions in advanced carcinoma of the cervix treated by radiation therapy: Results of a retrospective study of 386 patients. *Int J Radiat Oncol Biol Phys.* 1989;16:37–42.

39. **Grogan M, Thomas GM, Melamed I, et al.** The importance of hemoglobin levels during radiotherapy for carcinoma of the cervix. *Cancer.* 1999;86:1528–1536.

40. **Kapp KS, Poschauko J, Geyer E, et al.** Evaluation of the effect of routine packed red cell transfusion in anemic cervix cancer patients treated with radical radiotherapy. *Int J Radiat Oncol Biol Phys.* 2002;54:58–66.

41. **Sundfør K, Lyng H, Rofstad EK.** Tumour hypoxia and vascular density as predictors of metastasis in squamous cell carcinoma of the uterine cervix. *Br J Cancer.* 1998;78:822–827.

42. **Santin AD, Bellone S, Parrish RS, et al.** Influence of allogeneic blood transfusion on clinical outcome during radiotherapy for cancer of the uterine cervix. *Gynecol Obstet Invest.* 2003;56:28–34.

43. **Höckel M, Knoop C, Schlenger K, et al.** Intratumoral pO$_2$ predicts survival in advanced cancer of the uterine cervix. *Radiother Oncol.* 1993;26:45–50.

44. **Henke M, Laszig R, Rube C, et al.** Erythropoietin to treat head and neck cancer patients with anaemia undergoing radiotherapy: Randomised, double-blind, placebo-controlled trial. *Lancet.* 2003;362:1255–1260.

45. **Thomas G, Ali S, Hoebers FJ, et al.** Phase III trial to evaluate the efficacy of maintaining hemoglobin levels above 12.0 g/dL with erythropoietin vs above 10.0 g/dL without erythropoietin in anemic patients receiving concurrent radiation and cisplatin for cervical cancer. *Gynecol Oncol.* 2008;108:317–325.

46. **Fowler JF.** Rationales for high linear energy transfer radiotherapy. In: **Steel G, Adams GE, Peckham MJ, eds.** *The Biological Basis for Radiotherapy.* New York, NY: Elsevier; 1983:261.

47. **Perez CA, Gillespie B, Pajak T, et al.** Quality assurance problems in clinical hyperthermia and their impact on therapeutic outcome: A Report by the Radiation Therapy Oncology Group. *Int J Radiat Oncol Biol Phys.* 1989;16:551–558.

48. **Franckena M, Stalpers LJ, Koper PC, et al.** Long-term improvement in treatment outcome after radiotherapy and hyperthermia in locoregionally advanced cervix cancer: An update of the dutch deep hyperthermia trial. *Int J Radiat Oncol Biol Phys.* 2008;70:1176–1182.

49. **Steel GG, Peckham M.** Exploitable mechanisms in combined radiotherapy-chemotherapy: The concept of additivity. *Int J Radiat Oncol Biol Phys.* 1979;5:317–322.

50. **Fletcher GH.** Clinical dose response curves of human malignant epithelial tumours. *Br J Radiol.* 1973;46:1–12.

51. **Shukovsky LJ.** Dose, time, volume relationships in squamous cell carcinoma of the supraglottic larynx. *Am J Roentgenol Radium Ther Nucl Med.* 1970;108:27–29.

52. **Withers HR, Mason KA.** The kinetics of recovery in irradiated colonic mucosa of the mouse. *Cancer.* 1974;34(suppl):896–903.

53. **Peters LJ, Ang KK.** Unconventional fractionation schemes in radiotherapy. *Important Advances in Oncology.* Philadelphia, PA: J. B. Lippincott; 1986:269–285.

54. **Thames HD Jr., Withers HR, Peters LJ, et al.** Changes in early and late radiation responses with altered dose fractionation: Implications for dose-survival relationships. *Int J Radiat Oncol Biol Phys.* 1982;8:219–226.

55. **Thames HD Jr., Peters LJ, Withers HR, et al.** Accelerated fractionation vs hyperfractionation: Rationales for several treatments per day. *Int J Radiat Oncol Biol Phys.* 1983;9:127–138.

56. **Eifel PJ, Jhingran A, Bodurka DC, et al.** Correlation of smoking history and other patient characteristics with major complications of pelvic radiation therapy for cervical cancer. *J Clin Oncol.* 2002;20:3651–3657.

57. **Konski A, Sowers M.** Pelvic fractures following irradiation for endometrial carcinoma. *Int J Radiat Oncol Biol Phys.* 1996;35:361–367.

58. **National Institutes of Health Consensus Development Conference statement on cervical cancer.** April 1–3, 1996. *Gynecol Oncol.* 1997;66:351–361.

59. **Seider MJ, Peters LJ, Wharton JT, et al.** Safety of adjunctive transvaginal beam therapy in the treatment of squamous cell carcinoma of the uterine cervix. *Int J Radiat Oncol Biol Phys.* 1988;14:729–735.

60. **Maor MH, Gillespie BW, Peters LJ, et al.** Neutron therapy in cervical cancer: Results of a phase III RTOG study. *Int J Radiat Oncol Biol Phys.* 1988;14:885–891.

61. **Kahn F.** *The Physics of Radiation Therapy.* 3rd ed. Philadelphia, PA: Lipincott Williams & Wilkins; 2003.

62. **Eifel PJ, Moughan J, Owen JB, et al.** Patterns of radiotherapy practice for patients with squamous carcinoma of the uterine cervix. A Patterns of Care study. *Int J Radiat Oncol Biol Phys.* 1999;43:351–358.

63. **Fletcher GH.** Female pelvis. In: **Fletcher GH, ed.** *Textbook of Radiotherapy.* Philadelphia, PA: Lea & Febiger; 1980.

64. **Delclos L, Fletcher GH, Sampiere V, et al.** Can the Fletcher gamma ray colpostat system be extrapolated to other systems? *Cancer.* 1978;41:970–979.

65. **Viswanathan AN, Petereit DG.** Gynecologic Brachytherapy. In: **Devlin P, ed.** *Brachytherapy: Techniques and Applications.* Philadelphia, PA: Lippincott Williams and Wilkins; 2006:223–268.

66. **Delclos L, Fletcher GH, Moore EB, et al.** Minicolpostats, dome cylinders, other additions and improvements of the Fletcher-suit afterloadable system: Indications and limitations of their use. *Int J Radiat Oncol Biol Phys.* 1980;6:1195–1206.

67. **Haie-Meder C, Kramar A, Lambin P, et al.** Analysis of complications in a prospective randomized trial comparing two brachytherapy low dose rates in cervical carcinoma. *Int J Radiat Oncol Biol Phys.* 1994;29:1195–1197.

68. **Eifel PJ.** High dose-rate brachytherapy for carcinoma of the cervix: High tech or high risk? *Int J Radiat Oncol Biol Phys.* 1992;24:383–386.

69. **Kapp KS, Stuecklschweiger GF, Kapp DS, et al.** Dosimetry of intracavitary placements for uterine and cervical carcinoma: Results of orthogonal film, TLD, and CT-assisted techniques. *Radiother Oncol.* 1992;24:137–146.

70. **Petereit DG, Pearcey R.** Literature analysis of high dose rate brachytherapy fractionation schedules in the treatment of cervical cancer: Is there an optimal fractionation schedule? *Int J Radiat Oncol Biol Phys.* 1999;43:359–366.

71. **Petereit DG, Sarkaria JN, Potter DM, et al.** High-dose-rate versus low-dose-rate brachytherapy in the treatment of cervical cancer: Analysis of tumor recurrence–the University of Wisconsin experience. *Int J Radiat Oncol Biol Phys.* 1999;45:1267–1274.

72. **Lancker M, Storme G.** Prediction of severe late complications in fractionated, high-dose-rate brachytherapy in gynecological applications. *Int J Radiat Oncol Biol Phys.* 1991;20:1125–1129.

73. **Nag S, Orton C, Young D, et al.** The American Brachytherapy Society survey of brachytherapy practice for carcinoma of the cervix in the United States. *Gynecol Oncol.* 1999;73:111–118.

74. **Viswanathan AN, Thomadsen B.** American Brachytherapy Society consensus guidelines for locally advanced carcinoma of the cervix. Part I: General principles. *Brachytherapy.* 2012;11:33–46.

75. **Dimopoulos JC, Schmid MP, Fidarova E, et al.** Treatment of locally advanced vaginal cancer with radiochemotherapy and magnetic resonance image-guided adaptive brachytherapy: Dose-volume parameters and first clinical results. *Int J Radiat Oncol Biol Phys.* 2012;82:1880–1888.

76. **Höckel M, Baußmann E, Mitze M, et al.** Are pelvic side-wall recurrences of cervical cancer biologically different from central relapses? *Cancer.* 1994;74:648–655.

77. **Erickson B, Gillin MT.** Interstitial implantation of gynecologic malignancies. *J Surg Oncol.* 1997;66:285–295.

78. **Hughes-Davies L, Silver B, Kapp D.** Parametrial interstitial brachytherapy for advanced or recurrent pelvic malignancy: The Harvard/Stanford experience. *Gynecol Oncol.* 1995;58:24–27.

79. **Monk BJ, Tewari K, Burger RA, et al.** A comparison of intracavitary versus interstitial irradiation in the treatment of cervical cancer. *Gynecol Oncol.* 1997;67:241–247.

80. **Viswanathan AN, Szymonifka J, Tempany-Afdhal CM, et al.** A prospective trial of real-time magnetic resonance-guided catheter placement in interstitial gynecologic brachytherapy. *Brachytherapy.* 2013;12:240–247.

81. **Delclos L, Fletcher GH.** Gynecologic cancers. In: **Levitt SH, Kahn FM, Potish RA, eds.** *Technological Basis of Radiation Therapy: Practical Clinical Applications.* Philadelphia, PA: Lea & Febiger; 1992:193–227.

82. **Martinez A, Edmundson GK, Cox RS, et al.** Combination of external beam irradiation and multiple-site perineal applicator (MUPIT) for treatment of locally advanced or recurrent prostatic, anorectal, and gynecologic malignancies. *Int J Radiat Oncol Biol Phys.* 1985;11:391–398.

83. **Syed AMN, Puthwala AA, Neblett D, et al.** Transperineal interstitial-intracavitary "Syed-Neblett" applicator in the treatment of carcinoma of the uterine cervix. *Endocuriether Hyperther Oncol.* 1986;2:1–13.

84. **Rosenshein NB.** Radioisotopes in the treatment of ovarian cancer. *Clin Obstet Gynaecol.* 1983;10:279–295.

85. **Reed GW, Watson ER, Chesters MS.** A note on the distribution of radioactive colloidal gold following intraperitoneal injection. *Br J Radiol.* 1961;34:323–326.

86. **Klaassen D, Starreveld A, Shelly W, et al.** External beam pelvic radiotherapy plus intraperitoneal radioactive chromic phosphate in early stage ovarian cancer: A toxic combination. *Int J Radiat Oncol Biol Phys.* 1985;11:1801–1804.

87. **Young RC, Walton LA, Ellenberg SS, et al.** Adjuvant therapy in stage I and stage II epithelial ovarian cancer. Results of two prospective randomized trials. *N Engl J Med.* 1990;322:1021–1027.

88. Lanciano RM, Martz K, Coia LR, et al. Tumor and treatment factors improving outcome in stage III-B cervix cancer. *Int J Radiat Oncol Biol Phys.* 1991;20:95–100.

89. Chao C, Williamson JF, Grigsby PW, et al. Uterosacral space involvement in locally advanced carcinoma of the uterine cervix. *Int J Radiat Oncol Biol Phys.* 1998;40:397–403.

90. Kim RY, McGinnis LS, Spencer SA, et al. Conventional four-field pelvic radiotherapy technique without CT treatment planning in cancer of the cervix: Potential geographic miss. *Radiother Oncol.* 1994;30:140–145.

91. Mundt AJ, Roeske JC, Lujan AE. Intensity-modulated radiation therapy in gynecologic malignancies. *Med Dosim.* 2002;27:131–136.

92. Fletcher GH, Hamberger AD. Squamous cell carcinoma of the uterine cervix. Treatment technique according to size of the cervical lesion and extension. In: Fletcher GH, ed. *Textbook of Radiotherapy.* Philadelphia, PA: Lea & Febiger; 1980:720–778.

93. International Commission on Radiation Units and Measurements. *Dose and Volume Specification for Reporting Intracavitary Therapy in Gynecology.* Bethesda, MD: International Commission on Radiation Units and Measurements; 1985.

94. Pelloski CE, Palmer M, Chronowski GM, et al. Comparison between CT-based volumetric calculations and ICRU reference-point estimates of radiation doses delivered to bladder and rectum during intracavitary radiotherapy for cervical cancer. *Int J Radiat Oncol Biol Phys.* 2005;62:131–137.

95. Potter R, Haie-Meder C, Van Limbergen E, et al. Recommendations from gynaecological (GYN) GEC ESTRO working group (II): Concepts and terms in 3D image-based treatment planning in cervix cancer brachytherapy-3D dose volume parameters and aspects of 3D image-based anatomy, radiation physics, radiobiology. *Radiother Oncol.* 2006;78:67–77.

96. Morris M, Eifel PJ, Lu J, et al. Pelvic radiation with concurrent chemotherapy compared with pelvic and paraaortic radiation for high-risk cervical cancer. *N Engl J Med.* 1999;340:1137–1143.

97. Eifel PJ, Winter K, Morris M, et al. Pelvic irradiation with concurrent chemotherapy versus pelvic and para-aortic irradiation for high-risk cervical cancer: An update of Radiation Therapy Oncology Group trial (RTOG) 90-01. *J Clin Oncol.* 2004;22:872–880.

98. Keys HM, Bundy BN, Stehman FB, et al. Weekly cisplatin chemotherapy during irradiation improves survival and reduces relapses for patients with bulky stage IB cervical cancer treated with irradiation and adjuvant hysterectomy: Results of a randomized GOG trial. *Gynecol Oncol.* 1998;68:100.

99. Peters WA III, Liu PY, Barrett RJ II, et al. Concurrent chemotherapy and pelvic radiation therapy compared with pelvic radiation therapy alone as adjuvant therapy after radical surgery in high-risk early-stage cancer of the cervix. *J Clin Oncol.* 2000;18:1606–1613.

100. Whitney CW, Sause W, Bundy BN, et al. A randomized comparison of fluorouracil plus cisplatin versus hydroxyurea as an adjunct to radiation therapy in stages IIB–IVA carcinoma of the cervix with negative para-aortic lymph nodes: A Gynecologic Oncology Group and Southwest Oncology Group study. *J Clin Oncol.* 1999;17:1339–1348.

101. Roberts KB, Urdaneta N, Vera R, et al. Interim results of a randomized trial of mitomycin C as an adjunct to radical radiotherapy in the treatment of locally advanced squamous-cell carcinoma of the cervix. *Int J Cancer.* 2000;90:206–223.

102. Lorvidhaya V, Chitapanarux I, Sangruchi S, et al. Concurrent mitomycin C, 5-fluorouracil, and radiotherapy in the treatment of locally advanced carcinoma of the cervix: A randomized trial. *Int J Radiat Oncol Biol Phys.* 2003;55:1226–1232.

103. Wong LC, Ngan HY, Cheung AN, et al. Chemoradiation and adjuvant chemotherapy in cervical cancer. *J Clin Oncol.* 1999;17:2055–2060.

104. Duenas-Gonzalez A, Zarba JJ, Patel F, et al. Phase III, open-label, randomized study comparing concurrent gemcitabine plus cisplatin and radiation followed by adjuvant gemcitabine and cisplatin versus concurrent cisplatin and radiation in patients with stage iib to iva carcinoma of the cervix. *J Clin Oncol.* 2011;29(13):1678–1685.

105. Alvarez RD, Potter ME, Soong SJ, et al. Rationale for using pathologic tumor dimensions and nodal status to subclassify surgically treated stage IB cervical cancer patients. *Gynecol Oncol.* 1991;43:108–112.

106. van Bommel PF, van Lindert AC, Kock HC, et al. A review of prognostic factors in early-stage carcinoma of the cervix (FIGO I B and II A) and implications for treatment strategy. *Eur J Obstet Gynecol Reprod Biol.* 1987;26:69–84.

107. Rotman M, Sedlis A, Piedmonte MR, et al. A phase III randomized trial of postoperative pelvic irradiation in Stage IB cervical carcinoma with poor prognostic features: Follow-up of a gynecologic oncology group study. *Int J Radiat Oncol Biol Phys.* 2006;65:169–176.

108. Ijaz T, Eifel PJ, Burke T, et al. Radiation therapy of pelvic recurrence after radical hysterectomy for cervical carcinoma. *Gynecol Oncol.* 1998;70:241–246.

109. Thomas G, Dembo A, Beale F, et al. Concurrent radiation, mitomycin C, and 5-fluorouracil in poor prognosis carcinoma of the cervix: Preliminary results of a phase I-II study. *Int J Radiat Oncol Biol Phys.* 1984;10:1785–1790.

110. Hamberger AD, Unal A, Gershenson DM, et al. Analysis of the severe complications of irradiation of carcinoma of the cervix: Whole pelvis irradiation and intracavitary radium. *Int J Radiat Oncol Biol Phys.* 1983;9:367–371.

111. Kucera H, Enzelsberger H, Eppel W, et al. The influence of nicotine abuse and diabetes mellitus on the results of primary irradiation in the treatment of carcinoma of the cervix. *Cancer.* 1987;60:1–4.

112. Bruner DW, Lanciano R, Keegan M, et al. Vaginal stenosis and sexual function following intracavitary radiation for the treatment of cervical and endometrial carcinoma. *Int J Radiat Oncol Biol Phys.* 1993;27:825–830.

113. Eifel PJ, Levenback C, Wharton JT, et al. Time course and incidence of late complications in patients treated with radiation therapy for FIGO stage IB carcinoma of the uterine cervix. *Int J Radiat Oncol Biol Phys.* 1995;32:1289–1300.

114. Chassagne D, Sismondi P, Horiot JC, et al. A glossary for reporting complications of treatment in gynecological cancers. *Radiother Oncol.* 1993;26:195–202.

115. Heyman J. The so-called Stockholm method and the results of treatment of uterine cancer at the Radiumhemmet. *Acta Radiol.* 1935;22:129.

116. Eifel PJ, Ross J, Hendrickson M, et al. Adenocarcinoma of the endometrium. Analysis of 256 cases with disease limited to the uterine corpus: Treatment options. *Cancer.* 1983;52:1026–1031.

117. Jones HW. Treatment of adenocarcinoma of the endometrium. *Obstet Gynecol Surv.* 1975;30:147–169.

118. Calais G, Vitu L, Descamps P, et al. Preoperative or postoperative brachytherapy for patients with endometrial carcinoma stage I and II. *Int J Radiat Oncol Biol Phys.* 1990;19:523–527.

119. Piver MS, Yazigi R, Blumenson L, et al. A prospective trial comparing hysterectomy, hysterectomy plus vaginal radium, and uterine radium plus hysterectomy in stage I endometrial carcinoma. *Obstet Gynecol.* 1979;54:85–89.

120. Nout RA, Smit VT, Putter H, et al. Vaginal brachytherapy versus pelvic external beam radiotherapy for patients with endometrial cancer of high-intermediate risk (PORTEC-2): An open-label, non-inferiority, randomised trial. *Lancet.* 2010;375:816–823.

121. Hendrickson M, Ross M, Eifel P, et al. Uterine papillary serous carcinoma. A highly malignant form of endometrial adenocarcinoma. *Am J Surg Pathol.* 1982;6:93–108.

122. Mallipeddi P, Kapp DS, Teng NN. Long-term survival with adjuvant whole abdominopelvic irradiation for uterine papillary serous carcinoma. *Cancer.* 1993;71:3076–3081.

123. Scholten AN, van Putten WL, Beerman H, et al. Postoperative radiotherapy for Stage 1 endometrial carcinoma: Long-term outcome of the randomized PORTEC trial with central pathology review. *Int J Radiat Oncol Biol Phys.* 2005;63:834–838.

124. Corn BW, Lanciano RM, Greven KM, et al. Impact of improved irradiation technique, age and lymph node sampling on the severe complication rate of surgically staged endometrial cancer patients: A multivariate analysis. *J Clin Oncol.* 1994;12:510–515.

125. Greven KM, Lanciano RM, Herbert SH, et al. Analysis of complications in patients with endometrial carcinoma receiving adjuvant irradiation. *Int J Radiat Oncol Biol Phys.* 1991;21:919–923.

126. Dembo A. The sequential multiple modality treatment of ovarian cancer. *Radiother Oncol.* 1985;3:187–192.

127. **Fuller DB, Sause WT, Plenk HP, et al.** Analysis of postoperative radiation therapy in Stage I through III epithelial ovarian carcinoma. *J Clin Oncol.* 1987;5:897–905.

128. **Martinez A, Schray MF, Howes AE, et al.** Postoperative radiation therapy for epithelial ovarian cancer: The curative role based on a 24-year experience. *J Clin Oncol.* 1985;3:901–911.

129. **Lederman JA, Dembo AJ, Sturgeon JF, et al.** Outcome of patients with unfavorable optimally cytoreduced ovarian cancer treated with chemotherapy and whole abdominal irradiation. *Gynecol Oncol.* 1991;41:30–35.

130. **Bruzzone M, Repetto L, Chiara S, et al.** Chemotherapy versus radiotherapy in the management of ovarian cancer patients with pathological complete response or minimal residual disease at second look. *Gynecol Oncol.* 1990;38:392–395.

131. **Lambert HE, Rustin GJ, Gregory WM, et al.** A randomized trial comparing single-agent carboplatin with carboplatin followed by radiotherapy for advanced ovarian cancer: A North Thames Ovary Group study. *J Clin Oncol.* 1993;11:440–448.

132. **Lawton F, Luesley D, Blackledge G, et al.** A randomized trial comparing whole abdominal radiotherapy with chemotherapy following cisplatinum cytoreduction in epithelial ovarian cancer. West Midlands Ovarian Cancer Group Trial II. *Clin Oncol (R Coll Radiol).* 1990;2:4–9.

133. **Eifel PJ, Gershenson DM, Delclos L, et al.** Twice-daily, split course abdominopelvic radiation therapy after chemotherapy and positive second-look laparotomy for epithelial ovarian carcinoma. *Int J Radiat Oncol Biol Phys.* 1991;21:1013–1018.

134. **Hacker N, Berek J, Burnison C, et al.** Whole abdominal radiation as salvage therapy for epithelial ovarian cancer. *Obstet Gynecol.* 1985;65:60–66.

135. **Faul C, Miramow D, Gerszten K, et al.** Isolated local recurrence in carcinoma of the vulva: Prognosis and implications for treatment. *Int J Gynecol Cancer.* 1998;8:409–414.

136. **Faul CM, Mirmow D, Huang Q, et al.** Adjuvant radiation for vulvar carcinoma: Improved local control. *Int J Radiat Oncol Biol Phys.* 1997;38:381–389.

137. **Thomas GM, Dembo AJ, Bryson SC, et al.** Changing concepts in the management of vulvar cancer. *Gynecol Oncol.* 1991;42:9–21.

138. **Petereit DG, Mehta MP, Buchler DA, et al.** A retrospective review of nodal treatment for vulvar cancer. *Am J Clin Oncol.* 1993;16:38–42.

139. **Koh WJ, Chiu M, Stelzer KJ, et al.** Femoral vessel depth and the implications for groin node radiation. *Int J Radiat Oncol Biol Phys.* 1993;27:969–974.

140. **Eifel PJ, Morris M, Burke TW, et al.** Preoperative continuous infusion cisplatinum and 5-fluorouracil with radiation for locally advanced or recurrent carcinoma of the vulva. *Gynecol Oncol.* 1995;59:51–56.

141. **Koh WJ, Wallace HJ, Greer BE, et al.** Combined radiotherapy and chemotherapy in the management of local-regionally advanced vulvar cancer. *Int J Radiat Oncol Biol Phys.* 1993;26:809–816.

142. **Moore DH, Thomas GM, Montana GS, et al.** Preoperative chemoradiation for advanced vulvar cancer: A phase II study of the Gynecologic Oncology Group. *Int J Radiat Oncol Biol Phys.* 1998;42:79–85.

143. **Berek JS, Heaps JM, Fu YS, et al.** Concurrent cisplatin and 5-fluorouracil chemotherapy and radiation therapy for advanced-stage squamous carcinoma of the vulva. *Gynecol Oncol.* 1991;42:197–201.

144. **Levin W, Goldberg G, Altaras M, et al.** The use of concomitant chemotherapy and radiotherapy prior to surgery in advanced stage carcinoma of the vulva. *Gynecol Oncol.* 1986;25:20–25.

145. **Thomas G, Dembo A, DePetrillo A, et al.** Concurrent radiation and chemotherapy in vulvar carcinoma. *Gynecol Oncol.* 1989;34:263–267.

146. **Wahlen SA, Slater JD, Wagner RJ, et al.** Concurrent radiation therapy and chemotherapy in the treatment of primary squamous cell carcinoma of the vulva. *Cancer.* 1995;75:2289–2294.

147. **Frank SJ, Deavers MT, Jhingran A, et al.** Primary adenocarcinoma of the vagina not associated with diethylstilbestrol (DES) exposure. *Gynecol Oncol.* 2007;105(2):470–474.

5 Pathology

Christina S. Kong
Teri A. Longacre
Michael R. Hendrickson

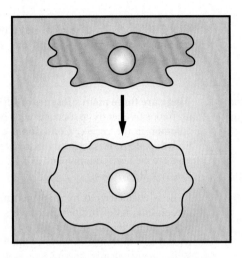

The individual organs within the genital tract make up an extended müllerian system that can give rise to a wide variety of histologically similar tumors. Because of this extended müllerian system, tumor classification and assignment of primary site can be problematic. This chapter provides an overview of the main tumors that are encountered in the female genital tract, emphasizing key histopathologic features and pertinent ancillary diagnostic studies.

To maximize the information provided by pathologic examination, it is important that the treating clinician understand basic concepts of gynecologic oncologic pathology. It is similarly important for the pathologist to understand basic clinical, radiologic, and serologic data. **The integration of clinical, radiologic, and pathologic information is central to intraoperative evaluation, and ultimately to treatment planning, and it occurs best within the framework of the multidisciplinary tumor board** conducted in most major cancer centers.

Cervix

Squamous Lesions of the Cervix

Terminology

Historically, there have been several systems for classifying preneoplastic lesions of the cervix, so it is useful to be familiar with all the systems because the terms can be used interchangeably (Table 5.1). Over the years, the classification systems have moved toward fewer, more clinically relevant categories. In 2012, the College of American Pathologists (CAP) and the American Society for Colposcopy and Cervical Pathology (ASCCP) sponsored a consensus conference to propose uniform terminology for HPV-related squamous intraepithelial lesions and early invasive carcinoma (1). **The Lower Anogenital Squamous Terminology (LAST) Project recommended a two-tiered nomenclature system—low-grade squamous intraepithelial lesion (LSIL) and high-grade squamous intraepithelial lesion (HSIL)—which can be further qualified by the grade of intraepithelial neoplasia (-IN).** The SIL terminology parallels the **Bethesda system,** which has been in use since 1988, and was developed for providing uniform diagnostic terminology for cervical cytologic specimens. The LSIL category encompasses condyloma and CIN 1, whereas the HSIL category encompasses CIN 2 and CIN 3. CIN 1 is equivalent to mild dysplasia,

Table 5.1 Terminology for Cervicovaginal Squamous Intraepithelial Lesions			
Low-grade Squamous Intraepithelial Lesion	*High-grade Squamous Intraepithelial Lesion*		
Cervical Intraepithelial Neoplasia (CIN)			
Condyloma	CIN 1	CIN 2	CIN 3
	Mild dysplasia	Moderate dysplasia	Severe dysplasia

CIN 2 to moderate dysplasia, and CIN 3 to severe dysplasia and carcinoma *in situ*. The LAST recommendations apply across the anogenital tract for HPV-related preneoplastic squamous lesions.

Low-grade Squamous Intraepithelial Lesion

There are three main subtypes of LSIL. Flat condylomas lack the exophytic growth pattern and are more frequently associated with intermediate and high-risk HPV types. These are the most common in the cervix. **Condyloma acuminatum** is the classic genital wart with an exophytic growth pattern. It is typically associated with low-risk HPV types 6 and 11. **Immature condylomas** are the least common and exhibit a filiform, papillary growth pattern; they are associated with low-risk HPV types.

LSIL is characterized by thickened mucosa with enlarged, dark cells that have low nuclear-to-cytoplasmic ratios in the upper layers (Fig. 5.1). Binucleation can be seen in 90% of LSIL, and when the nuclei are surrounded by an irregularly shaped and sharply punched out halo, they are known as *koilocytes*. However, binucleation and halos can be seen as part of a reactive process. With reactive change, the nucleus is minimally enlarged, not hyperchromatic, and the halo is less distinct, round, and uniform. Glycogen vacuoles can appear as round, uniform halos. In addition, LSIL can be mimicked by a squamous papilloma (also known as an *ectocervical* or *fibroepithelial polyp*). **Squamous papillomas lack koilocytes, and have central fibrovascular cores that are not typical of condylomas.**

The ASCUS-LSIL Triage Study investigated interobserver variability in the diagnosis of squamous intraepithelial lesion (SIL) on biopsy (2). More than 2,700 cervical biopsies and loop

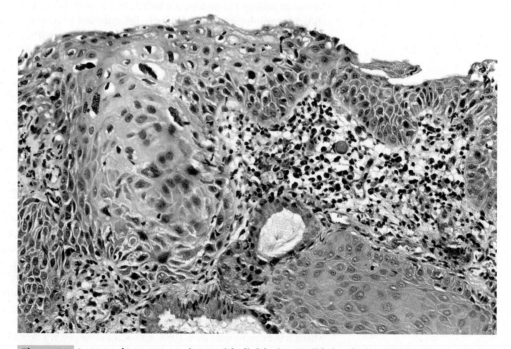

Figure 5.1 **Low-grade squamous intraepithelial lesion (mild dysplasia, CIN 1).** The mucosa is thickened with dysplastic cells and koilocytes in the upper layers.

electrosurgical excision procedure (LEEP) specimens were examined by one of two staff pathologists at one of four centers across the United States, and reviewed by one of four quality control (QC) pathologists. **There was agreement on the diagnosis of LSIL in 43% of cases, but 41% of the cases diagnosed by the staff pathologists as LSIL were downgraded by the QC pathologists to negative.** Most of the downgraded cases were positive for high-risk HPV, raising the question of which diagnosis was correct. The significance of this finding was not addressed by the study.

High-grade Squamous Intraepithelial Lesion

HSIL is characterized by atypical, dark cells with high nuclear-to-cytoplasmic ratios, which involve one-third to two-thirds of the epithelium in cases of CIN 2 (Fig. 5.2), **or more than two-thirds in cases of CIN 3** (Fig. 5.3). The involved mucosa is notable for disorderly arrangement of cells, with loss of polarity and crowding. Mitotic figures in the upper half of the mucosa are commonly identified.

Immature squamous metaplasia and atrophy can be difficult to distinguish from HSIL, because they are also characterized by cells with high nuclear-to-cytoplasmic ratios. However, the nuclei in squamous metaplasia and atrophy should lack crowding and appear uniform, with smooth nuclear membranes. Mitotic figures can be seen near the basal layer, but not in the upper half of the mucosa. In indeterminate cases, immunohistochemical staining for p16, a surrogate marker for high-risk HPV, can be helpful (3). In some cases, for various reasons (e.g., tangential sectioning, small dissociated fragments, cautery artifact), a distinction cannot be made between LSIL and HSIL. These are best characterized as SIL of indeterminate grade.

The ALT study found good reproducibility for the histologic diagnosis of CIN 3, with concordance in 72.8% of cases (4). The reproducibility for the diagnosis of CIN 2 was significantly lower at 43.4%. A separate joint National Cancer Institute (NCI)-Costa Rica study reported similar disparities in the rates of agreement: 13–31% for CIN 2 and 81–84% for CIN 3 (5). Recognizing that CIN 2 is an equivocal diagnosis that encompasses both CIN 1 and CIN 3, the CAP-ASCCP LAST Project recommended the use of p16 immunohistochemistry when considering a diagnosis of CIN 2. Strong and diffuse block positive p16 results support a diagnosis of HSIL (CIN 2), while negative p16 results support a LSIL (CIN 1) or a non-HPV–associated lesion (1). The presence of block positive p16 correlates with the presence of high-risk HPV that has integrated into the host genome, and correlates with a diagnosis of a precancerous lesion. Since LSIL can exhibit block positive p16 expression, grading of dysplasia is based primarily on H&E morphology.

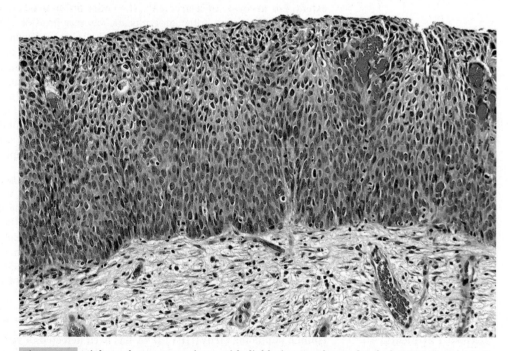

Figure 5.2 **High-grade squamous intraepithelial lesion (moderate dysplasia, CIN 2).** Dysplastic cells with high nuclear-to-cytoplasmic ratios involve less than two-thirds of the mucosa.

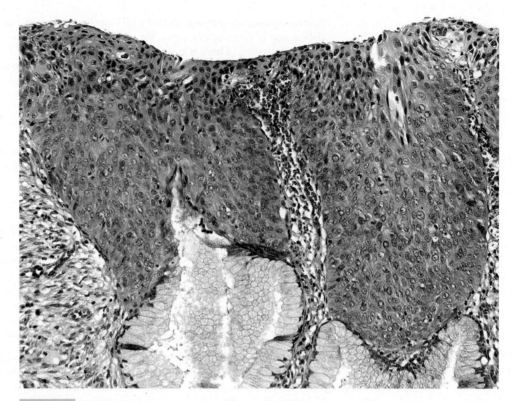

Figure 5.3 **High-grade squamous intraepithelial lesion (severe dysplasia, CIN 3).** The squamous mucosa is notable for full thickness atypia and extension of the dysplastic cells down into endocervical glands.

Squamous Cell Carcinoma

Cervical squamous cell carcinomas can be subdivided into two main groups: *superficially* invasive carcinomas and invasive carcinomas. ***Superficially invasive carcinoma* (FIGO* stage IA1) is defined as microscopic disease with ≤3 mm of stromal invasion and ≤7 mm of horizontal extent. For accurate measurements, the entire lesion needs to be visible, and requires negative surgical margins.** Although lymphatic-vascular invasion (LVI) is acknowledged as a poor prognostic factor, the presence or absence of LVI does not change the FIGO stage. The depth of invasion is measured from the basement membrane at the point of invasion to the deepest invasive focus (Fig. 5.4). Morphologically, superficially invasive carcinoma is characterized by jagged fingers extending from the base of HSIL into the submucosa, and surrounded by chronic inflammation and loose, fibroblastic stroma (i.e., desmoplasia). Often at the point of invasion, the neoplastic cells become more differentiated and have abundant eosinophilic cytoplasm that may be keratinizing. Superficially invasive carcinoma can be difficult to distinguish from HSIL, especially when HSIL involves endocervical glands, or is associated with previous biopsy site changes. Examining multiple level sections of the same focus can be helpful.

Squamous cell carcinomas that are clearly invasive can be keratinizing or nonkeratinizing, and range from well differentiated to poorly differentiated. Well- to moderately differentiated invasive squamous cell carcinoma is characterized by cohesive nests and sheets of neoplastic cells with abundant eosinophilic cytoplasm and distinct cell borders (Fig. 5.5). Keratin pearl formation, central keratinization, and necrosis within nests may also be identified. With poorly differentiated carcinomas, keratinization may be minimal or absent, and they may be difficult to distinguish from other types of poorly differentiated carcinomas (e.g., adenocarcinoma). **Grade and type have not been found to be prognostically significant.** Instead, depth of invasion, lymphatic or vascular invasion, and size are important prognostic variables.

Human Papilloma Virus

Human papilloma virus (HPV) DNA has been detected in virtually all cases of cervical dysplasia and carcinoma and is considered to be a necessary, but not sufficient cause for the development of the vast majority of invasive cervical carcinomas. Although a variety of HPV

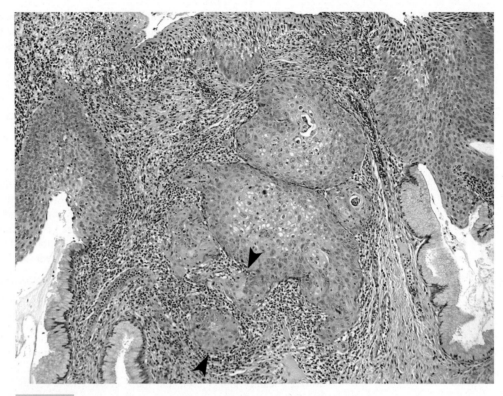

Figure 5.4 **Superficially invasive squamous cell carcinoma of the cervix.** Invasion is measured from the basement membrane at the point of invasion (upper arrow) to the deepest invasive focus (lower arrow). FIGO* Stage IA1 cervical cancer is defined by a depth of invasion ≤3 mm and horizontal extent ≤7 mm in a specimen with negative margins.

types may infect epithelial cells, the risk of oncogenic transformation is most strongly linked to several specific high-risk types. **In 2003, a large epidemiologic study by the International Agency for Research on Cancer (IARC) pooled data from nine countries, and identified 15 high-risk HPV types** (16, 18, 31, 33, 35, 39, 45, 51, 52, 56, 58, 59, 68, 73, and 82), 3 probable high-risk types (26, 53, and 66), and 12 low-risk types (6, 11, 40, 42, 43, 44, 54, 61, 70, 72, 81,

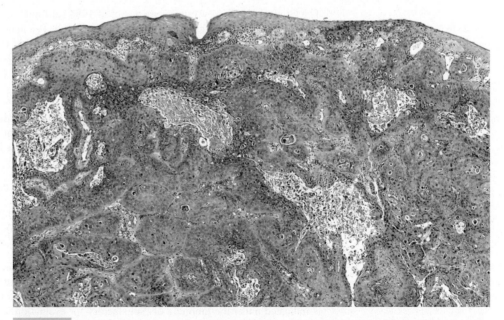

Figure 5.5 **Invasive squamous cell carcinoma of the cervix, moderately differentiated keratinizing.** Keratinization and necrosis within nests of malignant squamous cells are present.

127

and CP6108). **The IARC met again in 2005 to reassess the carcinogenicity of HPV, and revised the original list of high-risk types to include 13 types: 16, 18, 31, 33, 35, 39, 45, 51, 52, 56, 58, 59, and 66** (6). Most investigators now believe that persistent infection with high-risk HPV types is associated with the subsequent development of high-grade dysplasia and invasive carcinoma (7). A substantial proportion of LSIL is associated with infection by high-risk HPV types, but many infections are transitory (7,8).

Cervicovaginal Cytology–Pap Testing

Specimen Preparation Methods

There are two main specimen types for cervicovaginal cytology: conventional smear and liquid-based preparation. Conventional smears involve directly smearing material onto a glass slide, and immediately fixing the specimen with ethanol. The advantages of conventional smears are their low cost, and the lack of need for specialized equipment to process specimens. The disadvantages are lack of uniformity in specimen preparation, and unsatisfactory smears because of obscuring inflammation, blood, or thick areas in the smear.

Liquid-based preparations involve placing the cytologic material in a liquid fixative instead of directly smearing it on a glass slide. The two most commonly used are **ThinPrep** (Hologic, Bedford, MA) and **SurePath** (BD Diagnostics, Burlington, NC). ThinPrep uses a methanol-based fixative and a filter preparation for making the slide. SurePath uses an ethanol-based fixative and a Ficoll gradient. SurePath employs a detachable head for the collection device so that the entire specimen can be submitted for processing. **The advantages of liquid-based preparations are uniformity in slide preparation and fewer unsatisfactory specimens.** The disadvantages are significantly higher cost, and the necessity for specialized processing equipment for each liquid-based method.

Who Signs Out Pap Tests?

Cervicovaginal cytologic specimens are predominantly screened by board-certified cytotechnologists. In some small laboratories, the primary screening of the slides is performed by a pathologist. If the Pap test is negative for an intraepithelial lesion or malignancy and lacks reactive or reparative changes, the final report can be issued by the cytotechnologist. **Quality control review by a second senior cytotechnologist or a pathologist should be performed on at least 10% of all negative cases, and on all cases for patients with a history of an abnormal Pap test.** If any reactive, reparative, or epithelial abnormalities are found, the slide must be reviewed by a pathologist who will issue the final report.

The Clinical Laboratory Improvement Act of 1988 set limits on the number of Pap tests that can be reviewed by a cytotechnologist in a 24-hour period. The nationwide limit is 100 nonimaged or 200 imaged slides per day, but individual states can set lower limits (e.g., 80 nonimaged or 160 imaged slides in California). There is a requirement that all pathologists and cytotechnologists who interpret Pap tests pass an annual proficiency test.

The Bethesda System

In 1988, the National Cancer Institute sponsored a workshop in Bethesda, Maryland, to develop a uniform diagnostic terminology for Pap tests. The resulting classification system underwent multiple revisions and the system currently in use is Bethesda 2001 (9) (Table 5.2).

According to the Bethesda system, the Pap test report should include the following categories: specimen type (e.g., conventional, liquid based, or other), specimen adequacy, and interpretation or result. A general categorization section and educational notes and suggestions are optional. If automated screening is performed (e.g., ThinPrep Imager or BD FocalPoint), the device and result should also be reported. If ancillary testing is performed, the results may be indicated in the Pap test report or reported separately.

Specimen adequacy is divided into "**satisfactory for evaluation**" and "**unsatisfactory for evaluation.**" The presence or absence of transformation zone cells (i.e., endocervical cells or squamous metaplastic cells) and quality indicators (e.g., obscuring blood or inflammation, scant cellularity) is indicated under the umbrella of "satisfactory for evaluation." Specimens can be unsatisfactory for a variety of reasons, and this will be indicated on the report. Some specimens are rejected and not processed; these are usually the result of a broken slide or empty collection vial. Others are

Table 5.2 2001 Bethesda System

	Bethesda 2001
Specimen Type	Conventional Liquid-based (specify type: e.g., ThinPrep, SurePath) Other
Specimen Adequacy	Satisfactory for evaluation Unsatisfactory for evaluation
General Categorization (Optional)	Negative for intraepithelial lesion or malignancy Epithelial cell abnormality Other: Endometrial cells in a woman >40 yrs of age
Interpretation or Result	Negative for intraepithelial lesion or malignancy (specify organisms, other nonneoplastic findings)
Squamous	Atypical squamous cells of undetermined significance (ASC-US) or cannot exclude HSIL (ASC-H) Low-grade squamous intraepithelial lesion (LSIL) High-grade squamous intraepithelial lesion (HSIL) Squamous cell carcinoma
Glandular	Atypical endocervical, endometrial, or glandular cells (NOS or favor neoplastic) Endocervical adenocarcinoma *in situ* Adenocarcinoma
Other	Endometrial cells in a woman >40 yrs of age Other malignant neoplasms
Ancillary Testing	HPV, GC, Chlamydia: Include description of test method(s) and results
Automated Review	Specify device and result if slide is examined by an imaging system
Educational Notes and Suggestions (Optional)	Based on ASCCP management guidelines

found to be unsatisfactory after processing and examination of the slide. A common cause of unsatisfactory ThinPrep specimens is the use of lubricants containing carbomers or carbopol polymers when obtaining the sample. Cytyc has distributed a nonexhaustive list of lubricants that are less likely to interfere with processing (Table 5.3). Another common cause of unsatisfactory specimens is obscuring blood. Although liquid-based systems can remove blood from the sample, the ThinPrep system is able to handle less blood than the SurePath Ficoll gradient.

Squamous Cell Abnormalities

LSIL in cervical cytology specimens is characterized by enlarged, dark nuclei (more than three times the size of an intermediate cell nucleus), with irregular, thickened nuclear membranes. When the cells are binucleated and surrounded by a sharply defined, irregularly shaped halo with a peripheral rim of thickened cytoplasm, the cell is known as a *koilocyte* (Fig. 5.6). **Although koilocytes are pathognomonic for a diagnosis of LSIL, they are not required.** LSIL can be diagnosed based on cells with enlarged, dark, irregular nuclei and no cytoplasmic halo. Koilocytes can be mimicked by prominent glycogen vacuoles or inflammatory halos (Fig. 5.7). In these cases, the area of perinuclear clearing is not sharply demarcated, and tends to be round and regular with the nucleus centrally located. **When the findings fall short of LSIL, the diagnosis of *atypical***

Table 5.3 Lubricants Less Likely to Interfere with ThinPrep Samples

Brand	*Company*
KY Jelly	Johnson & Johnson
Surgilube	E. Fougera & Co.
Astroglide	Biofilm, Inc.
Crystelle	Deltex Pharmaceuticals

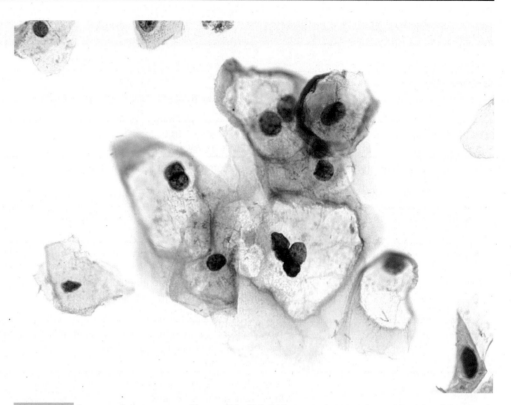

Figure 5.6 Low-grade squamous intraepithelial lesion. Koilocytes have sharply delineated, irregular halos and multiple, dark nuclei with irregular nuclear borders. (Papanicolaou stain)

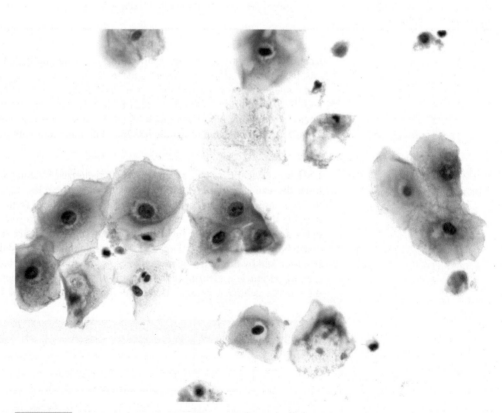

Figure 5.7 Inflammatory halos. Perinuclear clearing with a centrally located nucleus and hazy edges can be seen with infections (e.g., trichomonas) and can be mistaken for koilocytes. (Papanicolaou stain)

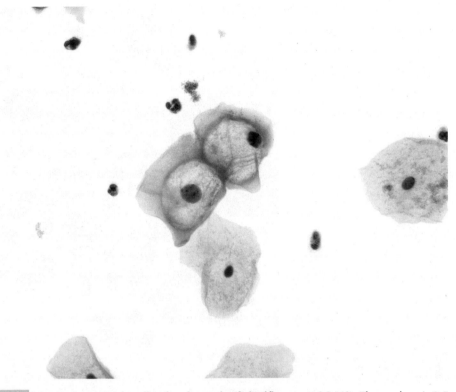

Figure 5.8 **Atypical squamous cells of undetermined significance (ASC-US).** The nucleus is 2.5 times the size of the intermediate cell nucleus, and the nuclear membranes are smooth. (Papanicolaou stain)

squamous cells of undetermined significance **(ASC-US) is used** (Fig. 5.8). Usually, this is because one of the nuclear features is lacking: The nuclei may be not quite large enough (2.5 to 3 times the size of an intermediate cell nucleus), dark enough, or irregular enough.

HSIL is characterized by cells with dark nuclei, irregular nuclear membranes, and high nuclear-to-cytoplasmic ratios (Fig. 5.9). The dysplastic cells can occur singly, in sheets, or as syncytial aggregates. The chromatin may range from coarse to bland, and the cytoplasm from delicate to dense. The nuclei vary in size, and are frequently smaller than those seen with LSIL. With liquid-based preparations, dispersed abnormal single cells are more common than aggregates. In addition, with ThinPrep, the nuclei may not be dark; the diagnosis relies on finding single cells with irregular nuclear membranes and high nuclear-to-cytoplasmic ratios.

Mimics of HSIL include squamous metaplasia, atrophy, repair, endometrial cells, histiocytes, and endocervical cells. Atrophy and squamous metaplasia can be especially difficult to distinguish from HSIL. With atrophic changes, the basal and parabasal cells have high nuclear-to-cytoplasmic ratios with enlarged, dark nuclei, and the background can resemble tumor diathesis (Fig. 5.10). The distinction from HSIL relies on finding smooth nuclear membranes, flat monolayer sheets, and lack of variability in the nuclear size and shape. **Squamous metaplastic cells have high nuclear-to-cytoplasmic ratios and dense cytoplasm, but smooth nuclear membranes. If the cytologic features fall short of a diagnosis of HSIL, the diagnosis of "atypical squamous cells–cannot exclude HSIL (ASC-H)" is used. If dysplastic cells are clearly present but do not quite meet criteria for HSIL, then the changes are characterized as "LSIL cannot exclude HSIL."**

The cytologic diagnosis of squamous cell carcinoma implies invasive carcinoma, because carcinoma *in situ* is encompassed within the category of HSIL. Keratinizing squamous cell carcinoma has single cells with dense, dark nuclei and dense, orangeophilic (i.e., orange-colored) cytoplasm. Nonkeratinizing squamous cell carcinoma has syncytial aggregates and single cells with coarse chromatin and poorly defined cell borders with delicate basophilic (i.e., blue-colored) cytoplasm. **Macronucleoli and tumor diathesis** (i.e., necrosis, degenerating blood, inflammation) can be seen with both, but more frequently with nonkeratinizing squamous cell carcinoma. **With liquid-based preparations, tumor diathesis is seen as necrotic material clinging to the edges of cell**

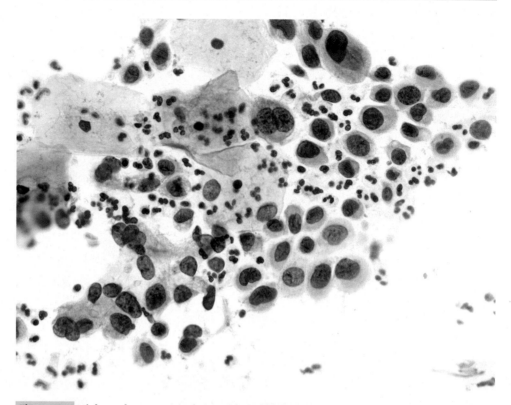

Figure 5.9 High-grade squamous intraepithelial lesion. The dysplastic cells have dark nuclei with focal nuclear membrane irregularities and high nuclear-to-cytoplasmic ratios. (Papanicolaou stain)

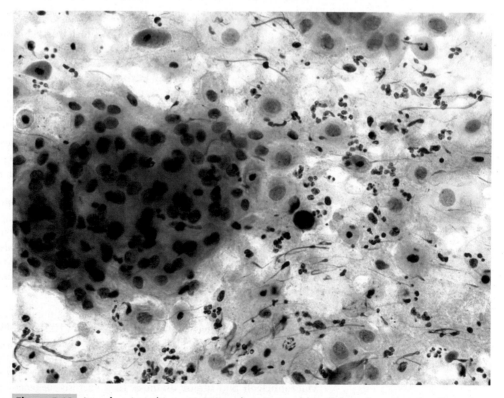

Figure 5.10 Atrophy. Atrophic vaginitis is characterized by sheets of parabasal cells and an inflammatory background that can mimic squamous cell carcinoma. (Papanicolaou stain)

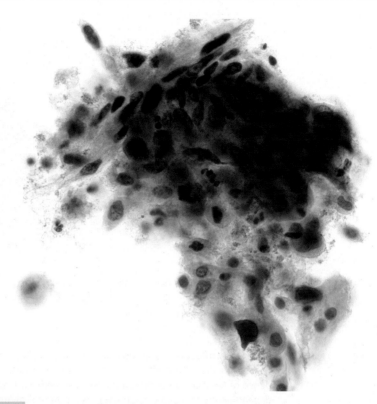

Figure 5.11 **Squamous cell carcinoma.** Necrosis in liquid-based preparations is characterized by granular debris that clings to the edges of tumor cell clusters. (Papanicolaou stain)

groups, and is less apparent than on conventional smears where it is spread across the background (Fig. 5.11). **Squamous cell carcinoma can be difficult to distinguish from HSIL,** because there is a significant morphologic overlap between these two entities. Because keratinization can be seen with both, the findings of macronucleoli and tumor diathesis are more reliable indicators of squamous cell carcinoma, but are not always present. For both HSIL and squamous cell carcinoma, the next step is colposcopy with biopsy, which will provide material for more definitive assessment of invasive carcinoma.

Glandular Cell Abnormalities

The diagnosis of "atypical glandular cells" accounts for less than 1% of all Pap tests. Significant disease is present in 9–38% of cases, with HSIL the most common abnormal finding (10). Other findings include endocervical adenocarcinoma *in situ* (AIS), endocervical adenocarcinoma, endometrial pathology including carcinoma, and extrauterine carcinoma. Postmenopausal women have a higher rate of abnormality, with a significant cervical or endometrial abnormality found in more than 30% of cases.

Endocervical AIS is characterized by enlarged, elongated nuclei, with irregular nuclear membranes and coarse chromatin arranged radially as rosettes or in strips as crowded palisades (Fig. 5.12). When the cytoplasm is partially stripped away, the palisading nuclei can resemble an array of feathers. This feature is referred to as *feathering,* and is considered characteristic of AIS. Mitotic figures are commonly present.

Endocervical AIS can be closely mimicked by tubal metaplasia, direct sampling of the endometrium, and HSIL involving endocervical glands. Tubal metaplasia is distinguished by the lack of nuclear crowding and smooth nuclear membranes. The presence of cilia is characteristic but not always seen. **Direct sampling of the endometrium** can yield strips and sheets of atypical glandular cells with feathering, rosette formation, and frequent mitotic figures. Identifying small, tightly cohesive endometrial stromal cells can help in the distinction from AIS. Sampling of endometrial glands can occur as the result of cervical endometriosis, or inadvertent sampling of the lower uterine segment or endometrial cavity (Fig. 5.13). The latter occurs more frequently in patients who have a shortened cervix because of previous LEEP or cone biopsy. The presence of glands embedded in stroma should raise the possibility of direct endometrial sampling. **HSIL**

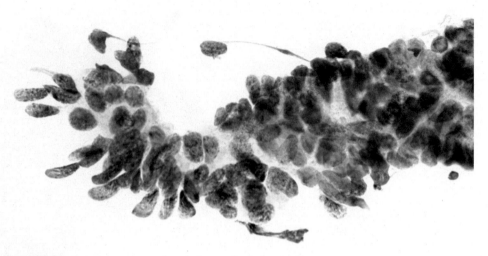

Figure 5.12 Endocervical adenocarcinoma *in situ*. Palisading nuclei stripped of cytoplasm ("feathering") is a characteristic feature. The nuclei are enlarged and elongated with coarse chromatin. (Papanicolaou stain)

involving endocervical glands can be distinguished from AIS by the lack of palisading, presence of single cells with high nuclear-to-cytoplasmic ratios and irregular nuclear membranes, or evidence of keratinization. AIS and HSIL can coexist. If the features fall short of a diagnosis of AIS, depending on the degree of atypia present, the following Bethesda diagnoses may be used: "Atypical endocervical cells, not otherwise specified (NOS)" or "Atypical endocervical cells, favor neoplastic." The latter diagnosis is associated with a higher likelihood of finding a clinically significant lesion on biopsy.

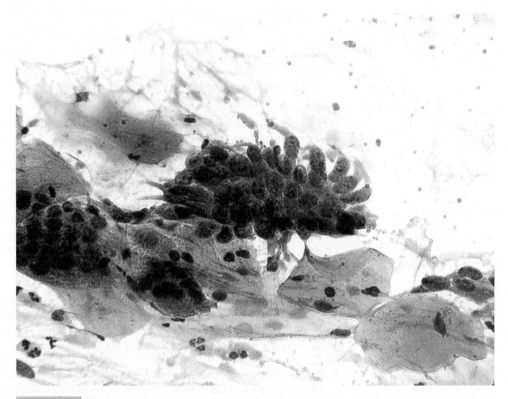

Figure 5.13 Endometriosis. Direct sampling of endometrial glands in cervical endometriosis can mimic endocervical adenocarcinoma *in situ*. The smooth nuclear membranes and lack of nuclear crowding support a benign process. (Papanicolaou stain)

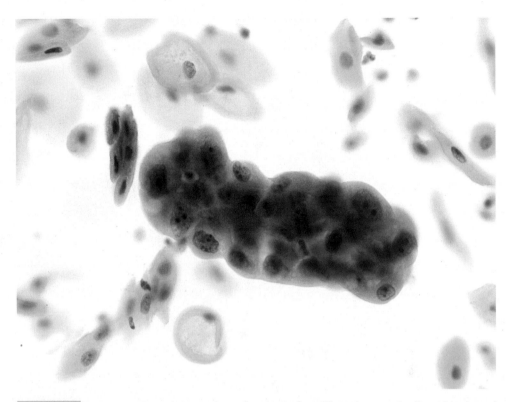

Figure 5.14 **Endometrial carcinoma.** Three-dimensional papillary clusters of cells with enlarged nuclei. (Papanicolaou stain)

Adenocarcinomas most commonly originate from the endocervix or endometrium, but malignant glandular cells on cervical cytology may represent spread from an extrauterine source (e.g., ovary, breast, stomach, colon, kidney, or bladder). Invasive endocervical adenocarcinomas resemble AIS, but are distinguished by the presence of a tumor diathesis in the background. Endometrial carcinoma is characterized by three-dimensional groups or papillary clusters of cells with enlarged nuclei, and often vacuolated cytoplasm (Fig. 5.14). Intracytoplasmic neutrophils are common. When the tumor cells have large cytoplasmic vacuoles and are associated with psammoma bodies, the findings are suggestive of a **serous carcinoma.** Adenocarcinoma cells in a clean background or with unusual morphology that is not typical of a uterine primary raise the possibility of metastatic disease (Fig. 5.15).

The diagnosis of **atypical endometrial cells** is used when endometrial cell clusters show mild nuclear enlargement, vacuolated cytoplasm, or cytoplasmic neutrophils. If it cannot be determined whether the atypical cells are endocervical or endometrial in origin, the diagnosis of **atypical glandular cells (NOS) or atypical glandular cells, favor neoplastic** can be used.

Other

The diagnosis of "**endometrial cells in a woman 40 years of age and older**" is used when benign-appearing exfoliated endometrial stromal or glandular cells are identified in a cervical cytologic specimen from a woman aged 40 or older. The age cutoff was set by the Bethesda system 2001 because menstrual data, menopausal status, hormonal therapy, and clinical risk factors are frequently unknown to the laboratory. For asymptomatic, premenopausal women, no further studies are recommended. Endometrial sampling is recommended for symptomatic premenopausal women and all postmenopausal women (10).

Ancillary Testing

HPV testing became routine after the ASCUS LSIL Triage (ALT) Study (11) and the publication of the American Society for Colposcopy and Cervical Pathology (ASCCP) *Consensus Guidelines for the Management of Women with Cervical Cytological Abnormalities.* Initially, **Digene Hybrid Capture II** (HC2) was the only commercially available HPV test, and had the additional distinction of being the assay used in the ALT study. In the intervening time, several different assays that use multiple different methodologies have become commercially available.

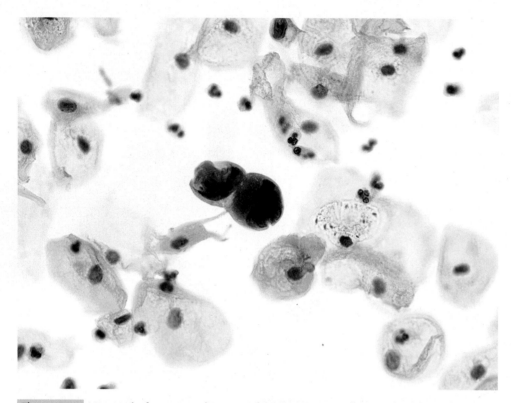

Figure 5.15 **Metastatic breast carcinoma.** Adenocarcinoma cells in a background without inflammation and necrosis raise the possibility of spread from an extrauterine source. (Papanicolaou stain)

There are four United States Food and Drug Administration (US FDA)-approved HPV assays for use in ASC-US triage and for co-testing in women over the age of 30: **HC2 (Qiagen), Cervista HPV HR (Hologic), cobas HPV Test (Roche), and Aptima HPV Assay (GenProbe).** The high-risk probes for all four assays target high-risk HPV types 16, 18, 31, 33, 35, 39, 45, 51, 52, 56, 58, 59, and 68. The probes for Cervista, cobas, and Aptima also target HPV type 66, which was classified as high risk by the IARC in 2005. Although the HC2 high-risk probe does not directly target HPV 66, studies showed that HPV 66 is detected through cross-reactivity. **One of the main criticisms of HC2 is decreased specificity because of cross-reactivity, but the benefit of cross-reactivity is increased clinical sensitivity.** As exemplified by HPV 66, cross-reactivity can allow for the detection of HPV types not classified as high risk.

The use of HPV genotyping has been incorporated into the ASCCP Consensus Guidelines since HPV types 16 and 18 were recognized as more carcinogenic and responsible for the majority of cervical cancers. The cobas HPV Test screens for 14 high-risk HPV types, and specifically identifies HPV types 16 and 18. Cervista has a separate HPV 16/18 probe that can be used for genotyping if the initial Cervista HPV HR screen is positive. **HPV testing was initially validated by the ALT study using HC2; the newer assays are required to show similar or better test characteristics.** In comparison with HC2, the other three systems exhibit similar sensitivity and offer the advantage of including an internal positive control.

Positive results with HC2 testing for high-risk HPV have been reported in many patients who have no cytologic or histologic evidence of dysplasia. False positive results with HC2 can occur as the result of cross-reactivity or signal leak. De Cremoux et al. (12) reported a false positive rate of 6.2%, with 1.9% because of cross-reactivity and 4.3% because of signal leak. **Cross-reactivity with high-risk HPV DNA can occur in cases that have very high loads of low-risk HPV;** similar cross-reactivity with low-risk types can occur with high loads of high-risk HPV. In addition, the chemiluminescent signal in cases with high viral loads can lead to false positive results in contiguous samples because of leaking of the signal.

HC2 results are reported as positive, negative, or equivocal based on the assigned cutoff of 1.0 RLU/PC. Although HC2 testing has been shown to have good interlaboratory reproducibility, there is poor reproducibility near the cutoff point of 1 RLU/PC (13). **In a significant portion of cases**

with borderline positive HC2 results, PCR analysis for HPV is negative (14). Cases that are near the cutoff point are reported as equivocal because they may represent a false positive result. The newer HPV assays exhibit less cross-reactivity and equivalent or better specificity than HC2.

Automated Screening

The main impetus behind developing automated screening systems has been to increase productivity and improve quality. Both **ThinPrep** and **SurePath** have imaging systems that can be used with their liquid-based preparations. **The ThinPrep Imaging System was approved by the US FDA in 2003** for dual review of ThinPrep cervical cytology slides. After the imaging system screens the slide, the cytotechnologist reviews 22 selected fields of view. If any abnormal cells are seen, the slide is manually rescreened by the cytotechnologist. **Studies have shown that the ThinPrep system has equivalent or better sensitivity than manual screening for the detection of LSIL and HSIL, and higher specificity for the diagnosis of HSIL** (15).

The BD FocalPoint Slide Profiler has been US FDA approved for primary screening of Sure-Path or conventional cervical cytologic slides. It functions as a triage device, allowing a portion of slides to be archived with no further review by a cytotechnologist, and identifying cases that are more likely to contain significant abnormalities, requiring further review. The BD Focal-Point GS Imaging System is an US FDA-approved location-guided screening system that can be used in conjunction with the Slide Profiler. The guided screener will direct the cytotechnologist to the fields of view containing the abnormal areas detected by image analysis.

Glandular Lesions of the Cervix

Terminology

A variety of terms have been used to describe preinvasive glandular lesions of the cervix, including atypia, dysplasia, and AIS. Unlike cervical squamous lesions, cervical glandular dysplasia is a poorly defined and controversial entity. Glandular lesions that exhibit some but not all the features of adenocarcinoma *in situ* have been associated with *in situ* and invasive adenocarcinoma, but the diagnostic criteria, clinical implications, prevalence, and progression rate of these lesions are not uniformly agreed upon (16).

Adenocarcinoma *In Situ*

The histologic diagnosis of AIS requires unequivocal dysplastic changes, which are typically manifested by low-power basophilia, nuclear hyperchromasia with either fine or coarsely granular chromatin, nuclear apoptotic or karyorrhectic debris, apical mitotic figures, and loss of polarity (which may be subtle) (Fig. 5.16). The involved glands exhibit a lobular architecture that may appear more pronounced than adjacent uninvolved endocervical glands, but irregular infiltration into the stroma is absent. Partial glandular involvement is common. **A superficial form of AIS has been described in the superficial columnar mucosa featuring similar cytologic alterations, but less pronounced atypia. This lesion is thought to occur more commonly in a younger age group (mean, 26 years)** and so is interpreted as an "early" form of AIS (17).

A variety of processes mimic AIS, including tubal or tuboendometrial metaplasia, endometriosis, reactive endocervical cells, and several endocervical cell alterations that do not necessarily appear to represent a reactive process (18). These latter alterations often pose the most diagnostic difficulty, and are classified on the basis of the abnormality present: endocervical glandular hyperplasia, mitotically active endocervical mucosa, stratified endocervical mucosa, and atypical oxyphilic metaplasia.

Biomarkers, particularly a combination of Ki-67 and p16, are helpful in the differential diagnosis of AIS. In general, strong, diffuse expression of p16 in conjunction with increased Ki-67 is more commonly associated with AIS, whereas weak or focal p16 expression with or without increased Ki-67 is more supportive of an AIS mimic (19). Exceptions occur, so it is important to be thoroughly aware of the variant expression patterns of these markers in the individual lesions, in order to prevent overinterpretation on the basis of staining patterns alone (20).

Invasive Adenocarcinoma

The diagnosis of invasive cervical adenocarcinoma can be very difficult in early or superficially invasive lesions, and in limited (superficial) biopsy specimens. Unlike squamous carcinoma of the cervix, invasion may not be associated with a significant stromal reaction; in

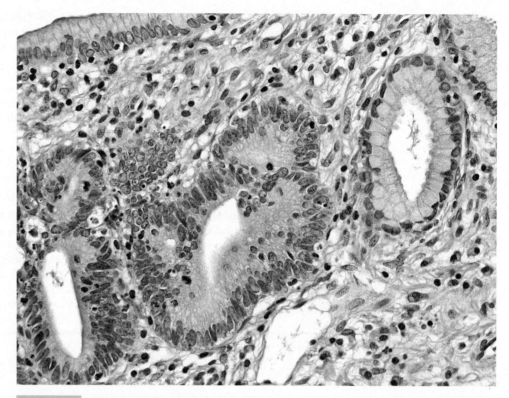

Figure 5.16 **Adenocarcinoma *in situ* of the cervix.** *In situ* carcinoma exhibits nuclear hyperchromasia, stratification, irregular chromatin, and apical mitotic figures. A normal endocervical gland is present on the right.

these instances, identification of invasion is based on the presence of significant glandular irregularity, an infiltrative glandular pattern, and the presence of enlarged, complex neoplastic glandular structures deep to the normal endocervical crypts (Fig. 5.17).

Because of the difficulties in diagnosing early invasive lesions, the concept of "microinvasive adenocarcinoma" is not as well accepted as it is for superficially invasive squamous cell carcinoma; nevertheless, a maximum depth of invasion of 3 mm with negative margins and no lymphovascular invasion is considered by most clinicians as the upper limit for consideration of conservative management. Measurements are made from the surface and expressed in millimeters.

Invasive adenocarcinoma of the usual or endocervical type accounts for 60–70% of cervical adenocarcinomas. Two variants—adenoma malignum (minimal deviation adenocarcinoma) and **villoglandular adenocarcinoma**—are very uncommon, but the source of frequent diagnostic problems. **Other named histologic subtypes include serous, clear cell, endometrioid, mesonephric, intestinal type, signet-ring cell type, adenosquamous, adenoid basal, adenoid cystic, and adenocarcinoma admixed with neuroendocrine carcinoma, and undifferentiated carcinoma** (18,21). Only those with distinctive clinical or differential diagnostic problems that affect prognosis or treatment are discussed.

Minimal Deviation Carcinoma—Adenoma Malignum

This tumor, which is characterized by a deceptively benign histologic appearance, accounts for <10% of all cervical adenocarcinomas. Patients present with irregular bleeding, diffuse cervical enlargement, or vaginal mucus discharge. Most minimal deviation carcinomas exhibit a gastric mucin phenotype. **An association with Peutz–Jeghers syndrome has been reported** (21). A wide age range has been reported, but virtually all patients are older than 20 years of age.

Microscopically, the tumor features cystically dilated, irregular (claw-shaped) glands with minimal cytologic atypia, and minimal stromal reaction (Fig. 5.18). The diagnosis is most easily established by careful search for foci of cytologic atypia, stromal reaction, or conventional-type adenocarcinoma. This tumor can replace normal endocervical and endometrial glandular tissue, mimicking mucinous metaplasia in uterine curettings and biopsy. Intracytoplasmic carcinoembryonic antigen (CEA) staining may be helpful in some cases, but not all adenoma malignum carcinomas are CEA

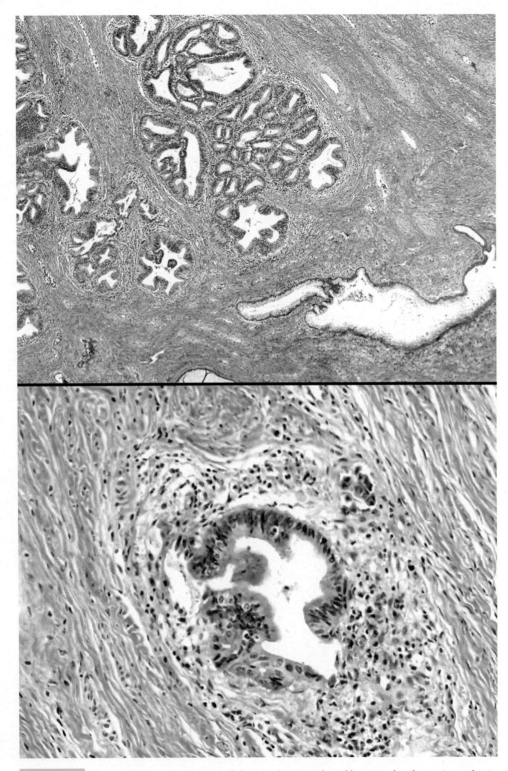

Figure 5.17 **Invasive adenocarcinoma of the cervix.** Deeply infiltrative glands are irregular in contour and surrounded by edematous stroma. (top, low power; bottom, high power)

positive and normal endocervical glands may express CEA on occasion, although usually only along the surface (glycocalyx). These carcinomas do not stain for p16.

| **Villoglandular Carcinoma** | **This tumor occurs predominantly in young women** and is characterized by villoglandular architectural growth pattern and low nuclear grade. These tumors have a good prognosis, but only if |

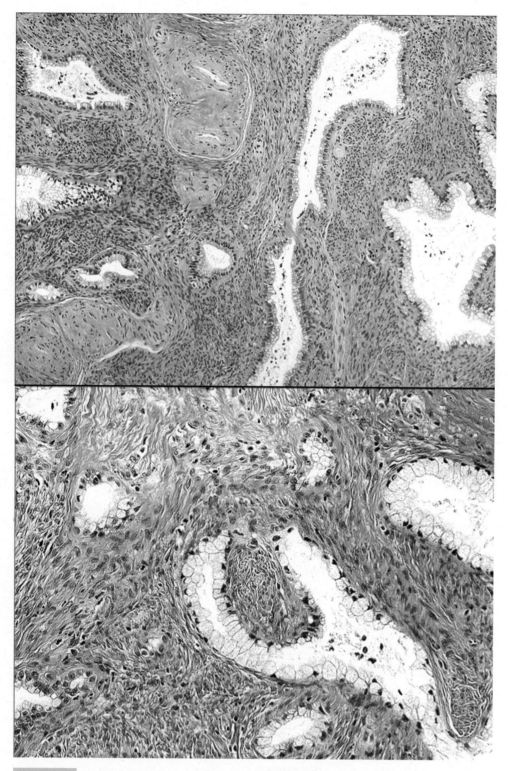

Figure 5.18 **Minimal deviation adenocarcinoma (adenoma malignum).** Large, irregular mucinous glands typically show bland or minimally atypical cytologic features. (top, low power; bottom, high power)

they are exophytic with minimal or no invasion (Fig. 5.19). **An association with HPV has been reported** and these tumors are p16 positive.

Clear Cell Carcinoma

Clear cell carcinoma may occur in young (*diethystilbestrol* exposure *in utero*) or older women, and may arise in the ectocervix (typically, associated with *diethystilbestrol*

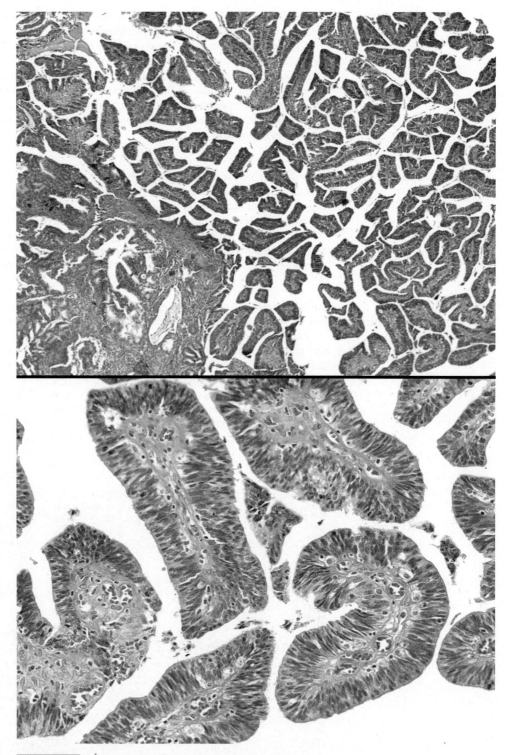

Figure 5.19 **Villoglandular adenocarcinoma of cervix.** Slender, elongated villi are lined by well-differentiated epithelium with an exophytic growth pattern. This tumor is associated with a good prognosis, provided there is minimal or no cervical stromal invasion. (top, low power; bottom, high power)

exposure) or endocervix. A variety of patterns—including tubulocystic or glandular, solid, and papillary—may be seen (21).

Mesonephric Carcinoma   **Mesonephric remnants may develop hyperplasia and carcinoma;** often a spectrum of these changes is seen in the carcinomas (21). The carcinomas often pose significant diagnostic difficulty because of their lateral and deep location within the cervix. **There may be no surface component.** Ductal, retiform, tubular, solid, and spindle patterns may be seen in the carcinomas. Most have low to moderate nuclear grade, so some cases may be difficult to distinguish from florid mesonephric hyperplasia. The distinction is often based on loss of lobular architecture and infiltrative pattern. Diagnosis of higher-grade mesonephric adenocarcinoma is based on identification of residual normal or hyperplastic mesonephric tubules with their characteristic eosinophilic luminal material. Prognosis is uncertain because of the limited numbers of cases, but probably similar to usual endocervical adenocarcinoma. **These tumors are not known to be associated with HPV and most are p16 negative.**

Neuroendocrine Carcinoma

Neuroendocrine carcinoma, small- and large-cell variants, accounts for less than 5% of all cervical carcinomas. These highly aggressive tumors may present as small lesions, but most are deeply invasive. They exhibit the usual features of a neuroendocrine carcinoma; high mitotic indices and necrosis are common (Fig. 5.20). **Neuroendocrine carcinoma is often associated with AIS, HSIL, and conventional invasive cervical adenocarcinoma.** Most harbor HPV-18 and are p16-positive. **Rarely, well-differentiated neuroendocrine tumors (carcinoid) may occur in the cervix** and the prognosis for these tumors may be better. Metastasis should always be ruled out.

Adenoid Basal Carcinoma—Adenoid Basal Epithelioma

Adenoid basal cell carcinoma (epithelioma) occurs in postmenopausal, elderly women (mean age 65 years). Most are asymptomatic and the tumor is discovered during evaluation of an atypical Pap smear. Indeed, it is often associated with HSIL. The cervix is often normal on colposcopic and physical examination. The tumor is cytologically bland (often looking like "bland squamous cell carcinoma"), and features basaloid, adenoid, and squamoid differentiation. The adenoid areas consist of small, closely packed tubules, occasionally with intraluminal secretions reminiscent of mesonephric tubules (Fig. 5.21). There is typically no stromal response. Mitotic figures are rare or absent. **The tumor has a favorable prognosis** and needs to be distinguished from the adenoid cystic pattern of cervical adenocarcinoma, which does not have a favorable prognosis (21). **Because of the extremely favorable prognosis associated with classic, superficial adenoid basal carcinoma, the diagnostic term** *adenoid basal epithelioma* **is preferred.**

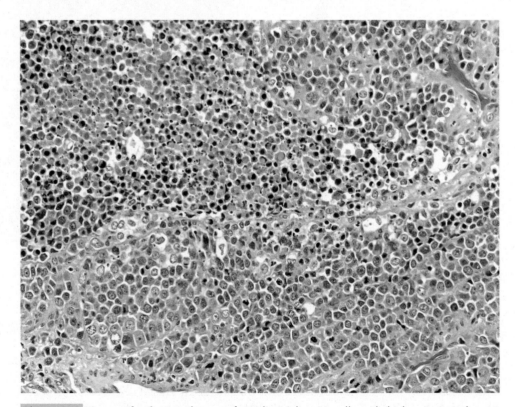

Figure 5.20 Neuroendocrine carcinoma of cervix. Malignant cells with high mitotic index are arranged in a sheetlike growth pattern. Necrosis is often present in these clinically aggressive tumors.

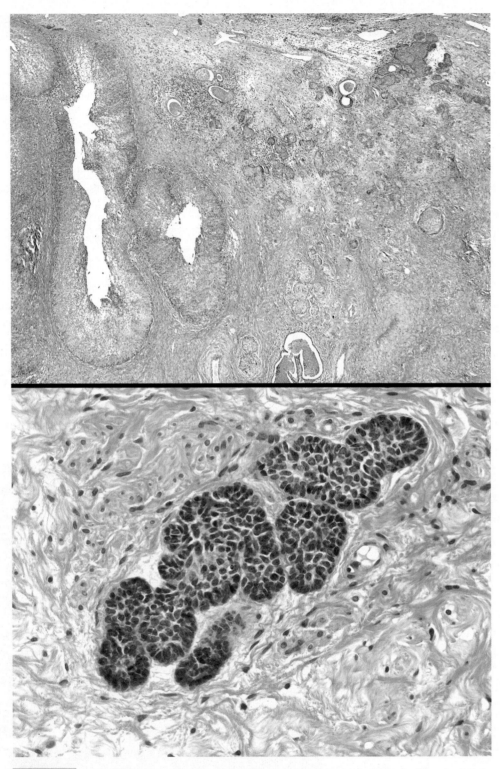

Figure 5.21 **Adenoid basal carcinoma (epithelioma).** This variant of cervical adenocarcinoma is characterized by nests of bland basaloid and squamoid cells in the cervical stroma. A squamous intraepithelial lesion is typically present in the overlying mucosa. This neoplasm is often referred to as *adenoid basal epithelioma* because it has a very favorable prognosis. (top, low power; bottom, high power)

Adenoid Cystic Carcinoma   Unlike adenoid basal carcinoma (epithelioma), **adenoid cystic carcinoma is a clinically aggressive neoplasm.** It is composed of cribriform nests containing eosinophilic hyaline material within the gland lumens, resembling adenoid cystic carcinoma of the salivary gland.

Table 5.4 Distinguishing Endometrial from Endocervical Adenocarcinoma

	Endocervical	Endometrial
Clinical or Radiologic	Dominant mass in cervix	Dominant mass in uterine fundus
H&E	Cancer containing fragments differ from endometrial functionalis fragments (dimorphic pattern) Adenocarcinoma *in situ* in associated endocervical glands Associated squamous intraepithelial lesion	Mergence of malignant fragments with less atypical patterns in other fragments (endometrial hyperplasia/metaplasia) Stromal foam cells No adenocarcinoma *in situ* in associated cervical fragments
Immunohistochemistry	ER-negative and PR-negative Vimentin-negative p16-positive	ER-positive and PR-positive Vimentin-positive p16-negative
HPV *in situ*	Positive	Negative

Localization of Adenocarcinoma: Cervix versus Corpus

Distinction between primary endometrial and primary endocervical adenocarcinoma may be difficult in biopsy and curettage specimens, especially when no precursor lesion is present. When clinical and histologic evaluation fails to clearly identify a carcinoma as cervical or endometrial in origin, an immunohistochemical panel that includes several markers, such as estrogen receptor (ER), progesterone receptor (PR), vimentin, and p16, is often useful (19,22,23). Using this particular panel (Table 5.4), glandular proliferations that are ER-positive and PR-positive, vimentin-positive, and p16-negative are almost always endometrial origin (Fig. 5.22), whereas those that are ER-negative and PR-negative, vimentin-negative, and p16-positive are very likely to be endocervical in origin (Fig. 5.23). Because the distinction between these two sites of origin may

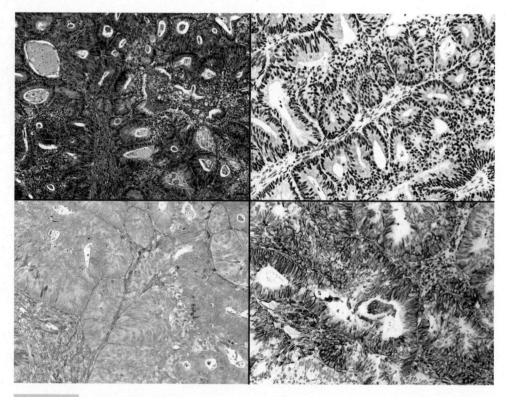

Figure 5.22 Endometrial adenocarcinoma (upper left). Endometrial adenocarcinoma is typically ER-positive/PR-positive (upper right), vimentin-positive (lower right), and p16-negative (lower left).

144

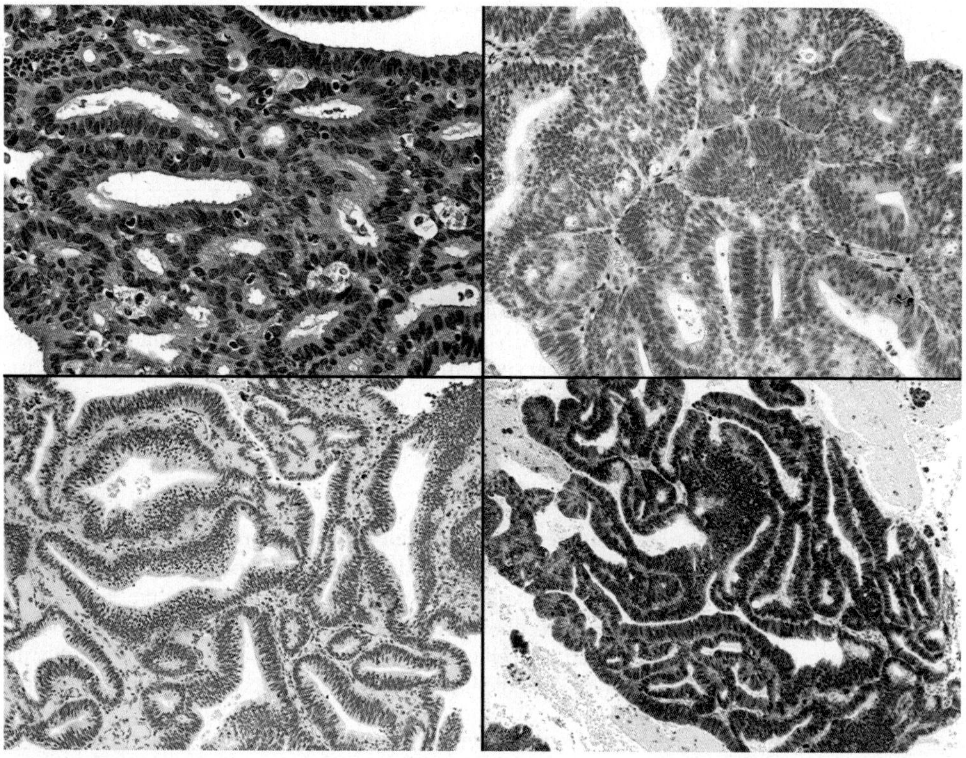

Figure 5.23 **Endocervical adenocarcinoma (upper left).** In contrast to endometrial adenocarcinoma (see **Figure 5.22**), **endocervical adenocarcinoma** is typically ER-negative/PR-negative (upper right), vimentin-negative (lower left), and p16-positive (lower right).

be based on whether a strong staining pattern with p16 is focal or diffuse in an individual case, this pattern of reactivity is most useful in whole tissue sections. In limited samplings, such as are encountered in routine biopsy and curettage specimens, these patterns may be misleading. In addition, overexpression of p16 can occur in a variety of other carcinomas independent of HPV status, including uterine serous carcinomas.

Mesenchymal Tumors

Stromal and smooth muscle tumors may occur in the cervix where they resemble their more common uterine counterparts. Although the vagina is the more common site, embryonal rhabdomyosarcoma may occur in the cervix; in contrast to vaginal rhabdomyosarcoma, which is more common in children, **cervical rhabdomyosarcomas tend to occur in young adults**. Most are embryonal, but alveolar variants may be seen.

Mixed Epithelial and Mesenchymal Tumors

The same mixed epithelial and mesenchymal tumors that occur in the uterine corpus may occur in the cervix. They tend to exhibit the same patient demographics as their uterine counterparts, but cervical adenosarcomas often occur at a younger age (24). Most present during the reproductive years with abnormal bleeding and recurrent polyps. Data are limited, but most appear to have a more favorable prognosis, possibly because of the early detection of low-stage disease in the majority of patients. As in uterine corpus tumors, deep invasion and sarcomatous overgrowth are adverse prognostic indicators.

Other Tumors

A variety of other neoplasms may arise in the uterine cervix. **These include alveolar soft part sarcoma, rhabdomyoma, and nerve sheath tumors.** Alveolar soft part sarcomas of the female genital tract appear to have a better prognosis than their counterparts in other sites. **Yolk sac tumors** may occur in the cervicovaginal region. **Melanoma, lymphoma, and leukemia** usually involve the cervix secondarily, either as metastases or in the setting of widespread disease (18).

Vagina

Squamous Lesions of the Vagina

Squamous Intraepithelial Lesion

The CAP-ASCCP LAST Project recommendations for standardized terminology apply across the anogenital tract for HPV-related preneoplastic squamous lesion. Consequently, preneoplastic lesions of the vagina are termed LSIL or HSIL with the corresponding *vaginal intraepithelial neoplasia* (VAIN) terminology in parentheses: LSIL (VAIN 1), HSIL (VAIN 2), HSIL (VAIN 3). **LSIL and HSIL in the vagina have the same morphologic features as those in the cervix.** LSIL can be mimicked by vaginal papillomatosis, which exhibits papillary architecture, parakeratosis, and cytoplasmic halos. However, papillomatosis lacks significant acanthosis and nuclear atypia. HSIL can be mimicked by atrophy and immature squamous metaplasia, but can be distinguished by a lack of nuclear atypia in the latter two entities.

Squamous Cell Carcinoma

Primary squamous cell carcinoma of the vagina is uncommon. Vaginal squamous cell carcinoma more frequently occurs as a result of secondary involvement by extension from the cervix or vulva. The morphologic features are the same as for the cervix. In patients with vaginal adenosis, immature squamous metaplasia involving areas of adenosis can be mistaken for invasive squamous cell carcinoma, but the two entities can be readily distinguished by the lack of cytologic atypia and the lack of desmoplastic response with the benign process.

Glandular Lesions of the Vagina

Clear cell adenocarcinoma is the most common malignant glandular lesion in the vagina, followed by endometrioid, mucinous, and mesonephric subtypes. The latter histologic subtypes occur predominantly in perimenopausal women.

Clear Cell Adenocarcinoma

Clear cell carcinoma of the cervicovaginal region is strongly linked to *in utero* exposure to diethylstilbestrol (DES) and has decreased in incidence with decreased use of this teratogen. It typically **occurs in association with adenosis.** Although the upper vagina is the most common site of involvement in DES-exposed women, the cervix is the most commonly affected site in non-DES–exposed women. The appearance is the same as the ovarian counterpart (Fig. 5.24), and prognosis is determined by tumor size, depth of invasion, and lymph node involvement.

Adenosis

The presence of ectopic glandular epithelium in the vagina is termed *adenosis*. Adenosis may exhibit mucinous endocervical-like epithelium or tuboendometrioid epithelium. It is often asymptomatic, but may be detected by colposcopic examination. Atypical adenosis, which exhibits architectural and cytologic atypia, is often seen in association with clear cell adenocarcinoma.

Fibroepithelial Stromal Polyp

Fibroepithelial stromal polyp is a common, typically small, exophytic polypoid lesion occurring in reproductive-aged women, most commonly in the vagina, but also in the vulva and cervix. Almost one-third occur during pregnancy. The polyps often occur in the anterior wall and range in size from 0.5 cm to 4 cm. Histologically, they are characterized by small spindle cells and enlarged, stellate, multinucleated cells in a myxoid stroma (Fig. 5.25). Mitotic figures can be prominent and may raise suspicion for a malignant process. Fibroepithelial stromal polyps are distinguished from sarcoma botryoides by the absence of a cambium layer.

Sarcoma Botyroides

Embryonal rhabdomyosarcoma is the most common vaginal sarcoma; it occurs almost always in infants and children, but rare cases have been reported in young adults and postmenopausal women. **The tumors present as polypoid vaginal masses, often protruding through the introitus,** that may vary in size from 0.2 cm to 12 cm. Microscopically, the tumor is composed of small, round to oval or spindle-shaped cells surrounded by an edematous, myxoid stroma (Fig. 5.26). A characteristically dense, cellular cambium layer can be seen in the subepithelial zone. Rhabdomyoblasts (strap cells) are present but may be sparse or ill defined. Identification of rhabdomyoblasts can be facilitated by immunostaining for myogenin or Myo-D1.

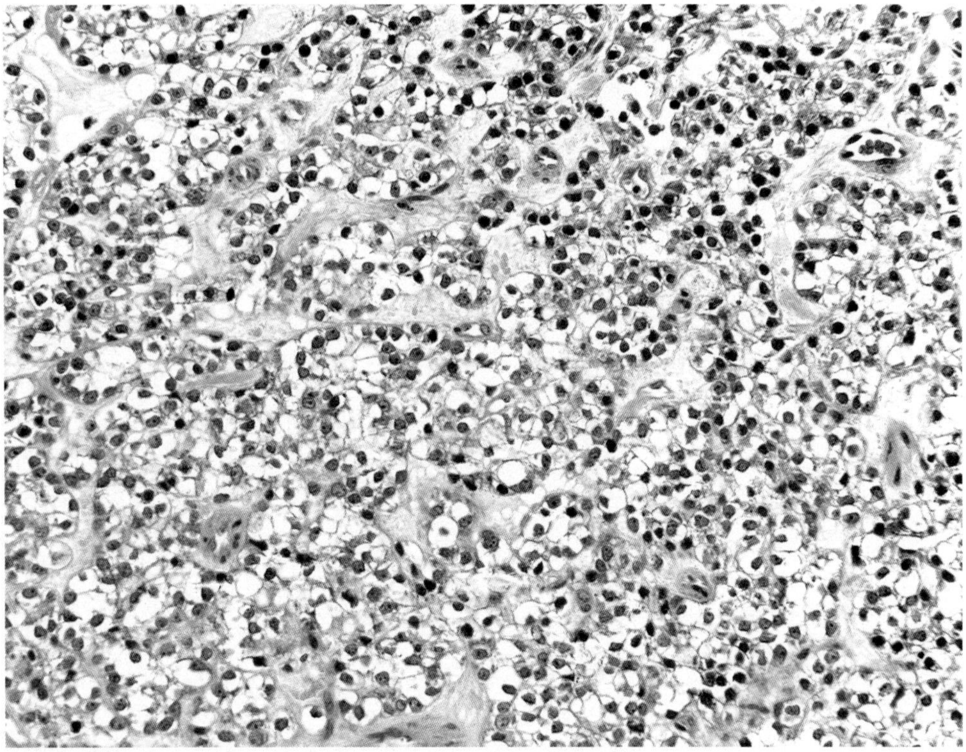

Figure 5.24 Clear cell adenocarcinoma of vagina. In this solid pattern of clear cell carcinoma, sheets of malignant cells with clear cytoplasm extensively replace normal tissue.

Wide local excision and combination chemotherapy is the preferred treatment for sarcoma botyroides. Staging in children is based on the Intergroup Rhabdomyosarcoma Study Group classification; adults are staged according to the TNM and FIGO system. Most rhabdomyosarcomas in the vulvovaginal region are of the embryonal type, but rare tumors are of the alveolar type, which has a worse prognosis.

Melanoma

Melanoma is the second most common malignancy to occur in the vagina (after squamous cell carcinoma). Affected patients are typically 60 years of age and present with vaginal bleeding. Most, but not all lesions are pigmented, nodular, or flat, and measure 2 to 3 cm in size at diagnosis; ulceration may be present. **The anterior wall of the lower third of the vagina is the most common site.** The diagnosis may be difficult on small biopsies because an *in situ* component or pagetoid spread is often absent. Epithelioid cell lesions may resemble carcinoma, whereas spindle cell lesions may create confusion with sarcoma. Immunohistochemical stains for melanoma markers are often required to establish a diagnosis. The prognosis is poor.

Postoperative Spindle Cell Nodule

A variety of reactive processes may occur within the vagina, particularly following surgical procedures. One such lesion is composed of a cellular, spindle cell proliferation that may simulate a neoplastic process. This lesion has been designated as postoperative spindle cell nodule.

Vulva

Squamous Cell Lesions of the Vulva

Terminology

Similar to the cervix, there are multiple terminology systems in use to describe preneoplastic lesions of the vulva (25) (Table 5.5). The main difference lies in whether VIN is graded. **The 2003**

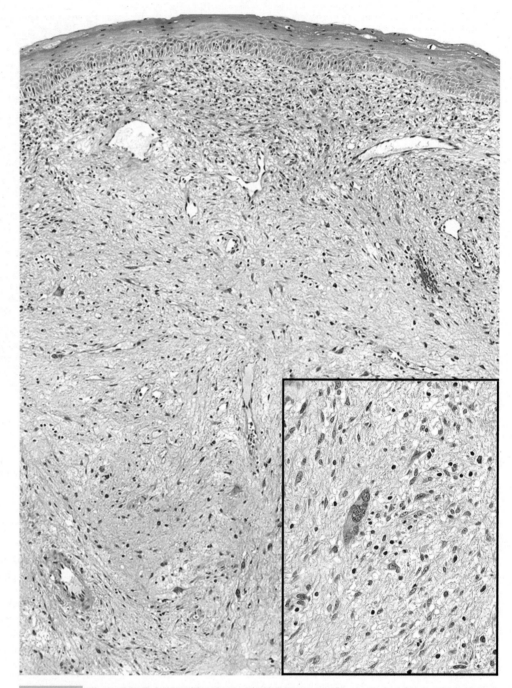

Figure 5.25 **Fibroepithelial stromal polyp.** Atypical stromal cells (inset) may simulate a malignancy, but this is a benign, probably reactive process. Although the lesion extends to the surface epithelium, there is no cellular condensation (forming a so-called cambium layer) at the surface; the absence of a cambium layer helps to distinguish this lesion from sarcoma botyroides on a limited sampling (see **Figure 5.26**). This polyp occurs most commonly in the vagina but can also be seen in the vulva and cervix.

World Health Organization (WHO) classification grades VIN on a scale of 1 to 3, with VIN 3 further subdivided into classic type and simplex type. In contrast, **the International Society for the Study of Vulvovaginal Disease (ISSVD) decided in 2004 to eliminate the category of VIN 1, and to abolish grading of VIN.** This decision was based on the lack of evidence that condylomas, which account for the majority of VIN 1 lesions, progress to carcinoma, and the lack of interobserver reproducibility for diagnosing VIN 1 or for distinguishing between VIN 2 and VIN 3 (26). The ISSVD retained the distinction between classic VIN and simplex (differentiated)

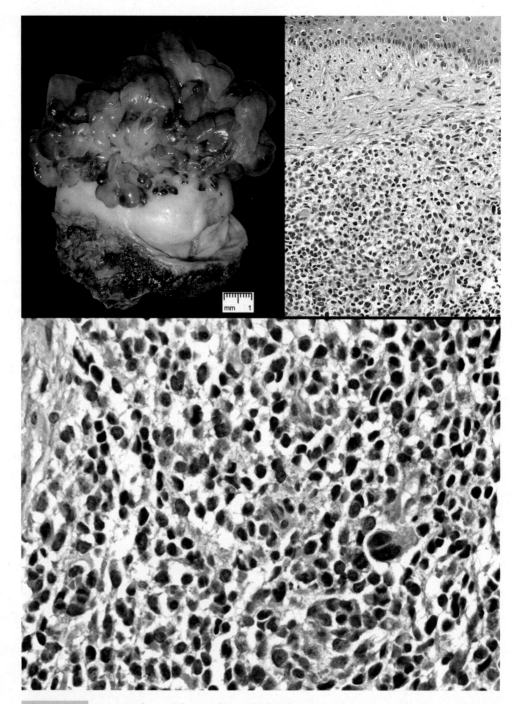

Figure 5.26 **Sarcoma botyroides (embryonal rhabdomyosarcoma).** Top left: Botyroid growth pattern of cervical embryonal rhabdomyosarcoma (Courtesy of Dr. Matthew Quick). Top right: Stellate cells set in myxoid stroma are more condensed beneath the surface epithelium, forming a distinct cambium layer. Bottom: Small cells with hyperchromatic nuclei are punctuated by larger cells with more abundant eosinophilic cytoplasm.

VIN. Given the variability in terminology, it is best to determine what terminology system the pathologist is using, especially if the diagnosis is "vulvar intraepithelial neoplasia (VIN)" with no further specification.

Vulvar Intraepithelial Neoplasia

In the vulva, there are two different pathways—HPV-related and HPV-unrelated—that lead to the development of squamous cell carcinoma. **The two-tiered CAP-ASCCP LAST**

	Table 5.5 Terminology for Precursor Lesions of Vulvar Squamous Cell Carcinoma		
LAST 2012	*WHO 2003*	*ISSVD 2004*	*Synonyms*
LSIL	Condyloma acuminatum	Condyloma acuminatum	n/a
LSIL	VIN 1	n/a	Flat condyloma, mild dysplasia
HSIL	VIN 2	VIN, usual type	Moderate dysplasia
HSIL	VIN 3		Severe dysplasia, carcinoma *in situ,* Bowen disease, bowenoid papulosis, bowenoid dysplasia
n/a	Carcinoma *in situ* (simplex type) VIN 3	VIN, differentiated type	n/a

LAST, Lower Anogenital Squamous Terminology; WHO, World Health Organization; ISSVD, International Society for the Study of Vulvar Disease; LSIL, low-grade squamous intraepithelial lesion; VIN, vulvar intraepithelial neoplasia; HSIL, high-grade squamous intraepithelial lesion.

Project terminology applies to HPV-related precursor lesions of the vulva (1). LSIL consists predominantly of condyloma acuminata, which are associated with low-risk HPV types 6 and 11 (Fig. 5.27). Flat condylomas are uncommon in the vulva, but may be associated with high-risk HPV. Fibroepithelial polyps (skin tags) and hymenal mucosa can be mistaken for exophytic condylomas. Nonspecific inflammatory atypia or psoriasis can be misdiagnosed as flat condylomas.

Vulvar HSIL can be qualified as VIN 2 or VIN 3. High-risk HPV is identified in 53–90% of cases of HSIL (VIN 3), with HPV 16 the most common type (27). HPV 18, 31, 33, 35, 51, 52, and 68 have also been isolated from cases of vulvar HSIL (28).

Vulvar HSIL is commonly multicentric, with extension to the perineum and involvement of the cervix and vagina. There are three patterns or subtypes of vulvar HSIL: warty, basaloid, and pagetoid. The **warty pattern** is characterized by prominent koilocytosis or warty architecture (Fig. 5.28), whereas the **basaloid** is more poorly differentiated (Fig. 5.29). The atypia involves two-thirds or more of the epithelium and is notable for disorganization, cells with high

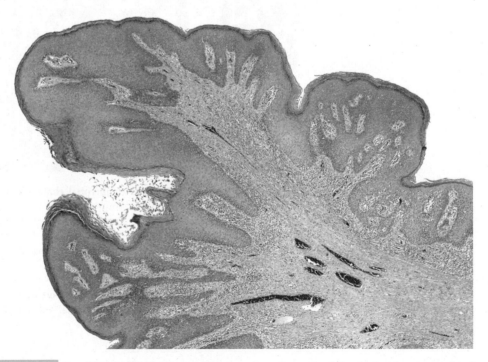

Figure 5.27 Condyloma. Exophytic condylomas are common in the vulva and are associated with low-risk HPV types 6 and 11.

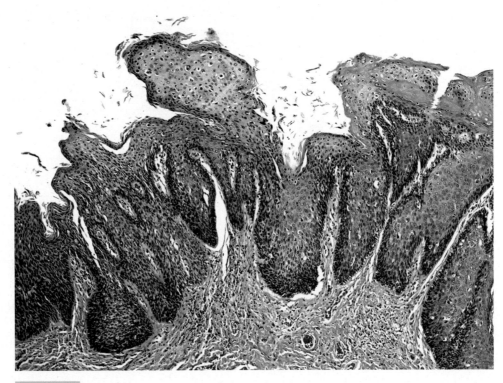

Figure 5.28 Classic VIN, warty. Prominent koilocytosis is present on the surface and overlies severe atypia involving two-thirds of the underlying epithelium.

nuclear-to-cytoplasmic ratios, dark irregular nuclei, and numerous mitotic figures, including abnormal forms. Dyskeratotic cells are often present, and the dysplastic cells frequently extend down pilosebaceous units, which can mimic invasive carcinoma.

The **pagetoid subtype** is rare but important to recognize because it can closely mimic extramammary Paget disease. The distinction between these two entities requires special stains, because

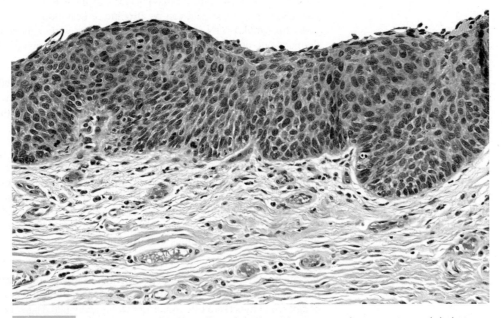

Figure 5.29 Classic VIN, basaloid. Cells with high nuclear-to-cytoplasmic ratios and dark, irregular nuclei involve the full thickness of the squamous epithelium.

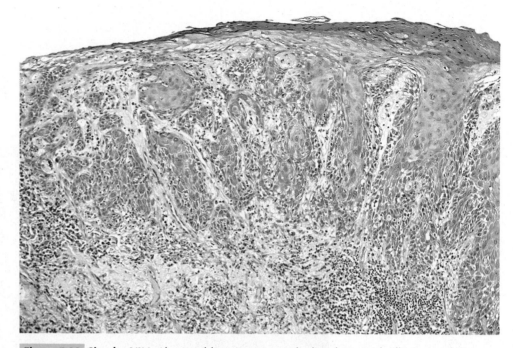

Figure 5.30 Simplex VIN. Abnormal keratinocytes with abundant, markedly eosinophilic cytoplasm involve the mid to superficial layers and extend into the elongated, branching rete ridges.

histologically, they both are characterized by single cells and clusters of cells with pale cytoplasm involving the squamous epithelium of the vulva.

Differentiated or simplex VIN is localized to the vulva and usually identified adjacent to areas of invasive carcinoma in elderly patients. It is rarely identified prospectively (29). In contrast to vulvar HSIL, **HPV is rarely identified in simplex VIN** (28). The morphologic changes of simplex VIN are subtle, and characterized by nuclear atypia of the basal cell layer and expansion of the basal layer into elongated, narrow, branching rete ridges (Fig. 5.30). The nuclei can range from relatively small, dark and irregular, to enlarged and pleomorphic. Maturation is abnormal, as exhibited by the presence of enlarged keratinocytes with large, pleomorphic nuclei and abundant, markedly eosinophilic cytoplasm in the mid- to superficial layers. These abnormal keratinocytes can extend into the basal layer and involve the rete ridges (29). The thickness of the epithelium is variable, and can be atrophic or acanthotic (i.e., thickened). The differential diagnosis for simplex VIN includes lichen sclerosus with squamous hyperplasia, and other benign dermatologic conditions such as lichen simplex chronicus, psoriasis, spongiotic dermatitis, and candida vulvitis.

Lichen sclerosus is a potential risk factor for the development of vulvar squamous cell carcinoma. It may play a role in the HPV-independent pathway. **Lichen sclerosus is negative for HPV** and is more frequently identified in association with simplex VIN than with classic VIN (27,28).

Squamous Cell Carcinoma

Primary invasive squamous cell carcinomas of the vulva can be subdivided into two main types: conventional squamous cell carcinoma and verrucous carcinoma. Conventional squamous cell carcinomas can exhibit different growth patterns, including warty, basaloid, and keratinizing (Fig. 5.31). Invasive squamous cell carcinomas that have warty or basaloid features are typically associated with classic VIN and high-risk HPV, whereas well-differentiated keratinizing squamous cell carcinomas are more commonly associated with simplex VIN (27).

Verrucous carcinoma is a rare special variant of squamous cell carcinoma that is slow growing and has minimal metastatic potential. It is typically exophytic, well circumscribed, and composed of hyperkeratotic fronds of cytologically bland squamous epithelium. The interface with the underlying stroma characteristically consists of a pushing border with associated chronic inflammation (Fig. 5.32).

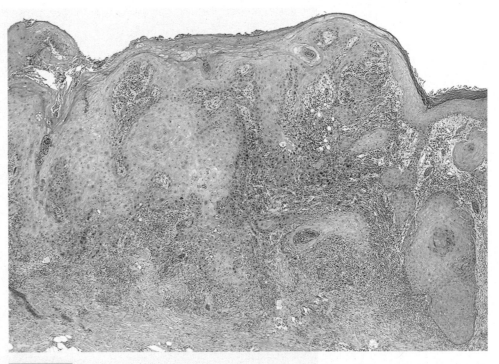

Figure 5.31 Conventional keratinizing squamous cell carcinoma of the vulva. Nests of well-differentiated tumor cells jaggedly invade into the stroma on microscopic examination.

Other Vulvar Lesions

Bartholin Cyst

Bartholin duct cyst is the most common cystic growth in the vulva. It occurs posteriorly in the vulvar vestibule. Excision is usually reserved for those lesions that fail to respond to conservative management. Some investigators recommend excision of Bartholin gland cysts to exclude adenocarcinoma when cysts or abscesses occur in patients more than 40 years of age. **The cyst lining is often variable: endocervical-like mucinous, squamous, and transitional epithelium is often present.** Cellular atypia, cellular stratification, and mitotic figures are concerning features, and should warrant full pathologic examination of the entire cyst wall to exclude carcinoma.

Bartholin Gland Adenocarcinoma

An uncommon tumor, this neoplasm affects women 50 years of age and older. The clinical impression is usually that of a Bartholin duct cyst. **Histologic types include adenocarcinoma, squamous cell carcinoma, adenoid cystic carcinoma, and hybrid types.** A transition zone adjacent to the Bartholin gland confirms the diagnosis. Approximately 20% of patients have ipsilateral groin lymph node metastases at initial diagnosis.

Fibroepithelial Stromal Polyp

Fibroepithelial stromal polyps occur on the vulva, but are most commonly seen in the vagina (30). They may be single or multiple. **Fibroepithelial stromal polyps probably represent a reactive lesion rather than a true neoplasm.**

Hidradenoma Papilliferum

A rare benign glandular neoplasm, papillary hidradenoma usually occurs in the region of the intralabial sulcus in adult women. The tumor is well circumscribed and composed of complex, branching papillae lined by a double layer of outer myoepithelial and inner epithelial cells (31).

Extramammary Paget Disease

Paget disease of the vulva is an intraepithelial neoplasm characterized by large, round cells with abundant, pale cytoplasm, often forming small intracytoplasmic lumina or glandlike structures (31). **Vulvar Paget disease may be primary or secondary, and presents clinically as a red, eczematous lesion. Postmenopausal women are most commonly affected.** Approximately 90% are primary and noninvasive (cutaneous), whereas 10% are associated with an underlying invasive

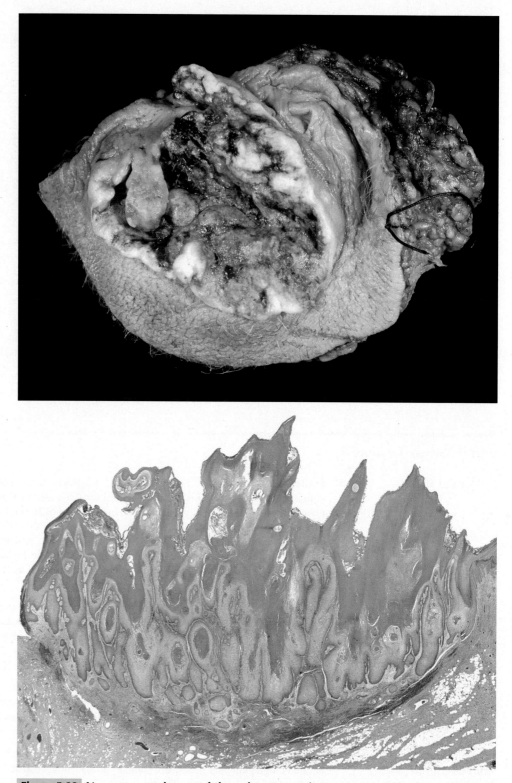

Figure 5.32 Verrucous carcinoma of the vulva. Top: Vulvectomy specimen shows exophytic verrucous tumor. Bottom: The tumor is exophytic with hyperkeratotic fronds of bland squamous epithelium and well circumscribed with a pushing border with the underlying stroma.

carcinoma (cutaneous, anorectal, urothelial). **All forms of Paget disease are immunoreactive for cytokeratin and epithelial membrane antigen.** Classic primary cutaneous vulvar Paget disease expresses CK7 and HER2 (Fig. 5.33), whereas secondary Paget's often exhibits an immunophenotype of the primary site of origin.

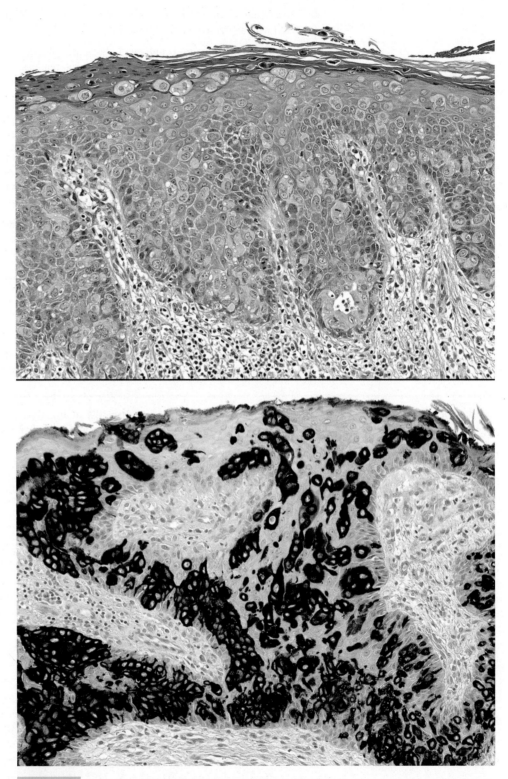

Figure 5.33 **Paget disease of vulva.** Top: Paget cells are confined to the intraepidermal compartment, forming small gland-like structures. Bottom: The Paget cells express cytokeratin 7.

Mesenchymal Tumors

A variety of specialized genital stromal neoplasms occur in the vulvovaginal region of reproductive-aged women (32). Most are small, hormonally responsive, and clinically indolent. The most common specialized genital stromal tumors are **angiomyofibroblastoma, cellular angiofibroma, and superficial angiomyxoma** (33). Often mistaken clinically for a Bartholin gland cyst, these specialized genital stromal lesions may recur locally if incompletely excised, but they are not associated with aggressive clinical behavior.

Prepubertal vulvar fibroma is unlikely to be confused with any of the typical vulvar mesenchymal lesions because of its predilection for prepubertal females. This lesion, which most commonly involves the labia majora, presents as a unilateral or rarely, bilateral, ill defined, and painless subcutaneous vulvar mass with microscopic features that suggest a hamartomatous process.

Other mesenchymal neoplasms that behave in a clinically benign fashion include lipoma, neurofibroma, schwannoma, granular cell tumor, glomus tumor, and hemangioma.

Dermatofibrosarcoma protuberans is a low-grade cutaneous tumor with a high risk for recurrence if incompletely excised. High-grade sarcomas that most commonly occur in the vulva include **rhabdomyosarcoma, proximal epithelioid sarcoma, alveolar soft part sarcoma, peripheral primitive neuroectodermal tumor, and postradiation angiosarcoma.**

Rarely, smooth muscle tumors may involve the vulvar region. Criteria for malignancy differ from those for uterine smooth muscle tumors, and are based on size (>5 cm), mitotic index (>5 mitotic figures per 10 high-power fields), infiltrative margins, and cellular atypia.

Aggressive Angiomyxoma

Aggressive angiomyxoma occurs in the deep vulvar and inguinal soft tissue and is characterized by a paucicellular spindle cell proliferation, separated by loose myxoid stroma (Fig. 5.34). Mitotic activity is low. Despite the bland histologic appearance, it is an infiltrative tumor that may locally invade deep pelvic structures if incompletely excised (31). Aggressive angiomyxoma occurs most commonly during the third to fifth decades. The clinical impression frequently includes Bartholin's gland cyst or hernia; the extent of disease is often underestimated.

Melanocytic Tumors

Malignant melanoma accounts for less than 10% of all vulvar malignancies, and consists of **three types: mucosal or acral lentiginous, nodular, and superficial spreading.** Up to 25% of tumors

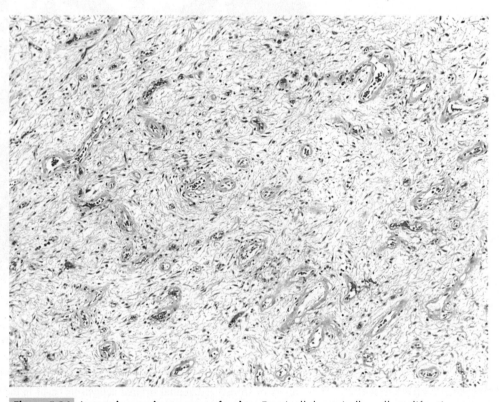

Figure 5.34 Aggressive angiomyxoma of vulva. Paucicellular spindle cell proliferation separated by loose myxoid stroma. Despite the bland appearance, this is an infiltrative tumor with a propensity for recurrence if incompletely excised.

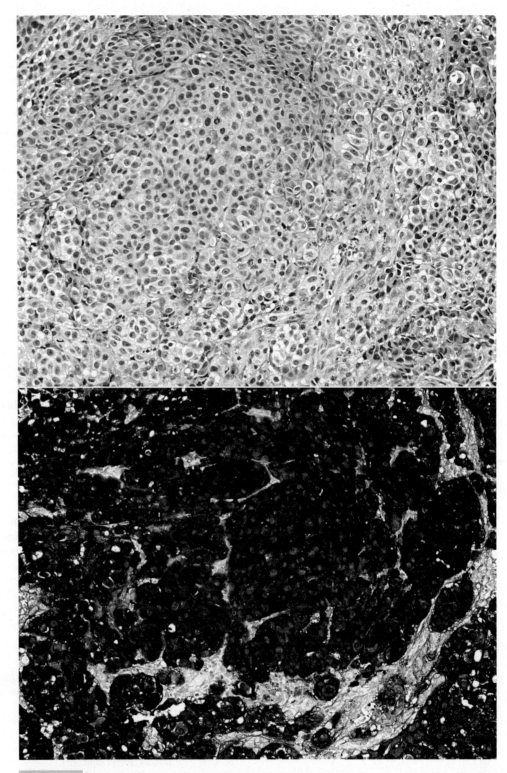

Figure 5.35 **Vulvar melanoma.** Top: Nests of epithelioid cells extensively replace normal vulvar tissue. Bottom: Strong expression of S100 protein.

are unclassified. Vulvar melanoma occurs more commonly in elderly, white women, and typically presents as a nodular mass that may be pigmented; satellite lesions are common. Melanomas express S-100 protein, HMB-45, and Melan A (Fig. 5.35). Clark levels and Breslow thickness should be reported for all vulvar melanomas.

Benign, atypical, and dysplastic nevi occur in the vulva. **Benign nevi** may be congenital or acquired. **Atypical vulvar nevi** (atypical melanocytic nevi of the genital type) occur primarily in young, reproductive-aged women and are characterized by atypical, superficial melanocytes, and variably sized junctional melanocytic nests. They are distinguished from melanomas on the basis of small size, circumscription, absence of pagetoid spread, significant cytologic atypia, and mitotic activity in the deeper dermal melanocytes. **Atypical vulvar nevi** may appear more atypical during pregnancy. **They are not associated with dysplastic nevi elsewhere.**

Dysplastic nevi occur predominantly in younger women and exhibit an irregular border; microscopically, clusters of atypical spindled and epithelioid nevus cells with prominent nucleoli and nuclear pleomorphism are seen. **Unlike atypical vulvar nevi, dysplastic vulvar nevi may be associated with dysplastic nevi elsewhere on the trunk and extremities.**

Uncommon Neoplasms

Other tumors that occur in the vulva include cutaneous adnexal tumors, tumors that arise from specialized anogenital mammary-like glands, and tumors of minor vestibulary gland and Skene gland origin (31).

Uterine Corpus

Endometrial Neoplasms

The endometrial morphologic changes with which the gynecologic oncologist is concerned are limited, and chiefly involve endometrial carcinoma and its precursors. This section focuses on these proliferations, and those that figure in their differential diagnosis.

In discussing endometrial nonsecretory proliferations, it is helpful to realize that **the endometrium can give rise to a variety of epithelial phenotypes that are more commonly encountered in other parts of the müllerian-derived system: the ovary, the fallopian tubes, and the endocervix. The term** *metaplasia* **is used for benign epithelial proliferations of this type, and** *special variant carcinoma* **is used for the malignant patterns.** Endometrial epithelial proliferations, whether benign or malignant, typically feature mixtures of these differentiated epithelial types. The carcinoma precursors feature this mixed epithelial phenotype in varying degrees, hence the full designation *hyperplasia/metaplasia,* which is to be understood when *hyperplasia* is used unmodified.

Endometrial Hyperplasia/Metaplasia

The term *endometrial hyperplasia* **denotes a proliferating endometrium featuring glandular architectural abnormalities that result in glandular crowding, and take the form of either cystic dilatation of glands (simple hyperplasia) or glandular budding (complex hyperplasia).** The current WHO taxonomy stratifies hyperplastic endometria on the basis of their cytologic features into **atypical endometrial hyperplasia** and **nonatypical endometrial hyperplasia,** the latter term implying that significant cytologic atypia is absent. The risk posed by hyperplasia for the subsequent development of endometrial carcinoma is roughly correlated with the degree of cytologic atypia present. The assessment of atypia is subject to observer disagreement. (Table 5.6) (Figs. 5.36 and 5.37).

Table 5.6 Features of Endometrial Hyperplasias		
	Hyperplasia Without Atypia	*Atypical Hyperplasia*[a]
Histology	Increased number of round glands, which may be cystically dilated ("Swiss cheese"). The glands are closely packed and have irregular contours; little stroma remains between glands. No cytologic atypia.[a]	Cytologic atypia (nuclear pleomorphism, loss of polarity, prominent nucleoli). Architecture may be either simple or (more commonly) complex.
Clinical	Perimenopausal and postmenopausal women	Postmenopausal
Premalignant potential	5–10%	≥30%

[a]Most atypical hyperplasia are complex.

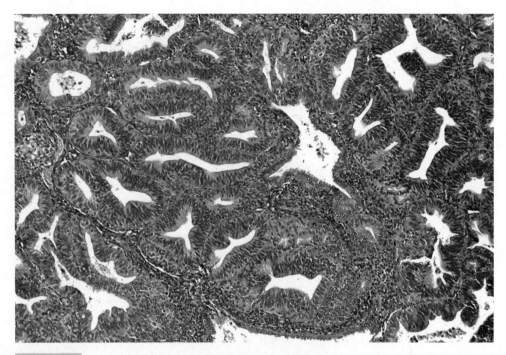

Figure 5.36 Simple endometrial hyperplasia without atypia. An increased number of round glands is seen, some of which are dilated. There is no cytologic atypia.

Differential Diagnosis

Atrophic or Weakly Proliferative Endometrium with the Architecture of Hyperplasia   When a complex hyperplasia is the last unshed endometrium of a postmenopausal woman and the epithelium subsequently becomes atrophic in the wake of estrogen withdrawal, the pattern often mimics hyperplasia. Confusion is avoided when it is noted that the epithelium is atrophic and not proliferating.

Well-differentiated Adenocarcinoma   This is the chief differential diagnostic consideration and, unfortunately, the one that exhibits one of the highest levels of expert disagreement in gynecologic pathology. The differential diagnosis is discussed below.

Endometrial Carcinoma

Histologic Types

First, carcinomas may be classified in terms of their differentiated histopathologic features (Table 5.7). The endometrium gives rise to a variety of differentiated carcinomas, but more than 80% are glandular neoplasms that resemble the epithelium found in endometrial hyperplasia. **Squamous or squamoid (*morular*) differentiation is commonly encountered in this endometrioid or usual adenocarcinoma.** The term *endometrioid* is used to denote this histologic pattern, and to distinguish it from *endometrial,* which is the generic term for carcinomas that originated anatomically in the endometrium. Other müllerian-differentiated types (e.g., serous, clear cell, mucinous) make up the remainder of the endometrial carcinomas, the so-called special variants.

Endometrial carcinomas may also be grouped with an eye to the hormonal (and associated epidemiologic) background in which they arise: **hyperestrogenic settings (type I) or hypoestrogenic settings (type II).**

Patients in the first group **(type I)** tend to be between 40 and 60 years of age (although carcinoma can develop in younger women, including, in rare instances, those in their 20s). **They may have a history of chronic anovulation or estrogen hormone-replacement therapy,** and the carcinomas are usually well differentiated, stage I, nonmyoinvasive tumors associated with endometrial hyperplasia/metaplasia (found either concurrently or in previous endometrial samplings). **Most of the**

159

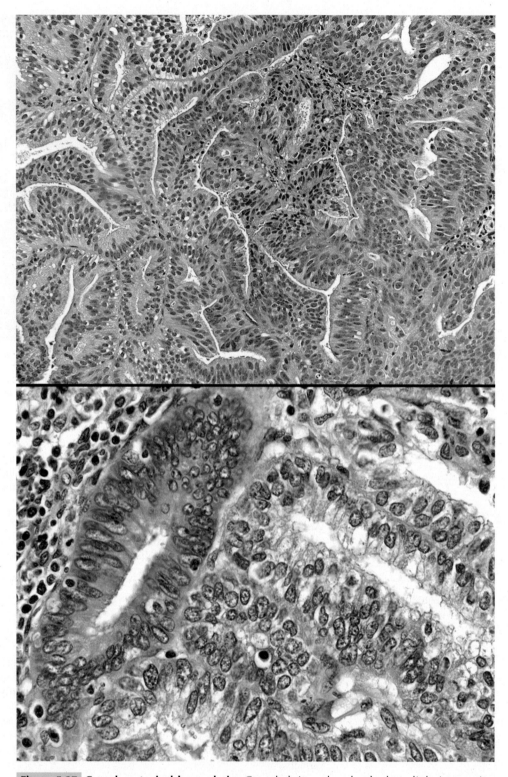

Figure 5.37 **Complex atypical hyperplasia.** Crowded, irregular glands show little intervening stroma. The glands show rounded, pleomorphic nuclei with prominent nucleoli. (top, low power; bottom, high power)

tumors are ER-positive and PR-positive and p53-negative and express low levels of the proliferation antigen Ki-67. Patients in this first group have a very favorable prognosis after hysterectomy.

In contrast, patients in the second group (**type II**) tend to be elderly, and typically have no history of hyperestrogenism. In these cases, the surrounding nonneoplastic endometrium is almost always

Table 5.7 Classification of Endometrial Carcinoma
Endometrioid Carcinoma (Usual)
a. Secretory
b. Villoglandular
c. With squamous differentiation (includes adenoacanthoma and adenosquamous carcinomas—see text)
Special Variant Carcinomas
a. Serous
b. Clear cell
c. Mucinous
d. Pure squamous cell
e. Mixed
f. Undifferentiated
g. Dedifferentiated
h. Neuroendocrine

atrophic or only weakly estrogen supported, but there may be an *in situ* component with high-grade cytologic features. **The carcinomas that develop in this group of patients are usually of the special variant type with a poor prognosis, or are high-grade endometrioid neoplasms that are high stage with deep myoinvasion. They tend to be ER-negative and PR-negative, strongly express p53, and show high Ki-67 labeling.**

Most endometrial adenocarcinomas are of endometrioid type. In these tumors, malignant glands are lined by stratified, often elongated, nuclei, reminiscent of benign endometrial epithelium. A distinct subtype of endometrioid carcinoma is **villoglandular carcinoma,** in which there are long, slender papillae lined by relatively bland cells with cigar-shaped nuclei (Fig. 5.38). Villoglandular carcinoma is a low-grade tumor, and the main reason for recognizing this subtype is that it should not be confused with serous carcinoma of the endometrium, which is papillary, but has a much worse prognosis.

Well-differentiated Endometrioid Adenocarcinoma versus Atypical Hyperplasia or Metaplasia

Several morphologic definitions of well-differentiated endometrioid adenocarcinoma have been published over the years, and they differ in various respects (34,35). Most require a certain level of cytologic atypia or architectural complexity. Architectural complexity usually takes the form of one or more of the following: extensive budding and branching of glands, papillary structures with superimposed secondary structures (buds or secondary papillae), and a cribriform pattern (Fig. 5.39). Expert disagreement over cases in this gray zone is common. This disagreement impedes clinical decision making in only a small subset of patients, including those with comorbidities or those for whom uterine conservation is important.

Endometrioid Adenocarcinoma with Squamous Elements

Squamous elements are very common in endometrioid adenocarcinoma of all grades (Fig. 5.40). The presence of squamous differentiation does not affect the prognosis. Of importance, the squamous areas (benign or malignant), which typically form sheets, are ruled out when determining architectural grade (see below).

Other subtypes of endometrioid adenocarcinoma include the rare secretory carcinoma and ciliated carcinomas. These are well differentiated and have a favorable prognosis. These morphologic patterns can be seen focally in an otherwise ordinary endometrioid carcinoma.

Mucinous Adenocarcinoma

Mucinous adenocarcinoma (Fig. 5.41) **is usually low grade and low stage and is frequently seen in women treated with *tamoxifen.*** If this pattern is seen in an endometrial sampling, the anatomic origin—cervix or endometrium—may be in doubt. Strategies for illuminating this issue are set out in Table 5.5.

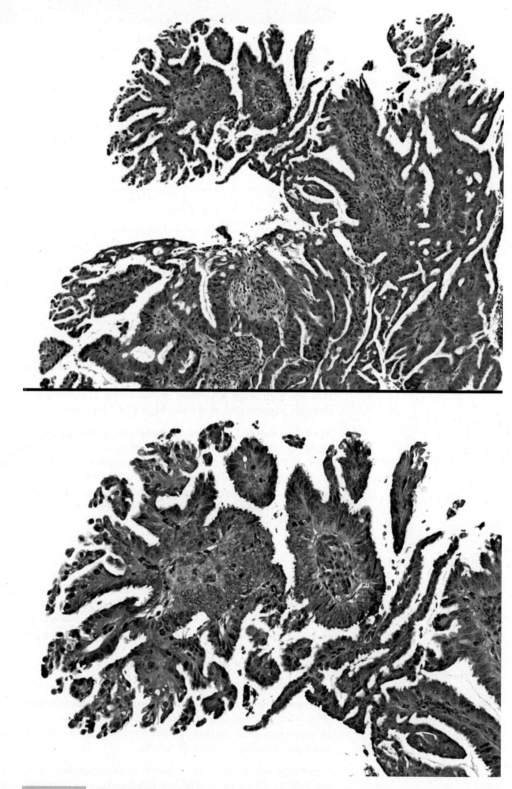

Figure 5.38 **Villoglandular carcinoma.** Delicate, elongated papillae (analogous to villous structures in villous adenomas of the large bowel) are lined by small, complex, epithelial buds. (top, low power; bottom, high power)

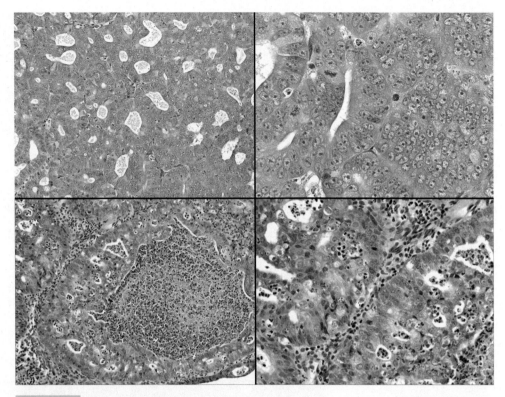

Figure 5.39 **Well-differentiated endometrioid adenocarcinoma.** Back-to-back glands with minimal or no intervening stroma (upper left) and cytologic atypia (note prominent nucleoli, upper right) are features of usual endometrial carcinoma. Glandular nests with extensive cribriforming are another common pattern seen in endometrioid adenocarcinoma (lower left and lower right). Note that in this example, the cytologic atypia is not significantly different from that seen in endometrial hyperplasia (lower right) and the diagnosis of carcinoma is based on complex architecture.

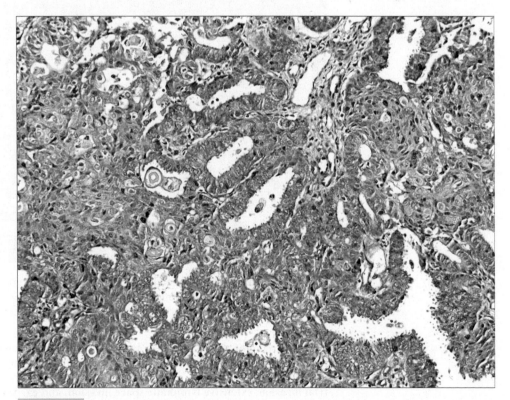

Figure 5.40 **Endometrioid adenocarcinoma with squamous elements.** A solid area of benign-appearing squamous cells is seen in the low center portion of the field.

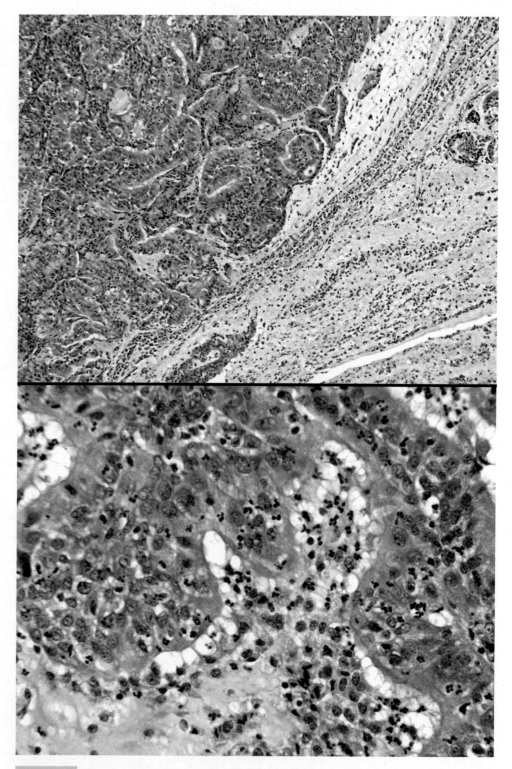

Figure 5.41 **Mucinous adenocarcinoma.** Confluent and cribriform glands are lined by mucinous epithelium. (top, low power; bottom, high power)

Serous Carcinoma

Serous carcinoma makes up between 5–10% of all endometrial carcinomas and is known for its aggressive behavior (36–38). It typically affects postmenopausal women and arises in the setting of endometrial atrophy. The hallmarks of this carcinoma are a **tendency for myometrial invasion, extensive lymphatic space invasion, and early, clinically inapparent dissemination** beyond the uterus (most often in the form of diffuse peritoneal involvement).

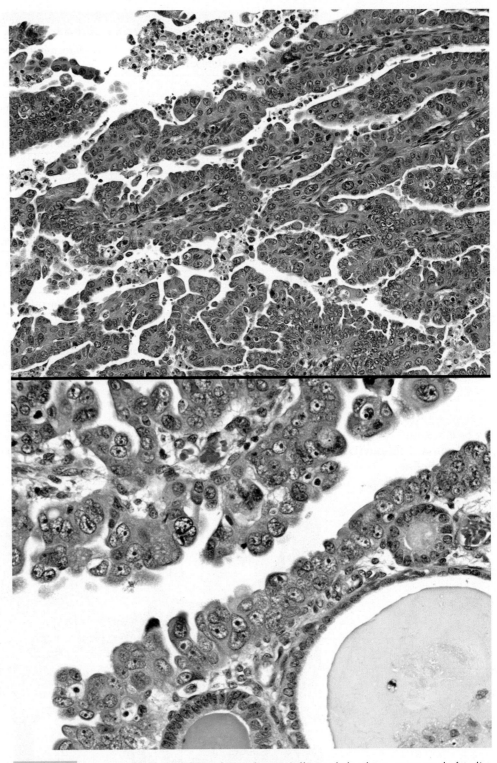

Figure 5.42 Serous carcinoma of the endometrium. Papillae and glands are composed of malignant cells with marked nuclear atypia. (top, low power; bottom, high power)

Microscopically, the tumor is composed of complex papillary fronds, lined by highly malignant cells possessing prominent, eosinophilic nucleoli (Fig. 5.42). Uterine serous carcinomas may express ER and/or PR, but the expression levels are generally lower than those seen in low-grade endometrioid carcinomas; uterine serous carcinomas are strongly immunoreactive for p53. **Serous carcinoma of the endometrium is not graded, but is regarded as a high-grade tumor by definition.**

Table 5.8 Papillary Proliferations of the Endometrium		
Anticipated Clinical Behavior	*Architecture of Connective Tissue Scaffolding*	*Cytologic Atypia*
Benign		
Papillary syncytial metaplasia	Epithelial stratification with a papillary configuration	Minimal
Papillary change	Three-dimensional papillae	Minimal
Villoglandular hyperplasia	Sheets or folia	Minimal to moderate
Type I carcinomas		
Villoglandular endometrioid carcinoma	Sheets or folia	Moderate to severe
Endometrioid carcinomas with small nonvillous papillae	Epithelial stratification with a papillary configuration	Minimal to moderate
Mucinous carcinoma	Sheets or folia	Moderate to severe
Type II carcinomas		
Uterine (papillary) serous carcinoma	Three-dimensional papillae	Markedly atypical

Most papillary proliferations of the endometrium are not serous carcinomas; more frequent are papillary hyperplasia/metaplasias and villoglandular endometrioid carcinomas. All of these are benign or low-grade proliferations (Table 5.8). Metastatic serous carcinoma to the endometrium must be ruled out.

In Situ Serous Carcinoma (Endometrial Intraepithelial Carcinoma)

This lesion is characterized by replacement of benign (often atrophic) endometrial epithelium by highly malignant cells resembling serous carcinoma (Fig. 5.43) (38). It is regarded as a precursor of serous carcinoma and is sometimes seen adjacent to it (39).

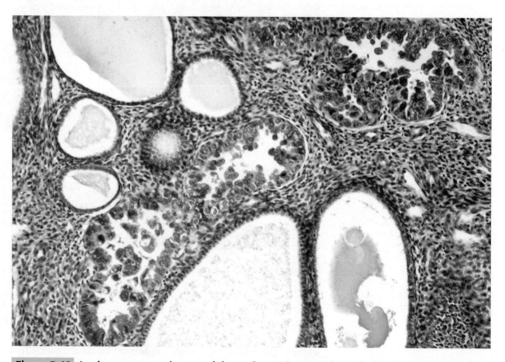

Figure 5.43 *In situ* **serous carcinoma of the endometrium.** High-grade nuclear atypia of serous carcinoma contrasts with benign, inactive glandular epithelium of the adjacent, nonhyperplastic endometrium.

Clear Cell Carcinoma

Primary clear cell carcinoma of the endometrium is very uncommon and is histologically indistinguishable from clear cell carcinoma of the ovary. This neoplasm combines high-grade cytologic features characterized by enlarged, angulated nuclei and large, irregular nucleoli, with cytoplasmic clearing (at least in focal areas). The architecture may be papillary, glandular, or sheetlike. When it is glandular, the tumor cell nuclei often protrude into the luminal space, giving rise to a **hobnail or tombstone appearance** (Fig. 5.44). **The differential diagnosis includes**

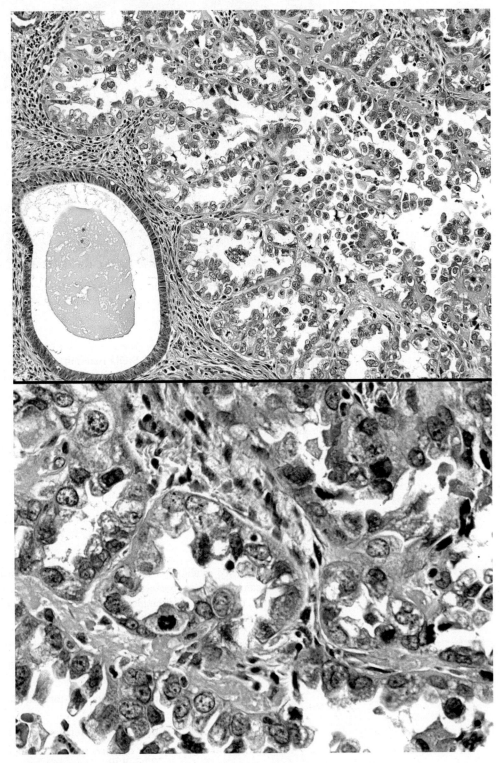

Figure 5.44 **Clear cell carcinoma of the endometrium.** Malignant glands are lined by anaplastic hobnail cells with clear cytoplasm. (top, low power; bottom, high power)

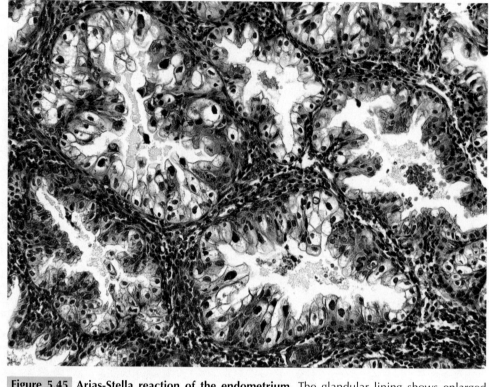

Figure 5.45 **Arias-Stella reaction of the endometrium.** The glandular lining shows enlarged hobnail cells with clear cytoplasm and "smudged" nuclei, a pattern that may mimic clear cell carcinoma.

(i) the hypersecretory change (**Arias-Stella reaction**) (Fig. 5.45) seen both in pregnancy and with the use of progestational medication and (ii) the clinically nonaggressive **secretory variant of endometrioid carcinoma.**

Squamous Cell Carcinoma	Primary squamous cell carcinoma of the endometrium is very rare and is much less common than extension of a primary uterine cervical carcinoma to the endometrium. Primary squamous cell carcinoma of the endometrium may be associated with cervical stenosis and pyometra.
Undifferentiated Carcinoma	This is a tumor that shows no glandular or squamous differentiation. It represents 1–2% of all endometrial carcinomas and has epidemiologic features similar to those of endometrioid carcinoma.
Mixed Carcinoma	Tumor heterogeneity is ubiquitous and a well-established consequence of tumor progression; endometrial carcinomas are no exception. When differences between components become sufficiently striking, the term *mixed* is employed. To qualify for this diagnosis, **the minor component(s) should compose 10% or more of the tumor**.

Histologic Grading of Endometrioid Carcinoma

The histologic grade is assigned according to the percentage of solid epithelial growth (not including areas of squamous differentiation).

1. **FIGO grade 1: The tumor exhibits well-formed glands and has 5% or less of solid growth pattern.**
2. **FIGO grade 2: The solid growth pattern occupies 6–50% of the tumor.**
3. **FIGO grade 3: The tumor displays more than 50% solid epithelial growth.**

Severe nuclear atypia raises the grade by one, but the possibility of a nonendometrioid (serous or clear cell) carcinoma should always be ruled out in this situation.

Pathologic Staging of Endometrial Carcinoma

Endocervical Involvement

Endocervical stromal involvement is usually diagnosed on the hysterectomy specimen. Infrequently, it may be diagnosed from an endocervical curettage, but the cancer present in the endocervical curettage is usually a contamination from the uterine cavity.

Myometrial Invasion

The depth of myometrial invasion is expressed as a proportion of the myometrium invaded by carcinoma. In the FIGO staging system, this is reported as inner or outer half. The presence of lymphatic or vascular space invasion is not used to determine the depth of invasion. Involvement of adenomyosis by adenocarcinoma may resemble myometrial invasion on intraoperative visual examination, but the presence of residual endometrial stroma or benign basalis glands between the tumor and myometrium is a helpful microscopic differentiating feature.

Ovarian Involvement

Simultaneous primary involvement should be considered before diagnosing ovarian metastases with well-differentiated uterine endometrioid carcinoma. In most such cases, the uterine tumor shows minimal or no myometrial invasion, and there is no lymphovascular or cervical stromal invasion.

Metastatic Carcinoma

The most common sites of origin for metastatic carcinomas presenting in the uterine corpus are breast, stomach, ovary, and colon. Most patients have a previous history of carcinoma, and the metastasis is not the first presentation of disease. Lymphoma and melanoma, although rare, continue to pose diagnostic problems when encountered in this location because of their mimicry of undifferentiated carcinoma or sarcoma. Use of a basic panel for undifferentiated tumors and a low threshold for suspecting metastasis will prevent most misclassifications.

Mesenchymal Neoplasms

Endometrial stromal tumors and smooth muscle tumors account for the majority of mesenchymal neoplasms in the uterine corpus. Although most endometrial stromal neoplasms are easily separated from smooth muscle neoplasms, there is a range over which clear distinction is not possible using conventional light microscopy and immunohistochemistry. These "mixed" tumors are occasionally referred to as stromomyomas. When such lesions remain ambiguous despite immunohistochemical analysis and the probability of an endometrial stromal proliferation is high on other grounds, they should be assigned to the endometrial stromal group for management purposes (40).

Smooth Muscle Tumors

Smooth muscle tumors are the most common mesenchymal neoplasm in the uterus. Most are composed of interlacing fascicles of spindle-shaped smooth muscle fibers (Fig. 5.46), but **epithelioid** (Fig. 5.47) and **myxoid** (Fig. 5.48) **variants** may be seen.

Leiomyoma

Leiomyomas represent the most common tumor of the uterus. They present during reproductive years and are often multiple. The typical gross appearance is that of a well-circumscribed, solid, white to tan myometrial nodule with a trabeculated surface on cut sections. Degenerative changes may alter this appearance, and edema, hemorrhage, fibrosis, and hyaline (infarction-type) necrosis are commonly seen. **Occasionally, mitotically active leiomyomas containing 15 or more mitotic figures per 10 high-power fields may be encountered, but in the absence of other atypical features** (i.e., coagulative tumor cell necrosis or significant cytologic atypia), **these neoplasms are clinically benign** (41).

Cellular Leiomyoma

Leiomyomas exhibiting dense cellularity without tumor cell necrosis or significant cytologic atypia are designated cellular leiomyomas. They are clinically benign, but may be confused with endometrial stromal neoplasms (Fig. 5.49). They are distinguished from stromal tumors by the

169

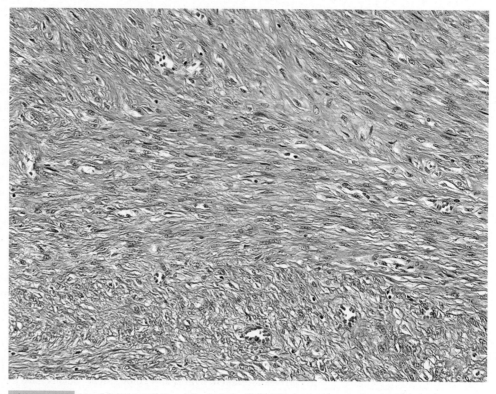

Figure 5.46 **Uterine smooth muscle tumor (leiomyoma), standard morphology.** The usual smooth muscle tumor forms a discrete intramyometrial fibrous mass. Bland spindle cell histology features ovoid, blunt-ended nuclei with no atypia.

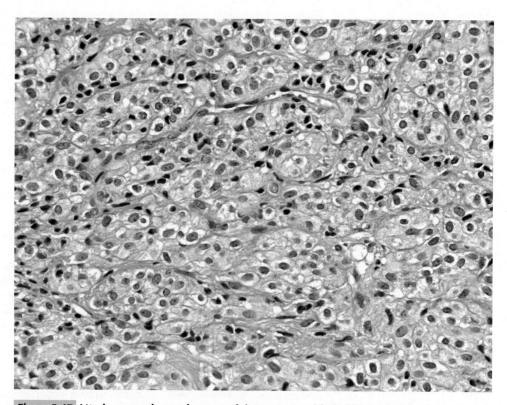

Figure 5.47 **Uterine smooth muscle tumor (leiomyoma), epithelioid morphology.** Some smooth muscle tumors exhibit pronounced epithelioid histology, mimicking epithelial processes.

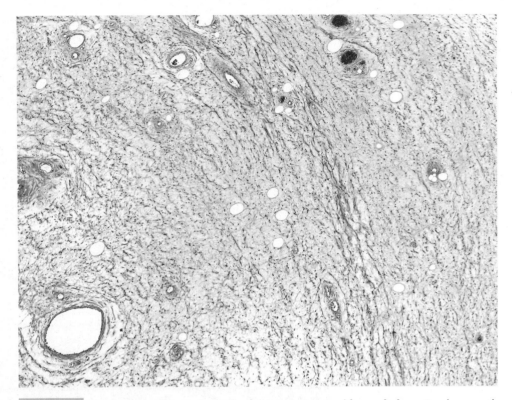

Figure 5.48 Uterine smooth muscle tumor (leiomyoma), myxoid morphology. Rarely, smooth muscle tumors undergo extensive myxoid change. In these cases, a myxoid leiomyosarcoma must be ruled out.

presence of diffuse expression of the smooth muscle markers desmin and h-caldesmon, with minimal or absent expression of CD10 (41).

Leiomyoma with Bizarre Nuclei (Atypical Leiomyoma)

Leiomyomas that exhibit diffuse or multifocal moderate to severe cytologic atypia, but no tumor cell necrosis or increased mitotic index (>10 mitotic figures per 10 high-power fields), are designated symplastic or bizarre leiomyomas. Most of these atypical leiomyomas (Fig. 5.50) are clinically benign, although local recurrence may rarely occur (42).

Leiomyosarcoma

Leiomyosarcomas are uncommon uterine tumors but are the most common sarcoma in the uterus. They typically affect adult women in the perimenopausal years. Leiomyosarcomas are typically solitary, fleshy, and necrotic intramural tumors. **The presence of coagulative tumor cell necrosis, moderate-to-severe cytologic atypia, and numerous mitotic figures distinguishes leiomyosarcomas from leiomyomas** (Fig. 5.51). Leiomyosarcoma is a highly malignant neoplasm and the prognosis is poor.

Epithelioid Leiomyosarcomas

These lesions exhibit patterns of epithelioid differentiation in addition to the usual features of malignancy seen in the more conventional leiomyosarcomas: cytologic atypia, tumor cell necrosis, and increased mitotic index (5 mitotic figures per 10 high-power fields) (41).

Myxoid Leiomyosarcoma

This is a large, gelatinous neoplasm that usually appears to be circumscribed on gross examination. Microscopically, the smooth muscle cells are usually widely separated by myxoid material (Fig. 5.52). The characteristic low cellularity partly accounts for the presence of only a few mitotic figures per 10 high-power fields in most myxoid leiomyosarcomas. Despite the low mitotic counts, myxoid leiomyosarcoma has the same unfavorable prognosis as typical leiomyosarcoma (41).

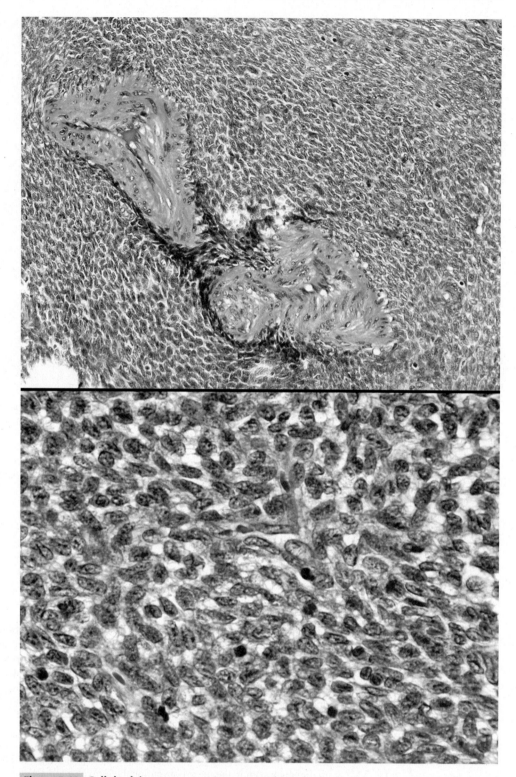

Figure 5.49 **Cellular leiomyoma.** Leiomyomas with marked cellularity may mimic endometrial stromal differentiation (see Figs. 5.53 and 5.54). (top, low power; bottom, high power)

Smooth Muscle Tumor of Uncertain Malignant Potential

Uterine smooth muscle tumors that cannot be reliably diagnosed as benign or malignant are designated as tumors of uncertain malignant potential. This diagnosis is used when there is uncertainty concerning the type of necrosis (hyaline versus coagulative), the subtype of smooth muscle differentiation (standard vs. epithelioid vs. myxoid), the degree of cytologic atypia, or the mitotic index (41).

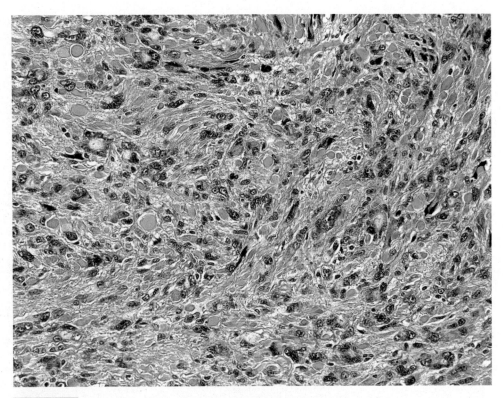

Figure 5.50 Leiomyoma with bizarre nuclei (atypical leiomyoma). Diffuse, marked nuclear atypia in the absence of tumor cell necrosis and increased mitotic index is classified as bizarre or symplastic leiomyoma (atypical leiomyoma), which has a very low risk of recurrence.

Smooth Muscle Neoplasms with Unusual Growth Patterns

Uterine smooth muscle tumors may demonstrate unusual patterns of distribution. As in other uterine smooth muscle neoplasms, the tumors showing these unusual patterns of distribution may exhibit standard spindle, epithelioid, or myxoid histology (41).

Diffuse Leiomyomatosis

Diffuse leiomyomatosis refers to the presence of numerous, histologically benign small smooth muscle nodules diffusely distributed throughout the uterus. The nodules range up to 3 cm in diameter, but most are less than 1 cm. This condition is benign.

Intravenous Leiomyomatosis

This condition is characterized by the presence of cords of histologically benign smooth muscle growing within venous channels beyond the confines of a leiomyoma. Extension into pelvic veins and, on occasion, the inferior vena cava and right heart may be seen.

Metastasizing Leiomyoma

This clinicopathologic condition consists of the presence of histologically benign smooth muscle tumors in the lung, pelvic lymph nodes, or abdomen in association with a histologically benign uterine smooth muscle tumor. Typically, the uterine tumor is removed years before the extrauterine tumors are detected.

Disseminated Peritoneal Leiomyomatosis

Disseminated peritoneal leiomyomatosis is a rare condition characterized by widespread nodules of histologically benign smooth muscle in the omentum and peritoneum, often numbering in the tens to hundreds. The nodules are usually small, firm, gray to white, and cover the peritoneal surfaces, clinically simulating a disseminated malignancy. This condition typically occurs during the reproductive years, and many patients are pregnant at the time of diagnosis. **Despite the alarming**

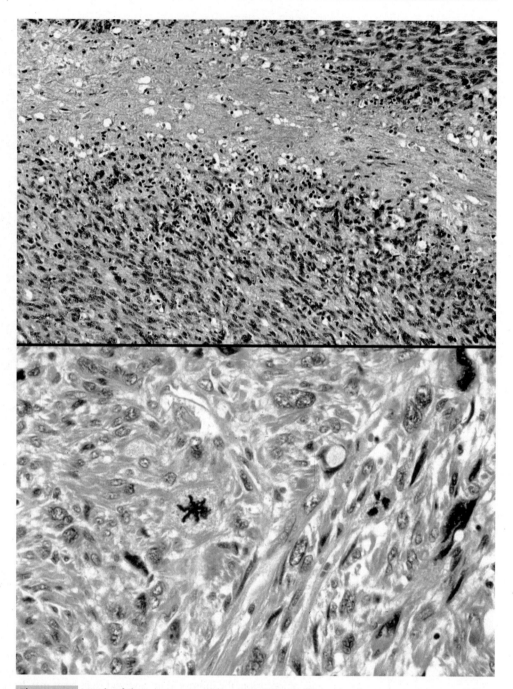

Figure 5.51 **Uterine leiomyosarcoma.** Diagnostic criteria for uterine leiomyosarcoma are diffuse atypia, tumor cell necrosis, and increased mitotic index. (top, low power; bottom, high power)

appearance, disseminated peritoneal leiomyomatosis is usually associated with an indolent clinical course, and can be treated conservatively with long-term follow-up.

Uterine Tumor Resembling Ovarian Sex Cord-Stromal Tumor

Mesenchymal neoplasms that resemble ovarian sex cord tumors are classified as uterine tumors resembling ovarian sex cord tumors provided there is no recognizable endometrial stromal component (41). Most are well-circumscribed; cytologic atypia is absent and mitoses are rare. These tumors are often immunoreactive for sex cord-stromal markers such as inhibin, calretinin; they also express keratin and/or desmin cases. Most tumors of this group have a benign clinical course.

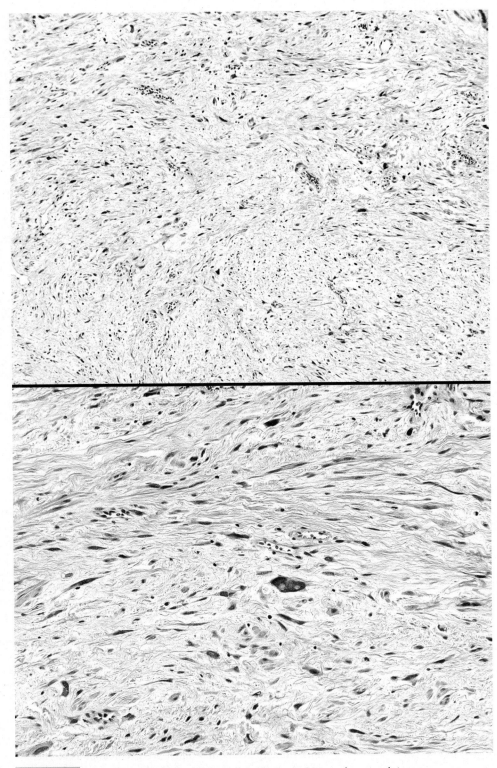

Figure 5.52 **Uterine myxoid leiomyosarcoma.** This rare variant of uterine leiomyosarcoma may exhibit clinically aggressive behavior in the absence of significant mitotic activity (>2 mitotic figures per 50 high-power fields). The presence of cytologic atypia and tumor cell necrosis distinguishes this infiltrative lesion from myxoid leiomyoma. (top, low power; bottom, high power)

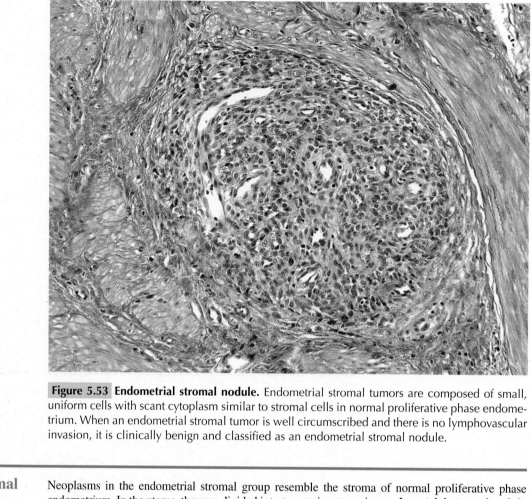

Figure 5.53 Endometrial stromal nodule. Endometrial stromal tumors are composed of small, uniform cells with scant cytoplasm similar to stromal cells in normal proliferative phase endometrium. When an endometrial stromal tumor is well circumscribed and there is no lymphovascular invasion, it is clinically benign and classified as an endometrial stromal nodule.

Endometrial Stromal Tumors

Neoplasms in the endometrial stromal group resemble the stroma of normal proliferative phase endometrium. In the uterus, they are divided into two main categories: **endometrial stromal nodule** and **endometrial stromal sarcoma.** Both are composed of a monomorphous population of ovoid to spindled cells possessing scanty cytoplasm and small, bland, uniform nuclei with evenly distributed chromatin. These cells are embedded in an abundant reticulin framework that contains a highly characteristic, delicate, arborizing vasculature. Focal hyaline thickening of the vessel walls and collagen bands may be present. Endometrial stromal nodules are clinically benign, whereas endometrial stromal sarcomas may recur, sometimes many years after the primary tumor has been removed.

Endometrial Stromal Nodule

Endometrial stromal nodules are well circumscribed, usually small and intramural (Fig. 5.53). Infiltration of the myometrium or uterine vasculature is absent. Because diagnosis is based on complete circumscription and absence of lymphovascular invasion, the distinction between stromal nodule and stromal sarcoma can usually be made only at the time of hysterectomy.

Low-grade Endometrial Stromal Sarcoma

Endometrial stromal sarcoma (low-grade) accounts for less than 20% of all uterine sarcomas, occurs almost exclusively in adults, and has a peak incidence in the fifth decade; more than three-quarters of women are premenopausal. There is no association with previous irradiation, and nor do patients share the risk profile of patients with endometrial carcinoma. Low-grade endometrial stromal sarcoma is **an indolent neoplasm with a protracted clinical course**. At the time of clinical presentation, most tumors are confined to the uterus. Extrauterine disease is associated with a higher risk for recurrence, but is still compatible with long-term survival.

Patients come to clinical attention because of a mass that may be associated with abdominal pain or uterine bleeding. When advanced, the uterus is asymmetrically enlarged by a typically yellow or tan tumor mass that infiltrates the surrounding normal myometrium, often extending into the endometrial cavity as a polypoid growth. **The neoplasm is distinguished from endometrial stromal nodule by (i) the presence of infiltrating margins or (ii) vascular invasion** (Fig. 5.54). In most cases,

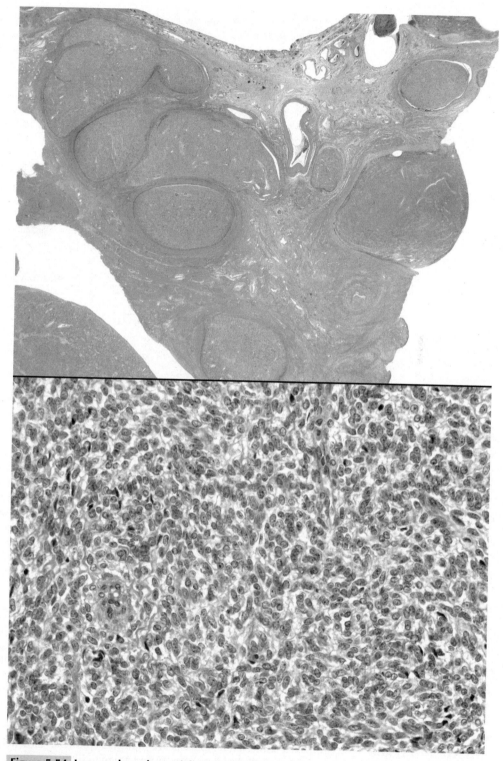

Figure 5.54 **Low-grade endometrial stromal sarcoma.** The presence of infiltrative margins and lymphovascular invasion distinguish low-grade endometrial stromal sarcoma from benign stromal nodule. (top, low power; bottom, high power)

mitotic figures are difficult to find, but occasional tumors have in excess of 10 mitotic figures per 10 high-power fields. Although it has been traditional to stratify low-grade endometrial stromal sarcoma based on the mitotic index, this classification has relatively little utility in diagnostic practice and patient management (43). **Low-grade endometrial stromal sarcoma should be distinguished from "high-grade endometrial stromal sarcoma" and "undifferentiated uterine sarcoma."**

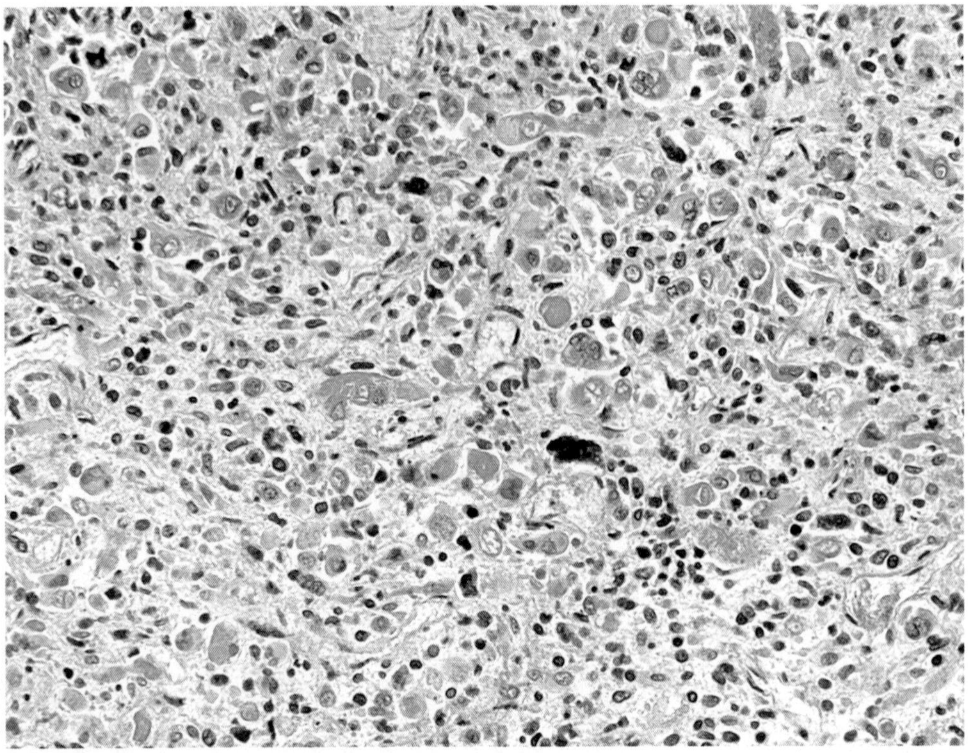

Figure 5.55 Undifferentiated uterine sarcoma. Mesenchymal tumors showing marked cellularity, cytologic atypia, and high mitotic index are classified as undifferentiated uterine sarcomas. Heterologous elements may also be present.

High-grade Endometrial Stromal Sarcoma

The term *high-grade endometrial stromal sarcoma* **has been reintroduced to identify a subset of uterine mesenchymal neoplasms** that demonstrate histologic and immunohistologic evidence of endometrial stromal cell differentiation, but possess cellularity, cytolgic atypia, and a mitotic index beyond that seen in the usual low-grade endometrial stromal sarcoma (44). These tumors harbor a *YWHAE-FAM22* gene fusion, are readily recognizable as malignant, but do not demonstrate the pleomorphism and anaplasia seen in undifferentiated uterine sarcomas. Histologically, they are characterized by a high-grade round to epithelioid cell component that is strongly and diffusely cyclin D1-positive. Expression of ER and PR is generally diminished in comparison to the usual low-grade endometrial stromal sarcoma.

Undifferentiated Uterine Sarcoma

Undifferentiated uterine sarcomas are much less common than low-grade endometrial stromal sarcomas. They are easily recognized as cytologically malignant, and are composed of highly cellular, often pleomorphic, undifferentiated rounded to spindled cells with a high mitotic index (Fig. 5.55). Most resemble the undifferentiated malignant stroma often encountered in carcinosarcomas. **Undifferentiated uterine sarcomas, in sharp contrast to endometrial stromal sarcomas, are aggressive neoplasms with a high incidence of metastases.**

Mixed Müllerian Neoplasms

Mixed müllerian neoplasms are biphasic, epithelial–mesenchymal proliferations that exhibit a range of clinical behaviors from benign to highly malignant. Adenofibroma, adenomyoma, and **atypical polypoid adenomyoma** are the common biphasic epithelial–mesenchymal lesions at the benign end of the spectrum, whereas **adenosarcoma** and **carcinosarcoma** represent the malignant end of the spectrum (Table 5.9).

Adenofibroma

Adenofibromas are considered to be clinically benign with little risk for recurrence after they are completely excised. They typically have broad, fibrotic to mildly cellular stroma, with intervening cleft-like epithelial-lined surfaces morphologically similar to phyllodes tumor of the breast (Fig. 5.56). Authorities differ on the appropriate mitotic index for distinguishing adenofibroma

Table 5.9 Mixed Müllerian Neoplasms

Epithelial Elements

Mesenchymal Elements		Benign	Malignant
	Benign	Adenomyoma Adenofibroma Atypical polypoid adenomyoma	
	Malignant	Adenosarcoma Endometrial stromal sarcoma with glandular elements	Carcinosarcoma • Homologous • Heterologous

from adenosarcoma. Zaloudek and Norris (45) advocate a threshold of 4 mitotic figures per 10 high-power fields, whereas Clement and Scully (46) suggest a threshold of 2 mitotic figures per 10 high-power fields. In most instances, the 4 mitotic figures per 10 high-power fields criterion is sufficient to diagnose adenosarcoma, but tumors with particularly cellular stroma or borderline mitotic counts are best regarded as being of uncertain malignant potential, particularly if subepithelial condensation is present (see **Adenosarcoma** below). Many pathologists believe that adenofibroma is not a distinct entity; instead it is considered to represent one end of a mixed glandular-stromal spectrum in which adenosarcoma with sarcomatous overgrowth represents the opposite end. Uterine curettings exhibiting features of adenofibroma may occasionally be associated with an intrauterine tumor more closely affiliated to adenosarcoma (and vice versa).

Atypical Polypoid Adenomyoma

Atypical polypoid adenomyoma is a polypoid endometrial proliferation composed of irregular glands set in a stroma composed of smooth muscle or, more commonly, smooth muscle and fibrous tissue (Fig. 5.57). Morular or squamous metaplasia is present in most cases and is often florid. The endometrial samplings typically consist of large fragments or chunks of tissue simulating carcinoma. The condition occurs in premenopausal or perimenopausal women; a clinical history of infertility is not uncommon. These lesions can recur locally, but do not have metastatic potential.

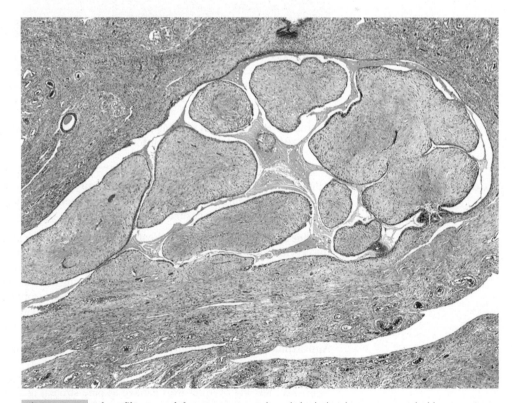

Figure 5.56 Adenofibroma of the uterus. Irregular, clefted glands are surrounded by prominent paucicellular and mitotically inactive stroma.

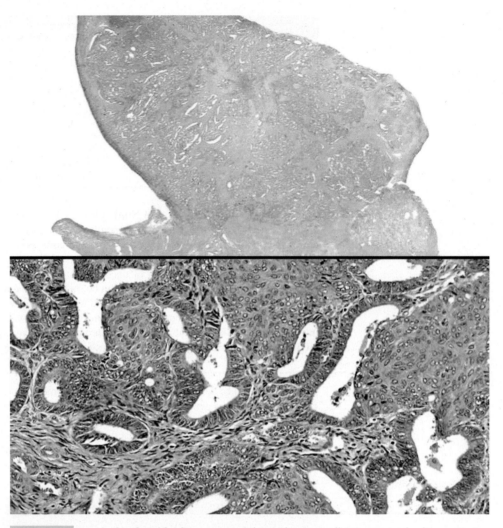

Figure 5.57 **Atypical polypoid adenomyoma.** This polyp typically occurs in the lower uterine segment and is composed of complex endometrioid glands with squamous metaplasia set in a fibromuscular stroma. (top, low power; bottom, high power)

Reproductive conservation utilizing procedures short of hysterectomy is warranted for the conventional APA, provided there is regular follow-up (47).

Adenosarcoma

Adenosarcoma is an uncommon, predominantly low-grade malignant biphasic tumor that is composed of benign epithelial elements and sarcomatous stroma. Most patients with uterine corpus adenosarcoma are postmenopausal.

Uterine corpus adenosarcoma typically presents as a polypoid growth that protrudes through the cervical os or appears to arise from the cervix or lower uterine segment; often there is a history of recurrent polyps, which in retrospect may represent early or subtle forms of adenosarcoma. Microscopically, the tumor consists of uniformly distributed, often cystic and irregularly contoured glandular elements, often with internal papillations scattered throughout a variably cellular stroma. The stroma forms a characteristic hypercellular collar or cuff (so-called cambium layer) around the glands, often producing irregular, stellate glandular configurations (Fig. 5.58).

Approximately 25% of adenosarcomas are myoinvasive. Most patients with uterine adenosarcoma are cured by hysterectomy. Deep myoinvasion, lymphovascular invasion, high-grade heterologous stroma, stromal overgrowth, and extrauterine spread are associated with disease recurrence. Stromal overgrowth is defined as pure stromal proliferation constituting greater than 25% of the tumor. **Approximately 10–25% of patients with uterine adenosarcoma die of their disease.** This figure rises to 50% for those whose tumors contain stromal overgrowth.

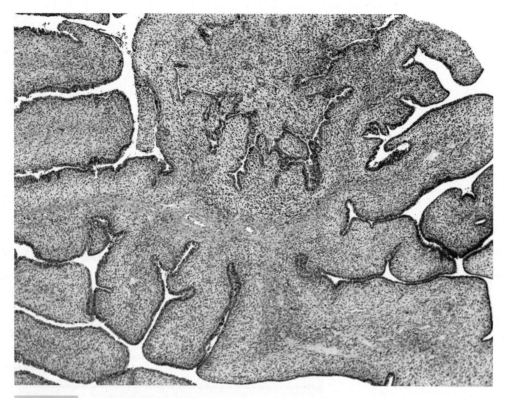

Figure 5.58 Adenosarcoma of uterus. In contrast to adenofibroma, the stroma in adenosarcoma is cellular and mitotically active. Stromal condensation around the glandular component forms a characteristic cambium layer.

Adenosarcoma often represents a challenge for the pathologist because of a significant overlap with adenofibroma and other forms of benign polyp. Most adenosarcomas arise in the uterine corpus, but cervical, vaginal, tubal, ovarian, and primary peritoneal adenosarcomas also occur. Involvement of additional extragenital sites in women is linked to endometriosis.

Carcinosarcoma

Despite the long entrenched terminology of "malignant mixed müllerian tumor," carcinosarcoma is the current preferred designation for mixed neoplasms composed of carcinoma and sarcoma. **With rare exceptions, carcinosarcoma is a disease of elderly menopausal women, and there is an association with prior pelvic radiation.** Most patients present with uterine bleeding, and the typical clinical appearance is that of a fleshy, necrotic and hemorrhagic, polypoid mass that fills the uterine cavity and extends through the cervical os.

The histologic diagnosis of carcinosarcoma requires the presence of a distinct biphasic neoplasm, composed of separate but admixed malignant-appearing epithelial and mesenchymal elements (Fig. 5.59). The mesenchymal and epithelial elements should not merge with one another. Both the high-grade nuclear features and the biphasic pattern of this neoplasm are obvious in the typical case. **The stromal components may be *homologous*** (leiomyosarcoma, stromal sarcoma, fibrosarcoma) or ***heterologous*** (chondrosarcoma, rhabdomyosarcoma, osteosarcoma, liposarcoma). Although tradition holds that heterologous elements do not bear on prognosis, a 2007 study from Memorial Sloan-Kettering suggests that surgical stage I uterine carcinosarcoma with heterologous elements may be more aggressive than those with homologous elements (48). Prognosis is dependent on the stage, the size of the tumor, and the depth of myometrial invasion.

Ovary

Four broad histogenetic categories of ovarian tumors are observed: surface epithelial–stromal tumors (65–70%), sex cord-stromal tumors (15–20%), germ cell tumors (5–10%), and metastases (5%).

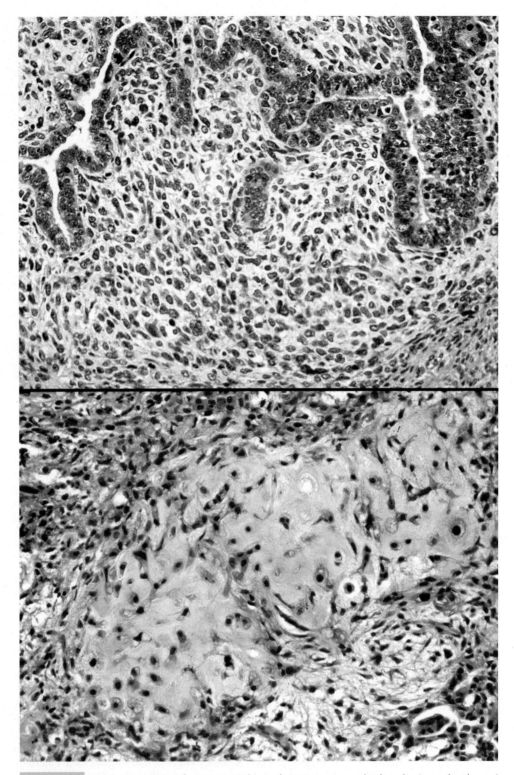

Figure 5.59 Carcinosarcoma of uterus. Biphasic lesion composed of malignant glands and stroma (top). Heterologous elements, such as cartilage depicted here, may be present in carcinosarcoma (bottom).

Surface Epithelial–Stromal Tumors

Surface epithelial–stromal tumors are the most common neoplasms of the ovary (Table 5.10). **They consist of six types: serous, mucinous, endometrioid, clear cell, transitional, and undifferentiated** (49,50). Tumors with squamous differentiation were historically included among the surface epithelial–stromal tumors, but pure squamous tumors are rare; most arise in teratomas.

Table 5.10 Histologic Classification of Surface-Epithelial Stromal Tumors	
Histologic Type[a]	Total (%)
Serous	46
Mucinous	36
Endometrioid	8
Clear	3
Transitional	2
Undifferentiated	2
Mixed	3

[a]Tumors with squamous differentiation have also been included among the surface epithelial–stromal tumors, but pure squamous tumors are rare. Most arise in an epidermoid or dermoid cyst (49,50).

Serous Tumors

Tumors with serous differentiation represent 45% of surface epithelial–stromal ovarian neoplasms; they are characterized by epithelial cells resembling those of the fallopian tube and encompass a group of three biologically distinct entities: benign serous cystadenofibroma, serous borderline tumor (low malignant potential), and serous carcinoma.

Benign Serous Tumors

Benign serous cystadenomas or cystadenofibromas constitute almost one-half of all serous ovarian neoplasms. Benign serous tumors occur over a wide age range but are most common in the reproductive age group. They are often bilateral and composed of varying amounts of fibrous stroma and cysts. They range in size from 1 cm to 10 cm (rarely as large as 30 cm). The cysts are unilocular or multilocular and may contain papillary projections. Surface papillomas may also be present. Microscopically, the cysts are lined by a simple layer of epithelium that recapitulates the ciliated epithelial cells of the fallopian tube.

Serous Borderline Tumors—Serous Tumors of Low Malignant Potential

Serous borderline tumors constitute approximately 15% of ovarian serous neoplasms and account for the vast majority of all borderline surface epithelial–stromal neoplasms. They occur at a slightly younger age than serous carcinoma (mean 45 years vs. 60 years). They are more often bilateral and larger than benign serous tumors, and may present with disease beyond the confines of the ovary. Serous neoplasms in the borderline group are predominately cystic with variable amounts of papillary epithelial projections, although solid tumors with surface papillary excrescences may occur. Microscopically, serous borderline tumors are composed of architecturally complex branching papillary and micropapillary structures, not unlike that of low-grade serous carcinomas, but they do not feature destructive invasion of the ovarian stroma. The nuclei are uniform or mildly atypical (Fig. 5.60). Mitotic activity is low. Psammoma bodies are often present but are not diagnostic.

Micropapillary Pattern

Approximately 10% of serous borderline tumors contain foci of significant micropapillary architecture, defined as nonhierarchical branching of slender, elongated papillae that are at least five times as long as they are wide (Fig. 5.61), *or* a sievelike cribriform pattern occupying a continuous 5-mm extent. The micropapillary variant is more frequently associated with bilaterality, ovarian surface involvement, and the presence of extraovarian disease (51). When the extraovarian disease is invasive, serous borderline tumors with micropapillary architecture have a poorer prognosis.

Stromal Microinvasion

Stromal microinvasion, defined as 5 mm in linear extent or 10 mm^2 in area, may be found in 10–15% of serous tumors of low malignant potential. Stromal microinvasion is characterized by eosinophilic cells or small micropapillae lying within stromal spaces beneath larger papillae (Fig. 5.62). It is seen more frequently during pregnancy. Although the overall prognosis is

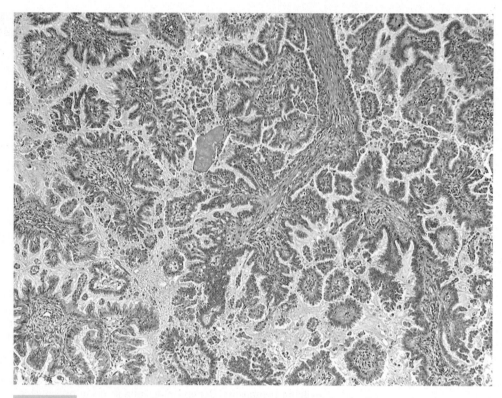

Figure 5.60 Serous borderline tumor (low malignant potential). Papillae are lined by stratified tubal type epithelium with tufting. Mitotic activity is minimal, and cytologic atypia is mild to moderate. There is no stromal invasion.

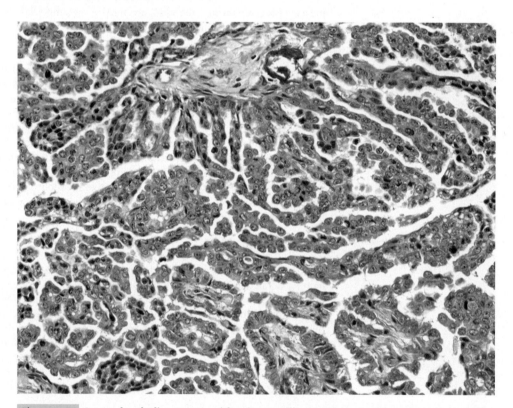

Figure 5.61 Serous borderline tumor with micropapillary pattern. In this variant, the papillae are elongated and at least fivefold longer than their width. Ovarian surface involvement, bilaterality, and extraovarian implants are more common in this variant than in the usual serous borderline tumor.

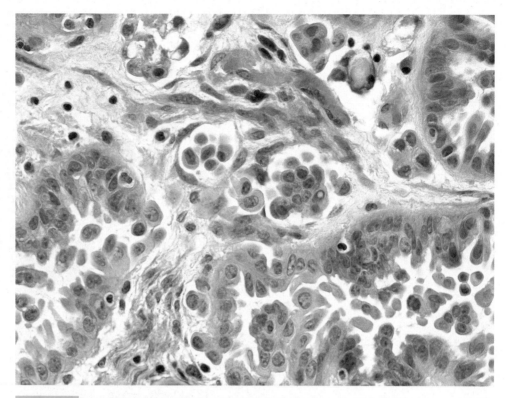

Figure 5.62 Stromal microinvasion in serous borderline tumor. Small foci of intrastromal single cells and small, nonbranching papillae may be seen in 10–15% of serous borderline tumors. Although such foci likely represent early stromal invasion, their presence does not warrant a diagnosis of carcinoma, provided they are small (<5 mm) and show no significant cytologic atypia.

favorable, stromal microinvasion appears to represent a histologic link between serous borderline tumors and low-grade serous carcinoma, and is likely a bona fide form of early invasion (52).

Extraovarian Disease

Approximately 30–40% of serous borderline tumors are associated with similar-appearing lesions in the pelvis and intra-abdominal sites, including lymph nodes. These lesions, termed *implants,* **may be microscopic or macroscopic, and are subclassified as noninvasive or invasive types, based on the presence of destructive infiltration into underlying normal tissue structures (Fig. 5.63). Noninvasive implants are divided into epithelial and desmoplastic types,** depending on whether or not there is an associated stromal response. **The distinction between noninvasive and invasive implants is important, because extraovarian invasive disease is associated with a significantly poorer prognosis (51).** At times, it is difficult to determine whether an implant is invasive or not; in these instances, the implants may be classified as indeterminate. **Implants that are indeterminate for invasion appear to have a prognosis that is intermediate to that of noninvasive and invasive implants (53).**

Lymph node involvement (Fig. 5.64) occurs in 20–30% of ovarian serous tumors of low malignant potential (54), but the presence of lymph node involvement does not confer a worse prognosis unless it exhibits an invasive pattern.

Endosalpingiosis frequently coexists with serous borderline lesions in the peritoneum and lymph nodes, but the presence of endosalpingiosis alone does not upstage the disease. The frequent coexistence of endosalpingiosis with "implants" of ovarian serous borderline tumor would seem to support the concept that serous tumors may arise in endosalpingiosis in at least a subset of cases.

Low-grade Serous Carcinoma

Ovarian serous carcinoma is graded using a two-tiered system based on the degree of nuclear atypia and the mitotic index (55,56). Low-grade (grade 1) serous carcinomas (Fig. 5.65) are much

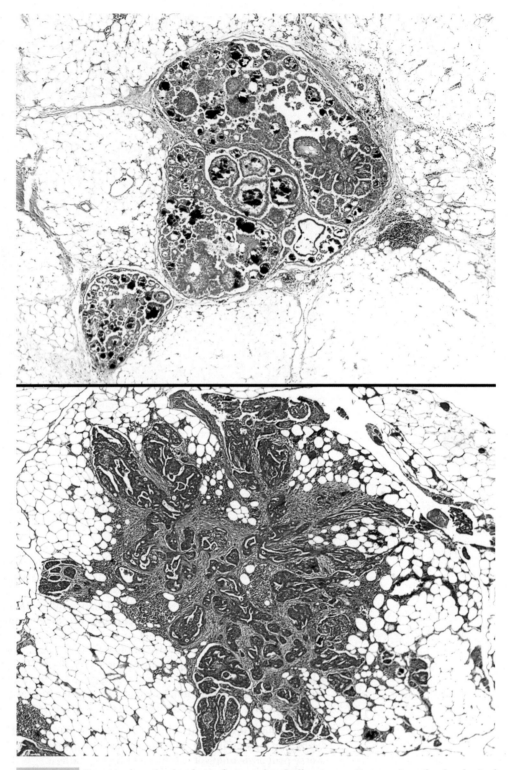

Figure 5.63 Top: **Noninvasive implant of serous borderline tumor.** Bottom: **Invasive implant of serous borderline tumor.** Unlike noninvasive implants, invasive implants have an irregular stromal interface.

less common than high-grade serous carcinomas (Fig. 5.66), accounting for less than 10% of serous carcinomas. The low-grade (grade 1) serous carcinomas exhibit mutations in *BRAF* and *KRAS*, similar to those seen in serous borderline tumors (57).

Serous psammocarcinoma, a very rare variant of low-grade serous carcinoma, is defined by the presence of massive psammomatous calcification (at least 75% of the tumor cell nests contain a

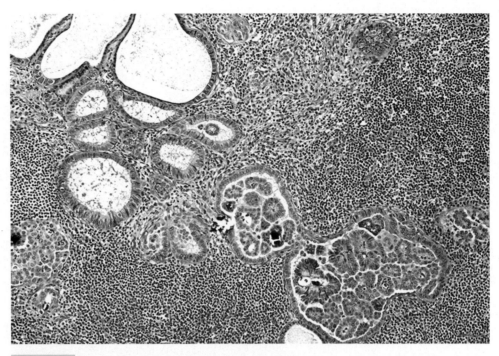

Figure 5.64 **Lymph node involvement by serous borderline tumor.** Lymph node involvement by serous borderline tumor can be florid but does not confer a poorer prognosis.

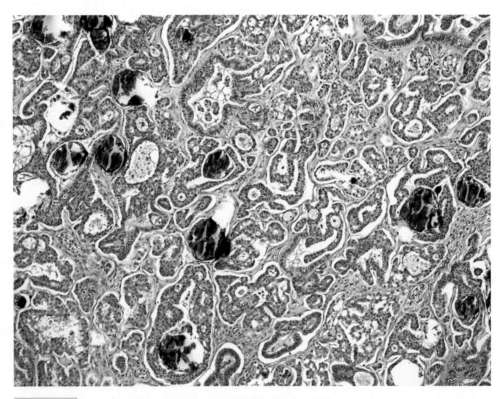

Figure 5.65 **Low-grade serous carcinoma of ovary.** Simple and branching papillae invade stroma but show moderate cytologic atypia and low mitotic activity.

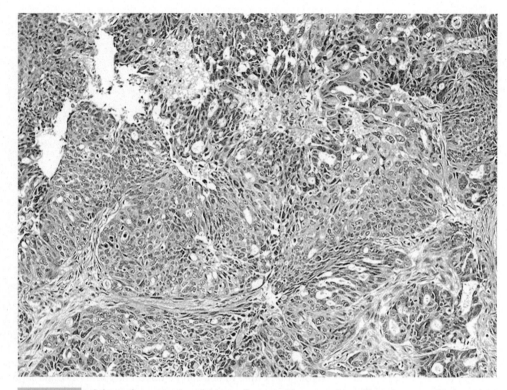

Figure 5.66 **High-grade serous carcinoma of ovary.** Sheets and papillae show marked nuclear pleomorphism and frequent mitotic figures.

psammoma body), predominant extraovarian disease distribution, and low-grade cytologic atypia. The prognosis for serous psammocarcinoma is favorable (58).

High-grade Serous Carcinoma

High-grade serous carcinoma accounts for 35–40% of all serous ovarian neoplasms and approximately 75% of ovarian surface epithelial–stromal carcinomas. Ovarian high-grade serous carcinoma tends to occur in the sixth to seventh decades (mean 56 years). Grossly, serous carcinoma is bilateral in 60% of cases, and is solid and cystic or mostly solid. Microscopically, serous carcinomas exhibit papillary structures that can become fused and form solid sheets of cells with slitlike spaces. Marked nuclear atypia and numerous mitotic figures, which may be atypical, are characteristic of the high-grade tumors (Fig. 5.66). **Psammoma bodies are often present** but are not specific.

High-grade serous carcinomas are the most common surface epithelial carcinomas, and are associated with *p53* mutations and somatic or germ-line abnormalities of *BRCA1* or *BRCA2*. High-grade serous carcinoma is the most common gynecologic tumor to occur in women with a germline *BRCA1* or *BRCA2* mutation; **serous carcinoma may also develop in the fallopian tubes and on the surface of the peritoneum.**

Mucinous Tumors

Surface epithelial tumors with mucinous differentiation account for 15% of all ovarian neoplasms in the United States and Europe. These tumors are characterized by epithelial cells resembling those of the endocervix (mullerian or endocervical like) or gastrointestinal tract (intestinal type). Like the serous tumors, they encompass a group of three distinct entities: benign mucinous cystadenoma or adenofibroma, mucinous borderline tumor (tumor of low malignant potential), and mucinous carcinoma (50,59).

Benign Mucinous Tumors

Almost 80% of all mucinous ovarian neoplasms are benign unilocular or multilocular cystadenomas. They occur in a wide age range, but are most commonly diagnosed in the reproductive age group. Benign mucinous tumors are typically unilateral, and can reach 30 cm or more in diameter. Microscopically, the tumors are composed of a columnar epithelial lining with abundant, pale-staining intracellular mucin that resembles endocervical or gastric-type epithelium. Goblet cells may be present but are uncommon in benign mucinous tumors (in contrast to intestinal-type mucinous borderline tumors or mucinous carcinomas).

Mucinous Borderline Tumors—Mucinous Tumors of Low Malignant Potential, Gastrointestinal Type	**Mucinous borderline tumors account for 10–15% of all mucinous ovarian tumors; the gastrointestinal type is most common. Mucinous borderline tumors of intestinal type are unilateral, and often larger than benign mucinous tumors.** They occur most commonly during the late reproductive years (mean 45 years). Microscopically, the multilocular cysts are lined by variably stratified mucinous epithelium forming complex papillary folds. The individual cells show mild to moderate cytologic atypia with increased mitotic figures (Fig. 5.67). Goblet cells are present. The presence of marked or severe nuclear atypia involving the full thickness of stratified epithelium (i.e., not limited to the crypts) is classified as *intraepithelial carcinoma.*
	Two patterns of microinvasion are recognized in mucinous borderline tumors of gastrointestinal type. **The first pattern consists of infiltration of stroma by individual cells or small nests of cells that are cytologically similar to the cells elsewhere in the borderline tumor.** Such foci must not exceed 5 mm in linear extent or 10 mm^2 in area. This is an uncommon finding in mucinous borderline tumors (in comparison to the frequency of microinvasion in serous borderline tumors). **The second, more common pattern of microinvasion consists of one or more small foci** (≤5 mm in linear extent or ≤10 mm^2 in area) **of nests, individual cells, and glands exhibiting cytologic features of high-grade carcinoma cells; this latter pattern is classified as *microinvasive* carcinoma.** Foci of microinvasive carcinoma are of uncertain prognostic significance, but their presence should prompt a search by the pathologist for larger foci of invasive carcinoma (49).
Mucinous Borderline Tumors—Mucinous Tumors of Low Malignant Potential, Müllerian (Seromucinous) Type	**Mucinous borderline tumors of müllerian (seromucinous) type are bilateral in up to 40% of cases, and have a strong association with endometriosis, which is present in up to 50% of cases** (49). The mean age of patients with müllerian mucinous borderline tumors is mid-30s. These tumors are composed of complex papillae, architecturally similar to those of serous borderline tumors, lined by columnar mucin-secreting epithelium and ciliated eosinophilic epithelium. Nuclear atypia is mild to moderate, and mitotic figures may be present. Typically, there is a prominent neutrophilic infiltrate in the stroma of the papillae. Stromal microinvasion, similar to that in serous borderline tumors, may be present. Extraovarian implants may be present in as many as 20% of cases, but their presence is not associated with a poorer prognosis.
Mucinous Carcinoma, Intestinal Type	Mucinous carcinomas account for less than 10% of all mucinous ovarian neoplasms. Two different patterns of invasion are recognized, both of which may coexist in a single tumor. The confluent glandular or expansile invasive pattern is recognized by marked glandular crowding, with little intervening stroma (Fig. 5.68). The destructive stromal invasive pattern, which is less common, is recognized by irregular nests and single cells with malignant cytologic features infiltrating the stroma (Fig. 5.69). The presence of stromal invasion, whether of destructive or confluent type, must exceed 5 mm in linear extent or 10 mm^2 in area in order to be classified as carcinoma; otherwise, a diagnosis of microinvasive carcinoma is warranted.
	Most primary mucinous carcinomas of the ovary are confined to the ovary at the time of diagnosis. An advanced stage mucinous carcinoma involving the ovary at first diagnosis should be evaluated as a possible metastasis from another site, particularly the gastrointestinal tract (49).
Mucinous Tumor with Pseudomyxoma Peritonei	Although ovarian mucinous tumors associated with pseudomyxoma peritonei are listed as a distinct category by the WHO, **most of these tumors are metastases from primary mucinous tumors of the vermiform appendix** (Fig. 5.70). Rarely, primary ovarian mucinous tumors of the intestinal type are associated with pseudomyxoma peritonei; these tumors typically have an associated teratomatous component in the ovary (60,61). The natural history of these tumors is not well understood.
Endometrioid Tumors	Surface epithelial tumors with endometrioid differentiation exhibit the glandular or stromal histologic features of endometrial glands and stroma. **Ovarian tumors showing endometrioid differentiation account for less than 10% of all surface epithelial–stromal tumors.**

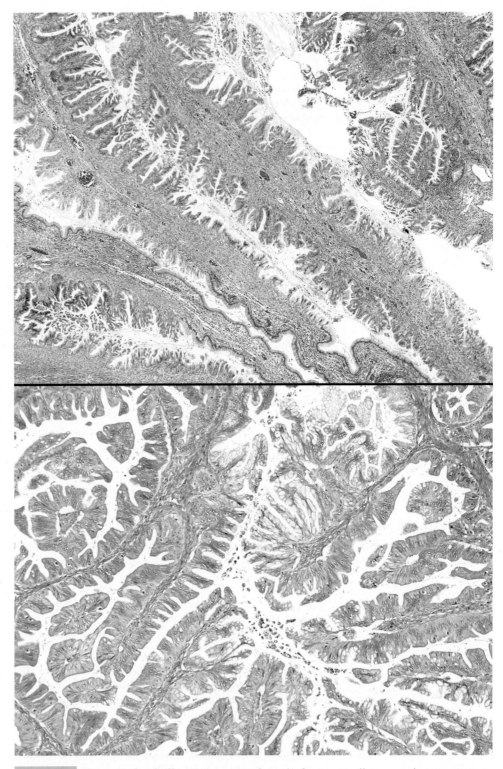

Figure 5.67 Mucinous borderline tumor, gastrointestinal type. Papillary growth pattern, stratification, and nuclear atypia distinguish these tumors from cystadenoma. Intestinal differentiation is exemplified by goblet cells and, in some cases, Paneth cells. There is no stromal invasion. (top, low power; bottom, high power)

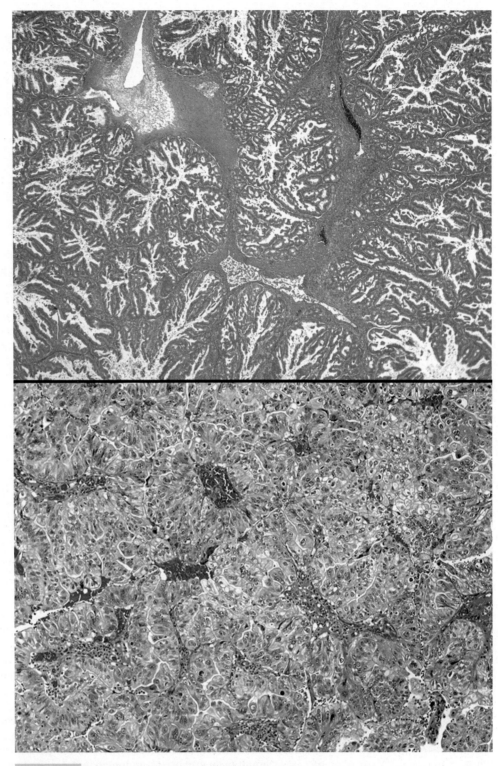

Figure 5.68 Mucinous adenocarcinoma of ovary. Expansile stromal invasion in a mucinous ovarian tumor is classified as mucinous carcinoma, but it does not appear to confer the same ominous prognosis as mucinous ovarian tumors with destructive stromal invasion **(Fig. 5.69)**. (top, low power; bottom, high power)

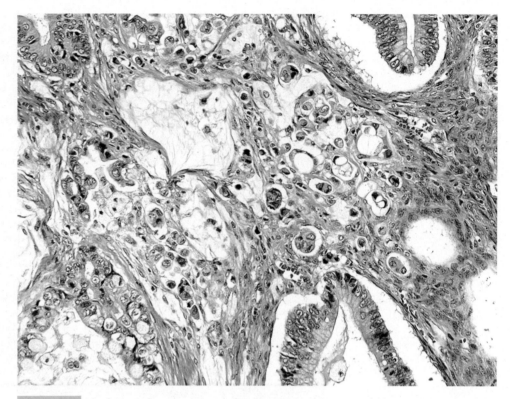

Figure 5.69 **Mucinous adenocarcinoma of ovary.** Destructive stromal invasion in a mucinous ovarian tumor is classified as mucinous carcinoma. Metastasis—for example, from the gastrointestinal tract—should always be considered, especially in the presence of high-stage disease or bilateral ovarian involvement.

Benign Endometrioid Tumors and Endometrioid Borderline Tumors—Endometrioid Tumors of Low Malignant Potential

Benign endometrioid tumors are rare and, when present, typically unilateral. Borderline endometrioid tumors may be bilateral (30%). Both are clinically benign. The tumors resemble their uterine counterparts and are composed of glandular or villoglandular proliferations, which may show cytoplasmic clearing or secretory-type changes with sub- or supranuclear vacuolization. Squamous metaplasia is common. The changes in borderline endometrioid tumors are analogous to those seen in complex atypical hyperplasia of the endometrium, in that there are cytologic and architectural atypia but no stromal invasion.

Endometrioid Ovarian Carcinoma

The typical ovarian endometrioid carcinoma is comparable to FIGO grade 1 or 2 endometrioid adenocarcinoma of the uterus, although occasional tumors have a higher-grade, with a more solid growth pattern (Figure 5.71). Squamous metaplasia is common, as are other metaplastic changes (secretory, ciliated cell, oxyphilic, or mucinous). Endometrioid carcinomas of the ovary exhibit a wide array of patterns that may pose differential diagnostic problems for the pathologist, including spindled, tubular, insular, trabecular, microglandular, adenoid basal, and adenoid cystic. When prominent, these patterns may mimic Sertoli cell or Sertoli–Leydig cell tumors, carcinoid tumors, or granulosa cell tumors. Metastases from the gastrointestinal tract may simulate a primary endometrioid carcinoma. **An association with endometriosis, either ovarian or elsewhere in the pelvis, is observed in as many as 40% of cases. Simultaneous primary endometrioid carcinomas in the uterus are present in 20% of cases** (49).

Clear Cell Tumors

Surface epithelial stromal tumors with clear cell differentiation are characterized by epithelial cells containing glycogen-rich clear cytoplasm, and hobnail cells with varying degrees of fibrous stroma. Once considered to be of mesonephric origin, clear cell surface epithelial tumors are now recognized as derivatives of the müllerian tract. **Clear cell tumors account for only 3% of surface epithelial stromal tumors, but almost all are malignant.**

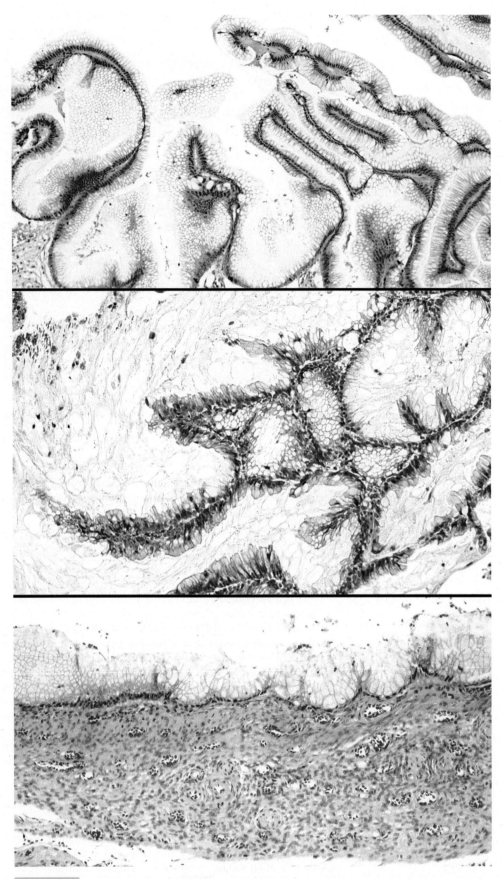

Figure 5.70 **Pseudomyxoma peritonei.** Cytologically low-grade mucinous epithelium is present within pools of mucin in the ovarian stroma (top), peritoneum (middle), and within the appendix (bottom) in this condition. Most cases are associated with an appendiceal mucinous neoplasm; rarely, this condition is encountered in mucinous ovarian tumors arising in a mature teratoma.

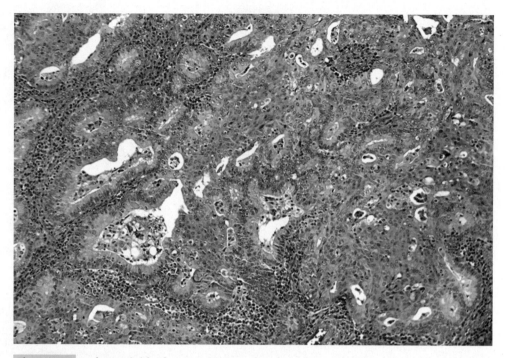

Figure 5.71 **Endometrioid adenocarcinoma of ovary.** Ovarian endometrioid carcinoma has similar morphology to endometrial endometrioid carcinoma, including squamous cell differentiation.

Benign Clear Cell Tumors and Borderline Clear Cell Tumors— Clear Cell Tumors of Low Malignant Potential

The benign and borderline clear cell adenofibromatous tumors are extremely rare (<1% of clear cell tumors) and present in the second to seventh decades of life.

Clear Cell Ovarian Carcinoma

Clear cell carcinomas tend to occur in the fifth to seventh decades (10% in the fourth decade). There is an unexplained increased prevalence of clear cell carcinoma in Japan relative to Western countries. Two-thirds of women with clear cell carcinomas are nulliparous. **More than one-half have associated endometriosis involving the ovary or other pelvic sites. When associated with endometriosis, mixed clear cell and endometrioid carcinoma may occur. Patients with clear cell carcinoma are at risk for developing paraneoplastic hypercalcemia or pelvic venous thromboses.** Most clear cell carcinomas, even when advanced stage, are unilateral (49). The tumors are composed of glands, tubules, papillae, or solid sheets of polyhedral cells with optically clear or eosinophilic granular cytoplasm (Fig. 5.72). Hobnail cells are characteristic. Psammoma bodies may be present, and as many as 25% contain eosinophilic hyaline bodies. Clear cell carcinomas of the ovary are not graded (49). Approximatley 45% of endometriosis-associated clear cell carcinomas (and 30% of endometriosis-associated endometrioid ovarian carcinomas) harbor mutations in *ARID1A* (62).

Transitional Cell (Brenner) Tumors

Transitional cell tumors are thought to arise through metaplasia of the ovarian surface epithelium and are analogous to Walthard nests, which are transitional-type epithelial inclusions occurring beneath the serosa of the fallopian tubes and in the hilar regions of the ovaries. They are uncommon (3% of all surface epithelial–stromal tumors). Most are clinically benign.

Benign Transitional Cell (Brenner) Tumor

Brenner tumors are the most common type of ovarian transitional cell tumor. They are often microscopic or incidental findings discovered at laparotomy for unrelated pelvic conditions. They affect patients during the fourth to eighth decades (mean age 50 years). They are typically solid, unilateral

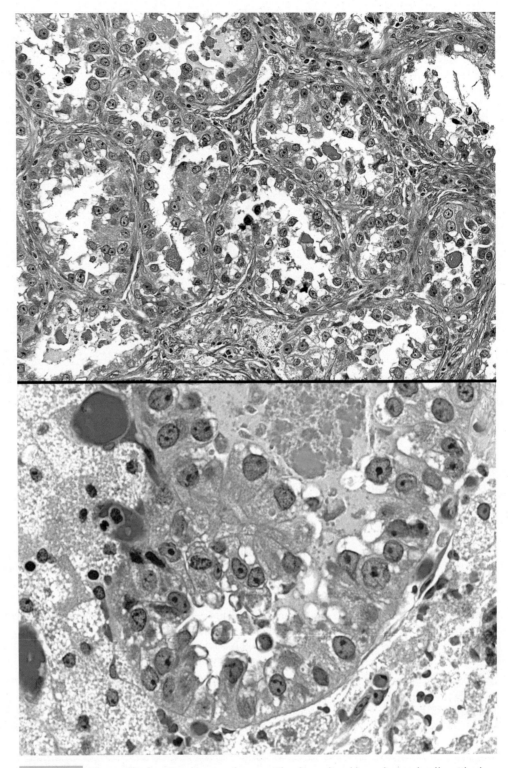

Figure 5.72 **Clear cell adenocarcinoma of ovary.** Glands are lined by polygonal cells with clear cytoplasm and enlarged, hyperchromatic, and pleomorphic nuclei. (top, low power; bottom, high power)

tumors with small cysts on cut section; most are less than 2 cm. A gritty consistency may be present because of flecks of calcification (Fig. 5.73). They may be associated with a mucinous cystic tumor. Microscopically, they contain nests of cytologically bland cells with an urothelial appearance, surrounded by a prominent fibromatous stroma. The individual nests may be solid or microcystic, with an inner mucinous epithelial lining.

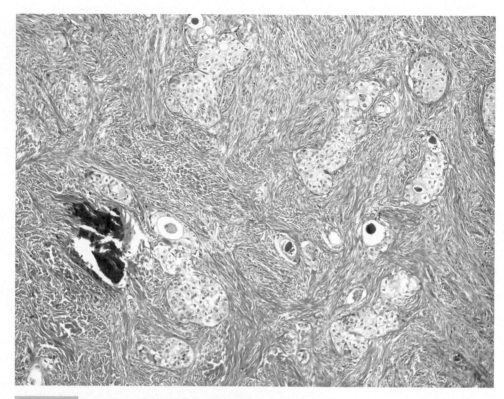

Figure 5.73 **Brenner tumor of ovary.** Nests of transitional epithelium are set in fibrous stroma. Stromal calcifications may impart a gritty texture.

Borderline Transitional Cell (Brenner) Tumor— Transitional Cell Tumor of Low Malignant Potential	**Borderline tumors are typically unilateral, solid, and cystic and usually larger (10 to 25 cm) than benign Brenner tumors.** Microscopically, they feature coarse papillary fronds lined by multilayered uroepithelium that resembles low-grade papillary urothelial carcinoma of the urinary tract. Despite their epithelial proliferation, these tumors are clinically benign.
Malignant Brenner Tumor	**Malignant transitional cell tumors *with* benign or atypical proliferating transitional elements are designated as malignant Brenner tumors.** These tumors show nuclear pleomorphism, hyperchromasia, numerous mitotic figures, and destructive stromal invasion.
Transitional Cell Carcinoma	**Malignant transitional cell tumors *without* benign or atypical proliferating transitional elements have been designated as transitional cell carcinomas.** The diagnosis of transitional cell carcinoma is highly subjective, and it is likely that most, if not all, such tumors are variants of high-grade serous carcinoma.
Undifferentiated Epithelial Tumors	Undifferentiated carcinomas lack histologic features of a specific müllerian cell type. They are invariably high grade. Because undifferentiated areas are common in high-grade ovarian carcinomas that contain specific features of serous, clear cell, or other differentiation elsewhere, pure undifferentiated carcinomas are infrequent (49).
Mixed Surface Epithelial–Stromal Tumors	Mixed surface epithelial–stromal tumors have two or more differentiated histologic cell types, each of which account for at least 10% of the tumor.
Sex Cord–Stromal Tumors	**Sex cord–stromal tumors demonstrate ovarian, testicular, or a mixture of ovarian and testicular cell differentiation (63). Many of the tumors of this subtype variably express inhibin,** a feature that is often used in confirming the presence of sex cord–stromal differentiation.

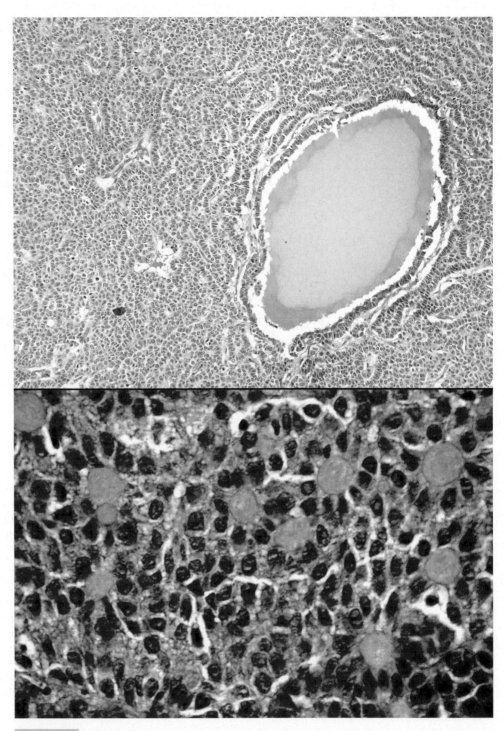

Figure 5.74 **Adult granulosa cell tumor.** Top: Ribbons of cells with coffee-bean nuclei surround a macrofollicle. The mitotic index is usually low in these tumors. Bottom: Microfollicular pattern with Call-Exner bodies.

Adult Granulosa Cell Tumors

Adult granulosa cell tumor is the most common sex cord–stromal tumor in the ovary. This tumor **occurs in females over a wide age range** (mean 52 years), but is more common in late reproductive years than in the pediatric age group. Patients often present with estrogenic symptoms (50).

Adult granulosa cell tumors are unilateral and solid, solid and cystic, or predominantly cystic. Microscopically, they are characterized by a proliferation of ovoid, predominantly uniform cells

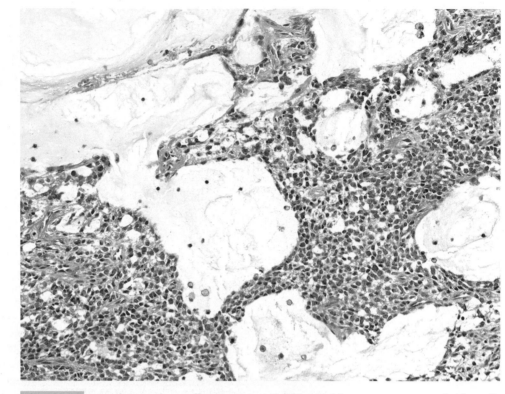

Figure 5.75 **Juvenile granulosa cell tumor.** Macrofollicles in this tumor are surrounded by cells with more hyperchromatic and often more mitotically active nuclei than those in the adult type.

with an open chromatin pattern and nuclear grooves (Fig. 5.74). Mitotic figures are present, but typically fewer in number. A variety of patterns can be observed, including trabecular, insular, diffuse, and **microfollicular,** featuring characteristic **Call-Exner bodies** (small round spaces filled with eosinophilic material formed by the surrounding granulosa cells). Macrofollicles are present in most adult granulosa cell tumors. Adult granulosa cell tumor is **a neoplasm of low malignant potential;** recurrences may occur many years after initial diagnosis. The most important prognostic feature is the stage of disease. Adult granulosa cell tumor is associated with a somatic mutation in *FOXL2* (64).

Juvenile Granulosa Cell Tumors

Ninety-seven percent of juvenile granulosa cell tumors occur in females younger than 30 years. Patients often present with isosexual pseudoprecocity or menstrual irregularities. Most are unilateral and low stage, with a macroscopic appearance similar to the adult granulosa cell tumor. They are distinguished from the adult variant by the presence of larger, more irregular follicles and rounded, more atypical nuclei that are euchromatic or hyperchromatic and non-grooved (Fig. 5.75). Mitotic figures are often numerous. **Most juvenile granulosa cell tumors are clinically benign,** but approximately 10% will develop recurrences, typically within the first 5 years (63).

Sertoli–Leydig Cell Tumors

Sertoli–Leydig cell tumors occur most commonly in women in their mid-20s, but can occur in females as young as 2 and as old as 75 years. Approximately one-third of patients present with virilization; estrogenic manifestations are less frequent. Almost one-half of patients exhibit no endocrinologic manifestations (65).

Sertoli–Leydig cell tumors are typically unilateral and low stage, but 10% may have ovarian surface involvement. Less than 5% exhibit extraovarian spread at diagnosis. Most are solid or solid and cystic, and pale yellow or tan in color. The characteristic features are tubules or cords of Sertoli cells, with interspersed nests of Leydig cells enmeshed in primitive gonadal stroma (Fig. 5.76). **Rarely, a Sertoli-only cell tumor can be seen.** Approximately 20% have heterologous elements, which may be epithelial or mesenchymal and include mucinous, cartilaginous, neuroendocrinologic (carcinoid tumor), or skeletal muscular (rhabdomyosarcoma) differentiation. Retiform elements

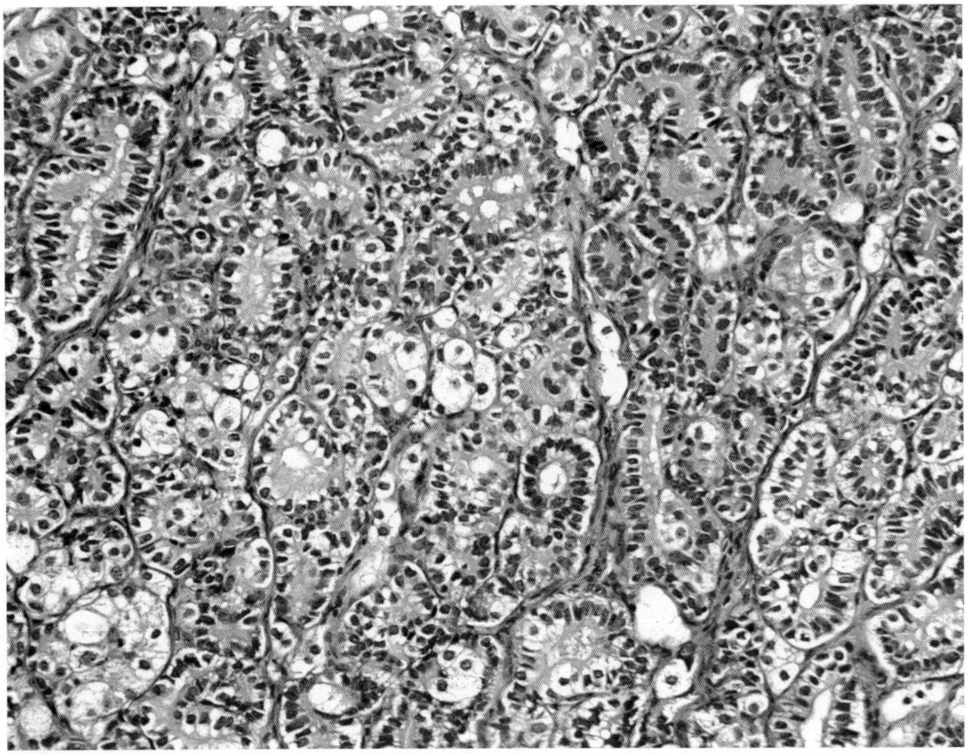

Figure 5.76 Sertoli–Leydig cell tumor. Sertoli tubules with interspersed Leydig cells form this well-differentiated tumor.

resembling rete testis are seen in 15% of cases. The tumors are graded on the basis of the degree of Sertoli tubule formation and the extent of primitive stroma. Well-differentiated tumors have a mitotic index of less than 5 mitotic figures per 10 high-power fields, whereas poorly differentiated tumors have a mitotic index greater than 10 mitoses per 10 high-power fields, and intermediate tumors have an intermediate mitotic index.

Sex-cord Tumor with Annular Tubules

A rare variant of Sertoli cell tumor, the sex-cord tumor with annular tubules, is distinguished by the presence of simple or complex annular tubules composed of Sertoli cells arranged antipodally around hyaline material (Fig. 5.77). Tumors are unilateral, and often associated with hormonal manifestations. Up to 25% are clinically malignant (50). **One-third occur in patients with Peutz–Jeghers syndrome,** when they are clinically benign, bilateral, small, and often incidental findings.

Gynandroblastoma

When sex cord–stromal tumors contain minor components of other types of sex cord–stromal tumor, the tumor is usually designated by the major component. However, when a tumor is composed of an admixture of well-differentiated Sertoli cell tubules and granulosa cell elements, and the second cell population makes up at least 10% of the tumor, the tumor is classified as a gynandroblastoma, and the relative contribution and subtypes are reported. Most such tumors are benign.

Fibroma–Thecoma

This group of stromal tumors is composed of spindle or oval cells, with scant (**fibroma**) or more abundant, pale, lipid-rich cytoplasm (**thecoma**), associated with varying degrees of collagen. **Estrogenic manifestations are generally absent in fibromas, but occur in as many as 60% of patients with thecomas.** Tumors in this group tend to occur in middle age (fibroma) or after menopause (thecoma). Most are unilateral, solid, or solid and microcystic, and they vary from gray or white (fibroma) to bright yellow (thecoma). Microscopically, the tumors are composed of cells arranged in fascicles or in a storiform pattern; calcification and hyaline plaques may be seen (Fig. 5.78). Patients with nevoid basal cell carcinoma syndrome develop ovarian fibromas at a younger age, and the tumors are bilateral, multinodular, and calcified. **Almost all fibromas and**

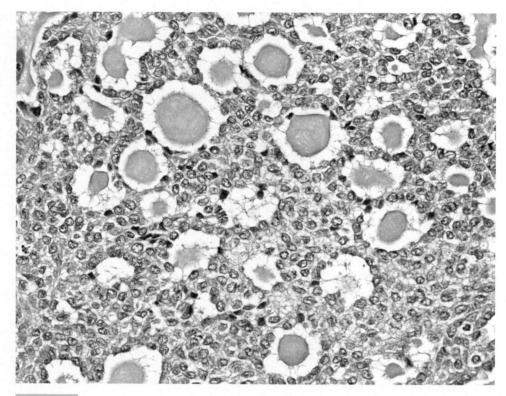

Figure 5.77 **Sex-cord tumor with annular tubules.** Prominent hyaline bodies are surrounded by a proliferation of complex annular tubules. This tumor may be associated with Peutz–Jeghers syndrome and is typically incidental and clinically benign in that setting. Those tumors that are not associated with the syndrome may recur and demonstrate clinically aggressive behavior.

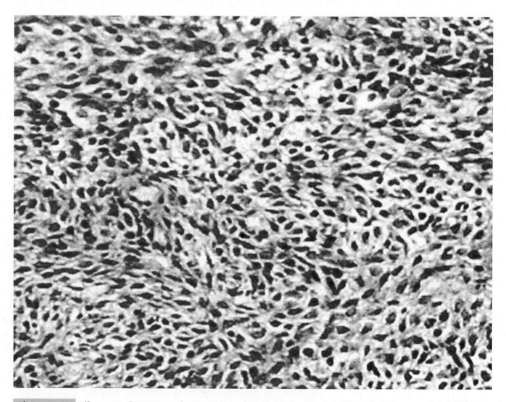

Figure 5.78 **Fibroma–thecoma of ovary.** Spindle-shaped cells are dispersed in a variably fibrous stroma.

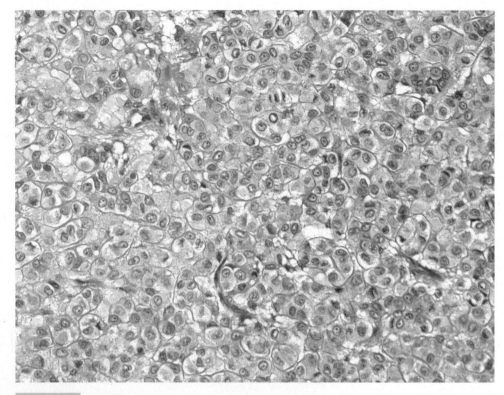

Figure 5.79 Steroid cell tumor of ovary. Nests of polygonal cells with central rounded nuclei may exhibit finely vacuolated, eosinophilic, or, less commonly, optically clear cytoplasm.

thecomas are benign. Some fibromas present with ascites and a pleural effusion (Meigs syndrome), which resolves on removal of the tumor.

Sclerosing Stromal Cell Tumors	These stromal tumors occur in young women and are rarely associated with endocrine manifestations. They are unilateral and clinically benign. Sclerosing stromal tumors are distinguished by the presence of alternating, relatively hypercellular and hypocellular areas of stromal proliferation, arranged in a pseudolobular pattern. An extensive, thin-walled vascular pattern is often present.
Steroid Cell Tumors, Not Otherwise Specified	Steroid cell tumors tend to occur in young, reproductive-aged women, and 25% occur before the age of 30 years. Most are confined to one ovary at diagnosis, but as many as 20% have extraovarian spread, and 30% are clinically malignant. **Endocrine manifestations, when present, tend to be androgenic,** although estrogenic, progestogenic, and Cushingoid manifestations may also be seen (63). Most are solid and pale yellow or orange, with the color depending on the steroid content. Microscopically, the tumors are composed of solid nests of uniform, round, or polygonal cells, with distinct cell borders, and central nuclei that contain small, but distinct nucleoli (Fig. 5.79). The cytoplasm may be finely vacuolated, or eosinophilic and granular. Most tumors are mitotically inactive with fewer than 2 mitotic figures per 10 high-power fields; tumors with a high mitotic index may be more aggressive.
Leydig Cell Tumors and Stromal Luteomas	Steroid cell tumors, not otherwise specified, must be distinguished from Leydig cell tumors and stromal luteomas, both of which tend to exhibit a benign clinical course. **Leydig cell tumors** are recognized by the presence of **Reinke crystals.** They are either small and typically hilar in location, or large and replacing most of the ovarian parenchyma. **Stromal luteomas** are typically small (less than 3 cm), well-circumscribed tumors that occur within the ovarian stroma. **A size criterion of 1 cm has been imposed to distinguish Leydig cell tumors and stromal luteomas from benign, nonneoplastic ovarian steroid cell proliferations.**

Germ Cell Tumors

These tumors are derived from the primordial germ cells of the ovary. Most are mature cystic teratomas and are clinically benign. The remaining germ cell tumors are malignant; most occur in children or adolescent girls (63).

Mature Cystic Teratoma

Mature teratomas are typically cystic, although solid variants do occur. They have a wide age range, occurring in females from 2 to 80 years (mean 32 years). Up to 15% are bilateral at presentation. **Mature teratomas are one of the most common ovarian neoplasms, accounting for 30–45% of all ovarian tumors, and as many as 60% of all benign ovarian tumors.** Recurrences may appear in the residual ipsilateral ovary following cystectomy, particularly when the tumors are multiple or ruptured. The presence of *mature glial implants* in the peritoneum (grade 0 implants) does not adversely affect prognosis (50) (Fig. 5.80).

Monodermal mature teratomas are not uncommon in the ovary, and include struma ovarii (thyroid), carcinoid, strumal carcinoid, ependymoma, and primitive neuroectodermal tumor.

The development of a secondary somatic carcinoma may rarely occur in mature teratomas in postmenopausal women. Squamous carcinoma and adenocarcinoma, usually of intestinal type, account for most cases of secondary carcinoma. **Secondary sarcomas** are less common, and tend to occur in younger patients.

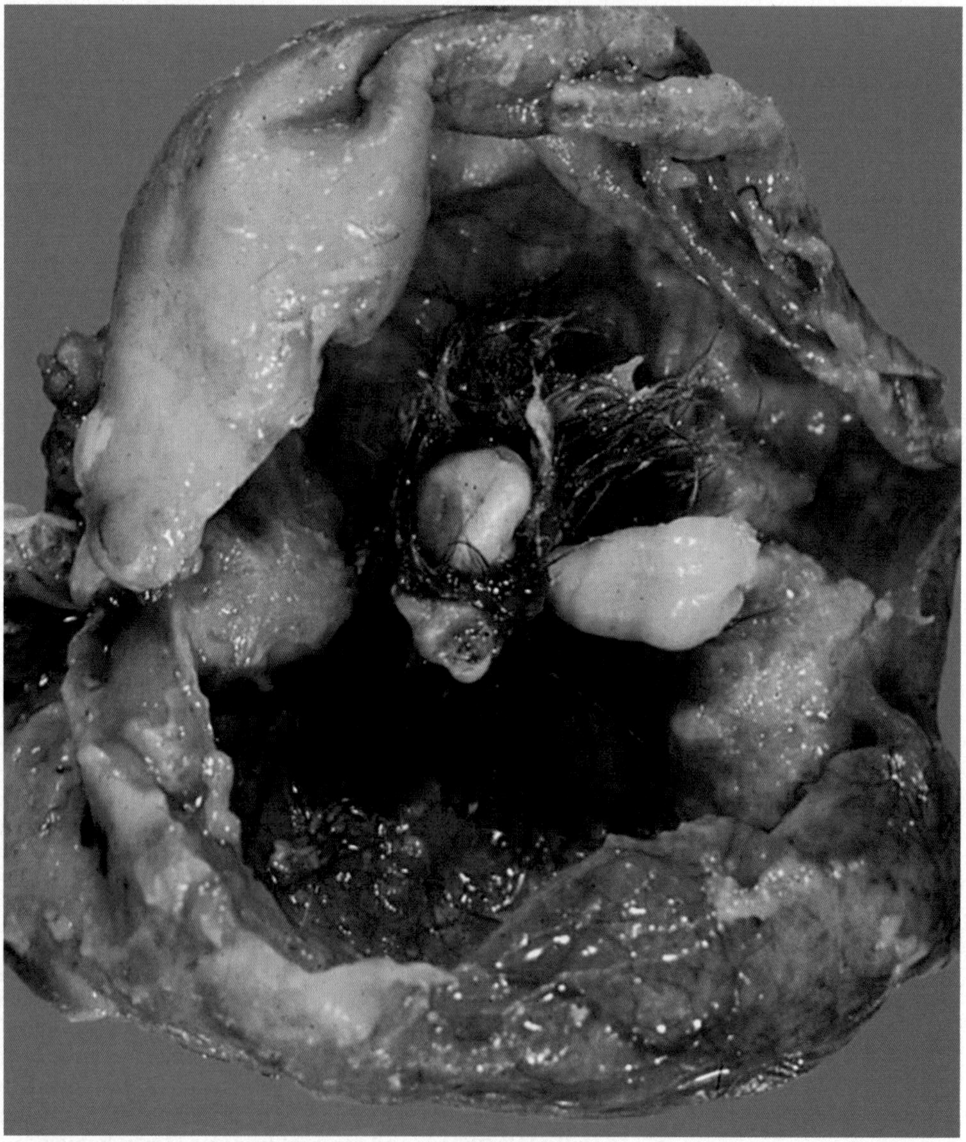

Figure 5.80 **Mature teratoma.** Cystic neoplasm contains teeth, hair, and sebaceous material.

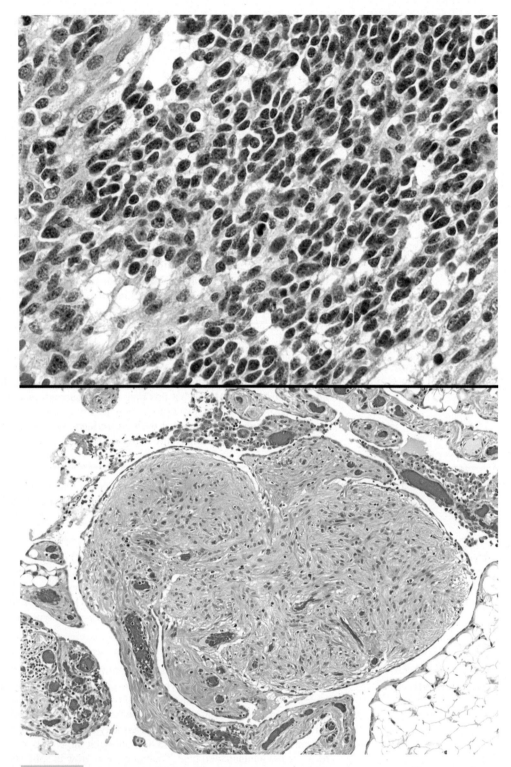

Figure 5.81 **Immature teratoma.** Top: Teratomas are graded on the amount of immature tissue, most commonly manifested by immature neural tissue, that is present. Bottom: In contrast, the presence of mature glial tissue does not affect prognosis, even when it forms nodular deposits throughout the peritoneum (gliomatosis).

Immature Teratoma

Immature teratomas are distinguished from mature teratomas by the presence of variable amounts of immature embryonal tissue, typically in the form of immature neuroectodermal tissue (Fig. 5.81). Prognosis is dependent on the grade and stage of disease. Tumors are graded on the basis of the amount of immature tissue present. **Grading is traditionally based on a three-tiered**

203

system, although a two-tiered system may be more reproducible. Treatment of immature teratomas has evolved. Surgery alone is considered curative in children and adolescent patients regardless of the grade. Chemotherapy is used for patients who relapse.

Dysgerminoma

Dysgerminoma is identical to its testicular counterpart, the seminoma. The ovarian tumors are unilateral in 80% of patients, large (mean 15 cm), solid, and tan in appearance; cyst formation is seen in areas of infarction. Most occur in the second and third decades, although 5% present in children less than 5 years of age. The tumors are composed of a diffuse proliferation of rounded cells with discrete cell membranes and central nuclei, with one to four prominent nucleoli (Fig. 5.82). Lymphocytes and granulomas are often present. Some tumors contain syncytiotrophoblastic cells, which may be associated with elevated serum beta-human chorionic gonadotropin. The neoplastic cells express placental alkaline phosphatase, CD117, and OCT 3/4. Calcifications should prompt consideration for the presence of concomitant gonadoblastoma (50).

Yolk Sac Tumor

Yolk sac tumor (endodermal sinus tumor) occurs in females from as young as 17 months to 43 years (mean 20 years). The tumor is usually unilateral, solid, and cystic with areas of hemorrhage and necrosis. A reticular or tubulocystic pattern with **Schiller–Duval bodies** is characteristic, but microcystic, macrocystic, solid, and glandular patterns can also be seen (Fig. 5.83). Yolk sac tumors are associated with elevated serum alpha fetoprotein (AFP), and the tumors express AFP, cytokeratin, glypigan-3, and SALL4 (66).

Gonadoblastoma

This tumor is composed of dysgerminoma cells admixed with sex-cord derivatives resembling Sertoli or granulosa cells. Gonadoblastoma is typically diagnosed in children or young adults. Most are bilateral, but this may not be macroscopically apparent. Calcifications within hyalinized bodies of the sex-cord component are seen in more than 80% of cases. **Almost all gonadoblastomas are associated with an underlying gonadal disorder, either pure or mixed dysgenesis, with a Y chromosome being detected.**

Embryonal Carcinoma

Pure embryonal carcinoma is rare in the ovary but may be admixed with other germ cell tumors; this appears to be particularly common in gonadoblastomas. Embryonal carcinomas express cytokeratin, CD117, OCT 3/4, and CD30.

Miscellaneous Ovarian Tumors

The ovary gives rise to a variety of other benign and malignant tumors that do not easily sort into one or another of the major ovarian tumor categories. Most of these tumors are extremely rare and include such diverse entities as **paraganglioma; myxoma; small cell carcinoma, hypercalcemic type; small cell carcinoma, pulmonary type;** and **large-cell neuroendocrine carcinoma,** among others (67). Only small cell carcinoma, hypercalcemic type, occurs with sufficient frequency to warrant discussion in this chapter.

Small Cell Carcinoma, Hypercalcemic Type

This is an uncommon, highly malignant tumor presenting in young women, often in association with paraneoplastic hypercalcemia. The tumors are usually large and unilateral, even in the presence of advanced stage disease. Approximately 50% of tumors are confined to the ovary at presentation, and these tumors appear to have a better prognosis than tumors with extraovarian spread. Small cell carcinoma, hypercalcemic type is typically composed of small, undifferentiated, and mitotically active cells (Fig. 5.84), although large cells may be present and, in some cases, form the predominant cell type. The tumor cells grow in solid sheets punctuated by variably sized follicle-like spaces. Mucinous epithelium may be seen in as many as 15% of cases (67).

Small cell carcinoma, hypercalcemic type should not be confused with small cell carcinoma, pulmonary type. The latter tumor occurs in postmenopausal women and is histologically and immunohistologically similar to small cell neuroendocrine carcinoma of the lung.

Secondary Tumors of the Ovary—Metastases

Tumors secondarily involving the ovary include **carcinoma, lymphoma or leukemia, melanoma, and sarcoma.** The tubular gastrointestinal tract, particularly **the colon, is the most common source of metastatic carcinoma** (Fig. 5.85), followed by the breast and pancreatobiliary tract.

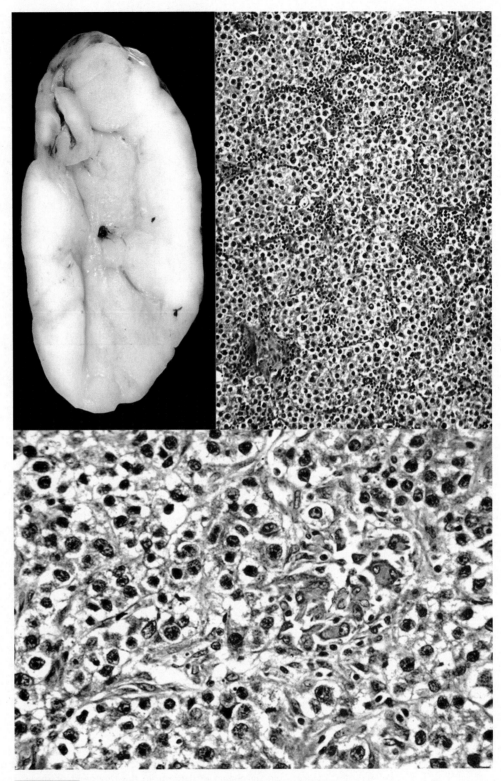

Figure 5.82 Dysgerminoma. Top left: Solid, pale tan lobulated growth pattern is characteristic of dysgerminoma. Top right and bottom: The tumor is composed of sheets of ovoid to polygonal cells with clear cytoplasm, prominent cell borders, and central nuclei with multiple small nucleoli. Interspersed mature lymphocytes are characteristic.

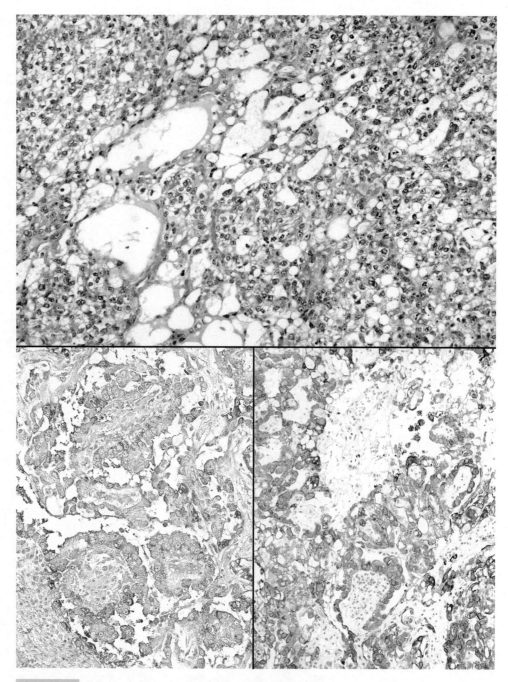

Figure 5.83 **Yolk sac tumor of ovary.** Top: Microcystic reticular pattern of yolk sac tumor. Bottom: These tumors express AFP (left) and glypican-3, as well as SALL4 (right).

Tumors arising in any site may secondarily spread to the ovary; the relative frequency of the primary site varies in different countries, depending on the relative incidence of various types of cancer, and on changing patterns in the treatment of these cancers. The classic **Kruckenberg tumor** refers to **metastatic signet-ring carcinoma** involving the ovaries (Fig. 5.86), which typically arises in the stomach, appendix, or large bowel. A variety of features may suggest an ovarian metastasis, including bilateral disease, surface nodules, extensive lymphatic involvement, and diameter smaller than 10 cm.

Nonneoplastic Lesions of the Ovary

Many nonneoplastic lesions of the ovary may mimic an ovarian neoplasm. Most occur during the reproductive years. Some are associated with infertility. These include **cysts of follicular origin,**

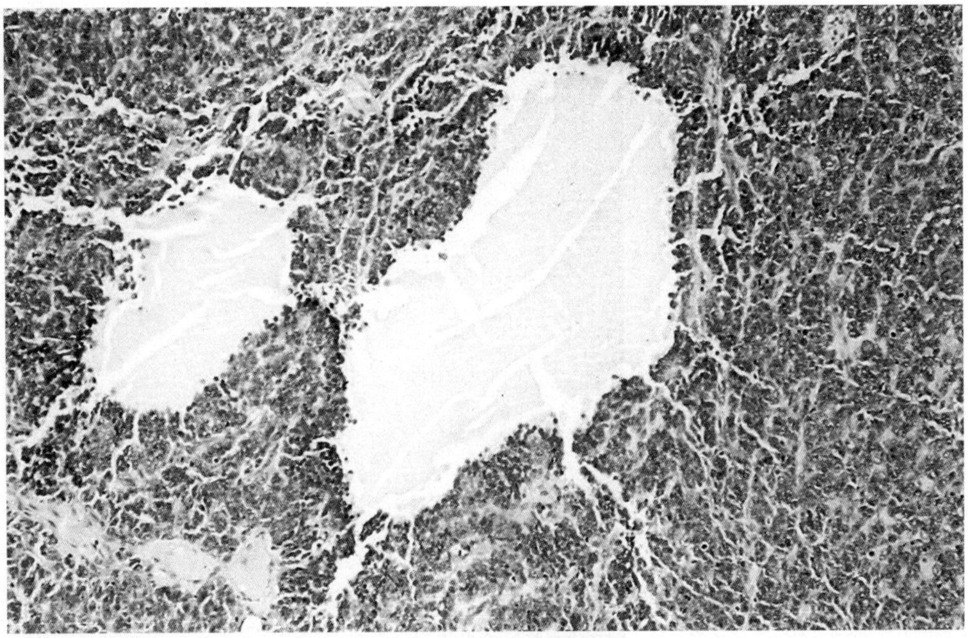

Figure 5.84 Small cell carcinoma, hypercalcemic type of ovary. Sheets of immature small cells with high mitotic index are punctuated by follicle-like spaces containing eosinophilic material.

massive ovarian edema, stromal hyperplasia and hyperthecosis, endometriosis, and a variety of pregnancy-associated changes (68).

Cysts of Follicular Origin	Cysts of follicular origin are classified as **follicular or luteal,** depending on whether the cyst lining is composed of nonluteinized or luteinized granulosa and theca cells. Larger than 3 cm by definition, most cysts of follicular origin do not exceed 8 cm in diameter. Rupture of a follicular or corpus luteal cyst may cause abrupt abdominal pain or hemoperitoneum.
Polycystic Ovarian Disease—Sclerocystic Ovaries	Sclerocystic ovaries show bilateral ovarian enlargement with numerous cortical cysts, most measuring less than 3 cm, underlying a white fibrous band of cortical tissue. The etiology of this relatively common condition is heterogeneous, but in many cases the underlying defect has been attributed to insulin resistance of peripheral tissue, or an abnormality of the hypothalamic-pituitary-ovarian axis. Patients present with anovulation, menstrual dysfunction, and hyperandrogenemia (**Polycystic Ovarian Syndrome, Stein–Leventhal syndrome**).
Massive Ovarian Edema	Massive ovarian edema occurs predominantly in children, adolescents, and young women. The etiology is uncertain, but is thought to be the result of partial lymphatic or venous obstruction leading to accumulation of edema fluid and ovarian enlargement. Patients present with abdominal pain, abdominal distention, or menstrual irregularities. Affected patients may show features of virilism, hirsutism, and, rarely, precocious pseudopuberty. The affected ovary is gelatinous because of fluid accumulation within the interstitium of the ovary, separating and sometimes involving pre-existing follicular structures (68).
Stromal Hyperplasia	Stromal hyperplasia is found predominantly in the postmenopausal age group. The ovaries are enlarged bilaterally by hyperplastic stroma, which may contain luteinized cells. **The condition is benign and generally asymptomatic,** often discovered incidentally during surgery for other causes.
Stromal Hyperthecosis	Stromal hyperthecosis may be seen in association with stromal hyperplasia in postmenopausal women, but can also occur in reproductive-aged women. Virilization, acne, obesity, hypertension, and glucose intolerance may be seen in association with stromal hyperthecosis in premenopausal women. **A small percentage of patients have HAIR-AN (hyperandrogenism, insulin resistance,**

207

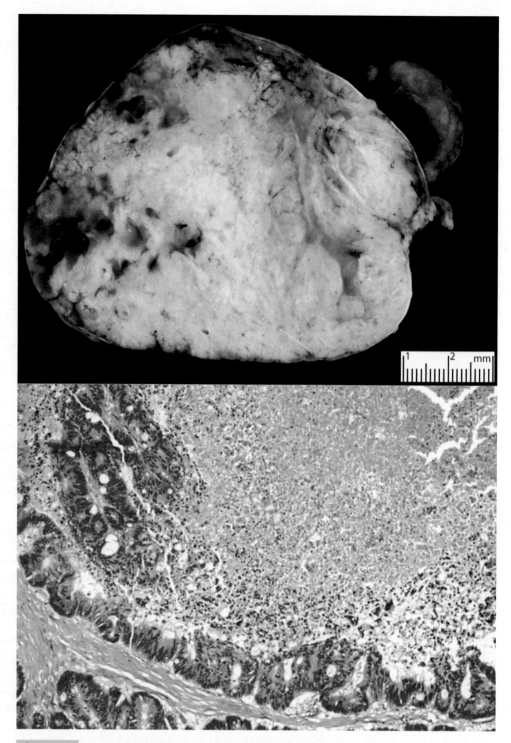

Figure 5.85 **Metastatic colorectal adenocarcinoma.** Top: Metastatic colorectal carcinoma often simulates a primary ovarian tumor. Note the smooth external capsule. Bottom: A garland gland pattern and the presence of extensive "dirty cell" necrosis secondary to the presence of necrotic cellular debris within gland lumens are characteristic of metastatic colorectal carcinoma.

and acanthosis nigricans) syndrome. The ovaries are bilaterally enlarged by a proliferation of theca cells, similar to those of the theca interna.

Endometriois

Endometriois commonly presents during the reproductive years and ranges from single or multiple microscopic deposits of ectopic endometrial glands and stroma to large hemorrhagic cysts

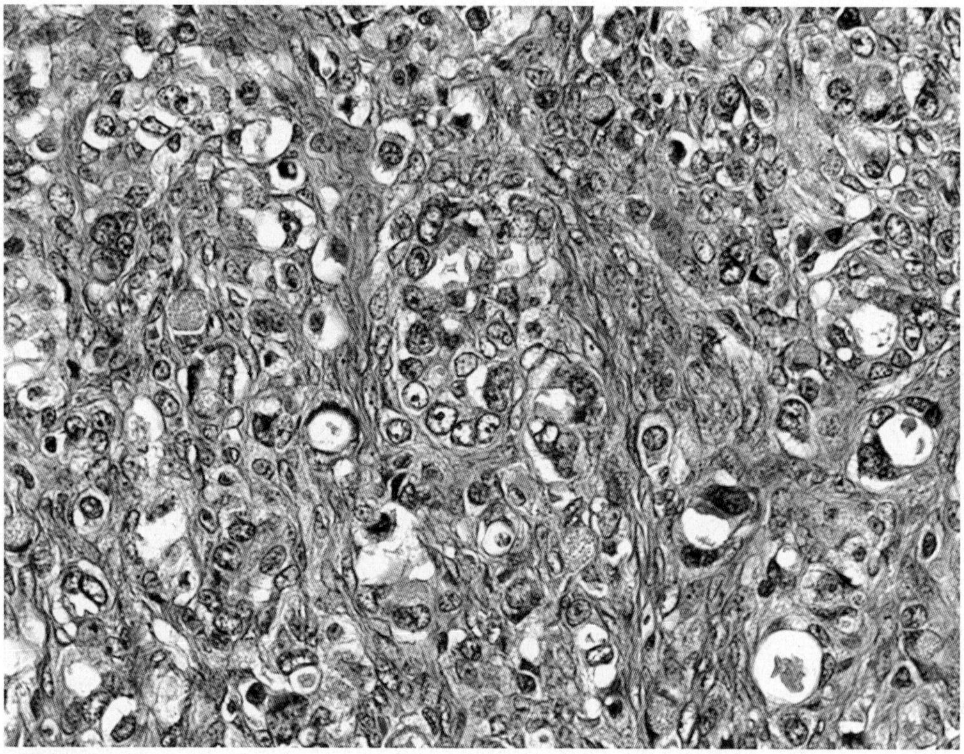

Figure 5.86 **Metastatic gastric signet-ring adenocarcinoma (Kruckenberg tumor).** Metastatic signet-ring carcinomas are often associated with ovarian stromal hyperplasia, which may mimic a stromal process.

(endometriomas) simulating a tumor mass. **The larger cysts should be carefully examined to exclude the presence of an occult clear cell or endometrioid carcinoma.**

Polypoid Endometriosis

Rarely, foci of endometriois may form large, polypoid masses on the ovary, fallopian tube, bowel, or peritoneum (Fig. 5.87). Most of the reported lesions have followed a benign clinical course (69), but complete excision and thorough microscopic examination should be performed to exclude adenosarcoma, stromal sarcoma, or adenocarcinoma arising in the setting of endometriosis.

Luteinized Ovarian Conditions

Pregnancy Luteoma

Pregnancy luteoma is a benign condition that occurs in the second half of pregnancy and regresses after delivery. One or both ovaries are enlarged by single or multiple nodules of steroid cells with abundant, eosinophilic cytoplasm. Necrosis and degenerative changes may be present. Most are discovered during cesarean section.

Large Solitary Luteinized Cyst of Pregnancy and the Puerperium

Large solitary luteinized follicular cyst of pregnancy and the puerperium is a rare, unilateral, thin-walled cyst lined by large cells with abundant cytoplasm with focal pleomorphic and hyperchromatic nuclei. These atypical cells are thought to be degenerative. A distinct theca layer is absent.

Hyperreactio Luteinalis

Hyperreactio luteinalis is characterized by bilateral ovarian enlargement secondary to the development of multiple luteinized cysts. This condition is rare in normal pregnancy, but may

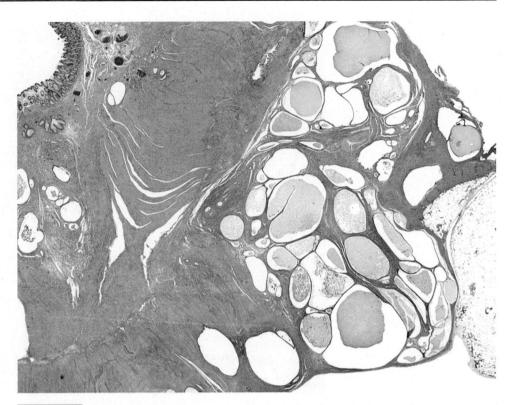

Figure 5.87 Polypoid endometriosis. When large and multifocal, these polypoid masses of ectopic endometrial tissue may simulate a neoplasm.

occur in 10–40% of women with gestational trophoblastic disease, and in women undergoing ovulation induction (especially those with pre-existing polycystic ovaries).

Fallopian Tube

The traditional, admittedly arbitrary, criteria to distinguish serous carcinoma of the ovary from serous carcinoma of the peritoneum are based on the presence of at least 5 mm of ovarian parenchymal involvement or, in the case of low-stage disease, by the exclusive presence of ovarian (surface or parenchymal) involvement. Primary serous carcinoma of the fallopian tube, once considered to be very rare, is based on the exclusion of primary ovarian and uterine disease. The historical basis for these distinctions rests largely on the hypothesis that most serous carcinomas arise either from the surface epithelium of the ovary or from inclusion glands within the ovarian parenchyma.

This hypothesis has been challenged by the revival of the **alternative theory that serous carcinoma arises from the epithelium of the fimbria of the fallopian tube.** The detection of tubal intraepithelial carcinoma (Fig. 5.88) in women undergoing risk-reducing salpingo-oophorectomy, or in women with an ovarian or peritoneal serous carcinoma buffeted this claim, and generated renewed interest in the tubal fimbria as a candidate source of serous carcinoma. Whether all such examples reflect primary tubal epithelium as the source of carcinoma or secondary involvement by carcinoma arising elsewhere is currently unanswerable, except in those cases in which the fallopian tube is the only site of involvement. **A p53 signature has been identified in the fimbriated tubal epithelium that may represent a precursor lesion of tubal intraepithelial carcinoma** (Fig. 5.89), but this requires further study (70). Metastases not uncommonly involve the fallopian tube mucosa and serosa.

The fallopian tubes from all risk-reducing salpingo-oophorectomy specimens should be serially sectioned and completely examined microscopically in order to exclude occult tubal intraepithelial carcinoma (71).

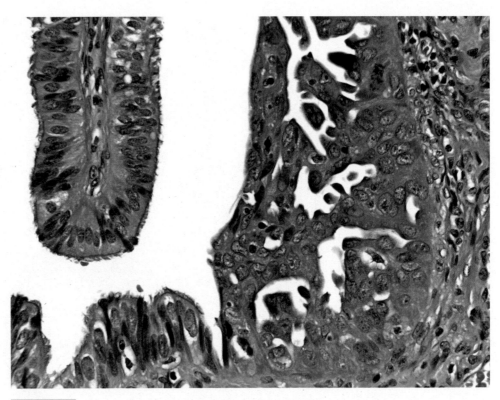

Figure 5.88 **Serous tubal intraepithelial carcinoma.** Tubal mucosa is focally replaced by stratified cells with markedly pleomorphic nuclei. The lesion is confined to the mucosa and typically occurs in the fimbria and distal fallopian tube in women with *BRCA* germ-line mutations.

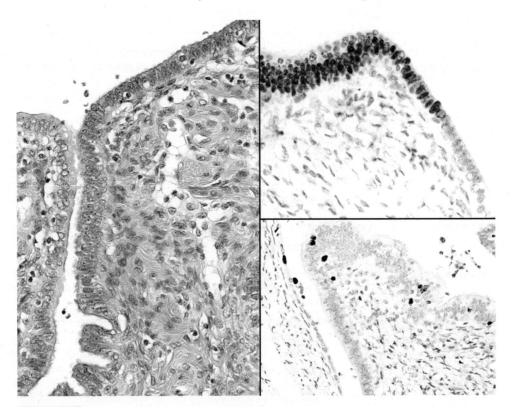

Figure 5.89 **Fallopian tube with "p53 signature."** Histologically normal tubal mucosa (left) may exhibit nuclear over-expression of p53 (top right), but low Ki-67 proliferation rate (bottom right). Although it has been proposed that this lesion may be a precursor to serous tubal carcinoma, it is not known to be associated with an adverse prognosis in the absence of morphologic carcinoma.

211

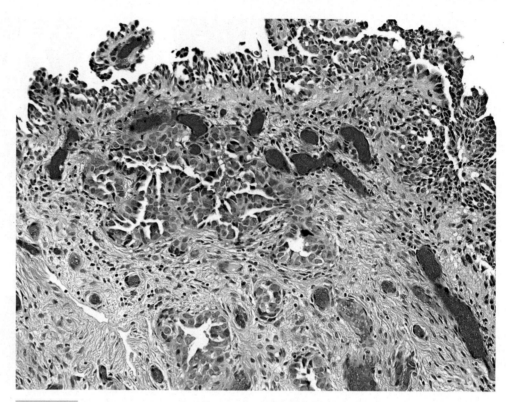

Figure 5.90 **Invasive serous carcinoma, fallopian tube.** Superficial invasion into the tubal stroma is seen in this early invasive serous tubal carcinoma.

Primary Tubal Carcinoma	**Serous carcinoma is the most common** histologic subtype of carcinoma to occur in the fallopian tube (Fig. 5.90), but **endometrioid neoplasms** (adenofibroma, borderline, and carcinoma) **may occur.** The distinction among the three types of endometrioid and serous tumors is based on the same criteria that are used elsewhere in the female genital tract.
Adenomatoid Tumor	Adenomatoid tumors are common, benign mesothelial neoplasms that arise in the subserosa of the paratubal region, but they may also be seen in the uterus and, rarely, in the ovary. When occurring in the fallopian tube, they are small, firm, tan white nodules, often measuring less than 1 cm in diameter. The uterine tumors are usually larger and arise in the myometrium. The presence of tubular and signet-ring–like cells may simulate a metastatic carcinoma (Fig. 5.91).

Gestational Trophoblastic Disease

Gestatational trophoblastic disease arises as a result of abnormal placental development, with a resultant proliferation of syncytiotrophoblastic, cytotrophoblastic, or intermediate trophoblastic tissue (72).

Hydatidiform Mole	Hydatidiform mole is the most common form of gestatational trophoblastic disease, and is divided into complete or partial moles. **The complete mole is diploid (46XX or 46XY)** and derived entirely from paternal chromosomes because of fertilization of an empty ovum by a single spermatozum, whereas a **partial mole is triploid (69XXX, 69XXY, or 69XYY)** and derived from fertilization of a normal egg by two spermatozoa.
Complete Hydatidiform Mole	**Complete moles exhibit uniformly enlarged, hydropic villi, with variable degrees of circumferential trophoblastic proliferation.** The well-developed, second trimester complete moles are

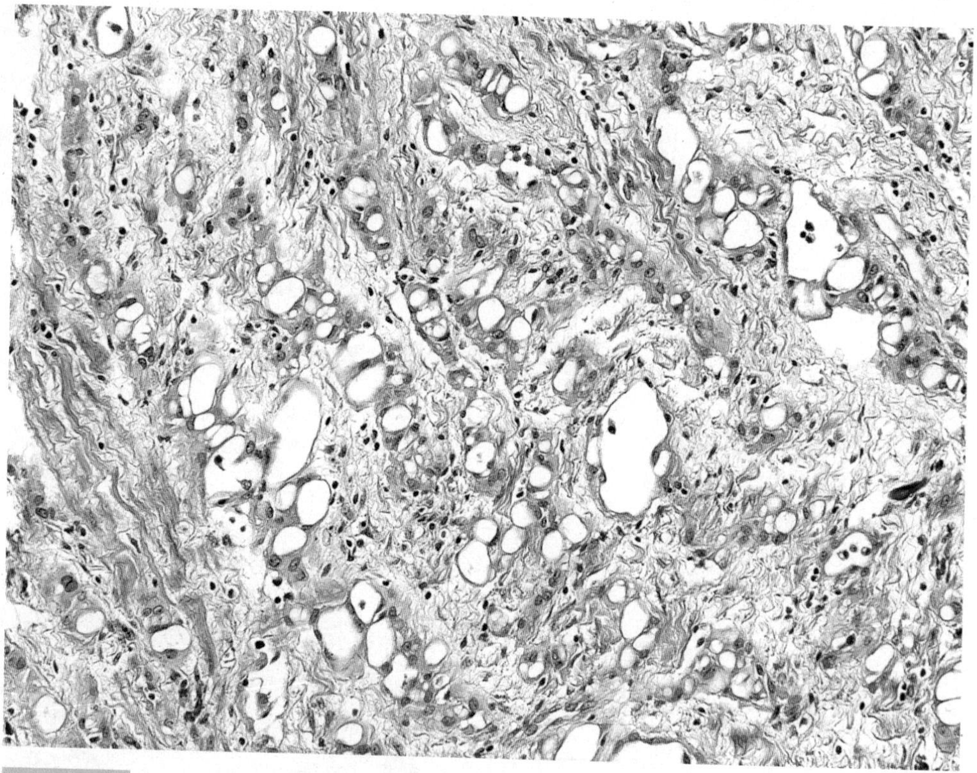

Figure 5.91 **Adenomatoid tumor, fallopian tube.** Signet-ring appearance may simulate metastatic carcinoma.

visualized as transparent, grapelike vesicles on macroscopic examination, but complete moles in early trimester abortuses may be difficult to detect, even on microscopic examination. Because complete moles are paternally derived, proteins encoded by paternally imprinted genes are not expressed in the villous stromal tissue or cytotrophoblast of complete moles. One of these proteins, p57, may be used to establish the diagnosis of complete moles in diagnostically more difficult cases (Fig. 5.92).

Complete moles may progress to invasive mole or choriocarcinoma. Progression is associated with progressively rising serum beta human chorionic gonadotropin levels.

Partial Hydatidiform Mole	**Partial moles exhibit a dimorphic population of small and larger villi, with lesser degrees of trophoblastic proliferation. Most are associated with a fetus.** Progression of partial mole to invasive mole or choriocarcinoma is rare or nonexistent.
Invasive Mole	**Invasive mole is diagnosed on the basis of invasion into myometrium or its blood vessels** (Fig. 5.93). Common sites of extrauterine spread include the vagina, vulva, and lung.
Choriocarcinoma	**Choriocarcinoma is a highly malignant tumor composed of syncytiotrophoblastic, intermediate trophoblastic and cytotrophoblastic cells arranged in a bilaminar configuration** (Fig. 5.94). Chorionic villi are almost always absent. Hemorrhage and necrosis are common. Patients often present with profuse vaginal bleeding. Distant lung, brain, or liver metastases may also be present.
Placental Site Trophoblastic Tumor	This very uncommon form of gestational trophoblastic disease is composed of intermediate trophoblastic cells (Fig. 5.95). The tumor may form a discrete mass or irregularly infiltrate the myometrium, causing uterine enlargement. **Although most placental site trophoblastic tumors follow a benign clinical course, the behavior is unpredictable, and occasional tumors spread throughout the uterus and metastasize to distant sites.**

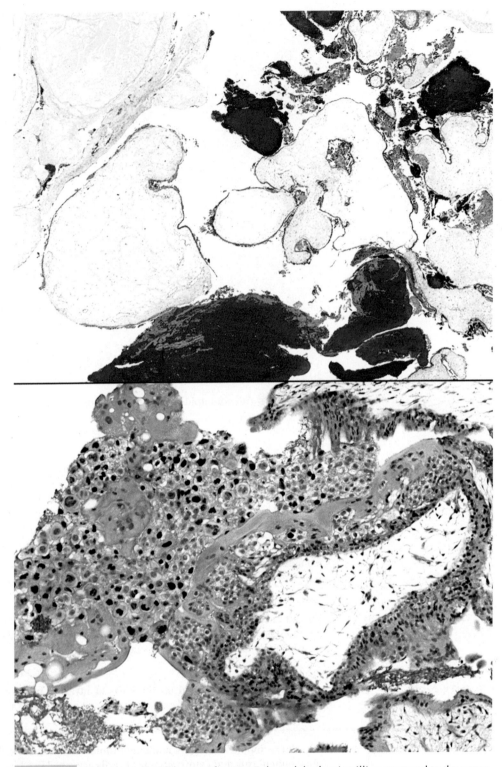

Figure 5.92 Complete hydatidiform mole. Top: Enlarged, hydropic villi correspond to the grape-like vesicles seen in curettage specimens. Bottom: Villous stromal cells and cytotrophoblast cells do not express paternally imprinted nuclear p57 in complete hydatidiform mole.

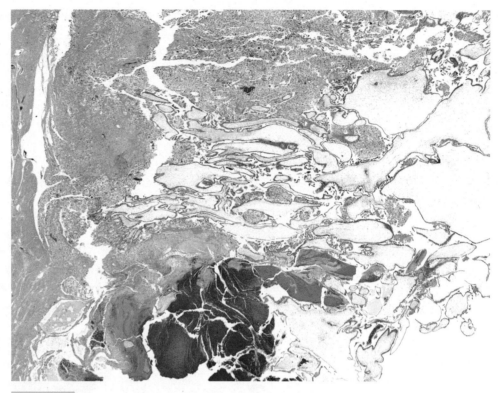

Figure 5.93 Invasive mole. Complete hydatidiform mole with exuberant trophoblastic proliferation invades the myometrium in this hysterectomy specimen.

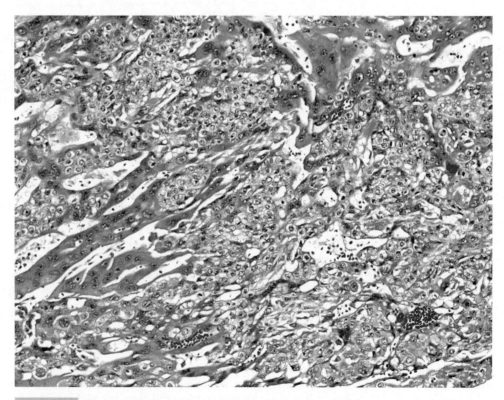

Figure 5.94 Choriocarcinoma. Bilaminar pattern of syncytiotrophoblastic and cytotrophoblastic cells is diagnostic of this tumor.

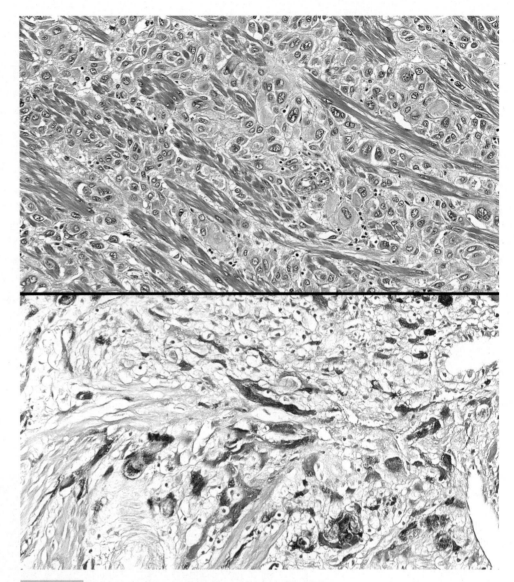

Figure 5.95 **Placental site trophoblastic tumor.** Top: Large, atypical eosinophilic and polygonal cells diffusely infiltrate the deep myometrium. Bottom: Human placental lactogen is expressed by the neoplastic intermediate trophoblastic cells.

An epithelioid variant, composed of smaller, more epithelioid cells resembling squamous cell carcinoma, appears to be more aggressive (72).

Exaggerated Placental Site

Exaggerated placental site is a benign condition marked by an exuberance of intermediate trophoblastic cells that may simulate placental site trophoblastic tumor. The lesion is no different from the usual implantation site, but the individual intermediate trophoblastic cells are larger and more numerous; nuclear hyperchromasia may also be present. Unlike placental site trophoblastic tumor, chorionic villi and syncytiotrophoblastic giant cells are typically present, mitotic figures are rare or absent, and there is no necrosis.

Placental Site Nodule and Plaque

Placental site nodules are essentially hyalinized implantation sites. They occur during the reproductive years, and may be a cause of uterine bleeding or an incidental finding. They are discrete lesions, forming nodules or plaques, but occasionally they may present as multiple fragments or lesions in a uterine sampling (Fig. 5.96). A history of pregnancy may be remote or even absent. Placental site nodule or plaque is a benign process, and not to be confused with placental site trophoblastic tumor.

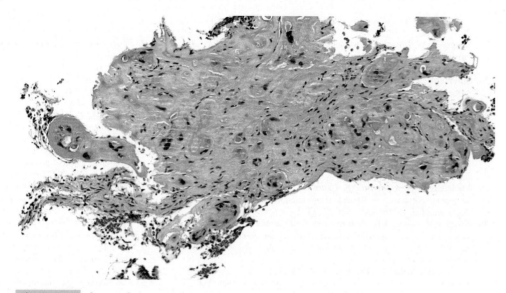

Figure 5.96 Placental site nodule. Discrete nodules or plaques of hyalinized intermediate trophoblastic tissue may be seen in curettage specimens.

References

1. **Darragh TM, Colgan TJ, Cox JT, et al.** The Lower Anogenital Squamous Terminology Standardization Project for HPV-Associated Lesions: Background and consensus recommendations from the College of American Pathologists and the American Society for Colposcopy and Cervical Pathology. *J Low Genit Tract Dis.* 2012;16(3): 205–242.
2. **Stoler MH, Schiffman M.** Interobserver reproducibility of cervical cytologic and histologic interpretations: Realistic estimates from the ASCUS-LSIL Triage Study. *JAMA.* 2001;285:1500–1505.
3. **Kong CS, Balzer BL, Troxell ML, et al.** p16INK4 A immunohistochemistry is superior to HPV *in situ* hybridization for the detection of high-risk HPV in atypical squamous metaplasia. *Am J Surg Pathol.* 2007;31:33–43.
4. **Castle PE, Stoler MH, Solomon D, et al.** The relationship of community biopsy-diagnosed cervical intraepithelial neoplasia grade 2 to the quality control pathology-reviewed diagnoses: An ALTS report. *Am J Clin Pathol.* 2007;127(5):805–815.
5. **Carreon JD, Sherman ME, Guillen D, et al.** CIN 2 is a much less reproducible and less valid diagnosis than CIN 3: Results from a histological review of population-based cervical samples. *Int J Gynecol Pathol.* 2007;26(4):441–446.
6. **Cogliano V, Baan R, Straif K, et al.** Carcinogenicity of human papillomaviruses. *Lancet Oncol.* 2005;6:204.
7. **Ho GY, Bierman R, Beardsley L, et al.** Natural history of cervicovaginal papillomavirus infection in young women. *N Engl J Med.* 1998;338:423–428.
8. **Human papillomavirus testing for triage of women with cytologic evidence of low-grade squamous intraepithelial lesions: Baseline data from a randomized trial.** The Atypical Squamous Cells of Undetermined Significance/Low-Grade Squamous Intraepithelial Lesions Triage Study (ALTS) Group. *J Natl Cancer Inst.* 2000;92: 397–402.
9. **Solomon D, Nayar R, eds.** *The Bethesda System for Reporting Cervical Cytology.* New York, NY: Springer; 2004.
10. **Massad LS, Einstein MH, Huh WK, et al.** 2012 updated consensus guidelines for the management of abnormal cervical cancer screening tests and cancer precursors. *J Low Genit Tract Dis.* 2013;17(5 Suppl 1): S1–S27.
11. **Solomon D, Schiffman M, Tarone R; ALTS Study Group.** Comparison of three management strategies for patients with atypical squamous cells of undetermined significance: Baseline results from a randomized trial. *J Natl Cancer Inst.* 2001;93:293–299.
12. **De Cremoux P, Coste J, Sastre-Garau X, et al.** Efficiency of the hybrid capture 2 HPV DNA test in cervical cancer screening. A study by the French Society of Clinical Cytology. *Am J Clin Pathol.* 2003; 120:492–499.
13. **Carozzi FM, Del Mistro A, Confortini M, et al.** Reproducibility of HPV DNA testing by hybrid capture 2 in a screening setting. *Am J Clin Pathol.* 2005;124:716–721.
14. **Castle PE, Lorincz AT, Mielzynska-Lohnas I, et al.** Results of human papillomavirus DNA testing with the hybrid capture 2 assay are reproducible. *J Clin Microbiol.* 2002;40:1088–1090.
15. **Biscotti CV, Dawson AE, Dziura B, et al.** Assisted primary screening using the automated ThinPrep Imaging System. *Am J Clin Pathol.* 2005;123:281–287.
16. **Ioffe OB, Sagae S, Moritani S, et al.** Proposal of a new scoring scheme for the diagnosis of noninvasive endocervical glandular lesions. *Am J Surg Pathol.* 2003;27:452–460.
17. **Witkiewicz A, Lee KR, Brodsky G, et al.** Superficial (early) endocervical adenocarcinoma *in situ*: A study of 12 cases and comparison to conventional AIS. *Am J Surg Pathol.* 2005;29:1609–1614.
18. **Crum CP, Nucci MR, Lee KR.** The cervix. In: **Mills SE, ed.** *Sternberg's Diagnostic Surgical Pathology.* New York, NY: Lippincott Williams & Wilkins; 2009.
19. **Ansari-Lari MA, Staebler A, Zaino RJ, et al.** Distinction of endocervical and endometrial adenocarcinomas: Immunohistochemical p16 expression correlated with human papillomavirus (HPV) DNA detection. *Am J Surg Pathol.* 2004;28:160–167.
20. **Kong CS, Beck AH, Longacre TA.** A panel of 3 markers including p16, ProExC, or HPV ISH is optimal for distinguishing between primary endometrial and endocervical adenocarcinomas. *Am J Surg Pathol.* 2010;34(7):915–926.
21. **Young RH, Clement PB.** Endocervical adenocarcinoma and its variants: Their morphology and differential diagnosis. *Histopathology.* 2002;41:185–207.
22. **Staebler A, Sherman ME, Zaino RJ, et al.** Hormone receptor immunohistochemistry and human papillomavirus *in situ* hybridization are useful for distinguishing endocervical and endometrial adenocarcinomas. *Am J Surg Pathol.* 2002;26:998–1006.
23. **Alkushi A, Irving J, Hsu F, et al.** Immunoprofile of cervical and endometrial adenocarcinomas using a tissue microarray. *Virchows Arch.* 2003;442:271–277.
24. **Park HM, Park MH, Kim YJ, et al.** Müllerian adenosarcoma with sarcomatous overgrowth of the cervix presenting as cervical polyp:

A case report and review of the literature. *Int J Gynecol Cancer.* 2004;14:1024–1029.

25. **Scurry J, Wilkinson EJ.** Review of terminology of precursors of vulvar squamous cell carcinoma. *J Low Genit Tract Dis.* 2006;10: 161–169.

26. **Sideri M, Jones RW, Wilkinson EJ, et al.** Squamous vulvar intraepithelial neoplasia: 2004 modified terminology, ISSVD Vulvar Oncology Subcommittee. *J Reprod Med.* 2005;50:807–810.

27. **Hart WR.** Vulvar intraepithelial neoplasia: Historical aspects and current status. *Int J Gynecol Pathol.* 2001;20:16–30.

28. **van der Avoort IA, Shirango H, Hoevenaars BM, et al.** Vulvar squamous cell carcinoma is a multifactorial disease following two separate and independent pathways. *Int J Gynecol Pathol.* 2006;25: 22–29.

29. **Medeiros F, Nascimento AF, Crum CP.** Early vulvar squamous neoplasia: Advances in classification, diagnosis, and differential diagnosis. *Adv Anat Pathol.* 2005;12:20–26.

30. **Nucci MR, Young RH, Fletcher CD.** Cellular pseudosarcomatous fibroepithelial stromal polyps of the lower female genital tract: An underrecognized lesion often misdiagnosed as sarcoma. *Am J Surg Pathol.* 2000;24:231–240.

31. **Stoler MH, Mills SE, Frierson HFJ.** The vulva and vagina. In: **Mills SE,** ed. *Sternberg's Diagnostic Surgical Pathology.* New York, NY: Lippincott Williams & Wilkins; 2009.

32. **Nielsen GP, Young RH.** Mesenchymal tumors and tumor-like lesions of the female genital tract: A selective review with emphasis on recently described entities. *Int J Gynecol Pathol.* 2001;20:105–127.

33. **Nucci MR, Fletcher CD.** Vulvovaginal soft tissue tumours: Update and review. *Histopathology.* 2000;36:97–108.

34. **Longacre TA, Chung MH, Jensen DN, et al.** Proposed criteria for the diagnosis of well-differentiated endometrial carcinoma. A diagnostic test for myoinvasion. *Am J Surg Pathol.* 1995;19:371–406.

35. **Kurman R, Norris H.** Evaluation of criteria for distinguishing atypical endometrial hyperplasia from well-differentiated carcinoma. *Cancer.* 1982;49:2547–2559.

36. **Hendrickson M, Ross J, Eifel P, et al.** Uterine papillary serous carcinoma: A highly malignant form of endometrial adenocarcinoma. *Am J Surg Pathol.* 1982;6:93–108.

37. **Hendrickson MR, Longacre TA, Kempson RL.** Uterine papillary serous carcinoma revisited. *Gynecol Oncol.* 1994;54:261–263.

38. **Sherman ME, Bitterman P, Rosenshein NB, et al.** Uterine serous carcinoma. A morphologically diverse neoplasm with unifying clinicopathologic features. *Am J Surg Pathol.* 1992;16:600–610.

39. **Soslow RA, Pirog E, Isacson C.** Endometrial intraepithelial carcinoma with associated peritoneal carcinomatosis. *Am J Surg Pathol.* 2000;24:726–732.

40. **Kempson RL, Hendrickson MR.** Smooth muscle, endometrial stromal, and mixed müllerian tumors of the uterus. *Mod Pathol.* 2000;13:328–342.

41. **Longacre TA, Atkins KA, Kempson RL, et al.** The uterine corpus. In: **Mills S,** ed. *Sternberg's Diagnostic Surgical Patholology.* Philadelphia, PA: Lippincott Williams & Wilkins; 2009.

42. **Bell SW, Kempson RL, Hendrickson MR.** Problematic uterine smooth muscle neoplasms. A clinicopathologic study of 213 cases. *Am J Surg Pathol.* 1994;18:535–558.

43. **Chang K, Crabtree G, Lim-Tan S, et al.** Primary uterine endometrial stromal neoplasms. A clinicopathologic study of 117 cases. *Am J Surg Pathol.* 1990;14:415–438.

44. **Lee CH, Marino-Enriquez A, Ou W, et al.** The clinicopathologic features of YWHAE-FAM22 endometrial stromal sarcomas: A histologically high-grade and clinically aggressive tumor. *Am J Surg Pathol.* 2012;36:641–653.

45. **Zaloudek C, Norris H.** Adenofibroma and adenosarcoma of the uterus: A clinicopathologic study of 35 cases. *Cancer.* 1981;48:354–366.

46. **Clement P, Scully R.** Müllerian adenosarcoma of the uterus: A clinicopathologic analysis of 100 cases with a review of the literature. *Hum Pathol.* 1990;21:363–381.

47. **Longacre TA, Chung MH, Rouse RV, et al.** Atypical polypoid adenomyofibromas (atypical polypoid adenomyomas) of the uterus.

A clinicopathologic study of 55 cases. *Am J Surg Pathol.* 1996; 20:1–20.

48. **Ferguson SE, Tornos C, Hummer A, et al.** Prognostic features of surgical stage I uterine carcinosarcoma. *Am J Surg Pathol.* 2007;31:1653–1661.

49. **Longacre TA, Gilks CB.** Surface epithelial stromal tumors. In: **Nucci M, Oliva E, eds.** *Gynecologic Pathology.* Philadelphia, PA: Elsevier; 2008.

50. **Lee KR, Tavassoli FA, Prat J, et al.** Tumours of the ovary and peritoneum. In: **Tavassoli FA, Devillee P, eds.** *Tumours of the Breast and Female Genital Organs.* Lyon: IARC Press; 2003;119–124.

51. **Bell DA, Longacre TA, et al.** Serous borderline (low malignant potential, atypical proliferative) ovarian tumors: Workshop perspectives. *Hum Pathol.* 2004;35:934–948.

52. **McKenney JK, Balzer BL, Longacre TA.** Patterns of stromal invasion in ovarian serous tumors of low malignant potential (borderline tumors): A re-evaluation of the concept of stromal microinvasion. *Am J Surg Pathol.* 2006;30:1209–1221.

53. **Longacre TA, McKenney JK, Tazelaar HD, et al.** Ovarian serous tumors of low malignant potential (borderline tumors): Outcome-based study of 276 patients with long-term (> or = 5-year) follow-up. *Am J Surg Pathol.* 2005;29:707–723.

54. **McKenney JK, Balzer BL, Longacre TA.** Lymph node involvement in ovarian serous tumors of low malignant potential (borderline tumors): Pathology, prognosis, and proposed classification. *Am J Surg Pathol.* 2006;30:614–624.

55. **Malpica A, Deavers MT, Lu K, et al.** Grading ovarian serous carcinoma using a two-tier system. *Am J Surg Pathol.* 2004;28:496–504.

56. **Shimizu Y, Kamoi S, Amada S, et al.** Toward the development of a universal grading system for ovarian epithelial carcinoma. I. Prognostic significance of histopathologic features—Problems involved in the architectural grading system. *Gynecol Oncol.* 1998;70:2–12.

57. **Shih Ie M, Kurman RJ.** Ovarian tumorigenesis: A proposed model based on morphological and molecular genetic analysis. *Am J Pathol.* 2004;164:1511–1518.

58. **Gilks CB, Bell DA, Scully RE.** Serous psammocarcinoma of the ovary and peritoneum. *Int J Gynecol Pathol.* 1990;9:110–121.

59. **Ronnett BM, Kajdacsy-Balla A, Gilks CB, et al.** Mucinous borderline ovarian tumors: Points of general agreement and persistent controversies regarding nomenclature, diagnostic criteria, and behavior. *Hum Pathol.* 2004;35:949–960.

60. **McKenney JK, Soslow RA, Longacre TA.** Ovarian mature teratomas with mucinous epithelial neoplasms: Morphologic heterogeneity and association with pseudomyxoma peritonei. *Am J Surg Pathol.* 2008;32:645–655.

61. **Vang R, Gown AM, Zhao C, et al.** Ovarian mucinous tumors associated with mature cystic teratomas: Morphologic and immunohistochemical analysis identifies a subset of potential teratomatous origin that shares features of lower gastrointestinal tract mucinous tumors more commonly encountered as secondary tumors in the ovary. *Am J Surg Pathol.* 2007;31:854–869.

62. **Wiegand KC, Shah SP, Al-Agha OM, et al.** ARID1A mutations in endometriosis-associated ovarian carcinomas. *N Engl J Med.* 2010; 363:1532–1543.

63. **Young RH, Clement PB, Scully RE.** Sex cord-stromal, steroid cell, and germ cell tumors of the ovary. In: **Mills SE, ed.** *Sternberg's Diagnostic Surgical Pathology.* Philadelphia, PA: Lippincott Williams & Wilkins; 2009.

64. **Shah SP, Köbel M, Senz J, et al.** Mutation of FOXL2 in granulosa-cell tumors of the ovary. *N Engl J Med.* 2009;360:2719–2729.

65. **Scully RE, Clement PB, Young RH.** Ovarian surface epithelial-stromal tumors. In: **Mills SE, ed.** *Sternberg's Diagnostic Surgical Pathology.* Philadelphia, PA: Lippincott Williams & Wilkins; 2009.

66. **Esheba GE, Pate LL, Longacre TA.** Oncofetal protein glypican-3 distinguishes yolk sac tumor from clear cell carcinoma of the ovary. *Am J Surg Pathol.* 2008;32:600–607.

67. **Clement PB, Young RH, Scully RE.** Miscellaneous primary tumors, secondary tumors, and non-neoplastic lesions of the ovary. In: **Mills SE, ed.** *Sternberg's Diagnostic Surgical Pathology.* Philadelphia, PA: Lippincott Williams & Wilkins; 2009.

68. **Longacre TA, Gilks CB.** Nonneoplastic lesions of the ovary. In: **Nucci M, Oliva E, eds.** *Gynecologic Pathology.* Philadelphia, PA: Elsevier, 2008.

69. **Parker RL, Clement PB, Chercover DJ, et al.** Early recurrence of ovarian serous borderline tumor as high-grade carcinoma: A report of two cases. *Int J Gynecol Pathol.* 2004;23:265–272.

70. **Folkins AK, Jarboe EA, Saleemuddin A, et al.** A candidate precursor to pelvic serous cancer (p53 signature) and its prevalence in ovaries and fallopian tubes from women with *BRCA* mutations. *Gynecol Oncol.* 2008;109:168–173. Epub 2008 Mar 14.

71. **Longacre TA, Oliva E, Soslow RA.** Recommendations for the reporting of fallopian tube neoplasms. *Virchows Arch.* 2007;450: 25–29.

72. **Shih IE, Mazur MT, Kurman RJ.** Gestational trophoblastic disease. In: **Mills SE, ed.** *Sternberg's Diagnostic Surgical Pathology.* Philadelphia, PA: Lippincott Williams & Wilkins; 2009.

6 Epidemiology and Biostatistics

Daniel W. Cramer
Kathryn L. Terry

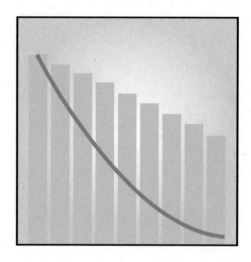

The disciplines of epidemiology and biostatistics apply to gynecologic oncology in defining cancer occurrence and survival, identifying risk factors, and implementing strategies for treatment or prevention, including the proper design of clinical trials. Epidemiology and biostatistics are essential to the practice of evidence-based medicine. Some key principles of epidemiology and biostatistics are considered under the headings of descriptive statistics, etiologic studies, statistical inference and validity, and cancer risk and prevention. Standard statistical and epidemiologic texts present more detailed discussions and computational formulas (1,2).

Descriptive Statistics

Cancer is described in populations by statistics related to its occurrence and patient survival. How cancer varies by age, ethnicity, and geography is of particular interest. Descriptive statistics about cancer in the United States can be obtained from the National Cancer Institute through its Web site: http://www.seer.cancer.gov/. Descriptive statistics about cancer in the world can be obtained from the International Agency for Research on Cancer through its Web site: http://www-dep.iarc.fr/.

Incidence

The incidence rate (IR) is defined as the number of new cases of disease in a population within a specified time period:

$$IR = \text{New cases/Person-time}$$

The fact that time is a component of the denominator should help clinicians avoid the misapplication of this term to **prevalence—another measure of disease occurrence that includes both old and new cases existing at a single point in time.**

Cancer Incidence and Mortality

Cancer incidence or mortality is usually stated as cases (or deaths) per 100,000 people per year, or as cases per 100,000 person-years. Incidence or mortality is measured in a specific population over a specific period. For example, country or state cancer registries count the number of new cancer cases diagnosed or cancer deaths among residents over a year, and divide that figure by census estimates of the total population in the region.

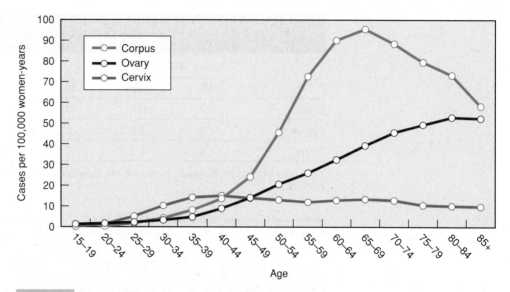

Figure 6.1 **Age-specific incidence curves for gynecologic cancers in women in the United States, 2006–2010.** (Modified from **Howlader N, Noone AM, Krapcho M, et al., eds.** *SEER Cancer Statistics Review, 1975–2010.* Bethesda, MD: National Cancer Institute. Available at http://seer.cancer.gov/csr/1975_2010/. Based on November 2012 SEER data submission, posted to the SEER web site, 2013.)

Crude Incidence or Mortality

Crude incidence or mortality is the total number of new cancers (or deaths) that occur over a specified time in the entire population.

Age-specific Incidence or Mortality

Age-specific incidence (or mortality) is the number of new cancers (or deaths) that occur over a specified time among individuals of a particular age group divided by the total population in that same age group. Age-specific incidence or mortality rates are the best way to describe the occurrence of cancer in a population and are commonly graphed in 5- or 10-year groups. Annual age-specific incidence and mortality curves for the common malignant gynecologic cancers in the United States based on all women in the **Surveillance, Epidemiology, and End Results (SEER) survey** area for 2006 to 2010 are shown in Figures 6.1 and 6.2 (3). Invasive cervical cancer

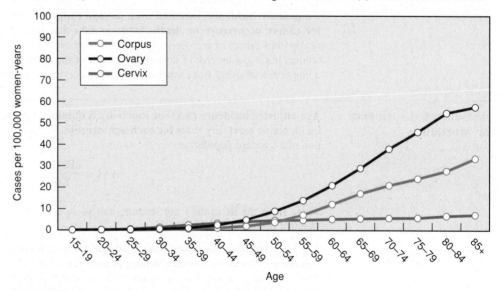

Figure 6.2 **Age-specific mortality curves for gynecologic cancers in women in the United States, 2006–2010.** (Modified from **Howlader N, Noone AM, Krapcho M, et al., eds.** *SEER Cancer Statistics Review, 1975–2010.* Bethesda, MD: National Cancer Institute. Available at http://seer.cancer.gov/csr/1975_2010/. Based on November 2012 SEER data submission, posted to the SEER web site, 2013.)

	Risk of Acquiring (%)			**Risk of Dying (%)**		
	All	White	Black	All	White	Black
Cervix	0.7	0.7	0.8	0.2	0.2	0.4
Corpus	2.7	2.8	2.3	0.6	0.5	0.8
Ovary	1.4	1.5	1	1	1	0.8

Table 6.1 Lifetime Risk of Acquiring or Dying from Gynecologic Cancers in White and Black U.S. Women[a]

[a]Data from 1975–2010. **Howlader N, Noone AM, Krapcho M, et al., eds.** SEER Cancer Statistics Review, 1975–2010.

shows a gradual rise and plateau after 40 years of age at approximately 15 cases per 100,000 women-years. Cancer of the corpus (largely endometrium) rises during the perimenopause and peaks at approximately 90 cases per 100,000 women-years after 60 years of age. Cancer of the ovary displays an increase during the perimenopause and peaks after 70 years of age at approximately 50 cases per 100,000 women-years. *In situ* cervical intraepithelial neoplasias (CIN) are no longer being tabulated by the SEER registries. The vast majority of these cases are seen between the ages of 20 and 50 years, with a peak occurrence of approximately 200 cases per 100,000 women per year at ages 25 to 29. **In addition, SEER is no longer counting ovarian tumors of borderline malignancy, accounting for a decline of 21% in incidence and 6% in mortality between 2004 and 2006.**

Cumulative Incidence or Mortality

Cumulative incidence (or mortality) may be thought of as the proportion of people who develop disease (or die from it) during some period of observation. Cumulative "incidence" is technically a misnomer because it does not contain time in the denominator but, rather, is expressed as a percentage.

The cumulative IR (CIR) may be crudely approximated from age-specific IRs by the following formula:

$$CIR = \Sigma IR_i(\Delta T_i)$$

where IR_i is the age-specific rate for the i age stratum and ΔT_i is the size of the age interval of the i stratum (usually 5 years).

Cumulative incidence, summed over the age range 0 to 85 years, yields the "lifetime risk" for cancer occurrence or death. Lifetime risks that a woman in the United States will have or die from cancer of the cervix, corpus, or ovary are shown in Table 6.1 and confirm that a US woman has a greater risk of developing cancer of the corpus than cervical or ovarian cancer, but a higher risk of dying from ovarian cancer than cervical or endometrial cancer combined.

Age-adjusted Incidence or Mortality

Age-adjusted incidence (AAI) or mortality is obtained by summing weighted averages of the incidence or mortality rates for each age stratum. The weight is derived from the age distribution of a standard population:

$$AAI = \frac{\Sigma IR_i(W_i)}{\Sigma W_i}$$

where IR_i is the IR in the i age stratum, and W_i is the number of people in the i stratum in the standard population.

Age-adjusted rates are better than crude rates for summarizing incidence or mortality when comparing cancer occurrence among populations that may differ in their age structure. An "old" population would have a higher crude incidence of ovarian cancer and a lower crude incidence of carcinoma in situ of the cervix than a "young" population, even though both populations might have identical age-specific incidences for each disease. Cancer rates adjusted to the "world population standard" are shown in Table 6.2.

Worldwide, cervical cancer is the most prevelant of the gynecologic cancers and is second only to breast cancer in overall occurrence. Cervical cancer is most frequent in southern Africa

Table 6.2 Age-adjusted Incidence Rate for the Gynecologic Cancers in Comparison with Other Major Cancers in Women in 2008[a]

Region	Breast	Colon	Lung	Stomach	Cervix	Corpus	Ovary
World	38.9	14.6	13.5	9	15.2	8.2	6.3
Northern Africa	32.7	5.8	2.2	2.4	6.6	2.2	4.8
Southern Africa	38.1	8.2	8	2.2	26.8	6.9	3.8
Eastern Africa	19.3	4.7	1.4	4	34.5	2.4	4
Western Africa	31.8	4.2	1.2	3.3	33.7	1.9	3.8
Northern America	76.7	25.7	35.8	2.8	5.7	16.4	8.7
Central America	26	6.4	5.5	9.3	22.2	6.1	5.2
South America	44.3	11.9	8.4	8.4	24.1	4.4	6.2
Eastern Asia	25.3	14.8	19.9	18.3	9.6	10.3	4.3
South-Eastern Asia	31	12.9	11.9	6.7	15.8	5.7	6.6
Western Asia	32.7	10.2	5.3	6.7	4.5	5.6	4.8
Northern Europe	85	25.6	23	4	8.4	13.8	11.8
Central and Eastern Europe	45.4	21.1	9.7	9.7	14.7	14.6	11
Western Europe	89.7	26.3	16.9	4.4	6.9	11.2	8.9
Southern Europe	68.9	24.5	10.5	6.8	8.1	10.4	8.4
Australia/New Zealand	85.5	33	19.9	3.4	5	11.5	7.8
Micronesia	57	20.7	17.2	6.7	9.5	8	6.1
Polynesia	59.1	7.2	14.9	6.4	16.7	11.5	5

[a]Age adjusted to the world standard in cases per 100,000.

Data from IARC Web site. Available at: http://globocan.iarc.fr/

and Central America and least frequent in North America and parts of Asia. Cancer of the corpus is least frequent in Africa and Asia and most frequent in North America. Ovarian cancer is least frequent in Africa and Asia and most frequent in northern Europe.

Prevalence

Prevalence (P) is the proportion of people who have a particular disease or condition at a specified time. Prevalence can be calculated by multiplying incidence times the average duration of disease:

$$\text{Prevalence} = \text{Incidence} \times \text{Average duration of disease}$$

More commonly, prevalence is derived from cross-sectional studies in which the number of individuals alive with a particular condition is identified from a survey and stated as a percentage of the total number of people who responded to the survey. Other examples of studies that yield prevalence data are those based on autopsy findings and screening tests. The frequency of previously unidentified cancers found in a series of autopsies yields data on the prevalence of occult cancer. The first application of a screening test in a previously unscreened population yields the prevalence of preclinical disease.

Cancer Survival

When the proportion of patients surviving cancer is plotted against time, the pattern often fits an exponential function, meaning that the rate of death is constant over time, which can be demonstrated by plotting the logarithm of the probability of survival against time and demonstrating a straight line. **Summary measures for a survival curve commonly include median survival time, or the point at which 50% of the patients have died, and the probability of survival at 1, 2, and 5 years.**

223

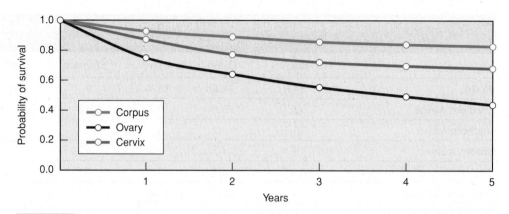

Figure 6.3 Relative Survival rates for invasive cancers of the cervix, corpus, and ovaries for women diagnosed in the United States in 2005. (Modified from **Howlader N, Noone AM, Krapcho M, et al., eds.** *SEER Cancer Statistics Review, 1975–2010.* Bethesda, MD: National Cancer Institute. Available at http://seer.cancer.gov/csr/1975_2010/. Based on November 2012 SEER data submission, posted to the SEER web site, 2013.)

Relative Survival

Relative survival is defined as the ratio of the observed survival rate for the patient group to the survival rate expected for a population with similar demographic characteristics. Relative survival rates for US women diagnosed in 2005 are shown in Figure 6.3 for the major gynecologic cancers and reveal that survival is best after cancer of the corpus, worst after cancer of the ovary, and intermediate after cancer of the cervix. Five-year relative survival rates are shown in Table 6.3 by type and stage of gynecologic cancer for US women. **Stage at presentation and 5-year survival are most favorable for cancer of the corpus and least favorable for cancer of the ovary. In general, African Americans tend to be diagnosed at more advanced stages and have poorer survival compared with whites, especially for cancer of the cervix and corpus.**

Table 6.3 Stage at Diagnosis for the Gynecologic Cancers and 5-Year Survival Rates for U.S. Women[a]

	Stage Distribution at Diagnosis (%)			5-Year Survival Rate (%)		
	All	**White**	**Black**	**All**	**White**	**Black**
Cervix						
All Stages				67.9	77.4	55.8
Localized	47	59	33	90.9	93.6	84.8
Regional	36	30	45	57.1	62.2	52.7
Distant	12	8	17	16.1	19.8	13.7
Corpus						
All Stages				81.5	89	80.1
Localized	68	72	67	95.3	96.5	95.1
Regional	20	17	21	67.5	82.3	65.1
Distant	8	7	9	16.9	28.2	15.2
Ovary						
All Stages				44.2	57	27.5
Localized	15	20	7	91.9	93.2	87.1
Regional	18	22	13	72	79.6	55.9
Distant	61	55	69	27.3	35.6	18.6

[a]Data from 2006–2010. Information insufficient to stage 4% cervical, 4% corpus, and 6% of ovarian cases.
Howlader N, Noone AM, Krapcho M, et al., eds. SEER Cancer Statistics Review, 1975–2010.

Etiologic Studies

In distinction to descriptive studies, etiologic studies examine the relationship between cancer occurrence and survival and personal factors such as diet and reproductive history. This relationship is often described by the epidemiologic parameters, relative risk, and attributable risk.

Relative Risk (RR) is the risk of disease or death in a population exposed to some factor of interest divided by the risk in those not exposed. Absence of association is indicated by an RR of 1 (null value); a number greater than 1 may indicate that exposure increases the risk of disease and a number less than 1 that exposure decreases the risk of disease.

Attributable risk is the risk of disease or death in a population exposed to some factor of interest minus the risk in those not exposed. The null value is 0; a number greater than 0 may indicate that exposure increases the risk of disease and a number less than 0 that exposure decreases the risk.

Case-control Study

In a case-control study, diseased and nondiseased populations are selected, and existing or past characteristics (exposures) are assessed to determine the possible relationship between exposure and disease. The investigator starts with diseased cases and nondiseased control subjects who are then studied to determine whether they had a particular exposure (before the illness). **The odds that the cases were exposed (a/b) are compared with the odds that the control subjects were exposed (c/d) in a measure called the *exposure odds ratio* (Fig. 6.4).**

Exposure Odds Ratio

The odds of exposure among cases divided by the odds of exposure among the control subjects is the exposure odds ratio; it approximates the RR. If an entire population could be characterized by its exposure and disease status, then the exposure odds ratio would be mathematically identical to the RR obtained in a cohort study. Because it is feasible to study only subsets of cases and control subjects, the exposure odds ratio in the sampled population approximates the RR, as long as the cases and control subjects actually sampled were not preferentially selected on the basis of their exposure status. **Attributable risk cannot be directly calculated in a case-control study but is often estimated by a term called the etiologic fraction (4).**

Cohort Studies

In a cohort study, the groups to be studied (the cohorts) are defined by characteristics (or exposures) that occur before the disease of interest, and the study groups are followed to observe the risk of disease in the cohorts. The investigator starts with exposed and nonexposed individuals who are monitored over time to identify the number of diseased cases that develop. The

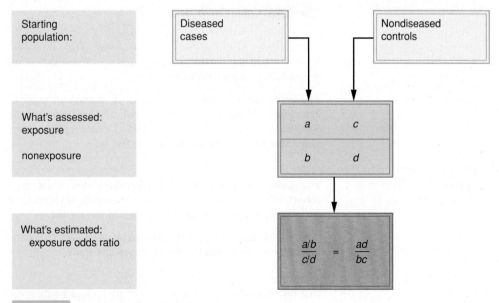

Figure 6.4 Case-control study design.

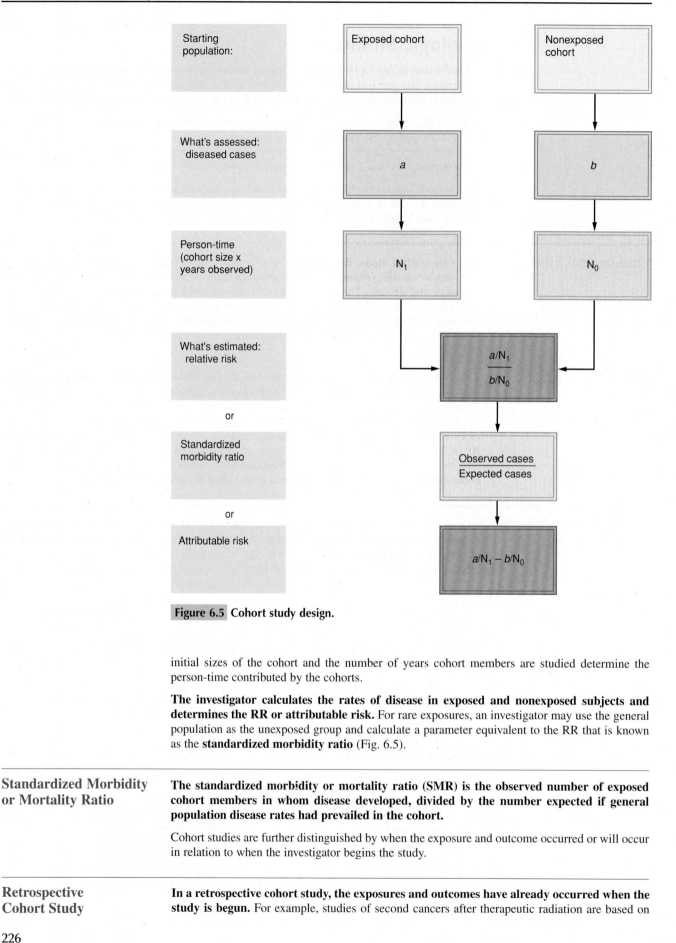

Figure 6.5 Cohort study design.

initial sizes of the cohort and the number of years cohort members are studied determine the person-time contributed by the cohorts.

The investigator calculates the rates of disease in exposed and nonexposed subjects and determines the RR or attributable risk. For rare exposures, an investigator may use the general population as the unexposed group and calculate a parameter equivalent to the RR that is known as the **standardized morbidity ratio** (Fig. 6.5).

Standardized Morbidity or Mortality Ratio

The standardized morbidity or mortality ratio (SMR) is the observed number of exposed cohort members in whom disease developed, divided by the number expected if general population disease rates had prevailed in the cohort.

Cohort studies are further distinguished by when the exposure and outcome occurred or will occur in relation to when the investigator begins the study.

Retrospective Cohort Study

In a retrospective cohort study, the exposures and outcomes have already occurred when the study is begun. For example, studies of second cancers after therapeutic radiation are based on follow-up of women irradiated for cervical cancer 10 to 30 years ago. Medical records and death certificates are used to determine those who subsequently died of cancers other than cervical.

Prospective Cohort Study	**In a prospective cohort study, the relevant exposure may or may not have occurred when the study began, but the outcome has not yet occurred.** After the cohort is selected, the investigator must wait for the disease or outcome to appear in the cohort members. The Nurses' Health Study is a good example of a prospective cohort study (5).
Clinical Trial	**A clinical trial is a special type of prospective cohort study in which the investigator assigns a therapy or preventive agent in randomized fashion to minimize the possibility of bias accounting for different outcomes subsequently observed between treatment cohorts.** Obviously, such studies cannot be used to assess a harmful effect of an exposure except as might occur as an unintended side effect of the therapy. Clinical trials are the only satisfactory way to assess the effect of different cancer therapies on disease recurrence or death because, in theory, they are able to overcome many of the biases that may affect case-control or cohort studies, as discussed in the next section.

Statistical Inference and Validity

Clinicians should understand issues affecting statistical significance and validity to evaluate studies claiming that some exposure causes cancer, a new therapy is superior to standard treatment, or a screening test can improve mortality.

Statistical Inference

Statistical inference is a process of drawing conclusions from data by hypothesis testing, during which a decision is made either to reject or not reject a null hypothesis. Hypothesis testing involves the following steps:

1. Observations are made and summarized by some statistical parameters, such as a mean, a proportion, or a relative risk.
2. A research question is stated in terms of a null hypothesis claiming no difference between the observed parameter and some theoretical value.
3. A statistical test is chosen based on the study design and nature of the parameters being studied.
4. The test statistic is calculated, and its associated p value is read from the appropriate statistical table or generated from a statistical program.
5. A p value less than the traditional 5% leads to the decision to reject the null hypothesis, whereas a value greater than 5% leads to the decision not to reject the null hypothesis. Errors are possible with either decision.
6. A confidence interval on the parameter may be constructed from the test results and defines the range in which the true value of the parameter is expected to fall. **Precision** refers to a characteristic of a parameter falling into a narrow confidence interval, a desirable feature of large studies.

Type I Error

The degree of conflict between the parameter observed and that assumed by the null hypothesis is summarized by the p value, alpha, or Type I error and indicates the probability of incorrectly rejecting the null hypothesis. In practice, an alpha level is chosen *a priori,* usually $p = 0.05$; and if the association tested has a p value less than the predetermined alpha level, then the results are considered statistically significant. It is important to note that when many tests are performed, some results will be observed by chance. One way to address this multiple testing issue, called **Bonferroni correction,** is to divide the alpha level by the number of tests being performed. If this method is used and 100 tests are performed, then the alpha level will be 0.05/100 or 0.0005.

Type II Error

A Type II or beta error indicates the probability of failing to reject the null hypothesis when, in reality, it is false. To calculate a beta error, an alternate hypothesis must be stated.

Power	**Power is 1 minus the beta error and reflects the ability of a study to detect an actual effect.** More precisely, power is the ability of a test statistic to detect differences of a specified size in test parameters. In planning a clinical trial, an investigator often calculates the power that a study will have to detect an association, given a certain study size and certain assumptions about the nature of the association. Small clinical trials that find no significant difference among therapies may be cited as evidence of "no effect of therapy" when the statistical power may have been well below the accepted target of 80% for a meaningful difference in response rates.
Statistical Distributions and Tests	**There are no simple rules for determining which statistical test is appropriate in every situation.** The choice depends on whether the variable is qualitative (nominal) or quantitative (numerical), what assumptions are made about the distribution of the parameter being measured, the nature of the study question, and the number of groups or variables being studied. For example, a **chi-square test** is used to test the null hypothesis that proportions are equal or that nominal variables are independent. The **unpaired *t*-test** is used to compare two means from independent samples, whereas the **paired *t*-test** compares the difference or change in a numerical variable for matched or paired groups or samples.
Validity	**Validity has two components: internal validity and external validity. Internal validity means freedom from bias.** *Bias* **refers to a systematic error in the design, conduct, or analysis of a study that results in a mistaken conclusion and is commonly divided into observation bias, selection bias, and confounding. The** *external validity* **of a study refers to the ability to generalize the results observed in one study population to another.** Although there is controversy about what characteristics of a study make for generalizability, it is clear that external validity is an issue only for those studies that possess internal validity, which is the main focus of this discussion.
Observation Bias	**Observation bias or misclassification occurs when subjects are classified incorrectly with respect to exposure or disease.** If misclassification was equally likely to occur whether the subject was a case or control or an exposed or nonexposed cohort member, then the observation bias would be nondifferential and would cause the RR to be biased toward the null value, 1. Alternatively, if misclassification was more likely to occur for case than control subjects or for exposed than nonexposed cohort members, then a falsely elevated (or decreased) RR might occur (e.g., if cases preferentially recalled or admitted to a particular exposure compared with control subjects).
	Criteria for exposure or disease should be clearly defined to minimize observation bias and, whenever possible, exposure or disease confirmed from medical records. Ideally, researchers recording the disease status in a cohort study or exposure status in a case-control study should be unaware of the subject's study group or blinded to key hypotheses. **In a clinical trial, observation bias may be minimized by double blindness,** when neither the subject nor the investigator knows which specific treatment the subject is receiving.
Selection Bias	**Selection bias is an error that results from systematic differences in the characteristics of subjects who are and are not selected for study.** For example, a selection bias might occur in a case-control study if exposed cases did much better or worse than nonexposed cases. If the case group consisted of long-term survivors, then they might have a different frequency of the exposure than newly diagnosed individuals. Selection bias may also occur in the process of selecting control subjects; for example, control subjects might be selected from hospitalized patients in a disease category that may, itself, relate to the exposure. Selection bias is less likely to occur in cohort studies or in population-based case-control studies, where most cases in a particular area are studied and control subjects are selected from the general population.
Confounding	**Confounding occurs when some factor not considered in the design or analysis accounts for an association because that factor is correlated with both exposure and disease.** Potential confounders for any cancer study are age, ethnicity, and socioeconomic status. Confounding may be controlled during the design of a study by matching cases to control subjects on key confounding variables, or during the analytic phase of the study by stratification or multivariate analysis.

Stratifying means examining the association of interest within groups that are similar with respect to a potential confounder, whereas multivariate analysis is a statistical technique that controls for a number of confounders simultaneously.

In a clinical trial, confounding is avoided by randomization; that is, subjects are allocated to treatment groups by a chance mechanism such that prejudices of the investigator or preferences by the subject do not influence allocation of treatment. In practice, participant randomization assignments can be determined using computer-generated random numbers or random number tables found in most statistic textbooks (6,7). The initial table in the report of a clinical trial usually shows how the treatment groups compared with respect to age, ethnicity, or other important variables to demonstrate whether randomization indeed balanced key variables. Similar tables are helpful in case-control and cohort studies.

Other Criteria for Judging an Epidemiologic Study

Besides the important exercise of ruling out potential biases in a study, other criteria are invoked to decide whether an epidemiologic association is likely to be causal. The well-known British statistician Sir Austin Bradford Hill is credited with establishing the criteria that epidemiologists often use in judging whether an association is likely to be causal (8). Hill originally listed nine criteria, which have been restated over the years, but in one form or another, are considered when regulatory or legal issues arise in connection with an epidemiologic association. **The following criteria are most important: Statistical significance, reverse causality, consistency, effect of removing the causal agent, bias and confounding, strength of the association, dose–response, and biologic credibility.**

Statistical Significance of the Association

Applying the steps listed under statistical inference allows one to address the question of whether chance could have accounted for the observation. Mostly a p value cutoff of 5% is used to answer this question. A different bar is required in genome wide association studies (GWAS), in which risk predisposing variants are searched for using gene chips that can profile hundreds of thousands of genetic variants. Typically, genetic variations called single nucleotide polymorphisms (SNPs) are searched for and may number half a million or more. In such studies, p values on the order of 10^{-7} are common, and external validation is sought by retesting the associations identified in another or even several additional datasets.

Exposure Precedes the Disease

That exposure precedes disease in an obvious requirement. As discussed under "Observation Bias," subjects are interviewed about exposures after their disease is diagnosed in a case-control study; therefore, cases may cite exposures that began because of symptoms or treatment of their illness resulting in "reverse causality." **Epidemiologists who conduct case-control studies generally censor exposures for some time period prior to disease diagnosis to minimize this limitation.**

Consistency

Measurements that are in close agreement when repeated are said to be consistent. In the context of an epidemiologic association, RRs that are consistent among studies, especially those in which different study methods have been used, provide evidence for a causal association. However, the possibility that a systematic bias has affected all the studies should be considered. Consistency can be assessed in a formal manner by performing a study called a *meta-analysis.*

In a meta-analysis, results from independent studies examining the same exposure (or treatment) and outcome are combined, so that a more powerful test of the null hypothesis may be conducted. As part of the meta-analysis, a test for heterogeneity is performed to indicate whether there have been any statistical differences among the results of different studies. The meta-analysis has become an important component of evidence-based medical reviews. For example, oral contraceptive use was less common in ovarian cancer cases compared to controls in 45 studies; when the results of all studies were combined in a meta-analysis, women who had ever used oral contraceptives had an estimated 17% reduction in ovarian cancer risk compared to women who had never used oral contraceptives (9).

Removal of the Agent Results in a Reduction of Disease Frequency

In diseases caused by infection, showing that treatment of the infection or protection by vaccination cured or prevented the disease would satisfy this criterion, and has been clearly demonstrated for HPV vaccination and high-grade CIN. In chronic disease epidemiology, this criterion might be addressed by showing a correlation between calendar year and disease occurrence for an exposure that was relatively limited in time or has changed over time. The increased incidence of endometrial cancer that followed the expanded use of estrogen therapy for the menopause and the decline that followed the addition of a progestogen satisfy this criterion. The decline in breast cancer occurrence following the Women's Health initiative study showing an increased incidence of the disease in women using combined hormone replacement therapy (HRT), and the subsequent decreased use of HRT, would be another example.

Strength of the Association

It is common to hear clinical epidemiologists argue that an RR or OR of 2 is a benchmark as the minimum for associations likely to be causal (10). Bradford-Hill himself said: "We must not be too ready to dismiss a cause-and-effect hypothesis merely on the grounds that the observed association appears to be slight. There are many occasions in medicine where this is in truth so." He cited the case of coronary thrombosis and smoking.

The argument that risks less than 2 cannot be causal should be rigorously challenged. An overall summary risk less than 2 does not rule out a stronger association for certain histologic types of gynecologic cancer, certain categories of exposure, or for women with certain characteristics. The question of whether an association less than 2 can be causal is addressed by recent genome-wide association studies (GWAS), which test hundreds of thousands of genetic variants called SNPs in cases and controls. GWAS studies have revealed genetic polymorphic variants that individuals are born with that may increase the risk for various cancers, including ovarian cancer. Thus, SNPs rs8170 and rs2363956 on chromosome 19 are associated with ORs of 1.16 and 1.18 for serous ovarian cancer, respectively. These associations are almost certain to be real, based on three phases of evaluation in over 5,900 cases and 13,000 controls, and p values of 10^{-9} and 10^{-11}, respectively (11).

Dose–Response

A dose–response (or biologic gradient) refers to a consistent increase (or decrease in the case of a protective exposure) in risk, corresponding to increasing levels of the exposure. Whether there is an association is addressed by a simple "yes" or "no" answer to a question about exposure. Individuals who answer "yes" and had a particular exposure should be asked additional questions about the frequency and duration of the exposure. To categorize dose–response as precisely as possible, it is necessary to combine both frequency and duration, similar to that which is done for smoking when a "pack-years" variable is calculated (i.e., the number of packs per day smoked multiplied by the number of years smoked). A key issue in calculating dose–response is whether those who have never had the exposure should be included in the calculation, or whether the dose–response should be calculated only for those who have had the exposure.

Biologic Credibility

Biologic credibility requires that we ask whether the association makes biologic sense in terms of what is known about the biology of the cancer or the exposure, and whether animal or cell line experiments support an association. Any epidemiologic study claiming a new association needs to address the biologic credibility of the association. Bradford-Hill cautioned against making this an essential criterion: "It will be helpful if the causation we suspect is biologically plausible. But this is a feature I am convinced we cannot demand. What is biologically plausible depends upon the biologic knowledge of the day" (8).

Cancer Risk and Prevention

Risk factors for the gynecologic cancers are presented, along with the application of this information to cancer prevention. Table 6.4 summarizes major epidemiologic risk factors for cervical, endometrial, and ovarian cancer.

Cervical Cancer

Invasive squamous cell carcinoma of the cervix is the end stage of a process beginning with atypical transformation of cervical epithelium at the squamocolumnar junction, leading to CIN of advancing grades, and eventually invasive disease. Risk factors for cervical cancer are those associated with atypical transformation and those that influence persistence and progression of disease.

Factors associated with atypical transformation largely relate to sexual practices that increase the opportunity for human papilloma virus (HPV) infection. Early age at first intercourse

Table 6.4 Risk Factors for Gynecologic Cancers

Factor	Cervix	Endometrium	Ovary
Sexual	Increased risk associated with coitus at an early age, multiple partners, or "high-risk men"	Increased risk in women who have never married	Increased risk in women who have never married
Contraception	Barrier methods protective; oral contraceptives may increase risk	Oral contraceptives protective IUD use protective	Oral contraceptives and tubal ligation protective
Childbirth	Increasing risk with increasing parity	Decreasing risk with increasing parity	Decreasing risk with increasing parity
Age at menopause	No clear association	Late menopause increases risk	No clear association
Menopausal hormones	No clear association	Increased risk from "unopposed estrogen"	Weak increased risk with "unopposed estrogen"
Family history	Weak evidence of familial tendency	Mutations of DNA mismatch repair genes increase risk	Mutations of BRCA1, BRCA2, and DNA mismatch repair increase risk
Body habitus, diet	Carotene, vitamin C, and folic acid potentially protective	Obesity a strong risk factor	No clear association
Smoking	Increased risk	Decreased risk	Varies by epithelial type; increased risk of mucinous type
Other exposures	Douching may increase risk	Association with estrogen-producing tumors of the ovary, liver disease, tamoxifen use	Foreign bodies (talc) per vagina may increase risk; acetaminophen may decrease risk

may be important, because adolescence is a period of heightened squamous metaplasia, and intercourse at this time may increase the likelihood of atypical transformation (12). The woman who has intercourse with multiple partners, or with a "high-risk" male who has had contact with multiple partners, increases the likelihood of her exposure to HPV and cervical cancer (13–15). An estimated 27% of US women aged 14 to 59 have a prevalent HPV infection, and the rate is 45% among women aged 20 to 24 years (16). Over a lifetime, an estimated 79% of women will be infected with HPV at least once (17). The link with HPV infection means that a woman can decrease her risk of cervical cancer by vaccination, safe sexual practices, and use of barrier methods of contraception (18). In addition, both observational studies and randomized trials suggest that male circumcision decreases the risk of HPV infection and cervical cancer in their partners (19–21).

The recent development of HPV vaccines offers an exciting approach to true primary prevention of this prevalent cancer worldwide (22). The available HPV vaccines target only oncogenic HPV types 16 and 18, which cause an estimated 70% of cervical cancers (23,24). The FDA approved HPV vaccines in 2006 and 2009, but vaccine coverage is low, with less than half of 13- to 17-year-old girls vaccinated in 2010 (25). Consequently, screening with Papanicolaou (Pap) tests continues to be an important cervical cancer preventive strategy (24,26). Vaccination does not accelerate clearance of prevalent HPV infections, so it is not effective for women who are already infected (27). Thus, females should receive the vaccine before becoming sexually active.

Vaccine trials in males are ongoing, because HPV vaccines may prevent anogenital warts a subset of anal, penile, oral, and head and neck cancers, as well as juvenile respiratory papillomatosis in their children (28). **Mathematical models suggest that male vaccination would reduce cervical cancer, but only slightly more than vaccination of females alone** (29,30). Although implementation of HPV vaccination has gone fairly smoothly in developed countries, the cost of the vaccine ($335–$360) has made distribution difficult in developing countries, where 80% of cervical cancers occur (31).

Given the high prevalence of HPV but relatively low incidence of cervical cancer, factors that distinguish those women infected with HPV who will go on to develop cervical cancer are important. **Smoking is associated with an increased risk for cervical cancer, even after adjustment** for a number of confounding factors (32,33). An association between smoking and cervical cancer has biologic credibility, because potentially mutagenic substances are secreted in the cervical mucus of smokers (34). In third world countries, chronic exposure to wood smoke may increase the risk for cervical cancer in HPV-infected women (35,36).

Besides factors that affect the risk for cervical cancer by initiating atypical transformation, other factors may modulate the risk by affecting the likelihood that a preinvasive lesion will persist or progress. **A factor indisputably related to the progression of CIN is the frequency of cervical cytologic screening. Population studies demonstrated a correlation between cytologic screening and declining mortality from cervical cancer** (37). Case-control studies demonstrate that women who have had Pap tests at least every 3 years have one-tenth the risk of developing invasive disease compared with women who have never had a Pap test (38). **The recent introduction of HPV testing has improved cervical cancer screening even further** (see Chapter 7).

Other factors that relate to disease progression may include oral contraceptive use and diet. Current oral contraceptive use is associated with an elevated cervical cancer risk, particularly for those who have used them for more than 5 years. However, the risk declines after cessation (39). Butterworth et al. (40) attributed the potential harmful effects of oral contraceptives to folate deficiency, and recommended supplementation. In addition, fruit and vegetable intake, particularly those rich in vitamin A, reduces cervical cancer risk (41–43). Finally, progression of CIN is likely to be greater in immunosuppressed women, such as those with HIV infection, or after kidney transplantation (44,45). Recent genome-wide studies of cervical cancer lend support to the role of immune function, having identified genetic variants in the major histocompatibility complex that are strongly associated with cervical cancer risk (46,47).

Endometrial Cancer

Cancer of the endometrium can be divided into Type I cancers, consisting of tumors with endometrioid histology, and the much less frequent Type II cancers, including serous and clear cell tumors. Risk for Type I adenocarcinoma of the endometrium is largely attributed to estrogen (48). States that lead to an excess of estrogen over progesterone or increase lifetime exposure to estrogen increase endometrial cancer risk. For instance, early age at menarche and late age at menopause increase endometrial cancer risk (49–55). **Furthermore, obesity, which leads to increased estrogen production through the peripheral conversion of androstenedione, accounts for an estimated 57% of all endometrial cancers in the United States** (56).

Alternatively, protective factors are those associated with decreased estrogen production. Surgical castration at an early age with retention of the uterus is a strong protective factor (57). Leanness and regular exercise lower estrogen levels and protect against endometrial cancer (58,59). Smoking lowers estrogen and protects against endometrial cancer but obviously cannot be encouraged as a preventive measure (60). Endometrial cancer as a consequence of decreased degradation of estrogen is illustrated by case reports of the disease in women with cirrhosis of the liver (61).

Endometrial cancer as a consequence of exogenous estrogen is demonstrated by the impressive evidence that unopposed estrogen administered for the menopause increases the risk of endometrial cancer in a dose–response fashion (62). *Tamoxifen,* with its estrogen antagonist effects in the breast and agonist effects in the uterus, has been shown to increase the risk of endometrial cancer in clinical trial data (63). Alternatively, menopausal estrogen taken with a progestin has not been shown to increase the risk, and past use of combination birth control pills decreases the risk of endometrial cancer (64,65). Clinical trials have suggested very low rates of hyperplasia occurring with a continuous regimen of 0.625 mg of *conjugated estrogen* and 2.5 mg of *medroxyprogesterone acetate* (66).

Fitting with key roles for estrogen and progesterone in this disease, the risk for endometrial cancer may be modified by genetic polymorphisms of the progesterone receptor, estrogen receptor alpha, estrogen metabolic genes, and aromatase, which catalyzes the conversion of androgens to estrogens (67–70). It is less clear how the DNA mismatch repair genes that are associated with an increased risk for colorectal and endometrial cancers, and the HNF1B locus recently identified in a genome-wide association study of endometrial cancer, would operate through the "estrogen excess" model (71,72).

Although the majority of risk factors for endometrial cancer are nicely explained by estrogen excess, some associations suggest other etiologic pathways warrant consideration. The consistent observation that even **inert intrauterine devices (IUDs) decrease the risk suggests that immune** factors related to the low-grade inflammation that occurs with IUDs may play a role, and the association with insulin resistance, even among nonobese women, suggests that insulin may also play a role (73–75).

Ovarian Cancer

Ovarian cancer is a very diverse set of cancers that can arise from the germ cell compartment, the hormonally active stromal compartment, or the surface epithelium of the ovary. Even for epithelial tumors of the ovary, there are various histologic types: serous, mucinous, endometrioid, clear cell cancers, undifferentiated, and others. Most of the information about risk factors for ovarian cancer relate to the epithelial tumors and are the focus of this discussion.

Invasive serous is the most common type, so most of the risk factors relate to this type and are less likely to pertain to mucinous types of ovarian cancer. With the recent observation that **some (if not the majority) of high-grade serous ovarian cancers may arise from the fimbriated end of the fallopian tube,** some pathologists have proposed a Type I/II analogy similar to endometrial cancer (76–79). **Type I cancers include those arising within the ovary. They include low-grade serous, mucinous, endometrioid, and clear cell tumors, while Type II cancers are the high-grade serous cancer, which are likely to come from the tube.**

Consistently observed risk factors for epithelial ovarian cancer include a protective effect of pregnancy, breast-feeding, and oral contraceptive use. A popular theory to account for these findings is that these events lead to a break in monthly ovulations and, therefore, repeated disruption and healing of the surface of the ovary (incessant ovulation), leading to ovarian cancer (80). With the new interest in the fallopian tubes, the effect of ovulation on fimbriae, including exposure to the cytokine-rich follicular fluid, should now be given attention.

An alternative theory to incessant ovulation is that ovarian cancer may arise from excessive gonadotropin stimulation of the ovary (81). Classic animal models for ovarian cancer have involved disruption of ovarian–pituitary feedback, either by prematurely destroying oocytes using radiation or chemical toxins or by transplanting the animal's ovary to its spleen, leading to enhanced metabolism of ovarian hormones before they can exert feedback inhibition (82–84). A role for gonadotropins was indicated by observations that ovarian tumors did not develop in rodents who were hypophysectomized before the experimental treatment, or who were given estrogen, which inhibited gonadotropin release (85,86). Gonadal stromal tumors invariably developed in mice with a targeted deletion of the gene for the gonadotropin down regulator, α-inhibin, unless the mice were also incapable of secreting gonadotropins (87,88).

Most of these experimental tumors are stromal in origin, and their relevance to the epithelial types observed in women is debated. Supporting data include the fact that **ovarian cancer incidence rises sharply between the ages of 45 and 54, and remains elevated for the remainder of a woman's life, paralleling gonadotropin levels over this period.** In addition, the strong protective association between oral contraceptives and ovarian cancer duplicates the effect of exogenous estrogen in the animal models (89). Also relevant to the animal models are cohort studies that demonstrate that ovarian cancer occurs after radiation for cervical cancer after a 10- to 15-year lag period (90,91). In contrast, as might be predicted by the gonadotropin theory, there does not appear to be a strong and consistent association between use of fertility drugs and ovarian cancer (92–94).

An alternate theory gaining credibility is that ovarian cancer relates to inflammatory processes involving the ovary (95). Under this theory, inflammation from incessant ovulation, or inflammation occurring from vaginal or uterine contaminants that reach the ovary, is viewed as the pathway to ovarian cancer. One such contaminant might be talc used in genital hygiene, which has been fairly consistently identified as a risk factor for ovarian cancer, and was recently declared a possible carcinogen by the International Agency for Research on Cancer (96–98).

Besides talc, another pelvic "contaminant" might be menstrual products, which are believed to flow out of the fallopian tubes during menstruation to explain endometriosis (99). Indeed, **prior endometriosis is a risk factor for ovarian cancer, especially the endometrioid and clear cell types** (100,101). The pelvic contamination theory might explain why tubal ligation decreases the risk of ovarian cancer (102). Another theory suggested is androgen excess and progesterone deficiency, but this does not explain the observations on talc or tubal ligation (103).

These theories do not accommodate the observation from earlier studies that a history of childhood mumps decreases the risk for ovarian cancer, or the recent observation that puerperal mastitis may lower the risk (104,105). These observations, and all described risk factors, are accommodated by a theory involving immune effects related to the surface glycoprotein and tumor marker, human mucin 1 (MUC1) (106). MUC1 is a high molecular weight protein expressed in a highly glycosylated form at low levels by many types of normal epithelial cells, and in an underglycosylated form at high levels by most epithelial adenocarcinomas, including endometrial, breast, and ovarian cancer (107). In cancer patients, anti-MUC1 antibodies may correlate with a more favorable prognosis (108,109). Interestingly, anti-MUC1 antibodies are found in healthy individuals, especially in women during pregnancy and lactation, leading to the **hypothesis that a natural immunity against tumor MUC1 might develop and account for the long-term protective effect of pregnancy or breast-feeding on the risk of breast cancer** (110). This has led to the broader theory that women who develop ovarian cancer may have had relatively fewer acute inflammatory events, such as mumps, a tubal ligation, mastitis, and others that may lead to anti-MUC1 antibodies, and an excess of chronic inflammatory events, such as incessant ovulation, endometriosis, and talc use that may down-regulate MUC1 immunity, thereby leading to the emergence of a MUC1-expressing cancer such as ovarian. The observation that anti-MUC16 (CA125) antibodies may be raised by mastitis suggests that immune events related to CA125 should be brought into the picture (105).

Finally, there are a number of genetic risk factors emerging for ovarian cancer. Having a mother or sister with the disease increases a woman's risk for ovarian cancer approximately two- to three-fold (111). **Specific genetic factors include mutations of the *BRCA1* and *BRCA2* and the DNA mismatch genes** (112). Although these genetic factors are more likely to be found in families in which a number of relatives were affected with breast or ovarian cancer, they may be found in up to 44% of women with no significant family history (113,114). Genome-wide association studies found small but significant increases in risk with genetic variants located at 9p22 (in the BNC2 gene), 8q24, 2q31, 3q25, and 17q21 (115,116).

Other Gynecologic Neoplasms

Other than clear cell adenocarcinomas of the vagina associated with maternal use of *diethylstilbestrol*, vaginal carcinoma is primarily a disease of women older than 50 years of age. Vulvar cancer has an age-incidence distribution similar to vaginal cancer. **HPV infection appears to play a role in both vaginal and vulvar cancers** (117–120). In a population-based case-control study, HPV was detected in more than 80% of the tumor blocks from patients with in situ vaginal cancer and in 60% of those from invasive vaginal cancers (118). For vulvar cancer, **two types of vulvar cancer were defined** (117,118,120). **The first, which affects younger women, is associated with HPV and has a preinvasive stage. The second type occurs in older women and arises in areas with nonneoplastic epithelial disorders such as lichen sclerosus. Risk factors known to exist for cervical neoplasms also pertain to vulvar and vaginal neoplasms, including sexual history and smoking** (118,121–123). Dietary studies suggest that alcohol may increase the risk while vegetable intake may decrease the risk, but validation of these studies is needed (124,125).

Trophoblastic neoplasms include complete and partial hydatidiform moles, invasive moles, and choriocarcinoma. The epidemiology of hydatidiform mole is probably better understood than that of other trophoblastic diseases, and it is likely to be relevant because of the association between molar pregnancy and subsequent invasive mole or choriocarcinoma. **The prevalence of molar pregnancy is 10 times more common in Asia, Indonesia, and other developing countries, than in the United States** (126). **The risk of having a molar pregnancy increases with maternal age,** but it is less certain whether adolescents are at increased risk (127–129). A previous hydatidiform mole is a strong risk factor; subsequent pregnancies have a 1% risk of being a choriocarcinoma (130). The peculiar cytogenetic patterns of complete and partial hydatidiform moles are discussed in Chapter 15 and may indicate the importance of aberrant germ cells in the origin of these disorders.

Berkowitz et al. (131) suggested that **deficiency of the vitamin A precursor, carotene, or of animal fats necessary for its absorption, might be a factor in the cause of this disease.** Vitamin A deficiency causes fetal wastage and aberrancy of epithelial development in female animals, and degeneration of seminiferous epithelium with poor gamete development in male animals (132–134). Geographic regions where molar pregnancy is common have a high incidence of night blindness (135).

Paternal blood group combinations may influence the risk of a molar pregnancy. Mothers with group A blood and fathers with group A or 0 have an increased risk compared with all other blood group combinations (136–138). Oral contraceptives are associated with an increased risk of hydatidiform mole that increases with duration of use. Ten or more years of use are associated with a more than twofold increase in risk (139). Smoking doubles the risk of hydatidiform mole, and quadruples the risk with 10 or more years of smoking (136,140,141). The roles of alcohol, asbestos, and infections (HPV, adeno-associated virus and tuberculosis) have also been considered (142,143).

Cancer Prevention

Cancer prevention may occur at the level of primary prevention (the identification and modification of risk factors for disease), secondary prevention (the detection of the disease at earlier, more treatable stages), or tertiary prevention (effective treatment of clinical disease). This section addresses primary and secondary measures of prevention.

Methods of primary prevention are by no means certain, but suggestions include the following:

1. **For cervical cancer,** use of barrier methods of contraception, avoidance of tobacco, and maintenance of a diet high in folates, B vitamins, and β-carotene may be beneficial. HPV vaccines have proven benefits, and should be used by women before sexual debut.

2. **For endometrial cancer,** maintenance of ideal body weight, avoidance of a high-fat diet, and avoidance of unopposed estrogen therapy during menopause may be beneficial.

3. **For ovarian cancer,** use of oral contraceptives, if not medically contraindicated, and avoidance of talc in genital hygiene may be beneficial. Women known to carry a predisposing mutation should undergo prophylactic salpingo-oophorectomy after they have completed childbearing. A proposal that women coming to hysterectomy who would not otherwise require oophorectomy have their tubes removed deserves further study (144).

Secondary Prevention

Detecting disease at a stage when it is more curable may prevent cancer deaths. The secondary prevention of cervical cancer is successful, and screening programs for the other gynecologic cancers may eventually be devised. To be successful, a screening program must be directed at a "suitable" disease with a "suitable" screening test (145). A suitable disease must be one that has serious consequences, as most cancers do. Treatment must be available so that when such therapy is applied to screen-detected (preclinical) disease, it will be more effective than when applied after symptoms of the disease have appeared. The preclinical phase of the disease must be long enough that the chances are good that a person will be screened. There must be a suitable screening test as defined by simplicity, acceptability to patients, low cost, and high validity (defined by the measures in Table 6.5).

Table 6.5 Measures of Validity for a Screening Procedure

Status Determined by Screening	True Disease Status		
	Positive	**Negative**	**Total**
Positive	a (true positives)	b (false positives)	$a + b$ (all screened positives)
Negative	c (false negatives)	d (true negatives)	$c + d$ (all screened negatives)
Total	$a + c$ (all diseased)	$b + d$ (all nondiseased)	N (all subjects)
Measure	*Definition*	*Formula[a]*	
Sensitivity	True positives; all diseased	$\dfrac{a}{a + c}$	
Specificity	True negatives; all nondiseased	$\dfrac{d}{b + d}$	
Predictive value of a positive screen	True positives; all screened positives	$\dfrac{a}{a + b}$ or $\dfrac{SN(P)}{[SN(P) + (1 - SP)(1 - P)]}$	

[a]SN, sensitivity; SP, specificity; P, prevalence of disease.

Test Definitions

Sensitivity

The sensitivity of a test is defined as the proportion of people with a true positive screening result of all those who have the disease.

Specificity

The specificity of a test is defined as the proportion of people with a true negative screening result of all those who do not have the disease.

Predictive Value

The predictive value of a positive test is defined as the proportion of true positives out of all those who screened positive. The alternate formula shown in Table 6.5 reveals that predictive value is a function of sensitivity, specificity, and disease prevalence. This function implies that a positive screening test is more likely to indicate disease in a high-risk population than in a low-risk population. Positive predictive value cannot be calculated from a case-control study, because the ratio of cases to controls is set by design, and does not reflect disease prevalence in the general population.

Screening Strategies

Cervical cytology represents one of the most effective screening tests for cancer ever developed; controversies relate to how to make it more efficient. Guidelines suggested by the American Cancer Society are that **the interval between screenings may be safely lengthened to 3 years in women who have at least three consecutive negative screens and are at otherwise low risk (e.g., no history of immunosuppression)** (146). Similar guidelines were proposed by the American College of Obstetricians and Gynecologists in 2000, although the less frequent intervals were to be at the discretion of the physician (147). An analysis of the potential effects of extending screening intervals from annually to once every 3 years concluded that an average excess risk of three cases of cervical cancer per 100,000 women screened would result (148). However, to avert one additional case of cancer by screening women annually for 3 years rather than once every 3 years would necessitate approximately 280,000 additional Pap tests and 15,000 colposcopic examinations.

HPV testing, which involves detection of HPV DNA in a cervical swab, can greatly improve the sensitivity of the traditional Pap test to identify high-grade CIN in women ages 30 to 69 years. In a study of 10,154 women aged 30 to 69 years, the HPV test had a much higher sensitivity (95%) than the Pap test (55%), and similar specificity (95% for HPV testing and 97% for the Pap test). Using HPV testing together with the Pap test increases the sensitivity to 100% (149). A cost-benefit analysis revealed that the maximum number of lives would be saved when combined HPV and Pap test screening was performed every 2 years until death (150). Further discussion of this topic is found in Chapter 7.

Screening for endometrial cancer in asymptomatic women in the general population is not justified, but endometrial biopsies or assessment of the endometrial stripe by transvaginal ultrasound may be appropriate for perimenopausal or postmenopausal women at risk for endometrial cancer, including those who are obese, are exposed to unopposed estrogen, use *tamoxifen*, or come from families with both colon and endometrial cancer.

Based on expert opinion only, women at high risk for ovarian cancer by virtue of a *BRCA1* or *BRCA2* mutation are recommended to have annual or semiannual screening with transvaginal ultrasound and CA125 measurements (151). A large randomized trial of annual screening with CA125 with transvaginal ultrasound showed no benefit (152). A similar trial is under way in the United Kingdom (153).

Acknowledgment   Kristina Williams for her assistance in updating the figures and tables.

References

1. **Rosner B.** *Fundamentals of Biostatistics.* 7th ed. Duxbury, Division of Thompson Learning, Pacific Grove, CA; 2010.
2. **Rothman KJ, Lash TL, Greenland S.** Modern epidemiology. In: **Wilkins LW, ed.** *Modern Epidemiology.* 3rd ed. Philadelphia, PA: Lippincott Williams & Wilkins; 2012.
3. **Howlader N, Noone AM, Krapcho M, et al.** *SEER Cancer Statistics Review 1975–2010, based on November 2012 SEER data submission, posted to the SEER Web site, April 2013.* Bethesda, MD: National Cancer Institute; 2012.
4. **Hennekens CH, Buring J.** *Epidemiology in Medicine.* 1st ed. **Mayrent SL, ed.** Boston/Toronto: Little, Brown and Company; 1987.
5. **Colditz GA, Hankinson SE.** The Nurses' Health Study: Lifestyle and health among women. *Nat Rev Cancer.* 2005;5:388–396.
6. **Altman DG.** *Practical Statistics for Medical Research.* London: Chapman and Hall CRC; 1991.
7. **Rosner B, ed.** *Fundamentals of Biostatistics.* 5th ed. Pacific Grove, CA: Duxbury Thompson Learning; 2000.
8. **Hill AB.** The Environment and Disease: Association or Causation? *Proc R Soc Med.* 1965;58:295–300.1898525.
9. **Collaborative Group on Epidemiological Studies of Ovarian Cancer, Beral V, Doll R, Hermon C, et al.** Ovarian cancer and oral contraceptives: Collaborative reanalysis of data from 45 epidemiological studies including 23,257 women with ovarian cancer and 87,303 controls. *Lancet.* 2008;371:303–314.
10. **Muscat JE, Huncharek MS.** Causation and disease: Biomedical science in toxic tort litigation. *J Occup Med.* 1989;31:997–1002.
11. **Bolton KL, Tyrer J, Song H, et al.** Common variants at 19p13 are associated with susceptibility to ovarian cancer. *Nat Genet.* 2010; 42:880–884.
12. **Singer A.** The cervical epithelium during puberty and adolescence. In: **Jordan JA, ed.** *The cervix.* London: WB Saunders; 1976: 87–104.
13. **International Collaboration of Epidemiological Studies of Cervical Cancer.** Cervical carcinoma and sexual behavior: Collaborative reanalysis of individual data on 15,461 women with cervical carcinoma and 29,164 women without cervical carcinoma from 21 epidemiological studies. *Cancer Epidemiol Biomarkers Prev.* 2009;18:1060–1069.
14. **Oakeshott P, Aghaizu A, Reid F, et al.** Frequency and risk factors for prevalent, incident, and persistent genital carcinogenic human papillomavirus infection in sexually active women: Community based cohort study. *BMJ.* 2012;344:e4168.
15. **Rositch AF, Burke AE, Viscidi RP, et al.** Contributions of recent and past sexual partnerships on incident human papillomavirus detection: Acquisition and reactivation in older women. *Cancer Res.* 2012;72:6183–6190.
16. **Dunne EF, Unger ER, Sternberg M, et al.** Prevalence of HPV infection among females in the United States. *JAMA.* 2007;297:813–819.
17. **Syrjanen K, Hakama M, Saarikoski S, et al.** Prevalence, incidence, and estimated life-time risk of cervical human papillomavirus infections in a nonselected Finnish female population. *Sex Transm Dis.* 1990;17:15–19.
18. **Hildesheim A, Brinton LA, Mallin K, et al.** Barrier and spermicidal contraceptive methods and risk of invasive cervical cancer. *Epidemiology.* 1990;1:266–272.
19. **Castellsague X, Bosch FX, Munoz N, et al.** Male circumcision, penile human papillomavirus infection, and cervical cancer in female partners. *N Engl J Med.* 2002;346:1105–1112.
20. **Albero G, Castellsague X, Giuliano AR, et al.** Male circumcision and genital human papillomavirus: A systematic review and meta-analysis. *Sex Transm Dis.* 2012;39:104–113.
21. **Davis MA, Gray RH, Grabowski MK, et al.** Male circumcision decreases high-risk human papillomavirus viral load in female partners: A randomized trial in Rakai, Uganda. *Int J Cancer.* 2013;133: 1247–1252.
22. **Koutsky LA, Ault KA, Wheeler CM, et al.** A controlled trial of a human papillomavirus type 16 vaccine. *N Engl J Med.* 2002;347: 1645–1651.
23. **Kahn JA, Burk RD.** Papillomavirus vaccines in perspective. *Lancet.* 2007;369:2135–2137.
24. **Savage L.** Proposed HPV vaccine mandates rile health experts across the country. *J Natl Cancer Inst.* 2007;99:665–666.
25. **Jemal A, Simard EP, Dorell C, et al.** Annual Report to the Nation on the Status of Cancer, 1975–2009, featuring the burden and trends in human papillomavirus (HPV)-associated cancers and HPV vaccination coverage levels. *J Natl Cancer Inst.* 2013;105:175–201.
26. **Kiviat NB, Hawes SE, Feng Q.** Screening for cervical cancer in the era of the HPV vaccine–The urgent need for both new screening guidelines and new biomarkers. *J Natl Cancer Inst.* 2008;100:290–291.
27. **Hildesheim A, Herrero R, Wacholder S, et al.** Effect of human papillomavirus 16/18 L1 viruslike particle vaccine among young women with preexisting infection: A randomized trial. *JAMA.* 2007; 298:743–753.
28. **Saslow D, Castle PE, Cox JT, et al.** American Cancer Society Guideline for human papillomavirus (HPV) vaccine use to prevent cervical cancer and its precursors. *CA Cancer J Clin.* 2007;57:7–28.
29. **Barnabas RV, Laukkanen P, Koskela P, et al.** Epidemiology of HPV 16 and cervical cancer in Finland and the potential impact of vaccination: Mathematical modelling analyses. *PLoS Med.* 2006; 3:e138.
30. **Choi YH, Jit M, Gay N, et al.** Transmission dynamic modelling of the impact of human papillomavirus vaccination in the United Kingdom. *Vaccine.* 2010;28:4091–4102.
31. **Editors.** Cheaper HPV vaccines needed. *Lancet.* 2008;371:1638, editorial.
32. **Brinton LA, Barrett RJ, Berman ML, et al.** Cigarette smoking and the risk of endometrial cancer. *Am J Epidemiol.* 1993;137: 281–291.
33. **Appleby P, Beral V, Berrington de Gonzalez A, et al.;** International Collaboration of Epidemiological Studies of Cervical Cancer. Carcinoma of the cervix and tobacco smoking: Collaborative reanalysis of individual data on 13,541 women with carcinoma of the cervix and 23,017 women without carcinoma of the cervix from 23 epidemiological studies. *Int J Cancer.* 2006;118:1481–1495.
34. **Schiffman MH, Haley NJ, Felton JS, et al.** Biochemical epidemiology of cervical neoplasia: Measuring cigarette smoke constituents in the cervix. *Cancer Res.* 1987;47:3886–3888.
35. **Ferrera A, Velema JP, Figueroa M, et al.** Co-factors related to the causal relationship between human papillomavirus and invasive cervcial cancer in Honduras. *Int J Epidemiology.* 2000;29:817–825.
36. **Velema JP, Ferrera A, Figueroa M, et al.** Burning wood in the kitchen increases the risk of cervical neoplasia in HPV-infected women in Honduras. *Int J Cancer.* 2002;97:536–541.
37. **Miller AB, Lindsay J, Hill GB.** Mortality from cancer of the uterus in Canada and its relationship to screening for cancer of the cervix. *Int J Cancer.* 1976;17:602–612.
38. **La Vecchia C, Franceschi S, Decarli A, et al.** "Pap" smear and the risk of cervical neoplasia: Quantitative estimates from a case-control study. *Lancet.* 1984;2:779–782.
39. **Appleby P, Beral V, Berrington de Gonzalez A, et al.** Cervical cancer and hormonal contraceptives: Collaborative reanalysis of individual data for 16,573 women with cervical cancer and 35,509 women without cervical cancer from 24 epidemiological studies. *Lancet.* 2007;370:1609–1621.
40. **Butterworth CE Jr., Hatch KD, Gore H, et al.** Improvement in cervical dysplasia associated with folic acid therapy in users of oral contraceptives. *Am J Clin Nutr.* 1982;35:73–82.
41. **Chih HJ, Lee AH, Colville L, et al.** A review of dietary prevention of human papillomavirus-related infection of the cervix and cervical intraepithelial neoplasia. *Nutr Cancer.* 2013;65:317–328.
42. **Gonzalez CA, Travier N, Lujan-Barroso L, et al.** Dietary factors and in situ and invasive cervical cancer risk in the European prospective investigation into cancer and nutrition study. *Int J Cancer.* 2011; 129:449–459.
43. **Zhang X, Dai B, Zhang B, et al.** Vitamin A and risk of cervical cancer: A meta-analysis. *Gynecol Oncol.* 2012;124:366–373.
44. **Alloub MI, Barr BB, McLaren KM, et al.** Human papillomavirus infection and cervical intraepithelial neoplasia in women with renal allografts. *BMJ.* 1989;298:153–156.
45. **Maiman M, Fruchter R, Seldis A, et al.** Prevalence, risk factors, and accuracy of cytologic screening for cervical intraepithelial

neoplasia in women with the human immunodeficiency virus. *Gynecol Oncol.* 1998;68:223–229.

46. **Chen D, Juko-Pecirep I, Hammer J, et al.** Genome-wide association study of susceptibility loci for cervical cancer. *J Natl Cancer Inst.* 2013;105:624–633.

47. **Shi Y, Li L, Hu Z, et al.** A genome-wide association study identifies two new cervical cancer susceptibility loci at 4q12 and 17q12. *Nat Genet.* 2013;45:918–922.

48. **Key TJ, Pike MC.** The dose-effect relationship between "unopposed" oestrogens and endometrial mitotic rate: Its central role in explaining and predicting endometrial cancer risk. *Br J Cancer.* 1988; 57:205–212.

49. **Elwood JM, Cole P, Rothman KJ, et al.** Epidemiology of endometrial cancer. *J Natl Cancer Inst.* 1977;59:1055–1060.

50. **Ewertz M, Schou G, Boice JD Jr.** The joint effect of risk factors on endometrial cancer. *Eur J Cancer Clin Oncol.* 1988;24:189–194.

51. **Kalandidi A, Tzonou A, Lipworth L, et al.** A case-control study of endometrial cancer in relation to reproductive, somatometric, and life-style variables. *Oncology.* 1996;53:354–359.

52. **Kelsey JL, LiVolsi VA, Holford TR, et al.** A case-control study of cancer of the endometrium. *Am J Epidemiol.* 1982;116:333–342.

53. **Koumantaki Y, Tzonou A, Koumantakis E, et al.** A case-control study of cancer of endometrium in Athens. *Int J Cancer.* 1989;43:795–799.

54. **Kvale G, Heuch I, Ursin G.** Reproductive factors and risk of cancer of the uterine corpus: A prospective study. *Cancer Res.* 1988;48:6217–6221.

55. **McPherson CP, Sellers TA, Potter JD, et al.** Reproductive factors and risk of endometrial cancer. The Iowa Women's Health Study. *Am J Epidemiol.* 1996;143:1195–1202.

56. **Calle EE, Kaaks R.** Overweight, obesity and cancer: Epidemiological evidence and proposed mechanisms. *Nat Rev Cancer.* 2004; 4:579–591.

57. **Jansen D, Ostergaard E.** Clinical studies concerning the relationship of estrogens to the development of cancer of the corpus uteri. *Am J Obstet Gynecol.* 1954;67:1094–1102.

58. **Frisch RE, Wyshak G, Albright NL, et al.** Lower prevalence of breast cancer and cancers of the reproductive system among former college athletes compared to non-athletes. *Br J Cancer.* 1985;52:885–891.

59. **Patel AV, Feigelson HS, Talbot JT, et al.** The role of body weight in the relationship between physical activity and endometrial cancer: Results from a large cohort of US women. *Int J Cancer.* 2008;123: 1877–1882.

60. **Lesko SM, Rosenberg L, Kaufman DW, et al.** Cigarette smoking and the risk of endometrial cancer. *N Engl J Med.* 1985;313:593–596.

61. **Speert H.** Endometrial cancer and hepatic cirrhosis. *Cancer.* 1949; 2:597–603.

62. **Grady D, Gebretsadik T, Kerlikowske K, et al.** Hormone replacement therapy and endometrial cancer risk: A meta-analysis. *Obstet Gynecol.* 1995;85:304–313.

63. **Fisher B, Constantino JP, Wickerham DL, et al.** Tamoxifen for prevention of breast cancer: Report of the National Surgical Adjuvant Breast and Bowel Project P-1 Study. *J Natl Cancer Inst.* 1998; 90:1371–1388.

64. **Beresford SA, Weiss NS, Voigt LF, et al.** Risk of endometrial cancer in relation to use of oestrogen combined with cyclic progestagen therapy in postmenopausal women. *Lancet.* 1997;349:458–461.

65. **Weiss NS, Sayvetz TA.** Incidence of endometrial cancer in relation to the use of oral contraceptives. *N Engl J Med.* 1980;302:551–554.

66. **The Writing Group for the PEPI Trial.** Effects of hormone replacement therapy on endometrial histology in postmenopausal women: The Postmenopausal Estrogen/Progestin Interventions (PEPI) Trial. *JAMA.* 1996;275:370–375.

67. **De Vivo I, Huggins GS, Hankinson SE, et al.** A functional polymorphism in the promoter of the progesterone receptor gene associated with endometrial cancer risk. *Proc Natl Acad Sci U S A.* 2002; 99:12263–12268.

68. **Doherty JA, Weiss NS, Freeman RJ, et al.** Genetic factors in catechol estrogen metabolism in relation to the risk of endometrial cancer. *Cancer Epidemiol Biomarkers Prev.* 2005;14:357–366.

69. **Paynter RA, Hankinson SE, Colditz GA, et al.** CYP19 (aromatase) haplotypes and endometrial cancer risk. *Int J Cancer.* 2005; 116:267–274.

70. **Sasaki M, Tanaka Y, Kaneuchi M, et al.** Polymorphisms of estrogen receptor alpha gene in endometrial cancer. *Biochem Biophys Res Commun.* 2002;297:558–564.

71. **Spurdle AB, Thompson DJ, Ahmed S, et al.** Genome-wide association study identifies a common variant associated with risk of endometrial cancer. *Nat Genet.* 2011;43:451–454.PMID:21499250.

72. **Watson P, Vasen HF, Mecklin JP, et al.** The risk of endometrial cancer in hereditary nonpolyposis colorectal cancer. *Am J Med.* 1994;96:516–520.

73. **Benshushan A, Paltiel O, Rojanksy N, et al.** IUD use and the risk for endometrial cancer. *Eur J Obstet Gynecol Reprod Biol.* 2002; 105:166–169.

74. **Burzawa JK, Schmeler KM, Soliman PT, et al.** Prospective evaluation of insulin resistance among endometrial cancer patients. *Am J Obstet Gynecol.* 2011;204:355.e1–e7.PMID:21324431.

75. **Friedenreich CM, Langley AR, Speidel TP, et al.** Case-control study of markers of insulin resistance and endometrial cancer risk. *Endocr Relat Cancer.* 2012;19:785–792.PMC3493985.

76. **Kindelberger DW, Lee Y, Miron A, et al.** Intraepithelial carcinoma of the fimbria and pelvic serous carcinoma: Evidence for a causal relationship. *Am J Surg Pathol.* 2007;31:161–169.

77. **Kurman RJ, Shih Ie M.** The origin and pathogenesis of epithelial ovarian cancer: A proposed unifying theory. *Am J Surg Pathol.* 2010; 34:433–443.2841791.

78. **Levanon K, Crum C, Drapkin R.** New insights into the pathogenesis of serous ovarian cancer and its clinical impact. *J Clin Oncol.* 2008;26:5284–5293.2652087.

79. **Piek JM, van Diest PJ, Zweemer RP, et al.** Dysplastic changes in prophylactically removed Fallopian tubes of women predisposed to developing ovarian cancer. *J Pathol.* 2001;195(4):451–456.

80. **Fathalla MF.** Incessant ovulation—A factor in ovarian neoplasia? *Lancet.* 1971;2:163.

81. **Cramer DW, Welch WR.** Determinants of ovarian cancer risk. II. Inferences regarding pathogenesis. *J Natl Cancer Inst.* 1983;71:717–721.

82. **Biskind M, Biskind G.** Development of tumors in the rat ovary after transplantation into the spleen. *Proc Soc Exp Biol Med.* 1944;55: 176–179.

83. **Furth J, Butterworth J.** Neoplastic diseases occurring among mice subjected to general irradiation with x-rays. *Am J Cancer.* 1936;71: 717–721.

84. **Howell JS, Marchant J, Orr JW.** The induction of ovarian tumours in mice with 9:10-dimethyl-1:2-benzanthracene. *Br J Cancer.* 1954;8: 635–646.

85. **Jull JW, Streeter DJ, Sutherland L.** The mechanism of induction of ovarian tumors in the mouse by 7,12-dimethylbenz-[alpha]anthracene. I. Effect of steroid hormones and carcinogen concentration in vivo. *J Natl Cancer Inst.* 1966;37:409–420.

86. **Marchant J.** The effect of hypophysectomy on the development of ovarian tumours in mice treated with dimethylbenzanthracene. *Br J Cancer.* 1961;15:821–827.

87. **Kumar TR, Wang Y, Matzuk MM.** Gonadotropins are essential modifier factors for gonadal tumor development in inhibin-deficient mice. *Endocrinology.* 1996;137:4210–4216.

88. **Matzuk MM, Finegold MJ, Su JG, et al.** Alpha-inhibin is a tumour-suppressor gene with gonadal specificity in mice. *Nature.* 1992;360:313–319.

89. **Schlesselman JJ.** Net effect of oral contraceptive use on the risk of cancer in women in the United States. *Obstet Gynecol.* 1995;85:793–801.

90. **Boice JD Jr., Day NE, Andersen A, et al.** Second cancers following radiation treatment for cervical cancer. An international collaboration among cancer registries. *J Natl Cancer Inst.* 1985;74:955–975.

91. **Pettersson F, Fotiou S, Einhorn N, et al.** Cohort study of the long-term effect of irradiation for carcinoma of the uterine cervix. Second primary malignancies in the pelvic organs in women irradiated for cervical carcinoma at Radiumhemmet 1914–1965. *Acta Radiol Oncol.* 1985;24:145–151.

92. **Rizzuto I, Behrens RF, Smith LA.** Risk of ovarian cancer in women treated with ovarian stimulating drugs for infertility. *Cochrane Database Syst Rev.* 2013;8:CD008215.

93. **Asante A, Leonard PH, Weaver AL, et al.** Fertility drug use and the risk of ovarian tumors in infertile women: A case-control study. *Fertil Steril.* 2013;99:2031–2036.

94. **Kurta ML, Moysich KB, Weissfeld JL, et al.** Use of fertility drugs and risk of ovarian cancer: Results from a U.S.-based case-control study. *Cancer Epidemiol Biomarkers Prev.* 2012;21:1282–1292. 3415595.

95. **Ness RB, Cottreau C.** Possible role of ovarian epithelial inflammation in ovarian cancer. *J Natl Cancer Inst.* 1999;91:1459–1467.

96. **Baan R, Straif K, Grosse Y, et al.** Carcinogenicity of carbon black, titanium dioxide, and talc. *Lancet Oncol.* 2006;7:295–296.

97. **Cramer DW, Liberman RF, Titus-Ernstoff L, et al.** Genital talc exposure and risk of ovarian cancer. *Int J Cancer.* 1999;81:351–356.

98. **Terry KL, Karageorgi S, Shvetsov YB, et al.** Genital powder use and risk of ovarian cancer: A pooled analysis of 8,525 cases and 9,859 controls. *Cancer Prev Res (Phila).* 2013;6:811–821.NIHMS492194.

99. **Sampson J.** The development of the implantatino theory for the origin of endometriosis. *Am J Obstet Gynecol.* 1940;40:549–557.

100. **Mostoufizadeh M, Scully RE.** Malignant tumors arising in endometriosis. *Clin Obstet Gynecol.* 1980;23:951–963.

101. **Pearce CL, Templeman C, Rossing MA, et al.** Association between endometriosis and risk of histological subtypes of ovarian cancer: A pooled analysis of case-control studies. *Lancet Oncol.* 2012;13(4):385–394.

102. **Sieh W, Salvador S, McGuire V, et al.** Tubal ligation and risk of ovarian cancer subtypes: A pooled analysis of case-control studies. *Int J Epidemiol.* 2013;42:579–589.PMC3619957.

103. **Risch HA.** Hormonal etiology of epithelial ovarian cancer, with a hypothesis concerning the role of androgens and progesterone. *J Natl Cancer Inst.* 1998;90:1774–1786.

104. **Cramer DW, Williams K, Vitonis AF, et al.** Puerperal mastitis: A reproductive event of importance affecting anti-mucin antibody levels and ovarian cancer risk. *Cancer Causes Control.* 2013;24(11):1911–1923.

105. **Menczer J, Modan M, Ranon L, et al.** Possible role of mumps virus in the etiology of ovarian cancer. *Cancer.* 1979;43:1375–1379.

106. **Cramer DW, Titus-Ernstoff L, McKolanis JR, et al.** Conditions associated with antibodies against the tumor-associated antigen MUC1 and their relationship to risk for ovarian cancer. *Cancer Epidemiol Biomarkers Prev.* 2005;14:1125–1131.

107. **Ho SB, Niehans GA, Lyftogt C, et al.** Heterogeneity of mucin gene expression in normal and neoplastic tissues. *Cancer Res.* 1993;53:641–651.

108. **Kotera Y, Fontenot JD, Pecher G, et al.** Humoral immunity against a tandem repeat epitope of human mucin MUC-1 in sera from breast, pancreatic, and colon cancer patients. *Cancer Res.* 1994;54:2856–2860.

109. **Richards ER, Devine PL, Quin RJ, et al.** Antibodies reactive with the protein core of MUC1 mucin are present in ovarian cancer patients and healthy women. *Cancer Immunol Immunother.* 1998;46:245–252.

110. **Agrawal B, Reddish MA, Krantz MJ, et al.** Does pregnancy immunize against breast cancer? *Cancer Res.* 1995;55:2257–2261.

111. **Kerlikowske K, Brown JS, Grady DG.** Should women with familial ovarian cancer undergo prophylactic oophorectomy? *Obstet Gynecol.* 1992;80:700–707.

112. **Claus EB, Schwartz PE.** Familial ovarian cancer. Update and clinical applications. *Cancer.* 1995;76:1998–2003.

113. **Alsop K, Fereday S, Meldrum C, et al.** BRCA mutation frequency and patterns of treatment response in BRCA mutation-positive women with ovarian cancer: A report from the Australian Ovarian Cancer Study Group. *J Clin Oncol.* 2012;30(21):2654–2663.3413277.

114. **Walsh T, Casadei S, Lee MK, et al.** Mutations in 12 genes for inherited ovarian, fallopian tube, and peritoneal carcinoma identified by massively parallel sequencing. *Proc Natl Acad Sci U S A.* 2011;108(44):18032–18037.

115. **Song H, Ramus SJ, Tyrer J, et al.** A genome-wide association study identifies a new ovarian cancer susceptibility locus on 9p22.2. *Nat Genet.* 2009;41:996–1000.

116. **Goode EL, Chenevix-Trench G, Song H, et al.** A genome-wide association study identifies susceptibility loci for ovarian cancer at 2q31 and 8q24. *Nat Genet.* 2010;42:874–879.

117. **Canavan TP, Cohen D.** Vulvar cancer. *Am Fam Physician.* 2002;66:1269–1274.

118. **Daling JR, Madeleine MM, Schwartz SM, et al.** A population-based study of squamous cell vaginal cancer: HPV and cofactors. *Gynecol Oncology.* 2002;84:263–270.

119. **Herbst AL, Kurman RJ, Scully RE, et al.** Clear-cell adenocarcinoma of the genital tract in young females. Registry report. *N Engl J Med.* 1972;287:1259–1264.

120. **Stehman FB, Look KY.** Carcinoma of the vulva. *Obstet Gynecol.* 2006;107:719–733.

121. **Brinton LA, Nasca PC, Mallin K, et al.** Case-control study of cancer of the vulva. *Obstet Gynecol.* 1990;75:859–866.

122. **Crum CP, Fu YS, Levine RU, et al.** Intraepithelial squamous lesions of the vulva: Biologic and histologic criteria for the distinction of condylomas from vulvar intraepithelial neoplasia. *Am J Obstet Gynecol.* 1982;144:77–83.

123. **Newcomb PA, Weiss NS, Daling JR.** Incidence of vulvar carcinoma in relation to menstrual, reproductive, and medical factors. *J Natl Cancer Inst.* 1984;73:391–396.

124. **Parazzini F, Moroni S, Negri E, et al.** Selected food intake and risk of vulvar cancer. *Cancer.* 1995;76:2291–2296.

125. **Weiderpass E, Ye W, Tamimi R, et al.** Alcoholism and risk for cancer of the cervix uteri, vagina, and vulva. *Cancer Epidemiol Biomarkers Prev.* 2001;10:899–901.

126. **Bagshawe K, Lawler S.** Choriocarcinoma. In: **Schottenfeld DJ, Fraumeni JF Jr., eds.** *Cancer Epidemiology and Prevention.* Philadelphia, PA: WB Saunders; 1982.

127. **Hayashi K, Bracken MB, Freeman DH Jr., et al.** Hydatidiform mole in the United States (1970–1977): A statistical and theoretical analysis. *Am J Epidemiol.* 1982;115:67–77.

128. **Jacobs PA, Hunt PA, Matsuura JS, et al.** Complete and partial hydatidiform mole in Hawaii: Cytogenetics, morphology and epidemiology. *Br J Obstet Gynaecol.* 1982;89:258–266.

129. **Stone M, Bagshawe KD.** An analysis of the influences of maternal age, gestational age, contraceptive method, and the mode of primary treatment of patients with hydatidiform moles on the incidence of subsequent chemotherapy. *Br J Obstet Gynaecol.* 1979;86:782–792.

130. **Salehi S, Eloranta S, Johansson AL, et al.** Reporting and incidence trends of hydatidiform mole in Sweden 1973–2004. *Acta Oncol.* 2011;50(3):367–372.

131. **Berkowitz RS, Cramer DW, Bernstein MR, et al.** Risk factors for complete molar pregnancy from a case-control study. *Am J Obstet Gynecol.* 1985;152:1016–1020.

132. **Evans HM, Murphy EA.** Vital need of the body for certain unsaturated fatty acids. VI. Male sterility on fat-free diets. *J Biol Chem.* 1934;106:445–450.

133. **Kim HL, Picciano MF, O'Brien W.** Influence of maternal dietary protein and fat levels on fetal growth in mice. *Growth.* 1981;45:8–18.

134. **O'Toole BA, Fradkin R, Warkany J, et al.** Vitamin A deficiency and reproduction in rhesus monkeys. *J Nutr.* 1974;104:1513–1524.

135. **McLaren DS.** Present knowledge of the role of vitamin A in health and disease. *Trans R Soc Trop Med Hyg.* 1966;60:436–462.

136. **La Vecchia C, Franceschi S, Parazzini F, et al.** Risk factors for gestational trophoblastic disease in Italy. *Am J Epidemiol.* 1985;121:457–464.

137. **Parazzini F, La Vecchia C, Franceschi S, et al.** ABO blood-groups and the risk of gestational trophoblastic disease. *Tumori.* 1985;71:123–126.

138. **Parazzini F, Mangili G, La Vecchia C, et al.** Risk factors for gestational trophoblastic disease: A separate analysis of complete and partial hydatidiform moles. *Obstet Gynecol.* 1991;78:1039–1045.

139. **Palmer JR, Driscoll SG, Rosenberg L, et al.** Oral contraceptive use and risk of gestational trophoblastic tumors. *J Natl Cancer Inst.* 1999;91:635–640.

140. **Baltazar JC.** Epidemiological features of choriocarcinoma. *Bull World Health Organ.* 1976;54:523–532.

141. **Ha MC, Cordier S, Bard D, et al.** Agent orange and the risk of gestational trophoblastic disease in Vietnam. *Arch Environ Health.* 1996;51:368–374.

142. **Altieri A, Franceschi S, Ferlay J, et al.** Epidemiology and aetiology of gestational trophoblastic diseases. *Lancet Oncol.* 2003;4:670–678.

143. **Reid A, Heyworth J, de Klerk N, et al.** Asbestos exposure and gestational trophoblastic disease: A hypothesis. *Cancer Epidemiol Biomarkers Prev.* 2009;18:2895–2898.

144. **Salvador S, Gilks B, Kobel M, et al.** The fallopian tube: Primary site of most pelvic high-grade serous carcinomas. *Int J Gynecol Cancer.* 2009;19:58–64.

145. **Cole P, Morrison AS.** Basic issues in population screening for cancer. *J Natl Cancer Inst.* 1980;64:1263–1272.

146. **Saslow D, Runowicz CD, Solomon D, et al.** American Cancer Society guideline for the early detection of cervical neoplasia and cancer. *CA Cancer J Clin.* 2002;52:342–362.

147. *ACOG Committee Opinion on Routine Cancer Screening.* Washington DC: American College of Obstetricians and Gynecologists; 2000.

148. **Sawaya GF, McConnell KJ, Kulasingam SL, et al.** Risk of cervical cancer associated with extending the interval between cervical-cancer screenings. *N Engl J Med.* 2003;349:1501–1509.

149. **Mayrand MH, Duarte-Franco E, Rodrigues I, et al.** Human papillomavirus DNA versus Papanicolaou screening tests for cervical cancer. *N Engl J Med.* 2007;357:1579–1588.

150. **Mandelblatt JS, Lawrence WF, Womack SM, et al.** Benefits and costs of using HPV testing to screen for cervical cancer. *JAMA.* 2002;287:2372–2381.

151. **Burke W, Daly M, Garber J, et al.** Recommendations for follow-up care of individuals with an inherited predisposition to cancer. II. BRCA1 and BRCA2. Cancer Genetics Studies Consortium. *JAMA.* 1997;277:997–1003.

152. **Buys SS, Partridge E, Black A, et al.** Effect of screening on ovarian cancer mortality: The Prostate, Lung, Colorectal and Ovarian (PLCO) Cancer Screening Randomized Controlled Trial. *JAMA.* 2011;305:2295–2303.

153. **Menon U, Jacobs IJ.** Ovarian cancer screening in the general population. *Curr Opin Obstet Gynecol.* 2001;13:61–64.

DISEASE SITES

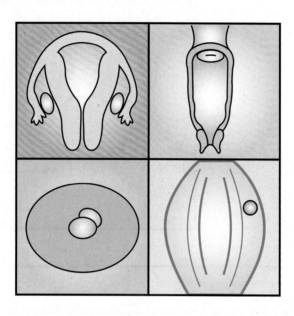

7 Cervical Cancer Screening and Preinvasive Disease

Michael J. Campion
Karen Canfell

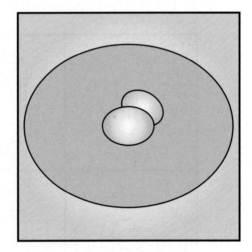

Cervix

Cervical cancer is the third most common cancer among women worldwide and is entirely attributable to infection with the Human Papillomavirus (HPV). Global estimates indicate that 610,000 newly incident HPV-related cancers occurred in 2008, including cancers at several sites in the female and male anogenital and oral tracts. Of these, cervical cancer was estimated to account for 530,000 new cases and 275,000 deaths. Rates of cervical cancer are estimated to be at least four-fold higher in low resource countries with a "low" ranking for Human Development Index compared with those in developed countries in the "very high" category (1).

Although differences in HPV exposure in various countries may play some role in explaining the differences between cervical cancer rates (2), **the higher incidence and death rates of cervical cancer in low resource settings are likely to result from the lack of organized cervical screening and inadequate access to treatment.** In many developed countries, screening with cervical cytology has resulted in large-scale reductions in cervical cancer incidence and mortality over time (3,4).

The primary goal of cervical screening is to prevent cervical cancer. This is achieved by the detection, treatment, and follow-up of preinvasive cervical lesions (3,5,6). Modern understanding that almost all cervical cancers are caused by persistent infection with approximately 15 types of HPV has led to important new approaches to primary and secondary cervical cancer prevention via prophylactic HPV vaccination and primary HPV-based screening.

Classification of Preinvasive Cervical Disease

The proposal that invasive squamous carcinoma of the cervix arises through progression of a pre-invasive lesion, as opposed to a *de novo* event, was initially postulated by Schauenstein in 1908 (7). The term "carcinoma *in situ*" was later introduced to describe cancerous changes confined to the epithelium (8). It is now understood that precancerous lesions arise from persisting HPV infection of the cervix, even though the majority of HPV infections regress (9).

The Dysplasia Terminology

Although referred to earlier by Papanicolaou and Traut (10), in 1956 Reagan and Hamonic (11) described cytologic differences between "carcinoma *in situ*" and a group of "less anaplastic" lesions, for which they introduced the term **dysplasia** (12). In 1975, the World Health Organization defined dysplasia as a "lesion in which part of the epithelium was replaced by cells showing varying degrees of atypia." Dysplastic changes were graded as mild, moderate, and severe, but precise guidelines for these subdivisions were not defined and grading always remained highly subjective (13–16).

A dual terminology developed, leading to inconsistencies in treatment policies. If a diagnosis of "dysplasia" was made, this was considered a nonspecific change and the patient was subjected to a cone biopsy. If the diagnosis of "carcinoma *in situ*" was made, this was considered a "preinvasive cancer" and the patient underwent an obligatory hysterectomy (15–17).

Cervical Intraepithelial Neoplasia

Invasive squamous cell carcinoma of the cervix was demonstrated to be the end result of progressive intraepithelial dysplastic atypia occurring within the metaplastic epithelium of the cervical transformation zone (18). The classification of lesions from mild dysplasia to carcinoma *in situ* did not truly reflect either the morphologic or biologic continuum of preinvasive cervical disease. The diagnosis was highly subjective and was not reproducible.

After pioneering research into the natural history of cervical cancer precursors, **Richart** (19) **proposed the term "cervical intraepithelial neoplasia" (CIN) in 1973** to describe the biologic spectrum of cervical preinvasive squamous disease. **Three grades of CIN were described, CIN 1 (mild dysplasia), CIN 2 (moderate dysplasia), and CIN 3 (severe dysplasia/carcinoma *in situ*).** This system was consistent with biologic evidence that strongly implied a single process of cervical squamous carcinogenesis (19–25).

Forty years' experience with the CIN terminology, coupled with recent advances in the understanding of the role of HPV in the causation of cervical neoplasia (24–30), has led to a critical reappraisal of this model and to further reclassification of the terminology for reporting cytologic abnormalities consistent with preinvasive disease (31–38).

The CIN grading is also very subjective. No reproducible cytologic or histologic distinction at the lower end of the CIN continuum exists between CIN 1 and HPV infection alone. Both interobserver and intraobserver consistency in diagnosis are poor (37–40). Separating CIN 2 from CIN 3 is often not reproducible (26,41–43). In reality, **the two critical questions in the assessment of the cervical epithelium are: (i) do the changes represent a cancer precursor; and (ii) is the lesion invasive cancer?**

In histologic terms, CIN 3 is clearly established as a *bona fide* cancer precursor, although there are few identified risk factors for progression of CIN 3 to cancer other than time (44). CIN 3 is a reliable and more highly reproducible morphologic diagnosis, with undifferentiated cells having fixed genetic abnormalities replacing almost the full thickness of the cervical epithelium (40,41). It is reliably distinguished from recently acquired HPV infection and is a genuine surrogate marker of subsequent cancer risk. **Uncertainty still exists in relation to the progressive potential of less severe dysplastic lesions** (45,46).

CIN 1 is increasingly viewed as an insensitive histologic marker of HPV infection. The diagnosis includes errors of processing and interpretation of colposcopically directed biopsies (40). **Standardized for positivity of a given high-risk HPV type, a diagnosis of CIN 1 does not predict a meaningfully higher risk of CIN 3 than does a negative biopsy** (44). By contrast, longitudinal outcomes after HPV infection have demonstrated higher risk of CIN 2+ and CIN 3+ in HPV-positive versus HPV-negative women, with follow-up times up to 18 years now reported (47). These studies have demonstrated that the risk of subsequent high-grade CIN is dependent on the initial HPV type, with types 16 and 18 being associated with a higher risk than the other oncogenic types (47,48).

There appears to be considerable heterogeneity in the microscopic diagnosis, biology and clinical behavior of CIN 2 lesions (49). CIN 2 can sometimes be produced by noncarcinogenic HPV types and is equivocal in its cancer potential (49). Some CIN 2 lesions represent acute HPV infection with a more severe microscopic appearance that is destined to regress. Others are incipient precancer (CIN 3) that will persist and progress with an attendant high risk of future invasion if left untreated.

The risk factor profiles (49–51) and HPV genotype distributions (52) in CIN 2 and CIN 3 are different. CIN 2 is more likely to spontaneously regress than CIN 3 (53), but current clinical management of CIN 2 and CIN 3 is similar in most settings. **The clinical dilemma remains the**

Terminology

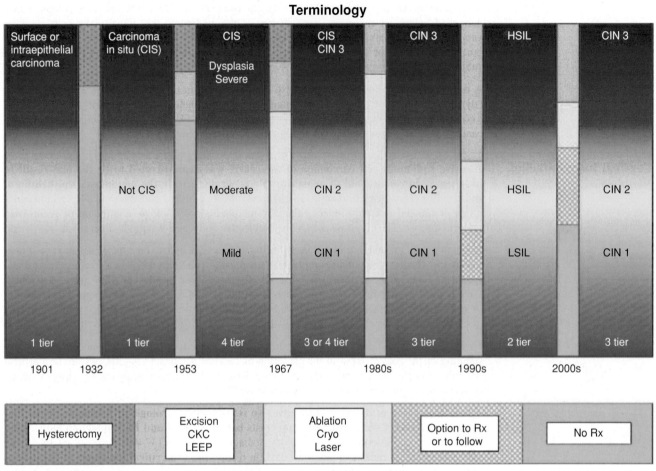

Figure 7.1 Changes to the terminology and number of tiers used to describe cervical precancer over time with corresponding management options (procedure). CKC, cold-knife conization; Cryo, cryotherapy; Rx, treatment. Modified with permission. Courtesy of J. Thomas Cox. Reproduced from **Darragh TM, Colgan TJ, Cox JT, et al.;** for members of the LAST Project Work Groups. The Lower Anogenital Squamous Terminology Standardization Project for HPV-associated Lesions: Background and consensus recommendations from the College of American Pathologists and the American Society for Colposcopy and Cervical Pathology. *Arch Pathol Lab Med.* 2012;136:1266–1297.

inability to reliably predict those lesions less severe than CIN 3 that are at greatest risk of progression to cancer.

New molecular markers hold promise in this regard (54–58) **and there is emerging evidence that technologies such as dual immunohistochemical (IHC) staining for the markers Ki-67 and p16 can improve histologic classification of CIN 3 abnormalities and resolve CIN 2 diagnoses** (58). The Lower Anogenital Squamous Terminology Standardization Project (**LAST nomenclature**) relies on p16 IHC staining to triage CIN 2 (58); p16 is a biomarker for disruption of the Rb pathway by HPV (57,59). **CIN 2 that is p16 positive is combined with CIN 3 as a high-grade lesion.** CIN 2 that is p16 negative is combined with CIN 1 as a low-grade lesion, the histologic diagnosis of HPV infection (Fig. 7.1).

Cervical Precancer—Modern Concepts

HPV infection is a necessary precursor of true precancer. A defined precancerous lesion remains the target of screening and preventive treatment programs and represents a genuine surrogate for cancer risk (60–62). CIN 3 is the most certain histologic surrogate marker of cancer risk. **CIN 3 lesions demonstrate the same aneuploid DNA** (63) **content and genetic instability** (64)

as seen in invasive cancer. Some CIN 3 lesions are small and a proportion may regress, particularly after biopsy, but at this time, all CIN 3 lesions should be managed as definite precancer lesions.

CIN 2 has demonstrated greater heterogeneity in biology and definition and has a greater potential for regression when compared to CIN 3 (49,50,65). Despite the emergence of biomarkers such as p16 IHC staining, it is recommended that CIN 2 lesions should be treated to provide a further safety margin against the development of cancer.

A histologic diagnosis of a low-grade cervical intraepithelial lesion (HPV infection/CIN 1) is increasingly viewed as not representing precancer. However, infection with oncogenic HPV types is strongly predictive of future risk of high-grade abnormalities/precancer (47,48,67). HPV infection might not be associated with any microscopic abnormality, while most low-grade abnormalities will regress (68,69), particularly among young women (70).

High-grade lesions are commonly found within a broader field of low-grade disease, suggesting that CIN 3 may develop in high-risk HPV-infected epithelium independent of, and within a CIN 1 lesion, rather than as a classical stepwise progression. **The reported progressive potential of histologically confirmed low-grade lesions varies from 12–33%** (17,18,71–73).

Lower Anogenital Squamous Terminology Standardization Project for HPV-Associated Lesions (LAST Project)

HPV interacts with genital tract squamous epithelia in two basic ways. Firstly, HPV infection may produce transient lesions, which support virion production. Such lesions have been variously described as low-grade lesions, intraepithelial neoplasia grade 1, mild dysplasia, or condyloma. Such lesions may be undetected clinically. **Secondly, HPV-epithelial interaction may produce lesions classified as precancerous.** Viral oncogenic overexpression drives cell proliferation to produce a clonal expansion of undifferentiated cells, characterized clinically by persistent viral detection, persistent and advancing colposcopic abnormalities, and increasing risk of malignant transformation. These precancerous lesions are not reliably distinguishable by routine histology, regardless of the site of the lesion or the sex of the individual (74–77).

On the basis of specified principles of HPV-associated disease (Table 7.1) and issues related to terminology, a consensus process was sponsored by the College of American Pathologists (CAP) and the American Society for Colposcopy and Cervical Pathology (ASCCP). In 2012, the **Lower Anogenital Squamous Terminology (LAST Project)** published a comprehensive reevaluation of the terminology of HPV-associated lesions of the lower anogenital tract including the cervix, vagina, vulva, perianal area, anus, penis, and scrotum (59).

The LAST Project recommendations include the following:

1. **There should be a unified histopathologic nomenclature** with a single set of diagnostic terms. A two-tiered nomenclature was recommended for noninvasive HPV-associated squamous proliferations of the lower anogenital tract, which may be further qualified

Table 7.1 General Principles Underlying the LAST Project

1. There is unified epithelial biology to HPV-related squamous disease

2. Each cytologic or histologic sample is only a statistical representation of the patient's true biology

3. The more samples or data points available, the more accurate the assessment of the patient's true biology

4. The true biology represents the risk for cancer at the current time and, to a lesser extent, the risk for cancer over time

5. Diagnostic variation can be improved by:

   a. Aligning the number of diagnostic terms with the number of biologically relevant categories and

   b. The use of biologic markers

Reproduced from **Darragh TM, Colgan TJ, Cox JT, et al.** The Lower Anogenital Squamous Terminology Standardization Project for HPV-associated lesions: Background and consensus recommendations from the College of American Pathologists and the American Society for Colposcopy and Cervical Pathology. *J Low Genit Tract Dis.* 2012;16:205–242.

with the appropriate –IN terminology. (–IN refers to the generic intraepithelial neoplasia terminology without specifying location.)

2. **HPV-associated squamous lesions of the lower anogenital tract should be classified as low-grade squamous intraepithelial lesion (LSIL) and high-grade squamous intraepithelial lesion (HSIL), which may be further classified by the –IN classification.**

3. **The biomarker p16 immunohistochemical (IHC) staining should be used when the hematoxylin and eosin (H&E) morphologic diagnosis is between precancer (–IN 2 or –IN 3) and a mimic of precancer** (e.g., processes known to be unrelated to neoplastic risk, such as immature squamous metaplasia, atrophy, reparative epithelial changes, tangential cutting). Strong and diffuse block-positive p16 results would support a categorization of precancerous disease.

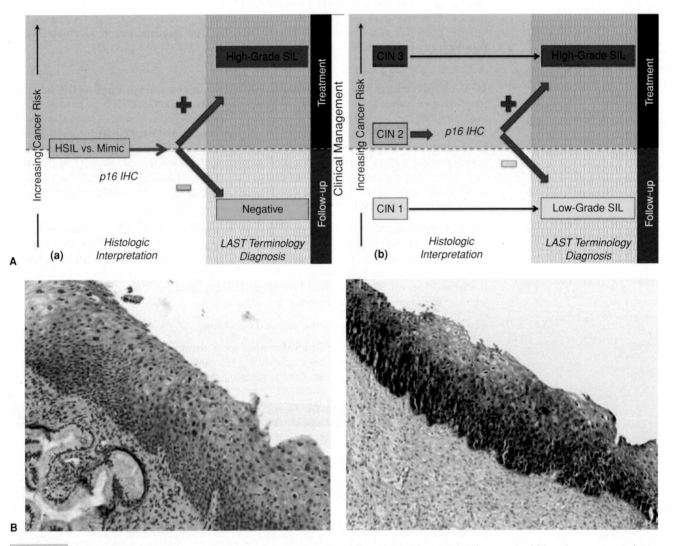

Figure 7.2 A: **Pathologic diagnoses using p16 and potential clinical management options for cervical biopsies.** (a) Use of p16 to evaluate the differential diagnosis of HSIL versus a mimic, such as immature squamous metaplasia and atrophy. (b) Use of p16 to evaluate morphologic CIN 2. The choice of clinical management for HSIL depends on the entire clinical scenario including patient's age, colposcopic findings, and biopsy diagnosis. (Modified with permission. Courtesy of Philip E. Castle.) B: Cervical biopsy with SIL showing partial maturation, and a CIN lesion that is challenging to classify as low-grade or high-grade SIL. H&E morphology at medium power shows atypical parabasal-like cells extending into the middle third of the epithelium. Corresponding p16 IHC stains reveals diffuse strong staining meeting the definition of p16 strong diffuse block-positive. This case is best interpreted as HSIL. Reproduced from: **Darragh TM, Colgan TJ, Cox JT, et al.;** for members of the LAST Project Work Groups. The Lower Anogenital Squamous Terminology Standardization Project for HPV-associated lesions: Background and consensus recommendations from the College of American Pathologists and the American Society for Colposcopy and Cervical Pathology. *Arch Pathol Lab Med.* 2012;136:1266–1297.

Table 7.2 LAST Terminology and the Three-tiered CIN System in Cytologic and Histologic Diagnoses

Natural History Model	Histology			Cytology	
	Dysplasia Nomenclature	CIN Nomenclature	LAST Nomenclature	Papanicolaou Classification	The Bethesda System
Infection	Negative	Negative		I	NILM
	Squamous atypia	Squamous atypia		II	ASC-US
Precancer	Mild dysplasia	CIN 1	LSIL	III	LSIL
	Moderate dysplasia	CIN 2			
	Severe dysplasia	CIN 3			HSIL
	Carcinoma *in situ*			IV	
Cancer	Carcinoma	Carcinoma	HSIL	V	Carcinoma

Terminology of cervical disease categories. The table shows histologic and cytologic terminologies of cervical disease categories.

NILM, negative for intraepithelial lesion or malignancy; ASC-US, atypical squamous cells of unknown significance; CIN, cervical intraepithelial neoplasia; LSIL, low-grade squamous intraepithelial lesion; HSIL, high-grade squamous intraepithelial lesion.

From **Mark Schiffman M, Wentzensen N**. Human papillomavirus infection and the multistage carcinogenesis of cervical cancer. *Cancer Epidemiol Biomarkers Prev.* 2013;22(4);553–560.

4. **If the pathologist is entertaining an H&E morphologic interpretation of –IN 2 (under the old terminology, which is a biologically equivocal lesion falling between the morphologic changes of HPV infection and precancer), p16 IHC is recommended to help clarify the situation.** Strong and diffuse block-positive p16 results support a categorization of precancer. Negative or nonblock-positive staining strongly favors an interpretation of low-grade disease or a non–HPV-associated pathology.

5. **p16 IHC should be used as an adjudication tool for cases in which there is a professional disagreement in histologic specimen interpretation, with the caveat that the differential diagnosis should include a precancerous lesion (–IN 2 or –IN 3).**

6. **p16 IHC should not be used as a routine adjunct to histologic assessment of biopsy specimens with morphologic interpretations of negative, –IN 1, and –IN 3.**

The LAST terminology for squamous HPV-associated lesions and associated p16 biomarker usage reflects modern clinical practice (Fig. 7.2A,B). If the LAST terminology is broadly accepted, squamous histology and cytologic reporting should be indistinguishable and consistent in the United States. Potential reconciliation of LAST terminology and the three-tiered CIN system in cytologic and histologic diagnoses is represented in Table 7.2.

Understanding the Cervical Transformation Zone

Embryogenesis

The cervix and vagina are derived from the müllerian ducts and are initially lined by a single layer of müllerian-derived columnar epithelium. At 18 to 20 weeks of gestation, the columnar epithelium lining the vaginal tube is colonized by the upward growth of stratified squamous epithelium derived from cloacal endoderm.

Original Squamo-columnar Junction

The junction in fetal life between the stratified squamous epithelium of the vagina and ectocervix, and the columnar epithelium of the endocervical canal is called the original squamocolumnar junction (78). Original squamous epithelium extends from Hart's line or the mucocutaneous, vulvovaginal junction to the original squamocolumnar junction. **The position of the original squamocolumnar junction is variable, lying on the ectocervix in 66%, within the endocervical canal in 30%, and on the vaginal fornices in 4% of female infants** (79). The position of the original squamocolumnar junction determines the extent of cervical squamous metaplasia (79,80). Embryogenesis, in determining the distribution of native squamous and columnar epithelia, is an important early

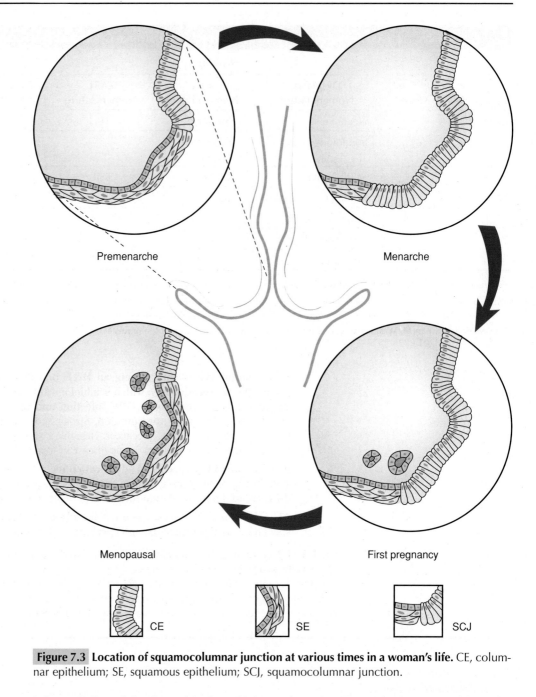

Premenarche

Menarche

Menopausal

First pregnancy

CE

SE

SCJ

Figure 7.3 Location of squamocolumnar junction at various times in a woman's life. CE, columnar epithelium; SE, squamous epithelium; SCJ, squamocolumnar junction.

influence in determining future risk of neoplastic transformation (Fig. 7.3), although **sexual behavior and subsequent exposure to HPV infection are the primary determinants of overall risk.**

New Squamocolumnar Junction

Increased estrogen secretion, particularly with puberty and with the first pregnancy, causes an increase in cervical volume and an eversion of endocervical columnar epithelium to an ectocervical location (79). **This eversion of columnar epithelium onto the ectocervix is called an ectropion.** An "ectropion" is often mistakenly referred to as an "erosion."

The estrogen surge of puberty results in the establishment of lactobacilli as part of the normal flora of the vagina. These microorganisms produce lactic acid, reducing the vaginal pH to 4 or less (79). Everted endocervical columnar epithelium is exposed in the postpubertal years to the acidity of the vaginal environment. Damage to the everted columnar epithelium caused by vaginal acidity results in proliferation of a stromal reserve cell underlying the columnar epithelium. This replaces the columnar epithelium with an immature, undifferentiated, stratified, squamous, metaplastic epithelium (79,80). **Immature squamous metaplasia then undergoes a maturation**

process, producing a mature, stratified squamous metaplastic epithelium, distinguishable only with difficulty from the original squamous epithelium.

The original linear junction between squamous and columnar epithelium is replaced by a zone of squamous metaplasia at varying degrees of maturation. At the upper or cephalad margin of this zone is a sharp demarcation between epithelium, which appears morphologically squamous, and villous epithelium, which appears colposcopically columnar. This colposcopic junction is called the **new squamocolumnar junction**.

The Transformation Zone

The transformation zone is defined as that area lying between the original squamocolumnar junction and the colposcopic new squamocolumnar junction (20,21). The initial clinical assessment for most women is in the postpubertal years, when mature squamous metaplastic epithelium has often replaced the distal or caudad limit of the columnar epithelium. As the transformation zone matures, the original squamocolumnar junction becomes impossible to delineate, and only the presence of nabothian follicles and gland openings hint at the original columnar origin of mature squamous metaplasia.

Cervical neoplasia almost invariably originates within the transformation zone (Fig. 7.4). For reasons that are poorly understood, persistent HPV infection causes cancers mainly at the transformation zone between different kinds of epithelia (e.g., cervix, anus, and oropharynx) (81). Carcinogenic HPV infection is equally common in the cervical and vaginal epithelia (82). However, cervical cancer is the third most common cancer among women worldwide, while vaginal cancer is rare. This reflects the pivotal importance of the metaplastic epithelium of the transformation zone in cervical carcinogenesis (83).

Research from Harvard Medical School has described **an embryonic cell population within the transformation zone with specific morphologic and molecular features that may represent the cells of origin for most cervical precancers and cancers** (84,85). Early in life, embryonic cervical epithelial cells are seen throughout the cervix. These cells subsequently diminish in number and concentrate at the SC junction in the adult. These cuboidal embryonic/SC junction cells

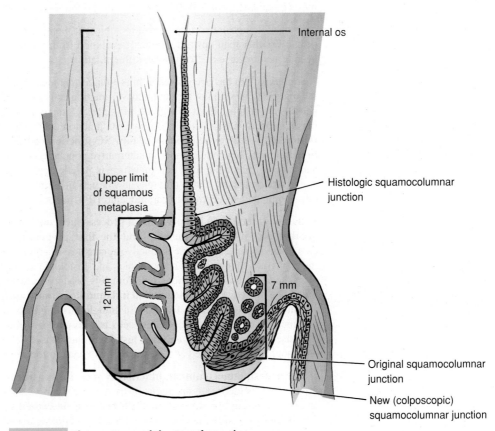

Figure 7.4 **The anatomy of the transformation zone.**

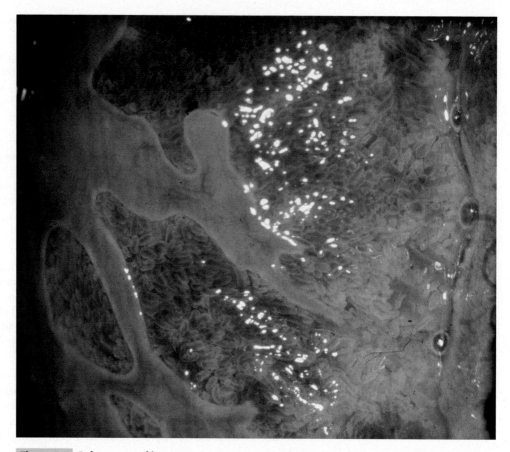

Figure 7.5 **Colposcopy of immature squamous metaplasia.** Note the tongues of pale grey squamous metaplastic epithelium growing over the fronds of native columnar epithelium.

have been demonstrated to give rise to subjacent metaplastic basal/reserve cells. This downward or basal (rather than upward or apical) evolution from progenitor cell to metaplastic progeny has been termed reverse or "top down" differentiation.

A similar pattern has been noted in high-grade squamous intraepithelial lesions (HSILs), suggesting that HPV infection of the cuboidal SC junction cells may initiate outgrowth of basally-oriented neoplastic progeny. Most low-grade SILs are SC junction-negative, implying infection of metaplastic progeny rather than the original SC junction cells. **This "model of "top down" differentiation may resolve the mystery of how SC junction cells remodel the cervix and participate in neoplasia.** The model defines an alternative population of metaplastic progeny (including basal and reserve cells), the infection of which is paradoxically less likely to produce a biologically aggressive precursor. It also provides new targets in animal models to determine why the SC junction is uniquely susceptible to carcinogenic HPV infection" (85).

Squamous metaplasia is a permanent process but is not continuous. It occurs in "spurts," with greatest activity during puberty and the first pregnancy. During the maturation phase, the columnar villi fuse, losing the distinctive appearance of columnar epithelium (Fig. 7.5) and producing a myriad of cytologic, colposcopic, and histologic appearances. The process fluctuates in response to hormonal influences, but ultimately produces a mature, glycogenated squamous epithelium. **The presence of a subepithelial inflammatory infiltrate in biopsy specimens of immature squamous metaplasia may lead to a histologic misdiagnosis of chronic cervicitis** (Fig. 7.6). The presence of such inflammatory white cells is a normal part of the metaplastic process and is not a response to an infectious organism. A histologic diagnosis of "chronic cervicitis" is often misleading and should not be accepted as a satisfactory explanation for an abnormal Papanicolaou (Pap) smear.

If the new squamocolumnar junction is seen in its entirety in the absence of premalignant disease, the incidence of squamous disease above the new squamocolumnar junction is very low and **the colposcopic examination of the cervix is described as** *adequate* **in the current ASCCP Guidelines** (86). If the new squamocolumnar junction is not seen in its entirety, the colposcopic examination is described as *inadequate.* The transformation zone further defines the distal limit of

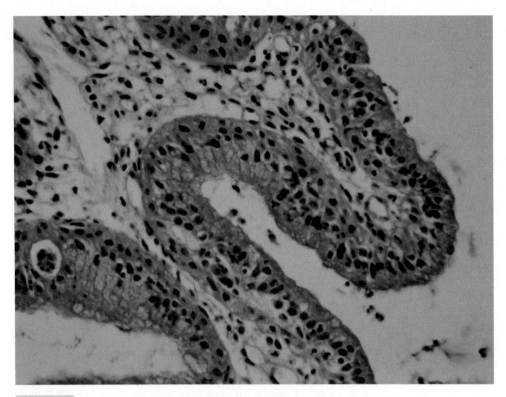

Figure 7.6 Histology of immature squamous metaplasia (chronic cervicitis).

high-grade glandular intraepithelial neoplasia, which is the precursor lesion to invasive adenocarcinoma of the cervix.

Upper Limit of Squamous Metaplasia	The new squamocolumnar junction is an unstable boundary. Serial colposcopic assessments of the cervix frequently show the new squamocolumnar junction to have moved cephalad. Careful colposcopic assessment of columnar villi immediately above the new squamocolumnar junction reveals opaque, opalescent tips, and early villous fusion (Fig. 7.5). Histologic study of colposcopically directed biopsy specimens reveals reserve cell hyperplasia and early immature squamous metaplasia occurring in epithelium, which appears colposcopically columnar. This early immature squamous metaplasia can extend as far as 10 mm above the new squamocolumnar junction.

The immature metaplastic epithelium cephalad to the new squamocolumnar junction is not included in the modern definition of the transformation zone, but represents the epithelium at greatest risk for future neoplastic transformation. During dynamic phases of metaplasia, occurring particularly with puberty and the first pregnancy, the immature metaplastic cells are actively phagocytic (79). The most critical phase is the initiation of squamous metaplasia at puberty and in early adolescence.

2011 IFCPC Colposcopic Terminology of the Cervix, Vagina, and Vulva	**The International Federation for Colposcopy and Cervical Pathology (IFCPC) has recently released the latest colposcopic nomenclature for cervical and vulvar disease** (Table 7.3), attempting to bring greater clarity to terminology in colposcopy practice (87,88). The most recent nomenclature has introduced a classification of transformation zone distribution, which shapes treatment of CIN lesions. It also includes vulvar and vaginal terminology for the first time.

The formalization of a classification of the cervical transformation zone according to its distribution and location of the new squamocolumnar junction is of clinical value (89). **A Type 1 Transformation Zone is fully visible with the new SCJ on the ectocervix** (Fig. 7.7A). **A Type 2 Transformation Zone is partially or totally endocervical but the new squamocolumnar junction is fully visible usually in the distal millimeters of the endocervical canal** (Fig. 7.7B). **A Type 3 Transformation Zone is partially or completely endocervical with the new squamocolumnar junction not fully visible as a result of its extension into the endocervical canal or the tightness of the canal** (Fig. 7.7C). The location of the transformation zone, and whether the new

Table 7.3 2011 IFCPC Terminology of the Cervix			
2011 IFCPC Colposcopic Terminology of the Cervix			
General assessment		• Adequate/inadequate for the reason (i.e., cervix obscured by inflammation, bleeding, scar) • Squamocolumnar junction visibility: Completely visible, partially visible, not visible • Transformation zone types 1, 2, 3	
Normal colposcopic findings		Original squamous epithelium • Mature • Atrophic Columnar epithelium • Ectopy Metaplastic squamous epithelium • Nabothian cysts • Crypt (gland) openings Deciduosis in pregnancy	
Abnormal colposcopic findings	**General principles**	**Location of the lesion:** Inside or outside the T-zone, Location of the lesion by clock position **Size of the lesion:** Number of cervical quadrants the lesion covers, Size of the lesion in percentage of cervix.	
	Grade 1 (Minor)	Thin acetowhite epithelium Irregular, geographic border	Fine mosaic, Fine punctation
	Grade 2 (Major)	Dense acetowhite epithelium, Rapid appearance of acetowhitening, Cuffed crypt (gland) openings	Coarse mosaic, Coarse punctuation, Sharp border, Inner border sign, Ridge sign
	Nonspecific	Leukoplakia (keratosis, hyperkeratosis), Erosion Lugol staining (Schiller test): Stained/nonstained	
Suspicious for invasion		Atypical vessels **Additional signs:** Fragile vessels, Irregular surface, Exophytic lesion, Necrosis, Ulceration (necrotic), tumor/gross neoplasm	
Miscellaneous finding		Congenital transformation zone Condyloma Polyp (Ectocervical/endocervical) Inflammation	Stenosis Congenital anomaly Posttreatment consequence Endometriosis
2011 IFCPC Colposcopic Terminology of the Cervix—Addendum			
Excision treatment types		**Excision type 1, 2, 3**	
Excision specimen dimensions		**Length**—the distance from the distal/external margin to the proximal/internal margin **Thickness**—the distance from the stromal margin to the surface of the excised specimen **Circumference** (Optional)—the perimeter of the excised specimen	

2011 IFCPC Nomenclature Accepted in Rio World Congress, July 5, 2011.

From **Bornstein J, Bentley J, Bosze P, et al.** The 2011 Colposcopic Terminology of the International Federation for Cervical Pathology and Colposcopy. *Obstet Gynecol.* 2012;120(1):166–172.

SCJ is seen in its entirety, influences the diagnostic completion of the colposcopic examination and the method of treatment (Table 7.4). In the current nomenclature, three transformation zone excision types have been introduced (Fig. 7.8A–C). A fully visible small, ectocervical transformation zone is easy to assess and simple to treat either by destruction or simple excision. **A large Type 3 Transformation Zone is not possible to completely assess colposcopically, as all or part of it is situated within the canal beyond colposcopic view. Treatment is more difficult and the risks of long-term morbidity and treatment failure are increased.**

The current nomenclature emphasizes the importance of the colposcopic findings of an internal margin (Fig. 7.9) (90,91) and the raised, rolled margin described as a "ridge-sign" (92) (Fig. 7.10). Each is an integral component of the assessment of the lesion margin in the discrimination of high-grade disease within the Reid Colposcopic Index (90) and they are highly sensitive colposcopic predictors of HSIL.

A

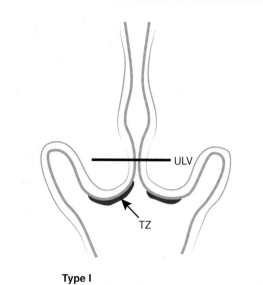

Type I

- Fully visible
- Completely ectocervical
- Small or large

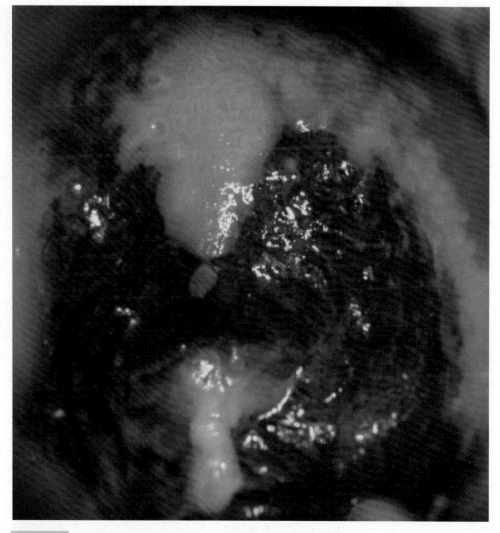

Figure 7.7 A: The Transformation Zone Classification—Type 1 TZ.

B

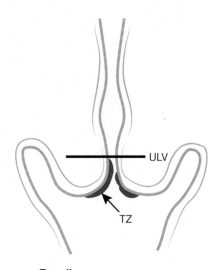

ULV

TZ

Type II

- **Fully visible**
- **Has endocervical component**
- **May have ectocervical component which may be small or large**

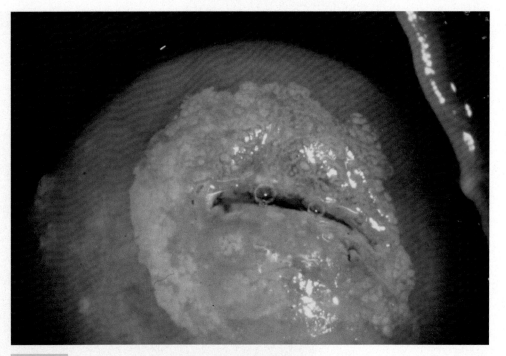

Figure 7.7 B: The Transformation Zone Classification—Type 2 TZ.

Human Papillomaviruses and Cervical Neoplasia

Extensive molecular biologic and epidemiologic research has confirmed certain HPV types to be carcinogenic in humans (9,64,65,77,93–99). The four major steps in the development of cervical cancer are (i) **infection of the metaplastic epithelium** of the transformation zone with one or more carcinogenic HPV types; (ii) **viral persistence** rather than clearance; (iii) **progression** of persistently infected epithelium to cervical precancer (CIN 3) (potentially reflecting the host immune response and/or exposure to the confirmed cofactors for HPV progression, which include multiparity, age at first full-term pregnancy, use of oral contraceptives, and current tobacco exposure) (51,100–103); and (iv) **invasion**.

C

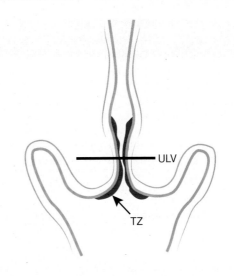

Type III

- Not fully visible
- Has endocervical component
- May have ectocervical component which may be small or large

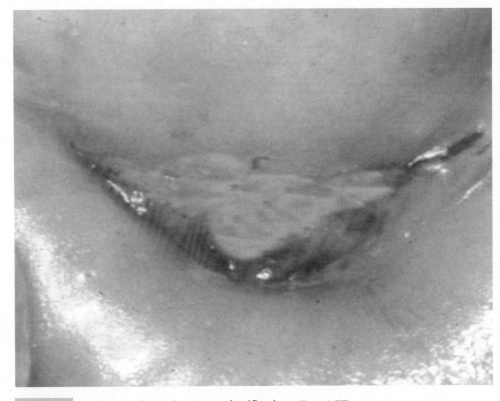

Figure 7.7 C: The Transformation Zone Classification—Type 3 TZ.

Table 7.4 2011 IFCPC Classification of Types of Excisional Procedures for Cervical Disease Based on Type of Transformation Zone

Excision Type	Type 1 Excision	Type 2 Excision	Type 3 Excision
Transformation Zone type	Type 1	Type 2	Type 3
Condition	Any grade of squamous CIN, serious consideration should be given to excising CIN 3 disease	Any grade of squamous CIN Glandular disease in women <36 yrs Suspected microinvasion	Any grade of squamous CIN Glandular disease in women >36 yrs Suspected microinvasion
Other circumstances		Previous treatment	Previous treatment
Techniques included in this category of excision	LLETZ/LEEP Laser excision	LLETZ/LEEP SWETZ Laser excision Cold knife cone biopsy/ cylindrical excision	LLETZ/LEEP SWETZ Cold knife cone biopsy/cylindrical excision
Alternative treatment choices	Type 1 ablation		

LLETZ, large loop excision of the transformation zone; LEEP, loop electrosurgical excision procedure; SWETZ, straight wire excision of the transformation zone.

From **Silvio Tatti S, Bornstein J, Prendiville W.** Colposcopy: A global perspective introduction of the new FCPC colposcopy terminology. *Obstet Gynecol Clin N Am.* 2013;40:235–250.

Taxonomy and Biology

Papillomaviruses are small, nonenveloped, double-stranded DNA viruses encased in a 72-sided icosahedral protein capsid. The HPV genome consists of circular, double-stranded DNA of approximately 7,900 nucleotide base pairs. Papillomaviruses are a divergent group of evolutionarily related viruses with similar biologic characteristics but enormous differences in species specificity, site of predilection, and oncogenic potential (104,105).

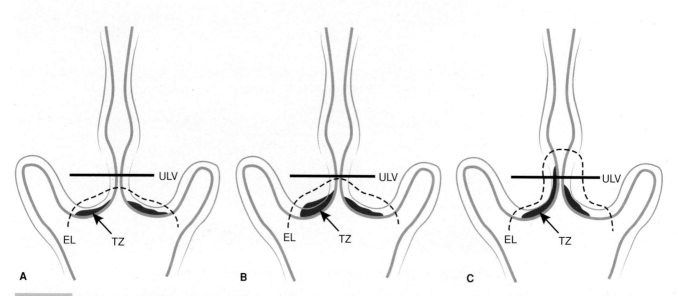

Figure 7.8 A: Type 1 Excision resects a completely ectocervical or type 1 Transformation Zone. The large loop excision of the TZ (LLETZ) procedure need not encroach the endocervical canal nor be greater than 8 mm thick throughout the resection. The excision margin is depicted by a dashed line. **B: A Type 2 excision resects a Type 2 Transformation Zone** (has an endocervical component but is fully visible). The excision margin is depicted by a *dashed green line.* **C: A Type 3 excision resects a Type 3 Transformation Zone.** A longer and larger amount of tissue of tissue is resected. The excision margin is depicted by a *dashed green line.* Adapted from **Silvio Tatti S, Bornstein J, Prendiville W.** Colposcopy: A global perspective introduction of the new IFCPC colposcopy terminology. *Obstet Gynecol Clin N Am.* 2013;40(2):235–250.

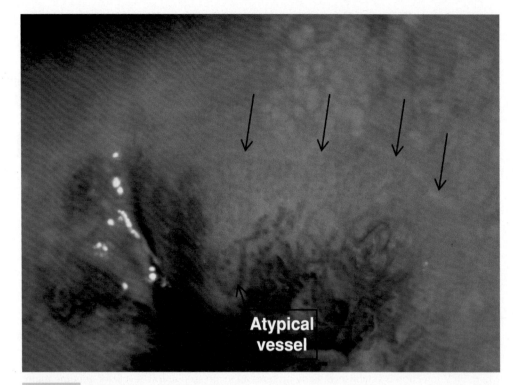

Figure 7.9 Colpophotograph of cervix of 25-year-old women with low-grade ectocervical SIL, an internal margin with a high-grade central lesion revealing an atypical vessel at a focus of microinvasive cancer.

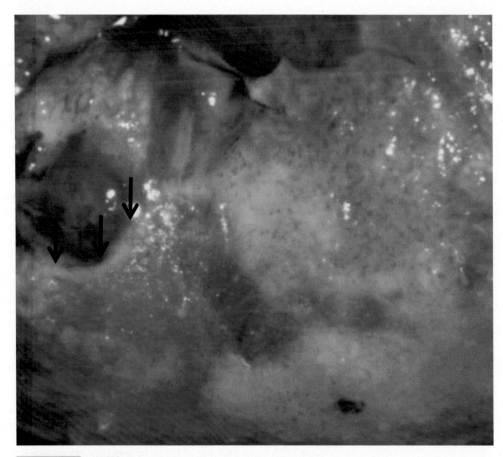

Figure 7.10 Colpophotograph of cervix of a 33-year-old woman with a high-grade SIL showing a "ridge" sign or raised, rolled, peeling margin at an area of early invasion.

257

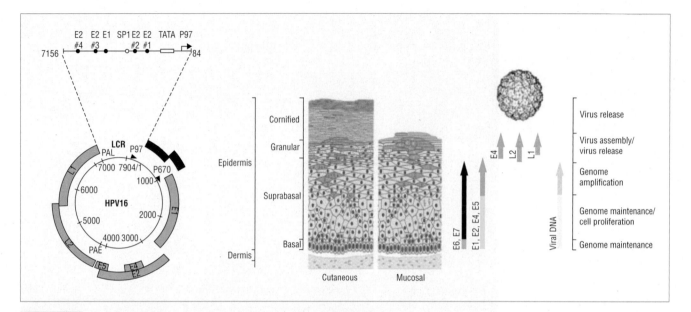

Figure 7.11 **The HPV genome and its expression within the epithelium.** The HPV genome consists of approximately 8,000 base pairs of single-stranded, circular DNA. HPV genes are designated as E or L according to their expression in early or late differentiation stage of the epithelium: *E1, E2, E5, E6,* and *E7* are expressed early in the differentiation, *E4* is expressed throughout, and *L1* and *L2* are expressed during the final stages of differentiation. The viral genome is maintained at the basal layer of the epithelium, where HPV infection is established. Early proteins are expressed at low levels for genome maintenance (raising the possibility of a latent state) and cell proliferation. As the basal epithelial cells differentiate, the viral life cycle enters successive stages of genome amplification, virus assembly and virus release, with a concomitant shift in expression patterns from early genes to late genes, including *L1* and *L2,* which assemble into viral capsid. (Reproduced with permission from **Schiffman M, Castle PE, Jeronimo J, et al**. Human papillomavirus and cervical cancer. *Lancet.* 2007;370;890–907.)

More than 100 types of HPV have been fully sequenced. HPV types are divided into phylogenetic trees, based on their DNA sequence and protein homologies. This assists in understanding HPV classification and behavior (106). The oncogenic HPV types infect the epithelium of the anogenital and oral tracts and are generally acquired through sexual contact.

Genetic sequencing has defined clades of viruses, which produce similar pathology (105). Viruses of clades alpha-7 and alpha-9 are most commonly associated with anogenital cancers and HPV 16 in particular (an alpha-9 species) appears to be a "uniquely powerful human carcinogen" (106), which is implicated in approximately 50% of cervical cancers and the majority of HPV-related cancers at other anogenital and oropharyngeal sites.

The HPV genome is usually maintained as a stable viral episome, independent of the host cell genome, in the nucleus of infected cells. It codes for only eight genes (107). In some high-grade CIN lesions, and more frequently in cervical cancer, HPV genomes are covalently bonded or integrated into the host chromosomes (108–112). This integration event involves the *E1* and *E2* genes with important consequences for regulation of viral gene expression (Fig. 7.11) (113). The late genes, *L1* and *L2,* the sequences of which are highly conserved among all papillomaviruses, encode the common capsid proteins. These viral proteins reflect late viral gene expression and are exclusively present in well-differentiated keratinocytes (114). Both proteins play an important role in mediating efficient virus infectivity.

The proteins encoded by the *E6* and *E7* genes of high-risk HPV types, particularly HPV 16 (clade alpha-9) and 18 (clade alpha-7), are directly involved in cellular transformation in the presence of an active oncogene (115). **E6 and E7 are the primary HPV oncoproteins with numerous cellular targets** (116,117). Both E6 and E7 proteins can immortalize primary keratinocytes from cervical epithelium and influence transcription from viral and cellular promoters (118). The activity of these viral oncoproteins results in genomic instability, leading to the malignant phenotype. **E6 proteins of high-risk HPV types bind the tumor suppressor protein p53** (119,120). This induces ubiquitination and degradation of p53, removing the p53-dependent control of the host cell cycle (121–123). The role of E6 as an antiapoptotic protein is of key significance in the development of cervical cancer.

E6 increases telomerase activity in keratinocytes through increased transcription of the *telomerase catalytic subunit* **gene (hTERT) via induction of** *c-myc* (124,125). Telomerase activity is usually absent in somatic cells, leading to shortening of *telomeres* with successive cell divisions and to eventual cell senescence. **E6 mediation of telomerase activity may predispose to long-term infection and the development of cancer.** *E6* and *E7* viral oncogenes have been shown to antagonize *BRCA*-mediated inhibition of the hTERT promoter (126).

The *E7* **gene product is a nuclear phosphoprotein that associates with the product of the** *retinoblastoma* **gene (pRb), which is a tumor suppressor gene important in the negative control of cell growth** (127–129). E7 is the primary transforming protein. Degradation of p53 by E6 and the functional inactivation of pRb by E7 represent the main mechanisms whereby expression of HPV E6 and E7 oncoproteins subverts the function of the negative regulators of the cell cycle (130–132). **Deregulated expression of the viral oncogenes is a predisposing factor to the development of HPV-associated cancers.**

The products of the *E2* gene are involved in transcriptional regulation of the HPV genome. The process of HPV integration into the cellular genome, which occurs in some high-grade CIN lesions and most invasive cervical cancers, disrupts the *E2* gene (133). This results in increased levels of E6 and E7 expression, correlating with increased immortalization activity (133–136).

Aberrant expression of high-risk viral oncogenes can predispose to the development of cervical cancer, but their expression alone is not sufficient (107). HPV-mediated oncogenesis requires accumulation of additional genetic mutations over time. The median age of women with invasive cervical cancer is approximately 45 to 50 years in an unscreened population, whereas the median age for women with CIN 3 is often under 30 years. This suggests a long precancerous state, which allows the accumulation of secondary genetic mutations. These mutations can occur randomly but may also reflect the influence of cofactors such as tobacco carcinogens and exogenous and endogenous hormonal influences (65).

Human Papillomavirus Type–Specific Disease Pattern

Over 100 HPV types have been identified, but 15 anogenital types are often termed "oncogenic"; these include HPV16, the most frequently involved, HPVs 18, 45, 31, 33, 35, 52, and 58, which are the next most commonly identified in cancer, and a further seven types with lower level and less certain contributions (HPVs 51, 56, 39, 59, 68, 73, and 66) (106) (Fig. 7.12).

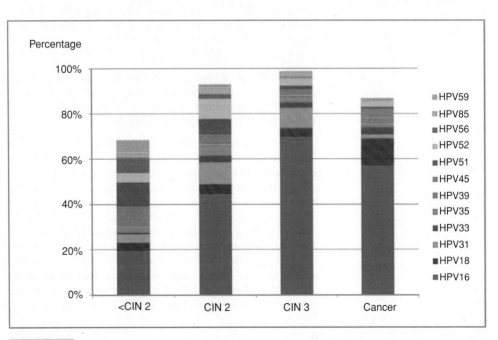

Figure 7.12 **Attribution of carcinogenic HPV types to cervical disease categories.** Expanded from the work of Wentzensen et al. The type attribution is based on the hierarchical attribution model for carcinogenic genotypes present in multiple infections. HPV genotyping is based on concurrent cytologic specimens, not on tissue specimens. From **Mark Schiffman M, Wentzensen N**. Human papillomavirus infection and the multistage carcinogenesis of cervical cancer. *Cancer Epidemiol Biomarkers Prev.* 2013;22(4):553–560.

Low-risk HPV types, particularly HPVs 6 and 11 (clade alpha-10), are associated with condylomata acuminata of the genital tract in both sexes. HPVs 6 and 11 are detected alone in low-grade cervical lesions (exophytic condylomata acuminata, subclinical HPV infection, CIN 1, and some CIN 2 lesions). These viruses are unable to integrate into the human genome. The E6 and E7 proteins of "low-risk" HPV types only weakly bind p53 and pRb, and thus do not immortalize keratinocytes *in vitro*.

Human papillomavirus 16 is the HPV type universally detected with greatest frequency in HPV-related invasive cancers. HPV16 is associated with 50% of cervical squamous cancers and about the same proportion of adenocarcinomas (137–140). It is present in a high proportion of high-grade cervical, vaginal, vulvar, perianal, and penile preinvasive lesions.

HPV18 is the second most common (20–25%) **HPV type in invasive cervical cancer** and is associated with the development of a substantial proportion of cervical adenocarcinomas. Organized cytologic screening programs have not been as effective against adenocarcinomas, rates of which have remained stable in some settings, while squamous cancers have declined (141).

Human Papillomavirus and Cervical Cancer: A Causal or Casual Association?

In the prevaccination era, most sexually active women were exposed to HPV infection (142) but **the majority of exposed women cleared a specific HPV-type within 2 years** (143,144). Humoral and cellular immune responses to natural infection with genital HPV types are inconsistently detected, possibly because the virus is nonlytic to infected cells and does not spread systemically. **Secondary peaks of HPV infection in older and postmenopausal women have suggested the possibility of reactivation of a latent viral reservoir caused by senescence of cell-mediated immunity,** although this could also potentially be explained by sexual behavior (of women or partners).

The longer a specific HPV type persists in the epithelium, the lower the probability of clearance within a defined period, and the greater the risk of precancer development (144). **HPV type is the strongest factor affecting risk of viral persistence** (66). A number of longitudinal studies have documented the long term risk of cervical precancer and cancer according to HPV type at baseline (47,48,67,145,146). Women exposed to HPV 16 are consistently documented to be at elevated risk. One of the longest reported follow-up periods has been for the Kaiser Permanente cohort in the USA, where the 16-year risk of developing CIN 3+ in women aged under 30 years was 14.6% (95% CI: 10 to 20.9) for women with HPV 16 at baseline; 7% (4.2 to 11.4), for women with other oncogenic HPV types, and 1.8% (1.2 to 2.5) for women with no HPV infection. For women over 30 years, the risks were 8.5% (95% CI: 4.1 to 17.2) for HPV 16, 3.1% (1.6 to 6.1) for other oncogenic types, and 0.7% (0.5 to 0.9) for HPV-negative women (47).

High viral loads do not generally imply an increased risk of progression, except for HPV16 (147,148). Recently acquired low-grade cervical lesions contain some of the highest viral loads, analogous to condylomata acuminata, and frequently regress (149). **In general terms, viral load measurement is not clinically useful** (9).

The median time from HPV infection to CIN 3 is short, often within 5 years (150). Infection occurs in the late teens or early twenties after the initiation of sexual activity (in unvaccinated populations) and the diagnosis of CIN 3 peaks at 25 to 30 years (138,150) or 20 to 24 years in some populations (141). CIN 3 has been diagnosed within 2 years of coitarche, and CIN 2 to 3 has been documented to rapidly develop within several months of an incident HPV infection (151,152). The biologic significance and risk of invasion associated with these early CIN 3 lesions is uncertain, but cytologic screening in women under 25 years is of limited effectiveness (153), and the International Agency for Research on Cancer (IARC) recommends starting screening at 25 years (3). The transit time from CIN 3 to invasive cancer is variable, **but long-term follow-up from an unethical experiment in women managed only by punch or wedge biopsy has suggested that about 30% of cases of CIN 3 will progress to invasive cancer over 30 years** (61). The major steps in the development of cervical cancer are summarized in Figure 7.13.

Cofactors in the Progression of Cervical Human Papillomavirus Infection

The established cofactors in progression of HPV infection to invasive cancer are the use of tobacco, multiparity, age at first full term pregnancy, and use of oral contraceptives (100–103). Host genetic factors influencing HPV infection control exist, but are poorly understood. There is a consistent human leucocyte antigen (HLA) association, reflecting the importance of T-cell responses in control of HPV infection and cervical cancer precursors (154). An earlier association between condom use and decreased persistence of high-risk and low-risk HPV types among high-risk

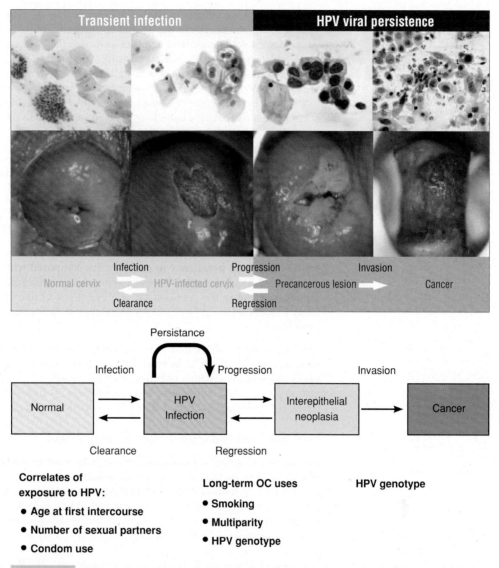

Figure 7.13 **Major steps in the development of cervical cancer.** Incident HPV infection is best measured by molecular tests. Most HPV infections show no concurrent cytologic abnormality. Approximately 30% of infections produce concurrent cytopathology, usually nonclassical (equivocal) changes. Most HPV infections clear within 2 years. Ten percent persist for 2 years and are highly linked to development of precancer. Top image reproduced with permission from **Schiffman M, Castle PE, Jeronimo J, et al.** Human papillomavirus and cervical cancer. *Lancet.* 2007;370:890–907; Bottom image reproduced with permission from **Mark Schiffman M, Wentzensen N.** Human papillomavirus infection and the multistage carcinogenesis of cervical cancer. *Cancer Epidemiol Biomarkers Prev.* 2013;22(4);553–560.

HPV-positive women has been confirmed (155,156). Increased HPV clearance and low-grade CIN regression with condom use has been reported (157).

Tobacco Use

Cigarette smoking has been demonstrated to be a risk factor for squamous cervical and vulvar carcinoma (100,158–163). An increased risk of developing a high-grade squamous intraepithelial lesion (HSIL) has been demonstrated among high-risk HPV positive women who smoke. It is uncertain whether smoking acts via an immunosuppressing or genotoxic pathway. The detection of high levels of genotoxic breakdown products of cigarette smoke—including nicotine, cotinine, hydrocarbons, and tars—in cervical secretions of smokers and the demonstration of mutagenic activity of these products in cervical cells, similar to that observed in lung cells, point to an important role for these compounds in cervical carcinogenesis.

Cigarette smoking influences epithelial immunity by decreasing the numbers of antigen-presenting Langerhans cells in the genital epithelium (164,165). Cervical HPV infection and CIN are associated with diminished numbers of intraepithelial Langerhans cells. Such local immunologic depletion could favor viral persistence, contributing to malignant transformation. Cigarette smoke concentrates have been demonstrated *in vitro* to transform HPV 16–immortalized endocervical cells (160). However, though squamous cervical cancer and adenocarcinoma share hormonal risk factors (increasing parity, younger age at first full-term pregnancy, and increasing duration of hormonal contraceptive use), smoking does not appear to be a risk factor for adenocarcinoma (103).

Sex Hormonal Influences

Condylomata acuminata may increase rapidly in size and number in pregnancy. This could suggest that maternal estrogen status is permissive for HPV replication, although it may reflect the immunosuppressive effect of pregnancy. Increased detection of HPV DNA in cervical cytologic samples in pregnancy, including detection of oncogenic HPV types in up to 27% of pregnant women, suggests hormonally induced active viral replication (166,167).

A pooled analysis of worldwide data has found that the relative risk of invasive cervical cancer for first full-term pregnancy under 17 years compared with 25 years or older is 1.77 (95% CI: 1.42 to 2.23). Independently of age at first full term pregnancy, parity has been shown to be a significant factor in the development of cervical cancer, the relative risk among parous women being 1.76 (95% CI: 1.53 to 2.02) for seven or more full-term pregnancies, compared with one or two (101).

The International collaboration of Epidemiologic Studies of Cervical Cancer has pooled the worldwide data and identified an increase in the relative risk of cervical cancer in current users of oral contraceptives, which declines after use ceases. Use for 10 years between the ages of 20 and 30 increased the cumulative incidence by age 50 from 7.3 to 8.3 per 1,000 women in less developed countries, and from 3.8 to 4.5 in more developed countries (102).

Exogenous and Endogenous Immunosuppression

Iatrogenic induction of immunosuppression in renal transplant recipients increases the rate of CIN to 16 times that of the general community (168). The risk of CIN and cervical cancer is increased in human immunodeficiency virus (HIV)–infected women and failure rates of treatment for preinvasive lesions are increased (169–173). Systemic immune suppression from diseases such as Hodgkin disease, leukemia, and collagen vascular diseases are associated with an increased incidence of HPV-associated disease (172,174).

Human Papillomavirus Vaccines

Over the last several years, prophylactic vaccination against HPV in young females has been introduced in most developed countries. The introduction of this intervention has been supported by evaluations of its cost-effectiveness, even in the context of cervical screening (175). Two vaccines are currently available—quadrivalent vaccine- *Gardasil* (Merck, USA) and bivalent vaccine- *Cervarix* (GSK, Belgium). These protect against HPV 16/18, together responsible for about 70% of invasive cervical cancers (176). HPV (predominantly HPV 16) has also been identified in varying fractions of vulval, vaginal, anal, penile, and oropharyngeal cancers (1) and thus the vaccines have the potential to prevent a proportion of these cancers. The quadrivalent vaccine also protects against HPV6/11 which is found to be associated with approximately 90% of anogenital warts.

HPV vaccination has been shown to be effective in preventing persistent infection and high-grade precancerous cervical intraepithelial neoplasia (CIN 2–3) in females naïve to HPV vaccine types (177) and at preventing persistent infection, external genital lesions, and anal intraepithelial neoplasia in males (178,179). In most countries, immunization programs have adopted the quadrivalent vaccine. Because the number of HPV-related cancers are lower in males than in females and heterosexual males benefit to some extent from female vaccination via herd immunity, inclusion of young males in vaccination programs is associated with a lower return on investment than female-only vaccination, especially if coverage in females is over 50%, because this increases the herd-immunity–induced protection to males (175,180,181).

Male vaccination has now been recommended in a few settings, including Australia, where publicly funded vaccination of 12- to 13-year-old boys commenced in 2013, with a 2-year catch-up to 14 to 15 years. **It has been recommended in the USA, Canada, and Austria,** but is not recommended in most other countries (175).

The HPV vaccine is a major scientific and public health advance in the prevention of HPV related cancer (182,183). **HPV prophylactic vaccines, designed to prevent HPV infection, are based on virus-like particle (VLP) technology** developed through the pioneering research of Zhou and Fraser in Brisbane, Australia, by Schiller and Lowy at the National Institutes of Health USA and by others (182–185). These DNA-free VLPs are empty capsids and contain no oncogenic or infectious materials. VLPs resemble the virus immunologically, and induce HPV type-specific antibody on administration (186,187). The immunogenicity of HPV involves presentation of the major capsid protein L1 to the immune system. L1 VLP vaccines induce strong, cell-mediated and humoral immune responses (188–191).

Vaccine Efficacy

Clinical trials have demonstrated that HPV vaccines are effective and safe (177,186–189,192,193). For ethical and scientific reasons, surrogate end points in efficacy trials have consisted of prevention of HPV acquisition and of persistent infection, development of high-grade precancerous lesions (CIN 2–3), and development of genital neoplasia and genital warts (as opposed to development of cervical cancer). Studies have been largely undertaken among sexually active women 16 to 25 years of age, although some studies have been extended to include women up to 45 years. Immunogenicity bridging studies have been carried out in young females and males aged 10 to 15 years, where antibody levels produced are substantially higher than in 16- to 23-year olds. A larger proportion of this population has been previously exposed to HPV, so that at a population level, effectiveness is lower. **For population effectiveness, and thus for cost-effectiveness reasons, vaccination of women aged over 26 years has not been routinely recommended within vaccination programs.** However, **novel "screen-and-vaccinate" strategies might be possible in settings where a transition to primary HPV based screening is taking place,** because women negative for particular HPV types could potentially be offered vaccination after screening. The cost-effectiveness of these new options requires detailed consideration.

In strict protocol studies, where only women naïve to the HPV types of interest have been considered, both the bivalent and quadrivalent vaccines have demonstrated efficacy approaching 98–100% in preventing high-grade cervical lesions among young sexually active women where the disease endpoints are associated with the vaccine-included types (177,182,183,186,192–199). In trial analyses that have included less strenuously defined criteria, such as including women with known infection or with disease associated with vaccine types prior to vaccination (and which are thus more likely to reflect actual population exposure in the relevant age group), vaccine efficacy is reduced. For example, the quadrivalent vaccine has been shown to be 44% effective in preventing CIN 2–3 associated with HPV 16 or HPV 18, in women aged 15 to 26 years (177).

No therapeutic effect has been demonstrated in women with vaccine-type existing HPV infection or HPV-related disease, with lesions regressing or progressing at similar rates in vaccine and placebo recipients (200). **Follow-up studies of women have demonstrated sustained efficacy for up to 10 years. Three doses of vaccine induce peak antibody levels many times higher than those seen with natural HPV infection** (182). Antibody levels fall significantly in the first 2 years after immunization, but remain above those stimulated by natural infection (201). A modeling study has suggested that antibody levels will remain above those associated with natural infection for 12 years or more (202). Immunologic memory is retained, and a single booster dose given 60 months postcompletion of the HPV vaccination protocol has been shown to produce a strong anamnestic increase in antibody titers, not seen in nonimmune subjects, with continued sustained efficacy typical of many vaccines (201). **There are indications that sustained vaccine-induced protection may be maintained with fewer than three doses** (203–205), and if confirmed, this has potential to reduce the cost of HPV vaccination (and thus to increase its cost-effectiveness), which will be of considerable importance in low resource settings. A recent Canadian trial found that the immunogenicity (geometric mean titres) for HPV 16 and HPV 18 one month after the last vaccine dose of a two-dose schedule at 0 and 6 months in girls 9 to 13 years was statistically noninferior to the immunogenicity in women receiving three doses (205). However, longer-term follow-up, more data on protection against disease endpoints for all HPV-related disease, and more extensive data in different age groups, will likely be needed before a recommendation to decrease the number of doses in routine vaccination schedules can be made (206). **Immunization with HPV 16 and 18 VLPs may provide some protection against other**

high-risk HPV types and development of associated disease, although the duration and degree of any cross-protection is not yet clear.

A next generation nonavalent vaccine from Merck is scheduled for market release (207). It will be based on the VLP technology used for the quadrivalent vaccine and will provide broad spectrum protection against HPV types responsible for 89% of cervical cancers by adding VLPs for types 31, 33, 45, 52, and 58 (208).

The nonavalent vaccine is currently in Phase III trials. There is uncertainty about whether high levels of efficacy against HPV 16/18 will be maintained, since increasing the valency may result in decreased effectiveness of the vaccine to individual HPV types through immune interference (209).

Vaccine Safety

No serious adverse effects attributable to vaccination have been seen in placebo controlled trials (177,192). Local reactogenicity at the immunization site, systemic malaise and fever have been slightly more common than with placebo, but have not led to discontinuation of the vaccination schedule. Since vaccine licensure, over 170 million doses of HPV vaccine have been given to young women. The product labeling has been revised to address issues for monitoring for anaphylaxis and syncope, outcomes previously identified as concerns (210).

A recent large scale data linkage study of approximately 300,000 girls vaccinated with quadrivalent vaccine in Sweden and Denmark compared them with almost 700,000 unvaccinated girls born from 1988 to 2000. It concluded that there was no evidence supporting associations between exposure to the vaccine and autoimmune, neurologic, or venous thromboembolic adverse events, and that although associations for three autoimmune events were initially observed, on further assessment these were weak and not temporally related to vaccine exposure (211).

A 2013 review of the worldwide experience by the WHO's Global Advisory Committee on Vaccine Safety (GAVCS) involved review of updated information about the safety of HPV vaccines. It concluded, **"In summary, 4 years after the last review of HPV vaccine safety and with more than 170 million doses distributed worldwide and more countries offering the vaccine through national immunization programs, the Committee continues to be reassured by the safety profile of the available products"** (210). Although vaccination in pregnancy is not recommended, HPV vaccination does not appear to be associated with increased rates of spontaneous pregnancy loss or adverse fetal outcomes (210,212,213).

Vaccine Deployment

The greatest public health benefit is achieved by vaccination of individuals prior to sexual initiation, as the vaccines are prophylactic (214). The US Advisory Committee on Immunization Practices (ACIP) has recommended routine vaccination of all 11- to 12-year-old girls with the quadrivalent HPV vaccine, and "catch-up" vaccination of all 13- to 26-year-old girls and women (215). Vaccination of 9- to 10-year-old girls should be at the providers' discretion.

Vaccination of young sexually active women may still provide some protection. Routine cytology or HPV DNA testing prior to vaccination is not currently recommended, although such screening may be appropriate for sexually active women as part of cervical screening practices. **Cervical cancer screening should continue for the immunized population, to screen for disease caused by nonvaccine HPV types,** and to screen HPV infected women, as the vaccine is not therapeutic.

The optimal vaccination-dosing schedule is three doses at 0, 2, and 6 months. Accelerated delivery schedules over 4 months are being used in some countries. **The US Advisory Committee on Immunization Practices (ACIP) has recommended** (215):

1. **First and second doses must be separated by at least 4 weeks.**
2. **Second and third doses must be separated by at least 12 weeks.**
3. **If the dosing schedule is interrupted, the vaccine series should not be restarted, but the required dose should be given as soon as possible.**

The vast majority of studies examining the cost-effectiveness of vaccination of preadolescent females suggest that vaccinating 12-year-old girls against HPV is cost-effective, even in the context of cervical screening (175). Cost savings are achieved by reducing abnormal Pap smears, colposcopy referrals, cervical biopsies, treatment procedures, and cancer-related treatment costs, as well as reducing the costs of diagnosis and treatment of genital warts. Reductions in these outcomes also increase quality of life, measured in cost-effectiveness analyses as Quality-Adjusted Life-Years Saved (QALYS). Vaccination will potentially reduce the costs and morbidity associated with the complications of treatment procedures among young women (216,217), although the association between cervical treatment and obstetric complications has not been confirmed in all studies and settings (218).

Some clinical trials have shown high levels of effectiveness of HPV vaccination in men (179). The decision regarding vaccination of men is more complex, because HPV causes fewer cancers in men, and vaccinating women offers some protection to men via herd immunity. Therefore **male HPV vaccination may not represent the best "value for money" compared to vaccinating more females or making other investments in health.** This determination in a particular setting will depend on vaccine price, coverage in females, achievable coverage in males, rates of HPV-related disease in males, and other factors.

HPV Vaccine Experience

Coverage rates achieved for vaccination of young females vary widely between countries. **The highest coverage rates have been achieved where national publicly funded school-based vaccination programs have been introduced,** including England (80%), Scotland (90%), and Australia (73%) (175). By contrast, coverage rates in countries that have implemented practitioner-based vaccination programs are lower; for example, in preadolescent girls in the USA, reported rates have been less than 50% (219).

Australia was the first country to introduce a national HPV vaccination program and it has achieved relatively high coverage rates in adolescent girls (220). In Australia, a 2-year vaccination catch-up was performed to age 26 years. The recommended age of first screening is 18 to 20 years in sexually active women, and participation rates in cervical screening are relatively high. This overlap between vaccinated and screened groups has led to early effects on the number of high-grade lesions identified through screening. An early postvaccination ecologic analysis identified a decreasing incidence of high-grade disease in women less than 18 years (221). For women under age 20 years, a decrease in CIN 2–3 from 7.8 to 7.1 per 1,000 women screened (9%) was observed between 2010 and 2011, corresponding to a total decrease from 13.2 to 7.1 (46%) between 2006 and 2011 (141). For women 20 to 24 years, rates were stable until 2010, and then decreased from 19.7 to 17.4 (12%) between 2010 and 2011 (141). **For the first time since the introduction of organized screening more than 20 years previously, the peak age for confirmed CIN 2–3 in Australia has shifted from 20 to 24 to 25 to 29 years.**

Australia uses the quadrivalent vaccine in its national program and a number of studies have documented substantial decreases in anogenital warts in Australia in cohorts of females who were eligible for HPV vaccination. Studies have documented lesser, but still substantial, reductions in anogenital warts in heterosexual males in the same age group, presumably as a result of herd immunity from female vaccination (222,223). By contrast, no substantial postvaccination changes in rates of anogenital warts in young men who have sex with men (MSM) or older women have been documented, which is consistent with the expected effect of female HPV vaccination.

In low resource settings, the Global Alliance for Vaccines and Immunization (GAVI) has announced that it will make the HPV vaccine available to females for under $5 per dose. It is hoped that this will drive increased vaccine utilization in some of those settings with the greatest need because of the high burden of HPV-related disease and the lack of organized cervical screening programs.

Screening for Cervical Neoplasia

Incidence and mortality rates for cervical cancer in the United States have steadily decreased since the 1950s (224,225). Although the overall incidence of cervical cancer in Western countries was beginning to decline before the introduction of screening efforts, the significant decreases in cervical cancer incidence and mortality can be largely attributed to the success of widespread screening (3,4,226–228).

A single Pap smear has limited sensitivity for the detection of cervical cancer and precancer. Strategies used in the past to compensate for this limited sensitivity include repeat screening at short intervals (such as annual Pap smears) and a low threshold for repeat smears or referral for colposcopy (Fig. 7.14). This approach is costly and generates many unnecessary follow-up examinations and tests. Prior to the introduction of 2012 changes in the recommendations,

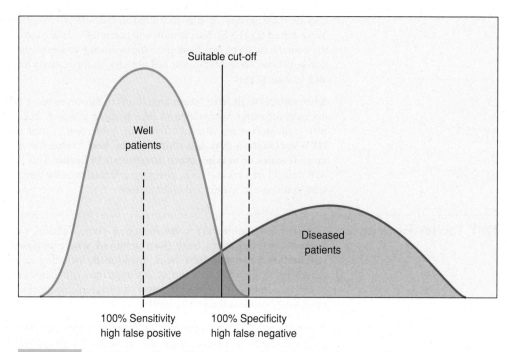

Suitable cut-off

Well patients

Diseased patients

100% Sensitivity
high false positive

100% Specificity
high false negative

Figure 7.14 Sensitivity and specificity of screening test as reciprocal ratios.

expenditure in the United States totaled $6 billion annually for more than 50 million screening tests and for the ongoing clinical care of women with mainly minor cytologic abnormalities (229).

The 2001 Bethesda System

The Bethesda System for reporting cervical/vaginal cytologic diagnoses was originally developed in 1988 at a US National Cancer Institute (Bethesda, MD) workshop (33). In 1991, a second NCI-sponsored workshop reviewed and modified the Bethesda System on the basis of laboratory and clinical experience (35).

A cervical–vaginal smear report using the revised 1991 Bethesda system had three components: (i) a description of smear adequacy; (ii) a general categorization (i.e., "within normal limits" or "not within normal limits"); and **(iii) description of the cytologic abnormality,** specifying whether squamous or glandular. Abnormal morphology that may represent preinvasive squamous disease fell into three descriptive categories: **ASC-US, LSIL, and HSIL.**

With the increased utilization of new cervical cancer screening technologies and in response to research findings, in 2001, the NCI sponsored a further multidisciplinary workshop to reevaluate and update the Bethesda System (TBS) (37) (See Chapter 5). This created standard reporting terms and criteria for each category of smear report, which has improved communication between pathologists and clinicians. TBS was designed to be consistent with current knowledge of HPV-associated disease and has enabled development of clinical management guidelines linked to standardized terminology.

Age at Start of Screening

In recent years, there has been a shift toward considering a later age to start cervical screening. **In 2006, the IARC recommended that cervical screening start at 25 years** (3). Population-based audit data have shown limited effectiveness of cytology in women younger than 25 years in preventing invasive cervical cancer before 30 years (153). HPV vaccination is expected to be a further factor driving a later age for commencement of screening.

A number of countries have raised, or are considering raising, the age for commencement of screening to 25 years. England implemented this change from 2004 and Wales from 2013; the Canadian Task Force recommended in 2012 that screening not start until age 25 years and Scotland will implement the change from 2015. In 2012, the revised guidelines in the USA recommended that screening should not start until age 21 years (230–232).

Table 7.5 Current US Cervical Cancer Screening Guidelines

Population	Screening Recommendation
Age group	
<21yr	Do not screen
21–29 yr	Perform cytologic testing alone every 3 yrs
30–65 yr	Perform cytologic and HPV co-testing every 5 yrs (preferred), or perform cytologic testing alone every 3 yrs (acceptable)[a]
>65 yr	Discontinue screening if there has been an adequate number of negative screening results previously (3 consecutive negative cytologic tests or 2 consecutive negative co-tests in the past 10 yrs, with the most recent test in the past 5 yrs) and if there is no history of HSIL,[b] adenocarcinoma *in situ,* or cancer.
Women who have undergone hysterectomy	Discontinue screening if the patient has undergone a total hysterectomy with removal of cervix and if there is no history of HSIL, adenocarcinoma *in situ,* or cancer.

The three major sets of screening guidelines were issued by the American Cancer Society, American Society for Colposcopy and Cervical Pathology, and American Society for Clinical Pathology Multisociety Guidelines Group; the American College of Obstetricians and Gynecologists; and the US Preventive Services Task Force (USPSTF). The guidelines agree on most recommendations, including the recommended age at the start of screening (21 years), the age at which screening can be discontinued if the history of negative screening is adequate (>65 years), and the recommended interval between tests. Specifically, co-testing at a 5-year interval is either preferred or acceptable for women 30 to 65 years of age, whereas cytologic testing alone every 3 years is acceptable for women 21 to 65 years of age. HSIL denotes high-grade squamous intraepithelial lesions.

[a]The terms "preferred" and "acceptable" are not included in the USPSTF Recommendation Statement.

[b]HSIL includes cervical intraepithelial neoplasia grade 3 and cases of grade 2 that stain positive for p16.

From: **Schiffman M, Solomon D**. Cervical cancer screening with human papillomavirus and cytologic cotesting. *N Engl J Med.* 2013;369:2324–2331. doi:10.1056/NEJMcpl210379.

Cervical Screening Interval

The IARC recommended that cervical screening with cytology should occur every 3 years in women 25 to 39 years, and every 5 years in women 50 to 65 years (3). This is underpinned by studies designed to assess the optimal interval at each age (233) and analysis of trends in various countries, which show similar outcomes in countries implementing three-yearly screening recommendations compared to those with more frequent screening (4,234).

The 2012 ACS/ASCCP/ASC guidelines in the USA and the 2012 Canadian Task Force guidelines recommend three-yearly cytologic screening. The ASCCP guidelines recommend that women should be screened every 3 years from 21 to 30 years with liquid-based cytology (LBC); and either thereafter every 3 years with LBC, or with co-testing with LBC and HPV DNA every 5 years (230) (Table 7.5). Evidence suggests that HPV-based primary screening can be safely performed at intervals of 5 years (235), and this is under consideration in a number of countries.

Test Performance Characteristics of Conventional Cervical Cytologic Screening

Cytologic screening has been highly successful in reducing the incidence and mortality from invasive cervical cancer in most industrialized countries. The Pap smear is associated with a significant false-negative rate, with an absolute sensitivity for detection of high-grade CIN 2–3 of the order of 50–60% in meta-analyses (236), although it can be up to 70% in some settings (237). A large US review previously concluded that the sensitivity of a single conventional smear was 51% (238). This reflects the inherent suboptimal sensitivity of conventional cytologic screening (Fig. 7.14). In nonindustrialized countries, many women in whom invasive cancer develops have never been screened or have been underscreened. The main factors contributing to the false-negative rate are (i) specimen collection; (ii) laboratory error; and (iii) deficiencies in laboratory quality assurance mechanisms.

Specimen Collection

The accuracy of cytologic diagnosis is highly sensitive to sample-to-sample variation in number of cells per smear. The cervix may desquamate unpredictably. A large, four-quadrant high-grade lesion may fail to provide representative cells despite conscientious sampling.

The patient should be informed to refrain from douching or using tampons or intravaginal medications for at least 48 hours before the scheduled examination. She should avoid intercourse for 48 hours before the visit and should reschedule if menstrual bleeding occurs. **Best results are obtained by paired use of the Ayre's spatula and cytobrush, or sampling devices that adequately sample both endocervix and ectocervix** (239).

Laboratory Error

A proportion of false-negative smear reporting is attributable to laboratory error. In response to medical and media pressure to address this problem, there has been a significant increase in the number of smears reported as showing minor abnormalities. Laboratory quality-assurance processes, including systematic review of a proportion of smears reported as negative, have been introduced in many countries to address laboratory error.

Specificity of Cervical Cytologic Screening

Competent laboratories operate with a false-positive rate between 2% and 5% for the diagnosis of high-grade disease (240).

Liquid-Based, Thin-Layer Cervical Cytology

Liquid-based cytology (LBC) is an alternate method for slide preparation. **Instead of smearing the sample onto a glass slide, the collection device is rinsed in a vial containing 20 mL of a buffered alcoholic liquid preservative.**

Two LBC technologies are available—*ThinPrep* method (Cytyc Corporation, Boxborough, MA) and *SurePath* (Becton Dickinson and Company, Franklin Lakes, NJ, USA). **The slide preparation technique is automated.** Slide evaluation is usually performed by cytotechnicians/cytologists, and both technologies have **automated image analysis systems** (Fig. 7.15).

In the United States and in many European countries, there has been rapid adoption of LBC for cervical screening over the past two decades, despite the lack of large randomized studies (242); although a randomized trial of LBC versus conventional cytology in the Netherlands was conducted (243). Technologic improvements, particularly the use of an automated imager, have increased this utilization. **The ability to test LBC specimens for HPV DNA and other sexually transmitted organisms further enhances the clinical appeal of this technology.** Furthermore, LBC has been shown to be associated with substantial reductions in the smear unsatisfactory (inadequate) rate (244). In England, this rate reduced from >7% to ~2% in the years since LBC was phased in as a replacement for conventional cytology.

A large scale meta-analysis of the comparative performance of LBC has suggested that its sensitivity for detection of CIN 2–3 is similar to that of conventional cytology, but its specificity for CIN 2–3 is somewhat lower at the ASCUS detection threshold (245); the Netherlands trial results were similar, finding that LBC does not perform better than conventional cytology in terms of relative sensitivity and positive predictive value for detection of CIN 2 or CIN 3 (243).

In most countries, LBC has been found to be cost-effective (246) and use of the liquid-based sample is an important transition to use of HPV DNA testing, for example, when used as a triage for low-grade cytologic results, which in many places is performed routinely from the LBC sample.

HPV DNA Testing

Understanding the central role of HPV in the development of cervical cancer has led to two effective preventive strategies in addition to Pap tests. These are primary prevention by vaccination and enhanced secondary prevention (screening) with the use of HPV-based molecular assays (247). There are various possible applications for HPV DNA testing in the cervical screening pathway. These include use of **HPV as a test-of-cure** following treatment of CIN 2–3 lesions; **HPV triage after LSIL cytology;** and **primary screening**. Several clinically positioned HPV testing systems allow large-scale automation and partial genotyping for HPV 16/18. This provides the potential for further risk stratification of HPV 16/18 positive women compared to women positive for other oncogenic types.

HPV Test-of-cure after CIN Treatment

High-risk HPV detection is implemented in many settings as a test-of-cure following treatment for high-grade disease. A recent meta-analysis of the international data has found that HPV has a 21–25% increase in the relative sensitivity for detection of recurrent or residual high-grade disease compared to follow-up cytology, but equivalent specificity (248). **HPV testing in posttreatment follow-up may result in earlier diagnosis of persistent or recurrent disease** (249).

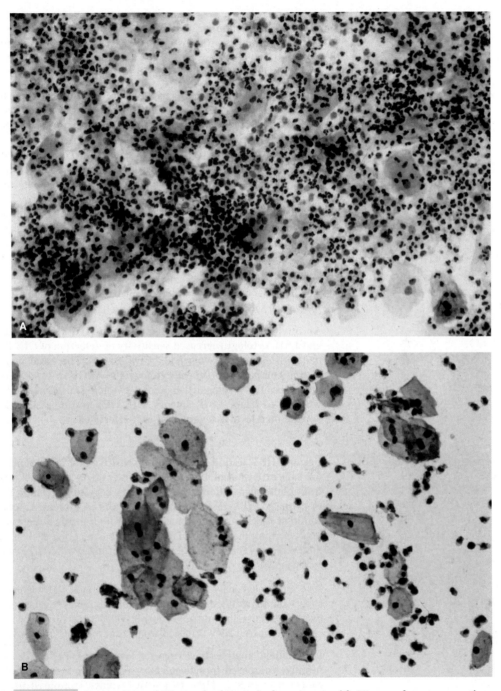

Figure 7.15 Comparison of (A) standard Papanicolaou smear with (B) monolayer preparation.

The recommendations for, and cost-effectiveness of, posttreatment HPV testing may vary by setting. A US study concluded that HPV testing after treatment was not cost-effective (250), and another US study concluded that although posttest risks were not sufficiently low to return women to 5-year routine screening, negative cytology and HPV co-testing after treatment provided more reassurance than using either test alone (251). However, a recent UK study and associated cost-effectiveness analysis, which took into account limitations in compliance with posttreatment attendance for annual cytologic follow-up, found that **a single posttreatment HPV test, after which women are discharged to routine screening if they are HPV negative, can be both more effective and more cost-effective than annual cytology after treatment** (252).

HPV Triage Testing after ASCUS and/or LSIL Cytology

The USA and a number of other countries have introduced recommendations for HPV triage testing for women with low-grade (ASCUS) cytology, to determine which women should be referred for colposcopy to identify the minority of women with clinically significant disease, while avoiding excessive intervention for others.

The US guidelines for HPV triage have been informed by the ASC-US/LSIL Triage Study (ALTS) (39,40,45,46,253–261) which was a multicenter, randomized trial comparing the sensitivity and specificity of the following management strategies to detect CIN 3 among women referred with ASC-US and LSIL smear reports: (i) Immediate colposcopy (considered to be the reference standard); (ii) triage to colposcopy based on enrollment HPV DNA testing results from Hybrid Capture 2 (HC2) and LBC results with a colposcopic referral threshold of HSIL; or (iii) conservative management, with triage based on repeat cytology alone at a referral threshold of HSIL. The trial had a majority of young women, with a median age of 25 years, and included 2-year follow-up with exit colposcopy. The overall percentage of CIN 2–3 in the ASCUS study population was 15.4% and in this group HPV triage was at least as sensitive as immediate colposcopy for detecting CIN 3: however, only half as many of these women required referral for colposcopy.

The ASCCP's 2001 Consensus Management Guidelines stated that reflex HPV testing was the preferred triage for an ASC-US smear result when LBC primary screening was used (255). This recommendation has been included as an acceptable option for ASCUS triage in the 2012 ASCCP guidelines for women aged 20 to 24 years and as a preferred option for ASCUS triage in older women (86).

An international meta-analysis found that HPV triage testing of women with both ASCUS and LSIL cytology increased sensitivity of detection of CIN 2–3 (248). However, the specificity trade-offs differed for women in the two groups. There was no loss of specificity for HPV triage testing compared to repeat cytology for ASCUS, whereas HPV testing was associated with lower specificity compared to repeat cytology in women with LSIL (248). The decision on whether to triage LSIL smears with HPV testing is therefore setting specific and should depend on a local assessment of cost-effectiveness.

Primary HPV Screening

Because HPV testing is both more sensitive and more reproducible than cytology, it allows for safe extension of the screening interval to at least 5 years at all ages (235,262). HPV testing has been endorsed as a primary cervical screening method by IARC (3). Compared to cytology, HPV testing generally results in increased detection of CIN 2–3 in the initial round of screening but reduced rates of high-grade disease in the follow-up round of screening. One trial, the UK's ARTISTIC trial, has reported decreased disease in the HPV arm over a third screening round (263). Lower rates of invasive cervical cancer have also been demonstrated following HPV screening (264,265).

A recent pooled analysis of longitudinal data on 175,000 women from European trials (266) has shown similar ability of HPV and cytology to protect against developing invasive cervical cancer over short term follow-up (2 years or less), but up to 60–70% increased protection against invasive cervical cancer in HPV screened women for intervals up to 5 years.

Longitudinal analyses have reported lower rates of CIN 3 or invasive cancer over time in HPV-negative compared to cytologically-negative women, and higher rates of CIN 3 or invasive cancer over time in HPV 16 positive women compared to other HPV types (47,48,67,267). Because vaccination does not affect the clearance of existing HPV infections (200), HPV testing can risk-stratify women irrespective of whether they have been offered vaccination, and if so, whether they were effectively vaccinated. The latter depends in part on dose completion (203–205,268), and for catch-up vaccination cohorts, on whether individuals were already exposed to HPV at the time of vaccination. Primary HPV testing as a stand-alone test should in future allow for the simplification of screening recommendations in the postvaccination era. However, in the US context HPV screening and cytology are used for co-testing. The key clinical points in relation to current HPV primary screening and contesting in the United States are summarized in Table 7.6.

The HPV test technology for which the most clinical evidence is available provides a pooled result for the presence of any oncogenic type; in most trials, these women have been triaged to colposcopy using cytology. A new generation of high-throughput automated HPV testing platforms are emerging which can perform partial genotyping, stratifying outputs with respect to whether HPV types 16,18 are present, which, in future primary HPV screening strategies, can potentially be used to further stratify management (269).

Table 7.6 Cervical Cancer Screening with Human Papillomavirus and Cytologic Contesting in the United States

- Cervical cancer screening in the United States should not start until the age of 21 yrs, since adolescents are at extremely low risk for cervical cancer but have high rates of transient human papillomavirus (HPV) infections and associated minor cytologic abnormalities.
- The risk of cervical precancer and cancer is very low in the years after a negative HPV test.
- For women in the United States who are 30 yrs of age or older (past the age at which new HPV infections peak), co-testing with HPV and cytologic tests every 5 yrs is an accepted alternative to cytologic testing alone every 3 yrs.
- Molecular testing for HPV, together with cytologic testing, yields multiple possible combinations of results, with varying associated risks of precancer and cancer; management strategies are guided by the magnitude of risk.

From: **Schiffman M, Solomon D**. Cervical-cancer screening with human papillomavirus and cytologic cotesting. *N Engl J Med.* 2013;369:2324–2331. doi:10.1056/NEJMcpl210379.

Effect of Vaccination on Cervical Screening

Preliminary modeled evaluations confirm that cervical screening, if recommendations remain unchanged, will be less cost-effective in vaccinated compared to unvaccinated cohorts (270–272). Cervical screening will likely need to change to maintain cost-effectiveness, but a recent review concluded "it is not yet clear whether there will be generalizable conclusions for optimizing screening, or whether differences in vaccination coverage, timing, catch-up ages, disparities in vaccination uptake, screening compliance, and the existing screening background will drive differing screening recommendations across settings" (175).

Revised strategies that reduce the number of primary tests but maintain overall screening effectiveness at a population level are a high priority; but it is likely that changes to cervical screening will occur over different time frames in different countries and this will depend in part on vaccination uptake. In the United States, one strategy for increasing the screening interval involves the use of co-testing in women 30 years of age and over (Fig. 7.16). The combination of cytologic screening with HPV testing produces many different result combinations. Each combination produces different risks of associated CIN 3 and invasive cancer. Management is determined by risk assessment (Table 7.7).

Systematic Approach to Colposcopy

Colposcopy is the examination of the epithelia of the cervix, lower genital tract, and anogenital area using magnified illumination after the application of specific solutions to detect abnormal appearances consistent with neoplasia, or to affirm normality. Integral to the procedure is targeting biopsies to areas of greatest abnormality.

Indications for Colposcopy

Colposcopy is most frequently performed in response to an abnormal cervical smear. Abnormal findings on adjunctive screening tests, such as HPV testing, can also be the indication for colposcopy. If the cervix is clinically abnormal or suspicious on naked-eye examination, colposcopy is indicated. Abnormal and unexplained intermenstrual or postcoital bleeding and unexplained, persistent vaginal discharge may be assessed by colposcopy to exclude a neoplastic cause. Other indications include a personal history of in utero *diethylstilbestrol (DES)* exposure (rare in modern practice), vulvar or vaginal neoplasia, or condylomata acuminata, and possibly in some settings, sexual partners of patients with genital tract neoplasia or condylomata acuminata.

There are no absolute contraindications to colposcopy. The examination may be deferred until after bleeding ceases for women who are menstruating. **Acute cervicitis or vulvovaginitis should be evaluated and treated before colposcopy is performed,** unless poor patient compliance is anticipated. The colposcopic procedure should be modified in pregnancy, with a less liberal use of biopsy in the absence of warning signs of high-grade disease or cancer, and avoidance of endocervical curettage. **Postmenopausal women who are not taking hormone replacement may benefit from a 3-week course of topical or oral estrogen before colposcopy.** Patients should avoid use of all intravaginal products for 24 hours before the examination.

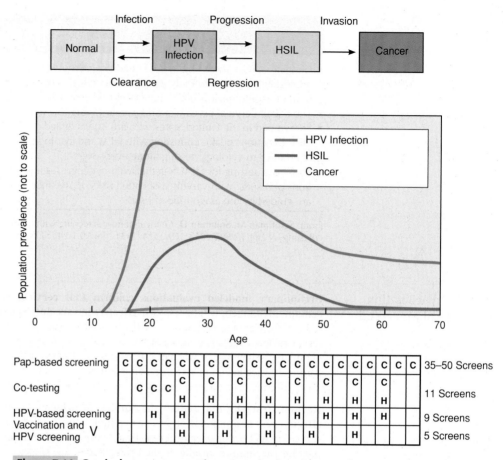

Figure 7.16 **Cervical cancer prevention strategies based on cytology, HPV testing, and HPV vaccination are shown with the effective total number of screens among screen-negative women per lifetime correlated against the prevalence of HPV infections, HSILs, and cancer by age.** The figure shows the natural history model and the corresponding prevalence of HPV infection, HSILs, and cancer in the population. Data on HPV infections are based on a summary of US-based HPV prevalence studies (50). The age distribution of HSIL is estimated on the basis of data on CIN 2 and CIN 3 from Kaiser Permanente Northern California (W. Kinney) and the data on cancers are from the SEER 17 database (http://seer.cancer.gov/). From: **Mark Schiffman M, Wentzensen N**. Human papillomavirus infection and the multistage carcinogenesis of cervical cancer. *Cancer Epidemiol Biomarkers Prev.* 2013;22(4):553–560.

Initial Clinical Workup

The patient should be prepared for the examination by a comprehensive explanation of the indication for colposcopy and a verbal description of the procedure. A complete medical history and general examination should be obtained. **A history of previous premalignant cervical disease or cervical treatment should be determined. A history of endogenous or exogenous immune suppression is relevant. A smoking history should be obtained.**

A clinical and speculum examination of the cervix, vagina, vulva, and perianal areas should be performed before the colposcopic examination. Squamous neoplasia may be **multicentric** (involving more than one genital tract site, i.e., cervix, vagina, or vulva) or **multifocal** (involving several areas at one site). A bimanual pelvic and rectal examination should be performed, usually on completion of the colposcopy, to exclude clinically apparent coexistent gynecologic or pelvic disease. Uncommonly, abnormal cervical smears are caused by palpable malignancies of the endocervix, uterine body, adnexae, or bowel.

Locating the Source of Abnormal Cells

Colposcopy is performed in the dorsal lithotomy position with a drape covering the patient's legs. The cervix is visualized using a standard speculum. The colposcopic examination involves the application of three standard solutions to the cervix:

Result on Cytologic Testing or Co-testing	Frequency of Screening Result (%)[a]	Risk of Histologic HSIL and Cancer (%)[b]	Suggested Management
Table 7.7 Ranked 5-Year Risk of HSIL and Cancer and Suggested Management According to Test Results			
SCC	0.0048	84	Immediate colposcopy
HPV+/HSIL	0.20	71	Immediate colposcopy
HSIL	0.21	69	Immediate colposcopy
HPV−/HSIL	0.013	49	Immediate colposcopy
HPV+/AGC	0.054	45	Immediate colposcopy
HPV+/ASC-H	0.12	45	Immediate colposcopy
ASC-H	0.17	35	Immediate colposcopy
HPV+/LSIL	0.81	19	Immediate colposcopy
HPV+/ASC-US	1.1	18	Immediate colposcopy
LSIL	0.97	16	Immediate colposcopy
AGC	0.21	13	Immediate colposcopy
HPV−/ASC-H	0.051	12	Immediate colposcopy
HPV+/Pap−	3.6	10	Repeat testing in 6–12 mo
ASC-US	2.8	6.9	Repeat testing in 6–12 mo
HPV−/LSIL	0.19	5.1	Repeat testing in 6–12 mo
HPV−/AGC[c]	0.16	2.2	Immediate colposcopy
HPV−/ASC-US	1.8	1.1	Repeat testing in 3 yr
Pap−	96	0.68	Repeat testing in 3 yr
HPV−/Pap−	92	0.27	Repeat testing in 5 yr

The data are based on cytologic testing and co-testing performed by Kaiser Permanente Northern California. Under the principle of similar management of similar risks, the management guidelines for co-testing results were "benchmarked" to the current management of cytologic-testing-only results. In accordance with the Bethesda System, AGC denotes atypical glandular cells, ASC-H atypical squamous cells (cannot rule out high-grade lesion), ASC-US atypical squamous cells of undetermined significance, LSIL low-grade squamous intraepithelial lesion, Pap Papanicolaou test, and SCC squamous-cell carcinoma. Minus signs denote negative, and plus signs positive

[a]The frequencies of cytologic-testing-only results are derived from data for all women with cytologic testing results, and the frequencies of co-testing results are derived from data for all women with co-testing results.

[b]The frequency of HSIL and cancer was estimated by the Kaiser histologic diagnoses of CIN 2, CIN 3, adenocarcinoma *in situ*, and cancer.

[c]For HPV−/AGC, the cancer risk remained high, justifying immediate colposcopy.

From: **Schiffman M, Solomon D**. Cervical-cancer screening with human papillomavirus and cytologic cotesting. *N Engl J Med*. 2013;369:2324–2331. doi:10.1056/NEJMcp1210379.

1. **Normal saline is initially applied to remove obscuring mucus and debris, to moisten the cervix, and to examine the cervix unaltered by subsequent solutions.** The two abnormal colposcopic findings detected after application of normal saline are **hyperkeratosis** (leukoplakia) and **atypical vessels**. Hyperkeratosis is a white, thickened epithelial area of the cervix (or lower genital tract) that is clinically apparent before application of acetic acid. Biopsy is indicated to exclude an underlying neoplastic process. Atypical vessels are the colposcopically apparent bizarre vascular abnormalities that occur in association with invasive cancer. **Green-filter examination of the cervix enhances the angioarchitecture.**

2. **A 3–5% acetic acid solution is then liberally applied to the cervix using soaked swabs or a spray technique. The abnormal colposcopic findings after application of acetic acid are acetowhite epithelium and abnormal vascular patterns.** Abnormal vascular patterns, reflecting the underlying capillary distribution, are mosaicism and punctation. Tissue swelling associated with the initial application of acetic acid compresses subepithelial capillaries, rendering vascular patterns less distinct. As the acetic

acid reaction fades, **mosaicism and punctation** become vivid against the whiter background.

3. **Lugol iodine (one-quarter strength) application to the cervix (if the patient is not allergic to iodine) is called a Schiller test.** Normal ectocervical and vaginal squamous epithelium contains glycogen, and stains mahogany brown after application of iodine solution. Normal columnar epithelium and immature squamous metaplastic or neoplastic epithelium do not contain glycogen, are not stained by iodine solution, and appear mustard yellow. Iodine solution application is considered an optional colposcopic procedure and is not uniformly performed, but is invaluable in the assessment of the vaginal mucosa.

Delineating the Margins of the Lesion

After the source of abnormal cells in a cervical smear has been located, the peripheral and distal margins of the lesion should be determined.

Distal Margin

The distal or peripheral margin of the lesion is usually readily identified. Occasionally, the lesion may extend onto the vaginal fornix.

Proximal Margin

Delineation of the proximal or upper margin of the lesion requires the colposcopic visualization of the new squamocolumnar junction, which establishes the colposcopy as adequate or inadequate using current ASCCP terminology. Failure accurately to delineate the position of the new squamocolumnar junction represents one of the most common colposcopic triage errors. An endocervical speculum may be helpful if the proximal margin is within the canal.

Endocervical Curettage

Endocervical curettage is performed to exclude an occult cancer in the canal (273). Cervical adenocarcinoma *in situ* (AIS) and invasive adenocarcinoma may be associated with squamous CIN lesions and endocervical curettage may provide a safeguard against missing such lesions.

Routine performance of endocervical curettage is controversial. When the entire new squamocolumnar junction can be visualized, it is reasonable to omit endocervical curettage. A negative endocervical curettage from a patient with an abnormal high-grade cytology and an unsatisfactory colposcopy does not exclude occult endocervical cancer, and excisional cone biopsy remains mandatory. **When specifically indicated, collection of an endocervical sample using a cytobrush may be a more sensitive sampling device than endocervical curettage for endocervical squamous and glandular disease.** Specificity, however, may be decreased (274–276).

Colposcopically Directed Cervical Biopsy

Cervical biopsies should be directed to the most significant lesions. Multiquadrant lesions may require multiple biopsies. Any area suspicious for occult invasion must be carefully sampled. The most reliable method of ensuring the accuracy of targeted biopsies is to grade lesions by deriving a colposcopic score. Cervical biopsies should be taken through the colposcope. The colposcopic grading score of the lesions and the biopsy sites should be recorded.

Documentation of Colposcopic Findings

The findings of the colposcopic examination should be carefully documented. **Photodocumentation can be extremely valuable.** A system for recording patient information, laboratory results, management plan, and tracking log should be established and maintained to ensure appropriate patient care and follow-up. **Modern computerized systems provide for many of these needs.**

The Abnormal Transformation Zone

If the transformation zone is deviated along a neoplastic pathway, epithelial, and vascular alterations produce the characteristic morphologic appearances of the abnormal transformation zone (87,277). The colposcopic signs of the abnormal transformation zone are described above in Table 7.3.

Squamous metaplasia, repair and regeneration, inflammation, and infection may all produce abnormal colposcopic transformation zone findings, such as acetowhite epithelium and abnormal vessels. Significant changes in the hormonal milieu such as accompany pregnancy, oral contraceptive pill use, estrogen withdrawal, and estrogen replacement can produce abnormal colposcopic signs in the absence of cervical disease. Atypical vessels, considered

one of the colposcopic hallmarks of invasive cancer, can occur in association with benign conditions, including immature metaplasia, nabothian follicles, inflammation, radiation treatment, and granulation tissue.

Colposcopic Grading Systems

The basis of colposcopic decision making is the process of cytologic–colposcopic–histologic correlation, with each component affording certain safeguards. **There are four basic colposcopic diagnoses: (i) Normal, (ii) low-grade disease (HPV infection/CIN 1), (iii) high-grade disease (CIN 2 or CIN 3), and (iv) invasive cancer.** Colposcopic grading systems have been developed to provide an objective, accurate, reproducible, and clinically meaningful prediction of the severity of CIN lesions based on discriminatory analysis of specific colposcopic signs (90,278–280).

The progress made in cervical cancer prevention over the past 60 years is largely a result of the detection and treatment of precancer, particularly CIN 3, before invasive cancer develops. **Over the past decade, the accuracy of colposcopy and colposcopically directed biopsy for detection of high-grade lesions has been widely studied** (281–291). However, several of these studies were not originally designed to assess colposcopic performance and several used static digitized cervigrams or colposcopic photographic images, which are not representative of the performance of "real-time" clinical colposcopy, particularly if it is performed in expert referral centers. Stoler et al. (289) compared the results of colposcopically directed biopsy with subsequent cervical excision (definitive therapy) among 737 women in the placebo arm of the quadrivalent HPV vaccine randomized controlled trials. The authors concluded that "colposcopy functioned well when allowed a one-degree difference between the biopsy and the surgical histologic interpretations, as done in clinical practice"; when CIN 2 was grouped together with CIN 3 and AIS as the diagnosis of high-grade disease, the overall agreement was 92% (289).

It has been suggested that the accuracy of colposcopic diagnosis could be improved by taking more than one biopsy at colposcopy (289,290), potentially including random biopsies from normal tissue. This would be essentially a return to the precolposcopy era of four-quadrant cervical biopsies. However, this suggestion needs to be balanced against the inevitable increase in patient discomfort, psychological trauma, and cost. It is likely that in many settings with comprehensively trained colposcopists and with quality assurance systems in place, current clinical management systems will be retained.

Routine determination of a colposcopic diagnosis has permitted quality control measures to be implemented in colposcopy (293–295). In colposcopic quality control programs, the colposcopist is required to achieve for example at least an 80% accuracy rate in colposcopic–histologic correlation or receive remedial training in colposcopic assessment of cervical lesions.

The Reid Colposcopic Index represents the most reproducible and clinically valid means of standardizing the evaluation of cervical lesions (90,279,280) (Table 7.8). A new colposcopic index, the Swede Index (295), based on, but modifying the Reid Index, has been demonstrated to produce a high level of colposcopic–histologic correlation (296) (Table 7.9).

Reid Colposcopic Index   The Reid Colposcopic Index uses four colposcopic features of premalignant cervical lesions to achieve predictive accuracy (Table 7.8). The colposcopic index permits accurate differentiation of low-grade from high-grade disease. It is not designed to differentiate premalignant from malignant cervical neoplasia. **The four colposcopic criteria used are (i) the margin of the lesion; (ii) the color of the acetowhitening; (iii) the type of vascular pattern; and (iv) the iodine staining reaction.**

The four colposcopic signs are scored individually and sequentially. The value of these colposcopic signs is maximized by combining them into a weighted scoring system. Scores of 0, 1, or 2 are assigned for each criterion. The four scores are added, and the total score is reported as a ratio, the denominator of which is constant at 8. **Scores of 0 to 2 are predictive of low-grade lesions (HPV infection/CIN 1;** Fig. 7.17). **Scores of 6 to 8 usually denote high-grade lesions** (CIN 2–3; Fig. 7.18). Scores of 3 to 5 represent an area of overlap between low-grade and high-grade lesions. **The overall predictive accuracy of the index exceeds 90% after a short training period.** The colposcopic index permits a significantly more accurate colposcopic–histologic agreement than can be achieved by less systematic approaches.

Swede Colposcopic Index   The Swede Colposcopic Index (developed by Strander et al. from Sweden) (295) is largely derived from the Reid Index, although the descriptive terms for color after application of acetic acid, margins of the lesion, and appearance after application of iodine are less accurate. **This scoring system adds lesion size as a further independent variable predictive of**

	Score		
Colposcopic Sign	**Zero Points**	**One Point**	**Two Points**

Table 7.8 Scoring System for Developing the Reid Colposcopic Index

Colposcopic Sign	Zero Points	One Point	Two Points
Margin	Exophytic condylomas; areas showing a micropapillary contour Lesions with distinct edges Feathered, scalloped edges Lesions with an angular, jagged shape "Satellite" areas and acetowhitening distal to the original squamocolumnar junction	Lesions with a regular (circular or semicircular) shape, showing smooth, straight edges	Rolled, peeling edges Any internal demarcation between areas of differing colposcopic appearance
Color	Shiny, snow-white color Areas of faint (semitransparent) whitening	Intermediate shade (shiny, but gray-white)	Dull reflectance with oyster-white color
Vessels	Fine-caliber vessels, poorly formed patterns	No surface vessels	Definite, coarse punctation or mosaic
Iodine	Any lesion staining mahogany brown; mustard-yellow staining by a minor lesion (by the first three criteria)	Partial iodine staining (mottled pattern)	Mustard-yellow staining of a significant lesion (an acetowhite area scoring 3 or more points by the first three criteria)

Adapted from **Reid R, Scalzi P**. Genital warts and cervical cancer: VII. An improved colposcopic index for differentiating benign papillomaviral infections from high-grade cervical intraepithelial neoplasia. *Am J Obstet Gynecol.* 1985;153:611–618.

disease severity (Table 7.9). The association between lesion size with CIN 3 and risk of occult invasion is well known. It is also well known that CIN 2–3 lesions often extend over several quadrants of the cervix. The implication of the Swede Index is that large low-grade lesions may harbor foci of evolving high-grade disease and that size of a low-grade lesion may be a predictor of risk of undetected high-grade disease. This will be determined by the location of the lesion. Large low-grade lesions outside the transformation zone or within already mature squamous metaplasia will rarely be high grade.

A large low-grade lesion within a large, immature transformation zone is very difficult to interpret colposcopically and multiple biopsies will frequently detect focal areas of evolving high-grade disease. This is a common source of the discrepancy between colposcopic prediction and ultimate disease severity. Accurate use of the Reid Index will often predict this evolving

Table 7.9 Scoring System for Developing the Swede Colposcopic Index

Swede Score	0	1	2
Aceto uptake	Zero or transparent	Shady, milky Neither transparent nor opaque	Distinct Opaque White
Margins/surface	Diffuse	Sharp but irregular, jagged, geographic satellites	Sharp, even difference in surface level, includes cuffing
Vessels	Fine, regular	Absent	Coarse or Atypical
Lesion size	<5 cm	5–15 cm or Two quadrants	>15 cm or Three to four quadrants or undefined endocervically
Iodine staining	Brown	Faintly or patchy yellow	Distinct yellow
Total score			

Adapted from: **Strander B, Ellstrom-Andersson A, Franzen S, et al.** The performance of a new scoring system for colposcopy in detecting high-grade dysplasia in the uterine cervix. *Acta Obstet Gynecol Scand.* 2005;84:1013–1017.

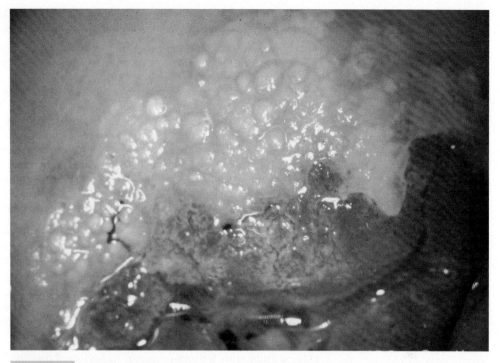

Figure 7.17 Colposcopy of a low-grade cervical lesion showing acetowhite epithelium with fine abnormal vascular pattern.

severity as the vessel pattern score will often be high grade reflecting the location of the lesion within immature metaplasia and, as a result, nonstaining with iodine will also be scored as high grade. The **addition of size of lesion as an independent predictor of disease severity is likely to be of value.** The suggestion by the authors that colposcopic scoring could be used to avoid biopsy for low scoring lesions should be interpreted with caution.

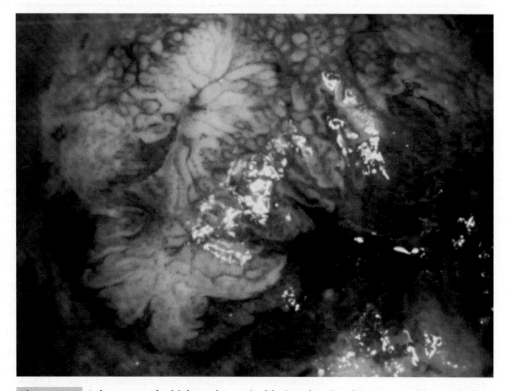

Figure 7.18 Colposcopy of a high-grade cervical lesion showing dense acetowhite epithelium and coarse abnormal vascular pattern.

Table 7.10 Colposcopic Warning Signs of Invasive Cancer

1. Yellow, degenerate, friable epithelium particularly with contact bleeding
2. Irregular surface contour, particularly when occurring in a high-grade colposcopic abnormality (RCI score > 6 points)
3. Surface ulceration or true "erosion," particularly when occurring in a high-grade colposcopic abnormality (RCI score > 6 points)
4. Atypical blood vessels (coarse, varicose, bizarre subepithelial vessels with irregular caliber and nondichotomous branching or long, unbranched course)
5. Extremely coarse abnormal vascular patterns (i.e., mosaicism and punctation), especially with wide and irregular intercapillary distances and umbilication
6. Large, complex, high-grade lesions (RCI score >6 points) occupying three or four cervical quadrants
7. High-grade colposcopic lesions extending into cervical canal either >5 mm or beyond colposcopic view

RCI, Reid Colposcopic Index.

Colposcopic Warning Signs of Invasive Cancer

Although most invasive cancers are clinically apparent and do not require colposcopy for identification, early invasive lesions may be clinically occult. Exclusion of invasive cancer demands both a high index of suspicion and knowledge of warning signs. Colposcopic warning signs are shown in Table 7.10.

Other warning signs for invasive cancer include the following:

1. **Any cytologic evidence of possible squamous carcinoma, adenocarcinoma, or AIS or recurrent high-grade cytologic findings in a patient previously treated for CIN 3.**
2. **Any histologic evidence of invasive cancer or CIN 2 or 3 in a tangentially sectioned punch biopsy** in which the basement membrane cannot be adequately defined.
3. **High-grade cytologic abnormality in a postmenopausal or previously irradiated woman.**

2012 Updated Consensus Guidelines for the Management of Abnormal Cervical Cancer Screening Tests and Cancer

Precursors

In 2001, the **ASCCP Consensus Guidelines** were developed to assist in the management of women with cytologic abnormalities (255) and in the management of cervical cancer precursors (297), in part in response to the 2001 Bethesda System. Improved understanding of the pathogenesis and natural history of cervical HPV infection and cervical cancer precursors, of the future pregnancy implications of treatment for CIN among young women and of the management of AIS led to a critical review of the earlier Guidelines (39,298). The ASCCP 2006 Consensus Guidelines (261) aligned management of minor cytologic abnormalities and CIN 1, incorporated the results of the ASCUS-LSIL Triage Study (ALTS), identified strategies for management of positive high-risk HPV DNA tests, and established guidelines for management of adolescents and young women.

Previous guidelines remain valid but knowledge has advanced. Screening recommendations have changed. **In 2012, national organizations published guidelines recommending longer screening intervals and commencement of screening at a later age (86). In the United States, co-testing with cytology and HPV-DNA testing at five-yearly intervals is now the preferred cervical cancer screening strategy for women 30 to 64 years of age.** Clinicians needed guidance on the incorporation of co-testing into management of women with cervical abnormalities (Table 7.7).

The 2006 ASCCP Guidelines for the management of abnormal cervical cancer screening tests, CIN, and AIS remain valid, with the exception of the specific areas reviewed (Table 7.11). These earlier guidelines have been combined with current revisions for cytology and histology to provide comprehensive management recommendations (Figs. 7.19A–K and 7.20A–F). Several of the 2006 ASCCP guidelines concluded by returning women to "routine screening." With the extended three-yearly cytologic or five-yearly co-testing screening intervals recommended in the 2011 screening

Table 7.11 Essential Changes from 2006 ASCCP Guidelines

- Cytology reported as negative but lacking endocervical cells can be managed without early repeat.
- CIN 1 on endocervical curettage should be managed as CIN 1 without a positive ECC.
- Cytology reported as unsatisfactory requires repeat even if HPV negative.
- Genotyping triages HPV-positive women with HPV type 16 or type 18 to earlier colposcopy only after negative cytology; colposcopy is indicated for all women with HPV and ASC-US, regardless of genotyping result.
- For ASC-US cytology, immediate colposcopy is not an option. The serial cytology option for ASC-US incorporates cytology at 12 mos, (not 6 mos and 12 mos), and then if negative, cytology every 3 yrs.
- HPV-negative and ASC-US results should be followed with co-testing at 3 yrs rather than 5 yrs.
- HPV-negative and ASC-US results are insufficient to allow exit from screening at age 65 yrs.
- The pathway to long-term follow-up of treated and untreated CIN 2 and CIN 3 is more clearly defined by incorporating co-testing.
- More strategies incorporate co-testing to reduce follow-up visits. Pap-only strategies are now limited to women younger than 30 yrs, but co-testing is expanded even to women younger than 30 yrs in some circumstances. Women aged 21–24 yrs are managed conservatively.

CIN, cervical intraepithelial neoplasia; ECC, endocervical curettage; HPV, human papillomavirus; ASC-US, atypical squamous cells of undetermined significance.

Prior management guidelines were from **Wright TC Jr., Massad LS, Dunton CJ, et al.** 2006 consensus guidelines for the management of women with cervical intraepithelial neoplasia or adenocarcinoma *in situ*. *Am J Obstet Gynecol.* 2007;197(4):340–345 (298). Prior guidelines not changed were retained.

Updated from: **Massad LS, Einstein MH, Huh WK, et al.** 2012 updated consensus guidelines for the management of abnormal cervical cancer screening tests and cancer precursors. *J Low Gen Tract Dis.* 2013;17(5):S1–S27.

guidelines, return to these screening intervals would be considered safe only if the risk of CIN 3 during the years between testing was low. This low level of risk exists for women with negative screening histories. **For women with some abnormalities, particularly those with histories of high-grade CIN, AIS, and microinvasive disease, the risk for CIN 3 remains elevated for years, even after treatment and even after initial negative surveillance** (299–302). In the United States context, it is considered that current follow-up data are insufficient to recommend return to 5-year routine screening intervals for these women and that even after treatment, the ongoing risk does not fall to a level consistent with 5-year retesting.

The role of endocervical sampling remains controversial. Endocervical brushing has better sensitivity than endocervical curettage with similar specificity, better tolerance and fewer insufficient samples, but grading is more difficult as a result of the absence of stroma (276). Either are considered acceptable for endocervical sampling. The indications defined in the 2006 Guidelines for endocervical sampling for women with ASCUS and LSIL smears are valid for women with ASC-H and HSIL smears as well.

Under earlier screening guidelines, women followed prospectively after a positive HPV test but negative cytology were referred for colposcopy only if they had LSIL or a more severe cytologic abnormality during surveillance co-testing (230). **For simplicity, current guidelines recommend colposcopy for any further positive HPV test or any abnormal cytology found during surveillance of women who had an initial positive HPV test but negative cytology.**

The 2006 Guidelines recommended conservative, prospective management of adolescents with cervical abnormalities. **The 2012 screening guidelines recommend not screening adolescents** (230–232). Cervical cancer risk remains low for women under 25 years (303). HPV infection is common (in unvaccinated females) (304) and lesions often regress (70,305–307). The rates of cervical cancer in the 21- to 24-year age group are low, but in the United States is 10-fold higher than the risk in adolescents (303). In the United States setting, the risk in the 21- to 24-year age group is considered high enough to justify screening, but is low enough to justify conservative, prospective follow-up of minor smear abnormalities. Guidelines for women 21 to 24 can be extrapolated to adolescents if they are screened.

HPV testing, despite attempts at public and patient education, can still elicit feelings of stigma and shame (308). The detection and management of screen-detected abnormalities can have adverse effects on work, relationships, and families (309,310). This potential for harm and the unintended negative impact from management of screen-detected abnormalities (311), reinforces the notion that colposcopy, biopsies, and treatment should be avoided if the risk of CIN 3, AIS or invasive cancer is low, or if identified screen abnormalities or diagnosed cervical lesions are likely to resolve. This philosophy is strongly reflected in the current Guidelines. **In the current**

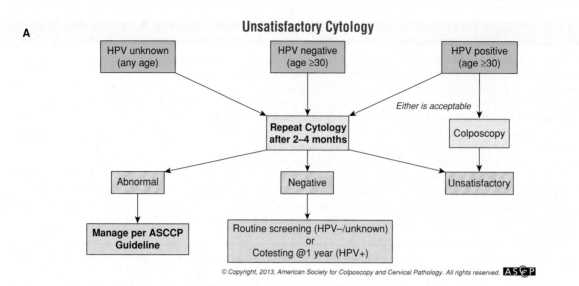

A

Unsatisfactory Cytology

© Copyright, 2013, American Society for Colposcopy and Cervical Pathology. All rights reserved.

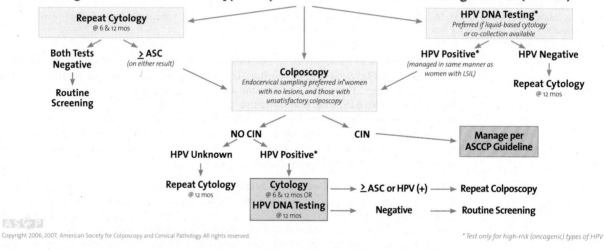

B   Management of Women with Atypical Squamous Cells of Undetermined Significance (ASC-US)

Copyright 2006, 2007, American Society for Colposcopy and Cervical Pathology. All rights reserved.

*Test only for high-risk (oncogenic) types of HPV

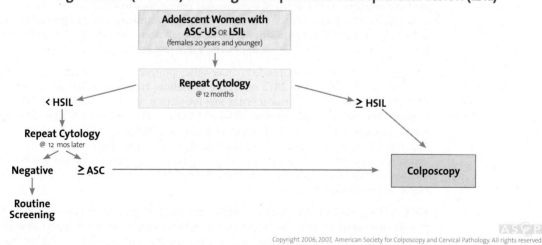

C   Management of Adolescent Women with Either Atypical Squamous Cells of Undetermined Significance (ASC-US) or Low-grade Squamous Intraepithelial Lesion (LSIL)

Copyright 2006, 2007, American Society for Colposcopy and Cervical Pathology. All rights reserved.

Figure 7.19 A–K: Algorithms from the Consensus Guidelines for the Management of Women with Cervical Cytological Abnormalities. Reprinted from *The Journal of Lower Genital Tract Disease* Vol. 11, Issue 4, with the permission of ASCCP © American Society for Colposcopy and Cervical Pathology 2007, 2013. No copies of the algorithms may be made without the prior consent of ASCCP.

D   Management of Women with Atypical Squamous Cells: Cannot Exclude High-grade SIL (ASC - H)

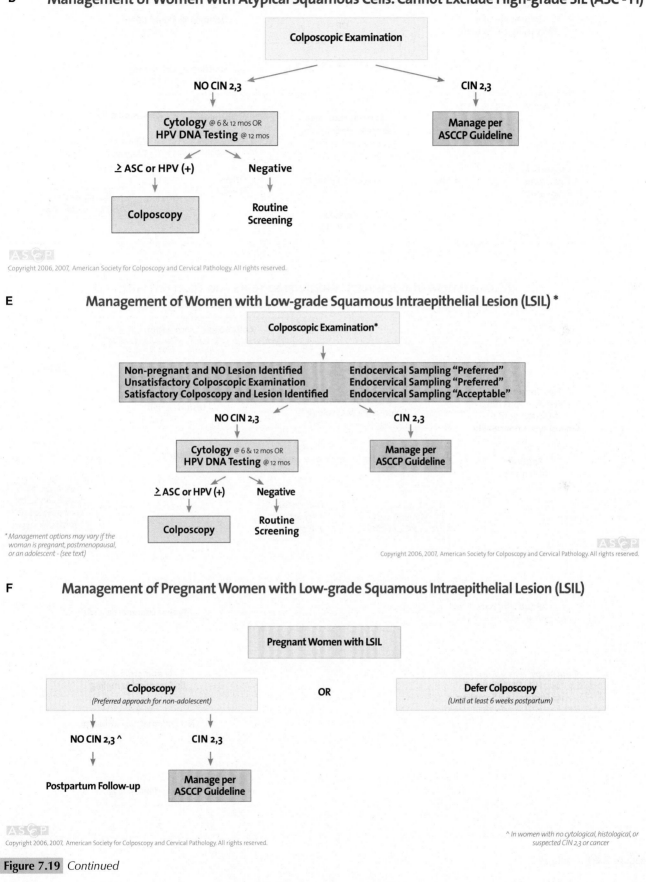

E   Management of Women with Low-grade Squamous Intraepithelial Lesion (LSIL) *

F   Management of Pregnant Women with Low-grade Squamous Intraepithelial Lesion (LSIL)

* Management options may vary if the woman is pregnant, postmenopausal, or an adolescent - (see text)

^ In women with no cytological, histological, or suspected CIN 2,3 or cancer

Copyright 2006, 2007, American Society for Colposcopy and Cervical Pathology. All rights reserved.

Figure 7.19 *Continued*

G

Management of Women with High-grade Squamous Intraepithelial Lesion (HSIL) *

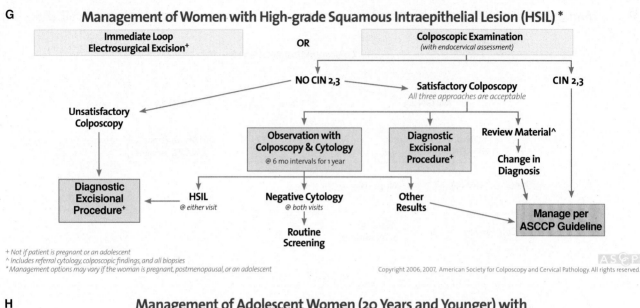

+ Not if patient is pregnant or an adolescent
^ Includes referral cytology, colposcopic findings, and all biopsies
* Management options may vary if the woman is pregnant, postmenopausal, or an adolescent

Copyright 2006, 2007, American Society for Colposcopy and Cervical Pathology. All rights reserved.

H

Management of Adolescent Women (20 Years and Younger) with High-grade Squamous Intraepithelial Lesion (HSIL)

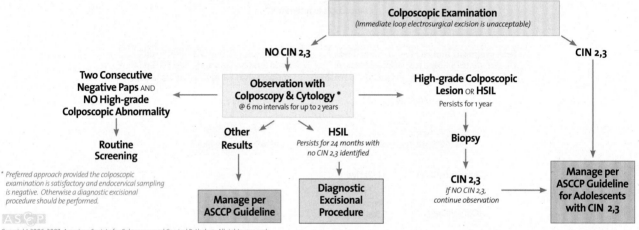

* Preferred approach provided the colposcopic examination is satisfactory and endocervical sampling is negative. Otherwise a diagnostic excisional procedure should be performed.

Copyright 2006, 2007, American Society for Colposcopy and Cervical Pathology. All rights reserved.

I

Initial Workup of Women with Atypical Glandular Cells (AGC)

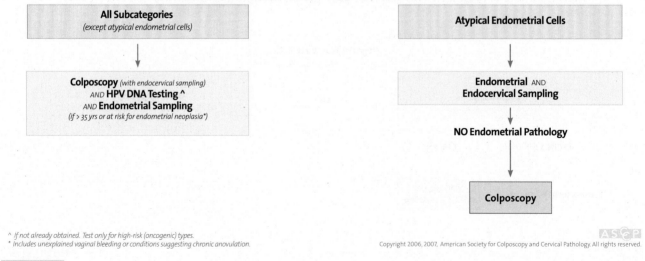

^ If not already obtained. Test only for high-risk (oncogenic) types.
* Includes unexplained vaginal bleeding or conditions suggesting chronic anovulation.

Copyright 2006, 2007, American Society for Colposcopy and Cervical Pathology. All rights reserved.

Figure 7.19 *Continued*

J   Subsequent Management of Women with Atypical Glandular Cells (AGC)

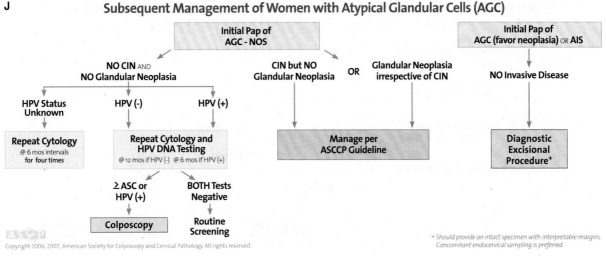

Copyright 2006, 2007, American Society for Colposcopy and Cervical Pathology. All rights reserved.

+ *Should provide an intact specimen with interpretable margins. Concomitant endocervical sampling is preferred.*

K   Use of HPV DNA Testing * as an Adjunct to Cytology for Cervical Cancer Screening in Women 30 Years and Older

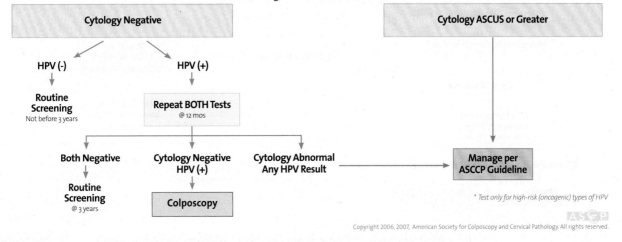

* *Test only for high-risk (oncogenic) types of HPV*

Copyright 2006, 2007, American Society for Colposcopy and Cervical Pathology. All rights reserved.

Figure 7.19 *Continued.* **A–K: Algorithms from the Consensus Guidelines for the Management of Women with Cervical Cytological Abnormalities.** Reprinted from *The Journal of Lower Genital Tract Disease* Vol. 11, Issue 4, with the permission of ASCCP © American Society for Colposcopy and Cervical Pathology 2007, 2013. No copies of the algorithms may be made without the prior consent of ASCCP.

Guidelines, immunosuppressed women, including HIV-infected women, are managed in the same manner as immunocompetent women.

Although these ASCCP Consensus Guidelines have an international influence, they are designed for the opportunistic cervical cancer screening system of the United States. Clinicians in other settings should consider the guidelines in the context in which they operate and adapt management appropriately. The Algorithms from the 2012 Consensus Guidelines have detailed explanatory notes, available from the relevant ASSCP publications and website (http://www.asccp.org/). The management discussion below summarizes the published recommendations (86).

Management of CIN and Histologic AIS

CIN 1 and No CIN Found at Colposcopy After Abnormal Cytology

CIN 1 is the histologic manifestation of HPV infection. Most CIN 1 lesions are associated with oncogenic HPV types, although HPV16 is less common than with CIN 3 lesions (69,312). **Regression rates are high particularly in younger women (45,70) and progression to CIN 2–3 is**

A Management of Women with a Histological Diagnosis of Cervical Intraepithelial Neoplasia
Grade 1 (CIN 1) Preceded by ASC-US, ASC-H, or LSIL Cytology

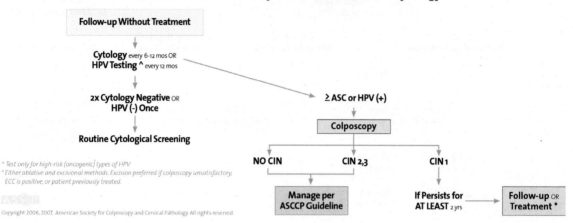

Copyright 2006, 2007, American Society for Colposcopy and Cervical Pathology. All rights reserved.

B Management of Women with a Histological Diagnosis of Cervical Intraepithelial Neoplasia - Grade 1 (CIN 1)
Preceded by HSIL or AGC-NOS Cytology

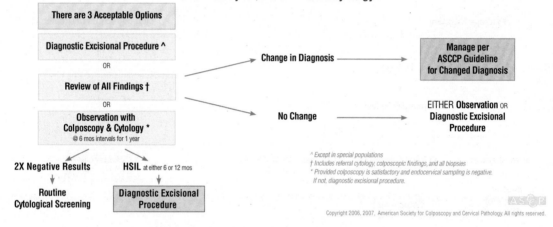

Copyright 2006, 2007, American Society for Colposcopy and Cervical Pathology. All rights reserved.

C Management of Adolescent Women (20 Years and Younger)
with a Histological Diagnosis of Cervical Intraepithelial Neoplasia - Grade 1 (CIN 1)

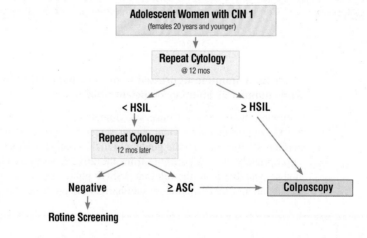

Copyright 2006, 2007, American Society for Colposcopy and Cervical Pathology. All rights reserved.

Figure 7.20 **A–F: Algorithms from the Consensus Guidelines for the Management of Women with Cervical Histological Abnormalities.** Reprinted from *The Journal of Lower Genital Tract Disease* Vol. 11, Issue 4, with the permission of ASCCP © American Society for Colposcopy and Cervical Pathology 2007, 2013. No copies of the algorithms may be made without the prior consent of ASCCP.

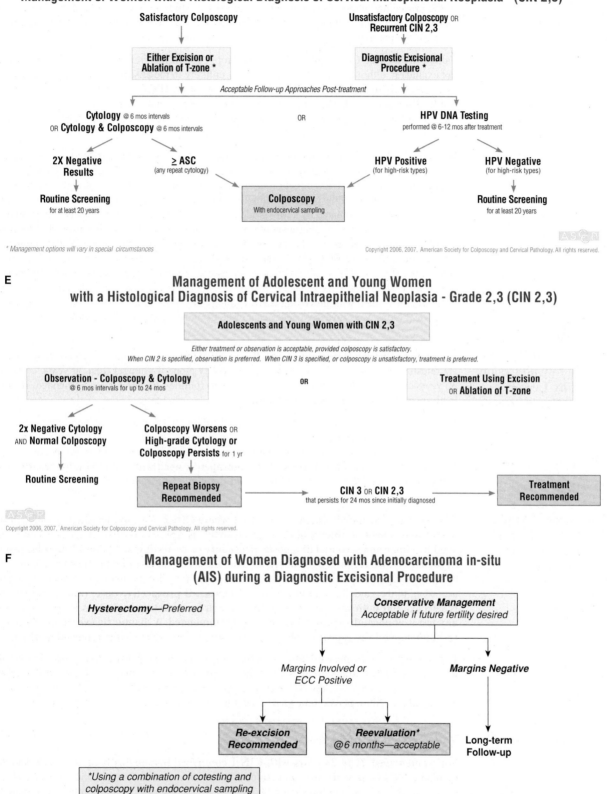

Figure 7.20 *Continued.* **A–F: Algorithms from the Consensus Guidelines for the Management of Women with Cervical Histological Abnormalities.** Reprinted from *The Journal of Lower Genital Tract Disease* Vol. 11, Issue 4, with the permission of ASCCP © American Society for Colposcopy and Cervical Pathology 2007, 2013. No copies of the algorithms may be made without the prior consentof ASCCP.

uncommon (45,313), **particularly after biopsy.** The risk of occult CIN 3 is linked to the severity of the preceding cytology leading to the diagnosis. A study in women aged 21 to 24 years found that if the preceding cytology was LSIL or ASCUS, the risk was low, but it was substantially higher if the preceding smear was HSIL, ASC-H, or AGC (307).

Failure to diagnose CIN 2–3 by colposcopic biopsy for women referred with an HSIL smear does not exclude it, although invasive cancer is very unlikely in the absence of warning signs of cancer. **Low-grade histology diagnosed after assessment of an HSIL smear is described as a "high-grade discrepancy."** If the smear is confirmed as high grade on review, this remains a strong indication for excisional treatment. If not treated, close follow-up is mandatory and safety relies on expert opinion.

Women with ASCUS and LSIL smears have a similar risk of CIN 3 whether colposcopic examination confirms CIN 1 or no lesion (45,307). CIN 3 risk is elevated for women with HPV16, HPV18, or persistent oncogenic HPV infection of any type, even with negative cytology. Detection of CIN 1 in endocervical sampling is associated with a low-risk of CIN 2–3 (314–316). The endocervical sample is often contaminated by a low-grade ectocervical lesion and CIN 1 lesions have high spontaneous regression rates. **A diagnosis of CIN 1 on endocervical sampling preceded by ASCUS or LSIL does not increase the risk of CIN 2–3 compared with women with ectocervical CIN 1 and a negative ECC** (316). The risk of CIN 2–3 in women followed up without an excisional procedure is sufficiently low that it is reasonable to offer conservative management similar to that for ectocervical CIN 1. This guideline does not apply if CIN 1 is detected on endocervical sampling for women with preceding HSIL cytology or if high-grade CIN is confirmed in histology of cervical biopsies as invasive cancer cannot be excluded without an excisional procedure.

Management of Women with CIN 1 or no Lesion Preceded by Lesser Abnormalities on Smear

Co-testing at 1 year is recommended. If both HPV test and cytology are negative, age appropriate retesting 3 years later is recommended (cytology alone if younger than 30 years, co-testing if 30 years or older). If all tests are negative, return to routine screening is recommended. **If any test is abnormal, colposcopy is recommended.**

If CIN 1 persists for 2 years or more, continued follow-up or treatment is appropriate. Treatment can be ablative or excisional. If colposcopy is inadequate, an endocervical sample is positive for high-grade or ungraded CIN, or the patient has been previously treated, a diagnostic excisional procedure is recommended. **Topical chemotherapeutic agents are unacceptable treatment as is hysterectomy for CIN 1 as the primary and principle treatment.**

Management of Women with CIN 1 or No Lesion Preceded by ASC-H or HSIL Cytology

Women with a histologic diagnosis of CIN 1 where CIN 2–3 is not identified histologically following assessment of abnormal cytology reported as ASC-H or HSIL (CIN 2–3) can be managed by either an excisional diagnostic procedure or co-testing at 12 and 24 months, provided in the latter case colposcopy is adequate and endocervical sampling is negative. A full review of the cytologic, colposcopic, and histologic results can also be undertaken with management according to the guidelines for any revised diagnosis. **If prospective observation with co-testing is selected and both co-tests are negative, return for retesting in 3 years is recommended. If any test is abnormal, repeat colposcopy is recommended. A diagnostic excisional procedure is recommended if the repeat cytology at either the 1- or 2-year visit is reported as HSIL.**

If histology of a colposcopically directed biopsy taken in prospective follow-up confirms high-grade CIN, management is according to guidelines irrespective of the cytologic result. If CIN 1 is preceded by ASC-H or HSIL cytology and colposcopy is inadequate, a diagnostic excisional procedure is recommended, except in special populations such as pregnant women.

CIN 1 in Special Populations

Women Aged 21 to 24 Years

For women aged 21 to 24 years with CIN 1 confirmed histologically after ASC-US or LSIL cytology, follow-up with annual cytology is recommended. Women with ASC-H, HSIL or greater at 12-month follow-up should be referred for colposcopy. At 24 months, those with ASC-US or greater should be referred. Prospective follow-up by **HPV testing in this age group is unacceptable, because of the frequency of positive results.** After two consecutive negative tests, routine screening is recommended.

For women aged 21 to 24 years with CIN 1 confirmed histologically after ASC-H or HSIL cytology, observation using colposcopy and cytology at six monthly intervals is recommended,

provided colposcopy is adequate, and endocervical assessment is negative. If CIN 2, CIN 3, or CIN 2–3 is diagnosed histologically, management should follow the guidelines for management of young women with CIN 2, CIN 3, or CIN 2–3. If during follow-up a high-grade lesion is identified at colposcopy, or if HSIL cytology persists for 1 year, biopsy is recommended. **If HSIL cytology persists for 24 months without identification of CIN 2–3, a diagnostic excisional procedure is recommended.** If colposcopy is inadequate or high-grade CIN or ungraded CIN is detected on endocervical sampling, a diagnostic excisional procedure is recommended.

Pregnant Women

Pregnant women with a histologic diagnosis of CIN 1 should be followed-up without treatment. Treatment of CIN 1 in pregnancy is unacceptable.

Management of Women with CIN 2 and CIN 3

The heterogeneity of CIN 2 lesions is significant. Regression rates are higher than for CIN 3 and progression rates to cancer are higher for CIN 3 (23,25). The histologic distinction between CIN 2 and CIN 3 remains subjective. CIN 2 remains the consensus threshold for treatment, except in special circumstances. **CIN 3 should not be observed regardless of age or fertility concerns.**

After treatment of high-grade CIN, recurrence risk remains greater than that of women with negative co-testing who have not been previously treated for CIN. After two negative co-tests in the first 2 years after treatment, the risk is similar to that of women with negative cytology, suggesting return to three-yearly screening (317). Whether routine screening is safe after three or more negative co-tests is considered to remain uncertain.

The objective of cervical screening during pregnancy is to exclude invasive cancer. CIN 3 is not a risk to the pregnancy, and is not an immediate risk to the mother. Treatment during pregnancy carries a substantial risk of complications including hemorrhage and pregnancy loss.

Management of Women with CIN 2, CIN 3, and CIN 2–3

Both excisional and ablative procedures are acceptable treatment modalities for women with histologically proven CIN 2, CIN 3, and CIN 2–3 with adequate colposcopy. An excisional procedure is recommended for residual/recurrent CIN 2–3. Ablation is unacceptable for women with a histologic diagnosis of CIN 2–3 and inadequate colposcopy or if endocervical sampling shows high-grade CIN or ungraded CIN. **Cytologic and colposcopic observation of CIN 2–3 without treatment is unacceptable except in pregnant women and young women.** Hysterectomy is unacceptable as primary treatment of high-grade CIN.

For women treated for CIN 2, CIN 3, or CIN 2–3, co-testing at 12 months and 24 months is recommended. If any test is abnormal, a very common situation particularly at the first posttreatment examination, referral for colposcopy and endocervical sampling is recommended. If all tests are negative, routine screening for at least 20 years is recommended, even if this extends beyond 65 years of age. The power of a negative HPV test as a predictor of normality posttreatment for CIN 2–3 should be emphasized but **repeat treatment or hysterectomy based on a positive HPV test in follow-up posttreatment is unacceptable.**

If CIN 2–3 is reported histologically at the margins of an excised cervical specimen or in an endocervical sample obtained immediately after the procedure, reassessment with four to six monthly cytology with endocervical sampling is preferred. The role of colposcopy in this follow-up option is not clearly defined in the Guidelines. In practice, cytology and colposcopy with endocervical sampling will be performed in most clinical settings. **A repeat diagnostic excisional procedure is acceptable.** The Guidelines allow for hysterectomy if a repeat diagnostic, excisional procedure is not feasible, although great care should be taken to exclude an undisclosed invasive cancer within the endocervical canal prior to hysterectomy.

The Guidelines permit a repeat excisional procedure or hysterectomy for women with histologically proven residual/recurrent CIN 2, CIN 3, or CIN 2–3. If a repeat excisional procedure is not feasible, our practice is to perform a modified radical hysterectomy. The specimen is evaluated intraoperatively, if necessary by frozen section, to determine any need for lymphadenectomy.

CIN 2, CIN 3, or CIN 2–3 in Special Populations

Young Women

For young women with a histologic diagnosis of CIN 2–3 not otherwise specified, the Guidelines state that either treatment or six-monthly observation by cytology and colposcopy for up to 12 months is acceptable, provided colposcopy is satisfactory. Allowing for the subjectivity in this histologic distinction, observation is preferred for a diagnosis of CIN 2 alone, but treatment is acceptable. If the colposcopic appearance of the lesion worsens, or if HSIL cytology or a high-grade colposcopic lesion persists for 1 year, repeat biopsy is recommended.

Treatment is recommended for a specified histologic diagnosis of CIN 3, if colposcopy is inadequate, if CIN 2 or CIN 2–3 persists for 24 months, or if specified CIN 3 subsequently develops in the prospective follow-up of a lesser high-grade lesion. Although invasive cervical cancer is very rare in this age group, prospective follow-up of a histologic diagnosis of CIN 2–3, not otherwise specified, in young women should be limited to those women likely to be compliant with the recommendations. Young women aged 21 to 24 years who are treated for high-grade CIN should be followed according to the ASCCP guidelines for treated high-grade CIN.

Pregnant Women

For pregnant women with a histologic diagnosis of CIN 2, CIN 3, or CIN 2–3 in the absence of invasive disease or advanced pregnancy, additional colposcopic and cytologic examinations are acceptable, at intervals not more frequent than every 12 weeks. Repeat biopsy is recommended only if the appearance of the lesion worsens, or if cytology suggests invasive cancer. **Deferring reevaluation until at least 6 weeks postpartum is acceptable. A diagnostic excisional procedure is recommended only if invasion is suspected.** Treatment is unacceptable unless invasive cancer is identified. Reevaluation with cytology and colposcopy is recommended no sooner than 6 weeks postpartum.

Cervical Adenocarcinoma In Situ (AIS)

The reported incidence of cervical glandular neoplasia is lower than that of squamous cancer (140,318–322). **Cytologic screening appears to have a lower prognostic value for adenocarcinoma than for squamous cancer** (103,323), which in some settings has resulted in an increase over time in the relative proportion of screen-detected adenocarcinomas, as rates of squamous cancers are reduced by the impact of screening (141).

There is convincing evidence that AIS is a precursor lesion (324–330). The mean age of diagnosis of AIS is 15 years younger than that for invasive adenocarcinoma (320,329,331). AIS frequently coexists with invasive adenocarcinoma in histologic specimens. **Patients who have a cone biopsy performed in response to cytologic evidence of AIS have invasive cancer diagnosed in up to one-third of cases.** Women diagnosed with cervical adenocarcinoma frequently have had previous cytologic evidence of endocervical atypia on smears for intervals of 2 to 10 years (332,333).

Specific HPV types, in particular HPV 16 and 18, are strongly implicated in the etiology of high-grade glandular neoplasia; HPV 16 and 18 are found in ~80% of cervical adenocarcinomas (140) and positivity for HPV 16 or 18 is associated with increased risk of subsequent development of adenocarcinoma (334). Cervical adenocarcinoma shares many of the same cofactors as squamous neoplasia, including increasing duration of use of oral contraceptives, younger age at first full term pregnancy and high parity, with the exception of current use of tobacco, which is associated with squamous neoplasia but not adenocarcinoma (103,140). **Widespread vaccination against HPV 16 and 18, which are associated with ~80% or more of glandular neoplasms** (140,329), **should significantly decrease the incidence of both AIS and adenocarcinoma** (335).

The relationship between AIS and lesser degrees of cervical glandular neoplasia is more uncertain and the neoplastic potential of these lesions remains uncertain. Glandular dysplasia, less than AIS, represents a heterogeneous group of lesions with variable progressive potential. Glandular dysplasia is less predictably associated with high-risk HPV types when compared to AIS.

Clinical Presentation

Adenocarcinoma *in situ* is usually diagnosed after an abnormal Pap test result (336). However, only 38–69% of AIS cases are detected by cytology prior to conization. The diagnosis increases to 85% following colposcopy, biopsy, and endocervical sampling. **Because AIS coexists**

with high-grade squamous CIN in 50% of cases, the abnormal smear will frequently predict only the squamous lesion (337). The diagnosis of AIS is often a coincidental finding in the histologic assessment of an excised specimen taken in the management of high-grade CIN, which is a compelling argument for the routine excision of high-grade CIN.

The 2001 Bethesda system includes a category for atypical glandular cells (AGC). Patients with AGC smear reports have a 30–50% risk of having high-grade cervical disease and are at much higher risk of significant disease than those with ASC smear reports (338–343). An AGC smear report is an indication for referral for colposcopy and careful endocervical assessment. According to the 2012 ASCCP Guidelines, for women with all subcategories of AGC and AIS, except atypical endometrial cells, colposcopy with endocervical sampling is recommended regardless of HPV result. Triage by reflex HPV testing is not recommended and triage using repeat cervical cytology is unacceptable. Endometrial sampling is recommended in conjunction with colposcopy and endocervical sampling in women 35 years of age and older with all subcategories of AGC and AIS. Endometrial sampling is also recommended for women younger than 35 years with clinical indications suggesting they may be at risk for endometrial neoplasia. These include unexplained vaginal bleeding or conditions suggesting chronic anovulation (86).

The underlying lesion, following colposcopic workup of women with AGC smears, is most frequently high-grade squamous CIN, which occurs in up to 25% of patients. AIS, cervical adenocarcinoma, and endometrial disease, including hyperplasia and carcinoma, occur in up to 20% of patients (333,340–343).

The colposcopic features of AIS and early adenocarcinoma are widely seen as nonspecific. A minority view is that most high-grade glandular lesions do have specific colposcopic features. Discrete or extensive stark acetowhitening of individual or fused columnar villi may be seen surrounded by normal villiform structures (Fig. 7.21). Prominent atypical vessels may also be seen, particularly in association with early invasion. Although colposcopy should be performed in response to cytologic or clinical suspicion of glandular neoplasia, excisional conization is mandatory for definitive diagnosis.

Management of AIS

Management is controversial. Many assumptions used to justify conservative management of high-grade CIN do not apply. Colposcopic features of AIS can be minimal. Determining the extent of the lesion can be difficult. AIS frequently extends into the endocervical canal or may involve the entire canal so determining the required depth of excision is complicated. Although AIS lesions are often unifocal and located at the transformation zone (344), AIS can be multifocal and discontinuous so negative excisional margins are not as reassuring for complete incision as for squamous lesions. There is a frequent association between AIS and invasive cancer. Cancer cannot be excluded without an excisional procedure (298).

An excisional cone biopsy is required to make the definitive diagnosis of AIS, and to exclude invasive cancer. Hysterectomy remains the preferred management recommendation for women with a histologic diagnosis of AIS on an excisional procedure (297). A histologic diagnosis of AIS from a punch biopsy or a cytologic diagnosis of AIS is not sufficient to justify hysterectomy. The difficulty in defining colposcopic limits of AIS lesions, the frequent extension of disease into the endocervical canal, and the presence of multifocal, "skip lesions" compromise conservative excisional procedures. The cone biopsy should usually be fashioned as a cylinder of at least 2.5 cm in depth and be performed with a cold knife to avoid thermal injury to the specimen.

If the conization margins are clear of disease, more than 80% of patients have negative cytologic and colposcopic follow-up beyond 12 months (345–349). Even when excision margins are clear, 6–25% of women who proceed to hysterectomy are reported to have persistent disease in the specimen (349). For this reason, hysterectomy is still considered the treatment of choice for women with AIS who do not desire fertility preservation (297,351,352).

Positive excisional margins or positive endocervical sampling at the time of excision predicts increased risk of residual disease. A negative HPV test after treatment identifies women at low risk for persistent or recurrent AIS whereas a positive HPV test result is the strongest predictor for recurrence after conservative management of AIS (353).

Younger women, and women wishing to maintain fertility, may be managed by excisional conization alone if margins of excision are clear. Careful cytologic and colposcopic follow-up

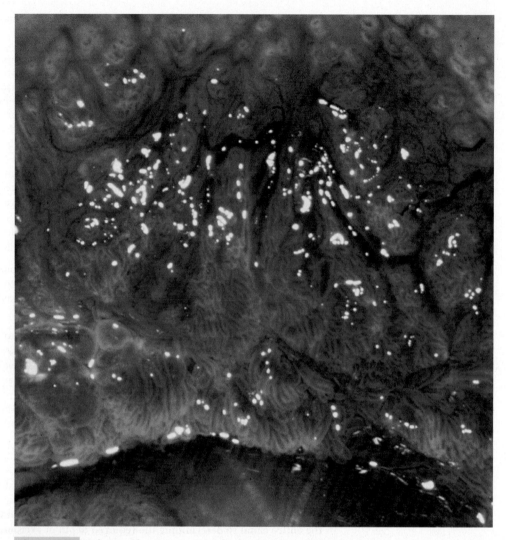

Figure 7.21 Colposcopic appearance of adenocarcinoma *in situ* lesion showing prominent atypical vessels.

is important. Even negative margins carry a less than 10% risk of persistent AIS and a small risk of cancer, which has been reported as late as 7 years postconization (348–357). Squamous and glandular preinvasive disease has been detected in as many as 33% of such patients during follow-up (348–356).

If the margins of excision of a cone biopsy performed for AIS are positive for AIS or high-grade CIN, more than 50% of patients will have residual disease at hysterectomy (351,353,355). Patients with positive conization margins and/or a positive endocervical curettage should have repeat excisional conization, with further endocervical sampling, to exclude invasive cancer. If the repeat cone biopsy is negative for invasive cancer, hysterectomy is indicated in the older patient, and should be seriously considered in the younger patient.

If conservative management by excisional cone biopsy alone is planned for women wishing to preserve fertility options and the excision margins are involved or the endocervical sample at the time of excision shows AIS or high-grade CIN, re-excision is recommended. Reassessment at 6 months using a combination of co-testing, colposcopy, and endocervical sampling is acceptable but these women remain at high-risk for AIS and invasive cancer (358,359).

Excisional cervical conization has been favored over loop or laser excision. Avoidance of thermal artifact at the margins and within glands of excised specimens aids the histologic assessment. **In the 2006 ASCCP Guidelines, wording was changed to allow diagnostic excision using any modality. Care must be taken, regardless of modality,** to avoid fragmentation of the

Table 7.12 Triage Rules for Ablative Treatment

1. Visualization of the entire new squamocolumnar junction, that is, 360 degrees of normal columnar epithelium seen with no significant disease extension within the endocervical canal

2. No colposcopic warning signs of invasive cancer

3. No cytologic or histologic evidence of invasive cancer

4. Concordance to within 1 degree of severity between the cytology and the histology of colposcopically directed biopsies

5. No evidence of high-grade disease on endocervical curettage

6. No cytologic or histologic suspicion of high-grade glandular neoplasia

specimen. This may require use of larger loops than those employed to excise visible squamous lesions.

In modern clinical practice, up to 50% of patients with AIS are diagnosed following the histologic assessment of a loop excision specimen. The standard approach in these circumstances has been to proceed to excisional conization regardless of margin status. **A number of studies have reported follow-up of these women if the margins were clear** (359–362). A meta-analysis comparing cold-knife conization and loop excision has shown no difference in the probability of obtaining negative margins, and no difference in the probability of residual disease or subsequent development of cervical adenocarcinoma (359). **HPV testing is a valuable test of cure following conservative treatment of cervical AIS** (353). **Long-term follow-up is recommended for women who do not undergo hysterectomy.**

Treatment of Cervical Intraepithelial Neoplasia

Historically, Anderson (363) from the United Kingdom in 1965 and Kolstad and Klem (364) from the Norwegian Radium Institute in 1969, demonstrated that **cone biopsy was as effective as hysterectomy in preventing the progression of carcinoma** *in situ* **to invasive cervical cancer.** In 1973, Stafl and Mattingly (365) from Wisconsin found that **colposcopically directed punch biopsies, taken by an experienced colposcopist, were as accurate as cone biopsy in obtaining a histologic diagnosis in women with an abnormal cervical smear.** This facilitated the use of physical modalities to destroy the abnormal transformation zone in selected patients.

Subsequently, high primary cure rates with minimal morbidity were reported for ablative techniques such as cryosurgery (366), **electrocoagulation diathermy** (367), **and the carbon dioxide laser** (368). Patient selection was based on a set of triage rules (Table 7.12). **Diagnostic excisional conization is now performed only for specific indications** in which there remains a genuine risk of undisclosed invasive cancer.

In the 1990s, loop electrosurgical excision procedures (LEEP) gained in popularity because of concerns regarding the occurrence of invasive cervical cancer in patients who had undergone ablative treatment (369). Invasive cancer has been reported after each of the ablative modalities (370). **When cancer occurred after ablative therapy, it occurred within 12 months in 66% of cases and within 2 years in 90%** (370). This suggested that a triage error was made in the initial assessment and invasive cancer was missed. Reports of misclassification of invasive cervical cancer or high-grade glandular neoplasia as squamous intraepithelial disease have raised concerns about the safety of ablation of high-grade squamous lesions (371–373).

LEEP allows for excision of the transformation zone with removal of a volume of tissue similar to that destroyed by ablative procedures, and with no greater morbidity. **When the procedure is performed by an inexperienced operator, adequate histologic evaluation can be difficult** because of diathermy artifact and orientation difficulties.

Treatment Modalities

The treatment modalities for preinvasive cervical disease are ablative procedures, including cryosurgery, electrocoagulation diathermy, and CO_2 laser; and excisional procedures, including LEEP, excisional conization, CO_2 laser excision, and hysterectomy. A Cochrane Systematic Review (updated in 2012) examined evidence from 29 randomized controlled trials, and reported that there was no obviously superior surgical technique in terms of treatment failures or operative morbidity, and that more research was needed (374).

Cryosurgery

Cryosurgery is a simple, effective, inexpensive, and relatively easy therapeutic option for treatment of selected patients with CIN. Cervical cryosurgery, which was first introduced in 1968, involves the destruction by cryonecrosis of the lesion, including the entire transformation zone. Hypothermia is produced by the evaporation of liquid refrigerants. Compressed nitrous oxide (N_2O) is allowed to expand through a small jet, producing an iceball at the surface of a metal probe placed in contact with the surface of the tissues to be frozen. **Crystallization of intracellular water results in cell death.**

The most appropriate cryoprobe tips are the 19- and 25-mm minicone. A water-soluble gel is used to coat the probe tip before the procedure. Temperatures achieved at the cryotip using N_2O are recorded at −65°C to −85°C. Cell death occurs in the range of −20°C to −30°C. **The lethal zone during cryosurgery begins 2 mm proximal to the iceball margin,** with the temperature at the margin of the iceball equal to 0°C. **To ensure a 5-mm depth of freezing, a total lateral spread of freeze of 7 mm is required.** For cervical cryosurgery, **the probe must cover the lesion and the entire transformation zone.**

If the transformation zone is large, successive overlapping treatments are required, increasing the duration and discomfort of the procedure. **Cryosurgery is therefore used mainly for smaller, ectocervical lesions.** It is usually used for low-grade lesions without extension into the endocervical canal.

Technique

The procedure is performed under colposcopic supervision without anesthesia. Prophylactic premedication with nonsteroidal anti-inflammatory drugs 30 to 60 minutes before the procedure may reduce pain and cramping associated with prostaglandin release from dying cells. The procedure should not be performed in pregnancy or during the menstrual period. The procedure is performed as follows:

1. **The cervix is exposed using a speculum, and a careful colposcopy is performed to check the topography of the lesion, and to ensure that the triage rules are fulfilled.**

2. **A warm cryotip is chosen that best conforms to the topography of the cervix, and a water-soluble gel is applied thinly to the tip.**

3. **The cryotip is positioned at room temperature on the cervix, with care taken to cover the entire lesion and the transformation zone. The probe must be clear of the vaginal walls. The procedure is initiated by activating a trigger on the cryogun. If the probe comes into contact with the vagina, the treatment is ceased and then reinitiated.**

4. **Crystallization begins on the back of the probe and proceeds until the ice ball is seen to extend 7 mm laterally beyond the edge of the probe.** This visual landmark is the indicator of the depth of the freeze (approximately 5 mm) and is the method for determining the duration of the procedure.

5. **The probe is defrosted completely and then disengaged from the cervix.**

A freeze–thaw–freeze technique is commonly used. This technique was reported by Creasman et al. (375) to reduce the failure rate from 29–7%, although others have claimed similar results from a single freeze (376,377). The second freeze is not commenced until the tissues have visibly thawed from the initial treatment.

Patients experience a watery, malodorous, blood-tinged discharge for 2 to 3 weeks after the procedure. This can be decreased by debridement of the bullous, necrotic tissue using a ring forceps and gauze 48 hours after the procedure. The patient should abstain from vaginal intercourse and tampon use for 4 weeks after the procedure.

Cryosurgery for large ectocervical lesions covering the ectocervix is associated with failure rates as high as 42%. Endocervical glandular involvement increases the failure rate from 9% to 27%. Decreasing cure rates with increasing severity of disease, specifically 94% for CIN 1, 93% for CIN 2, and 84% for CIN 3, have been reported (378). This may in part reflect the increased size of HGLs, which more frequently occupy two or more quadrants of the cervix (Table 7.13) (379).

Loop Electrosurgical Excision Procedure

To minimize the risk of failed detection of early invasive cancer and high-grade glandular neoplasia at the time of colposcopic triage, LEEP of the transformation zone has become a widely used and valuable therapeutic option. The LEEP equipment is relatively inexpensive, and the surgical

Table 7.13 Comparison of Treatment Modalities

Procedure Rates	Technical Ease	Equipment Cost	Complication Rates	Primary Cure (%)
Cryosurgery	+++	+++	++	80
Loop electrosurgical excision procedures	+++	++	+++	95
Laser ablation	++	+	+++	95
Laser excision	+	+	++	95
Cold-knife conization	++	+++	++	98

+, low benefit; ++, medium benefit; +++, high benefit.

skills are readily acquired. **The procedure combines the advantages of conservative ablative procedures in preserving cervical tissue with the safety of histologic assessment of the entire lesion.**

Cartier originally developed an electrosurgical method for management of CIN using 5-mm rectangular, thin wire loops to sample and treat the cervix by removing the epithelium and underlying stroma in multiple 5-mm strips (380). Prendiville et al. (381,382) introduced larger loop electrodes, 1 to 2 cm in width and 0.7 to 1.5 cm in depth, for excision of the entire transformation zone, usually in a single pass. The combination of very thin wire loops and modern electrosurgical generators capable of delivering high powers (35 to 55 W) has allowed electrosurgical cutting with little associated thermal injury.

The technique for electrosurgical loop excision is as follows:

1. **The cervix is visualized using a nonconductive nylon or plastic-coated speculum with suction attached.** For parous patients, a nonconductive vaginal lateral wall retractor is advisable to improve access to the cervix.

2. **The cervix is evaluated colposcopically to determine the distribution of the lesion and the transformation zone.** The appropriate loop size is chosen. Lugol's iodine solution helps demarcate the outer margin of excision. The procedure is performed under colposcopic control.

3. **The cervix is infiltrated with 4 to 6 mL of local anesthetic (1–2% *lidocaine* with *epinephrine*) using a dental syringe with a 27-gauge needle** at the 3, 6, 9, and 12 o'clock positions after a test dose of 1 mL is observed for side effects.

4. **A grounding pad is attached to the patient's thigh.**

5. **The electrosurgical generator is set at an appropriate power setting for the size of loop, usually 35 to 55 W of either pure cutting or blended current.**

6. **Suction is attached to the speculum.**

7. **The specimen is excised by activating the generator with a foot pedal or hand switch with the loop 2 mm from the tissue.** The loop is advanced perpendicularly into the cervix 2 to 3 mm lateral to the lesion and the transformation zone to a depth of 5 to 7 mm, and drawn across the cervix until 2 mm lateral to the opposite side. **Larger lesions may require more than a single pass with the electrode.** The central portion of the lesion should be excised first and remaining lesional tissue excised with additional passes. More peripheral CIN tissue can be destroyed with the ball electrode, provided a directed biopsy is taken and the triage rules for ablation are fulfilled.

8. **The base of the crater is lightly fulgurated using the 5-mm ball electrode with the electrosurgical generator at 40 to 60 W of coagulation current.** This is intended to stop bleeding, but not to char the tissue.

9. **An endocervical curettage, sampling, or "cowboy hat" biopsy should be performed if one has not been previously performed** (Fig. 7.22).

10. **Monsel solution should be applied to the cervix to maintain hemostasis.**

Complications are minimal, comparing favorably with those associated with CO_2 laser procedures (374). **Postoperative bleeding occurs in 2–5% of patients.** Postoperative infection is uncommon. **Clinically significant cervical stenosis and cervical incompetence are rare complications.**

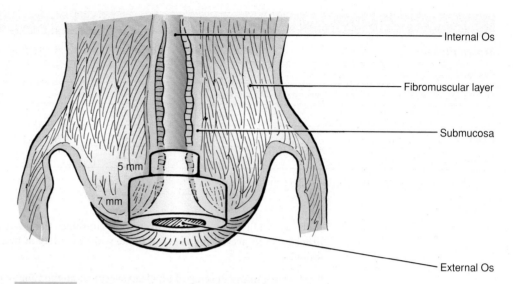

Internal Os

Fibromuscular layer

Submucosa

5 mm

7 mm

External Os

Figure 7.22 "Cowboy-hat" configuration for LEEP.

Cure rates appear comparable with those achieved with CO_2 laser procedures and with "cold-knife" conization (374).

Electrosurgical loop excision offers several advantages over CO_2 laser ablation. The procedure is **quicker and easier**. Patient acceptance is better and intraoperative pain is decreased. The entire specimen can be submitted for histologic study, and in many large studies, **the unsuspected invasive cancer and high-grade glandular disease rate has been as high as 1–2%** (383–386).

Another potential advantage of LEEP is the ability to "see-and-treat" at one visit. However, histologic study of loop-excised specimens removed at a "see-and-treat" approach have revealed no disease in 5–40% of specimens, particularly in young women referred with minor cytologic abnormalities (387).

Carbon Dioxide Laser Ablation of the Transformation Zone

The CO_2 laser is the ideal choice for vaporizing sharply defined tissue volumes to a precisely determined depth (388–390). To achieve optimal vaporization with minimal lateral thermal injury, the CO_2 laser should be used at the highest power output with which the surgeon is comfortable. This should be a minimum of 25 W but preferably above 60 W. The cautious use of low-power outputs is one of the most common CO_2 laser surgery errors causing thermal injury. For transformation zone ablative procedures, the average power density must be kept within the range of 750 to 2,000 W/cm^2 (391).

Surgical Control of the CO_2 Laser

For cervical transformation zone ablation, a high-power laser setting is selected. The spot diameter is progressively enlarged by defocusing the beam using the micromanipulator until a point is found where the impact crater (tested on a moistened wooden tongue blade) is hemispherical (Y-beam geometry). This permits controlled tissue vaporization with minimal lateral heat conduction. Controlled tissue vaporization is achieved by delivering the laser energy in short bursts, either by use of the mechanical timer in the laser console or, preferably, by gating the laser pulses using the foot pedal.

CO_2 laser ablation of the transformation zone should always be performed using a micromanipulator attached to a colposcope or operating microscope. Careful colposcopy is required at the time of transformation zone ablation to determine the lateral extent of disease. **The entire transformation zone must be treated, as selective ablation of areas of disease results in much lower primary cure rates.**

A major advantage of CO_2 laser ablation is the ability to destroy tissue to a precisely controlled depth. The maximum depth of gland involvement with CIN is 5.2 mm, whereas the maximum depth of uninvolved glands is 7.9 mm. **The transformation zone is usually destroyed to a depth of 7 to 10 mm.**

Control of Intraoperative Pain and Bleeding

CO_2 laser ablation of the transformation zone is usually performed under local anesthesia. The cervix is infiltrated with 4 to 6 mL of local anesthetic such as 1% *lidocaine,* with or without a vasospastic agent. A deeper, paracervical block does not always provide adequate anesthesia and its administration is associated with more discomfort and bleeding.

Should a small vessel such as an arteriole be encountered, hemostasis is readily achieved by using direct pressure from a moistened cotton-tipped applicator and lasing immediately onto the applicator tip at the site of the vessel. Monsel solution should be applied to the cervix on completion of the procedure, to minimize the risk of postoperative bleeding. CO_2 laser ablation of the transformation zone is an excellent treatment for selected patients with CIN, with minimal morbidity (374).

Excisional Cervical Conization

Excisional cervical conization performed with a scalpel, sometimes referred to as a "cold-knife conization," has been traditionally the standard response to cytologic abnormalities (392). It is both diagnostic and therapeutic. The geometry of the cervical conization should adapt to the size and shape of the lesion as well as the geometry of the cervix (Fig. 7.23). The procedure is performed in the following manner:

1. **Careful colposcopic examination is performed** to delineate the lateral margins of the lesion and transformation zone. Lugol's iodine solution aids in this determination.

2. **Lateral sutures may be placed** on the side of the cervix at the 3 and 9 o'clock positions to provide traction and hemostasis.

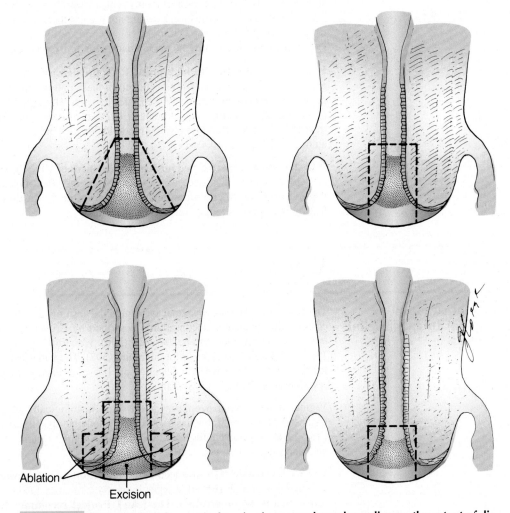

Ablation

Excision

Figure 7.23 **Tissue excised for cervical conization procedures depending on the extent of disease and the anatomy and shape of the cervix.**

295

3. **The cervix may be infiltrated with a vasospastic agent** to decrease intraoperative bleeding.

4. **The endocervical canal is sounded** to guide the direction and depth of the excision.

5. **The specimen is excised using a number 11 scalpel blade,** preferably with a cylinder-shaped geometry.

6. **The excised specimen is tagged at the 12 o'clock position** to allow for proper orientation by the pathologist.

7. **A fractional curettage (or biopsy) of the endocervical canal and endometrium is performed** to exclude residual squamous or glandular disease of the upper endocervical canal or disease of the endometrium.

8. **The base of the surgical site can be cauterized** to secure or maintain hemostasis. Simple U-sutures placed anteriorly and posteriorly may be used if bleeding persists.

Excisional cervical conization achieves high cure rates for high-grade CIN. **The risk of cervical stenosis and cervical incompetence is higher** for cervical conization performed with a scalpel than with CO_2 laser or electrosurgical excision. This in part reflects the fact that cervical conization performed with a scalpel has been traditionally used for the most severe lesions, often with significant disease extension to within the endocervical canal (393).

Hysterectomy

Hysterectomy is rarely indicated in the primary management of CIN. The most common indication is **coexistence of a gynecologic condition that warrants hysterectomy.** Such conditions include dysfunctional uterine bleeding, fibroids, uterovaginal prolapse, or patient request for sterilization. **Before any hysterectomy, colposcopic assessment should be performed.** If the entire lesion and transformation zone are not seen, if there is any evidence of high-grade glandular neoplasia, or if there is any cytologic, colposcopic, or histologic suspicion of invasive cancer, **an excisional conization must be performed prior to hysterectomy.**

In 2–3% of patients with high-grade CIN, the disease extends to the vaginal vault (394). If the vaginal cuff is not carefully fashioned in these patients, preferably using a vaginal approach, neoplastic epithelium may be sutured into the vault. High-grade vaginal intraepithelial neoplasia (VAIN) develops in the vaginal vault in 1–7% of patients who have undergone hysterectomy to treat CIN. Coppleson and Reid (395) reported 38 cases of invasive vault cancer after hysterectomy among 8,998 women (0.4%).

If hysterectomy is performed for the management of CIN, the patient should have a vault smear and colposcopy on two occasions in the 18 months after surgery. **She should be screened by vaginal vault smears on an annual basis thereafter. Co-testing with cytology and HPV DNA testing may permit longer screening intervals.**

Vagina

Classification of Vaginal Intraepithelial Neoplasia

The first description of a vaginal intraepithelial lesion was made at the Mayo Clinic in 1933, a century after vaginal cancer was first described by Cruveilhie. Described as vaginal carcinoma *in situ,* it was considered to be very rare (396). Woodruff's review of vaginal carcinoma *in situ* in 1981 found only 300 cases in the literature (397). The wider use of cytology and colposcopy has led to a significant increase in detection of HPV-associated lesions of the vagina, particularly less severe lesions than CIS (398–400).

Vaginal intraepithelial neoplasia is classified histologically in a manner similarly to cervical lesions: **VAIN 1** (mild dysplasia), **VAIN 2** (moderate dysplasia), and **VAIN 3** (severe dysplasia/CIS). **VAIN 3 is a premalignant lesion,** but the natural history of the lesser degrees of VAIN has not been submitted to prospective study.

VAIN 1 is often an HPV-induced change without an established progressive potential but is associated with high-risk HPV types in 64–84% of cases (401). Management should be conservative, that is, by observation. **The LAST Project recommended HPV Infection/VAIN 1 be classified as vaginal LSIL and VAIN 2–VAIN 3 be classified as vaginal HSIL** (59). This is consistent with clinical appearance and management.

Over 90% of high-grade VAIN 2–3 lesions and 70% of vaginal cancers are associated with HPV infections (401). HPVs 16 and 18 are associated with over 60% of high-grade VAIN and 40% of low-grade VAIN (401–404). Given the strong association of HPV with vaginal neoplasia, **prophylactic HPV vaccination against HPVs 16 and 18 should result in a decrease in the incidence of VAIN** (403).

Intraepithelial vaginal dysplasia of glandular origin, or atypical vaginal adenosis, is a separate entity. This lesion is associated with in utero DES exposure and may be a precursor to DES-associated clear-cell adenocarcinoma. This remains relevant, as cases have been reported of atypical adenosis and, rarely, vaginal adenocarcinomas in non–DES-exposed women (405).

Clinical Profile

Since the 1970s, the diagnosis of high-grade VAIN has been made with increasing frequency. The estimated frequency in the United States is 0.2 to 0.3 per 100,000 women (396,397). The median age at diagnosis is about 50 years although high-grade VAIN may be diagnosed in much younger women. Patients with high-grade VAIN are older on average than those diagnosed with high-grade CIN, but the notion that increasingly severe degrees of VAIN are associated with increasing age is not consistent with modern experience (399).

The increased rate of diagnosis of high-grade VAIN is a result of increased clinical awareness, improved screening and an absolute increase in incidence. The rarity of primary vaginal squamous cancer suggests that the malignant potential of VAIN is low, but progression to invasive cancer does occur (406). The lower malignant potential in part reflects the absence of a vulnerable squamocolumnar junction in the vagina, except in rare instances, and a lytic cell reaction, which enables the regression of vaginal HPV-induced lesions.

High-grade VAIN usually occurs in association with high-grade CIN, which extends onto the vaginal fornices in approximately 3% of cases, but primary foci of high-grade VAIN also occur (407,408). **VAIN 2–3 involves the upper third of the vagina in more than 70% of cases** and less commonly the lower third, with the middle third infrequently involved.

Occasionally, multifocal disease can extend throughout the vagina, particularly in the presence of extensive multicentric intraepithelial neoplasia. This reflects the **"field effect"** of squamous carcinogenesis in the lower genital tract related to HPV16 in particular (409). This is further supported by the more rapid development of VAIN among women with a prior history of **anogenital neoplasia** (406). A prior history of treatment for **cervical cancer and cigarette smoking** are risk factors for development of high-grade VAIN (406,410), as is **immunosuppression,** for example, following organ transplantation or due to concurrent HIV infection (406).

High-grade VAIN lesions are asymptomatic and are usually diagnosed by colposcopy and biopsy following abnormal cytologic screening (411). Among women who have not had a hysterectomy, concomitant or antecedent high-grade CIN is detected in over two-thirds of patients. Cervical cytologic testing is usually positive in the presence of VAIN. **The vaginal vault, in particular, and the vaginal walls, should be inspected at the time of colposcopy.** In addition, certain specific indications require careful vaginal colposcopy (Table 7.14). The IFCPC has recently

Table 7.14 Indications for Vaginal Colposcopy
1. Abnormal cytology after apparently successful treatment of CIN
2. Abnormal vaginal vault cytology posthysterectomy
3. Abnormal cytology at the presence of colposcopically normal cervix, particularly if colposcopy is satisfactory
4. Confirmed high-grade CIN in an immunosuppressed patient
5. Confirmed diagnosis of high-grade vulvar intraepithelial neoplasia
6. Abnormal gross vaginal examination
7. Confirmed or suspected intrauterine *diethylstilbestrol* exposure
8. Diagnosis and treatment of multicentric human papillomavirus infection, particularly if recalcitrant to conservative treatment
9. Confirmed diagnosis of invasive cervical cancer

CIN, cervical intraepithelial neoplasia.

Table 7.15 IFCPC Clinical/Colposcopic Terminology of the Vagina		
General assessment	Adequate/inadequate for the reason (i.e., inflammation, bleeding, scar) Transformation zone	
Normal colposcopic findings	Squamous epithelium: Mature Atrophic	
Abnormal colposcopic findings	General principles	Upper third /lower two-thirds, Anterior/posterior/lateral (right or left),
	Grade 1 (Minor)	Thin acetowhite epithelium Fine punctuation Fine mosaic
	Grade 2 (Major)	Dense acetowhite epithelium, Coarse punctuation Coarse mosaic
	Suspicious for invasion	Atypical vessels Additional signs: Fragile vessels, Irregular surface, Exophytic lesion, Necrosis, Ulceration (necrotic), tumor/gross neoplasm
	Nonspecific	Columnar epithelium (adenosis) Lesion staining by Lugol solution (Schiller test): Stained/nonstained, Leukoplakia
Miscellaneous findings	Erosion (traumatic), condyloma, polyp, cyst, endometriosis, inflammation, vaginal stenosis, congenital transformation zone	

From: **Bornstein J, Bentley J, Bosze P, et al.** The 2011 colposcopic terminology of the International Federation for Cervical Pathology and Colposcopy. *Obstet Gynecol.* 2012;120(1):166–172.

published terminology for clinical and colposcopic findings on examination of the vagina (Table 7.15). **Patients with VAIN have a 10% incidence of coexisting high-grade VIN** (406,409). Careful vulvar colposcopy should be performed for all women with VAIN.

Diagnosis

High-grade VAIN is generally diagnosed by histology of colposcopically directed biopsies. Lesions are usually flat and inconspicuous before application of acetic acid, although occasionally raised pink, red, or white lesions may be seen. **Clinically apparent hyperkeratosis or leukoplakia may represent an underlying VAIN lesion.** Peeling or ulceration of the vaginal epithelium, particularly in the perimenopausal and postmenopausal patient, may be an indicator of underlying high-grade VAIN. **Occasionally, recalcitrant condylomatous lesions of the vagina reveal a high-grade dysplastic morphology.**

VAIN 2–3 has a colposcopic appearance similar to that of high-grade CIN (Fig. 7.24) **after application of 5% acetic acid** (412). The reaction takes longer to develop than for CIN, and the rugosity of the vagina further impairs detection. **Vascular patterns are usually indistinct or absent.** A fine capillary punctation is often seen with high-grade VAIN as the acetic acid reaction fades. Prominent abnormal vascular patterns develop late in the neoplastic process. **Widely spaced, varicose punctation and, less frequently, mosaicism occurring in an area of high-grade VAIN, are highly suspicious for invasive cancer.**

The ability reliably to predict the probable histologic status of vaginal colposcopic lesions is a challenge for the most experienced colposcopist. **Examination under general or regional anesthesia may be required, particularly in the presence of extensive disease,** to permit accurate diagnostic workup.

The difficulty in colposcopic assessment of the vagina renders examination after application of aqueous iodine solution invaluable (Fig. 7.25). High-grade VAIN lesions appear mustard yellow against the mahogany-brown staining of normal surrounding mucosa. This assists in the mapping of significant lesions and in obtaining accurate biopsies. The application of aqueous iodine is mandatory for delineation of treatment margins.

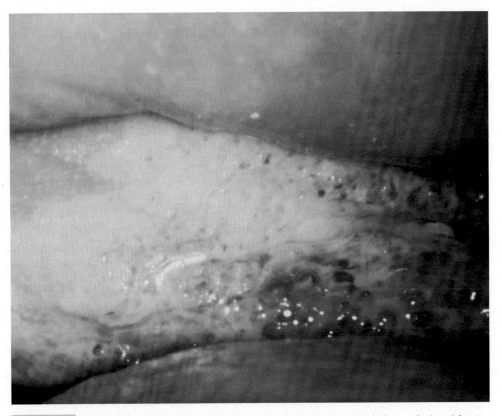

Figure 7.24 Colposcopic appearance of high-grade vaginal intraepithelial neoplasia with acetic acid.

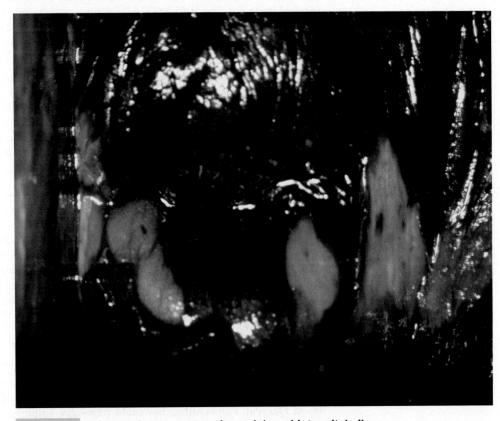

Figure 7.25 Colposcopic appearance after staining with Lugol's iodine.

Treatment of High-Grade Vaginal Intraepithelial Neoplasia

Vaginal intraepithelial neoplasia can be very difficult to treat, particularly in the presence of extensive, multifocal disease or when the vaginal vault is involved posthysterectomy. **Surgical excision, often requiring partial vaginectomy, or vaginal irradiation, were historically used as the main treatment modalities.** Significant morbidity was associated with both approaches.

The CO_2 laser is regarded as the treatment of choice for most VAIN cases (399,400,412,413). The vaginal wall is relatively thin compared with other genital tract sites, with vital organs in close proximity. Surgical access is, at times, difficult. The CO_2 laser provides the surgeon with the ability to treat to a precisely controlled depth and achieve very high cure rates for selected patients (415).

Topical 5-fluorouracil (5-FU) cream can be used with good effect for carefully selected patients (416–420). *5-FU* cream produces chemoinflammation and chemoulceration, which often adequately treats VAIN lesions. Care is required to protect the vulvar skin and to avoid persistent denudation of the vaginal mucosa, particularly in the posterior fornix.

Application of 5% *imiquimod* cream may be considered as an alternative treatment for high-grade VAIN where excision is not indicated. Although the data are limited, *imiquimod* cream has been demonstrated to achieve high clearance and response rates for VAIN. Recurrence rates are no greater than for other topical treatments and it appears to be safe and well tolerated by most patients. ***Imiquimod* has been used for management of extensive, multifocal VAIN lesions, as primary treatment and with the aim of decreasing the extent of disease before ablation** (420). Conservative ablative therapy requires expert colposcopy, liberal use of directed biopsies and no cytologic, colposcopic, or histologic evidence of invasive cancer.

Carbon dioxide laser treatment for high-grade VAIN is best performed using a high-powered superpulse or ultrapulse laser. The beam is defocused to an appropriate beam geometry (see vulvar section), and the vaginal mucosa is destroyed to the depth of the lamina propria, which is at most 2 to 3 mm. Because the vaginal mucosa contains no gland crypts or skin appendages, only superficial treatment is required. Conservatism is important, because delayed healing and scarring may occur after overenthusiastic destruction of vaginal mucosa.

Treatment of high-grade VAIN in the vaginal vault posthysterectomy represents a particular surgical challenge. The 2012 ASCCP Guidelines recommend vaginal cancer screening after hysterectomy be conducted only for women with a history of CIN 2 or worse (59,230). It is important to continue screening these at-risk women, because vaginal neoplasia may not develop for one to two decades or longer after the hysterectomy.

Woodman et al. (421) reported results of **vaginal vault laser surgery for VAIN following hysterectomy** in 23 patients who were followed for a mean period of 30 months. Only six patients remained disease free and invasive cancer developed in two patients. Hoffman et al. (422) reported 32 patients who underwent **upper vaginectomy for VAIN 3.** Occult invasive cancer was found in nine patients (28%). This very difficult problem is increasingly viewed as an indication for surgical excision (423), although CO_2 laser ablation may have a role if the patient is young and attendance at follow-up is likely to be reliable.

Vulva and Perianal Area

Since approximately 1970, there has been a marked increase in the incidence of high-grade preinvasive vulvar disease and a decrease in the modal age of diagnosis (424). Surveillance, Epidemiology, and End Results (SEER) data from the United States have shown a fourfold increase in diagnosis of VIN between 1973 and 2000 (425). There has been a much smaller increase in the incidence of invasive vulvar cancer, presumably because the preinvasive disease is actively treated (425–427). Although about 85% of high-grade VIN lesions are HPV-associated (401), **HPV DNA is detected only in approximately 40% of vulvar cancers** (401). Many of the HPV-negative cancers, particularly in older women, are associated with lichen sclerosus (428–434).

Classification

Preinvasive neoplasia of the vulva has been recognized for more than 75 years, but the descriptive terminology has been confusing. **Vulvar CIS has been described as Bowen disease, erythroplasia of Queyrat, CIS simplex, bowenoid papulosis, kraurosis vulvae, and leukoplakia.** This confusion has been compounded by the use of similar terms to describe a group of nonneoplastic vulvar diseases to which Jeffcoate in 1966 assigned the term **chronic vulvar dystrophy** (435). In 1986, the International Society for the Study of Vulvar Disease (ISSVD) recommended a new classification of vulvar epithelial disorders (436).

Although this classification represented a significant advance in rationalizing previously confusing terminology, significant shortcomings existed. The vulvar intraepithelial neoplasia (VIN) terminology was introduced for uniformity and consistency with the grade classification for CIN. Although this seemed logical, there was some basis for establishing a biologic continuum from CIN 1 to CIN 3. **The neoplastic biologic continuum from VIN 1 through VIN 3 to invasive cancer had not been established.**

Although the progression rate of VIN 3 to invasive cancer remains controversial, the malignant potential has been established (437–442). By contrast, **there is no direct evidence that VIN 1 has any malignant potential.** The detection of high-risk HPV-DNA types in a relatively high proportion of VIN 1 lesions (58%) (401), a considerably higher rate than in condylomata acuminata, has been advanced as an argument for retaining low-grade lesions within the VIN diagnosis. The inclusion of such lesions in the neoplastic continuum creates pressure for a more aggressive therapeutic approach. **There is a compelling argument for excluding low-grade VIN from the "intraepithelial neoplasia" category** (443). When mild squamous atypia is seen in vulvar skin, usually limited to the lower epidermis, the lesion is more likely to be nonneoplastic reactive atypia. Considerable interobserver and intraobserver variation occurs with the VIN 1 diagnosis and this diagnostic category is not reproducible (444).

Most histologic VIN lesions are categorized as VIN 2–3 and good histologic agreement is obtained when VIN 2–3 are combined as a single high-grade VIN diagnosis (444). **Careful histologic and molecular review in the 1990s,** particularly by Kurman and associates, **led to a reclassification of VIN 3 into three histologic subtypes, namely basaloid, warty (or bowenoid), and differentiated (or carcinoma simplex)** (445). Further clinical correlation refined the high-grade VIN diagnosis to include two distinct lesions, which have different morphology, biology, and clinical features (444).

VIN, *usual type,* is seen adjacent to 30% of both warty (condylomatous) and basaloid types of invasive squamous vulvar cancers. It is mostly high-risk HPV related, as are the associated cancers. It has a definite invasive potential, particularly in women over 30 years of age. **A variant of VIN, *usual type,* is the multifocal, pigmented, papular lesion seen in younger women,** often of non-European background, associated with genital warts and sometimes seen in pregnancy. These lesions can regress spontaneously and, although there is a definite potential to progress, close prospective follow-up is justified (446,447).

The less-common VIN, differentiated type, is seen in older women, often adjacent to invasive keratinizing squamous cell carcinoma of the vulva (444,445,448). It may occur with chronic vulvar dermatoses, particularly lichen sclerosus, but also with squamous cell hyperplasia, lichen simplex chronicus, and erosive lichen planus. **VIN, differentiated type, is neither HPV associated, nor is the associated keratinizing squamous cell cancer.** Clinically, these lesions are difficult to distinguish against a dystrophic background. A keratotic nodule or shallow ulcer may be the only clinical indicator.

In 2004, the ISSVD recommended the following modifications to the terminology for squamous vulvar intraepithelial neoplasia (444):

1. **The term VIN 1 should no longer be used,** being replaced with the terms flat condyloma acuminatum or HPV effect. The term "atypia" in this context is discouraged.

2. **The term VIN should apply to histologic high-grade squamous intraepithelial lesions (VIN 2–3).**

3. Two categories of VIN were described:

   a. The more common **VIN, usual type,** which encompasses VIN 2, VIN 3, and the older clinical and histologic terms: Bowen's disease, bowenoid papulosis, dysplasia, and CIS. These lesions are associated with high-risk HPV types, particularly HPV16. VIN, *usual type,* has been **subcategorized histologically as warty** (condylomatous), **basaloid, or mixed**.

   b. The less-common **VIN, differentiated type.** These lesions are not associated with HPV, but frequently occur against a background of a vulvar dermatosus, particularly lichen sclerosus.

Table 7.16 ISSVD Classification of Vulvar Diseases
Nonneoplastic epithelial disorders of skin and mucosa
Lichen sclerosus (formerly lichen sclerosus et atrophicus)
Squamous hyperplasia (formerly hyperplastic dystrophy)
Other dermatoses (e.g., psoriasis)
Intraepithelial neoplasia
Squamous intraepithelial neoplasia

VIN, usual type
  a. VIN, warty type
  b. VIN, basaloid type
  c. VIN, mixed (warty/basaloid) type
VIN, differentiated type

Nonsquamous intraepithelial neoplasia
Paget's disease
Tumors of the melanocytes, noninvasive (melanoma *in situ*)
Mixed nonneoplastic and neoplastic epithelial disorders
Invasive tumors

VIN, vulvar intraepithelial neoplasia.

From Committee on Terminology, International Society for the Study of Vulvar Disease, 2004.

4. The occasional VIN lesion that cannot be classified as VIN, *usual or differentiated* types is termed **VIN, *unclassified type*** (or VIN, NOS). (This includes the rare pagetoid VIN.)

5. Classification is on the basis of histologic morphology only, and not clinical appearance or HPV type.

The 2004 ISSVD classification of VIN is shown in Table 7.16.

Paget's Disease

Paget's disease of the vulva is an uncommon intraepithelial lesion. It is sometimes associated with underlying invasive carcinoma. These conditions are discussed in Chapter 13.

Clinical Profile of High-Grade Vulvar Intraepithelial Neoplasia

The increased incidence of VIN 3 in recent decades reflects increased clinical awareness, improved diagnostic accuracy and an absolute increase in disease incidence. **Specific genital HPV types, in particular HPV 16, are strongly implicated in the causation of high-grade VIN** (401,449–452). Other vulvar HPV-induced lesions, including condylomata acuminata and subclinical HPV infection, frequently either coexist with, or predate the diagnosis of VIN. **Cigarette smoking, endogenous and exogenous systemic immune suppression including HIV infection, previous radiation therapy, and pregnancy have been implicated as cofactors in the pathogenesis of VIN 3** (453–458). There is a strong association between VIN 3 and sexually transmitted disease, with rates varying from 20–60%.

Distribution

High-grade VIN lesions tend to be localized and unifocal in the older patient. A higher malignant potential is presumed for such lesions, because invasive vulvar cancer occurs predominantly in the older age groups. However, many of the invasive cancers in elderly women occur against a background of lichen sclerosus, without a prior history of VIN 3 or coexisting histologic evidence of VIN 3.

In younger patients, high-grade VIN lesions are frequently multifocal and extensive. Lesions may remain discrete or coalesce to develop a large field of disease. Lesions may extend laterally from the inner aspect of the mucous membranes of the labia minora to the hair-bearing skin of the labia majora and from the clitoris, periclitoral area, and mons pubis anteriorly to the perineum and perianal area posteriorly. Difficult-to-access sanctuary sites, such as the urethra, clitoris, vagina, and anal canal, need to be carefully inspected.

Symptoms

More than 30% of women with VIN 3 experience vulvar symptomatology. The most common symptoms are pruritus, burning, pain, and dysuria (458). Vulvar symptoms are often exacerbated by voiding. Patients may present reporting a localized lump or thickening in the vulvar skin, or they may notice an area of increased or decreased pigmentation. The patient may present with a history of recalcitrant vulvar condylomata acuminata.

Delay in diagnosis of high-grade VIN, even in symptomatic patients, is common. Opportunistic inspection of the vulva, particularly at the time of colposcopy for abnormal cervical cytology, is recommended.

Clinical Appearance

The clinical appearance of VIN lesions varies according to patient age and skin color, as well as the location of the lesions in the vulva and perianal region (Figs. 7.26 and 7.27). In both the hair-bearing and nonhair-bearing keratinized vulvar skin, **lesions tend to be raised or papular. They may be white, red, or brown in color.** White lesions are a result of hyperkeratosis or dehydration of the outer keratinized layer. Red lesions result from increased vascularity, reflecting either an inflammatory response or increased blood vessel formation secondary to angiogenic factors of neoplasia. Brown or pigmented lesions, which occur in more than 10% of patients, result from melanin incontinence, usually in the keratinized squamous epithelium.

On the mucosal surfaces and less frequently on the keratinized surfaces, VIN lesions may be flat or macular. Occasionally, such macular lesions are evident through associated erythema or pigmentation. **Usually, macular lesions are subclinical, and are detected on colposcopic examination** after application of 5% acetic acid solution.

The clinical appearance of VIN in dark-skinned women is similar when detected on mucosal surfaces, but may differ in keratinized and hair-bearing areas. Relative hypopigmentation may occur, producing pink or erythematous plaques. Such lesions may blanch densely acetowhite after application of acetic acid solution. Unifocal, localized lesions in older women less frequently involve the mucous membranes. **Care must be taken in the assessment of suspicious vulvar lesions in older women because of the increased risk of undisclosed invasive cancer.** Warning signs of an occult invasive lesion include yellow discoloration, nodularity, ulceration, thick scale, and abnormal vascularity.

VIN is reported in biopsies from 30% of patients with large, persistent condylomatous lesions, particularly if the lesions are pigmented, coalescent, or sessile with a micropapilliferous surface. Condylomatous lesions exhibiting a severely dysplastic morphology on biopsy

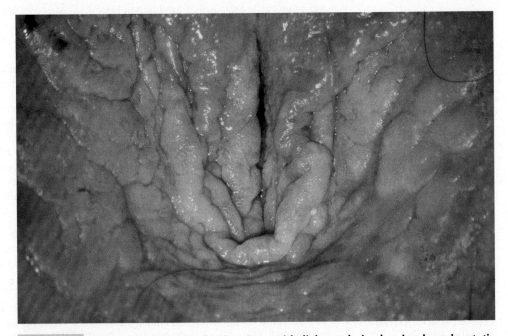

Figure 7.26 Clinical appearance of vulvar intraepithelial neoplasia showing hyperkeratotic papular lesions.

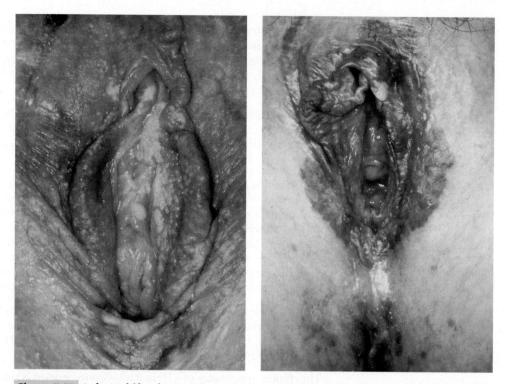

Figure 7.27 *Left:* **Multifocal VIN 3 lesion with multiple hyperpigmented and hyperkeratotic lesions.** *Right:* **Multifocal VIN 3 with confluent hyperpigmented areas on the vulva extending to the perineum and perianal areas.**

frequently harbor high-risk HPV types, with HPV 16 and 18 detected in more than 70% of such lesions (459).

Diagnosis

Colposcopy is now an accepted standard in the diagnostic assessment of preinvasive vulvar disease. The recently published 2011 IFCPC Nomenclature for clinical and colposcopic findings on vulvar examination (88) are shown in Table 7.17 and the definitions of secondary morphologic presentations on vulvar examination are shown in Table 7.18. After application of 5% acetic acid solution and colposcopic assessment, lesions appear as clearly demarcated, dense acetowhite areas. The multifocal distribution is usually evident. The acetic acid reaction is best seen in lesions that are nonpigmented or red. Pigmented lesions often develop an acetowhite hue or a rim of acetowhitening. Initial clinical examination may identify clinically apparent lesions. **Colposcopy may permit identification of previously unidentified, subclinical lesions** and better define the distribution of clinically evident disease.

In high-grade vulvar preinvasive lesions, vascular patterns are often inconspicuous or absent, particularly in the presence of hyperkeratosis. Macular lesions on the mucous membranes may reveal a capillary punctation pattern, and a fine punctation is sometimes observed in papular lesions. **Marked vascular abnormalities** characterized by a varicose, widely spaced punctation and, rarely, mosaicism **represent a definite warning sign of invasive cancer** and the lesion must be excised. Colposcopic warning signs of vulvar cancer occur late in the neoplastic process. **Histologic evidence of VIN may be seen outside colposcopically identified margins of disease, particularly laterally in the hair-bearing areas.**

Diagnosis ultimately depends on liberal use of directed biopsy. This is particularly the case if ablative treatment is being considered, either alone or in combination with excisional procedures. **Biopsies are best taken with a Keyes biopsy instrument** under local anesthesia in the office setting.

Natural History of High-Grade Vulvar Intraepithelial Neoplasia

Vulvar intraepithelial neoplasia coexists with invasive cancer in 30–50% of cases. Vulvar dystrophy occurs in up to 50% of specimens, with lichen sclerosus and squamous hyperplasia equally represented. There is no coexistent disease in 10–15% of specimens (424,439,458).

Table 7.17 The 2011 IFCPC Clinical/Colposcopic Terminology of the Vulva (Including the Anus)

Section	Pattern		
	Various structures Urethra, Skene duct openings, clitoris, prepuce, frenulum, pubis, labia majora, labia minora, interlabial sulci, vestibule, vestibular duct openings, Bartholin duct openings, hymen, fourchette, perineum, anus, anal squamocolumnar junction (dentate line)		
	Composition Squamous epithelium: Hairy/nonhairy, mucosa		
Normal findings	Micropapillomatosis, sebaceous glands (Fordyce spots), vestibular redness		
Abnormal findings	General principles: Size in centimeters, location		
	Lesion type	**Lesion color**	**Secondary morphology**
	Macule	Skin-colored	Eczema
	Patch	Red	Lichenification
	Papule	White	Excoriation
	Plaque	Dark	Purpura
	Nodule		Scarring
	Cyst		Uker
	Vesicle		Erosion
	Bulla		Fissure
	Pustule		Wart
Miscellaneous findings	Trauma Malformation		
Suspicion of malignancy	Gross neoplasm, ulceration, necrosis, bleeding, exophytic lesion, hyperkeratosis With or without white, gray, red, or brown discoloration		
Abnormal colposcopic/other magnification findings	Acetowhite epithelium, punctation, atypical vessels, surface irregularities Abnormal anal squamocolumnar junction (note location about the dentate line)		

From: **Bornstein J, Sideri M, Tatti S, et al.** 2011 Terminology of the Vulva of the International Federation for Cervical Pathology and Colposcopy. *J Low Gen Tract Dis.* 2012;16(3):290–295.

Table 7.18 Definitions of Secondary Morphologic Appearances on Vulvar Examination

Term	Definition
Eczema	A group of inflammatory diseases that are clinically characterized by the presence of itchy, poorly marginated red plaques with minor evidence of microvesiculation and/or, more frequently, subsequent surface disruption
Lichenification	Thickening of the tissue and increased prominence of skin markings. Scale may or may not be detectable in vulvar lichenification. Lichenification may be bright-red, dusky-red, white, or skin colored in appearance.
Excoriation	Surface disruption (notably excoriations) occurring as a result of the "itch-scratch cycle"
Erosion	A shallow defect in the skin surface; absence of some, or all, of the epidermis down to the basement membrane; the dermis is intact
Fissure	A thin, linear erosion of the skin surface
Ulcer	Deeper defect; absence of the epidermis and some, or all, of the dermis

From: **Bornstein J, Sideri M, Tatti S, et al.** 2011 Terminology of the vulva of the International Federation for Cervical Pathology and Colposcopy. *J Low Gen Tract Dis.* 2012;16(3):290–295.

Few studies have examined the natural history of untreated VIN. Jones and Rowan from New Zealand (438) reported in 1994 on the unethical follow-up of 113 women with VIN 3 diagnosed between 1961 and 1993. **Of eight untreated cases of VIN 3, progression to invasive cancer was reported in seven patients (87.5%)** within 8 years. **Other studies, with much shorter follow-up of untreated women, have suggested a lower progression rate** (437,441). A more recent study from New Zealand has reported 47 of 405 women who experienced spontaneous regression of VIN 2–3 (446). These women were young with a mean age of 24 years, often had an initial presentation through a sexual health clinic and a previous history of condylomata acuminata. Most had multifocal, pigmented lesions and median time to regression was 9.5 months. A further eight women in the 31- to 45-year age group with small VIN lesions had disease regression after a small diagnostic biopsy.

The occurrence, usually in younger women, of multifocal, pigmented, papular vulvar lesions reported histologically as VIN 3, has been described as **"bowenoid papulosis"** (460). Reports of spontaneous regression, especially associated with pregnancy, have suggested distinctive epidemiologic features, but the term has been abandoned by the ISSVD and the International Society for Gynecologic Pathologists. **High-grade VIN is a disease with a varied and individual clinical profile and histologic appearance.** This range encompasses the entity previously described as "bowenoid papulosis."

Treatment of High-Grade Vulvar Intraepithelial Neoplasia

Treatment is aimed at control of symptoms and prevention of progression to invasive cancer. Many treatment modalities have been used and, historically, vulvar CIS has been managed by simple vulvectomy (461). Such a radical approach is unjustified and is associated with significant morbidity, particularly for young women, including scarring, dyspareunia, urinary stream difficulties, loss of elasticity for vaginal delivery, and a "castration-like" self-image.

Since the 1970s, there has been a trend toward more conservative therapy, initially using excisional approaches, and more recently, ablative modalities (462,463). **The risk of occult malignancy occurring in association with VIN is too low to mandate complete excision of disease in all patients, but too high to allow routine ablation.** Women undergoing excisional treatment are reported to have a 15–23% incidence of unsuspected invasive squamous cell carcinoma (458,464,465).

The clinical profile of VIN, including a broad age range and marked variability in extent, distribution, and symptomatology, demands individualization of the therapeutic approach for each patient. Multifocality and immunocompromise are associated with an increased risk of recurrent disease. A period of close prospective follow-up without treatment may be appropriate for young, immunocompetent women with multifocal disease, particularly if they are pregnant.

Wide Local Excision, Skin Flap Procedures, and Superficial Vulvectomy

Localized high-grade VIN lesions are best managed by local, superficial ("skinning") excision. The lesion should be excised with a disease-free margin of at least 5 mm. Wide, local excision is ideal for unifocal and lateral lesions or for hemorrhoids involved with high-grade intraepithelial neoplasia. It is mandatory if a lesion has warning signs of possible invasive cancer. Primary closure of the defect usually achieves uncomplicated healing and a very satisfactory cosmetic and functional outcome. The elasticity of the vulvar skin permits preservation of sexual and reproductive functions.

The surgical specimen should be submitted to careful histologic evaluation to exclude invasive disease and to ensure clear surgical margins. **Surgical excision with disease-free margins achieves a 90% cure rate for localized disease. If the margins are involved with disease, the cure rate falls to 50%,** demanding very close follow-up (453). **As long as all macroscopic disease has been removed, re-excision is not justified for positive margins.** Most recurrences occur within 3 years of treatment, although late recurrence and progression to cancer can occur. Development of symptoms should prompt urgent review.

Large, confluent lesions or extensive multifocal disease, particularly in the presence of colposcopic warning signs of early invasion, require more extensive excisional procedures with rotational flaps to fill the defect, or superficial (skinning) vulvectomy with a split-thickness skin graft (466,467). Primary closure of a large vulvar wound may not be possible without undue tension, leading to wound breakdown or excessive scarring.

Cutaneous flaps with no muscle component have been used for cases of extensive excision of VIN (468–470). Perineal flaps of skin and fascial tissue rotated around a perforating branch of the internal iliac artery have been used to close larger vulvovaginal defects (468). Thin skin flaps with less than 1 cm of underlying fat can be raised from the buttock and rotated medially to close vulvar defects (469). Good postoperative healing is usually achieved without significant morbidity or long-term negative impact on sexual functioning.

"Skinning" vulvectomy was introduced by Rutledge and Sinclair (466) **for extensive VIN lesions,** particularly in the hair-bearing skin where the skin appendages may be involved. Lesions are carefully mapped and a shallow layer of vulvar skin is excised, preserving the subcutaneous tissues. The vulvar skin at risk is replaced with epidermis from a donor site on the inner aspect of the thigh or buttock. The clitoris is preserved, with lesions on the prepuce or glans being superficially excised or laser ablated. The epithelium regenerates without loss of sensation. DiSaia (467) reported a 39% recurrence rate in patients with VIN 3 treated by skinning vulvectomy with split-thickness skin grafting. There were no recurrences in grafted areas, although such recurrence has been reported.

CO$_2$ Laser Surgery

Vulvar intraepithelial neoplasia is occurring more frequently in young women, and the disease may be very extensive, involving the hair-bearing area of the labia majora in more than 30% of cases. **Excision of such wide areas, even with skin grafting, can cause significant scarring and anatomic distortion.** With careful, expert colposcopy and liberal use of directed biopsy, the undisclosed cancer risk in selected patients is low.

Some consider an ablative procedure in these young patients using the CO$_2$ laser to be the treatment of choice (471–475). The morbidity associated with ablation of large areas of VIN has been found to be unacceptable in some studies. The initial 2 weeks following more extensive laser ablative procedures will be associated with significant pain, particularly with micturition. The use of appropriate laser technology and settings, advanced surgical expertise with careful control of depth of ablation, and appropriate postoperative care will mitigate much of the potential morbidity. **CO$_2$ laser ablation is particularly useful in patients with periclitoral and perianal disease, where the preservation of anatomy and function is a substantial benefit.**

Physical Principles Governing Vulvar Laser Surgery

1. **Choice of appropriate laser wavelength.** The CO$_2$ laser is the only laser proven to be safe and effective for the management of high-grade VIN.

2. **Rapid delivery of the required energy dose.** Vulvar laser surgery demands minimization of lateral thermal injury to prevent scarring and morbidity. The surgeon must be able to control higher powers to permit precise, rapid ablation. For ablative procedures, **powers of less than 50 W in continuous mode are associated with an increased risk of thermal injury** and should be avoided.

3. **Choice of appropriate temporal mode.** The option of choosing **rapid super-pulse or the newer ultrapulse technology** affords a definite therapeutic advantage in CO$_2$ laser ablation of vulvar lesions. The ability precisely to vaporize diseased tissue under visual control with minimal heat propagation to adjacent tissue is the key to nonmorbid laser surgery.

4. **Choice of appropriate power density.** CO$_2$ laser ablation requires power densities in the range of 800 to 1,400 W/cm^2.

5. **Choice of appropriate beam geometry.** The incident laser beam produces a conical impact crater with marked variation in intensity of the beam from point to point in the focal spot. The clinical importance of the concept of beam geometry is that the crater shape mirrors the intensity profile of the incident energy (Fig. 7.28). When the incident laser beam is highly focused, the vaporization crater is a narrow, deep "drill hole." This reflects the high-power density and is arbitrarily designated as the *X-beam geometry.* The X-beam geometry is for cutting or for excisional procedures. If the incident laser beam is flattened completely, it will simply coagulate a broad zone of tissue at the impact site but will not have sufficient power to vaporize tissue. The wide, flattened spot size produces the *Z-beam geometry.* In contrast, **defocusing the laser beam to an intermediate, round beam geometry produces a round, shallow vaporization crater at the impact site. This is designated the *Y-beam geometry*** and permits controlled tissue vaporization to a relatively uniform and predictable depth. The laser should be first tested on a moistened tongue blade to defocus the beam to the hemispherical Y-beam geometry before use on the skin.

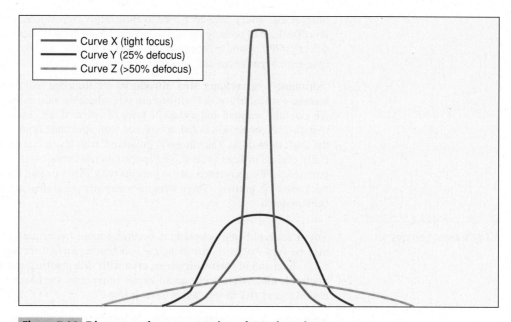

Curve X (tight focus)
Curve Y (25% defocus)
Curve Z (>50% defocus)

Figure 7.28 Diagrammatic representation of CO_2 laser beam geometry.

6. **Intermittent gated pulsing.** CO_2 laser surgery to the vulvar skin requires training and skill in the use of the foot pedal to deliver the laser energy in short bursts to control the depth of ablation.

Surgical Strategies Governing Vulvar CO_2 Laser Surgery

1. **Choice of appropriate beam delivery system.** For ablative procedures, the laser must be controlled using a micromanipulator through a colposcope or operating microscope with a 300-mm objective to produce a relatively large spot size with excellent depth of field. The angle of impact of the laser is controlled by traction on the skin. A handheld mirror may occasionally be required to reflect the beam to difficult-to-access sites.

2. **Minimization of thermal injury.** Thermal injury can be further minimized by chilling the vulvar skin, before and during surgery, with laparotomy packs soaked in iced saline solution. This simple strategy diminishes postoperative pain and swelling and promotes healing.

3. **Accurate delineation of treatment margins.** The laser is used under colposcopic control. The possible extension of high-grade VIN beyond areas that are colposcopically evident indicates the need for treatment margins of several spot sizes. The laser can be used initially to circumscribe the distribution of the lesions before the acetic acid reaction fades.

4. **Accurate depth control.** Determination of depth of ablation is best achieved by a precise understanding of the visual landmarks of the surgical planes of the vulva as described by Reid et al. (472,473) (Fig. 7.29).

5. **Control of intraoperative and postoperative pain and bleeding.** CO_2 laser procedures for high-grade VIN are performed under general or regional anesthesia unless the disease is localized. Subcutaneous injection of a long-acting local anesthetic on completion of the procedure diminishes pain in the immediate postoperative period. **Narcotic analgesia is usually required in the immediate postoperative period** or, alternatively, prolonged epidural analgesia can be used. Regular sitz baths followed by topical application of a mixture of equal parts 1% *lidocaine* and 2% *silver sulfadiazine* creams to the surgical site aid in pain relief. The postoperative discomfort is often most severe on the third to the sixth postoperative days. Patients should have available appropriate oral narcotic analgesics to provide relief after discharge from hospital.

Surgical Planes

First Surgical Plane   **Destruction to the first surgical plane removes the surface epithelium to the level of the basement membrane.** The laser beam is rapidly oscillated across the target

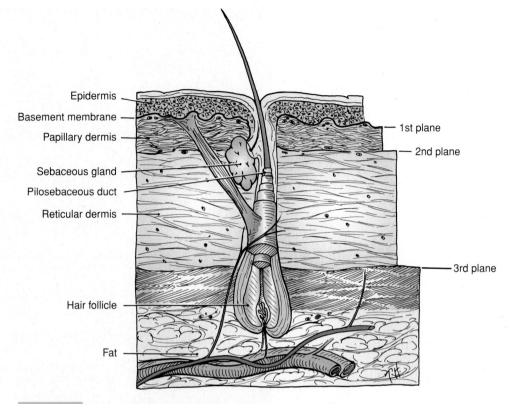

Figure 7.29 **Diagrammatic representation of three surgical planes.**

tissue with the spot describing a series of roughly parallel lines. When the impact debris is wiped away with a moistened swab, the moist "sand-grain" appearance of the papillary dermis will be evident (Fig. 7.30).

Second Surgical Plane   **Ablation to the second plane removes the epidermis and the superficial papillary dermis.** This plane is achieved by a slightly slower oscillation of the laser beam across the first surgical plane, scorching but not penetrating the papillary dermis. The visual effect is a shrinking of the target tissue because of dehydration and a finely roughened, yellowish surface similar in appearance to a chamois cloth is produced. Ablation extends to the deep papillary dermis with minimal thermal injury to the underlying reticular dermis. **The second surgical plane is the preferred depth of ablation for condylomata acuminata treated with the CO_2 laser.**

Third Surgical Plane   **Destruction to the third surgical plane removes the epidermis, papillary dermis, and superficial reticular dermis containing the upper portions of the skin appendages,** specifically the pilosebaceous ducts and hair follicles. This is achieved by a slower, purposeful movement of the laser beam across the second surgical plane. The tissue is seen to relax and separate as the midreticular dermis is exposed as moistened gray-white fibers representing coarse collagen bundles. **Healing occurs from the base of the skin appendages and scarring is absent or minimal. Ablative procedures for VIN should be carried to the depth of the third surgical plane** (Fig. 7.31). **The skin appendages are involved with the VIN process in more than 50% of cases** (473). Depth of hair follicle involvement is usually less than 1 mm but may extend to 2 mm. Measured sweat gland involvement has been more than 3 mm in depth. Beyond 3 mm, the equivalent of a third-degree thermal defect is created, resulting in delayed healing, scarring, and alopecia. The implications of residual disease after treatment of VIN are different from those of residual CIN, which may be buried and escape detection. Although the surgeon should be aware of vulvar skin appendage involvement, this is not an indication to destroy beyond the midreticular dermis.

Fourth Surgical Plane   Destruction of the reticular dermis creates a thermal injury extending to the subcutaneous tissues and must be avoided.

Long-Term Follow-up

Regardless of treatment modality, **recurrence of VIN is common** (453,454). Even with modern treatment and management, invasive cancer will still develop in 3–5% of women, considerably

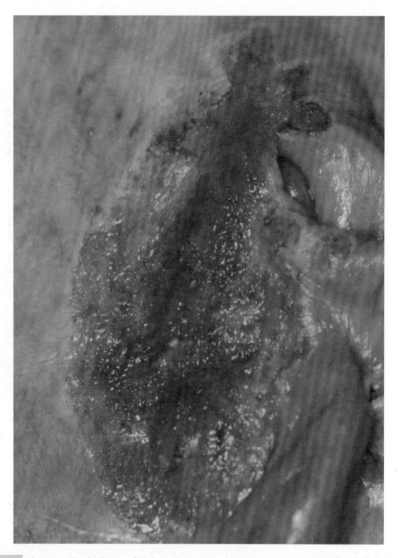

Figure 7.30 **First Surgical Plane of Vulvar CO$_2$ Laser Surgery—very superficial ablation of epidermis revealing the papillae of the papillary dermis.** The thermal effect extends into the superficial reticular dermis.

higher than the risk of cervical cancer posttreatment of CIN. Recurrent VIN is a significant problem and represents both incomplete primary treatment and disease recurrence. **Lifelong vigilance is an important component of the management of VIN.**

Immune Response Modifiers

Surgery is the treatment of choice for VIN, but the surgical margins will be positive in 24–68% of cases. Surgery does not eradicate HPV, the primary cause of most cases of VIN, which argues for the possible role of immune response modifiers in treatment (476–478).

Imiquimod   *Imiquimod (Aldara)* **is an imidazoquinoline, a novel synthetic compound that is a topical immune response stimulator.** It enhances both the innate and acquired immune pathways, particularly the T helper cell type 1–mediated immune response, resulting in antiviral, antitumor, and immunoregulatory activities (476,477). HPV exclusively infects epithelial keratinocytes. The virus does not elicit cell death and infection is not accompanied by inflammation, which would normally activate the immune system.

It is difficult for the host immune system to recognize the virus during the early stages of infection, which increases the risk for persistent infection. *Imiquimod* causes proinflammatory cytokine induction in the skin by binding on Toll-like receptors 7 and 8 on the cell surface of dendritic cells. This upregulates the host immune system to recognize the presence of a viral infection or tumor, theoretically leading to eradication of the lesion. It stimulates activation, maturation, and migration

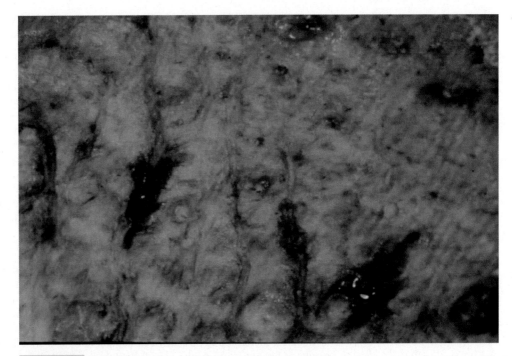

Figure 7.31 Third Surgical Plane of Vulvar CO_2 Laser Surgery—removes the epidermis, papillary dermis, and superficial reticular dermis containing the upper portions of the skin appendages, specifically the pilosebaceous ducts and hair follicles. The midreticular dermis is exposed as moistened gray-white fibers representing coarse collagen bundles.

of Langerhans cells, the major antigen-presenting cells of the skin, which are depleted by HPV infection (476,477). *Imiquimod* alters the local immune response in favor of clearance of a persistent HPV infection.

A patient-applied topical 5% *imiquimod* cream is clinically efficacious and safe in the management of condylomata acuminata (479–482). The beneficial effects, patient acceptability, and low morbidity have led to its recent evaluation in the treatment of VIN. Case reports demonstrated efficacy against VIN 2–3, including in an immune-suppressed lung transplant patient (483). Pilot studies, applying *imiquimod* one to three times a week at night, reported a 30% complete response rate and 60% partial response after 6 to 30 weeks of treatment (484–486). **In contrast to surgical treatment, *imiquimod* focuses on the cause of many VIN cases, and preserves the anatomy and function of the vulva (420).** Exclusion of invasive cancer is an important aspect of pretreatment assessment.

In a placebo controlled, randomized trial of *imiquimod* in the treatment of high-grade VIN, 26 women were treated with the active cream (487). Over an observation period of 1 year, 9 women (35%) showed complete response and 12 (46%) showed a partial response as opposed to none in the placebo group. All complete responders remained disease-free at 12 months follow-up. Regression from VIN 2–3 to low-grade disease was seen in 18 of 26 patients treated (69%) and 15 of these tested negative for HPV DNA after treatment. Three patients developed early invasive cancer to a depth less than 1 mm, two after placebo treatment and one after *imiquimod*, reinforcing the need for close follow-up. *Imiquimod* is well tolerated and less invasive than surgery. The authors subsequently reported on a median 7.2-year follow-up of the initial study group (488). If a patient had a complete response, there was only one later recurrence. Many of the complete responders had smaller lesions at the outset.

HPV Vaccination

The very strong association between usual-type VIN and HPV16 indicates that the current vaccination programs targeting HPV 16 and 18 should significantly impact the future incidence of VIN and vulvar cancer. The FUTURE I and FUTURE II trials of the quadrivalent vaccine against HPVs 6, 11, 16, and 18 have demonstrated very high levels of protection against future development of usual-type VIN (193). This protection applied to the population of women who may have been already exposed to high-risk HPV types. Although the modal age of diagnosis of usual-type VIN has fallen substantially, current trials still exclude the age groups at greatest risk of this disease. As the majority of HPV-associated vulvar and vaginal cancers occur in the older age-groups, the ultimate benefits of vaccination are likely to take some years to be fully realized.

The use of vaccination against HPV 16 oncoproteins as a therapeutic strategy for women with *usual-type* **VIN is very promising** (489). Kenter reported on 20 women with HPV 16-positive VIN who were vaccinated three or four times with a synthetic long-peptide that represented the entire length of the two HPV16 viral oncoproteins E6 and E7 (490). Three months after vaccination, 5 of 20 patients (25%) had a complete response. This increased to 9 of 19 (47%) at 12 months after last vaccination. Complete response was maintained at 24 months. Complete responders had a significantly stronger response of interferon-γ-associated proliferative CD4$^+$ T-cells, and a broader response of CD8$^+$ interferon-γ T-cells than did nonresponders. Complete response appeared to be correlated with induction of HPV 16-specific immunity. Smaller high-grade VIN lesions tended to respond better to vaccination. Of the 20 women followed prospectively after completion of the vaccination program, four women, who were all partial responders, were diagnosed with invasive cancer at between 1 and 3.5 years. Kenter et al. focused on HPV 16-positive VIN 3 lesions and HPV 16-specific immunotherapy. At least 14 common types of HPV (e.g., types 6, 11, 16, 18, 31, 33, 35, 39, 45, 51, 52, 56, 58, and 59) are detected in VIN lesions; many of these types are included in the next generation nonavalent HPV vaccine.

The combination of *imiquimod* **treatment with HPV vaccination may offer another nonsurgical approach to the treatment of VIN.** A recent British Phase II trial evaluated the treatment of VIN using *imiquimod* followed by an *HPV therapeutic vaccine* (TA-CIN, Fusion Protein HPV 16 E6E7L2) (491). There were 19 VIN patients treated with *imiquimod* for 8 weeks followed by three doses of *HPV therapeutic vaccine.* Complete histologic regression was observed in 32% of women at week 10, increasing to 58% at week 20, and 63% at week 52. These results are promising and results of larger trials and long-term follow-up are awaited.

No treatment modality is ideal for every woman. Treatment should be individualized according to age, distribution, severity, associated disease, and previous treatment. Close follow-up after treatment remains essential because of the risk of recurrent disease. Most recurrences occur within 3 years of treatment. Positive excision margins, multifocal disease, smoking, and immunosuppression are associated with increased recurrence rates.

Multicentric Lower Genital Tract Neoplasia

The concept of multicentricity of lower genital tract neoplasia is well established (492) reflecting the "field effect" of high-risk HPV types (493,494). Multiple primary preinvasive or invasive lesions involving the cervix, vagina, vulva, and/or anus can occur synchronously or metachronously in this region. **Multicentric preinvasive disease has a higher recurrence rate after treatment than unicentric disease** (495). Continued detection of high-risk HPV DNA results in a risk of recurrence of 45%. Other risk factors for recurrence include age, immunosuppression, smoking, choice of treatment modality, and positive surgical margins.

High-grade *perianal intraepithelial neoplasia* **(PAIN) occurs in more than 30% of patients with VIN** (496) (Fig. 7.32A) **or multicentric squamous neoplasia.** High-grade PAIN may occur in recalcitrant perianal condylomata acuminata, or as thickened, hyperkeratotic, often pigmented papular lesions usually visible to the naked eye. Proctoscopic examination using the colposcope after application of acetic acid may reveal high-grade squamous preinvasive disease extending to above the dentate line. **Men who have sex with men (MSM), especially if HIV positive, are at higher risk of anal cancer.** Viral analysis has confirmed a strong association between anal cancer and HPV16 (497–500). Women with HPV-related gynecologic neoplasms are at a higher risk of developing anal cancer compared to the general population (501), and may benefit from close observation and screening for anal cancer. **The incidence of anal cancer in women has risen by over 40% over the past 30 years** (502,503).

The frequency of progression of high-grade anal intraepithelial neoplasia to anal squamous cell cancer has not been fully elucidated, but is believed to be in the range of 8.5–13% (504,505). **High-grade PAIN is managed similarly to VIN.** Conservation of normal tissues by careful colposcopic delineation of diseased areas is important. The CO_2 laser may afford some therapeutic advantage, because disruption of nerve fibers with full-thickness excision can lead to incontinence of flatus. Disease may extend posteriorly onto the natal cleft. Although considerable postoperative care is required for pain control and wound care, **modern CO_2 laser surgery is usually the treatment of choice in this difficult situation,** after exclusion of invasive cancer (Fig. 7.32B). **Topical** *imiquimod* **cream may be a useful primary treatment** or adjuvant in difficult to access sites.

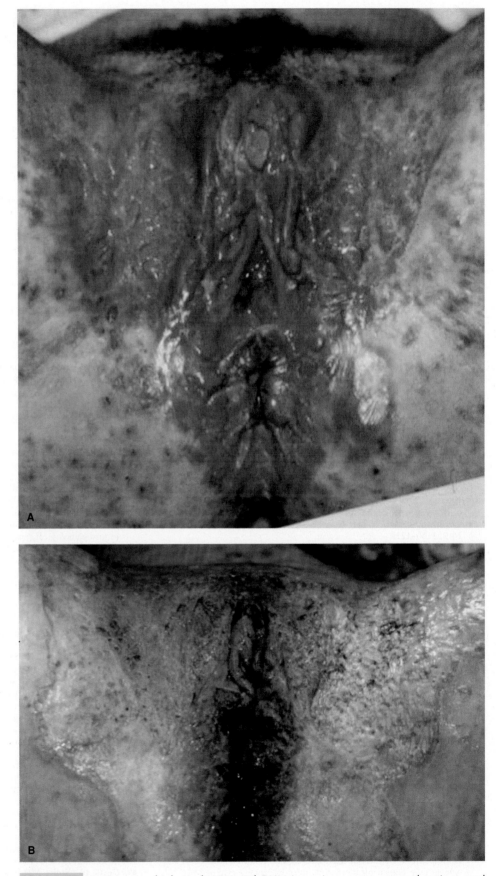

Figure 7.32 **A:** Extensive high-grade VIN and PAIN in an immunosuppressed patient, and **B:** following extensive laser treatment.

References

1. **Forman D, de Martel C, Lacey CJ, et al.** Global burden of human papillomavirus and related diseases. *Vaccine.* 2012;30(suppl 5):F12–F23.

2. **Maucort-Boulch D, Franceschi S, Plummer M, IARC HPV Prevalence Surveys Study Group.** International correlation between human papillomavirus prevalence and cervical cancer incidence. *Cancer Epidemiol Biomarkers Prev.* 2008;17(3):717–720.

3. **IARC.** Cervix cancer screening. In: Strategies IWGatEoCP, ed. *IARC Handbooks of Cancer Prevention.* Volume 10. Lyon: IARC Press; 2005.

4. **Simonella L, Canfell K.** The impact of a two- versus three-yearly cervical screening interval recommendation on cervical cancer incidence and mortality: An analysis of trends in Australia, New Zealand, and England. *Cancer Causes Control.* 2013;24(9):1727–1736.

5. **Barron BA, Richart RM.** Screening protocols for cervical neoplastic disease. *Gynecol Oncol.* 1981;12(2 Pt 2):S156–S167.

6. **Sasieni PD, Cuzick J, Lynch-Farmery E.** Estimating the efficacy of screening by auditing smear histories of women with and without cervical cancer. The National Co-ordinating Network for Cervical Screening Working Group. *Br J Cancer.* 1996;73(8):1001–1005.

7. **Schauenstein W.** Histologische untersuchunges uber atypisches plattienepithel an der portio an der innerflache der cervix uteri. *Arch Gynakol.* 1908;85:576.

8. **Weid GL ed.** *Exfoliative Cytology. Proceedings of the 1st International Congress on Exfoliative Cytology.* Philadephia, PA: JB Lippincott; 1961.

9. **Schiffman M, Castle PE, Jeronimo J, et al.** Human papillomavirus and cervical cancer. *Lancet.* 2007;370(9590):890–907.

10. **Papanicolaou GN, Traut HF.** *The Diagnosis of Uterine Cancer by the Vaginal Smear.* New York: Commonwealth Fund; 1943.

11. **Reagan JW, Hamonic MJ.** The cellular pathology in carcinoma in situ. A cytohistopathological correlation. *Cancer.* 1956;9(2):385–402.

12. **Reagan JW, Patten SF.** Dysplasia: A basic reaction to injury in the uterine cervix. *Ann N Y Acad Sci.* 1962;97(3):662–682.

13. **Reagan JW, Patten SFJ.** Analytic study of cellular changes in carcinoma in situ, squamous-cell cancer, and adenocarcinoma of uterine cervix. *Clin Obstet Gynecol.* 1961;4(4):1097–1127.

14. **Koss LG, Stewart FW, Foote FW, et al.** Some histological aspects of behavior of epidermoid carcinoma in situ and related lesions of the uterine cervix. A long-term prospective study. *Cancer.* 1963;16(9):1160–1211.

15. **Koss LG.** Dysplasia. A real concept or a misnomer? *Obstet Gynecol.* 1978;51(3):374–379.

16. **Langley FA.** In: Langley FA, Crompton AC, eds. *Epithelial Abnormalities of the Cervix Uteri.* Berlin, New York: Springer; 1973.

17. **Richart RM.** Natural history of cervical intraepithelial neoplasia. *Clin Obstet Gynecol.* 1968;10:748–784.

18. **Richart RM, Barron BA.** A follow-up study of patients with cervical dysplasia. *Am J Obstet Gynecol.* 1969;105(3):386–393.

19. **Richart RM.** Cervical intraepithelial neoplasia. *Pathol Annu.* 1973;8:301–328.

20. **Coppleson M, Reid, BL.** Aetiology of squamous carcinoma of the cervix. *Obstet Gynecol.* 1968;32:432–436.

21. **Coppleson M, Reid B.** Interpretation of changes in the uterine cervix. *Lancet.* 1969;2(7613):216–217.

22. **Richart RM.** Causes and management of cervical intraepithelial neoplasia. *Cancer.* 1987;60:1951–1959.

23. **Ostor AG.** Natural history of cervical intraepithelial neoplasia: A critical review. *Int J Gynecol Pathol.* 1993;12(2):186–192.

24. **Duggan MA, McGregor SE, Stuart GC, et al.** The natural history of CIN I lesions. *Eur J Gynaecol Oncol.* 1998;19(4):338–344.

25. **Holowaty P, Miller AB, Rohan T, et al.** RESPONSE: Re: Natural history of dysplasia of the uterine cervix. *J Natl Cancer Inst.* 1999;91(16):1420A–1421.

26. **Melnikow J, Nuovo J, Willan AR, et al.** Natural history of cervical squamous intraepithelial lesions: A meta-analysis. *Obstet Gynecol.* 1998;92(4 Pt 2):727–735.

27. **Hildesheim A, Schiffman MH, Gravitt PE, et al.** Persistence of type-specific human papillomavirus infection among cytologically normal women. *J Infect Dis.* 1994;169(2):235–240.

28. **Herrero R, Schiffman MH, Bratti C, et al.** Design and methods of a population-based natural history study of cervical neoplasia in a rural province of Costa Rica: The Guanacaste Project. *Rev Panam Salud Publica.* 1997;1(5):362–375.

29. **Manos MM, Kinney WK, Hurley LB, et al.** Identifying women with cervical neoplasia: Using human papillomavirus DNA testing for equivocal Papanicolaou results. *JAMA.* 1999;281(17):1605–1610.

30. **Moscicki AB, Schiffman M, Kjaer S, et al.** Chapter 5: Updating the natural history of HPV and anogenital cancer. *Vaccine.* 2006;24(suppl 3):S42–S51.

31. **Koutsky LA, Holmes KK, Critchlow CW, et al.** A cohort study of the risk of cervical intraepithelial neoplasia grade 2 or 3 in relation to papillomavirus infection. *N Engl J Med.* 1992;327(18):1272–1278.

32. **Ho GY, Bierman R, Beardsley L, et al.** Natural history of cervicovaginal papillomavirus infection in young women. *N Engl J Med.* 1998;338(7):423–428.

33. **The 1988 Bethesda System for reporting cervical/vaginal cytological diagnoses.** National Cancer Institute Workshop. *JAMA.* 1989;262(7):931–934.

34. **Schiffman MH.** Recent progress in defining the epidemiology of human papillomavirus infection and cervical neoplasia. *J Natl Cancer Inst.* 1992;84(6):394–398.

35. **The Bethesda System for reporting cervical/vaginal cytologic diagnoses.** Revised after the second National Cancer Institute Workshop, April 29–30, 1991. *Acta Cytol.* 1993;37(2):115–124.

36. **Kurman RJ, Henson DE, Herbst AL, et al.** Interim guidelines for management of abnormal cervical cytology. The 1992 National Cancer Institute Workshop. *JAMA.* 1994;271(23):1866–1869.

37. **Solomon D, Davey D, Kurman R, et al.** The 2001 Bethesda System: Terminology for reporting results of cervical cytology. *JAMA.* 2002;287(16):2114–2119.

38. **Stoler MH.** New Bethesda terminology and evidence-based management guidelines for cervical cytology findings. *JAMA.* 2002;287(16):2140–2141.

39. **Wright TC Jr., Massad LS, Dunton CJ, et al.** 2006 consensus guidelines for the management of women with abnormal cervical cancer screening tests. *Am J Obstet Gynecol.* 2007;197(4):346–355.

40. **Stoler MH, Schiffman M.** Interobserver reproducibility of cervical cytologic and histologic interpretations: Realistic estimates from the ASCUS-LSIL Triage Study. *JAMA.* 2001;285(11):1500–1505.

41. **Robertson AJ, Anderson JM, Beck JS, et al.** Observer variability in histopathological reporting of cervical biopsy specimens. *J Clin Pathol.* 1989;42(3):231–238.

42. **Mitchell MF, Tortolero-Luna G, Wright T, et al.** Cervical human papillomavirus infection and intraepithelial neoplasia: A review. *J Natl Cancer Inst Monogr.* 1996;(21):17–25.

43. **Wright TC.** CHAPTER 3 Pathology of HPV infection at the cytologic and histologic levels: Basis for a 2-tiered morphologic classification system. *Int J Gynaecol.* 2006;94(suppl 1):S22–S31.

44. **Schiffman M, Rodriguez AC.** Heterogeneity in CIN 3 diagnosis. *Lancet Oncol.* 2008;9:404–406.

45. **Cox JT, Schiffman M, Solomon D.** Prospective follow-up suggests similar risk of subsequent cervical intraepithelial neoplasia grade 2 or 3 among women with cervical intraepithelial neoplasia grade 1 or negative colposcopy and directed biopsy. *Am J Obstet Gynecol.* 2003;188(6):1406–1412.

46. **The ASCUS-LSIL Triage Study (ALTS) Group.** Results of a randomized trial on the management of cytology interpretations of atypical squamous cells of undetermined significance. *Am J Obstet Gynecol.* 2003;188(6):1383–1392.

47. **Schiffman M, Glass AG, Wentzensen N, et al.** A long-term prospective study of type-specific human papillomavirus infection and risk of cervical neoplasia among 20,000 women in the Portland Kaiser Cohort Study. *Cancer Epidemiol Biomarkers Prev.* 2011;20(7):1398–1409.

48. **Kjaer S, Hogdall E, Frederiksen K, et al.** The absolute risk of cervical abnormalities in high-risk human papillomavirus-positive, cytologically normal women over a 10-year period. *Cancer Res.* 2006;66(21):10630–10636.

49. **Castle PE, Stoler MH, Solomon D, et al.** The relationship of community biopsy-diagnosed cervical intraepithelial neoplasia grade 2 to

the quality control pathology-reviewed diagnoses: An ALTS report. *Am J Clin Pathol.* 2007;127(5):805–815.

50. **Wang SS, Zuna RE, Wentzensen N, et al.** Human papillomavirus cofactors by disease progression and human papillomavirus types in the study to understand cervical cancer early endpoints and determinants. *Cancer Epidemiol Biomarkers Prev.* 2009;18:113–120.

51. **Luhn P, Walker J, Schiffman M, et al.** The role of cofactors in the progression from human papillomavirus infection to cervical cancer. *Gynecol Oncol.* 2013;128:265–270.

52. **Wentzensen N, Schiffman M, Dunn T, et al.** Multiple human papillomavirus genotype infections in cervical cancer progression in the study to understand cervical cancer early endpoints and determinants. *Int J Cancer.* 2009;125:2151–2158.

53. **Castle PE, Schiffman M, Wheeler CM, et al.** Evidence for frequent regression of cervical intraepithelial neoplasia-grade 2. *Obstet Gynecol.* 2009;113:18–25.

54. **von Knebel Doeberitz M.** New markers for cervical dysplasia to visualise the genomic chaos created by aberrant oncogenic papillomavirus infections. *Eur J Cancer.* 2002;38(17):2229–2242.

55. **Sindos M, Ndisang D, Pisal N, et al.** Measurement of Brn-3 a levels in Pap smears provides a novel diagnostic marker for the detection of cervical neoplasia. *Gynecol Oncol.* 2003;90(2):366–371.

56. **Middleton K, Peh W, Southern S, et al.** Organization of human papillomavirus productive cycle during neoplastic progression provides a basis for selection of diagnostic markers. *J Virol.* 2003; 77(19):10186–10201.

57. **Wentzensen N, Schwartz L, Zuna RE, et al.** Performance of p16/Ki-67 immunostaining to detect cervical cancer precursors in a colposcopy referral population. *Clin Cancer Res.* 2012;18(15):4154–4162.

58. **Wentzensen N, von Knebel DM.** Biomarkers in cervical cancer screening. *Dis Markers.* 2007;23:315–330.

59. **Darragh TM, Colgan TJ, Cox JT, et al.** The Lower Anogenital Squamous Terminology Standardization Project for HPV-Associated Lesions: Background and consensus recommendations from the College of American Pathologists and the American Society for Colposcopy and Cervical Pathology. *J Low Genit Tract Dis.* 2012; 16:205–242.

60. **Castle PE, Sideri M, Jeronimo J, et al.** Risk assessment to guide the prevention of cervical cancer. *Am J Obstet Gynecol.* 2007; 197(4):1–6.

61. **McCredie MR, Sharples KJ, Paul C, et al.** Natural history of cervical neoplasia and risk of invasive cancer in women with cervical intraepithelial neoplasia 3: A retrospective cohort study. *Lancet Oncol.* 2008;9:425–434.

62. **McCredie MR, Paul C, Sharples KJ, et al.** Consequences in women participating in a study of the natural history of cervical intraepithelial neoplasia 3. *ANZJ Obstet Gynecol.* 2010;50:363–370.

63. **Melsheimer P, Vinokurova S, Wentzensen N, et al.** DNA aneuploidy and integration of human papillomavirus type 16 e6/e7 oncogenes in intraepithelial neoplasia and invasive squamous cell carcinoma of the cervix uteri. *Clin Cancer Res.* 2004;10:3059–3063.

64. **Chow LT, Broker TR.** Human papillomavirus infections: Warts or Cancer? *Cold Spring Harb Perspect Biol.* 2013;5:a012997.

65. **Schiffman M, Wentzensen N.** Human papillomavirus infection and the multistage carcinogenesis of cervical cancer. *Cancer Epidemiol Biomarkers Prev.* 2013;22(4):553–560.

66. **Schiffman M, Herrero R, Desalle R, et al.** The carcinogenicity of human papillomavirus types reflects viral evolution. *Virology.* 2005; 337(1):76–84.

67. **Khan MJ, Castle PE, Lorincz AT, et al.** The elevated 10-year risk of cervical precancer and cancer in women with human papillomavirus (HPV) type 16 or 18 and the possible utility of type-specific HPV testing in clinical practice. *J Natl Cancer Inst.* 2005;97(14):1072–1079.

68. **Nobbenhuis MA, Helmerhorst TJ, van den Brule AJ, et al.** Cytological regression and clearance of high-risk human papillomavirus in women with an abnormal cervical smear. *Lancet.* 2001; 358(9295):1782–1783.

69. **Schlecht NF, Platt RW, Duarte-Franco E, et al.** Human papillomavirus infection and time to progression and regression of cervical intraepithelial neoplasia. *J Natl Cancer Inst.* 2003;95(17):1336–1343.

70. **Moscicki AB, Shiboski S, Hills NK, et al.** Regression of low-grade squamous intra-epithelial lesions in young women. *Lancet.* 2004; 364(9446):1678–1683.

71. **Campion MJ, McCance DJ, Cuzick J, et al.** Progressive potential of mild cervical atypia: Prospective cytological, colposcopic, and virological study. *Lancet.* 1986;2(8501):237–240.

72. **Reid R.** Biology and colposcopic features of human papillomavirus-associated cervical disease. *Obstet Gynecol Clin North Am.* 1993; 20(1):123–151.

73. **Greenberg MD, Reid R, Schiffman M, et al.** A prospective study of biopsy-confirmed cervical intraepithelial neoplasia grade 1: Colposcopic, cytological, and virological risk factors for progression. *J Low Genit Tract Dis.* 1999;3(2):104–110.

74. **Doorbar J.** Papillomavirus life cycle organization and biomarker selection. *Dis Markers.* 2007;23:297–313.

75. **Doorbar J.** The papillomavirus life cycle. *J Clin Virol.* 2005;32 (suppl 1):S7–S15.

76. **Stoler MH.** The pathology of cervical neoplasia. In: **Rohan TE, Shah KV, eds.** *Cervical Cancer: From Etiology to Prevention.* New York, NY: Springer; 2004:3–60.

77. **Stoler MH.** Human papillomaviruses and cervical neoplasia: A model for carcinogenesis. *Int J Gynecol Pathol.* 2000;19:16–28.

78. **Pixley E.** Morphology of the fetal and prepubertal cervicovaginal epithelium. In: **Jordan JA, Singer A, eds.** *The Cervix.* Philadelphia, PA: WB Saunders; 1976:75–81.

79. **Coppleson M, Pixley E, Reid BL.** *Colposcopy: A Scientific Approach to the Cervix Uteri in Health and Disease.* Springfield, IL: Charles C Thomas; 1986.

80. **Kolstad P, Stafl A.** *Atlas of Colposcopy.* Oslo: Universitetsforlaget; 1982.

81. **Parkin DM, Bray F.** Chapter 2: The burden of HPV-related cancers. *Vaccine.* 2006;24(suppl 3):S3/11–S3/25.

82. **Castle PE, Schiffman M, Bratti MC, et al.** A population-based study of vaginal human papillomavirus infection in hysterectomized women. *J Infect Dis.* 2004;190(3):458–467.

83. **Castle PE, Jeronimo J, Schiffman M, et al.** Age-related changes of the cervix influence human papillomavirus type distribution. *Cancer Res.* 2006;66(2):1218–1224.

84. **Herfs M, Yamamoto Y, Laury A, et al.** A discrete population of squamocolumnar junction cells implicated in the pathogenesis of cervical cancer. *Proc Natl Acad Sci U S A* 2012;109:10516–10521.

85. **Herfs M, Vargas SO, Yamamoto Y, et al.** A novel blueprint for 'top down' differentiation defines the cervical squamocolumnar junction during development, reproductive life, and neoplasia. *J Pathol.* 2013; 229:460–468.

86. **Massad LS, Einstein MH, Huh WK, et al.** 2012 updated consensus guidelines for the management of abnormal cervical cancer screening tests and cancer precursors. *J Low Gen Tract Dis.* 2013;17(5):S1–S27.

87. **Bornstein J, Bentley J, Bosze P, et al.** The 2011 colposcopic terminology of the international federation for cervical pathology and colposcopy. *Obstet Gynecol.* 2012;120(1):166–172.

88. **Bornstein J, Sideri M, Tatti S, et al.** 2011 terminology of the vulva of the International Federation for Cervical Pathology and Colposcopy. *J Low Gen Tract Dis.* 2012;16(3):290–295.

89. **Tatti S, Bornstein J, Prendiville W.** Colposcopy: A global perspective. Introduction of the New IFCPC Colposcopy Terminology. *Obstet Gynecol Clin North Am.* 2013;40:235–250.

90. **Reid R, Scalzi P.** Genital warts and cervical cancer. VII. An improved colposcopic index for differentiating benign papillomaviral infections from high-grade cervical intraepithelial neoplasia. *Am J Obstet Gynecol.* 1985;153:611–618.

91. **Scheungraber C, Glutig K, Fechtel B, et al.** Inner border: A specific and significant colposcopic sign for moderate or severe dysplasia (cervical intra- epithelial neoplasia 2 or 3). *J Low Genit Tract Dis.* 2009;13:1–4.

92. **Scheungraber C, Koenig U, Fechtel B, et al.** The colposcopic feature ridge sign is associated with the presence of cervical intraepithelial neoplasia 2/3 and human papillomavirus 16 in young women. *J Low GenTract Dis.* 2009;13:13–16.

93. **Schiffman MH, Bauer HM, Hoover RN, et al.** Epidemiologic evidence showing that human papillomavirus infection causes most cervical intraepithelial neoplasia. *J Natl Cancer Inst.* 1993;85(12): 958–964.

94. **International Agency for Research on Cancer.** IARC monograph on the evaluation of carcinogenic risks to humans. Vol. 64. *Human Papillomaviruses.* Lyon: IARC Scientific Publications; 1995.

95. **zur Hausen H.** Immortalization of human cells and their malignant conversion by high risk human papillomavirus genotypes. *Semin Cancer Biol.* 1999;9(6):405–411.

96. **zur Hausen H.** Papillomaviruses causing cancer: Evasion from host-cell control in early events in carcinogenesis. *J Natl Cancer Inst.* 2000;92(9):690–698.

97. **zur Hausen H.** Papillomaviruses and cancer: From basic studies to clinical application. *Nat Rev Cancer.* 2002;2:342–350.

98. **Cogliano V, Baan R, Straif K, et al.** Carcinogenicity of human papillomaviruses. *Lancet Oncol.* 2005;6(4):204.

99. **Smith JS, Lindsay L, Hoots B, et al.** Human papillomavirus type distribution in invasive cervical cancer and high-grade cervical lesions: A meta-analysis update. *Int J Cancer.* 2007;121(3):621–632.

100. **International Collaboration of Epidemiological Studies of Cervical Cancer.** Carcinoma of the cervix and tobacco smoking: Collaborative reanalysis of individual data on 13,541 women with carcinoma of the cervix and 23,017 women without carcinoma of the cervix from 23 epidemiological studies. *Int J Cancer.* 2006;118(6):1481–1495.

101. **International Collaboration of Epidemiological Studies of Cervical Cancer.** Cervical carcinoma and reproductive factors: Collaborative reanalysis of individual data on 16,563 women with cervical carcinoma and 33,542 women without cervical carcinoma from 25 epidemiological studies. *Int J Cancer.* 2006;119:1108–1124.

102. **International Collaboration of Epidemiological Studies of Cervical Cancer.** Cervical cancer and hormonal contraceptives: Collaborative reanalysis of individual data for 16,573 women with cervical cancer and 35,509 women without cervical cancer from 24 epidemiological studies. *Lancet.* 2007;370(9599):1609–1621.

103. **International Collaboration of Epidemiological Studies of Cervical Cancer.** Comparison of risk factors for invasive squamous cell carcinoma and adenocarcinoma of the cervix: Collaborative reanalysis of individual data on 8,097 women with squamous cell carcinoma and 1,374 women with adenocarcinoma from 12 epidemiological studies. *Int J Cancer.* 2007;120(4):885–891.

104. **Bernard HU.** The clinical importance of the nomenclature, evolution and taxonomy of human papillomaviruses. *J Clin Virol.* 2005;32(suppl 1):S1–S6.

105. **de Villiers E-M, Fauquet C, Broker TR, et al.** Classification of papillomaviruses. *Virology.* 2004;324(1):17–27.

106. **Schiffman M, Clifford G, Buonaguro FM.** Classification of weakly carcinogenic human papillomavirus types: Addressing the limits of epidemiology at the borderline. *Infect Agent Cancer.* 2009;4:8.

107. **Doorbar J.** Molecular biology of human papillomavirus infection and cervical cancer. *Clin Sci (Lond).* 2006;110(5):525–541.

108. **Durst M, Kleinheinz A, Hotz M, et al.** The physical state of human papillomavirus type 16 DNA in benign and malignant genital tumours. *J Gen Virol.* 1985;66(Pt 7):1515–1522.

109. **Cullen AP, Reid R, Campion M, et al.** Analysis of the physical state of different human papillomavirus DNAs in intraepithelial and invasive cervical neoplasm. *J Virol.* 1991;65(2):606–612.

110. **Pirami L, Giache V, Becciolini A.** Analysis of HPV16, 18, 31, and 35 DNA in pre-invasive and invasive lesions of the uterine cervix. *J Clin Pathol.* 1997;50(7):600–604.

111. **Fujii T, Masumoto N, Saito M, et al.** Comparison between in situ hybridization and real-time PCR technique as a means of detecting the integrated form of human papillomavirus 16 in cervical neoplasia. *Diagn Mol Pathol.* 2005;14(2):103–108.

112. **Peter M, Stransky N, Couturier J, et al.** Frequent genomic structural alterations at HPV insertion sites in cervical carcinoma. *J Pathol.* 2010;221:320–330. doi: 10.1002/path.2713.

113. **Einstein MH, Goldberg GL.** Human papillomavirus and cervical neoplasia. *Cancer Invest.* 2002;20(7–8):1080–1085.

114. **Doorbar J, Ely S, Sterling J, et al.** Specific interaction between HPV-16 E1-E4 and cytokeratins results in collapse of the epithelial cell intermediate filament network. *Nature.* 1991;352(6338):824–827.

115. **Munger K, Phelps WC, Bubb V, et al.** The E6 and E7 genes of the human papillomavirus type 16 together are necessary and sufficient for transformation of primary human keratinocytes. *J Virol.* 1989;63(10):4417–4421.

116. **Munger K, Basile JR, Duensing S, et al.** Biological activities and molecular targets of the human papillomavirus E7 oncoprotein. *Oncogene.* 2001;20(54):7888–7898.

117. **Mantovani F, Banks L.** The human papillomavirus E6 protein and its contribution to malignant progression. *Oncogene.* 2001;20(54):7874–7887.

118. **McCance DJ, Kopan R, Fuchs E, et al.** Human papillomavirus type 16 alters human epithelial cell differentiation in vitro. *Proc Natl Acad Sci U S A.* 1988;85(19):7169–7173.

119. **Scheffner M, Werness BA, Huibregtse JM, et al.** The E6 oncoprotein encoded by human papillomavirus types 16 and 18 promotes the degradation of p53. *Cell.* 1990;63(6):1129–1136.

120. **Paquette RL, Lee YY, Wilczynski SP, et al.** Mutations of p53 and human papillomavirus infection in cervical carcinoma. *Cancer.* 1993;72(4):1272–1280.

121. **Scheffner M, Takahashi T, Huibregtse JM, et al.** Interaction of the human papillomavirus type 16 E6 oncoprotein with wild-type and mutant human p53 proteins. *J Virol.* 1992;66(8):5100–5105.

122. **Borresen AL, Helland A, Nesland J, et al.** Papillomaviruses, p53, and cervical cancer. *Lancet.* 1992;339(8805):1350–1351.

123. **Bosch FX, Lorincz A, Munoz N, et al.** The causal relation between human papillomavirus and cervical cancer. *J Clin Pathol.* 2002;55(4):244–265.

124. **Klingelhutz AJ, Foster SA, McDougall JK.** Telomerase activation by the E6 gene product of human papillomavirus type 16. *Nature.* 1996;380(6569):79–82.

125. **McMurray HR, McCance DJ.** Human papillomavirus type 16 E6 activates TERT gene transcription through induction of c-Myc and release of USF-mediated repression. *J Virol.* 2003;77(18):9852–9861.

126. **Zhang Y, Fan S, Meng Q, et al.** BRCA1 interaction with human papillomavirus oncoproteins. *J Biol Chem.* 2005;280(39):33165–33177.

127. **Dyson N, Howley PM, Munger K, et al.** The human papilloma virus-16 E7 oncoprotein is able to bind to the retinoblastoma gene product. *Science.* 1989;243(4893):934–937.

128. **Gage JR, Meyers C, Wettstein FO.** The E7 proteins of the nononcogenic human papillomavirus type 6b (HPV-6b) and of the oncogenic HPV-16 differ in retinoblastoma protein binding and other properties. *J Virol.* 1990;64(2):723–730.

129. **Berezutskaya E, Yu B, Morozov A, et al.** Differential regulation of the pocket domains of the retinoblastoma family proteins by the HPV16 E7 oncoprotein. *Cell Growth Differ.* 1997;8(12):1277–1286.

130. **Boyer SN, Wazer DE, Band V.** E7 protein of human papilloma virus-16 induces degradation of retinoblastoma protein through the ubiquitin-proteasome pathway. *Cancer Res.* 1996;56(20):4620–4624.

131. **Helt A-M, Galloway DA.** Mechanisms by which DNA tumor virus oncoproteins target the Rb family of pocket proteins. *Carcinogenesis.* 2003;24(2):159–169.

132. **Balsitis SJ, Sage J, Duensing S, et al.** Recapitulation of the effects of the human papillomavirus type 16 E7 oncogene on mouse epithelium by somatic Rb deletion and detection of pRb-independent effects of E7 in vivo. *Mol Cell Biol.* 2003;23(24):9094–9103.

133. **Fehrmann F, Laimins LA.** Human papillomaviruses: Targeting differentiating epithelial cells for malignant transformation. *Oncogene.* 2003;22(33):5201–5207.

134. **Woodworth CD, Doniger J, DiPaolo JA.** Immortalization of human foreskin keratinocytes by various human papillomavirus DNAs corresponds to their association with cervical carcinoma. *J Virol.* 1989;63(1):159–164.

135. **Barbosa MS, Schlegel R.** The E6 and E7 genes of HPV-18 are sufficient for inducing two-stage in vitro transformation of human keratinocytes. *Oncogene.* 1989;4(12):1529–1532.

136. **Nishimura A, Ono T, Ishimoto A, et al.** Mechanisms of human papillomavirus E2-mediated repression of viral oncogene expression and cervical cancer cell growth inhibition. *J Virol.* 2000;74(8):3752–3760.

137. **Muñoz N, Castellsagué X, de González AB, et al.** Chapter 1: HPV in the etiology of human cancer. *Vaccine.* 2006;24(suppl 3):S1–S10.

138. **Bosch FX, Manos MM, Munoz N, et al.** Prevalence of human papillomavirus in cervical cancer: A worldwide perspective. International biological study on cervical cancer (IBSCC) Study Group. *J Natl Cancer Inst.* 1995;87(11):796–802.

139. **Bosch FX, de Sanjose S.** The epidemiology of human papillomavirus infection and cervical cancer. *Dis Markers.* 2007;23(4):213–227.

140. **Castellsague X, Diaz M, de Sanjose S, et al.** Worldwide human papillomavirus etiology of cervical adenocarcinoma and its cofactors: Implications for screening and prevention. *J Natl Cancer Inst.* 2006;98(5):303–315.

141. **Australian Institute of Health and Welfare.** *Cervical screening in Australia 2010–2011.* Cancer series no. 76. Cat no. CAN 72. Canberra: AIHW; 2013.

142. **Burchell AN, Winer RL, de Sanjose S, et al.** Chapter 6: Epidemiology and transmission dynamics of genital HPV infection. *Vaccine.* 2006;24(suppl 3):52–61.

143. **Stanley M.** Immune responses to human papillomavirus. *Vaccine.* 2006;24(suppl 1):S16–S22.

144. **Plummer M, Schiffman M, Castle PE, et al.** A 2-year prospective study of human papillomavirus persistence among women with a cytological diagnosis of atypical squamous cells of undetermined significance or low-grade squamous intraepithelial lesion. *J Infect Dis.* 2007;195(11):1582–1589.

145. **Chen HC, You SL, Hsieh CY, et al.** Prevalence of genotype-specific human papillomavirus infection and cervical neoplasia in Taiwan: A community-based survey of 10,602 women. *Int J Cancer.* 2011; 128:1192–1203.

146. **Kjaer SK, Frederiksen K, Munk C, et al.** Long-term absolute risk of cervical intraepithelial neoplasia grade 3 or worse following human papillomavirus infection: Role of persistence. *J Natl Cancer Inst.* 2010;102:1478–1488.

147. **Ylitalo N, Sorensen P, Josefsson AM, et al.** Consistent high viral load of human papillomavirus 16 and risk of cervical carcinoma in situ: A nested case-control study. *Lancet.* 2000;355(9222):2194–2198.

148. **Josefsson AM, Magnusson PK, Ylitalo N, et al.** Viral load of human papilloma virus 16 as a determinant for development of cervical carcinoma in situ: A nested case-control study. *Lancet.* 2000; 355(9222):2189–2193.

149. **Sherman ME, Wang SS, Wheeler CM, et al.** Determinants of human papillomavirus load among women with histological cervical intraepithelial neoplasia 3: Dominant impact of surrounding low-grade lesions. *Cancer Epidemiol Biomarkers Prev.* 2003;12(10):1038–1044.

150. **Bosch FX, de Sanjose S.** Chapter 1: Human papillomavirus and cervical cancer–burden and assessment of causality. *J Natl Cancer Inst Monogr.* 2003;(31):3–13.

151. **Rodriguez AC, Burk R, Herrero R, et al.** The natural history of human papillomavirus infection and cervical intraepithelial neoplasia among young women in the Guanacaste cohort shortly after initiation of sexual life. *Sex Transm Dis.* 2007;34(7):494–502.

152. **Richardson H, Kelsall G, Tellier P, et al.** The natural history of type-specific human papillomavirus infections in female university students. *Cancer Epidemiol Biomarkers Prev.* 2003;12(6):485–490.

153. **Sasieni P, Castanon A, Cuzick J.** Effectiveness of cervical screening with age: Population based case-control study of prospectively recorded data. *BMJ.* 2009;339:b2968.

154. **Madeleine MM, Johnson LG, Smith AG, et al.** Comprehensive analysis of HLA-A, HLA-B, HLA-C, HLA-DRB1, and HLA-DQB1 loci and squamous cell cervical cancer risk. *Cancer Res.* 2008;68: 3532–3539.

155. **Richardson H, Abrahamowicz M, Tellier PP, et al.** Modifiable risk factors associated with clearance of type-specific cervical human papillomavirus infections in a cohort of university students. *Cancer Epidemiol Biomarkers Prev.* 2005;14(5):1149–1156.

156. **Shew ML, Fortenberry JD, Tu W, et al.** Association of condom use, sexual behaviors, and sexually transmitted infections with the duration of genital human papillomavirus infection among adolescent women. *Arch Pediatr Adolesc Med.* 2006;160(2):151–156.

157. **Tokudome S, Suzuki S, Ichikawa H, et al.** Condom use promotes regression of cervical intraepithelial neoplasia and clearance of human papillomavirus: A randomized clinical trial. *Int J Cancer.* 2004; 112(1):164; author reply 5.

158. **Slattery ML, Robison LM, Schuman KL, et al.** Cigarette smoking and exposure to passive smoke are risk factors for cervical cancer. *JAMA.* 1989;261(11):1593–1598.

159. **Coker AL, Bond SM, Williams A, et al.** Active and passive smoking, high-risk human papillomaviruses and cervical neoplasia. *Cancer Detect Prev.* 2002;26(2):121–128.

160. **Yang X, Jin G, Nakao Y, et al.** Malignant transformation of HPV 16-immortalized human endocervical cells by cigarette smoke condensate and characterization of multistage carcinogenesis. *Int J Cancer.* 1996;65(3):338–344.

161. **Ho GY, Kadish AS, Burk RD, et al.** HPV 16 and cigarette smoking as risk factors for high-grade cervical intra-epithelial neoplasia. *Int J Cancer.* 1998;78(3):281–285.

162. **Appleby P, Beral V, Berrington de Gonzalez A, et al.** Carcinoma of the cervix and tobacco smoking: Collaborative reanalysis of individual data on 13,541 women with carcinoma of the cervix and 23,017 women without carcinoma of the cervix from 23 epidemiological studies. *Int J Cancer.* 2006;118(6):1481–1495.

163. **Vaccarella S, Herrero R, Snijders PJ, et al.** Smoking and human papillomavirus infection: Pooled analysis of the International Agency for Research on Cancer HPV Prevalence Surveys. *Int J Epidemiol.* 2008;37(3):536–546.

164. **Hawthorn RJ, Murdoch JB, MacLean AB, et al.** Langerhans' cells and subtypes of human papillomavirus in cervical intraepithelial neoplasia. *BMJ.* 1988;297(6649):643–646.

165. **Viac J, Guerin-Reverchon I, Chardonnet Y, et al.** Langerhans cells and epithelial cell modifications in cervical intraepithelial neoplasia: Correlation with human papillomavirus infection. *Immunobiology.* 1990;180(4–5):328–338.

166. **Schneider A, Hotz M, Gissmann L.** Increased prevalence of human papillomaviruses in the lower genital tract of pregnant women. *Int J Cancer.* 1987;40(2):198–201.

167. **Rando RF, Lindheim S, Hasty L, et al.** Increased frequency of detection of human papillomavirus deoxyribonucleic acid in exfoliated cervical cells during pregnancy. *Am J Obstet Gynecol.* 1989; 161(1):50–55.

168. **Sillman F, Stanek A, Sedlis A, et al.** The relationship between human papillomavirus and lower genital intraepithelial neoplasia in immunosuppressed women. *Am J Obstet Gynecol.* 1984;150(3):300–308.

169. **Schafer A, Friedmann W, Mielke M, et al.** The increased frequency of cervical dysplasia-neoplasia in women infected with the human immunodeficiency virus is related to the degree of immunosuppression. *Am J Obstet Gynecol.* 1991;164(2):593–599.

170. **Conley LJ, Ellerbrock TV, Bush TJ, et al.** HIV-1 infection and risk of vulvovaginal and perianal condylomata acuminata and intraepithelial neoplasia: A prospective cohort study. *Lancet.* 2002; 359(9301):108–113.

171. **Harris TG, Burk RD, Palefsky JM, et al.** Incidence of cervical squamous intraepithelial lesions associated with HIV serostatus, CD4 cell counts, and human papillomavirus test results. *JAMA.* 2005; 293(12):1471–1476.

172. **Palefsky JM, Gillison ML, Strickler HD.** Chapter 16: HPV vaccines in immunocompromised women and men. *Vaccine.* 2006; 24(suppl 3):140–146.

173. **Clifford GM, Goncalves MA, Franceschi S.** Human papillomavirus types among women infected with HIV: A meta-analysis. *AIDS.* 2006;20(18):2337–2344.

174. **Dugué PA, Rebolj M, Garred P, et al.** Immunosuppression and risk of cervical cancer. *Expert Rev Anticancer Ther.* 2013;13(1):29–42. doi:10.1586/era.12.159

175. **Canfell K, Chesson H, Kulasingam SL, et al.** Modeling preventative strategies against human papillomavirus-related disease in developed countries. *Vaccine.* 2012;30 (suppl 5):F157–F167.

176. **de Sanjose S, Quint WG, Alemany L, et al.** Human papillomavirus genotype attribution in invasive cervical cancer: A retrospective cross-sectional worldwide study. *Lancet Oncol.* 2010;11(11):1048–1056.

177. **FUTURE II Study Group.** Quadrivalent vaccine against human papillomavirus to prevent high-grade cervical lesions. *N Engl J Med.* 2007;356(19):1915–1927.

178. **Giuliano AR, Palefsky JM, Goldstone S, et al.** Efficacy of quadrivalent HPV vaccine against HPV infection and disease in males. *N Engl J Med.* 2011;364(5):401–411.

179. **Palefsky JM, Giuliano AR, Goldstone S, et al.** HPV vaccine against anal HPV infection and anal intraepithelial neoplasia. *N Engl J Med.* 2011;365(17):1576–1585.

180. **Brisson M, van de Velde N, Franco EL, et al.** Incremental impact of adding boys to current human papillomavirus vaccination programs: Role of herd immunity. *J Infect Dis.* 2011;204(3): 372–376.

181. **Smith MA, Lew JB, Walker RJ, et al.** The predicted impact of HPV vaccination on male infections and male HPV-related cancers in Australia. *Vaccine.* 2011;29(48):9112–9122.

182. **Frazer IH.** HPV vaccines and the prevention of cervical cancer. *Update Cancer Ther.* 2008;3(1):43–48.

183. **Barr E, Sings HL.** Prophylactic HPV vaccines: New interventions for cancer control. *Vaccine.* 2008;26(49):6244–6257.

184. **Zhou J, Sun XY, Stenzel DJ, et al.** Expression of vaccinia recombinant HPV 16 L1 and L2 ORF proteins in epithelial cells is sufficient for assembly of HPV virion-like particles. *Virology.* 1991;185(1):251–257.

185. **Kirnbauer R, Taub J, Greenstone H, et al.** Efficient self-assembly of human papillomavirus type 16 L1 and L1-L2 into virus-like particles. *J Virol.* 1993;67(12):6929–6936.

186. **Harper DM, Franco EL, Wheeler CM, et al.** Sustained efficacy up to 4.5 years of a bivalent L1 virus-like particle vaccine against human papillomavirus types 16 and 18: Follow-up from a randomised control trial. *Lancet.* 2006;367(9518):1247–1255.

187. **Mao C, Koutsky LA, Ault KA, et al.** Efficacy of human papillomavirus-16 vaccine to prevent cervical intraepithelial neoplasia: A randomized controlled trial. *Obstet Gynecol.* 2006;107(1):18–27.

188. **Wideroff L, Schiffman M, Haderer P, et al.** Seroreactivity to human papillomavirus types 16, 18, 31, and 45 virus-like particles in a case-control study of cervical squamous intraepithelial lesions. *J Infect Dis.* 1999;180(5):1424–1428.

189. **Harro CD, Pang YY, Roden RB, et al.** Safety and immunogenicity trial in adult volunteers of a human papillomavirus 16 L1 virus-like particle vaccine. *J Natl Cancer Inst.* 2001;93(4):284–292.

190. **Pinto LA, Edwards J, Castle PE, et al.** Cellular immune responses to human papillomavirus (HPV)-16 L1 in healthy volunteers immunized with recombinant HPV-16 L1 virus-like particles. *J Infect Dis.* 2003;188(2):327–338.

191. **Jansen KU, Rosolowsky M, Schultz LD, et al.** Vaccination with yeast-expressed cottontail rabbit papillomavirus (CRPV) virus-like particles protects rabbits from CRPV-induced papilloma formation. *Vaccine.* 1995;13(16):1509–1514.

192. **Paavonen J, Naud P, Salmeron J, et al.** Efficacy of human papillomavirus (HPV)-16/18 AS04-adjuvanted vaccine against cervical infection and precancer caused by oncogenic HPV types (PATRICIA): Final analysis of a double-blind, randomised study in young women. *Lancet.* 2009;374(9686):301–314.

193. **Joura EA, Garland SM, Paavonen J, et al.** Effect of the human papillomavirus (HPV) quadrivalent vaccine in a subgroup of women with cervical and vulvar disease: Retrospective pooled analysis of trial data. *BMJ.* 2012;344:e1401.

194. **Block SL, Nolan T, Sattler C, et al.** Comparison of the immunogenicity and reactogenicity of a prophylactic quadrivalent human papillomavirus (types 6, 11, 16, and 18) L1 virus-like particle vaccine in male and female adolescents and young adult women. *Pediatrics.* 2006;118(5):2135–2145.

195. **Castellsague X, Schneider A, Kaufmann AM, et al.** HPV vaccination against cervical cancer in women above 25 years of age: Key considerations and current perspectives. *Gynecol Oncol.* 2009;115(3 suppl):S15–S23.

196. **Schwarz T, Dubin G.** Human papillomavirus (HPV) 16/18 l1 AS04 virus-like particle (VLP) cervical cancer vaccine is immunogenic and well-tolerated 18 months after vaccination in women up to age 55 years. *J Clin Oncol.* 2007;25(18 suppl):3007.

197. **Harper DM, Franco EL, Wheeler C, et al.** Efficacy of a bivalent L1 virus-like particle vaccine in prevention of infection with human papillomavirus types 16 and 18 in young women: A randomised controlled trial. *Lancet.* 2004;364(9447):1757–1765.

198. **Wright TC, Bosch FX, Franco EL, et al.** Chapter 30: HPV vaccines and screening in the prevention of cervical cancer; conclusions from a 2006 workshop of international experts. *Vaccine.* 2006;24(suppl 3):S3/251–S3/261.

199. **Ault KA.** Effect of prophylactic human papillomavirus L1 virus-like-particle vaccine on risk of cervical intraepithelial neoplasia grade 2, grade 3, and adenocarcinoma in situ: A combined analysis of four randomised clinical trials. *Lancet.* 2007;369(9576):1861–1868.

200. **Hildesheim A, Herrero R, Wacholder S, et al.** Effect of human papillomavirus 16/18 L1 viruslike particle vaccine among young women with preexisting infection: A randomized trial. *JAMA.* 2007;298(7):743–753.

201. **Olsson SE, Villa LL, Costa RL, et al.** Induction of immune memory following administration of a prophylactic quadrivalent human papillomavirus (HPV) types 6/11/16/18 L1 virus-like particle (VLP) vaccine. *Vaccine.* 2007;25(26):4931–4939.

202. **Fraser C, Tomassini JE, Xi L, et al.** Modeling the long-term antibody response of a human papillomavirus (HPV) virus-like particle (VLP) type 16 prophylactic vaccine. *Vaccine.* 2007;25(21):4324–4333.

203. **Kreimer AR, Rodriguez AC, Hildesheim A, et al.** Proof-of-principle evaluation of the efficacy of fewer than three doses of a bivalent HPV16/18 vaccine. *J Natl Cancer Inst.* 2011;103(19):1444–1451.

204. **Romanowski B, Schwarz TF, Ferguson LM, et al.** Immunogenicity and safety of the HPV-16/18 AS04-adjuvanted vaccine administered as a 2-dose schedule compared with the licensed 3-dose schedule: Results from a randomized study. *Hum Vaccin.* 2011;7(12):1374–1386.

205. **Dobson S, McNeil S, Dionne M, et al.** Immunogenicity of 2 doses of HPV vaccine in younger adolescents vs 3 doses in young women: A randomized clinical trial. *JAMA.* 2013;309(17):1793–1802.

206. **Kahn JA, Bernstein DI.** HPV vaccination: Too soon for 2 doses? *JAMA.* 2013;309(17):1832–1834.

207. **Peres J.** For cancers caused by HPV, two vaccines were just the beginning. *J Natl Cancer Inst.* 2011;103(5):360–362.

208. **Serrano B, Alemany L, Tous S, et al.** Potential impact of a nine-valent vaccine in human papillomavirus related cervical disease. *Infect Agent Cancer.* 2012;7(1):38.

209. **Schiller JT, Lowy DR.** Immunogenicity testing in human papillomavirus virus-like-particle vaccine trials. *J Infect Dis.* 2009;200(2):166–171.

210. **World Health Organisation, Global Advisory Committee on Vaccine Safety.** Global Advisory Committee on Vaccine Safety, report of meeting held 12–13 June 2013. *Wkly Epidemiol Rec.* 2013;29(88):301–312.

211. **Arnheim-Dahlström L, Pasternak B, Svanström H, et al.** Autoimmune, neurological, and venous thromboembolic adverse events after immunisation of adolescent girls with quadrivalent human papillomavirus vaccine in Denmark and Sweden: Cohort study. *BMJ.* 2013;347:f5906.

212. **Wacholder S, Chen BE, Wilcox A, et al.** Risk of miscarriage with bivalent vaccine against human papillomavirus (HPV) types 16 and 18: Pooled analysis of two randomised controlled trials. *BMJ.* 2010;340:c712.

213. **Canfell K.** Monitoring HPV vaccination programmes. *BMJ.* 2010;340:c1666.

214. **Wright TC, Jr., Huh WK, Monk BJ, et al.** Age considerations when vaccinating against HPV. *Gynecol Oncol.* 2008;109(2 suppl):S40–S47.

215. **Saslow D, Castle PE, Cox JT, et al.** American Cancer Society Guideline for human papillomavirus (HPV) vaccine use to prevent cervical cancer and its precursors. *CA Cancer J Clin.* 2007;57(1):7–28.

216. **Kyrgiou M, Koliopoulos G, Martin-Hirsch P, et al.** Obstetric outcomes after conservative treatment for intraepithelial or early invasive cervical lesions: Systematic review and meta-analysis. *Lancet.* 2006;367(9509):489–498.

217. **Bruinsma FJ, Quinn MA.** The risk of preterm birth following treatment for precancerous changes in the cervix: A systematic review and meta-analysis. *BJOG.* 2011;118(9):1031–1041.

218. **Castanon A, Brocklehurst P, Evans H, et al.** Risk of preterm birth after treatment for cervical intraepithelial neoplasia among women attending colposcopy in England: Retrospective-prospective cohort study. *BMJ.* 2012;345:e5174.

219. **Centers for Disease Control and Prevention.** National, State and Local Area Vaccination Coverage among Adolescents Aged 13 through 17 Years - United States 2010. *MMWR Morb Mortal Wkly Rep.* 2011;60(33):1117–1123.

220. **Brotherton JM, Murray SL, Hall MA, et al.** Human papillomavirus vaccine coverage among female Australian adolescents: Success of the school-based approach. *Med J Aust.* 2013;199(9):614–617.

221. **Brotherton JM, Fridman M, May CL, et al.** Early effect of the HPV vaccination programme on cervical abnormalities in Victoria, Australia: An ecological study. *Lancet.* 2011;377(9783):2085–2092.

222. **Donovan B, Guy R, Fairley CK.** Assessment of herd immunity from human papillomavirus vaccination - Authors' reply. *Lancet Infect Dis.* 2011;11(12):896–897.

223. Ali H, Donovan B, Wand H, et al. Genital warts in young Australians five years into national human papillomavirus vaccination programme: National surveillance data. *BMJ.* 2013;346:f2032.

224. Ponten J, Adami HO, Bergstrom R, et al. Strategies for global control of cervical cancer. *Int J Cancer.* 1995;60(1):1–26.

225. Siegel R, Naishadham D, Jemal A. Cancer statistics, 2013. *CA Cancer J Clin.* 2013;63:11–30.

226. Gustafsson L, Ponten J, Bergstrom R, et al. International incidence rates of invasive cervical cancer before cytological screening. *Int J Cancer.* 1997;71(2):159–165.

227. Kitchener HC, Castle PE, Cox JT. Chapter 7: Achievements and limitations of cervical cytology screening. *Vaccine.* 2006;24(suppl 3):S3/63–S3/70.

228. Ferlay J, Shin H, Bray F, et al. *GLOBOCAN 2008: Cancer Incidence and Mortality Worldwide:* Lyon: International Agency for Research on Cancer; 2008.

229. Solomon D, Breen N, McNeel T. Cervical cancer screening rates in the United States and the potential impact of implementation of screening guidelines. *CA Cancer J Clin.* 2007;57:105–111.

230. Saslow D, Solomon D, Lawson HW, et al. American Cancer Society, American Society for Colposcopy and Cervical Pathology, and American Society for Clinical Pathology screening guidelines for the prevention and early detection of cervical cancer. *CA Cancer J Clin.* 2012;62(3):147–172.

231. Moyer VA. Screening for cervical cancer: U.S. Preventive Services Task Force recommendation statement. *Ann Intern Med.* 2012;156:880–891.

232. Committee on Practice Bulletins—Gynecology. ACOG Practice Bulletin number 131: Screening for cervical cancer. *Obstet Gynecol.* 2012;120:1222–1238.

233. Sasieni P, Adams J, Cuzick J. Benefit of cervical screening at different ages: Evidence from the UK audit of screening histories. *Br J Cancer.* 2003;89(1):88–93.

234. Canfell K, Sitas F, Beral V. Cervical cancer in Australia and the United Kingdom: Comparison of screening policy and uptake, and cancer incidence and mortality. *Med J Aust.* 2006;185(9):482–486.

235. Schiffman M, Solomon D. Cervical-cancer screening with human papillomavirus and cytologic cotesting. *N Engl J Med.* 2013;369:2324–2331 .doi:10.1056/NEJMcp1210379.

236. Fahey MT, Irwig L, Macaskill P. Meta-analysis of Pap test accuracy. *Am J Epidemiol.* 1995;141(7):680–689.

237. Cuzick J, Clavel C, Petry KU, et al. Overview of the European and North American studies on HPV testing in primary cervical cancer screening. *Int J Cancer.* 2006;119(5):1095–1101.

238. Agency for Health Care Policy and Research. *Evaluation of Cervical Cytology: Evidence Report/Technology Assessment (no. 5).* Rockville, MD: AHCPR; 1999.

239. Martin-Hirsch P, Lilford R, Jarvis G, et al. Efficacy of cervical-smear collection devices: A systematic review and meta-analysis. *Lancet.* 1999;354(9192):1763–1770.

240. Nanda K, McCrory DC, Myers ER, et al. Accuracy of the Papanicolaou test in screening for and follow-up of cervical cytologic abnormalities: A systematic review. *Ann Intern Med.* 2000;132(10):810–819.

241. Davey E, Barratt A, Irwig L, et al. Effect of study design and quality on unsatisfactory rates, cytology classifications, and accuracy in liquid-based versus conventional cervical cytology: A systematic review. *Lancet.* 2006;367(9505):122–132.

242. Davey E, d'Assuncao J, Irwig L, et al. Accuracy of reading liquid based cytology slides using the ThinPrep Imager compared with conventional cytology: Prospective study. *BMJ.* 2007;335(7609):31.

243. Siebers AG, Klinkhamer PJ, Grefte JM, et al. Comparison of liquid-based cytology with conventional cytology for detection of cervical cancer precursors: A randomized controlled trial. *JAMA.* 2009;302(16):1757–1764.

244. NHS Cervical Screening Programme NHS Cervical Screening Programme Annual Review 2012. 2012.

245. Arbyn M, Bergeron C, Klinkhamer P, et al. Liquid compared with conventional cervical cytology: A systematic review and meta-analysis. *Obstet Gynecol.* 2008;111(1):167–177.

246. Canfell K. Models of cervical screening in the era of human papillomavirus vaccination. *Sex Health.* 2010;7(3):359–367.

247. Schiffman M, Wentzensen N, Wacholder S, et al. Human papillomavirus testing in the prevention of cervical cancer. *J Natl Cancer Inst.* 2011;103:368–383.

248. Arbyn M, Ronco G, Anttila A, et al. Evidence regarding human papillomavirus testing in secondary prevention of cervical cancer. *Vaccine.* 2012;30(suppl 5):F88–F99.

249. Kocken M, Uijterwaal MH, de Vries AL, et al. High-risk human papillomavirus testing versus cytology in predicting post-treatment disease in women treated for high-grade cervical disease: A systematic review and meta-analysis. *Gynecol Oncol.* 2012;125:500–507.

250. Melnikow J, Kulasingam S, Slee C, et al. Surveillance after treatment for cervical intraepithelial neoplasia: Outcomes, costs, and cost-effectiveness. *Obstet Gynecol.* 2010;116(5):1158–1170.

251. Katki HA, Schiffman M, Castle PE, et al. Five-year risk of recurrence after treatment of CIN 2, CIN 3, or AIS: Performance of HPV and Pap cotesting in posttreatment management. *J Low Genit Tract Dis.* 2013;17(5 suppl 1):S78–S84.

252. Legood R, Smith MA, Lew JB, et al. Cost effectiveness of human papillomavirus test of cure after treatment for cervical intraepithelial neoplasia in England: Economic analysis from NHS Sentinel Sites Study. *BMJ.* 2012;345:e7086.

253. Sherman ME, Solomon D, Schiffman M. Qualification of an ASCUS: A comparison of equivocal LSIL and equivocal HSIL cervical cytology in the ASCUS LSIL Triage Study. *Am J Clin Pathol.* 2001;116:386–394.

254. Sherman ME, Schiffman M, Cox JT. Effects of age and human papilloma viral load on colposcopy triage: Data from the randomized Atypical Squamous Cells of Undetermined Significance/Low-Grade Squamous Intraepithelial Lesion Triage Study (ALTS). *J Natl Cancer Inst.* 2002;94(2):102–107.

255. Wright TC, Cox JT, Massad LS, et al. 2001 Consensus guidelines for the management of women with cervical cytological abnormalities and cervical cancer precursors: Part 1: Cytological abnormalities. *JAMA.* 2002;287:2120–2129.

256. Schiffman M, Solomon D. Findings to date from the ASCUS-LSIL Triage Study (ALTS). *Arch Pathol Lab Med.* 2003;127:946–949.

257. Guido R, Schiffman M, Solomon D, et al. Postcolposcopy management strategies for women referred with low-grade squamous intraepithelial lesions or human papillomavirus DNA-positive atypical squamous cells of undetermined significance: A two-year prospective study. *Am J Obstet Gynecol.* 2003;188:1401–1405.

258. ASC-US-LSIL Triage Study (ALTS) Group. Results of a randomized trial on the management of cytology interpretations of atypical squamous cells of undetermined significance. *Am J Obstet Gynecol.* 2003;188:1383–1392.

259. ASC-US-LSIL Triage Study (ALTS) Group. A randomized trial on the management of low-grade squamous intraepithelial lesion cytology interpretations. *Am J Obstet Gynecol.* 2003;188:1393–1400.

260. Wright TC Jr, Cox JT, Massad LS, et al.; 2001 ASCCP-sponsored Consensus Workshop. 2001 consensus guidelines for the management of women with cervical intraepithelial neoplasia. *J Low Genit Tract Dis.* 2003;7(3):154–167.

261. Wright TC Jr, Massad LS, Dunton CJ, et al.; 2006 ASCCP-Sponsored Consensus Conference. 2006 consensus guidelines for the management of women with abnormal cervical screening tests. *J Low Genit Tract Dis.* 2007;11:201–222.

262. Schiffman M. Integration of human papillomavirus vaccination, cytology, and human papillomavirus testing. *Cancer.* 2007;111(3):145–153.

263. Kitchener HC, Gilham C, Sargent A, et al. A comparison of HPV DNA testing and liquid based cytology over three rounds of primary cervical screening: Extended follow up in the ARTISTIC trial. *Eur J Cancer.* 2011;47(6):864–871.

264. Rijkaart DC, Berkhof J, Rozendaal L, et al. Human papillomavirus testing for the detection of high-grade cervical intraepithelial neoplasia and cancer: Final results of the POBASCAM randomised controlled trial. *Lancet Oncol.* 2012;13(1):78–88.

265. Ronco G, Giorgi-Rossi P, Carozzi F, et al. Efficacy of human papillomavirus testing for the detection of invasive cervical cancers and cervical intraepithelial neoplasia: A randomised controlled trial. *Lancet Oncol.* 2010;11(3):249–257.

266. Ronco G, Dillner J, Elfstrom KM, et al. Efficacy of HPV-based screening for prevention of invasive cervical cancer: Follow-up of

four European randomised controlled trials. *Lancet.* 2014;383(9916): 524–532.

267. **Dillner J, Rebolj M, Birembaut P, et al.** Long term predictive values of cytology and human papillomavirus testing in cervical cancer screening: Joint European cohort study. *BMJ.* 2008;337: a1754.

268. **Safaeian M, Porras C, Pan Y, et al.** Durable antibody responses following one dose of the bivalent human papillomavirus L1 virus-like particle vaccine in the costa rica vaccine trial. *Cancer Prev Res (Phila).* 2013;6(11):1242–1250.

269. **Castle PE, Stoler MH, Wright TC, Jr., et al.** Performance of carcinogenic human papillomavirus (HPV) testing and HPV16 or HPV18 genotyping for cervical cancer screening of women aged 25 years and older: A subanalysis of the ATHENA study. *Lancet Oncol.* 2011;12(9):880–890.

270. **Canfell K, Lew JB, Clements M, et al.** Impact of HPV vaccination on cost-effectiveness of existing screening programs: Example from New Zealand 28th International Human Papillomavirus Conference & Clinical and Public Health Workshops; 2012 December; San Juan, Puerto Rico.

271. **Diaz M, De SS, Ortendahl J, et al.** Cost-effectiveness of human papillomavirus vaccination and screening in Spain. *Eur J Cancer.* 2010;46(16):2973–2985.

272. **Goldhaber-Fiebert JD, Stout NK, Salomon JA, et al.** Cost-effectiveness of cervical cancer screening with human papillomavirus DNA testing and HPV-16,18 vaccination. *J Natl Cancer Inst.* 2008; 100(5):308–320.

273. **Urcuyo R, Rome RM, Nelson JH.** Some observations on the value of endocervical curettage performed as an integral part of colposcopic examination of patients with abnormal cervical cytology. *Am J Obstet Gynecol.* 1977;128(7):787–792.

274. **Weitzman GA, Korhonen MO, Reeves KO, et al.** Endocervical brush cytology. An alternative to endocervical curettage? *J Reprod Med.* 1988;33(8):677–683.

275. **Mogensen ST, Bak M, Dueholm M, et al.** Cytobrush and endocervical curettage in the diagnosis of dysplasia and malignancy of the uterine cervix. *Acta Obstet Gynecol Scand.* 1997;76:69–73.

276. **Goksedef BP, Api M, Kaya O, et al.** Diagnostic accuracy of two endocervical sampling method: Randomized controlled trial. *Arch Gynecol Obstet.* 2013;287:117–122.

277. **Walker P, Dexeus S, De Palo G, et al.** International terminology of colposcopy: An updated report from the International Federation for Cervical Pathology and Colposcopy. *Obstet Gynecol.* 2003;101(1): 175–177.

278. **Coppleson M.** Colposcopic features of papillomaviral infection and premalignancy in the female lower genital tract. *Obstet Gynecol Clin North Am.* 1987;14(2):471–494.

279. **Reid R, Herschman BR, Crum CP, et al.** Genital warts and cervical cancer. V. The tissue basis of colposcopic change. *Am J Obstet Gynecol.* 1984;149(3):293–303.

280. **Reid R, Stanhope CR, Herschman BR, et al.** Genital warts and cervical cancer. IV. A colposcopic index for differentiating subclinical papillomaviral infection from cervical intraepithelial neoplasia. *Am J Obstet Gynecol.* 1984;149(8):815–823.

281. **Pretorius RG, Zhang WH, Belinson JL, et al.** Colposcopically directed biopsy, random cervical biopsy, and endocervical curettage in the diagnosis of cervical intraepithelial neoplasia II or worse. *Am J Obstet Gynecol.* 2004;191:430–434.

282. **Sideri M, Spolti N, Spinaci L, et al.** Interobserver variability of colposcopic interpretations and consistency with final histologic results. *J Low Genit Tract Dis.* 2004;8:212–216.

283. **Ferris DG, Litaker MS, ALTS Group.** Prediction of cervical histologic results using an abbreviated Reid Colposcopic Index during ALTS. *Am J Obstet Gynecol.* 2006;194:704–710.

284. **Gage JC, Hanson VW, Abbey K, et al.** Number of cervical biopsies and sensitivity of colposcopy. *Obstet Gynecol.* 2006;108:264–272.

285. **Jeronimo J, Massad LS, Castle PE, et al.**, NIH-ASCCP Research Group. Interobserver agreement in the evaluation of digitized cervical images. *Obstet Gynecol.* 2007;110:833–840.

286. **Massad LS, Jeronimo J, Schiffman M, NIH-ASCCP Research Group.** Interobserver agreement in the assessment of components of colposcopic grading. *Obstet Gynecol.* 2008;111: 1279–1284.

287. **TOMBOLA Group.** Biopsy and selective recall compared with immediate large loop excision in management of women with low grade abnormal cervical cytology referred for colposcopy: Multicentre randomised controlled trial. *BMJ.* 2009;339:b2548.

288. **Massad LS, Jeronimo J, Katki HA, et al.** The accuracy of colposcopic grading for detection of high-grade cervical intraepithelial neoplasia. *J Low Genit Tract Dis.* 2009;13:137–144.

289. **Stoler MH, Vichnin MD, Ferenczy A, et al.** The accuracy of colposcopic biopsy: Analyses from the placebo arm of the Gardasil clinical trials. *Int J Cancer.* 2011;128:1354–1362.

290. **Pretorius RG, Belinson JL, Burchette RJ, et al.** Regardless of skill, performing more biopsies increases the sensitivity of colposcopy. *J Low Genit Tract Dis.* 2011;15:180–188.

291. **Petry KU, Luyten A, Scherbring S.** Accuracy of colposcopy management to detect CIN 3 and invasive cancer in women with abnormal screening tests: Results from a primary HPV screening project from 2006 to 2011 in Wolfsburg, Germany. *Gynecol Oncol.* 2013;128: 282–287.

292. **Luesley DM.** *Standards and Quality in Colposcopy.* Sheffield: NHS Cervical Screening Programme; 1996.

293. **Ferris DG, Cox JT, Burke L, et al.** Colposcopy Quality Control: Establishing Colposcopy Criterion Standards for the National Cancer Institute ALTS Trial Using Cervigrams. *J Low Genit Tract Dis.* 1998;2(4):195–203.

294. **Arbyn M, Anttila A, Jordan J, et al.** European guidelines for quality assurance in cervical cancer screening. Second edition—summary document. *Ann Oncol.* 2010;21:448–458.

295. **Strander B, Ellstrom-Andersson A, Franzen S, et al.** The performance of a new scoring system for colposcopy in detecting high-grade dysplasia in the uterine cervix. *Acta Obstet Gynecol Scand.* 2005;84:1013–1017.

296. **Karrberg C, Ryd W, Strander B, et al.** Histological diagnosis and evaluation of the Swede score colposcopic system in a large cohort of pregnant women with atypical cervical cytology or cervical malignancy signs. *Acta Obstet Gynecol Scand.* 2012;91:952–958.

297. **Wright TC, Cox JT, Massad LS, et al.** 2001 consensus guidelines for the management of women with cervical intraepithelial neoplasia. *Am J Obstet Gynecol.* 2003;189(1):295–304.

298. **Wright TC Jr., Massad LS, Dunton CJ, et al.** 2006 consensus guidelines for the management of women with cervical intraepithelial neoplasia or adenocarcinoma in situ. *Am J Obstet Gynecol.* 2007;197(4):340–345.

299. **Soutter WP, Sasieni P, Panoskaltsis T.** Long-term risk of invasive cervical cancer after treatment of squamous cervical intraepithelial neoplasia. *Int J Cancer.* 2006;118:2048–2055.

300. **Strander B, Andersson-Ellstrom A, Milsom I, et al.** Long term risk of invasive cancer after treatment for cervical intraepithelial neoplasia grade 3: Population based cohort study. *BMJ.* 2007; 335:1077.

301. **Melnikow J, McGahan C, Sawaya GF, et al.** Cervical intraepithelial neoplasia outcomes after treatment: Long-term follow-up from the British Columbia Cohort Study. *J Natl Cancer Inst.* 2009;101: 721–728.

302. **Kocken M, Helmerhorst TJ, Berkhof J, et al.** Risk of recurrent high-grade cervical intraepithelial neoplasia after successful treatment: A long-term multi-cohort study. *Lancet Oncol.* 2011;12:441–450.

303. **Benard VB, Watson M, Castle PE, et al.** Cervical cancer rates among young females in the United States. *Obstet Gynecol.* 2012; 120:1117–1123.

304. **Winer RL, Lee SK, Hughes JP, et al.** Genital human papillomavirus infection: Incidence and risk factors in a cohort of female university students. *Am J Epidemiol.* 2003;157:218–226.

305. **Moscicki AB, Hills N, Shiboski S, et al.** Risks for incident human papillomavirus infection and low-grade squamous intraepithelial lesion development in young females. *JAMA.* 2001;285:2995–3002.

306. **Moscicki AB, Ma Y, Wibblesman C, et al.** Rate of and risks for regression of cervical intraepithelial neoplasia 2 in adolescents and young women. *Obstet Gynecol.* 2010;116:1373–1380.

307. **Katki HA, Schiffman M, Castle PE, et al.** Five-year risk of CIN 3 + to guide the management of women aged 21 to 24 years. *J Low Genit Tract Dis.* 2013;17:S64–S68.

308. **Kahn J, Slap G, Bernstein D, et al.** Psychological, behavioral, and interpersonal impact of human papillomavirus and Pap test results. *J Womens Health.* 2005;14:650–659.

309. **Kahn J, Slap G, Bernstein D, et al.** Personal meaning of human papillomavirus and pap test results in adolescent and young adult women. *Health Psychol.* 2007;26:192–200.

310. **Lerner D, Parsons SK, Justicia-Linde F, et al.** The impact of precancerous cervical lesions on functioning at work and work productivity. *J Occup Environ Med.* 2010;52:926–933.

311. **Sharp L, Cotton S, Carsin AE, et al.; TOMBOLA Group.** Factors associated with psychological distress following colposcopy among women with low-grade abnormal cervical cytology: A prospective study within the Trial Of Management of Borderline and Other Low-grade Abnormal smears (TOMBOLA). *Psychooncology.* 2013;22(2): 368–380. doi:10.1002/pon.2097.

312. **Sideri M, Iqidbashian S, Boveri S, et al.** Age distribution of HPV genotypes in cervical intraepithelial neoplasia. *Gynecol Oncol.* 2011; 212:510–513.

313. **Trimble CL, Piantadosi S, Gravitt P, et al.** Spontaneous regression of high-grade cervical dysplasia: Effects of human papillomavirus type and HLA phenotype. *Clin Cancer Res.* 2005;11:4717–4723.

314. **Petersen S, Belnap C, Larsen WI, et al.** Grading of squamous dysplasia in endocervical curettage specimens: The case for conservative management of mild endocervical dysplasia. *J Reprod Med.* 2007;52:917–921.

315. **Gage JC, Duggan MA, Nation JG, et al.** Comparative risk of high-grade histopathology diagnosis following a CIN 1 finding in endocervical curettage vs. cervical biopsy. *J Lower Genit Tract Dis.* 2012; 17:137–141.

316. **Fukuchi E, Fetterman B, Poitras N, et al.** Risk of cervical precancer and cancer in women with cervical intraepithelial neoplasia grade 1 on endocervical curettage. *J Low Genit Tract Dis.* 2013; 17(3):255–260.

317. **Katki HA, Schiffman M, Castle PE, et al.** Five-Year Risk of Recurrence After Treatment of CIN 2, CIN 3, or AIS: Performance of HPV and Pap Cotesting in Posttreatment Management. *J Low Genit Tract Dis.* 2013;17:S78–S84.

318. **Vizcaino AP, Moreno V, Bosch FX, et al.** International trends in the incidence of cervical cancer: I. Adenocarcinoma and adenosquamous cell carcinomas. *Int J Cancer.* 1998;75(4):536–545.

319. **Sasieni P, Adams J.** Changing rates of adenocarcinoma and adenosquamous carcinoma of the cervix in England. *Lancet.* 2001; 357(9267):1490–1493.

320. **Wang SS, Sherman ME, Hildesheim A, et al.** Cervical adenocarcinoma and squamous cell carcinoma incidence trends among white women and black women in the United States for 1976–2000. *Cancer.* 2004;100(5):1035–1044.

321. **Sherman ME, Wang SS, Carreon J, et al.** Mortality trends for cervical squamous and adenocarcinoma in the United States - relation to incidence and survival. *Cancer.* 2005;103:1258–1264.

322. **Bulk S, Visser O, Rozendaal L, et al.** Cervical cancer in the Netherlands 1989–1998: Decrease of squamous cell carcinoma in older women, increase of adenocarcinoma in younger women. *Int J Cancer.* 2005;113:1005–1009.

323. **Sasieni P, Castanon A, Cuzick J.** Screening and adenocarcinoma of the cervix. *Int J Cancer.* 2009;125(3):525–529.

324. **Schoolland M, Segal A, Allpress S, et al.** Adenocarcinoma in situ of the cervix. *Cancer.* 2002;96(6):330–337.

325. **Zaino RJ.** Symposium part I: Adenocarcinoma in situ, glandular dysplasia, and early invasive adenocarcinoma of the uterine cervix. *Int J Gynecol Pathol.* 2002;21:314–326.

326. **Smith HO, Padilla LA.** Adenocarcinoma in situ of the cervix: Sensitivity of detection by cervical smear: Will cytologic screening for adenocarcinoma in situ reduce incidence rates for adenocarcinoma. *Cancer.* 2002;96(6):319–322.

327. **Kinney W, Sawaya GF, Sung HY, et al.** Stage at diagnosis and mortality in patients with adenocarcinoma and adenosquamous carcinoma of the uterine cervix diagnosed as a consequence of cytologic screening. *Acta Cytol.* 2003;47(2):167–171.

328. **Syrjanen K.** Is improved detection of adenocarcinoma in situ by screening a key to reducing the incidence of cervical adenocarcinoma? *Acta Cytol.* 2004;48(5):591–594.

329. **Herzog TJ, Monk BJ.** Reducing the burden of glandular carcinomas of the uterine cervix. *Am J Obstet Gynecol.* 2007;197(6):566–571.

330. **Polterauer S, Reinthaller A, Horvat R, et al.** Cervical adenocarcinoma in situ: Update and management. *Curr Obstet Gynecol Rep.* 2013;2:86–93. doi:10.1007/s13669-013-0039-6

331. **Kjaer SK, Brinton LA.** Adenocarcinomas of the uterine cervix: The epidemiology of an increasing problem. *Epidemiol Rev.* 1993;15(2): 486–498.

332. **Duska LR.** Can we improve the detection of glandular cervical lesions: The role and limitations of the Pap smear diagnosis atypical glandular cells (AGC). *Gynecol Oncol.* 2009;114:381–382.

333. **Dunton CJ.** Management of atypical glandular cells and adenocarcinoma in situ. *Obstet Gynecol Clin North Am.* 2008;35:623–632.

334. **Dahlström LA, Ylitalo N, Sundström K, et al.** Prospective study of human papillomavirus and risk of cervical adenocarcinoma. *Int J Cancer.* 2010;127:1923–1930.

335. **Ault KA, Joura EA, Kjaer SK, et al.** Adenocarcinoma in situ and associated human papillomavirus type distribution observed in two clinical trials of a quadrivalent human papillomavirus vaccine. *Int J Cancer.* 2011;128:1344–1353.

336. **Di Bonito L, Bergeron C.** Cytological screening of endocervical adenocarcinoma. *Ann Pathol.* 2012;32:e8–e14.

337. **van Aspert-van Erp AJ, Smedts FM, Vooijs GP.** Severe cervical glandular cell lesions with coexisting squamous cell lesions. *Cancer.* 2004;102(4):218–227.

338. **Kennedy AW, Salmieri SS, Wirth SL, et al.** Results of the clinical evaluation of atypical glandular cells of undetermined significance (AGCUS) detected on cervical cytology screening. *Gynecol Oncol.* 1996;63(1):14–18.

339. **Nasuti JF, Fleisher SR, Gupta PK.** Atypical glandular cells of undetermined significance (AGUS): Clinical considerations and cytohistologic correlation. *Diagn Cytopathol.* 2002;26(3):186–190.

340. **Raab SS.** Can glandular lesions be diagnosed in pap smear cytology? *Diagn Cytopathol.* 2000;23(2):127–133.

341. **Jeng CJ, Liang HS, Wang TY, et al.** Cytologic and histologic review of atypical glandular cells (AGC) detected during cervical cytology screening. *Int J Gynecol Cancer.* 2003;13(4):518–521.

342. **Mattosinho de Castro Ferraz Mda G, Focchi J, Stavale JN, et al.** Atypical glandular cells of undetermined significance. Cytologic predictive value for glandular involvement in high grade squamous intraepithelial lesions. *Acta Cytol.* 2003;47(2):154–158.

343. **Diaz-Montes TP, Farinola MA, Zahurak ML, et al.** Clinical utility of atypical glandular cells (AGC) classification: Cytohistologic comparison and relationship to HPV results. *Gynecol Oncol.* 2007;104: 366–371.

344. **Bertrand M, Lickrish GM, Colgan TJ.** The anatomic distribution of cervical adenocarcinoma in situ: Implications for treatment. *Am J Obstet Gynecol.* 1987;157(1):21–25.

345. **Brand E, Berek JS, Hacker NF.** Controversies in the management of cervical adenocarcinoma. *Obstet Gynecol.* 1988;71(2):261–269.

346. **Poynor EA, Barakat RR, Hoskins WJ.** Management and follow-up of patients with adenocarcinoma in situ of the uterine cervix. *Gynecol Oncol.* 1995;57(2):158–164.

347. **Soutter W, Haidopoulos D, Gornall R, et al.** Is conservative treatment for adenocarcinoma in situ of the cervix safe? *BJOG.* 2001; 108(11):1184–1189.

348. **Bull-Phelps SL, Garner EI, Walsh CS, et al.** Fertility-sparing surgery in 101 women with adenocarcinoma in situ of the cervix. *Gynecol Oncol.* 2007;107(2):316–319.

349. **Dalrymple C, Valmadre S, Cook A, et al.** Cold knife versus laser cone biopsy for adenocarcinoma in situ of the cervix—a comparison of management and outcome. *Int J Gynecol Cancer.* 2008;18:116–120.

350. **Krivak TC, Rose GS, McBroom JW, et al.** Cervical adenocarcinoma in situ: A systematic review of therapeutic options and predictors of persistent or recurrent disease. *Obstet Gynecol Surv.* 2001; 56(9):567–575.

351. **Young JL, Jazaeri AA, Lachance JA, et al.** Cervical adenocarcinoma in situ: The predictive value of conization margin status. *Am J Obstet Gynecol.* 2007;197(2):195 e1–e7; discussion e7–e8.

352. **Dedecker F, Graesslin O, Bonneau S, et al.** [Persistence and recurrence of in situ cervical adenocarcinoma after primary treatment. About 121 cases]. *Gynecol Obstet Fertil.* 2008;36(6):616–622.

353. **Costa S, Venturoli S, Negri G, et al.** Factors predicting the outcome of conservatively treated adenocarcinoma in situ of the uterine cervix: An analysis of 166 cases. *Gynecol Oncol.* 2012;124:490–495.

354. **Cullimore JE, Luesley DM, Rollason TP, et al.** A prospective study of conization of the cervix in the management of cervical intraepithelial glandular neoplasia (CIGN)–a preliminary report. *Br J Obstet Gynaecol.* 1992;99(4):314–318.

355. **Wolf JK, Levenback C, Malpica A, et al.** Adenocarcinoma in situ of the cervix: Significance of cone biopsy margins. *Obstet Gynecol.* 1996;88(1):82–86.

356. **Hocking GR, Hayman JA, Ostor AG.** Adenocarcinoma in situ of the uterine cervix progressing to invasive adenocarcinoma. *Aust N Z J Obstet Gynaecol.* 1996;36(2):218–220.

357. **Cohn DE, Morrison CD, Zanagnolo VL, et al.** Invasive cervical adenocarcinoma immediately following a cone biopsy for adenocarcinoma in situ with negative margins. *Gynecol Oncol.* 2005;98(1): 158–160.

358. **El Masri WM, Walts AE, Chiang A, et al.** Predictors of invasive adenocarcinoma after conization for cervical adenocarcinoma in situ. *Gynecol Oncol.* 2012;125:589–593.

359. **Salani R, Puri I, Bristow RE.** Adenocarcinoma in situ of the uterine cervix: A meta-analysis of 1278 patients evaluating the predictive value of conization margin status. *Am J Obstet Gynecol.* 2009;200: 182.e1–e5.

360. **Purcell K, Cass I, Natarajan S, et al.** Cold knife cone superior to loop electrosurgical excision procedure for conservative management of cervical adenocarcinoma in situ. *Obstet Gynecol.* 2003; 101(4):104S–105S.

361. **Bryson P, Stulberg R, Shepherd L, et al.** Is electrosurgical loop excision with negative margins sufficient treatment for cervical ACIS? *Gynecol Oncol.* 2004;93(2):465–468.

362. **van Hanegem N, Barroilhet LM, Nucci MR, et al.** Fertility-sparing treatment in younger women with adenocarcinoma in situ of the cervix. *Gynecol Oncol.* 2012;124:72–77.

363. **Anderson AF.** Treatment and follow-up of non-invasive cancer of the uterine cervix. Report on 205 cases, (1948–1957). *J Obstet Gynaecol Br Commonw.* 1965;72:172–177.

364. **Kolstad P, Klem V.** Long-term followup of 1121 cases of carcinoma in situ. *Obstet Gynecol.* 1976;48(2):125–129.

365. **Stafl A, Mattingly RF.** Colposcopic diagnosis of cervical neoplasia. *Obstet Gynecol.* 1973;41(2):168–176.

366. **Andersen ES, Thorup K, Larsen G.** The results of cryosurgery for cervical intraepithelial neoplasia. *Gynecol Oncol.* 1988;30(1):21–25.

367. **Chanen W, Rome RM.** Electrocoagulation diathermy for cervical dysplasia and carcinoma in situ: A 15-year survey. *Obstet Gynecol.* 1983;61(6):673–679.

368. **Burke L.** The use of the carbon dioxide laser in the therapy of cervical intraepithelial neoplasia. *Am J Obstet Gynecol.* 1982;144(3):337–340.

369. **Luesley DM, Cullimore J, Redman CW, et al.** Loop diathermy excision of the cervical transformation zone in patients with abnormal cervical smears. *BMJ.* 1990;300(6741):1690–1693.

370. **Soutter WP, de Barros LA, Fletcher A, et al.** Invasive cervical cancer after conservative therapy for cervical intraepithelial neoplasia. *Lancet.* 1997;349(9057):978–980.

371. **Benedet JL, Anderson GH, Boyes DA.** Colposcopic accuracy in the diagnosis of microinvasive and occult invasive carcinoma of the cervix. *Obstet Gynecol.* 1985;65(4):557–562.

372. **Howe DT, Vincenti AC.** Is large loop excision of the transformation zone (LLETZ) more accurate than colposcopically directed punch biopsy in the diagnosis of cervical intraepithelial neoplasia? *Br J Obstet Gynaecol.* 1991;98(6):588–591.

373. **Andersen ES, Nielsen K, Pedersen B.** The reliability of preconization diagnostic evaluation in patients with cervical intraepithelial neoplasia and microinvasive carcinoma. *Gynecol Oncol.* 1995;59(1): 143–147.

374. **Martin-Hirsch PL, Paraskevaidis E, Bryant A, et al.** Surgery for cervical intraepithelial neoplasia. *Cochrane Database Syst Rev.* 2013;12:CD001318.

375. **Creasman WT, Weed JC, Curry SL, et al.** Efficacy of cryosurgical treatment of severe cervical intraepithelial neoplasia. *Obstet Gynecol.* 1973;41(4):501–506.

376. **Popkin DR, Scali V, Ahmed MN.** Cryosurgery for the treatment of cervical intraepithelial neoplasia. *Am J Obstet Gynecol.* 1978;130(5): 551–554.

377. **Kaufman RH, Irwin JF.** The cryosurgical therapy of cervical intraepithelial neoplasia. III. Continuing follow-up. *Am J Obstet Gynecol.* 1978;131(4):381–388.

378. **Benedet JL, Miller DM, Nickerson KG, et al.** The results of cryosurgical treatment of cervical intraepithelial neoplasia at one, five, and ten years. *Am J Obstet Gynecol.* 1987;157(2):268–273.

379. **Tidbury P, Singer A, Jenkins D.** CIN 3: The role of lesion size in invasion. *Br J Obstet Gynaecol.* 1992;99(7):583–586.

380. **Cartier R.** [The role of colposcopy in the diagnosis and treatment of dysplasias and intra-epithelial carcinomas of the uterine cervix (author's transl)]. *Bull Cancer.* 1979;66(4):447–454.

381. **Prendiville W, Cullimore J.** Excision of the transformation zone using the low voltage diathermy (LVD) loop: A superior method of treatment. *Colpose Gynecol Laser Surg.* 1987;122S:1–15.

382. **Prendiville W, Cullimore J, Norman S.** Large loop excision of the transformation zone (LLETZ). A new method of management for women with cervical intraepithelial neoplasia. *Br J Obstet Gynaecol.* 1989;96(9):1054–1060.

383. **Phipps JH, Gunasekara PC, Lewis BV.** Occult cervical carcinoma revealed by large loop diathermy. *Lancet.* 1989;2(8660):453–454.

384. **Chappatte OA, Byrne DL, Raju KS, et al.** Histological differences between colposcopic-directed biopsy and loop excision of the transformation zone (LETZ): A cause for concern. *Gynecol Oncol.* 1991; 43(1):46–50.

385. **Murdoch JB, Grimshaw RN, Morgan PR, et al.** The impact of loop diathermy on management of early invasive cervical cancer. *Int J Gynecol Cancer.* 1992;2(3):129–133.

386. **Burger MP, Hollema H.** The reliability of the histologic diagnosis in colposcopically directed biopsies. A plea for LETZ. *Int J Gynecol Cancer.* 1993;3(6):385–390.

387. **Howells RE, O'Mahony F, Tucker H, et al.** How can the incidence of negative specimens resulting from large loop excision of the cervical transformation zone (LLETZ) be reduced? An analysis of negative LLETZ specimens and development of a predictive model. *BJOG.* 2000;107(9):1075–1082.

388. **Reid R.** Physical and surgical principles governing expertise with the carbon dioxide laser. *Obstet Gynecol Clin North Am.* 1987;14(2): 513–535.

389. **Reid R.** Symposium on cervical neoplasia V. carbon dioxide laser ablation. *J Gynecol Surg.* 1984;1(4):291–297.

390. **Reid R.** Physical and surgical principles of laser surgery in the lower genital tract. *Obstet Gynecol Clin North Am.* 1991;18(3):429–474.

391. **Fuller TA.** Laser tissue interaction: The influence of power density. In: Baggish M, ed. *Basic and Advanced Laser Surgery and Gynecology.* New York: Appleton-Century-Crofts; 1985:51–60.

392. **Bjerre B, Eliasson G, Linell F, et al.** Conization as only treatment of carcinoma in situ of the uterine cervix. *Am J Obstet Gynecol.* 1976;125(2):143–152.

393. **Luesley DM, McCrum A, Terry PB, et al.** Complications of cone biopsy related to the dimensions of the cone and the influence of prior colposcopic assessment. *Br J Obstet Gynaecol.* 1985;92(2):158–164.

394. **Benedet JL, Sanders BH.** Carcinoma in situ of the vagina. *Am J Obstet Gynecol.* 1984;148(5):695–700.

395. **Coppleson M, Reid, B.** Treatment of preclinical carcinoma of the cervix. In: Coppleson M, Reid B, eds. *Preclinical Carcinoma of the Cervix.* Oxford: Pergamon Press; 1967:1–321.

396. **Wharton JT, Tortolero-Luna G, Linares AC, et al.** Vaginal intraepithelial neoplasia and vaginal cancer. *Obstet Gynecol Clin North Am.* 1996;23:325–345.

397. **Woodruff JD.** Carcinoma in situ of the vagina. *Clin Obstet Gynecol.* 1981;24:485–501.

398. **Hatch KD.** Vaginal intraepithelial neoplasia (VAIN). *Int J Gynecol Obstet.* 2006;94:S40–S43.

399. **Wee WW, Chia YN, Yam PK.** Diagnosis and treatment of vaginal intraepithelial neoplasia. *Int J Gynaecol Obstet.* 2012;117:15–17.

400. **Gunderson CC, Nugent EK, Elfrink SH, et al.** A contemporary analysis of epidemiology and management of vaginal intraepithelial neoplasia. *Am J Obstet Gynecol.* 2013;208:410.e1–e6.

401. **De Vuyst H, Clifford GM, Nascimento MC, et al.** Prevalence and type distribution of human papillomavirus in carcinoma and intraepithelial neoplasia of the vulva, vagina and anus: A meta-analysis. *Int J Cancer.* 2009;124(7):1626–1636.

402. **Srodon M, Stoler MH, Baber GB, et al.** The distribution of low and high-risk HPV types in vulvar and vaginal intraepithelial neoplasia (VIN and VaIN). *Am J Surg Pathol.* 2006;30(12):1513–1518.

403. **Smith JS, Backes DM, Hoots BE, et al.** Human papillomavirus type distribution in vulvar and vaginal cancers and their associated precursors. *Obstet Gynecol.* 2009;113:917–924.

404. **Brunner AH, Grimm C, Polterauer S, et al.** The prognostic role of human papillomavirus in patients with vaginal cancer. *Int J Gynecol Cancer.* 2011;21:923–929.

405. **Ballon SC, Lagasse LD, Chang NH, et al.** Primary adenocarcinoma of the vagina. *Surg Gynecol Obstet.* 1979;149:233–237.

406. **Sillman FH, Fruchter RG, Chen YS, et al.** Vaginal intraepithelial neoplasia: Risk factors for persistence, recurrence, and invasion and its management. *Am J Obstet Gynecol.* 1997;176(1 Pt 1):93–99.

407. **Dorsey J, Baggish M.** Multifocal vaginal intraepithelial neoplasia with uterus in situ. In: **Sharp F, Jordan J, eds.** *Gynaecological Laser Surgery.* Proceedings of the Fifteenth Study Group of the Royal College of Obstetricians and Gynaecologists. Ithaca, NY: Perinatology Press; 1986 (6):173.

408. **Dodge JA, Eltabbakh GH, Mount SL, et al.** Clinical features and risk of recurrence among patients with vaginal intraepithelial neoplasia. *Gynecol Oncol.* 2001;83(2):363–369.

409. **Campion M.** Clinical manifestations and natural history of genital human papillomavirus infection. *Dermatol Clin.* 1991;9(2):235–249.

410. **Sherman JF, Mount SL, Evans MF, et al.** Smoking increases the risk of high-grade vaginal intraepithelial neoplasia in women with oncogenic human papillomavirus. *Gynecol Oncol.* 2008;110(3):396–401.

411. **González BE, Torres A, Busquets M, et al.** Prognostic factors for the development of vaginal intraepithelial neoplasia. *Eur J Gynaecol Oncol.* 2008;29(1):43–45.

412. **Gagné HM.** Colposcopy of the vagina and vulva. *Obstet Gynecol Clin Nth Am.* 2008;35(4):659–669.

413. **Stafl A, Wilkinson EJ, Mattingly RF.** Laser treatment of cervical and vaginal neoplasia. *Am J Obstet Gynecol.* 1977;128(2):128–136.

414. **Yalcin OT, Rutherford TJ, Chambers SK, et al.** Vaginal intraepithelial neoplasia: Treatment by carbon dioxide laser and risk factors for failure. *Eur J Obstet Gynecol Reprod Biol.* 2003;106(1):64–68.

415. **Diakomanolis E, Stefanidis K, Rodolakis A, et al.** Vaginal intraepithelial neoplasia: Report of 102 cases. *Eur J Gynaecol Oncol.* 2002;23(5):457–459.

416. **Sillman FH, Sedlis A, Boyce JG.** A review of lower genital intraepithelial neoplasia and the use of topical 5-fluorouracil. *Obstet Gynecol Surv.* 1985;40(4):190–220.

417. **Krebs HB.** Prophylactic topical 5-fluorouracil following treatment of human papillomavirus-associated lesions of the vulva and vagina. *Obstet Gynecol.* 1986;68(6):837–841.

418. **Diakomanolis E, Haidopoulos D, Stefanidis K.** Treatment of high-grade vaginal intraepithelial neoplasia with imiquimod cream. *N Engl J Med.* 2002;347(5):374.

419. **Haidopoulos D, Diakomanolis E, Rodolakis A, et al.** Can local application of imiquimod cream be an alternative mode of therapy for patients with high-grade intraepithelial lesions of the vagina? *Int J Gynecol Cancer.* 2005;15(5):898–902.

420. **Iavazzo C, Pitsouni E, Athanasiou S, et al.** Imiquimod for treatment of vulvar and vaginal intraepithelial neoplasia. *Int J Gynecol Obstet.* 2008;101(1):3–10.

421. **Woodman C, Jordan J, WADE-EVANS T.** The management of vaginal intraepithelial neoplasia after hysterectomy. *Br J Obstet Gynaecol.* 1984;91(7):707–711.

422. **Hoffman M, DeCesare S, Roberts W, et al.** Upper vaginectomy for in situ and occult, superficially invasive carcinoma of the vagina. *Am J Obstet Gynecol.* 1992;166(1 Pt 1):30–33.

423. **Indermaur MD, Martino MA, Fiorica JV, et al.** Upper vaginectomy for the treatment of vaginal intraepithelial neoplasia. *Am J Obstet Gynecol.* 2005;193:577–581.

424. **Hart WR.** Vulvar intraepithelial neoplasia: Historical aspects and current status. *Int J Gynecol Pathol.* 2001;20(1):16–30.

425. **Judson PL, Habermann EB, Baxter NN, et al. Virnig BA: Trends in the incidence of invasive and in situ vulvar carcinoma.** *Obstet Gynecol.* 2006;107:1018–1022.

426. **Sturgeon S, Brinton L, Devesa S, et al.** In situ and invasive vulvar cancer incidence trends (1973 to 1987). *Am J Obstetrics Gynecol.* 1992;166(5):1482–1485.

427. **Joura EA, Losch A, Haider-Angeler MG, et al.** Trends in vulvar neoplasia. Increasing incidence of vulvar intraepithelial neoplasia and squamous cell carcinoma of the vulva in young women. *J Reprod Med.* 2000;45(8):613–615.

428. **Rodke G, Friedrich EG Jr, Wilkinson EJ.** Malignant potential of mixed vulvar dystrophy (lichen sclerosus associated with squamous cell hyperplasia). *J Reprod Med.* 1988;33(6):545–550.

429. **Bloss JD, Liao S-Y, Wilczynski SP, et al.** Clinical and histologic features of vulvar carcinomas analyzed for human papillomavirus status: Evidence that squamous cell carcinoma of the vulva has more than one etiology. *Hum Pathol.* 1991;22(7):711–718.

430. **Toki T, Kurman RJ, Park JS, et al.** Probable nonpapillomavirus etiology of squamous cell carcinoma of the vulva in older women: A clinicopathologic study using in situ hybridization and polymerase chain reaction. *Int J Gynecol Pathol.* 1991;10(2):107–125.

431. **Park J, Kurman R, Shiffman M.** Basaloid and warty carcinoma of the vulva: Distinctive types of squamous carcinoma with human papillomavirus. *Lab Invest.* 1991;1:62–68.

432. **Hording U, Junge J, Daugaard S, et al.** Vulvar squamous cell carcinoma and papillomaviruses: Indications for two different etiologies. *Gynecol Oncol.* 1994;52(2):241–246.

433. **Trimble CL, Hildesheim A, Brinton LA, et al.** Heterogeneous etiology of squamous cell carcinoma of the vulva. *Obstet Gynecol.* 1996;87(1):59–64.

434. **Kim YT, Thomas NF, Kessis TD, et al.** p53 mutations and clonality in vulvar carcinomas and squamous hyperplasias: Evidence suggesting that squamous hyperplasias do not serve as direct precursors of human papillomavirus-negative vulvar carcinomas. *Hum Pathol.* 1996;27(4):389–395.

435. **Jeffcoate T.** Chronic vulval dystrophies. *Am J Obstet Gynecol.* 1966;95(1):61–74.

436. **Committee on Terminology; International Society for the Study of Vulvar Disease.** New nomenclature for vulvar disease. *Int J Gynecol Pathol.* 1986;8:83–84.

437. **Herod J, Shafi M, Rollason T, et al.** Vulvar intraepithelial neoplasia: Long term follow up of treated and untreated women. *Br J Obstet Gynaecol.* 1996;103(5):446–452.

438. **Jones RW, Rowan DM.** Vulvar intraepithelial neoplasia III: A clinical study of the outcome in 113 cases with relation to the later development of invasive vulvar carcinoma. *Obstet Gynecol.* 1994;84(5):741–745.

439. **McNally O, Mulvany N, Pagano R, et al.** VIN 3: A clinicopathologic review. *Int J Gynecol Cancer.* 2002;12(5):490–495.

440. **Jones RW, Rowan DM, Stewart AW.** Vulvar intraepithelial neoplasia: Aspects of the natural history and outcome in 405 women. *Obstet Gynecol.* 2005;106(6):1319–1326.

441. **van Seters M, van Beurden M, de Craen AJ.** Is the assumed natural history of vulvar intraepithelial neoplasia III based on enough evidence? A systematic review of 3322 published patients. *Gynecol Oncol.* 2005;97(2):645–651.

442. **Preti M, Van Seters M, Sideri M, et al.** Squamous vulvar intraepithelial neoplasia. *Clin Obstet Gynecol.* 2005;48(4):845–861.

443. **Shylasree TS, Karanjgaokar V, Tristram A, et al.** Contribution of demographic, psychological and disease-related factors to quality of life in women with high-grade vulval intraepithelial neoplasia. *Gynecol Oncol.* 2008;110(2):185–189.

444. **Sideri M, Jones RW, Wilkinson EJ, et al.** Squamous vulvar intraepithelial neoplasia. *J Reprod Med.* 2005;50:807–810.

445. **Kurman RJ, Toki T, Schiffman MH.** Basaloid and warty carcinoma of the vulva. Distinctive types of squamous cell carcinoma frequently associated with human papillomaviruses. *Am J Surg Pathol.* 1993;17133–17145.

446. **Jones RW, Rowan DM.** Spontaneous regression of vulvar intraepithelial neoplasia 2–3. *Obstet Gynecol.* 2000;96(3):470–472.

447. **Jones RW, MacLean AB.** Re: "Is the assumed natural history of vulvar intraepithelial neoplasia III based on enough evidence? A systematic review of 3322 published patients". *Gynecol Oncol.* 2006;101(2):371–372.

448. **Kaufman RH.** Intraepithelial neoplasia of the vulva. *Gynecol Oncol.* 1995;56(1):8–21.

449. **Haefner HK, Tate JE, McLachlin CM, et al.** Vulvar intraepithelial neoplasia: Age, morphological phenotype, papillomavirus DNA, and coexisting invasive carcinoma. *Hum Pathol.* 1995;26(2):147–154.

450. **van Beurden M, ten Kate FW, Tjong-A-Hung SP, et al.** Human papillomavirus DNA in multicentric vulvar intraepithelial neoplasia. *Int J Gynecol Pathol.* 1998;17(1):12–16.

451. **Davidson EJ, Sehr P, Faulkner RL, et al.** Human papillomavirus type 16 E2- and L1-specific serological and T-cell responses in women with vulval intraepithelial neoplasia. *J GenVirol.* 2003;84(Pt 8): 2089–2097.

452. **Pearson JM, Feltman RS, Twiggs LB.** Association of human papillomavirus with vulvar and vaginal intraepithelial disease: Opportunities for prevention. *Womens Health (Lond Engl).* 2008;4(2):143–150.

453. **Wallbillich JJ, Rhodes HE, Milbourne AM, et al.** Vulvar intraepithelial neoplasia (VIN 2/3): Comparing clinical outcomes and evaluating risk factors for recurrence. *Gynecol Oncol.* 2012;127(2): 312–315.

454. **van Esch EM, Dam MC, Osse ME, et al.** Clinical characteristics associated with development of recurrence and progression in usual-type vulvar intraepithelial neoplasia. *Int J Gynecol Cancer.* 2013; 23(8):1476–1483.

455. **Petry KU, Kochel H, Bode U, et al.** Human papillomavirus is associated with the frequent detection of warty and basaloid high-grade neoplasia of the vulva and cervical neoplasia among immunocompromised women. *Gynecol Oncol.* 1996;60:30–34.

456. **Khan AM, Freeman-Wang T, Pisal N, et al.** Smoking and multicentric vulval intraepithelial neoplasia. *J Obstet Gynaecol.* 2009;29: 123–125.

457. **Meeuwis KA, van Rossum MM, van de Kerkhof PC, et al.** Skin cancer and (pre)malignancies of the female genital tract in renal transplant recipients. *Transpl Int.* 2010;23:191–199.

458. **Thuis YN, Campion M, Fox H, et al.** Contemporary experience with the management of vulvar intraepithelial neoplasia. *Int J Gynecol Cancer.* 2000;10(3):223–7.

459. **van Beurden M, ten Kate FJ, Smits HL, et al.** Multifocal vulvar intraepithelial neoplasia grade III and multicentric lower genital tract neoplasia is associated with transcriptionally active human papillomavirus. *Cancer.* 1995;75(12):2879–2884.

460. **Berger BW, Hori Y.** Multicentric Bowen's disease of the genitalia: Spontaneous regression of lesions. *Arc Dermatol.* 1978;114(11): 1698–1699.

461. **Forney J, Morrow C, Townsend D, et al.** Management of carcinoma in situ of the vulva. *Am J Obstet Gynecol.* 1977;127(8):801–806.

462. **Rodolakis A, Diakomanolis E, Vlachos G, et al.** Vulvar intraepithelial neoplasia (VIN): Diagnostic and therapeutic challenges. *Eur J Gynaecol Oncol.* 2003;24(3–4):317–322.

463. **McFadden K, Cruickshank M.** New developments in the management of VIN. *Rev Gynaecol Pract.* 2005;5(2):102–108.

464. **Modesitt SC, Waters AB, Walton L, et al.** Vulvar intraepithelial neoplasia III: Occult cancer and the impact of margin status on recurrence. *Obstet Gynecol.* 1998;92(6):962–966.

465. **Sykes P, Smith N, McCormick P, et al.** High-grade vulval intraepithelial neoplasia (VIN 3): A retrospective analysis of patient characteristics, management, outcome and relationship to squamous cell carcinoma of the vulva 1989–1999. *Aus N Z J Obstet Gynaecol.* 2002;42(1):75–80.

466. **Rutledge F, Sinclair M.** Treatment of intraepithelial neoplasia of the vulva by skin excision and graft. *Am J Obstet Gynecol.* 1968;102: 806–812.

467. **DiSaia P.** Management of superficially invasive vulvar carcinoma. *Clin Obstet Gynecol.* 1985;28(1):196–203.

468. **Yii N, Niranjan N.** Lotus petal flaps in vulvo-vaginal reconstruction. *Br J Plast Surg.* 1996;49(8):547–554.

469. **Davison PM, Sarhanis P, Shroff JF, et al.** A new approach to reconstruction following vulval excision. *Br J Obstet Gynaecol.* 1996; 103(5):475–477.

470. **Narayansingh G, Cumming G, Parkin D, et al.** Flap repair: An effective strategy for minimising sexual morbidity associated with the surgical management of vulval intra epithelial neoplasia. *J R Coll Surg Edinb.* 2000;45(2):81–84.

471. **Reid R.** Superficial laser vulvectomy. I. The efficacy of extended superficial ablation for refractory and very extensive condylomas. *Am J Obstet Gynecol.* 1985;151(8):1047–1052.

472. **Reid R, Elfont E, Zirkin R, et al.** Superficial laser vulvectomy. II. The anatomic and biophysical principles permitting accurate control over the depth of dermal destruction with the carbon dioxide laser. *Am J Obstet Gynecol.* 1985;152(3):261–271.

473. **Reid R.** Superficial laser vulvectomy. III. A new surgical technique for appendage-conserving ablation of refractory condylomas and vulvar intraepithelial neoplasia. *Am J Obstet Gynecol.* 1985; 152(5):504–509.

474. **Reid R, Greenberg MD, Lorincz AT, et al.** Superficial laser vulvectomy. IV. Extended laser vaporization and adjunctive 5-fluorouracil therapy of human papillomavirus-associated vulvar disease. *Obstet Gynecol.* 1990;76(3):439–448.

475. **Reid R, Greenberg M, Pizzuti D, et al.** Superficial laser vulvectomy. V: Surgical debulking is enhanced by adjuvant systemic interferon. *Am J Obstet Gynecol.* 1992;166(3):815–820.

476. **Hengge U, Benninghoff B, Ruzicka T, et al.** Topical immunomodulators—progress towards treating inflammation, infection, and cancer. *Lancet Infect Dis.* 2001;1(3):189–198.

477. **Tyring SK.** Immune-response modifiers: A new paradigm in the treatment of human papillomavirus. *Curr Ther Res.* 2000;61(9):584–596.

478. **Friedman-Kien AE, Eron LJ, Conant M, et al.** Natural interferon alfa for treatment of condylomata acuminata. *JAMA.* 1988;259(4): 533–538.

479. **Garland SM.** Imiquimod. *Curr Opin Infect Dis.* 2003;16(2):85–89.

480. **Beutner KR, Tyring SK, Trofatter KF, et al.** Imiquimod, a patient-applied immune-response modifier for treatment of external genital warts. *Antimicrob Agents Chemother.* 1998;42(4):789–794.

481. **Edwards L, Ferenczy A, Eron L, et al.** Self-administered topical 5% imiquimod cream for external anogenital warts. *Arch Dermatol.* 1998;134(1):25–30.

482. **Garland S, Sellors W, Wikstrom A, et al.** Imiquimod 5% cream is a safe and effective self-applied treatment for anogenital warts-results of an open-label, multicentre Phase IIIB trial. *Int J STD AIDS.* 2001;12(11):722–729.

483. **Travis LB, Weinberg JM, Krumholz BA.** Successful treatment of vulvar intraepithelial neoplasia with topical imiquimod 5% cream in a lung transplanted patient. *Acta Derm Venereol.* 2002;82(6):475–476.

484. **Diaz-Arrastia C, Arany I, Robazetti SC, et al.** Clinical and molecular responses in high-grade intraepithelial neoplasia treated with topical imiquimod 5%. *Clin Cancer Res.* 2001;7:3031–3033.

485. **Jayne CJ, Kaufman RH.** Treatment of vulvar intraepithelial neoplasia 2/3 with imiquimod. *J Reprod Med.* 2002;47:395–398.

486. **van Seters M, Fons G, van Beurden M.** Imiquimod in the treatment of multifocal vulvar intraepithelial neoplasia 2/3. Results of a pilot study. *J Reprod Med.* 2002;47(9):701–705.

487. **van Seters M, van Beurden M, ten Kate FJ, et al.** Treatment of vulvar intraepithelial neoplasia with topical imiquimod. *N Engl J Med.* 2008;358(14):1465–1473.

488. **Terlou A, Van Seters M, Ewing PC, et al.** Treatment of vulvar intraepithelial neoplasia with topical imiquimod: Seven years median follow-up of a randomized clinical trial. *Gynecol Oncol.* 2011;121: 157–162.

489. **Finn OJ, Edwards RP.** Human papillomavirus vaccine for cancer prevention. *N Engl J Med.* 2009;361(19):1899–1901.

490. **Kenter GG, Welters MJ, Valentijn AR, et al.** Vaccination against HPV-16 oncoproteins for vulvar intraepithelial neoplasia. *N Engl J Med.* 2009;361:1838–1847.

491. **Daayana S, Elkord E, Winters U, et al.** Phase II trial of imiquimod and HPV therapeutic vaccination in patients with vulval intraepithelial neoplasia. *Br J Cancer.* 2010;102(7):1129–1136.

492. **Campion M, Clarkson P, McCance DJ.** Squamous neoplasia of the cervix in relation to other genital tract neoplasia. *Clin Obstet Gynaecology.* 1985;12(1):265–280.

493. **Spitzer M, Krumholz BA, Seltzer VL.** The multicentric nature of disease related to human papillomavirus infection of the female lower genital tract. *Obstet Gynecol.* 1989;73(3 Pt 1):303–307.

494. **Vinokurova S, Wentzensen N, Einenkel J, et al.** Clonal history of papillomavirus-induced dysplasia in the female lower genital tract. *J Natl Cancer Inst.* 2005;97(24):1816–1821.

495. **Ait Menguellet S, Collinet P, Debarge VH, et al.** Management of multicentric lesions of the lower genital tract. *Eur J Obstet Gynecol Reprod Biol.* 2007;132(1):116–120.

496. **ElNaggar AC, Santoso JT.** Risk factors for anal intraepithelial neoplasia in women with genital dysplasia. *Obstet Gynecol.* 2013;122: 218–223.

497. **Ogunbiyi OA, Scholefield JH, Robertson G, et al.** Anal human papillomavirus infection and squamous neoplasia in patients with invasive vulvar cancer. *Obstet Gynecol.* 1994;83(2):212–216.

498. **Frisch M, Glimelius B, van den Brule AJ, et al.** Sexually transmitted infection as a cause of anal cancer. *N Engl J Med.* 1997;337: 1350–1358.

499. **Daling JR, Madeleine MM, Johnson LG, et al.** Human papillomavirus, smoking, and sexual practices in the etiology of anal cancer. *Cancer.* 2004;101:270–280.

500. **Bjørge T, Engeland A, Luostarinen T, et al.** Human papillomavirus infection as a risk factor for anal and perianal skin cancer in a prospective study. *Br J Cancer.* 2002;87:61–64.

501. **Saleem AM, Paulus JK, Shapter AP, et al.** Risk of anal cancer in a cohort with human papillomavirus–related gynecologic neoplasm. *Obstet Gynecol.* 2011;117:643–649.

502. **American Cancer Society.** Detailed guide: Anal cancer. Available online at: http://www.cancer.org/Cancer/AnalCancer/Detailed-Guide/anal-cancer-what-is-key-statistics. Retrieved December 27, 2013.

503. **Maggard MA, Beanes SR, Ko CY.** Anal canal cancer: A population-based reappraisal. *Dis Colon Rectum.* 2003;46:1517–1523; discussion 1523–1524; author reply 1524.

504. **Watson AJ, Smith BB, Whitehead MR, et al.** Malignant progression of anal intra-epithelial neoplasia. *ANZ J Surg.* 2006;76: 715–717.

505. **Devaraj B, Cosman BC.** Expectant management of anal squamous dysplasia in patients with HIV. *Dis Colon Rectum.* 2006;49(1): 36–40.

8

Cervical Cancer

Neville F. Hacker
Jan B. Vermorken

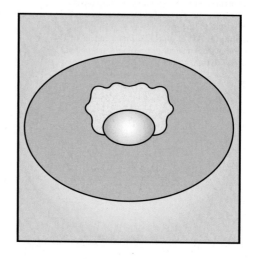

Cervical cancer is the third most common cancer in women worldwide, after breast and colorectal cancer. Annual global estimates for the year 2008 were 530,000 new cases and 275,000 deaths (1). It **is the most common cancer in women in Eastern Africa, South Central Asia, and Melanesia.** In the United States, 12,340 new cases with 4,030 deaths were anticipated in 2013 (2). **The median age at diagnosis is 48 years,** and the majority of cases are diagnosed between the ages of 35 and 55 years, when women are in the prime of their lives; 0.2% are diagnosed under the age of 20 (3).

Cervical cancer progresses slowly from preinvasive cervical intraepithelial neoplasia (CIN) to invasive cancer, and screening asymptomatic women with regular Papanicolaou (Pap) smears allows diagnosis of the readily treatable preinvasive phase. Hence, appropriate screening programs are an important public health issue. **In developed countries, most cases of cervical cancer occur in women who have not had regular Pap smear screening.**

In low-resource countries, facilities for screening asymptomatic women are not readily available. In addition, cultural attitudes and lack of public education discourage early diagnosis. Hence, **most patients in developing countries present with advanced disease that may have already invaded the bladder, rectum, pelvic nerves, or bone.** Because radiation therapy and palliative care facilities are also usually inadequate in these countries, many of these women die as social outcasts, with severe pain and a foul-smelling vaginal discharge. Most of these women have dependent children, so the social devastation caused by this disease is enormous.

Molecular biology has firmly established a **causal relationship between persistent infection with high-risk human papilloma virus (HPV) genotypes and cervical cancer.** In a study of almost 1,000 cases of cervical cancer worldwide, the prevalence of HPV infection was 99.7% (4). **This causal relationship has led to the opportunity for primary prevention through the development of vaccines.** The quadrivalent vaccine *Gardasil* and the bivalent vaccine *Cervarix* have been available for almost a decade, and one or other has been introduced into the school immunization program in many countries. **Secondary prevention, by screening directly for carcinogenic HPV, is likely to replace Pap smears for primary screening in older women.** Sankaranarayanan et al. (5) reported a large randomized trial from India which showed that **a single round of HPV testing dramatically reduced the incidence of advanced cervical cancer and cervical cancer mortality within 8 years,** when compared to traditional screening methods.

Nearly 9% of women in the United States have been estimated to receive no therapy for their disease. This neglect is more common in older, unmarried women, who present with late-stage disease. Obstacles to treatment include lack of access to treatment facilities, inability to pay, and inadequate social support (6).

Diagnosis

Early diagnosis of cervical cancer can be extremely challenging because of three factors:

1. **The frequently asymptomatic nature of early stage disease,** particularly in women who are not sexually active
2. **The origin of some tumors from within the endocervical canal or beneath the epithelium of the ectocervix,** making visualization on speculum examination impossible
3. **The significant false-negative rate for Pap smears,** even in women having regular screening

Symptoms

Abnormal vaginal bleeding is the most common presenting symptom of invasive cancer of the cervix. This may include postcoital, intermenstrual, or postmenopausal bleeding. Unlike endometrial cancer, which usually bleeds early, **cervical cancer often is asymptomatic until quite advanced in women who are not sexually active.** Large tumors commonly become infected and a vaginal discharge, sometimes malodorous, may occur before the onset of bleeding. In very advanced cases, pelvic pain, pressure symptoms pertaining to the bowel or bladder, and occasionally vaginal passage of urine or feces may be presenting symptoms.

In a review of 81 patients diagnosed with cervical cancer in southern California, Pretorius et al. (7) reported that 56% presented with abnormal vaginal bleeding, 28% with an abnormal Pap smear, 9% with pain, 4% with vaginal discharge, and 4% with other symptoms.

Signs

Physical examination should include palpation of the liver, supraclavicular, and groin nodes to exclude metastatic disease. On speculum examination, the primary lesion may be exophytic, endophytic, ulcerative, or polypoid. If the tumor arises beneath the epithelium or in the endocervical canal, the ectocervix may appear macroscopically normal. Direct extension to the vagina is usually grossly apparent, but the infiltration may be subepithelial and suspected only on the basis of obliteration of the vaginal fornices or the presence of apical stenosis. In the latter situation, it may be difficult to visualize the cervix. On palpation, the cervix is firm (except during pregnancy) and usually expanded. **The size of the cervix is best determined by rectal examination, which is also necessary for the detection of any extension of disease into the parametrium.**

Cytology

The presence of malignant cells in a background of necrotic debris, blood, and inflammatory cells is typical of invasive carcinoma (Fig. 8.1). Differentiation between squamous and glandular cells is usually possible except for poorly differentiated lesions. The Pap smear is basically a screening test for asymptomatic women, and **the false-negative rate for Pap smears in the presence of invasive cancer may be up to 50%** (8).

Biopsy

Any obvious tumor growth or ulceration should undergo office punch biopsy or loop excision for histologic confirmation. Any cervix that is unusually firm or expanded should also undergo biopsy and endocervical curettage (ECC).

If the patient has a normal-appearing cervix but is symptomatic or has an abnormal Pap smear, colposcopy should be performed. If a definitive diagnosis of invasive cancer cannot be made on the basis of an office biopsy, diagnostic conization may be necessary.

Colposcopy for Invasive Cancer

If a carcinoma is entirely within the endocervical canal, the ectocervix may be colposcopically normal. Ectocervical microcarcinomas are classically associated with atypical vessels, which are prone to bleed. **Atypical vessels show a completely irregular and haphazard disposition, great variation in caliber, and abrupt changes in direction, often forming acute angles** (Fig. 8.2). The intercapillary distance is increased and tends to be variable (9).

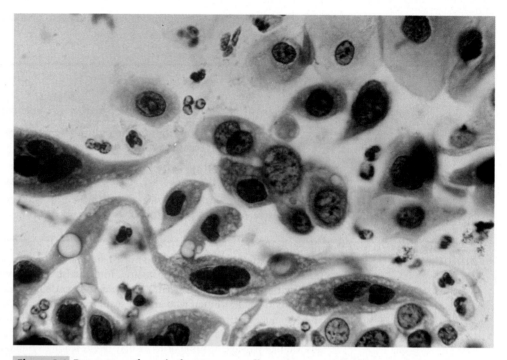

Figure 8.1 **Pap smear of cervical squamous cell carcinoma.** Malignant squamous cells, singly and in groups, show nuclear pleomorphism. A "tadpole" cell is present on the left. (Original magnification 165×.)

Frankly invasive cancers can usually be seen with the naked eye, but the colposcope highlights their surface irregularity and highly atypical, nonbranching, blood vessels (Fig. 8.3). Endophytic tumors may present as an "erosion," the true nature of which can be recognized only by their papillary surface and atypical vessels. A keratotic surface may mask the colposcopic features of an endophytic lesion, so biopsy of areas of keratosis is mandatory.

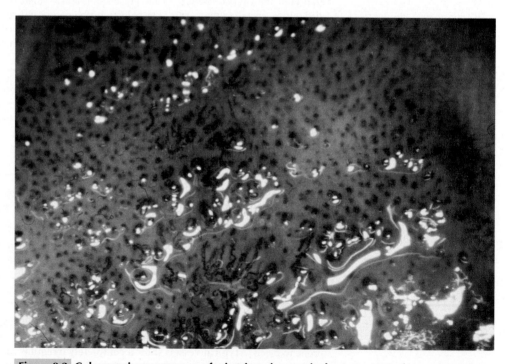

Figure 8.2 **Colposcopic appearance of microinvasive cervical cancer.** Note the severe varicose vascular abnormality with course punctation and transitional forms to atypical vessels.

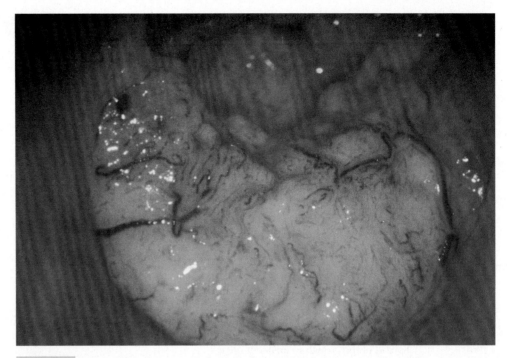

Figure 8.3 Colposcopic appearance of invasive cervical cancer. Note the surface irregularity and dilated atypical vessels.

Adenocarcinomas present no specific features. They often occur in association with squamous CIN, and all of the vascular changes described previously may be seen with these lesions.

Staging

Cervical cancer is staged clinically because most patients worldwide are treated only with radiation therapy.

In 2009, the FIGO Cancer Committee modified the staging (Table 8.1). **The main changes from the 1994 FIGO staging were the removal of stage 0, and the division of stage IIA into IIA1 (tumor ≤4 cm) and IIA2 (tumor >4 cm).** As expected, survival has been reported to be greater for IIA1 tumors (68% vs. 50%; $p = 0.0015$) (10).

Diagnostic imaging is now encouraged to assess tumor size. The ability of magnetic resonance imaging (MRI) to accurately determine not only tumor size, but also extension to surrounding organs, has made the need for examination under anesthesia (EUA), cystoscopy and sigmoidoscopy less frequent; they are now considered optional. A comparison of the FIGO staging and the TNM (tumor, nodes, metastasis) classification is shown in Table 8.2.

Clinical Staging

Clinical staging is often inaccurate in defining the extent of disease. The Gynecologic Oncology Group (GOG) (11), in a study of 290 patients with surgically staged cervical cancer, reported errors in FIGO clinical staging ranging from 24% in stage IB to 67% for stage IVA disease. **Most patients were upstaged on the basis of surgical exploration, with the most likely sites of occult metastases being the pelvic and para-aortic lymph nodes.** Other sites of occult disease were the parametrium, peritoneum, and omentum. **As many as 14% of patients may be downstaged** (12), typically because a benign pathologic process was discovered, such as pelvic inflammatory disease, endometriosis, or fibroids.

Noninvasive Diagnostic Studies

Because information about the extent of disease is critical for treatment planning, various imaging studies have been used to define more accurately the extent of disease.

Table 8.1 Carcinoma of the Cervix Uteri: FIGO Nomenclature (Capetown, 2009)	
Stage I	The carcinoma is strictly confined to the cervix (extension to the corpus would be disregarded)
IA	Invasive carcinoma that can be diagnosed only by microscopy, with deepest invasion ≤5 mm and largest extension ≤7 mm
IA1	Measured stromal invasion of ≤3 mm in depth and extension of ≤7 mm
IA2	Measured stromal invasion of >3 mm and not >5 mm with an extension of not >7 mm
IB	Clinically visible lesions limited to the cervix uteri or preclinical cancers greater than stage IA[a]
IB1	Clinically visible lesion ≤4 cm in greatest dimension
IB2	Clinically visible lesion >4 cm in greatest dimension
Stage II	Cervical carcinoma invades beyond the uterus, but not to the pelvic wall or to the lower third of the vagina
IIA	Without parametrial invasion
IIA1	Clinically visible lesion ≤4 cm in greatest dimension
IIA2	Clinically visible lesion >4 cm in greatest dimension
IIB	With obvious parametrial invasion
Stage III	The tumor extends to the pelvic wall and/or involves lower third of the vagina and/or causes hydronephrosis or nonfunctioning kidney[b]
IIIA	Tumor involves lower third of the vagina, with no extension to the pelvic wall
IIIB	Extension to the pelvic wall and/or hydronephrosis or nonfunctioning kidney
Stage IV	The carcinoma has extended beyond the true pelvis or has involved (biopsy proven) the mucosa of the bladder or rectum. A bullous edema, as such, does not permit a case to be allotted to Stage IV.
IVA	Spread of the growth to adjacent organs
IVB	Spread to distant organs

[a]All macroscopically visible lesions—even with superficial invasion—are allotted to stage IB carcinomas. Invasion is limited to a measured stromal invasion with a maximal depth of 5 mm and a horizontal extension of not >7 mm. Depth of invasion should not be >5 mm taken from the base of the epithelium of the original tissue—squamous or glandular. The depth of invasion should always be reported in mm, even in those cases with "early (minimal) stromal invasion" (~1 mm). The involvement of vascular/lymphatic spaces should not change the stage allotment.

[b]On rectal examination, there is no cancer-free space between the tumor and the pelvic wall. All cases with hydronephrosis or nonfunctioning kidney are included, unless they are known to be due to another cause.

FIGO Committee on Gynecologic Oncology. Revised FIGO staging for carcinoma of the vulva, cervix, and endometrium. *Int J Gynecol Obstet.* 2009;105:103–104.

Computed Tomography

Computed tomography (CT) has been used to help stage pelvic cancers since the mid-1970s. In addition to the lymph nodes, a pelvic and abdominal CT scan allows an evaluation of the liver, urinary tract, and bony structures. **A CT can detect only changes in the size of the nodes, those greater than 1 cm in diameter usually being considered positive.** Normal-sized nodes containing microscopic deposits give false-negative results, whereas nodal enlargement from inflammatory or hyperplastic changes gives false-positive results. If nodes greater than 1.5 cm in diameter are considered positive, then the sensitivity of the test is improved at the expense of the specificity.

In a review of the literature, Hacker and Berek (13) reported that the overall accuracy for the detection of para-aortic lymph node metastases was 84.4%, with a false-positive rate of approximately 21% (9 of 41 positive readings) and a false-negative rate of approximately 13% (13 of 99 negative readings).

Magnetic Resonance Imaging

Because CT cannot discriminate between cancer and normal soft tissue of the cervix and uterus, it is limited in the evaluation of early cervical cancer. MRI, which has been used since the early 1980s, has high-contrast resolution and multiplanar imaging capability and is **a valuable modality for determining tumor size, degree of stromal penetration, vaginal extension, corpus extension, parametrial extension, and lymph node status** (Fig. 8.4).

Subak et al. (14) evaluated CT or MRI before surgical exploration in 79 patients with FIGO stage IB, IIA, or IIB cervical carcinoma. They reported that **MRI estimated tumor size to within 0.5 cm of the surgical specimen in 64 of 69 patients (93%) and had an accuracy of 78% for measuring depth of stromal invasion.** By contrast, CT was unable to evaluate tumor size or depth of invasion. **For the evaluation of stage of disease, MRI had an accuracy of 90%**

Table 8.2 Carcinoma of the Cervix Uteri: *UICC* Stage Grouping

FIGO Stage	T	N	M
IA1	T_1a_1	N_0	M_0
IA2	T_1a_2	N_0	M_0
IB1	T_11b_1	N_0	M_0
IB2	T_1b_2	N_0	M_0
IIA1	T_2a_1	N_0	M_0
IIA2	T_2a_2		
IIB	T_{2b}	N_0	M_0
IIIA	T_{3b}	N_0	M_0
IIIB	T_1	N_1	M_0
	T_2	N_1	M_0
	T_{3a}	N_1	M_0
	T_{3b}	Any N	M_0
IVA	T_4	Any N	M_0
IVB	Any T	Any N	M_1

UICC, International Union Against Cancer; FIGO, International Federation of Gynecology and Obstetrics; T, tumor; N, nodes; M, metastasis.

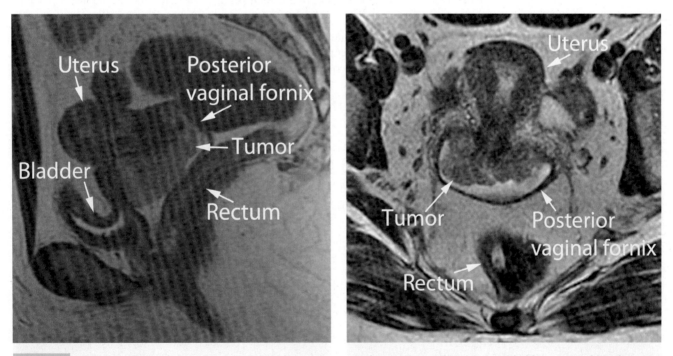

Figure 8.4 Pelvic MRI—6-cm cervical carcinoma with anterior vaginal extension and no uterine, bladder, or rectal involvement. **Left:** Sagittal view. **Right:** Coronal view. (Scans courtesy of Dr. Shreyas Vasanawala, Stanford University School of Medicine.)

compared with **65%** for **CT** ($p < 0.005$), **and it was more accurate in assessing parametrial invasion** (94% vs. 76%; $p < 0.005$). Both modalities were comparable for the evaluation of lymph node metastases (each 86% accurate). Narayan et al. (15) from Melbourne reported that the cervical diameter determined by EUA correlated poorly with the MRI diameter, but the MRI diameter correlated strongly with the pathologic diameter after surgical removal of the specimen ($p < 0.0001$).

The ability of MRI to more accurately determine tumor diameter and parametrial infiltration, particularly in patients with bulky cervical tumors, makes it an important adjunct to clinical evaluation in treatment planning. MRI is also important for the evaluation of pregnant patients because it poses no risk to the fetus (16).

A meta-analysis comparing the utility of lymphangiogram, CT, and MRI for the detection of pelvic and para-aortic lymph node metastases in patients with cervical cancer concluded that the three imaging modalities performed comparably (17).

Extension of cervical cancer into the uterus can be readily detected by MRI. In univariate analysis, Narayan et al. (18) reported a significant association between nodal involvement and both FIGO stage ($p = 0.018$) and uterine body involvement; in multivariate analysis, however, **only uterine body extension was independently related to the risk of lymph node involvement.** Positron emission tomography (PET)-documented pelvic node positivity was 75% (39 of 52) in patients with uterine extension compared to 11% (2 of 18) in those without ($p < 0.001$).

Positron Emission Tomography

The PET imaging technique has been available in some centers since the mid-1990s. **It depends on metabolic, rather than anatomic, alteration for the detection of disease.** PET uses radionuclides, which decay with the emission of positrons (positively charged particles). Because cancer cells are avid users of glucose, a radionuclide-labeled analogue of glucose, 2-[18F] fluoro-2-deoxy-d-glucose (FDG), can be used to detect sites of malignancy by identifying sites of increased glycolysis. **The PET scan has the potential to delineate more accurately the extent of disease, particularly in lymph nodes that are not enlarged** and in distant sites that are undetectable by conventional imaging studies (Fig. 8.5).

An Italian study evaluated the utility of PET scanning for preoperative staging in 159 patients with stages IB1–IIA1 cervical cancer undergoing radical hysterectomy and pelvic lymphadenectomy (19). Sensitivity of the PET scan was only 32.1% and positive predictive value only 69.2%. The authors

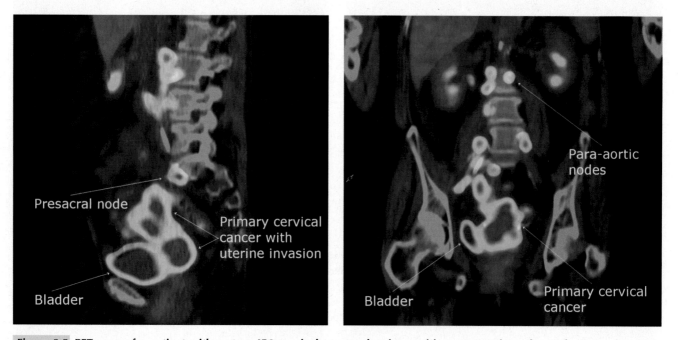

Figure 8.5 **PET scan of a patient with a stage IB2 cervical cancer showing positive para-aortic nodes. Left:** Coronal section. **Right:** Sagittal section. (Scan courtesy of Dr. Eva Wegner, Sydney, Australia.)

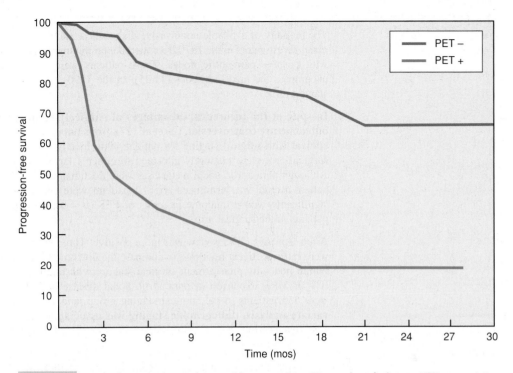

Figure 8.6 **Survival curves for patients with a negative CT scan in relation to PET scan status of the para-aortic lymph nodes.** (Reproduced with permission from **Grigsby PW, Siegel BA, Dehdashti F**. Lymph node staging by positron emission tomography in patients with carcinoma of the cervix. *J Clin Oncol.* 2001;19:3745–3749.)

concluded that **the PET scan had minimal clinical impact on the pretreatment planning of patients with early stage cervical cancer.**

In a study aimed at determining whether PET scanning could obviate the need for surgical staging in patients with locoregionally advanced cervical cancer, Narayan et al. (20) reported a sensitivity of 83%, specificity of 92%, positive predictive value of 91%, and negative predictive value of 85% in 24 patients evaluable for pelvic nodal status. However, PET detected only four of seven (57%) cases of positive para-aortic nodes. **All histologically confirmed nodes not visualized on PET were <1 cm in diameter.**

Grigsby et al. (21) retrospectively compared the results of CT lymph node staging with whole-body FDG–PET in 101 consecutive patients with cervical cancer who were referred for primary radiation therapy. CT demonstrated abnormally enlarged pelvic lymph nodes in 20 patients (20%) and para-aortic lymph nodes in 7 patients (7%). PET demonstrated abnormal FDG uptake in pelvic nodes in 67 patients (67%), in para-aortic nodes in 21 patients (21%), and in supraclavicular nodes in 8 patients (8%). For the 94 patients with negative para-aortic nodes on CT scan, the 2-year progression-free survival (PFS) was 64% in PET-negative patients and 18% in PET-positive patients ($p < 0.0001$) (Fig. 8.6). **A multivariate analysis demonstrated that the most significant factor for PFS was the presence of positive para-aortic lymph nodes as detected by PET imaging** ($p = 0.025$).

An analysis of 15 published PET studies in cervical cancer reported that the pooled sensitivity of FDG–PET for para-aortic lymph node metastases was 84% (95% confidence interval [CI], 68–94%), **and the specificity 95%** (95% CI, 89–98%) (22).

Fine-Needle Aspiration Cytology	If pelvic or abdominal masses or enlarged lymph nodes are detected during physical examination or imaging studies, fine-needle aspiration may be performed under CT or ultrasonic guidance. The procedure is performed under local anesthesia and is free of major complications, even in the presence of clotting problems or perforation of a hollow viscus. The reported accuracy for abdomino-pelvic nodes ranges from 74–95% (23,24). **Only a positive cytologic diagnosis should be used as a basis for therapeutic decision making.**

Surgical Staging

The inability of available noninvasive diagnostic tests to detect small lymph node metastases led many investigators in the 1970s to undertake pretreatment staging laparotomies to identify patients with positive para-aortic nodes. These patients were treated with extended-field radiation to encompass the involved nodes (11,25). In the 1990s, some investigators proposed laparoscopic staging (26).

In spite of the theoretical advantages of surgical staging, the benefits in terms of patient outcomes are controversial. Lai et al. (27), from Taipei, conducted a randomized trial to compare clinical with surgical staging for patients with locally advanced cervical cancer. Patients in the surgical arm were randomly allocated to either a laparoscopic or an extraperitoneal approach. Although para-aortic nodal metastases were documented in 25% of patients in the surgical arm, patient accrual was terminated after 61 patients were entered because interim analysis showed a significantly worse outcome in terms of PFS ($p = 0.003$) and overall survival ($p = 0.024$) for patients in the surgical arm.

A retrospective GOG review was more positive. Three phase III studies (GOG 85, 120, and 165) were retrospectively reviewed to compare the outcome for patients who had negative para-aortic lymph nodes by pretreatment surgical staging with that of patients who had only radiographic (CT or MRI) exclusion of para-aortic nodal disease before pelvic chemoradiation (28). There were 555 patients in the surgical staging group, and 130 in the radiographic group. **In multivariate analysis, radiographic staging was associated with a poorer prognosis both for disease progression** (hazard ratio [HR] 1.35; 95% CI, 1.01 to 1.81) and for death (HR 1.46; 95% CI, 1.08 to 1.99).

The results from the ongoing collaborative study of PET, MRI, and surgical staging being conducted by the American College of Radiology Imaging network and the GOG will help clarify whether or not there is any ongoing role for surgical staging in the PET scan era. By constructing a mathematical model from the available literature, Petereit et al. (29) predicted that surgical staging and tailored postoperative radiation would save 2.6, 6, and 7 lives per 100 patients treated, for stages IB, IIB, and IIIB, respectively.

At the Royal Hospital for Women in Sydney, PET/CT scanning is used prior to chemoradiation for staging patients with locally advanced disease. If positive nodes ≥1.5 cm diameter are identified below the inferior mesenteric artery, an extraperitoneal approach via a lower midline incision is used to resect the nodes before treatment begins. The peritoneum is stripped off the anterior and lateral abdominal walls to expose each pelvic sidewall. The round ligaments must be transected extraperitoneally to facilitate exposure. The dissection may be extended cephalad as far as necessary by extending the lower midline incision above the umbilicus (30).

Patterns of Spread

Cervical cancer spreads by the following means:

1. **Direct invasion** of the cervical stroma, corpus, vagina, and parametrium
2. **Lymphatic permeation and metastasis**
3. **Hematogenous dissemination**

Direct Infiltration

Invasive cervical cancer, whether squamous or glandular, arises from intraepithelial neoplasia. Malignant cells penetrate the basement membrane, and then progressively infiltrate the underlying stroma. They may progressively infiltrate laterally to involve the cardinal and uterosacral ligaments, superiorly to involve the uterine corpus, inferiorly to involve the vagina, anteriorly to involve the bladder, and posteriorly to involve the peritoneum of the pouch of Douglas and the rectum.

Lymphatic Spread

Cervical cancer can spread to all pelvic node groups, although the obturator nodes are most frequently involved. The parametrial nodes are not necessarily involved before the nodes on the pelvic sidewall. Although tumor cells can reach the common iliac and para-aortic nodes directly by the posterior cervical trunk (31), this is very uncommon, and **lymph node spread in cervical cancer almost invariably occurs in an orderly fashion from the nodes on the pelvic sidewall**

Table 8.3 Incidence of Pelvic Lymph Node Metastases in Patients with Stage IB Cervical Cancer Treated by Radical Hysterectomy

Authors	Patients	Positive Nodes	%
Zander et al., 1981 (32)	860	163	18.9
Fuller et al., 1982 (33)	280	42	15
Timmer et al., 1984 (34)	119	18	15.1
Inoue and Okamura, 1984 (35)	362	47	13
Creasman et al., 1986 (36)	258	36	14
Artman et al., 1987 (37)	153	13	8.5
Monaghan et al., 1990 (38)	494	102	20.6
Finan et al., 1996 (39)	229	49	21.4
Samlal et al., 1997 (40)	271	53	19.6
Total	3,026	523	17.3

to the common iliac and then the para-aortic group. From the para-aortic nodes, spread can occasionally occur through the thoracic duct to the left scalene nodes (41). The incidence of pelvic lymph node metastases in patients with stage IB cervical cancer treated by radical hysterectomy is shown in Table 8.3. The incidence of para-aortic nodal metastases in patients with stages II and III cervical cancer undergoing surgical staging is shown in Table 8.4.

Lymphatic invasion by tumor cells is commonly seen in the primary tumor, and tumor cells are also seen occasionally in lymphatic channels in the parametrium. Burghardt and Girardi (42) believe that tumor emboli may be held up in lymphatic vessels and grow to become foci of discontinuous parametrial involvement.

Ovarian involvement by cervical cancer is rare but most likely occurs through the lymphatic connection between the uterus and the adnexal structures (43). In a study of patients with clinical stage IB cervical cancer, the GOG reported ovarian spread in 4 of 770 patients (0.5%) with squamous carcinoma and in 2 of 121 patients (1.7%) with adenocarcinoma. All six patients with ovarian metastases had other evidence of extracervical spread (44).

Table 8.4 Incidence of Para-aortic Lymph Node Metastases in Patients Undergoing Surgical Staging for Stages II and III Cervical Cancer

Authors	Stage II			Stage III		
	Explored	Positive	%	Explored	Positive	%
Nelson et al., 1977 (25)	63	9	14.3	39	15	38.5
Delgado et al., 1977 (45)	18	8	44.4	13	5	38.5
Piver and Barlow, 1977 (46)	46	6	13	49	18	36.7
Sudarsanam et al., 1978 (47)	43	7	16.3	19	3	15.8
Buchsbaum, 1979 (48)	19	1	5.3	104	34	32.7
Hughes et al., 1980 (49)	80	14	17.5	96	23	24
Ballon et al., 1981 (50)	48	9	18.8	24	4	16.7
Welander et al., 1981 (51)	63	13	20.6	38	10	26.3
Berman et al., 1984 (52)	265	43	16.2	180	45	25
Potish et al., 1985 (53)	47	5	10.6	11	4	36.4
La Polla et al., 1986 (12)	47	6	12.8	38	14	36.8
Total	739	121	16.4	611	175	28.6

Hematogenous Spread

Although spread to virtually all parts of the body has been reported, the most common organs for hematogenous spread are the lungs, liver, and bone.

Treatment

Treatment of invasive cancer involves appropriate management for both the primary lesion and potential sites of metastatic disease. Both surgery and radiation therapy may be used for primary treatment, although definitive surgery is usually limited to patients with stages I or early IIA disease. Some European and Asian centers also treat patients with stage IIB disease with primary surgery (54–56).

Microinvasive Carcinoma

The term **microcarcinoma of the uterine cervix** was first introduced by Mestwerdt (57) in the German literature in 1947. He suggested that 5 mm was the deepest penetration acceptable. Since then, both terminology and treatment have been the subject of much debate.

In 1961, the Cancer Committee of FIGO recommended that clinical stage I cervical cancer should be subdivided into stage IA and stage IB. Stage IA was vaguely defined as a preclinical cancer with early stromal invasion. This did little to clarify even the definition.

In 1974, the Committee on Nomenclature of **the Society of Gynecologic Oncologists (SGO) in the United States proposed that microinvasive carcinoma should be defined as a lesion that invaded below the basement membrane to a depth of 3 mm or less, and in which there was no evidence of lymph-vascular space invasion (LVSI).** Although this definition provided no horizontal dimension, patients whose disease fulfilled these criteria were shown to have virtually no risk of lymph node metastases and to be adequately treated by either hysterectomy or cone biopsy (58–60).

A precise definition of microinvasive carcinoma was not adopted by FIGO until 1995. Stage IA1 was defined as a tumor that invaded to a depth of 3 mm or less, whereas stage IA2 referred to a tumor that invaded to a depth greater than 3 mm and up to 5 mm. In both stages, the horizontal spread should not exceed 7 mm. LVSI was not included as part of the definition. The official FIGO staging remains unchanged.

Stage IA1 Squamous Carcinoma

Although stromal invasion can be seen in small punch biopsies, a definitive diagnosis of microinvasion can be made only in conization (or hysterectomy) specimens. The conization specimen must be thoroughly sampled to make the correct diagnosis and to be certain about the margins.

In an extensive review of the literature, Ostor (61) reported that of 2,274 squamous lesions with invasion of less than 1 mm, only three cases had lymph node metastases (0.1%); invasive recurrence developed in 8 cases (0.4%). Among 1,324 squamous lesions invading between 1 and 3 mm, there were 7 cases with lymph node metastases (0.5%) and 26 cases in which invasive recurrence developed (2%). No horizontal limitation was placed on these lesions, so they do not strictly fit the current FIGO definition of stage IA1 disease, and most of the cases were treated without lymph node dissection.

Studies of stage IA disease in patients meeting the 1995 FIGO definition are shown in Table 8.5. This table includes patients with squamous and adenocarcinomas. The largest single institution series was reported by Elliott et al. (62) from Sydney. They reported 476 such patients, of whom 418 (88%) had squamous and 58 (12%) glandular tumors. Of 180 patients undergoing lymphadenectomy, the incidence of positive nodes in patients with stage IA1 disease was 0.8% (1 of 121 cases). **For the cumulative series of 1,127 patients, the overall incidence of positive nodes or pelvic side wall recurrence was 1.2%, and 0.9% of patients died of disease.**

Roman et al. (63) reported 87 cases of microinvasive carcinoma diagnosed on cone biopsy and followed by either repeat cone biopsy or hysterectomy. Significant predictors of residual invasion included status of the internal margin (residual invasion present in 22% of women with dysplasia at the margin vs. 3% with a negative margin; $p < 0.03$) and the combined status of the internal margin and the postconization ECC (residual invasion 4% if both negative, 13% if one positive,

Table 8.5 Lymph Node and Recurrence Status of patients with
FIGO Stage IA1 Cervical Cancer

Authors	Number	Positive Nodes or Sidewall Recurrence	Invasive Recurrence	DOD
Takeshima et al., 1999 (64)	297	1	0	0
Elliott et al., 2000 (62)	387	7	12	8
Lee et al., 2006 (65)	174	3	3	2
Costa et al., 2009 (66)	173	2	0	0
Yahata et al., 2010 (67)	27	0	0	0
Baalbergen et al., 2011 (68)	33	1	1	0
Al-Kalbani et al., 2012 (69)	36	0	0	0
Total	1,127	1.2%	1.4%	0.9%

DOD, dead of disease.

and 33% if both positive; $p < 0.015$). Depth of invasion and the number of invasive foci were not significant. The researchers concluded that **if either the internal margin or the postconization ECC contained dysplasia or carcinoma, then the risk of residual invasion was high and warranted repeat conization before definitive treatment planning.**

A study from Chang Mai, Thailand, confirmed these findings (70). Histopathology slides were reviewed from 129 patients who underwent hysterectomy following a cone biopsy that showed microinvasive squamous cell carcinoma. All had high-grade CIN or invasive carcinoma at the cone margins. Of the 129 patients, 77 (59.7%) had residual disease in the hysterectomy specimen, of whom 20 patients (15.5%) had residual invasive cancer: 18 were microinvasive and 2 were frankly invasive. **Factors that significantly affected the risk of residual disease included positive postconization ECC ($p = 0.001$), positive cone margins for invasive cancer ($p = 0.003$), and depth of stromal invasion >1 mm ($p = 0.014$). They also recommended repeat conization to determine the exact severity of the lesion before planning definite treatment.**

In view of these considerations, **a cone biopsy with clear surgical margins and a negative ECC should be considered adequate treatment for a patient with stage IA1 squamous carcinoma of the cervix.** If future childbearing is not required, then extrafascial hysterectomy may be considered. This should be the treatment of choice in postmenopausal women because stenosis of the endocervical canal is common after conization, which limits the ability to obtain endocervical cytology (71). **If the cone margins or postconization ECC reveals high-grade dysplasia or microinvasive carcinoma, then a repeat conization should be performed before proceeding to simple hysterectomy because more extensively invasive disease may be present.**

LVSI is uncommon in stage IA1 lesions. Elliott et al. (62) reported LVSI in 8.5% of tumors invading 1 mm or less, 19% between 1.1 and 2 mm, 29% between 2.1 and 3 mm, and 53% between 3.1 and 5 mm. Lee et al. (65) found a **positive correlation between depth of invasion and the presence of LVSI** but found **no definite correlation between LVSI and lymph node metastases,** only two of their four patients with positive nodes having LVSI. Its significance in microinvasive cervical cancer remains controversial, and it is not mentioned in the FIGO definition. It probably should be disregarded when planning treatment, unless it is extensive, although Rob et al. (71) recommend sentinel lymph node mapping, and removal of only the sentinel nodes, for patients with LVSI. A proposed algorithm for the management of microinvasive cervical cancer is shown in Figure 8.7.

Stage IA2 Squamous Carcinoma

Reports of nodal status and outcome for patients with FIGO stage IA2 cervical cancer are shown in Table 8.6. **There are a limited number of reported cases, but the incidence of positive nodes (3.2%) and death from disease (1.8%) are low when the horizontal spread is limited to 7 mm.** Takeshima et al. (64) reported that, of 73 patients with depth of invasion between 3 and 5 mm, the incidence of lymph node metastasis was 3.4% for tumors with a horizontal spread of 7 mm or less and 9.1% for those with greater than 7 mm spread.

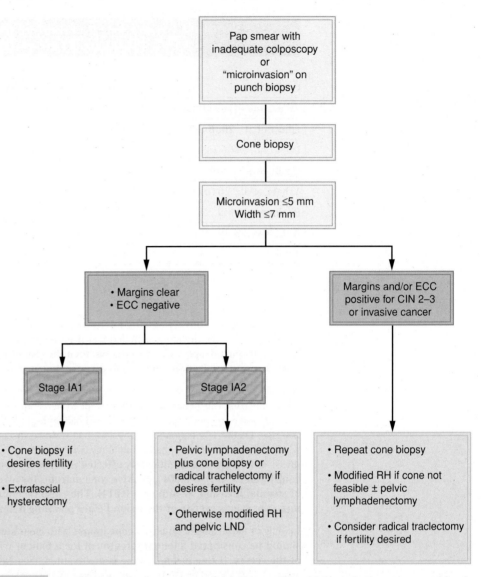

Figure 8.7 **Algorithm for the management of patients with a high-grade Pap smear and inadequate colposcopy or with microinvasive cervical carcinoma on punch biopsy.**

Many patients with early cervical cancer are young, and preservation of fertility is a major concern. Consequently, surgical approaches that remove the primary lesion and regional lymph nodes, while conserving the corpus for future childbearing, have been explored.

In 1994, Dargent et al. (72) pioneered the use of **radical trachelectomy and laparoscopic pelvic lymphadenectomy.** A nonabsorbable cervical cerclage was placed around the uterine isthmus at the time of the trachelectomy. Subsequent studies have confirmed that the operation is feasible in experienced hands, cure rates are high, and subsequent pregnancies can be carried to viability in many cases (see Table 21.3). **Radical abdominal trachelectomy was first reported** by Smith et al. (73) **in 1997**. One advantage of this approach is that the anatomy is more familiar to most gynecologic oncologists.

Less radical procedures, such as large cone biopsy or simple trachelectomy, combined with laparoscopic pelvic lymphadenectomy, are possible alternatives to radical trachelectomy, particularly in patients without vascular space invasion (74). The less radical procedures have less morbidity, but the small number of patients with stage IA2 cervical cancer makes it impractical to conduct prospective randomized trials to compare the two approaches.

There are some long-term morbidities associated with radical trachelectomy. In a retrospective review of 29 patients undergoing radical trachelectomy, the group from St. Bartholomew's

Table 8.6 Lymph Node and Recurrence Status of Patients with FIGO Stage IA2 Cervical Cancer				
Authors	Number	Positive Nodes or Sidewall Recurrence	Invasive Recurrence	DOD
Buckley et al., 1996 (75)	94	7	5	4
Creasman et al., 1998 (76)	51	0	0	0
Takeshima et al., 1999 (64)	33	1	1	1
Elliott et al., 2000 (62)	89	2	4	1
Lee et al., 2006 (65)	28	1	0	0
Costa et al., 2009 (66)	57	5	4	2
Suri et al., 2009 (77)	42	1	NS	NS
van Meurs et al., 2009 (78)	14	0	0	0
Baalbergen et al., 2011 (68)	26	0	0	0
Al-Kalbani et al., 2012 (69)	9	0	0	0
Smrkolj et al., 2012 (79)	89	0	1	1
Total	532	17 (3.2%)	15 (3.1%)	9 (1.8%)

DOD, dead of disease.

Hospital in London reported **dysmenorrhea in 24%, irregular menstruation in 17%, recurrent candidiasis in 14%, cervical suture problems in 14%, isthmic stenosis in 10%, and prolonged amenorrhea in 7% of patients** (80).

If the patient does not require fertility preservation, **the recommended treatment for stage IA2 squamous carcinoma of the cervix is modified radical hysterectomy and pelvic lymph node dissection.** In a medically unfit patient, intracavitary radiation may be used.

Microinvasive Adenocarcinoma

Although the concept of microinvasive squamous carcinoma has long been accepted, the concept for the glandular counterpart has been more controversial. Only recently have reports looked specifically at microinvasive adenocarcinoma as now defined by the FIGO staging (67–69,81), and the incidence of lymph node metastases appears to be comparable.

Most cases arise adjacent to the transformation zone, although Teshima et al. (82) reported that 3 of 30 cases (10%) arose outside the transformation zone. Adenocarcinoma in situ may extend up the entire endocervical canal, and invasion may occur at any point (82). Lee and Flynn (83), in a study of 40 cases of adenocarcinoma invasive to 5 mm or less, reported that in 78% of the cases, the midpoint of the invasive focus was in the region of the transformation zone. **The endometrioid variant is particularly likely to arise higher in the canal** (83), **and this variant has been reported to be associated with late recurrence and a worse survival for both stages IA1 and IA2 disease** (81).

Whereas squamous lesions are usually unifocal, glandular lesions are sometimes multifocal. Ostor et al. (84) reported that 21 of 77 cases (27.3%) were multicentric, meaning that both cervical lips were affected, without continuity around the "edges" at 3 and 9 o'clock. They reported no "skip" lesions, which they arbitrarily defined as separation between discrete microinvasive adenocarcinomas in the same lip of greater than 3 mm. More than one focus of invasive disease was present in 4 of 40 cases (10%) reported by Lee and Flynn (83).

Positive lymph nodes have rarely been reported in FIGO stage IA1 lesions, although Elliott et al. (62) reported a solitary nodal metastasis in a patient with <1 mm stromal invasion. Kaku et al. (85) reported recurrences at the vaginal vault in 2 of 30 patients (6.7%) with less than 5 mm of invasion. One patient had a tumor volume of 1,222 mm^3, but the other had a tumor with a depth of 3.9 mm and a width of 4.9 mm (i.e., FIGO stage IA2). The only adenocarcinoma recurrence in the 77 patients reported by Ostor et al. (84) involved a patient whose tumor invaded to a depth of 3.2 mm but was 21 mm in length (i.e., stage IB1).

A study from Melbourne reported 29 patients with stage IA1 and 9 with stage IA2 microinvasive adenocarcinoma of the cervix (86). A variety of treatment methods were used. Cone biopsy of the cervix was performed in 18 patients, including 2 with stage IA2 disease. No recurrences were noted during an average follow-up of 72 months. **In a literature review,** the same authors noted **positive nodes in 12 of 814 patients (1.5%) undergoing pelvic lymph node dissection for microinvasive adenocarcinoma of the cervix.** LVSI was present in 25 patients (3%), all without lymph node involvement (86).

The Surveillance, Epidemiology, and End Results (SEER) database was used to identify 131 cases of stage IA1 and 170 cases of stage IA2 adenocarcinoma of the cervix treated between 1988 and 1997 (87). There was no histologic review, and patients were treated in a variety of ways from cone biopsy to radical hysterectomy and pelvic lymphadenectomy. Simple hysterectomy alone was used for 118 patients (39.2%). With a mean follow-up of 46.5 months, the censored survival was 99.2% for patients with stage IA1 disease and 98.2% for stage IA2.

In view of these observations, **it seems reasonable to treat the disease in a similar manner to its squamous counterpart. For patients desiring fertility preservation, a cone biopsy with negative margins appears to be adequate treatment for stage 1A1** (88). **Ideally, the cone biopsy should be a cold knife procedure** (89), although loop excision procedures in expert hands may also be acceptable (90). For stage 1A2 disease, radical trachelectomy and resection of pelvic lymph nodes is desirable. Following childbearing, it seems reasonable to recommend hysterectomy because Pap smears and colposcopy are less reliable, and Poynor et al. (91) reported that ECC was positive before cervical conization in only 43% of patients with glandular lesions.

Stage IB1 and Early Stage IIA1 Cervical Cancer

In 1994, FIGO recognized the prognostic significance of tumor size by subdividing stage IB disease into stage IB1 (primary lesion ≤4 cm diameter) and stage IB2 (primary lesion >4 cm diameter). This same subdivision was applied to patients with stage IIA2 disease in 2009.

Patients with stage IB1 are universally regarded as being ideal candidates for radical hysterectomy and pelvic lymphadenectomy, although equal cure rates may be obtained with primary radiation therapy (92). The choice of modality should depend mainly on the availability of the appropriate expertise. Since the introduction of fellowship training in gynecologic oncology, expertise in radical pelvic surgery has become widely available in the United States and most developed countries. The Patterns of Care study in the United States suggests that the same may not be true for radiation oncology, particularly outside of tertiary referral units (93). If both surgical and radiotherapeutic expertise are available, radiation is usually reserved for the medically unfit patient. **Chronologic age should not be considered a contraindication to radical surgery, because elderly patients experience morbidity similar to that of younger patients** (94).

Primary surgery has the advantage of removing the primary disease and allowing accurate surgical staging, thereby allowing any adjuvant therapy to be more accurately targeted. In addition, it avoids possible chronic radiation damage to the bladder, small and large bowel, and vagina, which is difficult to manage. Surgical injuries to the same organs are more readily repaired because the blood supply is not compromised. **Sexual dysfunction is, in general, underreported, but is a problem for many patients who have had both external-beam therapy and brachytherapy because of vaginal atrophy, fibrosis, and stenosis** (95). Although the vagina is shortened by approximately 1.5 cm after radical hysterectomy, it is more elastic; in premenopausal patients, ovarian function can be preserved. In postmenopausal patients, the nonirradiated vagina responds much better to estrogen therapy.

Influence of Diagnostic Conization

The influence of previous cone biopsy on the morbidity of radical hysterectomy is controversial. Samlal et al. (96) reported no significant difference in morbidity, but the conization–radical hysterectomy interval in their study was 6 weeks. They believed that delaying the definitive surgery might allow the tissue reaction to subside, thereby decreasing morbidity. Others have found that the interval between the conization and radical hysterectomy has no influence on morbidity, and they recommend proceeding without delay (97). **The primary author prefers to proceed immediately with radical hysterectomy if the surgical margins of the cone biopsy are involved, but to postpone surgery for 6 weeks if the cone margins are clear.**

Types of Radical Hysterectomy

In 1974, Piver et al. (98) described the following **five types of hysterectomy: extrafascial, modified radical, radical, extended radical, and partial exenteration.**

Types I–V

Extrafascial Hysterectomy (Type I)   This is a simple hysterectomy and is suitable for stage IA1 cervical carcinoma.

Modified Radical Hysterectomy (Type II)   This is basically the hysterectomy described by Ernst Wertheim (99). The uterine artery is ligated where it crosses the ureter, and the medial halves of the cardinal ligaments and proximal uterosacral ligaments are resected. Piver et al. (98) described removal of the upper one-third of the vagina, but this is rarely necessary unless vaginal intraepithelial neoplasia (VAIN) 3 is extensive. The operation described by Wertheim involved selective removal of enlarged nodes rather than systematic pelvic lymphadenectomy. **The modified radical hysterectomy is appropriate for stage IA2 cervical cancer.**

Radical Hysterectomy (Type III)   The most commonly performed operation for stage IB cervical cancer is that originally described by Meigs in 1944 (100). The uterine artery is ligated at its origin from the superior vesicle or internal iliac artery, allowing removal of the entire width of the cardinal ligaments. Piver (98) originally described resection of the uterosacral ligaments at their sacral attachments and resection of the upper half of the vagina. Such extensive dissection of the uterosacral ligaments and vagina is not required for stage IB cervical cancer.

Extended Radical Hysterectomy (Type IV)   This differs from the type III operation in three aspects: (i) The ureter is completely dissected from the vesicouterine ligament, (ii) the superior vesicle artery is sacrificed, and (iii) three-fourths of the vagina is excised. The risk of ureteric fistula is increased with this procedure, which Piver (98) used for selected small central recurrences after radiation therapy.

Partial Exenteration (Type V)   The indication for this procedure was removal of a central recurrence involving a portion of the distal ureter or bladder. The relevant organ was partially excised and the ureter reimplanted into the bladder. This procedure is occasionally performed if cancer is found to be unexpectedly encasing the distal ureter at the time of radical hysterectomy. Alternatively, the operation may be aborted and the patient treated with primary radiation.

Kyoto Classification

A new classification for radical hysterectomy was described by Querleu and Morrow (101) following a consensus meeting in Kyoto, Japan, which was arranged by Shingo Fujii in February 2007. **The classification is based only on the lateral extent of the resection.** Four basic types are described, A to D, adding when necessary a few subtypes that consider nerve preservation and paracervical lymphadenectomy. **Lymph node dissection is considered separately,** and four levels (1 to 4) are defined according to the corresponding arterial anatomy and the radicality of the procedure.

A three-dimensional anatomic template for the parametrial resection has been described by Cibula et al. (102), and is included in Chapter 20. A description of the procedures from the original paper by Querleu and Morrow (101) is given below.

Type A: Minimum Resection of Paracervix   This is an extrafascial hysterectomy. The paracervix is transected medial to the ureter but lateral to the cervix. The uterosacral and vesicouterine ligaments are not transected at a distance from the uterus. Vaginal resection is generally at a minimum, routinely less than 10 mm, without removal of the vaginal part of the paracervix (paracolpos).

Type B: Transection of the Paracervix at the Ureter   This type has two levels:

> **B1—Without removal of lateral paracervical lymph nodes**
> **B2—With removal of lateral paracervical nodes**

Partial resection of the uterosacral and vesicouterine ligaments is a standard part of this category. The ureter is unroofed and rolled laterally, permitting transection of the paracervix at the level of the ureteral tunnel. The neural component of the paracervix caudal to the deep uterine vein is not resected. At least 10 mm of the vagina from the cervix or tumor is resected.

The operation corresponds to the modified or proximal radical hysterectomy and is adapted to early cervical cancer. The radicality of this operation can be improved without increasing postoperative morbidity by lymph node dissection of the lateral part of the paracervix, thus defining two subtypes—B1 and B2.

The border between paracervical and iliac or parietal lymph node dissection is defined arbitrarily as the obturator nerve: Paracervical nodes are medial and caudal. The combination of paracervical and parietal dissections is simply a comprehensive pelvic node dissection.

The morbidity of type B2 does not differ from that of B1, although the combination of B1 with paracervical lymph node dissection may be equivalent to that of type C1 resection.

Type C   In type C, the paracervix is transected at the junction with the internal iliac vascular system and has two types:

C1—With nerve preservation
C2—Without preservation of autonomic nerves

This type involves transection of the uterosacral ligament at the rectum and vesicouterine ligament at the bladder. The ureter is mobilized completely, and 15 to 20 mm of vagina from the tumor or cervix and the corresponding paracolpos is resected routinely, depending on vaginal and paracervical extent and on surgeon choice.

Type C corresponds to variants of classical radical hysterectomy. By contrast with types A and B, in which the autonomic nerve supply to the bladder is not threatened, the issue of nerve preservation is crucial. Two subcategories are defined: C1 with nerve preservation and C2 without preservation of autonomic nerves. In C1, the uterosacral ligament is transected after separation of the hypogastric nerves. The bladder branches of the pelvic plexus are preserved in the lateral ligament of the bladder (i.e., lateral part of bladder pillar). If the caudal part of the paracervix is transected, then careful identification of bladder nerves is needed.

For C2, the paracervix is transected completely, including the part caudal to the deep uterine vein.

Type D   In type D, the entire paracervix is resected:

D1—Resection of the entire paracervix along with the hypogastric vessels
D2—Resection of the entire paracervix, along with the hypogastric vessels and adjacent fascial or muscular structure

This group of rare operations features additional ultraradical procedures, mostly indicated at the time of pelvic exenteration. Type D1 is resection of the entire paracervix at the pelvic sidewall along with the hypogastric vessels, exposing the roots of the sciatic nerve. There is total resection of the vessels of the lateral part of the paracervix. These vessels (i.e., inferior gluteal, internal pudendal, and obturator vessels) arise from the internal iliac system.

Type D2 is D1 plus resection of the entire paracervix with the hypogastric vessels and adjacent fascial or muscular structures. This resection corresponds to the LEER (laterally extended endopelvic resection) procedure (103).

Lymph Node Dissection

Lymph node dissection has four levels:

Level 1—External and internal iliac
Level 2—Common iliac (including presacral)
Level 3—Aortic inframesenteric
Level 4—Aortic infrarenal

This classification ignores the widely used pelvic versus para-aortic dissection, in which the limit of the pelvis dissection is around the midcommon iliac area.

Within every level, and independently from each other, **several types of lymphadenectomy must be defined** to describe adequately the radicality of the procedure: **diagnostic** (minimum sampling of sentinel node only, removal of enlarged nodes only, or random sampling), **systematic lymphadenectomy,** and **debulking** (resection of all nodes ≥2 cm) (104).

Technique for Radical Hysterectomy

The patient is given prophylactic antibiotics on induction of anesthesia, and pneumatic calf compressors are used during and after surgery until the patient is fully mobilized. Prophylactic anticoagulants are given for at least 5 days postoperatively.

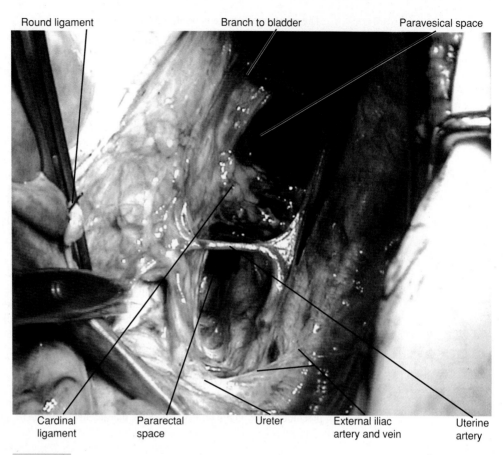

Round ligament   Branch to bladder   Paravesical space

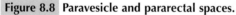

Cardinal   Pararectal   Ureter   External iliac   Uterine
ligament   space   artery and vein   artery

Figure 8.8 Paravesicle and pararectal spaces.

Incision

The abdomen may be opened either through a lower midline incision extending to the left of the umbilicus or through a low transverse **Maylard or Cherney** incision. The low transverse incision, which is described in Chapter 20, requires division of the rectus abdominus muscle, but provides excellent exposure of the primary tumor and pelvic sidewalls. The midline incision, which can be readily extended, provides better exposure of the para-aortic region if necessary.

Exploration

After entering the peritoneal cavity, all organs are systematically palpated, and any evidence of metastatic spread is documented by frozen section. The vesicouterine fold and pouch of Douglas peritoneum are examined for evidence of tumor infiltration, and the tubes and ovaries are examined for any abnormalities. Any bulky pelvic or para-aortic nodes are removed and frozen sections obtained to differentiate between inflammatory and malignant changes.

Radical Hysterectomy

With the uterus under traction, the retroperitoneum is entered through the round ligaments bilaterally. The ureter is identified as it crosses the pelvic rim, and the pelvic sidewall spaces are developed by a combination of sharp and blunt dissection.

The **paravesicle space** (Fig. 8.8) is bordered by the following:

1. The obliterated umbilical artery (a continuation of the superior vesicle artery) running along the bladder medially
2. The obturator internus muscle laterally
3. The cardinal ligament or paracervix posteriorly
4. The pubic symphysis anteriorly

The **pararectal space** is bordered by the following:

1. The rectum medially
2. The hypogastric artery laterally
3. The cardinal ligament or paracervix anteriorly
4. The sacrum posteriorly

The floor of the spaces is formed by the levator ani muscle.

Bladder Takedown

The vesicouterine fold of peritoneum is opened and the bladder dissected off the anterior cervix and upper vagina. This should be done before any blood supply is ligated, because occasionally tumor may infiltrate into the bladder base, making hysterectomy impossible. Rather than resecting the relevant section of the bladder in this situation, the abdomen is usually closed and the patient treated with primary chemoradiation.

Ligation of the Uterine Artery

The uterine artery usually arises from the superior vesicle artery, close to its origin from the hypogastric artery. The artery is ligated at its origin in a type III or type C radical hysterectomy, or at the point where it crosses the ureter in the modified or type B radical hysterectomy, then mobilized over the ureter by gentle traction and dissection. The superficial uterine veins must be identified and clipped or troublesome bleeding will occur.

Dissection of the Ureter

The roof of the ureteric tunnel is the anterior vesicouterine ligament. This can be taken down in a piecemeal fashion bilaterally (Fig. 8.9), thereby avoiding the troublesome venous bleeding that can

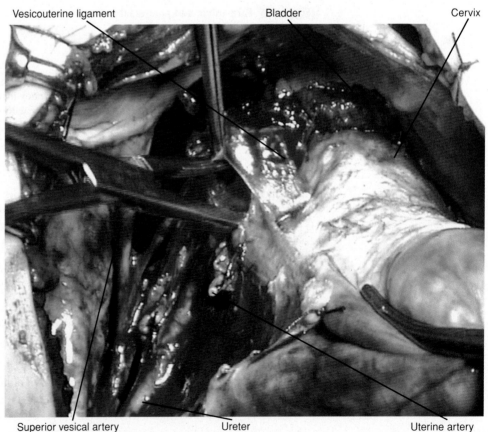

Figure 8.9 Piecemeal dissection of anterior vesicouterine ligament.

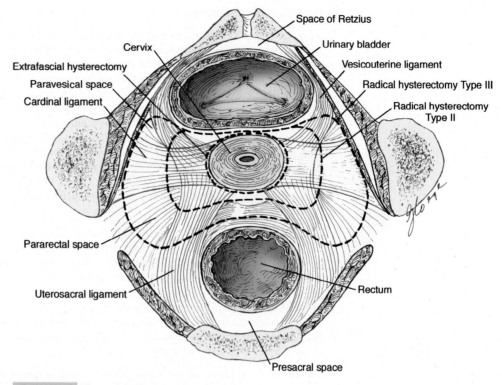
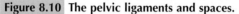

Figure 8.10 The pelvic ligaments and spaces.

occur by blindly advancing a right-angled forceps into the tunnel. Each ureter is mobilized off its peritoneal attachment fairly low in the pelvis to avoid unnecessary stripping from its peritoneal blood supply. It is also mobilized off the side of the uterus. This exposes the posterior or caudal vesicouterine ligament, which is also divided in a type III hysterectomy but not in a type II procedure. The anterolateral surface of the distal ureter is left attached to the bladder in a further effort to preserve the blood supply. If the caudal vesicouterine ligament is transected, it is desirable to identify and preserve the bladder branch from the inferior hypogastric plexus (105,106).

Posterior Dissection

The peritoneum across the pouch of Douglas is incised and the rectovaginal space identified by posterior traction on the rectum. The rectum is taken off the posterior vagina and the uterosacral ligaments using sharp and blunt dissection, and the latter are divided at the rectum (type III or C) or closer to the cervix (type II or B) (Fig. 8.10).

Lateral Dissection

After division of the uterosacral ligaments, the cardinal ligaments (paracervix) are clamped at the level of the pelvic sidewall (type III or C) or more medially (type II or B), after which two more clamps are usually required across the paravaginal tissues to reach the vagina. In a C1 procedure, only the paracervical tissue above the deep uterine vein is taken, which preserves the autonomic nerves at this point.

If the ovaries are to be removed, the infundibulopelvic ligaments are divided at this stage. If they are to be retained, they are freed from the fundus by transecting the ovarian ligament and fallopian tube. The tube should be removed from the ovary on each side.

Vaginal Resection

The length of vagina to be removed depends on the nature of the primary lesion and the colposcopic findings in the vagina. If the primary lesion is confined to the cervix and there is no evidence of VAIN, it suffices to resect only about 1.5 cm of upper vagina. This is achieved by entering the vagina anteriorly and transecting it circumferentially. The vault is closed, making sure to avoid "dog ears." The vaginal angles are sutured to the paravaginal tissues and uterosacral ligaments to avoid vault prolapse.

Pelvic Lymphadenectomy

After the uterus has been removed, the pelvic sidewall exposure is excellent. **If there are any bulky pelvic or para-aortic lymph nodes that are confirmed to be positive by frozen section, only the enlarged nodes should be removed, and external-beam radiation and concurrent chemotherapy relied on to sterilize any micrometastases (104).** A Surveillance, Epidemiology and End Results (SEER) study of 5,522 women having lymphadenectomy for early cervical cancer supports this policy (107). Among women with positive nodes, a more extensive lymphadectomy had no effect on survival. By contrast, for women with negative nodes, a more extensive lymphadenectomy was associated with improved survival. **Compared with node-negative patients with less than 10 nodes removed, patients with 21 to 30 nodes removed were 24% less likely to die** (HR = 0.76; CI = 0.53 to 1.09), **while patients with more than 30 nodes removed were 37% less likely to die of disease** (HR = 0.64; CI = 0.43 to 0.96) (107). These data suggest that a **thorough pelvic lymphadenectomy is of therapeutic value for patients with early cervical cancer.**

Using sharp dissection with Metzenbaum scissors, all fatty tissue is stripped off the vessels from the midcommon iliac region to the circumflex iliac vein distally, preserving the genitofemoral nerve on the psoas muscle. The obturator fossa is entered by retracting the external iliac artery and vein medially, then stripping the fatty tissue off the pelvic sidewall. All fatty tissue, both above and below the obturator nerve, is sharply dissected out of the obturator fossa. In order to avoid nerve injury, care must be taken to identify the obturator nerve, and this is best done where it enters the fossa at the bifurcation of the common iliac vein. Another hazard in the obturator fossa is the accessory obturator vein, which is seen in at least 30% of patients. It enters the distal external iliac vein inferiorly.

The anatomical relations of the pelvic and para-aortic lymph nodes are shown in Figure 8.11.

Technique for Radical Abdominal Trachelectomy

The operation proceeds in the same manner as a radical hysterectomy, except that upward traction on the uterus is with a suture through the fundus, rather than with clamps down each side of the fundus, which would damage the fallopian tubes. The infundibulopelvic ligaments are spared, and the tubes and ovaries are left attached to the fundus. The uterine arteries are ligated at their point of origin, and the ureters are dissected from their tunnels. The parametrium, paracolpos, and upper 1.5 cm of vagina are resected, following which the radical trachelectomy is completed by separating the corpus and proximal cervix from the bulk of the cervix and upper vagina (Fig. 8.12). A cerclage suture is placed around the upper cervix, and the latter is reanastomosed to the upper vagina with 0 *vicryl* sutures.

Sentinel Node Identification

Since its first description by Dargent et al. (108) in 2000, several authorities have evaluated the concept of sentinel node identification in patients with cervical cancer (109–113) (see also Chapter 21). **The cervix is theoretically an attractive target for lymphatic mapping, because unlike vulvar cancer, the disease is relatively common, and the cervix is readily accessible for submucosal injections of blue dye and radioisotopes.** On the other hand, lower limb lymphedema, the major morbidity to be avoided, is much less common than following groin dissection. **From 20 published reports of 802 patients having sentinel node biopsy for cervical cancer, Levenback reported a false-negative rate of 6.8%, which is unacceptably high** (112).

In a multicenter review of 645 patients with FIGO stages IA to IIB cervical cancer, in whom at least one sentinel node was identified and systemic pelvic lymphadenectomy performed, Cibula et al. (113) reported that sentinel nodes were detected bilaterally in 72% of cases. Patients with bilateral sentinel node detection were more likely to have any metastases detected (33.3% vs. 19.2%; $p < 0.001$), as well as micrometastases detected in their sentinel nodes (39.6% vs. 11.4%). With ultrastaging, the false-negative rate was 2.8% for the whole group, and 1.3% for patients with bilateral sentinel nodes identified.

The authors concluded that sentinel node mapping and ultrastaging should become standard practice in the surgical management of patients with early cervical cancer. These false-negative rates are much lower than those usually reported (112), but **even with a false-negative rate of 1.3%, there is still a 1 in 77 chance of the patient developing a pelvic sidewall recurrence, which is very likely to be fatal. Most women are not prepared to take this chance of death as a trade-off for a lower incidence of lymphedema** (114).

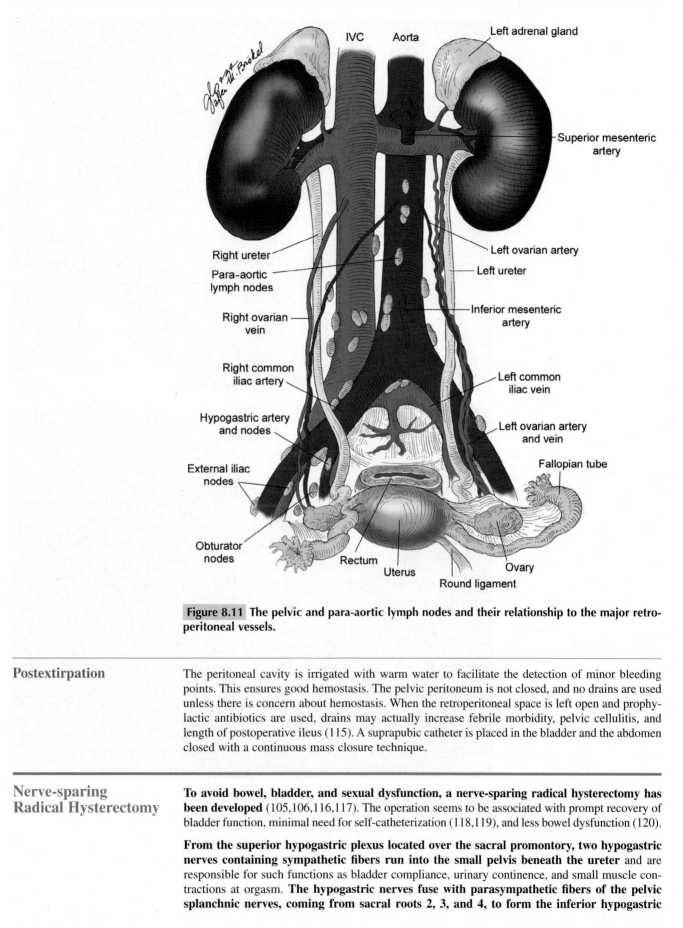

Figure 8.11 The pelvic and para-aortic lymph nodes and their relationship to the major retro-peritoneal vessels.

Postextirpation

The peritoneal cavity is irrigated with warm water to facilitate the detection of minor bleeding points. This ensures good hemostasis. The pelvic peritoneum is not closed, and no drains are used unless there is concern about hemostasis. When the retroperitoneal space is left open and prophylactic antibiotics are used, drains may actually increase febrile morbidity, pelvic cellulitis, and length of postoperative ileus (115). A suprapubic catheter is placed in the bladder and the abdomen closed with a continuous mass closure technique.

Nerve-sparing Radical Hysterectomy

To avoid bowel, bladder, and sexual dysfunction, a nerve-sparing radical hysterectomy has been developed (105,106,116,117). The operation seems to be associated with prompt recovery of bladder function, minimal need for self-catheterization (118,119), and less bowel dysfunction (120).

From the superior hypogastric plexus located over the sacral promontory, two hypogastric nerves containing sympathetic fibers run into the small pelvis beneath the ureter and are responsible for such functions as bladder compliance, urinary continence, and small muscle contractions at orgasm. **The hypogastric nerves fuse with parasympathetic fibers of the pelvic splanchnic nerves, coming from sacral roots 2, 3, and 4, to form the inferior hypogastric**

347

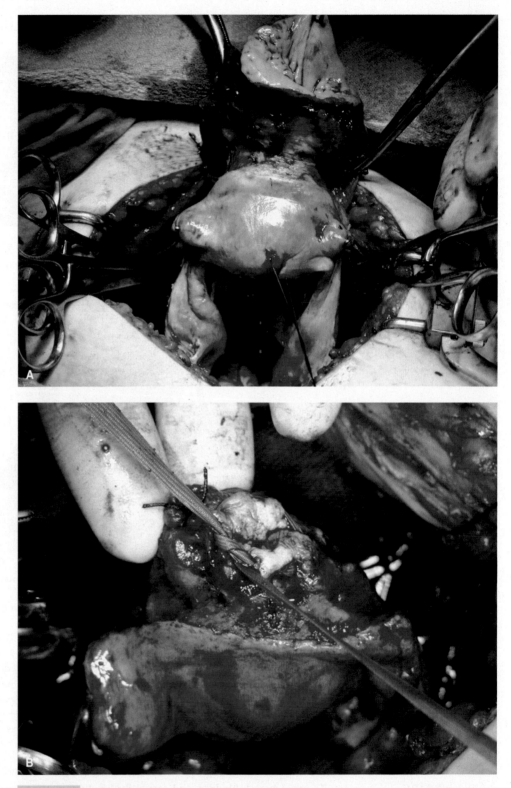

Figure 8.12 Radical abdominal trachelectomy. A: The uterus and upper upper vagina have been mobilized on the infundibulopelvic ligaments, **B:** most of the cervix has been amputated and a mersiline suture has been placed around the proximal end.

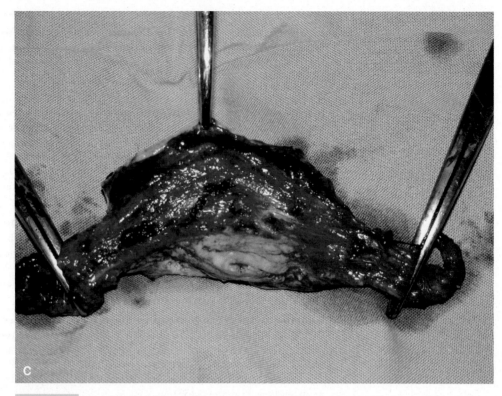

Figure 8.12 *Continued.* **C:** The specimen, showing the proximal cervical canal. Clamps are on the parametrium and and resected upper vagina.

plexus, which is situated in the dorsal part of the parametrium and the dorsal vesicouterine ligament. The parasympathetic fibers are responsible for vaginal lubrication and genital swelling during sexual arousal, detrusor contractility, and various rectal functions.

Performance of the nerve-sparing operation, as described by the Leiden group (121), involves two critical steps: (i) The dissection of the uterosacral ligament and (ii) the dissection of the parametrium. The hypogastric nerves run 1 to 2 cm dorsal to the ureter in the same peritoneal leaf. The hypogastric nerves are identified, dissected from the peritoneal leaf in a similar manner to the ureter, then lateralized as the uterosacral ligaments are clamped and cut. The splanchnic nerves in the parametrium are preserved by dissecting only the the parametrium above the deep uterine vein.

Nerve sparing occurs inevitably with a more conservative type of radical hysterectomy. A prospective, randomized study of type II versus type III radical hysterectomy for stages IB to IIA cervical cancer was reported by Landoni et al. (122). There was no significant difference in recurrence rate (24% type II vs. 26% type III) or the number of patients dead of disease (18% type II vs. 20% type III) for the two procedures, but urologic morbidity was significantly reduced with the less radical operation (13% vs. 28%).

Tailored Surgery for Cervical Cancer

Some authorities have investigated the possibility of less radical surgery, for example, omission of parametrectomy, in patients with small stage IB1 cervical cancers.

Parametrial involvement in patients with small, node-negative tumors is rare (123–126), and Rob's group in Prague have investigated the utility of using sentinel lymph node mapping to individually tailor surgery (127). They reported a prospective study of 158 patients with cervical cancer up to 30 mm diameter and not more than two-thirds stromal invasion, who all underwent sentinel lymph node biopsy, followed by radical hysterectomy and pelvic lymphadenectomy. **There was no parametrial invasion among the 133 patients with negative sentinel nodes,** but of the 25 patients (15.8%) with positive nodes, 28% had parametrial involvement.

Individualization of radicality for frankly invasive cervical cancer remains controversial. Modified radical hysterectomy is a low morbidity operation, and further studies are needed before it is replaced by less radical approaches.

Fertility-sparing Surgery for Stage IB1 Tumors

Fertility-sparing surgery has been widely used for patients with microinvasive cervical cancer, but the indications have been extended to patients with stage IB1 tumors. The literature has been reviewed by Rob et al. (128) in 2011, Schneider et al. (129) in 2012, and Pareja et al. (130) in 2013.

A critical issue when dealing with Stage IB1 patients is the actual extent of the cancer. Preoperatively, this may be defined by an MRI scan, or by transvaginal or transrectal ultrasound. A prospective, multicenter European Study reported that the agreement between histology and ultrasound was significantly better than that for MRI in assessing parametrial extension and residual tumor (after cone biopsy) ($p < 0.001$); ultrasound was comparable to MRI for assessing tumor size and depth of stromal invasion (131). Intraoperatively, surgical margins after trachelectomy can be effectively assessed by intraoperative frozen section (132); the minimum acceptable margin is considered to be 5 mm (128).

All authorities agree that ideally, fertility-sparing surgery should be limited to patients with tumors 2 cm or less in diameter. For these small lesions, both vaginal and abdominal radical trachelectomies have comparable outcomes, and both are considered safe surgical procedures (128). The overall recurrence rate is 3–6% and the death rate is 2–5% (128). Oncologic outcomes are also identical between the vaginal and abdominal approach for tumors larger than 2 cm, but the results cannot be considered satisfactory (128).

Following a radical trachelectomy, patients have impaired fertility caused by cervical stenosis, surgical adhesions, and decreased cervical mucus production. However, 41–79% of patients attempting to conceive are eventually successful. The rate of first trimester miscarriage is comparable to the healthy population, but second trimester deliveries are more common. Preterm delivery (<37 weeks) occurs in approximately 28% of patients, but only 12% have significant prematurity (<32 weeks) (133).

Even more conservative approaches have been tried, with apparently good outcomes in selected cases. **Simple extrafascial trachelectomy and pelvic lymphadenectomy have been reported to be successful in a limited number of patients** with tumors up to 2 cm in diameter, no LVSI, and no evidence of nodal metastases (128,134). A multicenter Italian study of **simple conization and pelvic lymphadenectomy** reported 36 patients with a median tumor size of 11.7 mm (range 8–25 mm). Adenocarcinoma was present in 12 patients (33%) and LVSI in 5 (14%). After a median follow-up of 66 months, one patient (2.8%) had recurred in a pelvic lymph node (135).

For larger stage IB cervical cancers, neoadjuvant chemotherapy to "downstage" the tumor has been reported (127,136–138). TIP (*paclitaxel* 175 mg/m^2 plus *cisplatin* 75 mg/m^2 plus *ifosfamide* 5 gm/m^2) or TEP (*paclitaxel* 175 mg/m^2 plus *cisplatin* 75 mg/m^2 plus *epirubicin* 80 mg/m^2) has been most commonly used, although the Prague protocol utilizes a high-dose density regime of three cycles of *cisplatin* (75 mg/m^2) plus either ifosfamide (2 gm/m^2) or doxorubicin (35 mg/m^2) every 10 days (138). Successful deliveries have been achieved (137,138).

Complications of Radical Hysterectomy

Intraoperative

The average blood loss reported is usually between 500 (139) and 1,500 mL (140). Intraoperative injuries occasionally occur to the pelvic blood vessels, ureter, bladder, rectum, or obturator nerve. These injuries should be recognized immediately and repaired. Even complete severance of the obturator nerve does not usually cause significant problems with walking.

Postoperative Complications

Detailed information about postoperative morbidity is infrequently supplied. Table 8.7 gives data from four series from which detailed information is available. Urinary tract infection is the most common complication, related to the need for prolonged catheter drainage. Other febrile morbidity from such causes as atelectasis or wound infection is also relatively common. **Prolonged ileus occasionally occurs and may result from lymphatic ascites that can develop following lymphadenectomy** (141). The ascites may require repeated paracenteses but will eventually settle completely. Venous thrombosis is undoubtedly underdiagnosed; but with proper prophylactic measures, pulmonary embolism is infrequent. Vesicovaginal or ureterovaginal fistulas occur in less than 1% of cases.

	Pikaat et al., 2007 (139)	Samlal et al., 1996 (140)	Sivanesaratnam et al., 1993 (142)	Hacker et al., 2013 (Stage IB2) (143)	
Complication	n = 156 (%)	n = 271 (%)	n = 397 (%)	n = 93 (%)	Total (%)
Early					
Urinary tract infection	10 (6.4)	NS	36 (9.1)	NS	46/553 (8.3)
Venous thrombosis	1 (0.6)	6 (2.2)	9 (2.3)	2 (2.2)	18/917 (2)
Pulmonary embolism	2 (1.2)	1 (0.4)	2 (0.5)	2 (2.2)	7/917 (0.8)
Ureterovaginal fistula	1 (0.6)	5 (1.8)	1 (0.3)	0 (0)	7/917 (0.8)
Vesicovaginal fistula	0 (0)	2 (0.7)	2 (0.5)	0 (0)	4/917 (0.4)
Fever[a]	11 (7.1)	10 (3.7)	2 (0.5)	5 (5.4)	28/917 (3.1)
Lymphocyst	1 (0.6)	8 (3)	3 (0.8)	1 (1.1)	10/917 (1.1)
Ileus	3 (1.9)	9 (3.3)	NS	3 (3.2)	15/520 (2.9)
Burst abdomen	0 (0)	1 (0.4)	1 (0.2)	0 (0)	2/917 (0.2)
Ureteral obstruction	2 (1.2)	1 (0.4)	0 (0)	0 (0)	3/917 (0.3)
Late					
Bladder atony	13 (8.3)	14 (5.2)	3 (0.8)	NS	30/824 (3.6)
Lymphedema	1 (0.6)	20 (7.4)	4 (1)	8 (8.6)	33/917 (3.6)
Sexual dysfunction	NS	6 (2.2)	NS	NS	6/271 (2.2)

Table 8.7 Postoperative Complications of Radical Hysterectomy

[a]Pelvic abscess, pelvic cellulitis, atelectasis, wound infection, psoas abscess.

NS, not stated.

Late Complications

Bladder Dysfunction   **A distressing late complication is prolonged bladder dysfunction, necessitating voiding by the clock with the aid of the abdominal muscles, and, in some cases, self-catheterization.** Covens et al. (144) reported a significant difference in the incidence of bladder dysfunction at 3 months among different surgeons at the University of Toronto. Twenty-one percent of patients reported objective or subjective bladder dysfunction, but the range among the eight surgeons concerned varied from 0–44%. Samlal et al. (140) from Amsterdam, using a more radical dissection of the paracervical tissues than is usually done in the United States (Okabayashi technique), reported a 5.2% incidence of this complication.

Voiding difficulties and bowel dysfunction are inevitable in the immediate postoperative period, and suprapubic or urethral catheter drainage and laxatives are desirable for at least the first 4 days. Nerve-sparing techniques have decreased the incidence of these complications in recent times (see above).

If cystometry is performed to evaluate bladder dysfunction, two abnormal patterns are found (145). **The hypertonic bladder with elevated urethral pressure is most common.** The hypotonic bladder occurs much less frequently. Patients with a hypertonic pattern have the normal bladder-filling sensation and the usual discomfort of a full bladder. The condition is self-limiting, and voiding usually occurs within 3 weeks of surgery. **The prognosis is much worse for patients with a hypotonic bladder, and some of these patients eventually require lifelong self-catheterization.**

Sexual Dysfunction   **A large Swedish study of sexuality in cervical cancer survivors reported sexual dysfunction in 55% of patients treated by radical hysterectomy alone** (146). Problems included insufficient lubrication, reduced genital swelling at arousal, reduced vaginal length and elasticity, and dyspareunia. The addition of preoperative brachytherapy or external-beam radiation yielded no excess risk of sexual dysfunction.

This is in marked contrast to the experience at the Royal Hospital for Women, where Grumann et al. (147), in a more detailed study of a much smaller group of patients, reported that radical hysterectomy was not associated with major sexual sequelae.

The differences between the two groups may be explained by the radicality of the surgery. At the Royal Hospital for Women, no more than 1.5 cm of normal vagina is taken at radical hysterectomy, so reports of vaginal shortness and dyspareunia are very unusual. Other studies have also reported a favorable outcome in terms of sexual function following radical hysterectomy (148,149), and the nerve-sparing operation is likely to further enhance sexual function, particularly in terms of orgasmic sensation and vaginal lubrication.

Lymphedema   As a late complication of pelvic lymphadenectomy, lymphedema is underreported in the medical literature. In a study of 233 patients having pelvic lymphadenectomy in our center, 47 (20.2%) developed lymphedema (150). The onset of the swelling was within 3 months in 53%, within 6 months in 71%, and within 12 months in 84% of patients. The addition of pelvic radiation postoperatively increased the risk of lymphedema.

Stage IB2 Cervical Carcinoma

Optimal management of patients with primary tumors greater than 4 cm in diameter is controversial. **Primary chemoradiation, neoadjuvant chemotherapy followed by radical hysterectomy, and primary radical hysterectomy followed by tailored adjuvant radiation therapy are the major options.** Overall survival is good, but local, regional, and distant failure are more likely than for stage IB1 lesions whatever primary modality is chosen. **Many of these patients are premenopausal, so quality-of-life issues, including preservation of sexual function, is important.**

Primary Chemoradiation Therapy

This has become the preferred treatment option in many centers because of concern about both increased morbidity when surgery is combined with radiation, and the technical difficulties associated with operating on large tumors.

There is a strong correlation between tumor size and outcome for patients with stage IB cervical cancer (151). For radiation without concurrent chemotherapy, Perez et al. (152) from St. Louis reported 10-year disease-free survival rates of 90% for stage IB tumors <2 cm, 76% for 2–4 cm, 61% for 4.1–5 cm, and 47% for >5 cm. For lesions <2 cm, doses of 75 Gray (Gy) to point A resulted in pelvic failure rates of 10%, whereas for more extensive lesions, even doses of 85 Gy resulted in 35–50% pelvic failure rates (151). **Bulky tumors require aggressive radiotherapy, and complication rates are high.** Perez et al. (153), in a study of 552 patients with stages IB to IIA cervical cancer treated with radiation alone, reported grade 3 morbidity in 7% of cases, with grade 2 morbidity in a further 10%. Grade 3 morbidity included 6 rectovaginal fistulae, 1 recto-uterine fistula, 5 vesicovaginal fistulae, 1 enterocolic fistula, 1 enterocutaneous fistula, 1 sigmoid perforation, 7 rectal strictures, 10 ureteral strictures, and 10 small bowel obstructions.

Since the introduction of chemoradiation, there has been a significant improvement in survival, but also a significant increase in morbidity. A systematic review and meta-analysis of 18 randomized trials indicated that toxity data are frequently underreported, particularly vaginal toxity, which was recorded in only 22% of the studies (154). A recent report from University College Hospital, London, noted a 3.3% incidence of total vaginal necrosis following chemoradiation for cervical cancer (155).

Radiation and Extrafascial Hysterectomy

The GOG have conducted two studies of primary radiation followed by extrafacial hysterectomy. In the first study, published in 2003, 256 patients with tumors ≥4 cm diameter were randomized between radiation alone (*n* = 124) and attenuated radiation followed by extrafascial hysterectomy (*n* = 132) (156). Twenty-five percent of patients had tumors ≥7 cm diameter. There was a lower incidence of local relapse in the hysterectomy group (27% vs. 14% at 5 years), although outcomes were not statistically different. Their conclusions were somewhat ambiguous: "Overall, there was no clinically important benefit with the use of extrafascial hysterectomy. However, there is good evidence to suggest that patients with 4, 5, and 6 cm tumors may have benefited from extrafascial hysterectomy."

In a subsequent trial of patients with bulky (≥4 cm) cervical cancers, all 374 patients were treated with pelvic radiation therapy followed by adjuvant extrafascial hysterectomy 3 to 6 weeks later. The patients were randomized between no chemotherapy and weekly *cisplatin* (40 mg/m²/wk) during the 6 weeks of external radiation. **Residual cancer in the hysterectomy specimen was significantly reduced in the group receiving *cisplatin* (47% vs. 57%). Survival at 24 months (89% vs. 79%) and recurrence-free survival (81% vs. 69%) were both significantly improved by the addition of *cisplatin*. Grades 3 and 4 hematologic and gastrointestinal toxicities were more frequent in the chemoradiation arm** (157).

Neoadjuvant Chemotherapy

In 1993, Sardi et al. (158) reported the results of a randomized trial of neoadjuvant chemotherapy for patients with bulky stage IB cervical cancer. In the control arm (75 patients), a Wertheim–Meigs operation followed by adjuvant whole-pelvic radiation was carried out, whereas in the neoadjuvant group (76 patients), the same procedures were preceded by three cycles of chemotherapy with **the *"quick" vincristine, bleomycin,* and *cisplatin (VBP)* regimen.** The chemotherapy protocol consisted of *cisplatin* 50 mg/m^2 on day 1, *vincristine* 1 mg/m^2 on day 1, and *bleomycin* 25 mg/m^2 on days 1, 2, and 3 (the latter given as a 6-hour infusion). Three cycles were given at 10-day intervals. **Survival and progression-free interval were significantly improved for patients with an echographic volume greater than 60 dL,** mainly because of a decrease in the incidence of locoregional failures. In the control group, pelvic recurrences were observed in 24.3% of patients compared with 7.6% of patients in the neoadjuvant group.

A recent Prague study reported 151 patients with bulky stage IB cervical cancer, including 119 (78.8%) with stage IB2 disease, who were treated with high-dose neoadjuvant chemotherapy (159). Squamous cancers were treated with *cisplatin* 75 mg/m^2 and *ifosfamide* 2 g/m^2, while adenocarcinomas received *cisplatin* 75 mg/m^2 plus *doxorubicin* 35 mg/m^2. Both regimens were given every 10 days for 3 or 4 cycles. **A complete response to chemotherapy was seen in 19 patients (12.6%), while 9 (6%) progressed on treatment.** Radical hysterectomy was performed in the 94% of patients who had at least a partial response, and 26 of these (18.3%) had positive nodes. Postoperative radiation was given to 36 patients (26.7%). **With a median follow-up of 88.5 months, the 5-year disease-specific survival was 83.6%.**

At the Royal Hospital for Women, **neoadjuvant chemotherapy is considered to be the treatment of choice for cervical cancer occurring during pregnancy if the patient wishes to retain the pregnancy, as it usually allows the pregnancy to be prolonged until fetal maturity has been achieved. Radical caesarean hysterectomy can then be performed at a time determined in consultation with the obstetrician and neonatologist.**

As is the case with ovarian cancer, neoadjuvant chemotherapy often makes the surgery more difficult because of the inflammatory reaction it creates. This is a particular problem if bulky positive lymph nodes are attached to veins. In addition, there is a low complete pathologic response rate, so radiation therapy is often given 6 weeks after the radical hysterectomy, which significantly prolongs treatment time.

Primary Radical Hysterectomy and Tailored Postoperative Radiation

The other option for medically fit patients is primary radical hysterectomy and tailored postoperative radiation, with or without chemotherapy (Fig. 8.13) (37,143,160–166). **At the Royal Hospital for Women in Sydney, primary surgery is preferred, and this philosophy is also applied to**

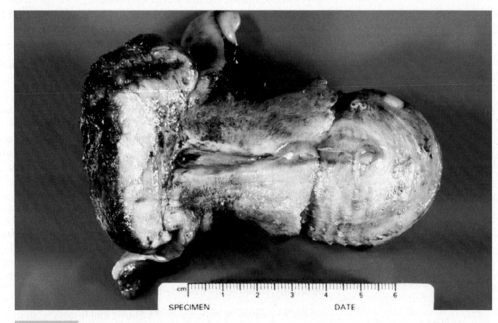

Figure 8.13 Radical hysterectomy specimen from a patient with an exophytic stage IB2 cervical cancer.

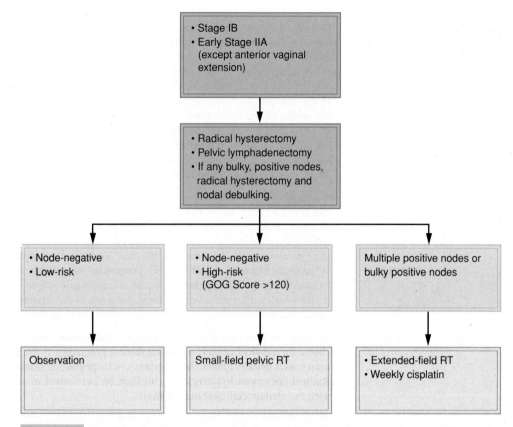

Figure 8.14 **Algorithm for the management of stages IB and early IIA carcinoma of the cervix.** RT, radiation therapy; GOG, Gynecologic Oncology Group.

patients with stage IIA disease, provided the tumor does not extend down the anterior vaginal wall; the algorithm for this approach is shown in Figure 8.14.

Older patients frequently tolerate radical surgery better than radiation therapy, although approximately 10% of patients older than 70 years of age have a medical contraindication to surgery (94). Radiation tolerance in elderly patients is controversial. Although comparable outcomes to younger patients have been reported (167), others have indicated that comorbid conditions in the elderly necessitate more frequent treatment breaks and less ability to deliver intracavitary therapy, thereby impairing overall prognosis (168).

There are several advantages to a primary surgical approach. First, it allows for accurate staging of the disease, thereby allowing adjuvant therapy to be modified according to needs (168). **Second, it allows resection of bulky positive lymph nodes,** thereby improving the prognosis significantly (104,170). **Third, it allows removal of the primary cancer,** thereby avoiding the difficulty of determining whether there is viable residual disease after the cervix has responded to radiation. **Fourth, for most premenopausal patients, it allows preservation of ovarian function,** which improves both quality and duration of life (171). **Finally, and very importantly, it obviates the need for brachytherapy, so virtually eliminates the risk of vaginal fistulae and vaginal stenosis.** A primary surgical approach is the treatment of choice in patients with acute or chronic pelvic inflammatory disease, or anatomic problems making optimal radiation therapy difficult.

The Royal Hospital for Women results with a primary surgical approach to patients with stage IB2 cervical cancer have been published (143). **An MRI was performed preoperatively to ensure that there was no spread to the bladder or parametrium, and other important features of this approach include (i) the use of small-field pelvic radiation for high-risk, node-negative patients and (ii) resection of bulky, positive lymph nodes without systematic pelvic lymphadenectomy, followed by extended-field radiation.**

Of the 93 patients in our series, 21 (22.6%) had tumors 6 cm or more in diameter, 28 (30.2%) had adenocarcinomas, 73 (78.5%) had deep stromal invasion, and 15 (16.1%) had occult parametrial extension. Positive pelvic nodes were present in 42 patients (45.2%) and bulky positive para-aortic

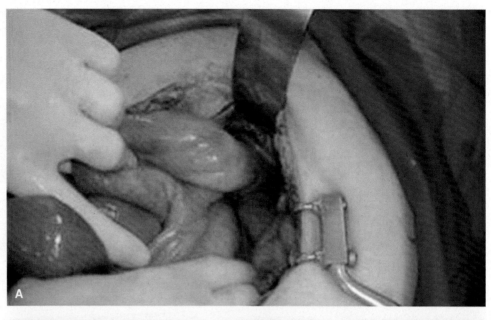

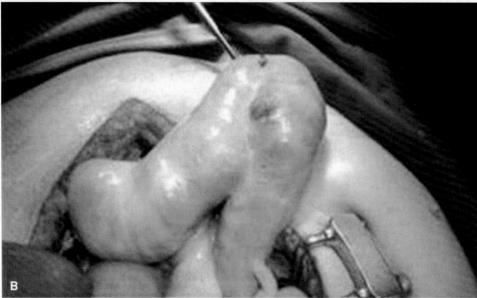

Figure 8.15 Distal small bowel obstruction following primary radical hysterectomy and adjuvant external pelvic chemoradiation for stage 1B2 cervical cancer. **A:** Site of obstruction in distal small bowel localized to the pelvis. **B:** Terminal ileum, showing marked radiation fibrosis, mobilized from the pelvis. (*continued*)

nodes in 5 (5.4%). Nineteen patients (20.4%) received no postoperative radiation, 29 (31.2%) small-field radiation, 17 (18.3%) pelvic chemoradiation, and 28 (30.1%) extended-field chemoradiation. **With a median follow-up of 96 months, the overall 5-year survival was 80.7%, being 85% for node-negative patients and 75% if node-positive** (143).

The major long-term surgical morbidity was lymphedema, which occurred in 8 patients (8.9%), while grade 3 or 4 radiation toxicity occurred in 3 (3.2%). Two of the patients had radiation enteritis and a small bowel obstruction that could be resected (Fig. 8.15), while the third patient developed a rectal stricture and required a colostomy (143). Published results of primary surgery for stage IB2 cervical cancer over the past decade are shown in Table 8.8.

In the only randomized, prospective study looking at radical surgery versus primary radiation for stages IB to IIA cervical cancer, Landoni et al. (92) reported that for patients with a cervical diameter larger than 4 cm, the rate of pelvic relapse in the group treated with radiation

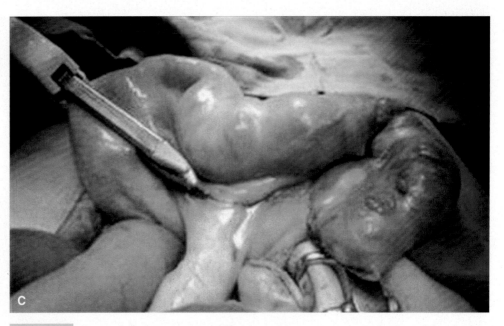

Figure 8.15 *Continued.* **C:** Resection and subsequent reanastomosis facilitated by stapling devices.

therapy was more than twice the rate of distant relapse (30% vs. 13%). In addition, **there was a significantly higher rate of pelvic relapse among those who had radiation alone (16 of 54; 30%) compared with those who had surgery plus adjuvant radiation (9 of 46; 20%).** This study did not utilize chemoradiation, and **properly randomized trials comparing primary surgery, primary chemoradiation, and neoadjuvant chemotherapy will be necessary in the future to determine the best approach. Such studies will need to evaluate quality of life for each approach,** so that patients can make a properly informed decision about their best treatment option.

Part of the question might be answered by an ongoing EORTC protocol (No. 55994; NCT00039338), comparing the results of neoadjuvant *cisplatin*-based chemotherapy followed by radical hysterectomy versus standard therapy, comprising concurrent radiotherapy and *cisplatin*-based chemotherapy in stages IB2, IIA, and IIB cervical cancer. Quality of life in that study will be assessed at baseline, and at 6, 12, 18, and 24 months.

Cost-effectiveness Analysis

Rocconi et al. (172) created a decision analysis model to determine the cost-effectiveness of the three common strategies for managing stage IB2 squamous carcinoma of the cervix. **They chose a hypothetical cohort of 10,000 patients, which they estimated to be the number of new cases of stage IB2 cervical cancer diagnosed in the United States every 5 years.** They assumed all patients were diagnosed and clinically staged by a gynecologic oncologist, and that each patient

Table 8.8 Primary Surgery and Tailored Adjuvant Radiation Therapy for Patients with Stage IB2 Cervical Cancer

Study	Number	Positive Nodes (%)	Adjuvant RT (%)	DFS (%)	5-Year Survival (%)
Rutledge et al., 2004 (162)	86	27.9	52	74.3	NS
Yessaian et al., 2004 (163)	58	28	62	NS	62.1
Havrilesky et al., 2004 (164)	72	17	31	63	72
Micha et al., 2006 (165)	47	25.5	76.6	NS	75
Zivanovic et al., 2008 (166)	27	7	52	52[a]	72[a]
Hacker et al., 2013 (143)	93	45	79.6	76.5	80.7

[a]3-year survival

RT, Radiation therapy; DFS, disease-free survival; NS, not stated.

underwent a CT scan of the pelvis and abdomen to exclude advanced disease. A literature review was undertaken to determine grade 3 and 4 complication rates and disease-free survival for each modality.

Radical hysterectomy with pelvic and para-aortic lymphadenectomy and tailored chemoradiation for high-risk patients was the least expensive strategy, with an estimated cost of $284 million per 10,000 women, and an estimated 5-year disease-free survival of 69% (172). Primary chemoradiation had an estimated cost of $299 million and a disease-free survival of 69.3%, while neoadjuvant chemotherapy followed by radical hysterectomy and tailored chemoradiation for high-risk patients had an estimated cost of $508 million (DFS 70%). **They concluded that primary surgery was the most cost-effective strategy and that primary chemoradiation would cost approximately $500,000 per additional survivor. Neoadjuvant chemotherapy would cost $2.24 million per additional survivor.**

Prognostic Factors for Stages IB to IIA

The major prognostic factors for patients having radical hysterectomy and pelvic lymphadenectomy for stages IB to IIA cervical cancer are as follows:

1. **Status of the lymph nodes**
2. **Size of the primary tumor**
3. **Depth of stromal invasion**
4. **Presence or absence of LVSI**
5. **Presence or absence of parametrial extension**
6. **Histologic cell type**
7. **Status of the vaginal margins**

Using clinical and histologic factors from 710 consecutive patients having primary surgery for stage IA2–IIA disease, a Dutch group has developed a prognostic model for disease-specific survival, which they believe should be used in clinical trials investigating the effectiveness of various adjuvant treatments on high-risk patients (173).

Lymph Node Status

The most important prognostic factor is the status of the lymph nodes. Survival data for patients with positive nodes are shown in Table 8.9. The influence of the number of positive nodes is shown in Table 8.10. **Patients with a single positive node below the common iliac bifurcation have a prognosis similar to that of patients with negative nodes** (174–176). A large Korean study has shown that **node-positive patients are a heterogenous group. Histologic type (adeno and adenosquamous variants do worse), tumor size, and parametrial involvement are all significant factors for recurrence-free and overall survival** in multivariate analysis of node-positive patients after radical hysterectomy and pelvic lymphadenectomy (177). Recent information has suggested that **micrometastases in sentinel nodes in patients with early cervical cancer cause a reduction in survival equivalent to that of macrometastases,** whereas no prognostic significance could be found for the presence of isolated tumor cells (178).

Table 8.9 Survival Versus Nodal Status after Radical Hysterectomy for Stages IB and IIA Cervical Cancer

Authors	Number	5-Year Survival Rate (%)		
		Negative Nodes	Positive Nodes	Overall
Kenter et al., 1989 (179)	213	94	65	87
Lee et al., 1989 (180)	954	88	73	86
Monaghan et al., 1990 (181)	498	91	51	83
Ayhan et al., 1991 (182)	278	91	63	84
Averette et al., 1993 (183)	978	96	64	90
Samlal et al., 1997 (40)	271	95	76	90
Kim et al., 2000 (174)	366	95	78	88

		No. of Positive Nodes		
Authors	**Patients**	**1**	**1–3**	**>4**
Noguchi et al., 1987 (184)	177	—	54	43
Lee et al., 1989 (180)	954	62	—	44
Inoue and Morita, 1990 (185)	484	91	—	50

Table 8.10 Five-Year Survival Rate (%) Versus Number of Positive Pelvic Nodes in Stage IB Cervical Carcinoma

Tumor Size, Depth of Stromal Invasion, Lymph-Vascular Space Invasion

In 1989, the GOG (176) published the results of a prospective clinicopathologic study of 732 patients with stage IB cervical carcinoma treated by radical hysterectomy and bilateral pelvic lymphadenectomy. Of these, 645 patients had no gross disease beyond the cervix or uterus and negative para-aortic nodes. One hundred patients had micrometastases in pelvic nodes, but their survival was not significantly different from patients with negative nodes.

There were three independent prognostic factors:

1. **The clinical size of the tumor**
2. **The presence or absence of LVSI**
3. **The depth of tumor invasion**

A relative risk (RR) was calculated for each prognostic variable and an overall estimate of risk determined by multiplying the appropriate RR for the three independent variables. For example, a tumor 4 cm in diameter was estimated to have a RR of 2.9. If it invaded 12 mm into the outer third of the cervix, then the RR was estimated to be 37. LVSI conferred a RR of 1.7. The overall estimate of risk was therefore $2.9 \times 37 \times 1.7 = 182.4$. At the Royal Hospital, the latter figure has been termed the *GOG score*. Disease-free survival curves were constructed for several RR groups (Fig. 8.16). **The likelihood of recurrence for a patient with a GOG score greater than 120 was 40% at 3 years.**

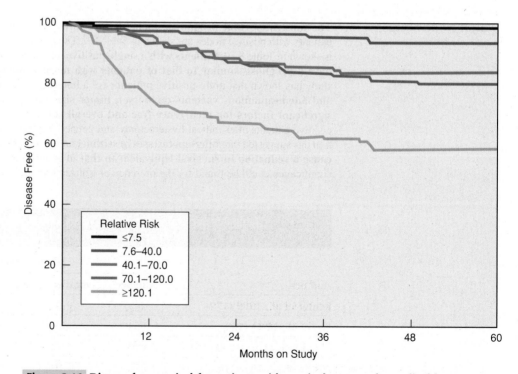

Figure 8.16 Disease-free survival for patients with cervical cancer after radical hysterectomy and bilateral pelvic lymphadenectomy. (From **Delgado G, Bundy B, Zaino R, et al.** Prospective surgical-pathological study of disease-free interval in patients with stage IB squamous cell carcinoma of the cervix: A Gynecologic Oncology Group study. *Gynecol Oncol.* 1990;38:352–357, with permission.)

The quantity of LVSI correlates significantly with the risk of nodal metastases in women with early stage cervical cancer (186), and it has been shown to be an independent prognostic factor for time to recurrence in women with early stage squamous carcinoma of the cervix (187).

Parametrial Invasion

Burghardt et al. (188) analyzed 1,004 cases of stages IB, IIA, or IIB cervical carcinoma treated by radical hysterectomy at Graz, Munich, and Erlangen, with all surgical specimens processed as giant sections. This processing technique allows accurate assessment of tumor volume and parametrial extension. The 5-year survival rate for 734 patients with no parametrial extension was 85.8%, compared with 62.4% for 270 patients with parametrial extension.

The group at Yale (189) reported that patients with parametrial extension, regardless of lymph node status, had a significantly shorter disease-free interval than patients with positive nodes alone, with 12 of 19 such patients (63%) recurring in the pelvis. By contrast, a Japanese study of 117 patients with stages IB to IIB disease and parametrial invasion after radical hysterectomy were divided into two groups based on the status of the pelvic lymph nodes. Five-year overall survival for node-positive and node-negative patients was 52% and 89%, respectively ($p = 0.0005$) (190). Extrapelvic recurrence was more common in patients with positive nodes ($p = 0.005$).

Histologic Cell Type

Small-cell carcinoma of the cervix is uncommon but has an unequivocally poor prognosis (191).

The prognostic significance of adenocarcinoma histologic type is more controversial. These tumors usually arise in the endocervical canal and diagnosis is often delayed, so it is difficult to be certain that lesions of comparable size are being compared. Many centers report adenocarcinoma histologic type as a poor prognostic factor in multivariate analysis (174,191,193), but Shingleton et al. (194) were unable to confirm this. In a patient care evaluation study of the American College of Surgeons, they evaluated 11,157 patients from 703 hospitals with cervical cancer treated between 1984 and 1990. There were 9,351 cases of squamous carcinoma (83.8%), 1,405 cases of adenocarcinoma (12.6%), and 401 cases of adenosquamous carcinoma (3.6%). In a multivariate analysis of patients with clinical stage IB disease, histologic type had no significant effect on survival.

The prognostic significance of adenosquamous carcinoma of the cervix is controversial, with some authors reporting a significantly worse prognosis for patients with these tumors (195–197), whereas others report no difference from adenocarcinomas with respect to metastatic potential or outcome (198,199).

Close Vaginal Margins

Investigators at the Jackson Memorial Hospital in Miami, Florida, reviewed the charts of 1,223 patients with stages IA2, IB, or IIA cervical cancer who had undergone radical hysterectomy (183). Fifty-one patients (4.2%) had positive or close vaginal margins, the latter being defined as tumor no more than 0.5 cm from the vaginal margin of resection. Twenty-three (45%) of these cases had negative nodes and no parametrial involvement, and 16 of the 23 (69.6%) received postoperative radiation. The 5-year survival rate was significantly improved by the addition of adjuvant radiation (81.3% vs. 28.6%; $p < 0.05$). They recommended that close vaginal margins without other high-risk factors should be considered a poor prognostic variable.

Tumor Markers

Several tumor markers have been reported to have prognostic value in early stage cervical cancer, but these are not yet used routinely in most clinical practices.

Serum Squamous Cell Carcinoma Antigen

Increased pretreatment serum squamous cell carcinoma antigen (SCC-Ag) levels, and failure of the levels to normalize at the completion of treatment, are associated with a decreased PFS (200). A Chinese study has demonstrated that the serum SCC-Ag level is more reliable for evaluating response to neoadjuvant chemotherapy than MRI (201), while a Japanese study has recommended routine SCC-Ag monitoring following treatment. They reported that the overall survival was higher when recurrence was predicted on the basis of tumor marker elevation than when diagnosed by other modalities ($p = 0.03$) (202).

Human Papilloma Virus Genotype

Cervical tumors associated with HPV type 18 appear to be associated with an increased risk of recurrence and death (203). This has been demonstrated in patients with early stage disease treated surgically (204,205), and in patients with advanced disease treated with radiotherapy (206).

Microvessel Density

Because angiogenesis is considered essential for tumor growth and the development of metastases, it is not surprising that high microvessel density has been reported adversely to influence survival in clinical stage IB cervical cancer and has been used to identify patients with negative nodes at risk for relapse (207).

Epidermal Growth Factor Receptor (EGFR)

High protein expression of genes involved in the EGFR pathway, particularly EGFR and C-erbB-2, are markers for poor survival in cervical cancer patients treated primarily with chemoradiation (208).

Postoperative Radiation

Adjuvant pelvic radiation following radical hysterectomy should be given in two circumstances: (i) patients with positive nodes, positive parametria, or positive surgical margins; and (ii) patients with negative nodes but high-risk features in the primary tumor.

Patients with Positive Nodes, Positive Parametria, or Positive Surgical Margins

In 2000, the Southwest Oncology Group (SWOG) and the GOG reported results of a randomized study of women with FIGO stages IA2, IB, and IIA carcinoma of the cervix found to have positive pelvic lymph nodes, positive parametrial involvement, or positive surgical margins at the time of primary radical hysterectomy and pelvic lymphadenectomy (209). Patients had to have confirmed negative para-aortic nodes. The regimens were as follows.

> **Regimen I**—external pelvic radiation with *cisplatin* and *5-fluorouracil* (5-FU) infusion
> **Regimen II**—external pelvic radiation

Patients on regimen I received intravenous *cisplatin* 70 mg/m^2 followed by a 96-hour continuous intravenous infusion of 5-FU (4,000 mg/m^2) every 3 weeks for four courses, with the first and the second cycles given concurrent with the radiation. Radiation therapy in both arms delivered 4,930 centiGray (cGy) to the pelvis using a four-field box technique. Patients with metastatic disease in high common iliac nodes also received 4,500 cGy to a para-aortic field.

Long-term follow-up was published in 2005 (210). **The absolute improvement in 5-year survival for adjuvant chemotherapy in patients with tumors ≤2 cm was only 5%** (77% vs. 82%), whereas for tumors >2 cm it was 19% (58% vs. 77%). Similarly, **the absolute 5-year survival benefit for patients with one nodal metastasis was only 4% (79% vs. 83%) compared to 20% when at least two nodes were positive (55% vs. 75%).**

Patients with Negative Nodes but High-Risk Features in the Primary Tumor

Although patients with negative nodes have an 85–90% survival rate after radical hysterectomy and pelvic lymphadenectomy, they contribute approximately 50% of the recurrences, with most (about 70%) occurring in the pelvis (211).

In 1999, the GOG reported the results of a randomized study of adjuvant whole-pelvic radiation at a dose of 50.4 Gy versus no further treatment after radical hysterectomy for patients with high-risk, node-negative stage IB cervical cancer (212). To be eligible for the study, patients had to have at least two of the following risk factors: Greater than one-third stromal invasion, LVSI, and large tumor size (usually ≥4 cm). There were 277 patients entered into the study. **The addition of radiation significantly reduced the risk of recurrence, with a disease-free rate of 88% for radiation versus 79% for observation at 2 years.** Severe (GOG grades 3 to 4) gastrointestinal or urologic toxicity occurred in 6.2% of patients receiving radiation versus 1.4% of controls.

An update of this GOG study was reported in 2006, which included seven additional recurrences and 19 additional deaths (213). **The radiation therapy arm continued to show a statistically significant reduction in risk of recurrence, but the improvement in the overall survival with**

Table 8.11 Anteroposterior and Lateral Portals for Standard and Small-Field Pelvic Radiation Used for Patients from the Royal Hospital for Women, Sydney

	Standard Field	*Small Field*
Anteroposterior		
Superior	L4–L5 junction	S1–S2 junction
Inferior	Inferior obturator foramen	Midobturator foramen
Lateral	1.5 cm lateral to pelvic brim	Bony pelvic brim
Lateral		
Anterior	Outer edge of pubic symphysis	1 cm posterior to pubic tubercle
Posterior	Ischial tuberosities	Anterior sacral plane

radiation did not reach statistical significance (HR = 0.70, 90% CI 0.45 to 1.05; $p = 0.074$). Postoperative radiation appeared to be particularly beneficial for patients with adeno or adenosquamous histologies.

The group from Leiden University in the Netherlands identified 51 patients (13%) who had two of the three high-risk factors identified by the GOG, among 402 patients who underwent radical hysterectomy for early stage cervical cancer (214). They compared 34 patients (66%) who received postoperative pelvic radiation with 17 patients (33%) who did not. **A statistically significant difference was found in 5-year cancer-specific survival in favor of the high-risk group treated with pelvic radiation (86% vs. 57%).**

Radiation morbidity is highly correlated with the target volume, and a clinical audit of patients with stage IB, node-negative, cervical cancer treated at the Royal Hospital for Women in Sydney revealed that 87% of recurrences occurred in the central pelvis (vaginal vault or paravaginal soft tissues). It was therefore decided to pilot a study involving a radiation field focused on the central pelvis to see if the central recurrence rate could be decreased without causing significant morbidity. The results were reported in 1999 (215). The portals for the standard and small pelvic radiation fields used on patients treated at the Royal Hospital for Women are shown in Table 8.11 (Fig. 8.17). **The small pelvic field decreases the amount of small and large bowel that is irradiated.**

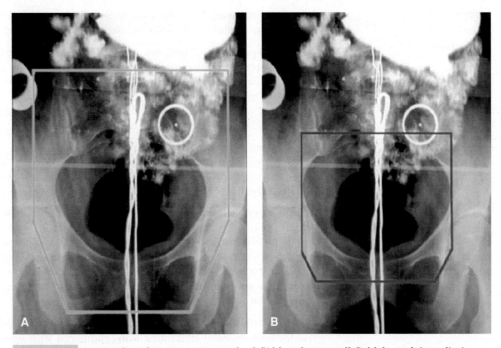

Figure 8.17 Comparison between (A) standard field and (B) small field for pelvic radiation.

High-risk, node-negative patients were selected on the basis of a GOG score of at least 120 (Fig. 8.16). Twenty-five consecutive patients were selected with a mean GOG score of 166 (range 120 to 263). **With a mean follow-up of 32 months (range 12 to 64 months), there was only one recurrence (4%) at 16 months.** A log-rank analysis demonstrated a significant improvement in the 5-year disease-free survival rate when this group was compared with the high-risk patients in the GOG study (GOG score ≥ 120) who were observed without postoperative radiation ($p = 0.005$) (214). No major morbidity occurred, but minor morbidity was recorded in four patients: Lymphedema in three and mild rectal incontinence in one.

A **2003 Japanese study compared adjuvant small-field pelvic radiation** for 42 patients with high-risk, node-negative stage I or II cervical cancer **with whole-pelvic radiation** for 42 patients with node-positive disease (216). **The 5-year pelvic control rate was 93% in the small pelvic field cohort and 90% in the whole-pelvic field group.** The same group subsequently reported decreased hematologic and gastrointestinal toxicity with the small-field technique (217). A more recent study of small-field radiation compared to standard-field radiation from Singapore confirmed the high pelvic control rates, and demonstrated **significantly less lower limb lymphedema in the small-field group** (218).

Stages IIB to IVA Disease

Primary Radiation Therapy

Radiation therapy can be used to treat all stages of cervical cancer, but for early stage disease, it is usually reserved for medically unfit patients. **Radical external-beam radiation therapy plus brachytherapy has been the gold standard for advanced disease,** but as the volume of the primary lesion increases, the likelihood of sterilizing it with radiation decreases. Increasing the dose of radiation increases the late morbidity to the bowel, bladder, and vaginal vault, so **various strategies have been investigated to try to improve local control.**

Strategies that have been investigated include the following:

1. **Hyperfractionation** of the radiation (219)
2. **Neoadjuvant chemotherapy before radiation (220)**
3. **Use of hypoxic cell radiation sensitizers (221)**
4. **Concurrent use of chemotherapy and radiation (chemoradiation)** (222–225)

Concurrent Chemotherapy and Radiation

Three large randomized prospective trials, all reported in 1999, have established chemoradiation as the treatment of choice for patients with advanced cervical cancer.

The GOG reported the results of a phase III randomized study of external-beam pelvic radiation and intracavitary radiation combined with concomitant *hydroxyurea* versus weekly *cisplatin* versus 5 FU-*cisplatin* and *hydroxyurea* (HFC) in 526 patients with stages IIB, III, and IVA cervical cancer who had undergone extraperitoneal surgical sampling of the para-aortic lymph nodes. Women with intraperitoneal disease or disease metastatic to the para-aortic lymph nodes were ineligible (222). Chemotherapy regimens were as follows.

Regimen I—weekly *cisplatin* 40 mg/m^2/wk for 6 weeks
Regimen II—*hydroxyurea* orally 2 mg/m^2 twice weekly for 6 weeks, *5-FU* 1,000 mg/m^2/d as a 96-hour infusion on days 1 and 29, and *cisplatin* 50 mg/m^2 days 1 and 29 (*HFC*)
Regimen III—*hydroxyurea* orally 3 g twice weekly

Both platinum-containing regimens improved the PFS compared with *hydroxyurea* alone ($p < 0.005$). The percentage of patients recurrence-free at 24 months was 70% for weekly *cisplatin*, 67% for *HFC*, and 50% for *hydroxyurea*. Grade 3 or 4 leukopenia and grade 4 gastrointestinal toxicity were increased with *HFC* compared with weekly *cisplatin* or *hydroxyurea* ($p = 0.0001$ and $p = 0.02$, respectively). The investigators concluded that **weekly *cisplatin* was more effective than *hydroxyurea* and more tolerable than *HFC* as a concomitant chemoradiation regimen for locally advanced cervical cancer.**

Long-term follow-up of these patients confirmed improved progression-free and overall survival for both *cisplatin*-containing arms compared with *hydroxyurea* ($p < 0.001$) (223). The

relative risk of progression of disease or death was 0.57 (95% CI, 0.43 to 0.75) with *cisplatin* and 0.51 (95% CI, 0.38 to 0.67) with *cisplatin*-based combination chemotherapy compared with *hydroxyurea* alone. The improved survival occurred collectively and individually for patients with stages IIB and III disease.

The Radiation Therapy Oncology Group (RTOG) randomized 403 patients with advanced cervical cancer confined to the pelvis (stages IIB through IVA, or IB/ IIA with a tumor of at least 5 cm or positive pelvic nodes) between pelvic and para-aortic radiation, and pelvic radiation with concurrent *cisplatin* and *5-fluorouracil* (224). With a median follow-up of 43 months, the actuarial survival at 5 years was 73% among patients having chemoradiation and 58% among those having radiation alone ($p = 0.004$). Disease-free 5-year survivals were 67% in the chemoradiation arm and 40% in the radiation alone arm, respectively ($p < 0.001$). **The rates of distant metastases and locoregional recurrences were significantly higher among patients treated with radiation alone.**

The GOG–SWOG groups randomized 388 patients with FIGO stages IIB, III, or IVA disease and negative para-aortic nodes at retroperitoneal para-aortic lymph node sampling between standard pelvic radiation with *hydroxyurea* and standard pelvic radiation with *5-fluorouracil* and *cisplatin* (225). **Both progression-free ($p = 0.03$) and overall survival ($p = 0.02$) were significantly better for patients randomized to receive *5 FU-cisplatin*.**

Since publication of these clinical trials and the NCI clinical announcement in 1999, there has been a significant change in the management of cervical cancer in the United States, with the number of patients receiving concurrent chemoradiation increasing from 20% in 1997 to 72% in 2001 (226). Underweight patients (BMI <18.5 kg/m^2) undergoing chemoradiation for locally advanced cervical cancer have been reported to have diminished survival and increased toxicity compared with normal weight and obese patients (227).

A systematic review and meta-analysis of data from 18 randomized chemoradiation trials, conducted by Medical Research Council Clinical Trials Unit in London, **endorsed the recommendations of the 1999 NCI alert**. There was a 6% absolute survival benefit, and an 8% disease-free survival benefit at 5 years. However, acute toxicity was increased, **late toxicity was poorly reported,** and only one trial reported quality-of-life outcomes (228).

The optimal regimen for the chemotherapy is yet to be defined, but single-agent *cisplatin* at a dose of 40 mg/m^2 given weekly during external-beam therapy is widely used. The high rates of chemotherapy completion achieved in multi-institutional trials can be difficult to reproduce in standard practice, and toxicity may be higher than reported, possibly because patients on trials are younger and have less comorbidity (229).

Nothing in the past 15 years has been shown to give better results than concurrent *cisplatin*-based chemoradiation, with the possible exception of radiation plus hyperthermia (230,231). However, that approach is not available in most centers, and it has never been directly compared with concurrent chemoradiation.

Another important issue is the role of adjuvant chemotherapy after concurrent chemoradiation. In a study reported by Dueñas-González et al. (232), patients with stages IIB to IVA cervical cancer were randomized between concurrent *gemcitabine* plus *cisplatin* and radiation followed by adjuvant *gemcitabine* and *cisplatin*, versus concurrent *cisplatin* and radiation. There was a signficiant benefit for the first approach. In the abovementioned meta-analysis (228), larger benefit was seen for the two studies in which chemotherapy was administered after concurrent chemoradiation. These data need to be confirmed.

This might be done in an ongoing Gynecologic Cancer InterGroup (GCIG) trial (The **OUTBACK trial**), which is being performed in Australia, New Zealand, India, the United States, and Canada (233). Patients with FIGO stages IB1 and positive nodes, IB2, IIA, IIB, and IVA, are being randomized to either (a) standard *cisplatin*-based concurrent chemoradiation or (b) standard *cisplatin*-based concurrent chemoradiation followed by four cycles of *paclitaxel/carboplatin*. **The primary objective of the trial is to determine whether the addition of adjuvant chemotherapy to standard *cisplatin*-based concurrent chemoradiation improves overall survival.** Secondary objectives are to compare PFS, treatment-related toxicity, patterns of disease-recurrence, quality of life, psychosexual health, and the association between radiation protocol compliance and outcomes.

Tumor Heterogeneity of Stage III Cervical Cancer

Stage III cervical cancer is a heterogeneous disease. Stage IIIA disease involves extension to the lower third of the vagina, without extension to the pelvic sidewall, while **there are two criteria for the diagnosis of stage IIIB: (i) tumor fixation to the pelvic sidewall** or **(ii) the presence of hydronephrosis.** The latter may be due to ureteric obstruction from tumor extension or from enlarged lymph nodes.

A study of 407 patients with stage III cervical cancer from South Korea reported that **more than half the patients with stage IIIA disease had involvement of only the lower third of the vagina, without parametrial extension** (234). **They also had smaller tumor size (<6 cm) than patients with stage IIIB disease.**

In a study of 539 patients with stage IIIB disease, the GOG reported that hydronephrosis was present in 238 patients (44.2%). Relief of ureteric obstruction was associated with improved outcome (235).

When the tumor is not fixed to the pelvic sidewall and the level of ureteric obstruction is above the main tumor mass, it is most likely the result of external ureteric compression from enlarged pelvic or para-aortic lymph nodes. **Resection of these nodes via an extraperitoneal approach before radiation therapy can markedly improve survival** (104,170).

If bulky nodal metastases are not resected, survival is significantly compromised. The Mallindk-rodt Institute of Radiology in St. Louis reported that PFS at 5 years was 35% in patients with hydronephrosis and tumor fixed to the pelvic sidewall but decreased to 23% for 16 patients who presented with hydronephrosis without sidewall fixation ($p < 0.001$) (236). **When the level of ureteric obstruction was below the pelvic brim, 5-year PFS was 39%, but this fell to 22% when the obstruction was above the brim ($p = 0.02$).**

Patients with bilateral hydronephrosis and a creatinine clearance <50 mL/min should be considered for elective ureteral stenting before the commencement of radiation therapy (237).

Extended-Field Radiation

Clinical staging fails to detect extension of disease to the para-aortic lymph nodes in approximately 17% of patients with stage IIB disease and 29% with stage III (Table 8.4). Such patients will have a "geographic" treatment failure if standard radiation therapy ports are used, so **pretreatment identification of positive para-aortic nodes is important so that extended-field radiation can be given.**

Surgical staging has been largely replaced by scanning with PET and MRI for locally advanced cervical cancer (247). Narayan reported that nodal status on PET was the best prognostic factor in locally advanced disease treated with chemoradiation, and was superior to FIGO staging. Tumor volume measured from MRI was an important predictor of locoregional relapse.

Chemoradiation and intensity-modulated radiation techniques have replaced standard extended-field radiation. **Distant spread remains a problem for this group of patients but a significant proportion with positive para-aortic nodes can be salvaged** (Table 8.12). Disease-free survival appears to be higher when compared to historical controls (243–246).

The RTOG in the United States conducted a randomized trial of prophylactic para-aortic radiation (4,500 cGy) in 330 patients with stages IB and IIA (>4 cm) or IIB cervical cancer (248). Patients with lymphangiographic or surgical evidence of para-aortic nodal involvement were excluded. **Significantly better 5-year survival rates (66% vs. 55%) were demonstrated for the patients receiving extended-field radiation therapy.** In addition, patients treated with pelvic radiation alone had a higher risk of distant failure (32% vs. 25%). Severe gastrointestinal morbidity was more common in the group receiving extended-field therapy but was mainly seen in patients having previous abdominal surgery. As mentioned earlier, **for patients without proven para-aortic nodal disease, the RTOG study reported in 1999 demonstrated that pelvic radiation plus concurrent chemotherapy was superior to prophylactic extended-field radiation without chemotherapy** (224).

The GOG conducted a trial of extended-field chemoradiation for patients with biopsy-proven para-aortic lymph node metastases (238). The radiation dose to the para-aortic area was 4,500 cGy, and the chemotherapeutic regime was *5-fluorouracil* 1,000 mg/m^2/d for 96 hours and

Table 8.12 Extended-Field Chemoradiation for Patients with Positive Common or Para-aortic Lymph Nodes

Author	Number of Patients	Pelvic Recurrence	Distant Recurrence	Overall Survival
Varia et al., 1998 (238)	86	27 (31.4%)	36 (41.9%)	39% at 36 mos
Grigsby et al., 2001 (239)	30	NS	NS	29% at 48 mos
Small et al., 2007 (240)	26	2 (7.7%)	14 (53.8%)	60% at 18 mos
Beriwal et al., 2007 (241)	10	0 (0%)	5 (50%)	50% at 24 mos
Kim et al., 2009 (242)	33	6 (18.2%)	6 (18.2%)	47% at 60 mos
Walker et al., 2009 (243)	27	NS	10 (37%)	45% at 60 mos
Rajasooriyar et al., 2011 (244)	39	11 (28.2%)	19 (48.7%)	26% at 60 mos
Kazumoto et al., 2011 (245)	16	1 (6.3%)	8 (50%)	56% at 48 mos
Zhang et al., 2012 (246)	58	2 (3.4%)	16 (27.6%)	71% at 34 mos
Total	325	49/268 (18.3%)	114/295 (38.6%)	

NS, not stated.

cisplatin 50 mg/m^2 in weeks 1 and 5. There were 86 evaluable patients with stages IB to IVA disease, and **the 3-year overall survival and PFS were 39% and 34%, respectively**. Severe acute toxicity was mainly gastrointestinal (18.6%) and hematologic (15%), and the major late morbidity was gastrointestinal (14% actuarial risk at 4 years).

Subsequently, the GOG reported a phase I/II study of extended-field chemoradiation in patients with para-aortic metastases to determine the maximum tolerated dose (MTD) of concomitant weekly *paclitaxel* and *cisplatin*. The MTD was determined to be *cisplatin* 40 mg/m^2 (maximum dose of 70 mg) and *paclitaxel* 40 mg/m^2 for 6 weeks. They were encouraged by improved survival compared to historical controls, but suggested that central radiation dose reduction should be considered in the next trial to decrease late toxicity (243).

Plan of Management for Advanced Cervical Cancer

In view of the aforementioned results, the current approach to patients with advanced cervical cancer at the Royal Hospital for Women in Sydney is summarized in Figure 8.18. All patients are subjected to a PET/CT scan. If there are distant metastases, palliative pelvic radiation is given. **Pretreatment laparotomy is undertaken if there is (i) adnexal pathology, (ii) pelvic or para-aortic lymph nodes at least 2 cm diameter, and (iii) no distant metastases. Enlarged nodes are resected via an extraperitoneal approach because of the evidence strongly suggesting that such an approach converts the prognosis to that of patients with micrometastases** (104,143,170). Patients with proven positive para-aortic nodes are given extended-field radiation with weekly *cisplatin* 30 to 40 mg/m^2, and all other patients are given pelvic chemoradiation.

Stage IVA Disease with Vesicovaginal or Rectovaginal Fistula

An occasional patient in developed countries has a vesicovaginal or rectovaginal fistula at presentation. If a PET scan demonstrates no evidence of systemic disease, these patients are suitable for primary pelvic exenteration.

Prognosis

The survival of patients with cervical cancer according to the *Annual Report on the Results of Treatment in Gynaecological Cancer* is shown in Table 8.13 (249). Older patients have a lower survival for any given stage.

Posttreatment Surveillance

After chemoradiation, the patient should be monitored monthly for the first 3 months. Regression may continue throughout this period, but if any progression of disease occurs, histologic confirmation should be obtained and consideration given to surgery. **Some authorities have recommended a postchemoradiation PET scan at about 3 to 4 months** (250,251). A Melbourne group has reported a low rate of recurrence in patients with a complete metabolic response on PET (251).

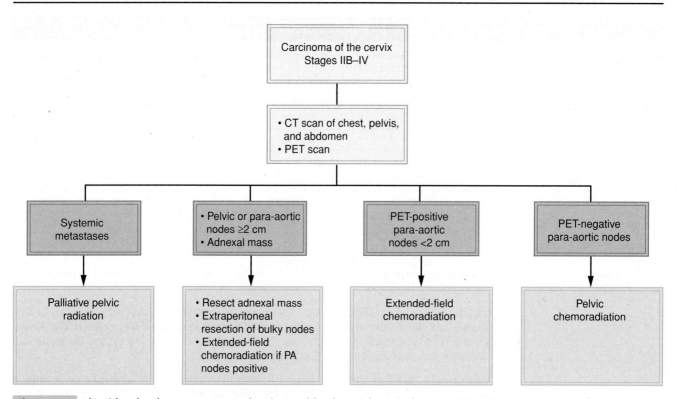

Figure 8.18 **Algorithm for the management of patients with advanced cervical cancer.** RT, radiation therapy.

After the immediate postradiation surveillance or postoperative checkup, patients are usually seen every 3 months until 2 years, and every 6 months until 5 years. Continued annual cytologic screening provides a low yield in women who have remained disease-free for 5 years (252), but these patients remain at increased risk for vulvar and vaginal neoplasia, so should probably be seen by their local doctor for a vaginal smear every 2 or 3 years.

Table 8.13 Carcinoma of the Cervix Uteri: Patients Treated in 1999 to 2001: Survival by FIGO Stage (*n* = 11,639)

		Overall Survival Rates (%)				
Stage	**Patients**	**1-Year**	**2-Year**	**3-Year**	**4-Year**	**5-Year**
Stage IA1	829	99.8	99.5	98.3	97.5	97.5
Stage IA2	275	98.5	96.9	95.2	94.8	94.8
Stage IB1	3,020	98.2	95	92.6	90.7	89.1
Stage IB2	1,090	95.8	88.3	81.7	78.8	75.7
Stage IIA	1,007	96.1	88.3	81.5	77	73.4
Stage IIB	2,510	91.7	79.8	73	69.3	65.8
Stage IIIA	211	76.7	59.8	54	45.1	39.7
Stage IIIB	2,028	77.9	59.5	51	46	41.5
Stage IVA	326	51.9	35.1	28.3	22.7	22
Stage IVB	343	42.2	22.7	16.4	12.6	9.3

From **Quinn MA, Benedet J, Odicino F, et al.** Carcinoma of the cervix uteri: FIGO 26th annual report on the results of treatment in gynecological cancer. *Int J Gynecol Obstet.* 2006;95:S43–S103, with permission.

The role of routine follow-up has been questioned because most recurrences are detected at self-referral because of symptoms. Nevertheless, follow-up allows psychosocial support for the patient, as well as data collection; in a Dutch study, 32% of all cases of recurrence were diagnosed at routine follow-up (253). The mean disease-free interval was 18 months.

At each visit, patients should be questioned about symptoms, and physical examination should include assessment of the supraclavicular and inguinal nodes, as well as abdominal and recto-vaginal examination. A Pap smear should be obtained at each visit. Chen et al. (254) reported that **72% of vaginal recurrences were asymptomatic,** and most had an abnormal cytologic smear. The others were detected by noting ulceration on visual inspection or by palpation of a nodule or cuff induration.

Whole-body FDG–PET appears to be a sensitive and specific tool for the detection of recurrent cervical cancer in patients who have clinical findings suspicious for recurrence (255,256). It has also been reported to be a **sensitive modality for the detection of recurrent cervical cancer in asymptomatic patients** (256), **and these patients may have a more favourable prognosis** (250). A study of 121 consecutive patients from the Republic of Korea reported a sensitivity of 96.1%, a specificity of 84.4%, and an accuracy of 91.7% for detection of recurrent disease (256).

Nonsquamous Histologic Types

Adenocarcinoma

Adenocarcinomas represent 20–25% of cervical cancers in the industrialized countries. In the United States, the age-adjusted incidence rates for adenocarcinoma have increased by 29.1% since the mid-1970s, and the proportion of adenocarcinomas relative to squamous carcinomas has increased by 95.2% (257). Age-adjusted cervical adenocarcinoma incidence rates have also increased throughout Europe, particularly in younger women (258).

Most of this relative increase is related to a decreasing incidence of squamous carcinomas secondary to screening programs, which are more effective in detecting squamous precursors (258,259). In contrast to squamous lesions, **smoking does not increase the risk of adenocarcinomas, but obesity does** (259,260). Squamous and adenocarcinomas also differ in their HPV status. Castellsague et al. (260) reported that HPV-16 and HPV-18 were present in 82% of adenocarcinomas worldwide, while **in the United States, data suggest that HPV-18 accounts for about 50% of adenocarcinomas, compared to only 15% of squamous lesions** (261). Management of adenocarcinomas has generally been the same as for their squamous counterpart. **There are no randomized trials specifically of adenocarcinomas.**

Whereas squamous cancers disseminate mainly via lymphatics, **there may be a greater tendency for adenocarcinomas to disseminate hematogenously** (259,262–264). This seems to be particularly true *after* lymphatic dissemination, because **among patients with positive nodes, adenocarcinomas have a significantly reduced survival compared to squamous lesions** (257,259,265). Other evidence in support of increased hematogenous spread includes (i) the largest series of surgically treated cervical cancers demonstrated **a significantly higher rate of ovarian metastases in patients with adenocarcinomas (5% vs. 0.8%; $p < 0.01$)** (263), and **(ii)** a study of 367 adenocarcinomas from the M D Anderson Hospital reported **higher rates of distant metastases for patients with stages II (46% vs. 13%) and stage III disease (38% vs. 21%), when compared to squamous cancers of a similar stage** (262).

Adenocarcinomas are generally regarded as being more radioresistant than squamous carcinomas. In the Italian randomized study of radical surgery versus radiation therapy for stages IB to IIA cervical cancer, 46 of 343 patients (13.4%) had adenocarcinomas (92). Surgery and radiation therapy were found to be identical in terms of 5-year survival and disease-free survival rates for the entire group, but for patients with adenocarcinomas, surgery was significantly better in terms of both overall survival (79% vs. 59%, $p = 0.05$) and disease-free survival rates (66% vs. 47%, $p = 0.02$). When chemotherapy is added to the radiation, survival seems to be comparable, and the greater the number of cycles of chemotherapy, the better the survival (209).

Researches in the Netherlands have shown that pretreatment serum CA125 levels are of prognostic significance for adenocarcinomas (266). The 5-year survival rate for stage IB adenocarcinomas was 52.4% when CA125 levels were elevated versus 95.6% when normal levels were present ($p < 0.01$). Similarly, 42% of patients with elevated serum CA125 levels had lymph node metastases versus 4% when normal levels were found ($p = 0.012$). **The presence of positive peritoneal cytology has also been reported to be an independent prognostic factor for patients with adenocarcinomas** (267).

Adenosquamous Carcinoma

Adenosquamous carcinomas represent approximately 20–30% of all adenocarcinomas of the cervix. **Some studies report a poorer outcome** (195–197). Farley et al. (197) investigated 185 women with pure adenocarcinomas (AC) and 88 women with adenosquamous carcinomas (ASC). They reported no difference in survival for patients with FIGO stage I disease (AC, 89%; ASC 86%; $p = 0.64$), but a significantly decreased median and overall survival for adenosquamous carcinoma in patients with advanced disease (FIGO stages II to IV).

In a series of surgically staged IB cases, Helm et al. (268) matched 38 patients with adenosquamous carcinomas with patients with other histologic subtypes of adenocarcinoma with respect to stage, lesion size, nodal status, grade of adenocarcinoma, and age at diagnosis. Diagnosis was based on hematoxylin and eosin staining without use of mucin staining. Glassy cell carcinomas were included. **Overall 5-year survival and disease-free survival rates for the matched adenosquamous and adenocarcinomas were not significantly different (83% vs. 90% and 78% vs. 81%, respectively), but the mean time to recurrence was significantly shorter in the adenosquamous group: 11 versus 32 months ($p = 0.003$).** In addition, six patients with adenosquamous carcinomas could not be matched. Five of these had positive nodes in association with lesions measuring between 2 and 4 cm in diameter, and one had an 8-cm lesion with negative nodes.

Similar findings were reported from the M.D. Anderson Cancer Center comparing 29 patients with stage IB1 adenosquamous carcinoma with 97 patients with stage IB1 adenocarcinoma of the cervix undergoing radical hysterectomy. The authors reported no difference in recurrence rates between the two histologic groups, but the **time to recurrence was shorter for patients with adenosquamous carcinoma (7.9 months vs. 15 months; $p = 0.01$)** (198).

A study of 163 adenocarcinomas and adenosquamous carcinomas with Stages IA2 to IIB disease treated by radical hysterectomy, with or without adjuvant radiation, found no difference in recurrence rates or patterns of recurrence between the two groups, in both the low-risk and intermediate-/high-risk groups (199).

Glassy Cell Carcinoma

In 1956, Glucksman and Cherry (269) defined "glassy cell" carcinoma of the cervix as **a poorly differentiated adenosquamous carcinoma, the cells of which had a moderate amount of cytoplasm and a typical "ground glass" appearance.** Survival was poor, regardless of the mode of therapy.

Other small series have suggested that survival is not significantly decreased when compared to other adenocarcinomas (270,271). A 2002 series of 22 patients from the University of Washington reported an overall survival of 73%, with the survival for patients having stage I disease being 86% (12 of 14) (271). Pelvic relapse was associated with LVSI, deep stromal invasion, and large tumor size.

Chemotherapy may play a role in the management of these tumors. Adjuvant chemotherapy with *carboplatin* and *paclitaxel* after radical hysterectomy and pelvic lymphadenectomy has been reported to be successful in a small number of patients (272,273), while neoadjuvant chemotherapy followed by postpartum chemoradiation and chemotherapy for consolidation has been reported to have successfully treated a 30-year-old woman diagnosed with stage IIIB glassy cell carcinoma at 24 weeks' gestation. The patient received weekly *cisplatin* and second weekly *vincristine* for 6 weeks, and three cycles of *carboplatin* and *paclitaxel* following her postpartum chemoradiation (274).

Radical vaginal trachelectomy or cone biopsy and laparoscopic pelvic lymphadenectomy has been reported in a limited number of patients with early stage disease (275,276).

Adenoma Malignum

The term **adenoma malignum of the cervix** was first used in 1870 by Gusserow to describe a very highly differentiated adenocarcinoma. McKelvey and Goodlin (277) reported five cases in 1963, four of which were fatal within 4 years of presentation. They pointed out the deceptively benign histologic appearance of the tumor and stated: **"If a lesion can be recognized as malignant by the usual criteria for adenocarcinoma of the cervix, it should be excluded from the adenoma malignum group."** McKelvey and Goodlin suggested that these tumors were radioresistant.

In 1975, Silverberg and Hurt (278) reported five additional cases. All patients were treated by modern radiotherapeutic techniques, and four of the five were long-term survivors. The authors believed that, with proper therapy, the tumor was no more malignant than might be expected for a highly differentiated adenocarcinoma, and they suggested the name **minimal deviation adenocarcinoma**.

An association has been noted with Peutz–Jeghers syndrome, as well as with sex-cord tumors with annular tubules, a distinctive ovarian neoplasm with features intermediate between those of the granulosa and Sertoli cell type (279).

These tumors represent approximately 1% of adenocarcinomas of the cervix and occur mainly in the fifth and sixth decades (280). **Diagnosis is often delayed because Pap smears may be normal or show very minor abnormalities.** A recent meta-analysis reported precancerous or malignant cells present in Pap smears in only one-third of patients (281).

Clinically, **patients usually present with a watery or mucous discharge** or with abnormal uterine bleeding. On physical examination, the cervix is usually firm and indurated (281,282). **Ultrasonic examination reveals a multiloculated tumor in about two-thirds of cases** (283,284). Punch biopsy is not helpful, and **deep wedge or cone biopsy is necessary to demonstrate the depth of glandular penetration.** The disease is often misdiagnosed as some benign condition, and the true diagnosis becomes apparent only after the patient has undergone an extrafascial hysterectomy (284).

Radical hysterectomy, bilateral salpingo-oophorectomy, and pelvic lymphadenectomy are the treatments of choice for operable cases, and the prognosis for such cases appears to be very good (281,282,284). Adjuvant (chemo)radiation may be given postoperatively for high-risk features, such as positive nodes (284). For more advanced cases, lymph node metastases are common, and the overall prognosis is poor (281,285).

Adenoid Cystic Carcinoma

Adenoid cystic carcinoma is a rare tumor that occurs most frequently in the salivary glands but also in the respiratory tract, skin, mucous membranes of the head and neck, and the breast. **In the female genital tract, it occurs in Bartholin gland, the endometrium, and the cervix** (286). **These tumors usually occur in postmenopausal black women of high parity** (286,287). Most present with postmenopausal bleeding, but some may be suspected by the presence of small "undifferentiated" cells on a routine Pap smear (286). **Approximately half the cases are stage I at presentation, but overall survival is poor** (287).

For patients with stage IB disease, adjuvant radiation should be given for high-risk features after radical hysterectomy and pelvic lymphadenectomy (288). Prempree et al. (287), in a review of the literature, reported a 3- to 5-year survival rate of only 56.3% (9 of 16) for patients with stage I disease, regardless of the type of treatment. The survival rate for stage II disease was 27.3% (3 of 11), and no patient with stage III or IV disease survived. **Lung metastases were common, whereas the tumors spread locally by direct tissue invasion and perineural infiltration.**

Adenoid Basal Carcinoma

This is a rare tumor with an excellent prognosis. Most adenoid basal carcinomas have coexistent **in situ** or invasive squamous carcinoma, and 50% have coexistent in situ or invasive adenocarcinoma (289). The prognosis and treatment is usually dependent on any associated malignancy (290). **In its pure form, the disease is almost invariably confined to the cervix, invasion is usually superficial, and extrafascial or radical hysterectomy without lymphadenectomy is a reasonable treatment option.** In a review of 26 cases reported in the literature, only 1 died of disease (with lung metastases) (291).

Clear Cell Adenocarcinoma

Clear cell adenocarcinoma of the cervix was rare until 1970, when the incidence rose because of **its association with *in utero* exposure to *diethylstilbestrol* and related nonsteroidal estrogens before the eighteenth week of pregnancy** (292). These cancers affected particularly adolescents and young women, and among DES-exposed women, clear cell adenocarcinoma occured with an incidence of 1 in 1,000 (293).

A multi-institutional review of 34 cases in the post-DES era reported a median age of 53 years; DES exposure was confirmed in only 2 cases (6%) (294). All 26 patients with stage I or IIA disease underwent surgery, with or without adjuvant radiotherapy or chemotherapy, and 6 (23%) had positive lymph nodes. PFS for node-negative patients was 92% versus 31% for node-positive ($p < 0.001$).

Treatment should be similar to that for other adenocarcinomas. **Unlike clear cell carcinoma of the endometrium, which carries a much worse prognosis, clear cell adenocarcinoma of the cervix has a prognosis comparable to that of other adenocarcinomas** (294,295).

Villoglandular Papillary Adenocarcinoma

This uncommon lesion tends to occur in younger women and to have a more favorable prognosis. Young and Scully (296) reviewed their consultation files to report 13 cases. The patients' ages ranged from 23 to 54 years (average 33 years). Two of the patients were pregnant. Both were asymptomatic, both had a grossly abnormal-appearing cervix, and one had an abnormal Pap smear. Treatment ranged from cone biopsy for very superficial cases to radical hysterectomy and pelvic lymphadenectomy. With follow-up of 2 to 14 years, no recurrences were seen.

In the largest reported series by Jones et al. (297), **none of 24 cases had lymph-vascular invasion or lymph node metastases, and all patients remained free of disease with 7 to 77 months of follow-up.** However, lymph-vascular invasion, lymph node metastases, and death from disease have been reported, and these patients should generally be managed in the same way as other adenocarcinomas of the cervix (298,299).

Because of their generally excellent prognosis and young age at presentation, conservative management may be justified in selected patients who want to retain fertility (297).

Small-Cell, including Small-Cell Neuroendocrine Carcinoma

Small-cell cancers are a rare, heterogeneous group of tumors, representing 0.5–1% of all invasive cervical cancers (300). In a thorough evaluation of 2,201 invasive cervical cancers at the University of Kentucky Medical Center, Van Nagell et al. (191) noted 25 cases (1.1%) of small-cell carcinoma. They were characterized by a nuclear area of 160 μm^2 or less and a maximum nuclear diameter of 16.2 μm. **Thirty-three percent of the small-cell carcinomas stained positively for the neuroendocrine markers (neuron-specific enolase and chromogranin),** whereas the remainder stained only for epithelial markers such as cytokeratin and epithelial membrane antigen. **Both types of small-cell cancers had a higher frequency of LVSI, a significantly higher rate of recurrence, particularly to extrapelvic sites, and a lower survival rate.**

The neuroendocrine tumors arise from the argyrophil cells or APUD cells (amine precursor uptake and decarboxylation) in the cervix (300). None of the neuroendocrine tumors in the Kentucky series had clinical signs of a paraendocrine syndrome, although **these tumors may sometimes present with carcinoid syndrome,** and those patients have elevated levels of 5-hydroxy-indoleacetic acid in the urine.

An epidemiologic study using population-based data reported to the SEER program in the United States compared 239 cases of endocrine tumors of the cervix with 18,458 squamous cell carcinomas (301). Mean age at diagnosis was 49 years for the endocrine tumors versus 52 years for the squamous carcinomas ($p < 0.01$). **Endocrine tumors were more likely to present at a later FIGO stage ($p < 0.01$) and to have lymph node involvement at diagnosis** (57% vs. 18%, $p < 0.01$). **At all stages of disease, survival was worse for the women with endocrine tumors.**

A later study reviewing **SEER data from 1977 to 2003** identified 290 women (0.9%) with small-cell carcinoma of the cervix, 27,527 (83.3%) with squamous cell carcinoma, and 5,231 patients (15.8%) with adenocarcinoma (302). **Five-year survival for small-cell carcinoma (35.7%) was worse compared with squamous cell carcinoma (60.5%) and adenocarcinoma (69.7%).** They noted that small-cell carcinomas had a predilection for nodal and distant metastases, but there was decreased survival even in early stage, node-negative patients.

Because of the propensity of small-cell carcinoma for early systemic spread, chemotherapy is usually advocated in addition to surgery or radiation therapy. The group at the **Chang Gung Memorial Hospital in Taiwan** administered adjuvant chemotherapy to 23 consecutive patients with stage IB to II small-cell cervical cancer who had been treated primarily with radical hysterectomy (303). **Ten of 14 patients (71.4%) who received a combination of *vincristine*, *doxorubicin*, and *cyclophosphamide* alternating with *cisplatin* and *etoposide* had no evidence of disease during a median follow-up of 41 months,** whereas only 3 of 9 (33.3%) who received *cisplatin, vinblastine,* and *bleomycin (PVB)* survived. The survival rate was 70% for patients with negative lymph nodes and 35% for those with positive nodes ($p = 0.05$). All patients who died of disease had extrapelvic metastases.

A study from Ohio State University reported 26 patients with neuroendocrine cervical carcinomas diagnosed between 1990 and 2012 (304). **Small-cell histology was presented in 21 cases (80%), and mixed small and large-cell histology in 1 case (4%).** Eleven patients (42%) had stage 1 disease, 5 of whom were treated with neoadjuvant chemotherapy, (mainly *platinum/ etoposide* based), followed by radical hysterectomy and pelvic lymphadenectomy, and 6 of whom had primary surgery followed by chemotherapy. Four patients received adjuvant postoperative radiation. Nine of the 11 patients (82%) were free of disease at the last follow-up. One of the patients who died declined adjuvant therapy, and the other had peritoneal metastases. Patients with stages II to IV had an overall survival of about 12%.

Large-Cell Neuroendocrine Carcinoma

Large-cell neuroendocrine carcinomas of the cervix are a rare and aggressive type of cervical cancer. A recent literature review identified 62 cases in the English literature and SEER database (305). The median age of the patients was 37 years (range 21 to 75), and 58% had stage I disease. Seventy-three percent underwent primary surgery and 62% recurred or died of disease. **Earlier stage ($p < 0.00001$) and the addition of chemotherapy ($p = 0.04$) were associated with improved survival.** Both platinum agents ($p = 0.034$) and the combination of platinum and etoposide ($p = 0.027$), given pre- or postoperatively, were associated with improved survival.

Serous Carcinoma

This tumor resembles microscopically its serous counterparts elsewhere in the female genital tract and peritoneum. Zhou et al. (306) reported a series of 17 cases. There was a bimodal age distribution, with one peak occurring before the age of 40 years and the second peak after 65 years. Eight patients (47%) had a polypoid or exophytic mass, two patients (12%) had an ulcerated lesion, and no abnormality was detected in seven patients (41%). Two tumors were stage IA, 12 were stage IB, 2 were stage II, and 1 was stage III. Seven tumors (41%) were mixed with another histologic subtype of cervical adenocarcinoma, most commonly low-grade villoglandular adenocarcinoma. Eight patients (47%) were alive without evidence of disease with a mean follow-up of 56 months. The researchers concluded that **the tumors can behave aggressively with supradiaphragmatic metastases and a rapidly fatal course when diagnosed at an advanced stage, but the outcome for patients with stage I tumors was similar to that of patients with cervical adenocarcinomas of the usual type.** A similar conclusion was reached in a recent Japanese study of 12 patients (307).

Sarcoma

Cervical sarcomas are a rare, heterogeneous group of tumors with a generally poor prognosis. The **SEER database** was used by a New York group to identify all women with a primary cervical sarcoma diagnosed between 1988 and 2005, and to compare them to patients with cervical squamous and adenocarcinomas (308). **Among 33,074 patients with invasive cervical neoplasms, 323 (1%) had a sarcoma. Carcinosarcomas were the most common, accounting for 40% of the cases ($N = 128$). Adenosarcomas and leiomyosarcomas each accounted for 21% of cases ($N = 67$),** rhabdomyosarcomas for 9% (30 cases), and sarcomas not otherwise stated (NOS) for 7% (22 cases). Endometrial stromal, spindle cell, epithelioid and fibrosarcomas each had fewer than 5 cases.

Patients with cervical sarcomas tended to be younger, and to have more advanced disease at diagnosis. Women with carcinosarcomas were the oldest group (median age 64 years), followed by leiomyosarcomas (49 years), adenosarcomas (45 years), and rhabdomyosarcomas (27 years). Among patients undergoing lymphadenectomy, 19% with carcinosarcomas had nodal metastases, compared to 3% with adenosarcomas and none of the patients with leiomyosarcomas. **In multivariate analysis, there was no difference in cancer-specific survival among any of the sarcoma subtypes, but sarcomas generally carried a worse prognosis than squamous cancers.**

The 5-year survival for patients with stage IB squamous carcinoma was 80%, which was significantly better than the 67% for patients with a sarcoma (308).

A molecular analysis of eight cervical carcinosarcomas identified human papillomavirus DNA in all eight cases, supporting the theory that like uterine carcinosarcomas, the cervical counterpart may represent a metaplastic tumor (308).

Rhabdomyosarcoma, including Sarcoma Botryoides

Rhabdomyosarcomas are malignant skeletal muscle tumors. They are rare in adults, but account for about 50% of soft tissue sarcomas in children (309). The Intergroup Rhabdomyosarcoma Study Group has divided these tumors into **three major histologic subtypes: Embryonal, alveolar, and undifferentiated. The embryonal subtype has been further subdivided into classic, botryoid, and spindle cell** (310). **Most cervical embryonal rhabdomyosarcomas have the gross and microscopic features of the sarcoma botryoides variant** (311).

A recent review of the database at the M.D. Anderson Cancer Center from 1980 to 2010 revealed 11 cases of cervical rhabdomyosarcoma (310). The median age was 18.4 years, and the commonest presenting symptom was vaginal bleeding. Eight patients (73%) presented with stage 1B disease, and **8 (73%) presented with the embryonal (botryoid) histologic subtype.** Nine patients (82%) received multimodal therapy consisting of conservative surgery with chemotherapy, radiation therapy, or both, and all patients were without evidence of disease at the completion of treatment. Only two patients (18%) recurred, and one (9%) died of disease, confirming the **good prognosis for patients with cervical rhabdomyosarcoma treated with multimodal therapy. Two (18%) of the patients had Sertoli–Leydig tumors, and the authors suggested that there may be a genetic link between these two rare tumors.**

A series of 14 cervical embryonal rhabdomyosarcomas was recently reported from St Louis (311). The median age of the patients was 13 years, with a range of 9 months to 32 years. **Twelve cases (86%) presented as a polyp, and had the histologic pattern of the sarcoma botryoides variant;** two patients had an infiltrative mass in the cervix. Two patients had a pleuropulmonary blastoma and one a Sertoli–Leydig cell tumor and nodular hyperplasia of the thyroid. The latter two conditions are part of the **familial pleuropulmonary blastoma tumor predisposition and dysplasia syndrome.** Twelve of the 14 patients (86%) were disease free after conservative surgery and chemotherapy.

In 1988, Daya and Scully (312) **reviewed 13 cases of sarcoma botryoides.** Their ages ranged from 12 to 26 years, with a mean of 18 years. All had polypoid lesions and presented with vaginal bleeding, "something" protruding from the introitus, or both. The patients were treated with a variety of operative procedures, with or without adjuvant chemotherapy, the operative procedures ranging from cervical polypectomy to hysterectomy with pelvic and para-aortic node dissection. **Twelve of the 13 patients (92%) were alive and well 1 to 8 years after surgery.**

Results from the **Intergroup Rhabdomyosarcoma Study Group's** four treatment protocols were summarized by Arndt et al. (313) in 2001. There were 151 patients entered into the four protocols, and 23 tumors (15%) arose from the cervix. **The recommended approach to management was conservative surgery and chemotherapy—primarily** *vincristine, actinomycin D,* **and** *cyclophosphamide*—**with or without radiation therapy.** The overall 5-year survival for the 151 patients was 82%. For patients with localized embryonal botryroid tumors, there was no significant difference in 5-year survival among patients with tumors at different sites. **Patients with more advanced disease should be treated initially with chemotherapy, and surgical excision should attempt to conserve the function of the bladder, rectum, vagina, and ovaries if possible** (314).

Lymphoma

Cervical lymphomas are rare. Of 9,500 women with lymphomas reported by the Armed Forces Institute of Pathology, only 6 (0.06%) arose primarily in the cervix (315).

Patients usually present with abnormal vaginal bleeding, and clinically the cervix is expanded by a subepithelial mass without ulceration or fungation.

Histologic diagnosis can be difficult (316), but it is important to distinguish malignant lymphoma from undifferentiated carcinoma or sarcoma because **cervical lymphoma can be successfully treated in spite of locally advanced disease** (317). **There is no evidence that radical gynecologic surgery is advantageous** (318).

An Australian study identified 43 cases of cervical lymphoma from 2000 to 2010. **Diffuse large B-cell lymphomas were the most frequently seen** (319). No optimal treatment could be defined, but chemotherapy alone was considered a good option, particularly for young women who wanted to retain fertility. **The recommended regimen was R-CHOP, which is** *rituximab,* a monoclonal antibody to CD20, *cyclophosphamide, doxorubicin, vincristine,* and *prednisolone.* **Prognosis was good and comparable with nodal lymphomas.**

Verrucous Carcinoma

This **slow-growing, locally aggressive, papillomatous lesion** was first reported in the cervix in 1972 (320).

In a **literature review** in 1988, Crowther et al. (321) reported 34 cases of cervical verrucous carcinoma. The age of the women ranged from 30 to 84 years (average 51 years), and only two had a past history of genital warts. Symptoms included vaginal discharge (42%) and abnormal bleeding (50%); **only 35% had an abnormal Pap smear. Colposcopy was not helpful because the lesion looked like a large condyloma acuminatum.** The lesions were confined to the cervix in 41% of cases, involved the vagina in 36%, and the parametrium in 23%. One case invaded the bladder.

Radical surgery is the mainstay of treatment. Radicality of surgery varied in the cases reviewed by Crowther et al. (321), but of 14 patients having radical hysterectomy (with vaginectomy in 3 cases), recurrence occurred in 6 (43%). Three of the recurrences were cured with radiation therapy or exenterative surgery. **Radiation therapy was used as a primary or secondary treatment in 17 cases, and recurrences occurred in 10 of these (59%).** Lymph node metastases were found in two patients and pulmonary metastases in a third, but careful histologic evaluation at autopsy showed nests of classic squamous carcinoma cells invading the stroma in two of these cases. Overall, recurrent or persistent disease was noted in 21 of the 34 cases (62%), with 82% of relapses occurring within 8 months.

Melanoma

Melanoma of the cervix originates from melanocytes that are present in the urogenital epithelium in about 3% of women (322). It is a rare entity, and a metastatic lesion must be excluded. Literature reviews and case studies have been reported by Mordel et al. (323) in 1989, Santosa et al. (324) in 1990, and Piura (322) in 2008. These tumors have in general been reported to occur in the seventh and eighth decades of life, and most lesions present with abnormal vaginal bleeding. **Macroscopically, the tumors are strongly colored, polypoid masses, and most patients have FIGO stage I or II disease at diagnosis. Recommended treatment is usually radical hysterectomy with or without pelvic lymphadenectomy. Adjuvant radiation may improve local control if the surgical margins are close.** The 5-year survival rate is poor, not exceeding 40% for stage I disease and reaching only 14% in stage II (323).

Metastatic Carcinoma

Metastasis of malignant epithelial tumors to the uterine cervix from extragenital sites is a rare occurrence. **A study of 149 tumors metastatic to the female genital tract from extragenital primaries reported that the ovary (75.8%) and vagina (13.4%) were the most common sites of spread, while only 3.4% involved the cervix** (325).

Lemoine and Hall (326) reviewed the **surgical pathology files of the London Hospital for 65 years** from 1919 to 1984 and found only 33 cases of cervical metastases. Cases that involved direct extension from a primary site, such as the endometrium or rectum, were excluded. They also reviewed the literature for individual case reports and small series. **Documented primary sites of diseases included stomach (25 cases), ovary (23), colon (21), breast (14), kidney (1), renal pelvis (1), carcinoid (1), and pancreas (1).**

The patients almost invariably present with vaginal bleeding, and the histologic features of the cervical biopsy lead to a search for an asymptomatic primary tumor.

Cancer of the Cervical Stump

Subtotal hysterectomy is less commonly performed today than in the past. However, a 2004 study from Brazil reported 14 cases (3.6%) out of 363 cervical cancers seen between 1985 and 1999 (327). Fibroids were the main reason for the subtotal hysterectomy, but the authors commented that **leaving the cervix should be avoided whenever possible in populations with restricted access to cervical screening programs** (327).

When invasive cancer arises in a cervical stump, the principles of treatment are the same as those for an intact uterus. The technique for abdominal radical trachelectomy is essentially the same as for radical hysterectomy, the only difficulty being the maintenance of adequate traction on the stump. Sometimes the bladder may be adherent over the stump, necessitating careful dissection.

The ability to deliver an adequate dose of radiation to patients with advanced disease depends on the length of the cervical canal and is compromised if the canal is less than 2 cm long. Although 5-year survival rates compare favorably to those in patients with an intact uterus, complication rates are higher because of the previous surgery and the sometimes compromised methods of radiation therapy (328).

Invasive Cancer Found after Simple Hysterectomy

When invasive cervical cancer is discovered after simple hysterectomy, **the treatment options include full pelvic radiation or radical surgery consisting of radical parametrectomy, upper vaginectomy, and pelvic lymphadenectomy.**

At the Royal Hospital for Women, radical surgery is preferred as long as a CT scan of the chest, pelvis, and abdomen or a PET scan shows no evidence of metastatic disease, and there are no high-risk features in the hysterectomy specimen (i.e., positive surgical margins, tumor deeply infiltrating, or prominent vascular space invasion), for which adjuvant radiation would otherwise be recommended. In these cases, primary pelvic chemoradiation is preferable.

The operation is considerably more difficult than a radical hysterectomy, the main difficulty being the identification of the bladder, which is usually adherent over the vaginal vault. Operating in the low lithotomy position to allow use of a metal instrument (e.g., narrow malleable retractor) to push up on the vault from below facilitates identification of the bladder. The Mayo Clinic reporteded 27 patients undergoing reoperation (329). Ureterovaginal fistulas developed in 2 of the 27 cases (7%), but the 5-year absolute survival rate was 82%. The group at Irvine, California, reported 18 patients, with a median follow-up of 72 months (330). The overall actuarial survival was 89%. Morbidity was comparable to that of patients undergoing primary radical hysterectomy.

Hopkins et al. (331) **reported 92 patients who were treated by primary radiation therapy.** Fifty-seven patients with stage I squamous cell carcinoma had a 5-year survival rate of 85%, whereas 27 patients with stage I adenocarcinoma had a 5-year survival rate of 42%. **The researchers suggested that alternative approaches should be investigated for adenocarcinomas.**

A study from Chandigarh, India, reported 105 patients who were found to have invasive cervical cancer following total ($n = 82$) or subtotal ($n = 23$) hysterectomy (332). All patients were treated with external-beam radiation, with or without intracavitary radiation. The 5-year overall survival, disease-free survival, and pelvic control rates for all patients were 55.2%, 53.3%, and 72%, respectively. **Adverse prognostic factors included absence of brachytherapy, hemoglobin <10 g%, and interval between surgery and radiation longer than 80 days.**

Coexistent Pelvic Mass

A pelvic mass may be identified clinically or on a staging CT scan of the pelvis and abdomen.

Uterine Masses

Solid masses of uterine origin are usually leiomyomas and do not need further investigation. **If the uterus is expanded by a pyometra or hematometra, the uterus must be drained if the preferred treatment is radiation.** Repeated dilatation of the cervix and aspiration of pus may be necessary every 2 to 3 days if there is ultrasonic evidence of a further collection. Broad-spectrum antibiotics should be used to cover *Bacteroides,* anaerobic *Streptococcus,* and aerobic coliforms. **Active infection decreases the response to radiation and may be exacerbated into a systemic infection if brachytherapy rods are packed into the uterus.**

Adnexal Masses

Coexistent adnexal masses must be explored and a histologic diagnosis obtained. A laparoscopic approach may be appropriate, particularly if the risk of malignancy is low. Benign adnexal masses can be surgically excised. Inflammatory masses can be excised and an omental carpet used to prevent bowel adhesions. Malignant masses require surgical staging or cytoreductive surgery, depending on the individual case.

Cervical Bleeding

Torrential bleeding may occasionally follow biopsy or pelvic examination, particularly with friable, advanced cancer. **A wide gauze bandage, soaked in Monsel solution (ferric subsulfate) and**

tightly packed against the cervix, usually controls the bleeding. It should be changed after 48 hours. If control of the bleeding is not achieved, consideration should be given to embolization of the uterine arteries (333), although this approach may increase tumor hypoxia, thereby decreasing radiosensitivity.

Commencement of external-beam therapy controls the bleeding within a few days. Daily fractions may be increased to 300 to 500 cGy for 2 or 3 days.

Recurrent Cervical Cancer

Treatment of recurrent disease depends on the mode of primary therapy and the site of recurrence. **If the disease recurs in the pelvis after primary radiation therapy, most patients require some type of pelvic exenteration** (see Chapter 23), although an occasional patient may be cured by radical hysterectomy.

Eifel et al. investigated the time course of central pelvic recurrence in 2,997 patients treated with radiation therapy for stages I and II squamous cell carcinoma of the cervix at the M.D. Anderson Cancer Center in Houston (334). Recurrence rates were 6.8%, 7.8%, and 9.6% at 5, 10, and 20 years, respectively. **The risk of central pelvic recurrence was independently correlated with tumor size ($p < 0.0001$) but not with FIGO stage.** Although after 3 years the risk of central recurrence was low, it continued to be slightly greater for patients with tumors ≥5 cm diameter ($p = 0.001$). **Patients with recurrence after 36 months had a significantly better survival following subsequent therapy.**

With pelvic recurrence after primary surgery, radiation therapy is the treatment of first choice. Grigsby (335) reported 36 patients who received external beam and brachytherapy for recurrent cervical cancer following radical hysterectomy. Tumor was recurrent in the central pelvis in 33 patients (92%) and on the pelvic sidewall in 3 cases. The overall 5- and 10-year survivals were 74% and 50%, respectively. Ten patients (28%) developed a further recurrence after irradiation, and seven (70%) of these had a pelvic component to the failure. Severe complications developed in four patients (11.1%), including one hip fracture, one bowel obstruction requiring a colostomy, and two fistulae. Using radiation with concurrent chemotherapy (*5-fluorouracil* with or without *mitomycin C*), Thomas et al. reported 8 of 17 patients (47%) alive and disease-free 21 to 58 months after therapy. The recurrent disease was present in the pelvis alone or pelvis and para-aortic nodes, and seven of the eight survivors had a component of pelvic sidewall disease (336).

Pulmonary metastases following primary radical hysterectomy have been reported in 6.4% of patients (24 of 377) with negative pelvic nodes and 11.3% of patients (16 of 142) with positive pelvic nodes (337). **When the lung was the only site of recurrence, a 5-year survival of 46% was achieved by surgical resection followed by chemotherapy in 12 patients who initially had negative pelvic nodes** and who now had one to three pulmonary metastases. Surgery was performed in the presence of unilateral or bilateral metastases.

Radical Hysterectomy for Recurrence

Selected patients with limited persistent or recurrent disease in the cervix after primary radiation therapy may be suitable for radical hysterectomy, with or without partial resection of bowel, bladder, or ureter. **The morbidity rate is high, but some patients can be cured without the need for a stoma.**

Rutledge et al. (338) from London, Ontario, reported data on 41 patients who underwent conservative surgery for postradiation recurrent or persistent cervical cancer. Thirteen patients who initially had FIGO stage IB or IIA disease underwent radical abdominal or radical vaginal hysterectomy. The 5-year survival rate for this group was 84%, and major morbidity occurred in 31% of cases. A second group of 20 patients had more advanced initial disease, and all underwent radical abdominal hysterectomy. This group had a 49% 5-year survival rate and a major morbidity rate of 50%. A third group of eight patients required an extended Wertheim's operation to encompass locally advanced disease involving the bladder base or parametrium. This group had a 5-year survival rate of 25% but experienced a 75% rate of major morbidity, including two treatment-related deaths. Fistula formation occurred in 26% of patients overall.

An Italian study of 34 patients reported an actuarial 5-year survival of 49% for the whole group, with major complications in 44% of cases and a fistula rate of 15% (339). Patients with FIGO stage IB–IIA disease at primary diagnosis, no clinical parametrial involvement, and small (≤4 cm) tumor diameter at the time of recurrence had a survival of 65% (11 of 17).

Conservative surgery is realistic only for patients with small disease confined to the cervix, preferably detected on PET scan or biopsy 4 to 6 months after primary radiation for bulky stage IB or IIA cervical cancer.

Chemotherapy

Patients with recurrent or metastatic cervical cancer are commonly symptomatic and may experience pain, anorexia, weight loss, vaginal bleeding, cachexia, and dyspnoea, among other symptoms. **The role of chemotherapy in such patients is palliation, with the primary objective to relieve symptoms and improve quality of life. A secondary objective is to prolong survival.**

Many factors influence the likelihood of response to chemotherapy, and these include performance status, patient age, histologic subtype, site of recurrence (lung vs. pelvis), number of metastatic sites, previous radiotherapy or chemotherapy, and interval from initial radiotherapy or chemoradiation (340–342). These factors should be taken into consideration when making treatment decisions because they can all influence the choice of treatment as well as the response rate.

A large number of chemotherapeutic agents from different classes have shown activity in patients with recurrent and/or metastatic cervical cancer, and a summary of the most relevant drugs is given in Table 8.14. These studies span the last 30 years and are a composite of many trials that have included very different patient subsets, making interpretation difficult.

Cisplatin **is the most active single agent, but** *paclitaxel, topotecan, vinorelbine, gemcitabine,* **and** *ifosfamide* **are also considered to be worthy of use in patients who would not be candidates for combination chemotherapy because of poor health.** Moreover, *paclitaxel, topotecan, vinorelbine, gemcitabine,* and *ifosfamide* are considered adequate candidates to be tested in combination with *cisplatin.* Although *gemcitabine* has not shown impressive activity as a single agent (<10% response rate), subjective improvement has been a universal finding; this, along with its attractive toxicity profile, has led to it being studied in combination with *cisplatin.*

Single agent *cisplatin* **became the standard of care after an initial study with 50 mg/m^2, given intravenously every 3 weeks, showed a response rate of 38%;** later studies did not lead to better outcomes, but showed more toxicity, when the dose intensity increased to more than 50 mg/m^2 every 3 weeks (342,343). In addition, a randomized study of two platinum analogs, *iproplatin* and *carboplatin,* suggested that these compounds were less active than *cisplatin* (344). Therefore, this 3-weekly low-dose *cisplatin* initially became the reference arm in randomized trials (Table 8.15).

The duration of the objective responses with *cisplatin* **has been disappointing (4 to 6 months), as has been the duration of survival. Median survival was only in the order of 7 months.** Nevertheless, there was a suggestion that treatment with *cisplatin* had a positive effect on survival. In a direct comparison of *cisplatin* (plus *methotrexate*) versus single agent treatment with *hydroxyurea* (an inactive drug), a significant survival advantage was observed in those treated with *cisplatin* (345).

A large number of phase II studies and a smaller number of phase III studies have investigated a variety of *cisplatin*-based combinations in the treatment of patients with metastatic cervical cancer, and there have been several reviews (340–342,346–351). Traditionally, response rates or time to progression have been the end points of phase II studies, whereas progression-free and overall survival have been the primary end points of phase III trials. With respect to the phase III trials, quality-of-life assessment and patient-reported outcomes have received increasing attention in recent trials.

Response rates with combinations generally have been higher than with single agent chemotherapy, but a survival benefit has been difficult to demonstrate, whether the trials concerned doublets, triplets, or quadruplets (Table 8.15). A randomized comparison of *cisplatin* plus *paclitaxel* versus *cisplatin* alone demonstrated a doubling of the response rate and progression-free survival, but no difference in overall survival (352). Interestingly, despite being a more intensive regimen, the quality-of-life scores were not inferior with *cisplatin* plus *paclitaxel,* and therefor this regimen has become the preferred regimen in the United States. **Only the randomized trial investigating the combination of** *cisplatin* **plus topotecan versus** *cisplatin* **alone showed an overall survival benefit** (353).

Individual patients may show an exceptional sensitivity to platinum. Such patients, whether treated with single agent platinum or platinum combinations, may achieve a complete response that can be long-lasting. An occasional patient may even be cured (340,354).

Table 8.14 Active Single Chemotherapeutic Agents in Cervical Carcinoma (≥10% Response Rate)

Classes and Drugs	No. Response/No. Treated	Response Rate (%)	References
Alkylating agents			
Cyclophosphamide	36/271	13	340
Ifosfamide	45/171	26	340, 355, 356
Platinum compounds			
Cisplatin	238/968	24.5	340
Carboplatin	50/260	19	340
Antimetabolites			
5-Fluorouracil	36/270	13	340, 357
Capecitabine	4/26	15	358, 359
Tegafur (S-1)	11/36	30.5	360
Methotrexate	12/73	16	340
Pemetrexed	16/104	15	361–363
Antibiotics			
Doxorubicin	32/172	19	340
Epirubicin	24/88	27	340, 364
Pirarubicin	6/31	19	365
Bleomycin	19/176	11	340
Mitomycin C	11/75	15	340–366
Plant Alkaloids			
Vincristine	10/58	17	340
Vindesine	13/49	26.5	340
Vinorelbine	21/146	14	367–370
Paclitaxel (every 3 wks)	30/116	26	371–373
Docetaxel	4/39	10	374, 375
Topotecan (daily × 5 schedule)	13/83	16	376, 377
Irinotecan	36/209	17	378–382
Etoposide	6/61	10	383, 384
Teniposide	7/32	18	385

Other interesting observations from the randomized trials, as shown in Table 8.15, are (1) **the decline in response rate with *cisplatin* alone in recent trials,** which appears to parallel the number of patients who have been treated initially with *cisplatin*-based chemoradiation for their primary disease, possibly reflecting *cisplatin*-resistance in patients who relapse relatively early (342); (2) **a gradual improvement in overall survival over time,** probably a result of stricter eligibility criteria for entry into successive GOG trials (386,387); and (3) **the substitution of *carboplatin* for *cisplatin* (in the combination with *paclitaxel*),** as evaluated in the Japanese JCOG 0505 trial, without apparently compromising outcome (388). However, a secondary analysis of 117 patients from the same trial who had not received prior platinum revealed the *cisplatin/paclitaxel* doublet to be superior to *carboplatin/paclitaxel,* with a median overall survival of 23.2 months versus 13 months (HR 1.57; 95% CI 1.06 to 2.32).

Active research toward the development of efficacious non–*cisplatin*-based combinations is ongoing (351).

Table 8.15 Relevant Phase III Trials in Recurrent/Metastatic Cervical Cancer

First Authors (References)	Treatment	Number	RR % (CR %)	PFS (mos)	OS (mos)
Bonomi et al., 1985 (343)	P: 50 mg/m^2, q3w	150	20.7 (10)	3.7	7.1
	P: 100 mg/m^2, q3wks	166	31.4 (13)	4.6	7
	P: 20 mg/m^2/d × 5, q3wks	128	25 (9)	3.9	6.1
Omura et al., 1997 (390)	IP	151	31.1 (12.6)	4.6	8.3
	MP	140	17.8 (6.4)	3.2	8
	P	147	21.1 (9.5)	3.3	7.3
Vermorken et al., 2001 (389)	BEMP	143	42 (11)	5.3	10.1
	P	144	25 (7)	4.5	9.3
Bloss et al., 2002 (391)	IP	146	32 (NS)	4.6	8.5
	BIP	141	31.2 (NS)	5.1	8.4
Moore et al., 2004 (352)	PP	130	36 (15)	4.8	9.7
	P	134	19 (6)	2.8	8.8
Long et al., 2005 (353)	TP	147	27 (10.4)	4.6	9.4
	P	146	13 (2.9)	2.9	6.5
Monk et al., 2009 (386)	PP	103	29.1 (2.9)	5.8	12.9
	TP	111	23.4 (1.8)	4.6	10.3
	GP	112	22.3 (0.9)	4.7	10.3
	VP	108	25.9 (7.4)	4	10
Kitagawa et al., 2012 (388)	PP	123	58.8 (3.9)	6.9	18.3
	PC	121	62.6 (7.1)	6.21	17.5
Tewari et al., 2013 (GOG 240) (387)	PP	114	45	—	14.3
	PP + Bevacizumab	115	50	—	17.5
	PC	111	27	—	12.7
	PC + Bevacizumab	112	47	—	16.2

RR, response rate; CR, complete response; PFS, progression-free survival; OS, overall survival; NS, not stated; P, *cisplatin* (in all control arms and combinations 50 mg/m^2); BEMP, *bleomycin/vindesine/mitomycin/cisplatin; IP, ifosfamide/cisplatin; MP, mitolactol/cisplatin; PP, paclitaxel/cisplatin; TP, topotecan/cisplatin; BIP, bleomycin/ifosfamide/cisplatin; GP, gemcitabine/cisplatin; VP, vinorelbine/cisplatin; PT, paclitaxel/topotecan; PC, paclitaxel/carboplatin.*

Targeted Therapies

There is an urgent need for more effective therapies in recurrent/metastatic cervical cancer, and clinical trials have suggested that biologic therapies may be helpful. **Two promising targets in cervical cancer are EGFR and the VEGF signaling pathway, which play critical roles in tumor growth and angiogenesis.** Several review articles have mainly focused on the role of EGFR inhibitors and angiogenesis inhibitors, but have mentioned other drugs of particular interest, such as mammalian target of rapamycin (mTOR) inhibitors, DNA-damaging anticancer agents, therapeutic targeting of apoptosis, and immunologic approaches (349–351,392). Most data are available for angiogenesis inhibitors and EGFR inhibitors.

Angiogenesis Inhibitors

Angiogenesis is central to cervical cancer development and progression. **The dominant role of angiogenesis in cervical cancer is thought to be directly related to HPV inhibition of p53 and stabilization of HIF-1 alpha, both of which increase VEGF** (393). VEGF is found markedly upregulated in human squamous carcinoma cells, and several authors have reported a strong association between overexpression of VEGF and poorer prognosis in cervical cancer (392). As angiogenesis is pivotal in cervical cancer, it seems a rational target for therapy in this disease.

Table 8.16 shows data from three studies with angiogenesis inhibitors, *bevacizumab, pazopanib, and sunitinib. Bevacizumab,* **a humanized monoclonal antibody directed against VEGF-A, was**

Table 8.16 Clinical Trials with Single Agent Molecular Targeted Agents in Recurrent/Metastatic Cervical Cancer

First Authors (References)	Number	Treatment	Prior Regimens (%)	RR (%)	PFS (mos)
Goncalves et al., 2008 (401)	28	Gefitinib	100	0	1.2
Monk et al., 2009 (394)	46	Bevacizumab	100	11	3.4
Kurtz et al., 2009 (399)	19	PT+cetuximab	—	32	5.6
Schilder et al., 2009 (400)	25	Erlotinib	100	0	1.8
Monk et al., 2010 (395)	74	Pazopanib	95	9	4.1
McKay et al., 2010 (396)	19	Sunitinib	100	0	3.5
Santin et al., 2011 (397)	35	Cetuximab	100	0	2
Farley et al., 2011 (398)	69	P+cetuximab	—	12	3.9
Monk et al., 2011 (395, 402)	76	Lapatinib	92	5	3.9

RR, response rate; PFS, progression-free survival; *P, cisplatin; PT, cisplatin* and *topotecan.*

first studied as a single agent by the GOG in protocol 227 C (393). The study accrued 46 patients with previously treated persistent or recurrent squamous cell cervical cancer. Prior treatment included radiation in 82.6% of patients and cytotoxic chemotheraqpy 100%. *Bevacizumab* was administered at a dose of 15 mg/kg intravenously every 3 weeks. Five patients (11%) had a partial response; however, 11 patients (24%) survived progression-free for at least 6 months. **Median PFS and overall survival times were 3.4 and 7.3 months, respectively.** These efficacy results compared favorably with historical controls of other cytotoxic single-agent compounds in this patient population (393). Median grade 3 or 4 adverse events, considered at least possibly related to *bevacizumab,* included hypertension (7 cases), thromboembolism (5), gastrointestinal toxicity (4), anemia (2), other cardiovascular toxicity (2), vaginal bleeding (1), neutropenia (1), and urinary fistula (1). One grade 4 infection was observed. There were no new or unexpected toxicities observed beyond what could have been expected from earlier studies in other solid tumors.

This trial has been followed by GOG protocol 240, which studied the role of *bevacizumab* in advanced cervical cancer (387). Using a 2×2 factorial design, **patients are randomly assigned to chemotherapy, with or without *bevacizumab.*** The chemotherapeutic regimens include the standard *cisplatin* plus *paclitaxel* regimen (*cisplatin* 50 mg/m^2, *paclitaxel* 135 to 175 mg/m^2) and a non–platinum-containing regimen (*topotecan* 0.75 mg/m^2, day 1 to 3, and *paclitaxel* 175 mg/m^2 on day 1). Cycles are repeated every 21 days until disease progression, unacceptable toxicity, or complete response occurs. Overall survival was the primary end point with a reduction in hazard of death by 30% using *bevacizumab* considered important (90% power, one-sided alpha = 2.5%).

The study was reported in 2013 at the 49th Annual Meeting of the Amercian Society of Clinical Oncology. From April 2009 to January 2012, 452 patients were accrued. A scheduled interim analysis after 174 patients had died showed that the *topotecan-paclitaxel* backbone was not superior to the *cisplatin-paclitaxel* backbone. **A second interim analysis after 271 deaths and a median follow-up of 20.8 months showed that the median survival of the 225 patients who were treated with chemotherapy alone was 13.3 months, while for the 227 patients treated with chemotherapy plus *bevacizumab*, it was 17 months.** The *bevacizumab* versus no *bevacizumab* HR of death was 0.71 (97% CI 0.54 to 0.94, one-sided $p = 0.0035$). **The median PFS was 5.9 months without *bevacizumab* and 8.2 months with *bevacizumab*** (HR 0.67; 95% CI 0.54 to 0.82, two-sided $p = 0.00807$). The response with *bevacizumab* was higher than without *bevacizumab* (48% vs. 36%, two-sided $p = 0.0078$). **Treatment with *bevacizumab* was associated with more grade 3 to 4 bleeding (5% vs. 1%), thromboembolic events (9% vs. 2%), and gastrointestinal fistulae (3% vs. 0%).** Despite the increased toxicity, the gain in efficacy was considered to be clinically important.

The phase II studies with *pazopanib* (395) and *sunitinib* (396), both oral receptor tyrosine kinase inhibitors with an antiangiogentic effect, have confirmed the beneficial effects on PFS that were observed with single-agent *bevacizumab* in phase II studies. In the study with *sunitinib*, a 26% fistula rate was observed, which was unexpectedly high. In the *pazopanib* study, which was a randomized phase II study versus **lapatinib** (a dual tyrosine kinase inhibitor of EGFR and ErbB2), fistula formation was seen only in 4% of the 74 accrued patients. The most commonly observed toxicities were diarrhea (54%), nausea (36%), hypertension (30%), and anorexia (28%) (395). In the direct comparison of *pazopanib* and *lapatinib,* the HR for progression favored *pazopanib* (HR 0.66; 90% CI 0.48 to 0.91, $p = 0.013$), which also had a more favorable toxicity profile (395,402).

Epidermal Growth Factor Receptor (EGFR) Inhibitors

In patients with squamous cell carcinoma of the uterine cervix, EGFR is overexpressed in up to 85% of cases, but studies evaluating the association between EGFR protein expression and prognosis have yielded conflicting results (403,404). However, EGFR has been shown to modulate tumor chemosensitivity and radiosensitivity (405). For example, EGFR blockade with EGFR-blocking antibodies has synergic effects with *cisplatin* in human tumor xenografts (406). In addition, radiotherapy increases the expression of EGFR in tumor cells, and blockade of EGFR signaling with EGFR-blocking antibodies sensitizes cells to the effects of radiation (407). Expression of HER2 in cervical cancer has been reported in only 3–9% of cases and is more frequent in adenocarcinomas than in squamous cell cancers (404,408). Moreover, the prognostic value of HER2 positivity is controversial, which for some investigators make the rationale to test anti-HER2 monotherapies questionable (405).

Single-agent *cetuximab* (given at 250 mg/m^2 weekly after a loading dose of 400 mg/m^2) in patients with persistent or recurrent cervical cancer has been well tolerated, but **has shown limited activity in a phase II GOG trial** (397). Nearly 70% of the tumors were of the squamous type, and all patients who were without progression at 6 months harbored tumors with squamous cell histology. Another GOG study, using *cisplatin* (30 mg/m^2 on days 1 and 8) **plus *cetuximab*** (loading dose 400 mg/m^2 followed by 250 mg/m^2 on days 1, 8, and 15) in a 21-day cycle, **showed considerable toxicity** (grade 4 anemia, allergy, metabolic, and vascular one case each; grade 3 metabolic [15], dermatologic [8], fatigue [6], and gastrointestinal [6]), but this was reported as being acceptable. However, **the study did not suggest additional benefit beyond what could have been expected from *cisplatin* therapy alone** (398). **The GINECO group in France tested the combination of *cetuximab* plus *cisplatin/topotecan*. This study was stopped early due to excessive toxicity.** Severe infection and febrile neutropenia occurred in 56% of patients, and five patients died on study (28%), three of them considered to be treatment-related (399).

A plethora of new agents are in early stages of development. The implementation of these new agents into the existing armamentarium should get high priority, taking into account that the majority of cervical cases occur in less developed countries. In order to reach this goal, global cooperation is needed, and the Gynecological Cancer InterGroup (GCIG) has proved to be an excellent platform for this (409,410).

References

1. **Globocan 2008 database.** Available online at: http://globocan.iarc.fr/fact sheets/cancers/cervix.asp
2. **Siegal R, Naishadham D, Jemal A.** Cancer statistics 2013. *CA Cancer J Clin.* 2013;63:11–30.
3. **Howlander N, Noone AM, Krapcho M, et al.** eds. *SEER Cancer Statistics Review, 1975–2009.* Bethesda, MD: National Cancer Institute. Available online at: http://seer.cancer.gov/statfacts/html/cervix.html
4. **Walboomers JM, Jacobs MV, Manos MM.** Human papillomavirus is a necessary cause of invasive cervical cancer worldwide. *J Pathol.* 1999;189:12–19.
5. **Sankaranarayanan R, Nene BM, Shastri SS, et al.** HPV screening for cervical cancer in rural India. *N Engl J Med.* 2009;360:1385–1394.
6. **Pretorius R, Harlan LG, Clegg LX.** Untreated cervical cancer in the United States. *Gynecol Oncol.* 2005;96:217–277.
7. **Pretorius R, Semrad N, Watring W, et al.** Presentation of cervical cancer. *Gynecol Oncol.* 1991;42:48–52.
8. **Sasieni PD, Cuzick J, Lynch-Farmery E.** Estimating the efficacy of screening by auditing smear histories of women with and without cervical cancer. The National Co-ordinating Network for Cervical Screening Working Group. *Br J Cancer.* 1996;73:1001–1005.
9. **Burghardt E, Pickel H, Girardi F.** *Colposcopy and Cervical Pathology: Textbook and Atlas.* Stuttgart: Thieme; 1998:138–192.
10. **Horn IC, Fischer U, Raptisb G, et al.** Tumor size is of prognostic value in surgically treated FIGO stage II cervical cancer. *Gynecol Oncol.* 2007;107:310–315.
11. **Lagasse LD, Creasman WT, Shingleton HM, et al.** Results and complications of operative staging in cervical cancer: Experience of the Gynecology Oncology Group. *Gynecol Oncol.* 1980;9:90–98.
12. **La Polla JP, Schlaerth JB, Gaddis O, et al.** The influence of surgical staging on the evaluation and treatment of patients with cervical carcinoma. *Gynecol Oncol.* 1986;24:194–199.
13. **Hacker NF, Berek JS.** Surgical staging of cervical cancer. In: **Surwit EA, Alberts DS,** eds. *Cervix Cancer.* Boston, MA: Martinus Nijhoff; 1987:43–47.
14. **Subak LL, Hricak H, Powell B, et al.** Cervical carcinoma: Computed tomography and magnetic resonance imaging for preoperative staging. *Obstet Gynecol.* 1995;86:43–50.
15. **Narayan K, McKenzie K, Fisher R, et al.** Estimation of tumor volume in cervical cancer by magnetic resonance imaging. *Am J Clin Oncol.* 2003;26:e163–e168.
16. **Sahdev A, Sohaib SA, Wenaden AET, et al.** The performance of magnetic resonance imaging in early cervical carcinoma: A long-term experience. *Int J Gynecol Cancer.* 2007;17:629–636.
17. **Scheidler J, Hricak H, Yu KK, et al.** Radiological evaluation of lymph node metastases in patients with cervical cancer: A meta-analysis. *JAMA.* 1997;278:1096–1101.
18. **Narayan K, McKenzie AF, Hicks RJ, et al.** Relation between FIGO stage, primary tumor volume, and presence of lymph node metastases in cervical cancer patients referred for radiotherapy. *Int J Gynecol Cancer.* 2003;13:657–663.
19. **Signorelli M, Guerra L, Montanelli L, et al.** Preoperative staging of cervical cancer: Is 18-FDG-PET/CT really effective in patients with early stage disease? *Gynecol Oncol.* 2011;123:236–240.
20. **Narayan K, Hicks RJ, Jobling T, et al.** A comparison of MRI and PET scanning in surgically staged locoregionally advanced cervical cancer: Potential impact on treatment. *Int J Gynecol Cancer.* 2001; 11:263–271.

21. **Grigsby PW, Siegel BA, Dehdashti F.** Lymph node staging by positron emission tomography in patients with carcinoma of the cervix. *J Clin Oncol.* 2001;19:3745–3749.

22. **Havrilesky LJ, Kulasingam SL, Matchar DB, et al.** FDG-PET for management of cervical and ovarian cancer. *Gynecol Oncol.* 2005; 97:183–191.

23. **McDonald TW, Morley GW, Choo YL, et al.** Fine needle aspiration of paraaortic and pelvic nodes showing lymphangiographic abnormalities. *Obstet Gynecol.* 1983;61:383–388.

24. **Ewing TL, Buchler DA, Hoogerland DL, et al.** Percutaneous lymph node aspiration in patients with gynecologic tumors. *Am J Obstet Gynecol.* 1982;143:824–830.

25. **Nelson JH Jr, Boyce J, Macasaet M, et al.** Incidence, significance and follow-up of paraaortic lymph node metastases in late invasive carcinoma of the cervix. *Am J Obstet Gynecol.* 1977; 128:336–340.

26. **Querleu D, Leblanc E, Castelain B.** Laparoscopic pelvic lymphadenectomy in the staging of early carcinoma of the cervix. *Am J Obstet Gynecol.* 1991;164:579–585.

27. **Lai C-H, Huang K-G, Hong J-H, et al.** Randomized trial of surgical staging (extraperitoneal or laparoscopic) versus clinical staging in locally advanced cervical cancer. *Gynecol Oncol.* 2003;89:160–167.

28. **Gold MA, Tian C, Whitney CW, et al.** Surgical versus radiographic determination of paraaortic lymph node metastases before chemoradiation for locally advanced cervical carcinoma. A Gynecologic Oncology Study. *Cancer.* 2008;112:1954–1963.

29. **Petereit DG, Hartenbach EM, Thomas GM.** Paraaortic lymph node evaluation in cervical cancer: The impact of staging upon treatment decisions and outcome. *Int J Gynecol Cancer.* 1998;8:353–364.

30. **Berman ML, Lagasse LD, Watring WG, et al.** The operative evaluation of patients with cervical carcinoma by an extraperitoneal approach. *Obstet Gynecol.* 1977;50:658–664.

31. **Plentyl AA, Friedman EA.** *Lymphatic System of the Female Genitalia: The Morphologic Basis of Oncologic Diagnosis and Therapy.* Philadelphia, PA: WB Saunders, 1971.

32. **Zander J, Baltzer J, Lobe KJ, et al.** Carcinoma of the cervix: An attempt to individualize treatment. *Am J Obstet Gynecol.* 1981;139: 752–759.

33. **Fuller AF, Elliott N, Kosloff C, et al.** Lymph node metastases from carcinoma of the cervix, stage IB and IIA: Implications for prognosis and treatment. *Gynecol Oncol.* 1982;13:165–174.

34. **Timmer PR, Aalders JG, Bouma J.** Radical surgery after preoperative intracavitary radiotherapy for stage IB and IIA carcinoma of the uterine cervix. *Gynecol Oncol.* 1984;18:206–212.

35. **Inoue T, Okamura M.** Prognostic significance of parametrial extension in patients with cervical carcinoma stages IB, IIA, and IIB. *Cancer.* 1984;54:1714–1719.

36. **Creasman WT, Soper JT, Clarke-Pearson D.** Radical hysterectomy as therapy for early carcinoma of the cervix. *Am J Obstet Gynecol.* 1986;155:964–969.

37. **Artman LE, Hoskins WJ, Birro MC, et al.** Radical hysterectomy and pelvic lymphadenectomy for stage IB carcinoma of the cervix: 21 years experience. *Gynecol Oncol.* 1987;28:8–13.

38. **Monaghan JM, Ireland D, Mor-Yosef S, et al.** Role of centralization of surgery in stage IB carcinoma of the cervix: A review of 498 cases. *Gynecol Oncol.* 1990;37:206–209.

39. **Finan MA, De Cesare S, Fiorica JV, et al.** Radical hysterectomy for stage IB1 vs IB2 carcinoma of the cervix: Does the new staging system predict morbidity and survival? *Gynecol Oncol.* 1996;62: 139–147.

40. **Samlal RA, van der Velden J, Ten Kate FJW, et al.** Surgical pathologic factors that predict recurrence in stage IB and IIA cervical carcinoma patients with negative pelvic nodes. *Cancer.* 1997;80: 1234–1240.

41. **Burke TW, Heller PB, Hoskins WJ, et al.** Evaluation of the scalene lymph nodes in primary and recurrent cervical carcinoma. *Gynecol Oncol.* 1987;28:312–317.

42. **Burghardt E, Girardi F.** Local spread of cervical cancer. In: **Burghardt E, ed.** *Surgical Gynecologic Oncology.* New York, NY: Thieme, 1993:203–212.

43. **Shingleton HM, Orr JW.** *Cancer of the Cervix.* Philadelphia, PA: JB Lippincott, 1995.

44. **Sutton GP, Bundy BN, Delgado G, et al.** Ovarian metastases in stage IB carcinoma of the cervix: A Gynecologic Oncology Group study. *Am J Obstet Gynecol.* 1992;166:50–53.

45. **Delgado G, Chun B, Calgar H, et al.** Paraaortic lymphadenectomy in gynecologic malignancies confined to the pelvis. *Obstet Gynecol.* 1977;50:418–423.

46. **Piver MS, Barlow JJ.** High dose irradiation to biopsy confirmed aortic node metastases from carcinoma of the uterine cervix. *Cancer.* 1977;39:1243–1248.

47. **Sudarsanam A, Charyulu K, Belinson J, et al.** Influence of exploratory celiotomy on the management of carcinoma of the cervix. *Cancer.* 1978;41:1049–1053.

48. **Buchsbaum H.** Extrapelvic lymph node metastases in cervical carcinoma. *Am J Obstet Gynecol.* 1979;133:814–824.

49. **Hughes RR, Brewington KC, Hanjani P, et al.** Extended field irradiation for cervical cancer based on surgical staging. *Gynecol Oncol.* 1980;9:153–161.

50. **Ballon SC, Berman ML, Lagasse LD, et al.** Survival after extraperitoneal pelvic and paraaortic lymphadenectomy and radiation therapy in cervical carcinoma. *Obstet Gynecol.* 1981;57:90–95.

51. **Welander CE, Pierce VK, Nori D, et al.** Pretreatment laparotomy in carcinoma of the cervix. *Gynecol Oncol.* 1981;12:336–347.

52. **Berman ML, Keys H, Creasman WT, et al.** Survival and patterns of recurrence in cervical cancer metastatic to periaortic lymph nodes: A Gynecologic Oncology Group study. *Gynecol Oncol.* 1984;19:8–16.

53. **Potish RA, Twiggs LB, Okagaki T, et al.** Therapeutic implications of the natural history of advanced cervical cancer as defined by pretreatment surgical staging. *Cancer.* 1985;56:956–960.

54. **Suprasert P, Srisomboon J, Kasamatsu T.** Radical hysterectomy for stage IIB cervical cancer: A review. *Int J Gynecol Cancer.* 2005; 15:995–1001.

55. **Kim JH, Kim HJ, Hong S, et al.** Post-hysterectomy radiotherapy for FIGO stage IB–IIB uterine cervical carcinoma. *Gynecol Oncol.* 2005;96:407–414.

56. **Hockel M, Horn L-C, Fritsch H.** Association between the management compartment of uterovaginal organogenesis and local tumor spread in stage IB–IIB cervical cancer: A prospective study. *Lancet Oncol.* 2005;6:751–756.

57. **Mestwerdt G.** Die Fruhdiagnose des Kollumkarzinoms. *Zentralbl Gynakol.* 1947;69:198–202.

58. **Creasman WT, Fetter BF, Clarke-Pearson DL, et al.** Management of stage IA carcinoma of the cervix. *Am J Obstet Gynecol.* 1985;153: 164–172.

59. **Van Nagell JR, Greenwell N, Powell DF, et al.** Microinvasive carcinoma of the cervix. *Am J Obstet Gynecol.* 1983;145:981–991.

60. **Simon NL, Gore H, Shingleton HM, et al.** Study of superficially invasive carcinoma of the cervix. *Obstet Gynecol.* 1986;68:19–24.

61. **Ostor AG.** Studies on 200 cases of early squamous cell carcinoma of the cervix. *Int J Gynecol Pathol.* 1993;12:193–207.

62. **Elliott P, Coppleson M, Russell P, et al.** Early invasive (FIGO stage IA) carcinoma of the cervix: A clinicopathologic study of 476 cases. *Int J Gynecol Cancer.* 2000;10:42–52.

63. **Roman LD, Felix JC, Muderspach LI, et al.** Risk of residual invasive disease in women with microinvasive squamous cancer in a conization specimen. *Obstet Gynecol.* 1997;90:759–764.

64. **Takeshima N, Yanoh K, Tabata T, et al.** Assessment of the revised International Federation of Gynecology and Obstetrics staging for early invasive squamous cervical cancer. *Gynecol Oncol.* 1999;74: 165–169.

65. **Lee KBM, Lee JM, Park CY, et al.** Lymph node metastases and lymphatic invasion in microinvasive squamous carcinoma of the uterine cervix. *Int J Gynecol Cancer.* 2006;16:1184–1187.

66. **Costa S, Marra E, Martinelli GN, et al.** Outcome of conservatively treated microinvasive squamous cell carcinoma of the uterine cervix during 10-year follow-up. *Int J Gynecol Cancer.* 2009;19:33–38.

67. **Yahata T, Nishino K, Kashima K, et al.** Conservative treatment of stage 1A1 adenocarcinoma of the uterine cervix with long-term follow-up. *Int J Gynecol Cancer.* 2010;20:1063–1066.

68. **Baalbergen A, Smedts F, Helmerhorst TJM.** Conservative therapy in microinvasive adenocarcinoma of the uterine cervix is justified. An analysis of 59 cases and a review of the literature. *Int J Gynecol Cancer.* 2011;21:1640–1645.

69. **Al-Kalbani M, McVeigh G, Nagar H, et al.** Do FIGO stage 1 A and small (≤2 cm) 1B1 cervical adenocarcinomas have a good prognosis and warrant less radical surgery? *Int J Gynecol Cancer.* 2012;22: 291–295.

70. **Phongnarisorn C, Srisomboon J, Khumamornpong S, et al.** The risk of residual neoplasia in women with microinvasive squamous cell carcinoma and positive cone margins. *Int J Gynecol Cancer.* 2006; 16:655–659.

71. **Rob L, Robova H, Chmel R, et al.** Surgical options in cervical cancer. *Int J Hyperthermia.* 2012;28:489–500.

72. **Dargent D, Brun JL, Roy M, et al.** Pregnancies following radical trachelectomy for invasive cervical cancer. *Gynecol Oncol.* 1994; 52:105(abst).

73. **Smith JR, Boyle DC, Corless DJ, et al.** Abdominal radical trachelectomy: A new surgical technique for the conservative management of cervical carcinoma. *BJOG.* 1997;104:1196–1200.

74. **Rob L, Charvat M, Robova H, et al.** Less radical fertility-sparing surgery than radical trachelectomy in early cervical cancer. *Int J Gynecol Cancer.* 2007;17:304–310.

75. **Buckley SL, Tritz DM, van Le L, et al.** Lymph node metastases and prognosis in patients with stage IA2 cervical cancer. *Gynecol Oncol.* 1996;63:4–9.

76. **Creasman WT, Zaino RJ, Major FJ, et al.** Early invasive carcinoma of the cervix (3 to 5 mm invasion): Risk factors and prognosis. A GOG study. *Am J Obstet Gynecol.* 1998;178:62–65.

77. **Suri A, Frumovitz M, Milam MR, et al.** Preoperative pathological findings associated with residual disease at radical hysterectomy in women with stage 1A2 cervical cancer. *Gynecol Oncol.* 2009;112: 110–113.

78. **van Meurs H, Visser O, Buist MR, et al.** Frequency of pelvic lymph node metastases and parametrial involvement in stage 1A2 cervical cancer. A population-based study and literature review. *Int J Gynecol Cancer.* 2009;19:21–26.

79. **Smrkolj S, Pogacnik RK, Slabe N, et al.** Clinical outcome of patients with stage 1A2 squamous cell carcinoma of the uterine cervix. *Gynecol Oncol.* 2012;124:68–71.

80. **Alexander-Sefre F, Chee N, Spencer C, et al.** Surgical morbidity associated with radical trachelectomy and radical hysterectomy. *Gynecol Oncol.* 2006;101:450–454.

81. **Hou J, Goldberg GL, Qualls CR, et al.** Risk factors for poor prognosis in microinvasive adenocarcinoma of the uterine cervix (1A1 and 1A2): A pooled analysis. *Gynecol Oncol.* 2011;121: 135–142.

82. **Teshima S, Shimosata Y, Kishi K, et al.** Early stage adenocarcinoma of the cervix. *Cancer.* 1985;56:167–172.

83. **Lee KR, Flynn CE.** Early invasive adenocarcinoma of the cervix: A histopathologic analysis of 40 cases with observations concerning histogenesis. *Cancer.* 2000;89:1048–1055.

84. **Ostor A, Rome R, Quinn M.** Microinvasive adenocarcinoma of the cervix: A clinicopathologic study of 77 women. *Obstet Gynecol.* 1997; 89:88–93.

85. **Kaku T, Kamura T, Sakai K, et al.** Early adenocarcinoma of the uterine cervix. *Gynecol Oncol.* 1997;65:281–285.

86. **Bisseling KCHM, Bekkers RLM, Rome RM, et al.** Treatment of microinvasive adenocarcinoma of the uterine cervix: A retrospective study and review of the literature. *Gynecol Oncol.* 2007;107:424–430.

87. **Webb JC, Key CR, Qualls CR, et al.** Population-based study of microinvasive adenocarcinoma of the uterine cervix. *Obstet Gynecol.* 2001;97:701–706.

88. **Poynor EA, Marshall D, Sonoda Y, et al.** Clinicopathologic features of early adenocarcinoma of the cervix initially managed with cervical conization. *Gynecol Oncol.* 2006;103:960–965.

89. **Ostor AG.** Early invasive adenocarcinoma of the cervix. *Int J Gynecol Pathol.* 2000;19:29–38.

90. **Suri A, Frumovitz M, Milan MR, et al.** Preoperative pathologic findings associated with residual disease at radical hysterectomy in women with stage 1A2 cervical cancer. *Gynecol Oncol.* 2009;112: 110–113.

91. **Poynor EA, Barakat RR, Hoskins WJ.** Management and follow-up of patients with adenocarcinoma *in situ* of the uterine cervix. *Gynecol Oncol.* 1995;57:158–164.

92. **Landoni F, Maneo A, Colombo A, et al.** Randomized study of radical surgery versus radiotherapy for stage IB–IIa cervical cancer. *Lancet.* 1997;350:535–540.

93. **Eifel PJ, Moughan J, Erickson B, et al.** Patterns of radiotherapy practice for patients with carcinoma of the uterine cervix: A patterns of care study. *Int J Radiat Oncol Biol Phys.* 2004;60:1144–1153.

94. **Lawton FG, Hacker NF.** Surgery for invasive gynecologic cancer in the elderly female population. *Obstet Gynecol.* 1990;76:287–291.

95. **Brand AH, Bull CA, Cakir B.** Vaginal stenosis in patients treated with radiotherapy for carcinoma of the cervix. *Int J Gynecol Cancer.* 2006;16:288–293.

96. **Samlal RAK, van der Velden J, Schilthuis MS, et al.** Influence of diagnostic conization on surgical morbidity and survival in patients undergoing radical hysterectomy for stage IB and IIA cervical carcinoma. *Eur J Gynaecol Oncol.* 1997;18:478–481.

97. **Orr JW, Shingleton HM, Hatch KD, et al.** Correlation of perioperative morbidity and conization to radical hysterectomy interval. *Obstet Gynecol.* 1982;59:726–731.

98. **Piver M, Rutledge F, Smith J.** Five classes of extended hysterectomy for women with cervical cancer. *Obstet Gynecol.* 1974;44:265–272.

99. **Wertheim E.** The extended abdominal operation for carcinoma uteri (based on 500 operative cases). *Am J Obstet.* 1912;66:169–174.

100. **Meigs J.** Carcinoma of the cervix: The Wertheim operation. *Surg Gynecol Obstet.* 1944;78:195–199.

101. **Querleu D, Morrow CP.** Classification of radical hysterectomy. *Lancet Oncol.* 2008;9:297–303.

102. **Cibula D, Abu Rustum NR, Benedetti-Panici P, et al.** New classification system of radical hysterectomy: Emphasis on a three-dimensional anatomic template for parametrial resection. *Gynecol Oncol.* 2011;122:264–268.

103. **Hockel M.** Laterally extended endopelvic resection: Surgical treatment of infrailiac pelvic wall recurrences of gynecologic malignancies. *Am J Obstet Gynecol.* 1999;180:306–312.

104. **Hacker NF, Wain GV, Nicklin JL.** Resection of bulky positive lymph nodes in patients with cervical cancer. *Int J Gynecol Cancer.* 1995;5:250–256.

105. **Fujii S, Tanakura K, Matsumura N, et al.** Anatomic identification and functional outcomes of the nerve sparing Okabayashi radical hysterectomy. *Gynecol Oncol.* 2007;107:4–13.

106. **Trimbos JB, Maas CP, Derviter MC, et al.** A nerve-sparing radical hysterectomy: Guidelines and feasibility in Western patients. *Int J Gynecol Cancer.* 2001;11:180–186.

107. **Shah M, Lewin SN, Deutsch I, et al.** Therapeutic role of lymphadenectomy for cervical cancer. *Cancer.* 2011;117:310–317.

108. **Dargent D, Martin X, Mathevet P.** Laparoscopic assessment of sentinel lymph nodes in early cervical cancer. *Gynecol Oncol.* 2000; 79:411–415.

109. **Rob L, Strnad P, Robova H, et al.** Study of lymphatic mapping and sentinel node identification in early stage cervical cancer. *Gynecol Oncol.* 2005;98:281–288.

110. **Wydra D, Sawicki S, Wojtylak S, et al.** Sentinel node identification in cervical cancer patients undergoing transperitoneal radical hysterectomy: A study of 100 cases. *Int J Gynecol Cancer.* 2006;16:649–654.

111. **Altgassen C, Hertel H, Brandstadt A, et al.** Multicenter validation study of sentinel lymph node concept in cervical cancer: AGO Study Group. *J Clin Oncol.* 2008;26:2943–2951.

112. **Levenback CF, van der Zee AGJ, Rob L, et al.** Sentinel lymph node biopsy in patients with gynecological cancers: Expert panel statement from the International Sentinel Node Society meeting, February 21, 2008. *Gynecol Oncol.* 2009;114:151–156.

113. **Cibula D, Abu-Rustum NR, Dusek L, et al.** Bilateral ultrastaging of sentinel lymph nodes in cervical cancer: Lowering the false-negative rate and improving the detection of micrometastasis. *Gynecol Oncol.* 2012;127:462–466.

114. **Farrell R, Gebski V, Hacker NF.** Quality of life after complete lymphadenectomy for vulvar cancer: Do women prefer sentinel node biopsy? *Int J Gynecol Cancer.* 2014;24:813–819.

115. **Jensen JK, Lucci JA, Di Saia PJ, et al.** To drain or not to drain: A retrospective study of closed-suction drainage following radical hysterectomy with pelvic lymphadenectomy. *Gynecol Oncol.* 1993; 51:46–49.

116. **Yabuki Y, Asamoto A, Hoshiba T, et al.** Radical hysterectomy: An anatomic evaluation of parametrial dissection. *Gynecol Oncol.* 2000; 77:155–163.

117. **Possover M, Stober S, Phaul K, et al.** Identification and preservation of the motoric innervation of the bladder in radical hysterectomy type III. *Gynecol Oncol.* 2000;79:154–157.

118. **Raspagliesi F, Ditto A, Fontanelli R, et al.** Type II versus type III nerve-sparing radical hysterectomy: Comparison of lower urinary tract dysfunctions. *Gynecol Oncol.* 2006;102:256–262.

119. **Todo Y, Kuwabara M, Watari H, et al.** Urodynamic study on post-surgical bladder function in cervical cancer treated with systematic nerve-sparing radical hysterectomy. *Int J Gynecol Cancer.* 2006;16: 369–375.

120. **Cibula D, Velechovska P, Slama J, et al.** Late morbidity following nerve-sparing radical hysterectomy. *Gynecol Oncol.* 2010;116:506–511.

121. **De Kroon CD, Gaarenstroom KN, van Poelgeest MI, et al.** Nerve sparing in radical surgery for early-stage cervical cancer. *Int J Gynecol Oncol.* 2010;20:S39-S41.

122. **Landoni F, Maneo A, Cormio G, et al.** Class II versus class III radical hysterectomy in stage IB–IIA cervical cancer: A prospective randomized study. *Gynecol Oncol.* 2001;80:3–12.

123. **Stegman M, Louwen M, van der Velden J, et al.** The incidence of parametrial tumor involvement in select patients with early cervix cancer is too low to justify parametrectomy. *Gynecol Oncol.* 2007; 105:475–480.

124. **Wright JD, Grigsby PW, Brooks R, et al.** Utility of parametrectomy for early stage cervical cancer treated with radical hysterectomy. *Cancer.* 2007;110:1281–1286.

125. **Covens A, Rosen B, Murphy J, et al.** How important is removal of the parametrium at surgery for carcinoma of the cervix? *Gynecol Oncol.* 2002;84:145–149.

126. **Winter R, Haas J, Reich O, et al.** Parametrial spread of cervical cancer in patients with negative pelvic lymph nodes. *Gynecol Oncol.* 2002;84:252–257.

127. **Strnad P, Robova H, Skapa P, et al.** A prospective study of sentinel lymph node status and parametrial involvement in patients with small tumour volume cervical cancer. *Gynecol Oncol.* 2008;109:280–284.

128. **Rob L, Skapa P, Robova H.** Fertility-sparing surgery in patients with cervical cancer. *Lancet Oncol.* 2011;12:192–200.

129. **Schneider A, Erdemoglu E, Chiantera V, et al.** Clinical recommendation radical trachelectomy for fertility preservation in patients with early-stage cervical cancer. *Int J Gynecol Oncol.* 2012;22: 659–666.

130. **Pareja R, Rendon GJ, Sanz-Lomana CM, et al.** Surgical, oncological, and obstetrical outcomes after abdominal radical trachelectomy—A systematic literature review. *Gynecol Oncol.* 2013;131: 77–82.

131. **Epstein E, Testa A, Gaurilcikas A, et al.** Early-stage cervical cancer: Tumor delineation by magnetic resonance imaging and ultrasound – A European multicenter trial. *Gynecol Oncol.* 2013;128: 449–453.

132. **Ismiil N, Ghorab Z, Covens A, et al.** Intraoperative margin assessment of the radical trachelectomy specimen. *Gynecol Oncol.* 2009; 113:42–46.

133. **Gien LT, Covens A.** Fertility-sparing options for early stage cervical cancer. *Gynecol Oncol.* 2010;117:350–357.

134. **Palaia I, Musella A, Bellati F, et al.** Simple extrafascial trachelectomy and pelvic bilateral lymphadectomy in early stage cervical cancer. *Gynecol Oncol.* 2012;126:78–81.

135. **Maneo A, Sideri M, Scambia G, et al.** Simple conization and lymphadenectomy for the conservative treatment of stage 1B1 cervical cancer. An Italian experience. *Gynecol Oncol.* 2011;123:557–560.

136. **Plante M, Lau S, Brydon L, et al.** Neoadjuvant chemotherapy followed by vaginal radical trachelectomy in bulky stage 1B1 cervical cancer: A case report. *Gynecol Oncol.* 2006;101:367–370.

137. **Maneo A, Chiari S, Bonazzi C, et al.** Neoadjuvant chemotherapy and conservative surgery for stage 1B1 cervical cancer. *Gynecol Oncol.* 2008;111:438–443.

138. **Robova H, Pluta M, Hrehorcak M, et al.** High dose density chemotherapy followed by simple trachelectomy: Full-term pregnancy. *Int J Gynecol Cancer.* 2008;18:1367–1371.

139. **Pikaat DP, Holloway RW, Ahmad S, et al.** Clinico-pathologic morbidity analysis of types 2 and 3 abdominal radical hysterectomy for cervical cancer. *Gynecol Oncol.* 2007;107:205–210.

140. **Samlal RAK, van der Velden J, Ketting BW, et al.** Disease-free interval and recurrence pattern after the Okabayashi variant of Wertheim's radical hysterectomy for stage IB and IIA cervical carcinoma. *Int J Gynecol Cancer.* 1996;6:120–127.

141. **Krishnan CS, Grant PT, Robertson G, et al.** Lymphatic ascites following lymphadenectomy for gynecological cancer. *Int J Gynecol Cancer.* 2001;11:392–396.

142. **Sivanesaratnam V, Sen DK, Jayalakshmi P, et al.** Radical hysterectomy and pelvic lymphadenectomy for early invasive cancer of the cervix: 14 years experience. *Int J Gynecol Cancer.* 1993;3:231–238.

143. **Hacker NF, Barlow E, Scurry J, et al.** Primary surgical management with tailored adjuvant radiation for stage 1 B2 cervical cancer. *Obstet Gynecol.* 2013;121:765–772.

144. **Covens A, Rosen B, Gibbons A, et al.** Differences in the morbidity of radical hysterectomy between gynecological oncologists. *Gynecol Oncol.* 1993;51:39–45.

145. **Lee RB, Park RC.** Bladder dysfunction following radical hysterectomy. *Gynecol Oncol.* 1981;11:304–308.

146. **Bergmark K, Avall-Lundqvist E, Dickman PW, et al.** Vaginal function and sexuality in women with a history of cervical cancer. *N Engl J Med.* 1999;340:1383–1389.

147. **Grumann M, Robertson R, Hacker NF, et al.** Sexual functioning in patients following radical hysterectomy for stage IB cancer of the cervix. *Int J Gynecol Cancer.* 2001;11:372–380.

148. **Frumovitz M, Sun CC, Schover LR, et al.** Quality of life and sexual functioning in cervical cancer survivors. *J Clin Oncol.* 2005; 23:7428–7436.

149. **Greenwald HP, McCorkle R.** Sexuality and sexual function in long-term survivors of cervical cancer. *J Women's Health.* 2008;17: 955–963.

150. **Ryan M, Stainton C, Slaytor EK, et al.** Aetiology and prevalence of lower limb lymphoedema following treatment for gynaecological cancer. *Aust N Z J Obstet Gynaecol.* 2003;143:148–151.

151. **Eifel PJ, Morris M, Wharton TJ, et al.** The influence of tumor size and morphology on the outcome of patients with FIGO stage IB squamous cell carcinoma of the uterine cervix. *Int J Radiat Oncol Biol Phys.* 1994;29:9–16.

152. **Perez CA, Grigsby PW, Chao KSC, et al.** Tumor size, irradiation dose, and long term outcome of carcinoma of the cervix. *Int J Radiat Oncol Biol Phys.* 1998;41:307–317.

153. **Perez CA, Grigsby PW, Camel HM, et al.** Irradiation alone or combined with surgery in stage IB, IIA and IIB carcinoma of the uterine cervix: Update of a nonrandomized comparison. *Int J Radiat Oncol Biol Phys.* 1995;31:706–716.

154. **MRC Clinical Trials Unit.** Reducing uncertainties about the effects of chemoradiotherapy for cervical cancer: A systematic review and meta-analysis of individual patient data from 18 randomized trials. *J Clin Oncol.* 2008;26:5802–5812.

155. **Guth U, Ella WA, Olaitan A, et al.** Total vaginal necrosis. A representative example of underreporting severe late toxic reaction after concomitant chemoradiation for cervical cancer. *Int J Gynecol Cancer.* 2010;20:54–60.

156. **Keys HM, Bundy BN, Stehman FB, et al.; for the Gynecology Oncology Group.** Radiation therapy with and without extrafascial hysterectomy for bulky stage IB cervical carcinoma: A randomized trial of the Gynecologic Oncology Group. *Gynecol Oncol.* 2003;89: 343–353.

157. **Stehman FB, Ali S, Keys HM, et al.** Radiation therapy with or without weekly cisplatin for bulky Stage IB cervical carcinoma: Follow-up of a Gynecologic Oncology Group trial. *Am J Obstet Gynecol.* 2007; 197:503e1–503e6.

158. **Sardi J, Sananes C, Giaroli A, et al.** Results of a prospective randomized trial with neoadjuvant chemotherapy in stage IB, bulky, squamous carcinoma of the cervix. *Gynecol Oncol.* 1993;49:156–165.

159. **Robova H, Rob L, Halaska MJ, et al.** High-dose density neoadjuvant chemotherapy in bulky 1B cervical cancer. *Gynecol Oncol.* 2013; 128:49–53.

160. **Bloss JD, Berman ML, Mukhererjee J, et al.** Bulky stage IB cervical carcinoma managed by primary radical hysterectomy followed by tailored radiotherapy. *Gynecol Oncol.* 1992;47:21–27.

161. **Boronow RC.** The bulky 6 cm barrel-shaped lesion of the cervix: Primary surgery and postoperative chemoradiation. *Gynecol Oncol.* 2000;78:313–317.

162. **Rutledge TL, Kamelle S, Tillmanns TD, et al.** A comparison of stage IB1 vs IB2 cervical cancers treated with radical hysterectomy. Is size the real difference? *Gynecol Oncol.* 2004;95:70–76.

163. **Yessaian A, Magistris A, Burger RA, et al.** Radical hysterectomy followed by tailored postoperative therapy in the treatment of stage IB2

cervical cancer: Feasibility and indications for adjuvant therapy. *Gynecol Oncol.* 2004;94:61–66.

164. **Havrilesky LJ, Leath CA, Huh W, et al.** Radical hysterectomy and pelvic lymphadenectomy for stage IB2 cervical cancer. *Gynecol Oncol.* 2004;93:429–434.

165. **Micha JP, Goldstein BH, Rettermaier MA, et al.** Surgery alone or surgery with combination radiation or chemoradiation for management of patients with bulky stage 1 B2 cervical cancer. *Int J Gynecol Cancer.* 2006;16:114–119.

166. **Zivanovic O, Alektiar KM, Sonda Q, et al.** Treatment patterns of FIGO stage 1 B2 cervical cancer: A single-institution experience of radical hysterectomy with individualized postoperative therapy and definitive radiation therapy. *Gynecol Oncol.* 2008;111:265–270.

167. **Ikushima H, Takegawa Y, Osaki K, et al.** Radiation therapy for cervical cancer in the elderly. *Gynecol Oncol.* 2007;107:339–343.

168. **Mitchell PA, Waggoner S, Rotmensch J, et al.** Cervical cancer in the elderly treated with radiation therapy. *Gynecol Oncol.* 1998;71:291–298.

169. **Hacker NF.** Clinical and operative staging of cervical cancer. *Baillieres Clin Obstet Gynaecol.* 1988;2:747–759.

170. **Cosin JA, Fowler JM, Chen MD, et al.** Pretreatment surgical staging of patients with cervical carcinoma: The case for lymph node debulking. *Cancer.* 1998;82:2241–2248.

171. **Parker WH, Feskanich D Broder MS, et al.** Long-term mortality associated with oophorectomy compared with ovarian conservation in the Nurses' Health Study. *Obstet Gynecol.* 2013;121:1–8.

172. **Rocconi RP, Estes JM, Leath CA III, et al.** Management strategies for stage IB2 cervical cancer: A cost effectiveness analysis. *Gynecol Oncol.* 2005;97:387–394.

173. **Biewenga P, van der Velden J, Mol BWJ, et al.** Prognostic model for survival in patients with early stage cervical cancer. *Cancer.* 2011;117:768–776.

174. **Kim SM, Choi HS, Byun JS.** Overall 5-year survival rate and prognostic factors in patients with stage IB and IIA cervical cancer treated by radical hysterectomy and pelvic lymph node dissection. *Int J Gynecol Cancer.* 2000;10:305–312.

175. **Tsai C-S, Lai C-H, Wang C-C, et al.** The prognostic factors for patients with early cervical cancer treated by radical hysterectomy and postoperative radiotherapy. *Gynecol Oncol.* 1999;75:328–333.

176. **Delgado G, Bundy B, Zaino R, et al.** Prospective surgical-pathological study of disease-free interval in patients with stage IB squamous cell carcinoma of the cervix: A Gynecologic Oncology Group study. *Gynecol Oncol.* 1990;38:352–357.

177. **Park J-Y, Kim D-Y, Kim J-H, et al.** Further stratification of risk groups in patients with lymph node metastasis after radical hysterectomy for early stage cervical cancer. *Gynecol Oncol.* 2010;117:53–58.

178. **Cibula D, Abu-Rustum NR, Dusek L, et al.** Prognostic significance of low volume sentinel lymph node disease in early-stage cervical cancer. *Gynecol Oncol.* 2012;124:496–501.

179. **Kenter GG, Ansink AG, Heintz APM, et al.** Carcinoma of the uterine cervix stage IB and IIA: Results of surgical treatment: Complications, recurrence and survival. *Eur J Surg Oncol.* 1989;15:55–60.

180. **Lee Y-N, Wang KL, Lin CH, et al.** Radical hysterectomy with pelvic lymph node dissection for treatment of cervical cancer: A clinical review of 954 cases. *Gynecol Oncol.* 1989;32:135–142.

181. **Monaghan JM, Ireland D, Shlomo MY, et al.** Role of centralization of surgery in stage IB carcinoma of the cervix: A review of 498 cases. *Gynecol Oncol.* 1990;37:206–209.

182. **Ayhan A, Tuncer ZS.** Radical hysterectomy with lymphadenectomy for treatment of early stage cervical cancer: Clinical experience of 278 cases. *J Surg Oncol.* 1991;47:175–177.

183. **Averette HE, Nguyen HN, Donato DM, et al.** Radical hysterectomy for invasive cervical cancer: A 25-year prospective experience with the Miami technique. *Cancer.* 1993;71:1422–1437.

184. **Noguchi H, Shiozawa I, Sakai Y, et al.** Pelvic lymph node metastases in uterine cervical cancer. *Gynecol Oncol.* 1987;27:150–155.

185. **Inoue T, Morita K.** The prognostic significance of number of positive nodes in cervical carcinoma stage IB, IIA, and IIB. *Cancer.* 1990;65:1923–1928.

186. **Roman LD, Felix JC, Muderspach LI, et al.** Influence of quantity of lymph-vascular space invasion on the risk of nodal metastases in women with early-stage squamous cancer of the cervix. *Gynecol Oncol.* 1998;68:220–225.

187. **Chernofsky MR, Felix JC, Muderspach LI, et al.** Influence of quantity of lymph vascular space invasion on time to recurrence in women with early-stage squamous cancer of the cervix. *Gynecol Oncol.* 2006;100:288–293.

188. **Burghardt E, Baltzer J, Tulusan AH, et al.** Results of surgical treatment of 1028 cervical cancers studied with volumetry. *Cancer.* 1992;70:648–655.

189. **Zreik TG, Chambers JT, Chambers SK.** Parametrial involvement, regardless of nodal status: A poor prognostic factor for cervical cancer. *Obstet Gynecol.* 1996;87:741–746.

190. **Uno T, Ho H, Isobe K, et al.** Post operative pelvic radiotherapy for cervical cancer patients with positive parametrial invasion. *Gynecol Oncol.* 2005;96:335–340.

191. **van Nagell JR Jr, Powell DE, Gallion HH, et al.** Small cell carcinoma of the uterine cervix. *Cancer.* 1988;62:1586–1593.

192. **Lee Y-Y, Choi CH, Kim T-J, et al.** A comparison of pure adenocarcinoma and squamous cell carcinoma of the cervix after radical hysterectomy in stage 1B-IIA. *Gynecol Oncol.* 2011;120:439–441.

193. **Galic V, Herzog TJ, Lewin SN, et al.** Prognostic significance of adenocarcinoma histology in women with cervical cancer. *Gynecol Oncol.* 2012;125:278–291.

194. **Shingleton HM, Bell MC, Fremgen A, et al.** Is there really a difference in survival of women with squamous cell carcinoma, adenocarcinoma and adenosquamous cell carcinoma of the cervix? *Cancer.* 1995;76:1948–1955.

195. **Adcock LL, Potish RA, Julian TM, et al.** Carcinoma of the cervix, FIGO stage IB: Treatment failures. *Gynecol Oncol.* 1984;18:218–225.

196. **Gallup DG, Harper RH, Stock RJ.** Poor prognosis in patients with adenosquamous cell carcinoma of the cervix. *Obstet Gynecol.* 1985;65:416–422.

197. **Farley JH, Hickey KW, Carlson JW, et al.** Adenosquamous histology predicts a poor outcome for patients with advanced-stage, but not early-stage cervical carcinoma. *Cancer.* 2003;97:2196–2202.

198. **Dos Reis R, Frumovitz M, Milam MR, et al.** Adenosquamous carcinoma versus adenocarcinoma in early-stage cervical cancer patients undergoing radical hysterectomy: An outcome analysis. *Gynecol Oncol.* 2007;107:458–463.

199. **Mabuchi S, Okazawa M, Kinose Y, et al.** Comparison of the prognosis of FIGO stage I to stage II adenosquamous carcinoma and adenocarcinoma of the uterine cervix treated with radical hysterectomy. *Int J Gynecol Cancer.* 2012;22:1389–1397.

200. **Olsen JRR, Dehdashti F, Siegel BA, et al.** Prognostic utility of squamous cell carcinoma antigen in carcinoma of the cervix: Association with pre- and posttreatment FDG-PET. *Int J Radiat Oncol Biol Phys.* 2011;81:772–777.

201. **Yin M, Hou Y, Zhang T, et al.** Evaluation of chemotherapy response with serum squamous cell carcinoma antigen level in cervical cancer patients: A prospective cohort study. *PLoS One.* 2013;8:1–7.

202. **Ogino I, Nakayama H, Kitamura T, et al.** The curative role of radiotherapy in patients with isolated paraaortic node recurrence from cervical cancer and the value of squamous cell carcinoma antigen for early detection. *Int J Gynecol Cancer.* 2005;15:630–638.

203. **Lombard I, Vincent-Salomon A, Validire P, et al.** Human papilloma genotype as a major determinant of the course of cervical cancer. *J Clin Oncol.* 1998;16:2613–2619.

204. **Rose BR, Thompson CH, Simpson JM, et al.** Human papillomavirus deoxyribonucleic acid as a prognostic indicator in early stage cervical cancer: A possible role for type 18. *Am J Obstet Gynecol.* 1995;173:1461–1468.

205. **Lai C-H, Chang C-J, Huang H-J, et al.** Role of human papillomavirus genotype in prognosis of early-stage cervical cancer undergoing primary surgery. *J Clin Oncol.* 2007;25:3628–3634.

206. **Wang C-C, Lai C-H, Huang H-J, et al.** Clinical effect of human papillomavirus genotypes in patients with cervical cancer undergoing primary radiotherapy. *Int J Radiat Onco Biol Phys.* 2010;78:1111–1120.

207. **Obermair A, Warner C, Bilgi S, et al.** Tumor angiogenesis in stage IB cervical cancer: Correlation of microvessel density with survival. *Am J Obstet Gynecol.* 1998;178:314–319.

208. **Noordhuis MG, Eijsink JJH, Roossink F, et al.** Prognostic cell biological markers in cervical cancer patients primarily treated with

(chemo)radiation: A systematic review. *Int J Radiat Oncol Biol Phys.* 2011;79:325–334.

209. **Peters WA 3rd, Liu PY, Barrett RJ, et al.** Cisplatin and 5-FU plus radiation therapy are superior to radiation therapy as adjunctive in high-risk early-stage carcinoma of the cervix after radical hysterectomy and pelvic lymphadenectomy: Report of a phase III intergroup study. *J Clin Oncol.* 2000;18:1606–1613.

210. **Monk BJ, Wang J, Im S, et al.** Rethinking the use of radiation and chemotherapy after radical hysterectomy: A clinical-pathologic analysis of a Gynecologic Oncology Group/Southwest Oncology Group/Radiation Therapy Oncology Group trial. *Gynecol Oncol.* 2005;96:721–728.

211. **Thomas GM, Dembo AJ.** Is there a role for adjuvant pelvic radiotherapy after radical hysterectomy in early stage cervical cancer? *Int J Gynecol Cancer.* 1991;1:1–8.

212. **Sedlis A, Bundy BN, Rotman M, et al.** A randomized trial of pelvic radiation therapy versus no further therapy in selected patients with stage IB carcinoma of the cervix after radical hysterectomy and pelvic lymphadenectomy: A Gynecologic Oncology Group study. *Gynecol Oncol.* 1999;73:177–183.

213. **Rotman M, Sedlis A, Piedmonte MR, et al.** A phase III randomized trial of postoperative pelvic irradiation in stage IB cervical carcinoma with poor prognostic features: Follow-up of a Gynecologic Oncology Group study. *Int J Radiat Oncol Biol Phys.* 2006;65:169–176.

214. **Pieterse QD, Trimbos JBMZ, Dijkman A, et al.** Postoperative radiation therapy improves prognosis in patients with adverse risk factors in localized, early-stage cervical cancer: A retrospective comparative study. *Int J Gynecol Cancer.* 2006;16:1112–1118.

215. **Kridelka FJ, Berg DO, Neuman M, et al.** Adjuvant small field pelvic radiation for patients with high-risk stage IB node negative cervical cancer after radical hysterectomy and pelvic lymph node dissection: A pilot study. *Cancer.* 1999;86:2059–2065.

216. **Ohara K, Tsunoda H, Nishida M, et al.** Use of small pelvic field instead of whole pelvic field in postoperative radiotherapy for node-negative, high-risk stage I and II cervical squamous carcinoma. *Int J Gynecol Cancer.* 2003;13:170–176.

217. **Ohara K, Tsunoda H, Satoh T, et al.** Use of the small pelvic field instead of the classic whole pelvic field in postoperative radiotherapy for cervical cancer: Reduction of adverse events. *Int J Radiat Oncol Biol Phys.* 2004;60:258–264.

218. **Yeo RMC, Chia YN, Namuduri RPD, et al.** Tailoring adjuvant radiotherapy for stage 1B-IIa node negative cervical hysterectomy after radical hysterectomy and pelvic lymph node dissection using the GOG score. *Gynecol Oncol.* 2011;123:225–229.

219. **Thomas G, Dembo A, Ackerman I, et al.** A randomized trial of standard versus partially hyperfractionated radiation with or without concurrent 5-fluorouracil in locally advanced cervical cancer. *Gynecol Oncol.* 1998;69:137–145.

220. **Tierney JF, Stewart LA.** Neoadjuvant chemotherapy followed by radiotherapy for locally advanced cervix cancer: A meta-analysis using individual patient data from randomized controlled trials. *Int J Gynecol Cancer.* 2002;12:576(abst).

221. **Stehman FB, Bundy BN, Thomas G, et al.** Hydroxyurea versus *misonidazole* with radiation in cervical carcinoma: Long term follow-up of a Gynecologic Oncology Group trial. *J Clin Oncol.* 1993;11:1523–1528.

222. **Rose PG, Bundy B, Watkins EB, et al.** Concurrent cisplatin-based radiotherapy and chemotherapy for locally advanced cervical cancer. *N Engl J Med.* 1999;340:1144–1153.

223. **Rose PG, Ali S, Watkins E, et al.** Long term follow-up of a randomized trial comparing concurrent single agent cisplatin or cisplatin-based combination chemotherapy for locally advanced cervical cancer: A Gynecologic Oncology Group Study. *J Clin Oncol.* 2007;25:1–7.

224. **Morris M, Eifel PJ, Lu J, et al.** Pelvic radiation with concurrent chemotherapy compared with pelvic and paraaortic radiation for high-risk cervical cancer. *N Engl J Med.* 1999;340:1137–1143.

225. **Whitney CW, Sause W, Bundy BN, et al.** Randomized comparison of fluorouracil plus cisplatin vs hydroxyurea as an adjunct to radiation therapy in stage IIB–IVA carcinoma of the cervix with negative paraaortic nodes: A Gynecologic Oncology Group and Southwest Oncology Group study. *J Clin Oncol.* 1999;17:1339–1348.

226. **Trimble EL, Harlan LC, Gius D, et al.** Patterns of care for women with cervical cancer in the United States. *Cancer.* 2008;113:743–749.

227. **Kizer NT, Thaker PH, Gao F, et al.** The effects of body mass index on complications and survival outcomes in patients with cervical carcinoma undergoing curative chemoradiation therapy. *Cancer.* 2011;117:948–956.

228. **Medical Research Council Clinical Trials Unit.** Reducing uncertainties about the effects of chemoradiotherapy for cervical cancer: A systematic review and meta-analysis of individual patient data from 18 randomized trials. *J Clin Oncol.* 2008;26:5802–5812.

229. **Torres MA, Jhingran A, Thames HD, et al.** Comparison of treatment tolerance and outcomes in patients with cervical cancer treated with concurrent chemoradiotherapy in a prospective randomized trial or with standard treatment. *Int J Radiat Oncol Biol Phys.* 2008;70:118–125.

230. **van der Zee J, González GD.** The Dutch Deep Hyperthermia trial: Results in cervical cancer. *Int J Hyperthermia.* 2002;18:1–12. (Erratum in *Int J Hyperthermoa.* 2003;19:213.)

231. **Lutgens L, van der Zee J, Pijls-Johannesma M, et al.** Combined use of hyperthermia and radiation therapy for treating locally advanced cervix carcinoma. *Cochrane Database Syst Rev.* 2010;(3): CD006377.doi: 10.1002/14651858.CD006377.pub3.Review.

232. **Dueñas-González A, Zarbá JJ, Patel F, et al.** Phase III, open label, randomized study comparing concurrent gemcitabine and cisplatin versus concurrent cisplatin and radiation in patients with stages IIB to IVA carcinoma of the cervix. *J Clin Oncol.* 2011;29: 1678–1685.

233. **Mileshkin LR, Narayan K, Moore KN, et al.** A phase III trial of adjuvant chemotherapy following chemoradiation as primary treatment for locally advanced cervical cancer compared to chemoradiation alone: The OUTBACK TRIAL. *J Clin Oncol.* 2012;30(suppl: abstr TPS5116).

234. **Kim BK, Lee IJ, Kim SK, et al.** Tumor heterogeneity of FIGO stage III carcinoma of the uterine cervix. *Int J Radiat Oncol Biol Phys.* 2009;75:1323–1328.

235. **Rose PG, Ali S, Whitney CW.** Impact of hydronephrosis on outcome of stage IIIB cervical cancer patients with disease limited to the pelvis, treated with radiation and concurrent chemotherapy: A Gynecologic Oncology Group study. *Gynecol Oncol.* 2010;117:270–275.

236. **Clifford KS, Leung W, Grigsby PW, et al.** The clinical implications of hydronephrosis and the level of ureteral obstruction in stage IIIB cervical cancer. *Int J Radiat Oncol Biol Phys.* 1998;40:1095–1100.

237. **Horan G, McArdle O, Martin J, et al.** Pelvic radiotherapy in patients with hydronephrosis in stage IIIB cancer of the cervix: Renal effects and the optimal timing of urinary diversion. *Gynecol Oncol.* 2006;101:441–444.

238. **Varia MA, Bundy BN, Deppe G, et al.** Cervical carcinoma metastatic to paraaortic nodes: Extended field radiation therapy with concomitant 5-fluorouracil and cisplatin chemotherapy. A Gynecologic Oncology Group study. *Int J Radiat Oncol Biol Phys.* 1998;42: 1015–1023.

239. **Grigsby PW, Heydon K, Mutch DG, et al.** Long term follow-up of RTOG 92–10: Cervical cancer with positive paraaortic nodes. *Int J Radiat Oncol Biol Phys.* 2001;51:982–987.

240. **Small W Jr, Winter K, Levenback C, et al.** Extended field irradiation and intracavitary brachytherapy combined with cisplatin chemotherapy for cervical cancer with positive paraaortic or high common iliac lymph nodes: Results of arm 1 of RTOG 0116. *Int J Radiat Oncol Biol Phys.* 2007;68:1081–1087.

241. **Beriwal S, Gan GN, Heron DE, et al.** Early clinical outcome with concurrent chemotherapy and extended-field, intensity-modulated radiotherapy for cervical cancer. *Int J Radiat Oncol Biol Phys.* 2007; 68:166–171.

242. **Kim YS, Kim JH, Ahn SD, et al.** High-dose extended field irradiation and high-dose-rate brachytherapy with concurrent chemotherapy for cervical cancer with positive paraaortic lymph nodes. *Int J Radiat Oncol Biol Phys.* 2009;74:1522–1528.

243. **Walker JL, Morrison A, DiSilvestro P, et al.** A phase I/II study of extended field radiation therapy with concomitant paclitaxel and cisplatin chemotherapy in patients with cervical carcinoma metastatic to paraaortic lymph nodes: A Gynecologic Oncology Group study. *Gynecol Oncol.* 2009;112:78–84.

244. **Rajasooriyar C, Van Dyk S, Bernshaw D, et al.** Patterns of failure and treatment-related toxicity in advanced cervical cancer patients treated using extended field radiotherapy with curative intent. *Int J Radiat Oncol Biol Phys.* 2011;80:422–428.

245. **Kazumoto T, Kato S, Yokota H, et al.** Is a low dose of concomitant chemotherapy with extended-field radiotherapy acceptable as an efficient treatment for cervical cancer patients with metastases to the para-aortic lymph nodes? *Int J Gynecol Oncol.* 2011;21:1465–1471.

246. **Zang G, Fu C, Zang Y, et al.** Extended-field intensity-modulated radiotherapy and concurrent cisplatin-based chemotherapy for postoperative cervical cancer with common iliac or paraaortic lymph node metastases. *Int J Gynecol Cancer.* 2012;22:1220–1225.

247. **Narayan K, Fisher RJ, Bernshaw D, et al.** Patterns of failure and prognostic factor analyses in locally advanced cervical cancer patients staged by positron emission tomography and treated with curative intent. *Int J Gynecol Cancer.* 2009;19:912–918.

248. **Rotman M, Choi K, Guze C, et al.** Prophylactic irradiation of the paraaortic lymph node chain in stage IIB and bulky stage IB carcinoma of the cervix: Initial treatment results of RTOG 7920. *Int J Radiat Oncol Biol Phys.* 1990;19:513–521.

249. **Quinn MA, Benedet JL, Odicino F, et al.** Carcinoma of the cervix uteri: FIGO 26th annual report on the results of treatment in gynaecological cancer. *Int J Gynecol Obstet.* 2006;95:S43–S103.

250. **Brooks RA, Rader JS, Dehdashti F, et al.** Surveillance FDG-PET detection of asymptomatic recurrences in patients with cervical cancer. *Gynecol Oncol.* 2009;112:104–109.

251. **Silva S, Herschtal A, Thomas JM, et al.** Impact of post-therapy Positron Emission Tomography on prognostic stratification and surveillance after chemoradiotherapy for cervical cancer. *Cancer.* 2011;117:3981–3988.

252. **Orr JM, Barnett JC, Leath CA III.** Incidence of subsequent abnormal cytology in cervical cancer patients completing five years of post treatment surveillance without evidence of recurrence. *Gynecol Oncol.* 2011;122:501–504.

253. **Duyn A, van Eijkeran M, Kenter G, et al.** Recurrent cervical cancer: Detection and prognosis. *Acta Obstet Gynecol Scand.* 2002; 81:759–763.

254. **Chen N-J, Okuda H, Sekiba K.** Recurrent carcinoma of the vagina following Okabayashi's radical hysterectomy for cervical cancer. *Gynecol Oncol.* 1985;20:10–16.

255. **Havrilesky LJ, Wong TZ, Secord AA, et al.** The role of PET scanning in the detection of recurrent cervical cancer. *Gynecol Oncol.* 2003;90:186–190.

256. **Chung HH, Kim S-K, Kim TH, et al.** Clinical impact of FDG-PET imaging in post-therapy surveillance of uterine cervical cancer: From diagnosis to prognosis. *Gynecol Oncol.* 2006;103:165–170.

257. **Smith HO, Tiffany MF, Qualls CR, et al.** The rising incidence of adenocarcinoma relative to squamous cell carcinoma of the uterine cervix in the United States: A 24 year population-based study. *Gynecol Oncol.* 2000;78:97–105.

258. **Bray F, Carstensen B, Møller H, et al.** Incidence trends of adenocarcinoma of the cervix in 13 European countries. *Cancer Epidemiol Biomarkers Prev.* 2005;14:2191–2199.

259. **Gien LT, Beauchemin M-C, Thomas G.** Adenocarcinoma: A unique cervical cancer. *Gynecol Oncol.* 2010;116:140–146.

260. **Castellsague X, Diaz M, De Sanjose S, et al.** Worldwide human papillomavirus etiology of cervical adenocarcinoma and its cofactors: Implications for screening and prevention. *J Natl Cancer Inst.* 2006;98:303–315.

261. **Sherman ME, Wang SS, Carreon J, et al.** Mortality trends for cervical squamous and adenocarcinoma in the United States. *Cancer.* 2005;103:1258–1264.

262. **Eifel JP, Morris M, Oswald MJ, et al.** Adenocarcinoma of the uterine cervix: Prognosis and patterns of failure in 367 cases. *Cancer.* 1990;65:2507–2514.

263. **Shimada M, Kiwaga J, Nishimura R, et al.** Ovarian metastasis in carcinoma of the uterine cervix. *Gynecol Oncol.* 2006;101:234–237.

264. **Berek JS, Hacker NF, Fu Y-S, et al.** Adenocarcinoma of the uterine cervix: Histologic variables associated with lymph node metastasis and survival. *Obstet Gynecol.* 1985;65:46–52.

265. **Nakanishi T, Ishikawa H, Suzuki Y, et al.** A comparison of prognoses of pathologic stage IB adenocarcinoma and squamous cell carcinoma of the uterine cervix. *Gynecol Oncol.* 2000;79:289–293.

266. **Duk JM, De Bruijn HWA, Groenier KH, et al.** Adenocarcinoma of the cervix. *Cancer.* 1990;65:1830–1837.

267. **Takahiro T, Onda T, Sasajima Y, et al.** Prognostic significance of positive peritoneal cytology in adenocarcinoma of the uterine cervix. *Gynecol Oncol.* 2009;115:488–492.

268. **Helm CW, Kinney WK, Keeney G, et al.** A matched study of surgically treated stage IB adenosquamous carcinoma and adenocarcinoma of the uterine cervix. *Int J Gynecol Cancer.* 1993;3:245–249.

269. **Glucksman A, Cherry C.** Incidence, histology and response to radiation of mixed carcinomas (adenoacanthomas) of the uterine cervix. *Cancer.* 1956;9:976–983.

270. **Hopkins MP, Morley GW.** Glassy cell adenocarcinoma of the uterine cervix. *Am J Obstet Gynecol.* 2004;190:67–70.

271. **Gray HJ, Garcia R, Tamimi HK, et al.** Glassy cell carcinoma of the cervix revisited. *Gynecol Oncol.* 2002;85:274–277.

272. **Takahashi Y, Sasaki H, Mogami H, et al.** Adjuvant combined paclitaxel and carboplatin chemotherapy for glassy cell carcinoma of the uterine cervix: Report of three cases with clinicopathological analysis. *J Obstet Gynaecol Res.* 2011;37:1860–1863.

273. **Nasu K, Takai N, Narahara H.** Multimodal treatment for glassy cell carcinoma of the uterine cervix. *J Obstet Gynaecol Res.* 2009; 35:584–587.

274. **Seamon LG, Downey GO, Harrison CR, et al.** Neoadjuvant chemotherapy followed by postpartum chemoradiotherapy and chemoconsolidation for stage IIIB glassy cell cervical carcinoma during pregnancy. *Gynecol Oncol.* 2009;114:540–541.

275. **Ferrandina G, Salutari V, Petrillo M, et al.** Conservatively treated glassy cell carcinoma of the cervix. *World J Surg Oncol.* 2008;6:92–93.

276. **Plante M, Renaud MC, Francois H, et al.** Vaginal radical trachelectomy: An oncologically safe fertility preserving surgery. An updated series of 72 cases and review of the literature. *Gynecol Oncol.* 2004;94:614–623.

277. **McKelvey JL, Goodlin RR.** Adenoma malignum of the cervix: A cancer of deceptively innocent histological pattern. *Cancer.* 1963;16:549–557.

278. **Silverberg SG, Hurt WG.** Minimal deviation adenocarcinoma ("adenoma malignum") of the cervix: A reappraisal. *Am J Obstet Gynecol.* 1975;121:971–975.

279. **McGowan L, Young RH, Scully RE.** Peutz-Jeghers syndrome with "adenoma malignum" of the cervix: A report of two cases. *Gynecol Oncol.* 1980;10:125–133.

280. **Hart WR.** Special types of adenocarcinomas of the uterine cervix. *Int J Gynecol Pathol.* 2002;21:327–346.

281. **Li G, Jang W, Gui SXUC.** Minimal deviation adenocarcinoma of the uterine cervix. *Int J Gynecol Obstet.* 2010;110:89–92.

282. **Hirai Y, Takeshima N, Haga A, et al.** A clinicocytopathologic study of adenoma malignum of the cervix. *Gynecol Oncol.* 1998;70:219–223.

283. **Park SB, Moon MH, Hong SR, et al.** Adenoma malignum of the uterine cervix: Ultrasonographic findings in 11 patients. *Ultrasound Obstet Gynecol.* 2011;38:716–721.

284. **Lim K-T, Lee I-H, Kim T-J, et al.** Adenoma malignum of the uterine cervix: Clinicopathologic analysis of 18 cases. *Kaohsiung J Med Sci.* 2012;28:161–164.

285. **Gilks CB, Young RH, Aguirre P, et al.** Adenoma malignum (minimal deviation adenocarcinoma) of the uterine cervix: A clinicopathological and immunohistochemical analysis of 26 cases. *Am J Surg Pathol.* 1989;13:717–729.

286. **Musa AG, Hughes RR, Coleman SA.** Adenoid cystic carcinoma of the cervix: A report of 17 cases. *Gynecol Oncol.* 1985;22:167–173.

287. **Prempree T, Villasanta U, Tang C-K.** Management of adenoid cystic carcinoma of the uterine cervix (cylindroma). *Cancer.* 1980; 46:1631–1635.

288. **Koyfman SA, Abidi A, Ravichandran P, et al.** Adenoid cystic carcinoma of the cervix. *Gynecol Oncol.* 2005;99:477–480.

289. **Ferry JA, Scully RE.** "Adenoid cystic" carcinoma and adenoid basal carcinoma of the uterine cervix: A study of 28 cases. *Am J Surg Pathol.* 1988;12:134–140.

290. **Viriyapak B, Park ST, Lee AW, et al.** Cervical adenoid basal carcinoma associated with invasive squamous cell carcinoma: A report of rare co-existence and review of the literature. *World J Surg Oncol.* 2011;9:132–138.

291. **Brainard JA, Hart WR.** Adenoid basal epithelioma of the uterine cervix. *Am J Surg Pathol.* 1998;22:965–972.

292. Herbst AL, Kurman RJ, Scully RE, et al. Clear cell adenocarcinoma of the genital tract in young females. *N Engl J Med.* 1972;287:1259–1264.

293. Herbst AL. Behavior of estrogen-associated female genital tract cancer and its relation to neoplasia following intrauterine exposure to diethylstilbestrol (DES). *Gynecol Oncol.* 2000;76:147–156.

294. Thomas MB, Wright JD, Leiser AL, et al. Clear cell carcinoma of the cervix: A multi-institutional review in the post-DES era. *Gynecol Oncol.* 2008;109:335–339.

295. Reich O, Tamussino K, Lauhousen M, et al. Clear cell carcinoma of the uterine cervix: Pathology and prognosis in surgically treated stage IB–IIB disease in women not exposed to *in utero* diethylstilbestrol. *Gynecol Oncol.* 2000;76:331–335.

296. Young RH, Scully RE. Villoglandular papillary adenocarcinoma of the uterine cervix. *Cancer.* 1989;63:1773–1779.

297. Jones MW, Silverberg SG, Kurman RJ. Well differentiated villoglandular adenocarcinoma of the uterine cervix: A clinicopathologic study of 24 cases. *Int J Gynecol Pathol.* 1993;12:1–7.

298. Kaku T, Kamura T, Shigematsu T, et al. Adenocarcinoma of the uterine cervix with predominantly villoglandular papillary growth pattern. *Gynecol Oncol.* 1997;64:147–152.

299. Utsugi K, Shimizu Y, Akiyama F, et al. Clinicopathologic features of villoglandular papillary adenocarcinoma of the uterine cervix. *Gynecol Oncol.* 2004;92:64–70.

300. Scully RE, Aguirre P, De Lellis RA. Argyrophilia, serotonin, and peptide hormones in the female genital tract and its tumors. *Int J Gynecol Pathol.* 1984;3:51–70.

301. McCusker ME, Cote TR, Clegg LX, et al. Endocrine tumors of the uterine cervix: Incidence, demographics, and survival with comparison to squamous cell carcinoma. *Gynecol Oncol.* 2003;88:333–339.

302. Chen J, Macdonald K, Gaffey DK. Incidence, mortality, and prognostic factors of small cell carcinoma of the cervix. *Obstet Gynecol.* 2008;111:1394–1402.

303. Chang T-C, Lai C-H, Tseng C-J, et al. Prognostic factors in surgically treated small cell cervical carcinoma followed by adjuvant chemotherapy. *Cancer.* 1998;83:712–718.

304. McCann GA, Boutsicaris CE, Preston MM, et al. Neuroendocrine carcinoma of the uterine cervix: The role of multimodality therapy in early-stage disease. *Gynecol Oncol.* 2013;129:135–139.

305. Embry JR, Kelly MG, Post MD, et al. Large cell neuroendocrine carcinoma of the cervix: Prognostic factors and survival advantage with platinum chemotherapy. *Gynecol Oncol.* 2011;120:444–448.

306. Zhou C, Gilks CB, Hayes M, et al. Papillary serous carcinoma of the uterine cervix: A clinicopathologic study of 17 cases. *Am J Surg Path.* 1998;22:113–120.

307. Togami S, Kasamatsu T, Sasajima Y, et al. Serous adenocarcinoma of the uterine cervix: A clinicopathological study of 12 cases and a review of the literature. *Gynecol Obstet Invest.* 2012;73:26–31.

308. Bansal S, Lewin SN, Burke WM, et al. Sarcoma of the cervix: Natural history and outcomes. *Gynecol Oncol.* 2010;118:134–138.

309. Ries LAG, Mariotto KM, Miller BA, et al., eds. *SEER Cancer Statistics Review, 1975–2003.* Bethesda, MD: National Cancer Institute; 2006.

310. Kriseman ML, Wang W-L, Sullinger J, et al. Rhabdomyosarcoma of the cervix in adult women and younger patients. *Gynecol Oncol.* 2012;126:351–356.

311. Dehner LP, Jarzembowski JA, Hill DA. Embryonal rhabdomyosarcoma of the uterine cervix: A report of 14 cases and a discussion of its usual clinicopathological associations. *Mod Pathol.* 2012;25:602–614.

312. Daya DA, Scully RE. Sarcoma botryoides of the uterine cervix in young women: A clinicopathological study of 13 cases. *Gynecol Oncol.* 1988;29:290–304.

313. Arndt CA, Donaldson SS, Anderson JR, et al. What constitutes optimal therapy for patients with rhabdomyosarcoma of the female genital tract? *Cancer.* 2001;91:2454–2468.

314. Brand E, Berek JS, Nieberg RK, et al. Rhabdomyosarcoma of the uterine cervix: Sarcoma botryoides. *Cancer.* 1987;60:1552–1560.

315. Chorlton I, Karnei RF, King FM, et al. Primary malignant reticuloendothelial disease involving the vagina, cervix and corpus uteri. *Obstet Gynecol.* 1974;44:735–748.

316. Harris NL, Scully RE. Malignant lymphoma and granulocytic sarcoma of the uterus and vagina. *Cancer.* 1984;52:2530–2545.

317. Komaki R, Cox JD, Hansen RM, et al. Malignant lymphoma of the uterine cervix. *Cancer.* 1984;54:1699–1704.

318. Perrin T, Farrant M, McCarthy K, et al. Lymphomas of the cervix and upper vagina: A report of five cases and a review of the literature. *Gynecol Oncol.* 1992;44:87–95.

319. Upanal N, Enjeti A. Primary lymphoma of the uterus and cervix: Two cases and review of the literature. *Aust NZ J Obstet Gynaecol.* 2011;51:559–562.

320. Jennings RH, Barclay DL. Verrucous carcinoma of the cervix. *Cancer.* 1972;30:430–433.

321. Crowther ME, Lowe DG, Shepherd JH. Verrucous carcinoma of the female genital tract: A review. *Obstet Gynecol Surv.* 1988;45:263–280.

322. Piura B. Management of primary melanoma of the female urogenital tract. *Lancet Oncol.* 2008;9:973–981.

323. Mordel N, Mor-Yosef S, Ben-Baruch N, et al. Malignant melanoma of the uterine cervix: Case report and review of the literature. *Gynecol Oncol.* 1989;32:375–380.

324. Santosa JT, Kucora PR, Ray J. Primary malignant melanoma of the uterine cervix: Two case reports and a century's review. *Obstet Gynecol Surv.* 1990;45:733–744.

325. Mazur MT, Hsuch S, Gersell DJ. Metastases to the female genital tract: Analysis of 325 cases. *Cancer.* 1984;53:1978–1984.

326. Lemoine NR, Hall PA. Epithelial tumors metastatic to the uterine cervix. *Cancer.* 1986;57:2002–2005.

327. Silva CS, Cardoso CO, Menegaz RA, et al. Cervical stump cancer: A study of 14 cases. *Acta Gynecol Obstet.* 2004;270:126–128.

328. Miller BE, Copeland LJ, Hamberger AD, et al. Carcinoma of the cervical stump. *Gynecol Oncol.* 1984;18:100–108.

329. Kinney WK, Egorshin EV, Ballard DJ, et al. Long-term survival and sequelae after surgical management of invasive cervical carcinoma diagnosed at the time of simple hysterectomy. *Gynecol Oncol.* 1992;44:24–27.

330. Chapman JA, Mannel RS, Di Saia PJ, et al. Surgical treatment of unexpected invasive cervical cancer found at total hysterectomy. *Obstet Gynecol.* 1992;80:931–934.

331. Hopkins MP, Peters WA III, Andersen W, et al. Invasive cervical cancer treated initially by standard hysterectomy. *Gynecol Oncol.* 1990;36:7–12.

332. Saibishkumar EP, Patel FD, Ghoshal S, et al. Results of salvage radiotherapy after inadequate surgery in invasive cervical carcinoma patients: A retrospective analysis. *Int J Radiat Oncol Biol Phys.* 2005;63:828–833.

333. Pisco JM, Martins JM, Correia MG. Internal iliac artery embolization to control hemorrhage from pelvic neoplasms. *Radiology.* 1989;172:337–343.

334. Eifel PJ, Jhingran A, Brown J, et al. Time course and outcome of central recurrence after radiation therapy for carcinoma of the cervix. *Int J Gynecol Cancer.* 2006;16:1106–1111.

335. Grigsby PW. Radiotherapy for pelvic recurrence after radical hysterectomy for cervical cancer. *Radiat Med.* 2005;23:327–330.

336. Thomas GM, Dembo AJ, Black B, et al. Concurrent radiation and chemotherapy for carcinoma of the cervix recurrent after radical surgery. *Gynecol Oncol.* 1987;27:254–260.

337. Shiromizu K, Kasamatsu T, Takahashi M, et al. A clinicopathological study of postoperative pulmonary metastases of uterine cervical carcinomas. *J Obstet Gynaecol Res.* 1999;25:245–249.

338. Rutledge S, Carey MS, Pritchard H, et al. Conservative surgery for recurrent or persistent carcinoma of the cervix following irradiation: Is exenteration always necessary? *Gynecol Oncol.* 1994;52:353–359.

339. Maneo A, Landoni F, Cormio G, et al. Radical hysterectomy for recurrent or persistent cervical cancer following radiation therapy. *Int J Gynecol Cancer.* 1999;9:295–301.

340. Vermorken JB. The role of chemotherapy in squamous cell carcinoma of the uterine cervix: A review. *Int J Gynecol Cancer.* 1993;3:129–142.

341. Hogg R, Friedlander M. Role of systemic chemotherapy in metastatic cervical cancer. *Expert Rev Anticancer Ther.* 2003;3:234–240.

342. Long HJ III. Management of metastatic cervical cancer: Review of the literature. *J Clin Oncol.* 2007;25:2966–2974.

343. Bonomi P, Blessing JA, Stehman FB, et al. Randomized trial of three cisplatin dose schedules in squamous cell carcinoma of the cervix: A Gynecologic Oncology Group study. *J Clin Oncol.* 1985;3:1079–1085.

344. **McGuire WP III, Arseneau J, Blessing JA, et al.** A randomized comparative trial of carboplatin and iproplatin in advanced squamous carcinoma of the uterine cervix: A Gynecologic Oncology Group study. *J Clin Oncol.* 1989;7:1462–1468.

345. **Bezwoda WR, Nussenbaum M, Med M, et al.** Treatment of metastatic and recurrent cervix cancer with chemotherapy: A randomized trial comparing cis-diamminedichloro-platinum plus methotrexate. *Med Pedriatic Oncol.* 1986;14:17–19.

346. **Leath CA, III, Straughn JM Jr.** Chemotherapy for advanced and recurrent cervical carcinoma: Results from cooperative group trials. *Gynecol Oncol.* 2013;129:251–257.

347. **Hirte HW, Strychowsky JE, Oliver T, et al.** Chemotherapy for recurrent, metastatic, or persistent cervical cancer: A systematic review. *Int J Gynecol Cancer.* 2007;17:1194–1204.

348. **Cadron I, Van Gorp T, Amant F, et al.** Chemotherapy for recurrent cervical cancer. *Gynecol Oncol.* 2007;107(1 suppl 1):S113–S118.

349. **Tao X, Hu W, Ramirez PT, Kavanagh JJ.** Chemotherapy for recurrent and metastatic cervical cancer. *Gynecol Oncol.* 2008;110;S67–S71.

350. **Movva S, Rodriguez L, Arias-Pulido H, et al.** Novel chemotherapy approaches for cervical cancer. *Cancer.* 2009;115:3166–3180.

351. **Mountzios G, Soultati A, Pectasides D, et al.** Developments in the systemic treatment of metastatic cervical cancer. *Cancer Treat Rev.* 2013;39:430–443.

352. **Moore DH, Blessing JA, McQuellon RP, et al.** Phase III study of cisplatin with or without paclitaxel in stage IVB, recurrent, or persistent squamous cell carcinoma of the cervix: A gynecologic oncology group study. *J Clin Oncol.* 2004;22:3113–3119.

353. **Long HJ III, Bundy BN, Glendys ED, et al.** Randomized phase III trial of cisplatin with or without topotecan for carcinoma of the uterine cervix: A Gynecologic Oncology Group study. *J Clin Oncol.* 2005;23:4626–4633.

354. **Khoury-Collado F, Bowes RJ, Jhamb N, et al.** Unexpected long-term survival without evidence of disease after salvage chemotherapy for recurrent metastatic cervical cancer: A case series. *Gynecol Oncol.* 2007;105:823–825.

355. **Sutton GP, Blessing JA, Adcock L, et al.** Phase II study of ifosfamide and mesna in patients with previously-treated carcinoma of the cervix: A Gynecologic Oncology Group study. *Invest New Drugs.* 1989;7:341–343.

356. **Sutton GP, Blessing JA, McGuire WP, et al.** Phase II trial of ifosfamide and mesna in patients with advanced or recurrent squamous carcinoma of the cervix who had never received chemotherapy: A Gyenclogic Oncology group study. *Am J Obstet Gynecol.* 1993;168:805–807.

357. **Look KY, Blessing JA, Muss HB, et al.** 5-fluorouracil and low-dose leucovorin in the treatment of recurrent squamous cell carcinoma of the cervix. A phase II trial of the Gyencologic Oncology group. *Am J Clin Oncol.* 1992;15:497–499.

358. **Garcia AA, Blessing JA, Darcy KM, et al.** Phase II clinical trial of capecitabine in the treatment of advanced, persistent or recurrent squamous carcinoma of the cervix with translational research: A Gynecologic Oncology Group study. *Gynecol Oncol.* 2007;104:572–579.

359. **Lorvidhaya V, Chitapanarux I, Phromratanapongse P, et al.** Phase II study of capecitabine (Ro 09–1978) in patients who have failed first line treatment for locally advanced and/or metastatic cervical cancer. *Gan to Kagaku Ryoho.* 2010;37:1271.

360. **Katsumata N, Hirai Y, Kamiura S, et al.** Phase II study of S-1, an oral fluoropyrimidine, in patients with advanced or recurrent cervical cancer. *Ann Oncol.* 2011;22:1353–1357.

361. **Miller DS, Blessing JA, Bodurka DC, et al.** Evaluation of pemetrexed (Alimta, LY231514) as second line chemotherapy in persistent or recurrent carcinoma of the cervix: A phase II study of the Gynecologic Oncology Group. *Gynecol Oncol.* 2008;110:65–70.

362. **Lorusso D, Ferrandina G, Pignata S, et al.** Evaluation of pemetrexed (Alimta, LY231514) as second-line chemotherapy in persistent or recurrent carcinoma of the cervix: The CERVIX 1 study of the MITO (Multicentre Italian trials in Ovarian Cancer and Gyenclogic malignancies) group. *Ann Oncol.* 2010;21:61–66.

363. **Goedhals L, van Wyck AL, Smith BL, et al.** Pemetrexed (Alimta, LY231514) demonstrates clinical activity in chermonaive patients with cervical cancer in a phase II single-agent trial. *Int J Gynecol Cancer.* 2006;16:1172–1178.

364. **Van der Burg ME, Monfardini S, Guastalla JP, et al.** Phase II study of weekly 4-epidoxorubicin in patients with metastatic squamous cell cancer of the cervix: Sn EORTC Gynaecologic Cancer Cooperative Group study. *Eur J Cancer.* 1992;29A:147–148.

365. **Chauvergne J, Fumoleau P, Cappeleare P, et al.** Phase II study of pirarubicin (THP) in patients with cervical, endometrial and ovarian cancer: Study of the Clinical Screening group of the European Organization for Research and treatment of cancer (EORTC). *Eur J Cancer.* 1993;29A:350–354.

366. **Thigpen T, Blessing JA, Gallip DG, et al.** Phase II trial of mitomycin-C in squamous cell carcinoma of the uterine cervix: A Gynecologic Oncology Group study. *Gynecol Oncol.* 1995;57:376–379.

367. **Lhommé C, Vermorken JB, Mickiewicz E, et al.** Phase II trial of vinorelbine in patients with advanced cervical carcinoma: An EORTC Gynaecological Cancer Cooperative group study. *Eur J Cancer.* 2000; 36:194–199.

368. **Morris M, Brader KR, Levenback C, et al.** Phase II study of vinorelbine in advanced and recurrent squamous cell carcinoma of the cervix. *J Clin Oncol.* 1998;16:1094–1098.

369. **Muggia FM, Blessing JA, Method M, et al.** Evaluation of vinorelbine in persistent or recurrent squamous cell carcinoma of the cervix: A Gynecologic Oncology Group study. *Gynecol Oncol.* 2004;92:639–643.

370. **Muggia FM, Blessing JA, Waggoner S, et al.** Evaluation of vinorelbine in persistent or recurrent nonsquamous carcinoma of the cervix: A Gynecologic Oncology Group study. *Gynecol Oncol.* 2005;96:108–111.

371. **McGuire WP, Blessing JA, Moore D, et al.** Paclitaxel has moderate activity in squamous cervix cancer. A Gynecologic Oncology Group study. *J Clin Oncol.* 1996;14:792–795.

372. **Curtin JP, Blessing JA, Webster KD, et al.** Paclitaxel, an active agent in nonsquamous carcinomas of the uterine cervix: A Gynecologic Oncology Group study. *J Clin Oncol.* 2001;19:1275–1278.

373. **Kudelka AP, Winn R, Edwards CL, et al.** An update of a phase II study of paclitaxel in advanced or recurrent squamous cell cancer of the cervix. *Anticancer Drugs.* 1997;8:657–661.

374. **Garcia AA, Blessing JA, Vaccarello L, et al.** Phase II clinical trial of docetaxel in refractory squamous cell carcinoma of the cervix: A Gynecologic Oncology group study. *Am J Clin Oncol.* 2007;30:428–431.

375. **Kudelka AP, Verschraegen CF, Levy T, et al.** Preliminary report of the activity of docetaxel in advanced or recurrent squamous cell cancer of the cervix. *Anticancer Drugs.* 1996;7:398–401.

376. **Muderspach LI, Blessing JA, Levenback C, et al.** A phase II study of topotecan in patients with squamous cell carcinoma of the cervix: A Gynecologic Oncology Group study. *Gynecol Oncol.* 2001;81:213–215.

377. **Bookman MA, Blessing JA, Hanjani P, et al.** Topotecan in squamous cell carcinoma of the cervix: A phase II study of the Gynecologic Oncology Group. *Gynecol Oncol.* 2000;77:446–449.

378. **Look KY, Blessing JA, Levenback C, et al.** A phase II trial of CPT-11 in recurrent squamous carcinoma of the cervix: A Gynecologic Oncology Group study. *Gynecol Oncol.* 1998;70:334–338.

379. **Irvin WP, Price FV, Bailey H, et al.** P phase II study of irinotecan (CPT-11) in patients with advanced squamous cell carcinoma of the cervix. *Cancer.* 1998;82:328–333.

380. **Lhommé C, Fumoledau P, Fargeot P, et al.** Results of a European Organization for Research and Treatment of Cancer/Early Clinical Studies group phase II trial of first-line irinotecan in patients with advanced or recurrent squamous cell carcinoma of the cervix. *J Clin Oncol.* 1999;17:3136–3142.

381. **Verschraegen CF, Levy T, Kudelka AP, et al.** Phase II study if irinotecan in prior chemotherapy-treated squamous cell carcinoma of the cervix. *J Clin Oncol.* 1997;15:625–631.

382. **Takeuchi S, Dobashi K, Fujimoto S, et al.** A late phase II study of CPT-11 on uterine cervical cancer and ovarian cancer. *Gan To Kagaku Ryoho.* 1991;18:1681–1689.

383. **Rose M, Blessing JA, Van Le L, et al.** Prolonged oral etoposide in recurrent or advanced squamous cell carcinoma of the cervix. A Gynecologic Oncology Group study. *Gynecol Oncol.* 1998;70:263–266.

384. **Morris M, Brader KR, Burke TW, et al.** A phase II study of prolonged oral etoposide in advanced or recurrent carcinoma of the cervix. *Gynecol Oncol.* 1998;70:215–218.

385. **Pfeiffer P, Cold S, Bertelsen K, et al.** Teniposide in recurrent or advanced cervical carcinoma: A phase II trial in patients not previously treated with cytotoxic therapy. *Gynecol Oncol.* 1990;37:230–233.

386. **Monk BJ, Sill MW, McMeekin DS, et al.** Phase III trial of four cisplatin containing doublet combinations in stage IVB, recurrent, or persistent cervical carcinoma: A Gynecologic Oncology Group study. *J Clin Oncol.* 2009;27:4649–4655.

387. **Tewari KS, Sill M, Long HJ, et al.** Incorporation of bevacizumab in the treatment of recurrent and metastatic cervical cancer: A phase III randomized trial of the Gynecologic Oncology Group. *J Clin Oncol.* 2013;31(suppl); abstr 3.

388. **Kitagawa R, Katsumata N, Shibata T, et al.** A randomized phase III trial of paclitaxel plus carboplatin (TC) versus paclitaxel plus cisplatin (TP) in Stage IVb, persistent or recurrent cervical cancer: Japan Clinical Oncology Group study (JCOG0505). *J Clin Oncol.* 2012;30(suppl); abstr 5006.

389. **Vermorken JB, Zanetta G, De Oliveira CF, et al.** Randomized phase III trial of bleomycin, vindesine, mitomycin-C, and cisplatin (BEMP) versus cisplatin (P) in disseminated squamous-cell carcinoma of the uterine cervix: An EORTC Gynecological Cancer Cooperative Group study. *Ann Oncol.* 2001;12:967–974.

390. **Omura GA, Blessing JA, Vaccarello L, et al.** Randomized trial of cisplatin versus *cisplatin* plus mitolactol (Dibromodulcitol) versus cisplatin plus ifosfamide in advanced squamous carcinoma of the cervix: A Gynecologic Oncology group study. *J Clin Oncol.* 1997;15:165–171.

391. **Bloss JD, Blessing JA, Behrens BC, et al.** Randomized trial of cisplatin and ifosfamide with or without bleomycin in squamous carcinoma of the cervix: A gynecologic oncology group study. *J Clin Oncol.* 2002;20:1832–1837.

392. **Diaz-Padilla I, Monk BJ, Mackay HJ, et al.** Treatment of metastatic cervical cancer: Future directions involving targeted agents. *Crit Rev Oncol/Hematol.* 2013;85:303–314.

393. **Monk BJ, Willmott LJ, Sumner DA.** Anti-angiogenesis agents in metastatic or recurrent cervical cancer. *Gynecol Oncol.* 2010;116:181–186.

394. **Monk BJ, Sill MW, Burger RA, et al.** Phase II trial of bevacizumab in the treatment of persistent or recurrent squamous cell carcinoma of the cervix: A Gynecologic Oncology Group study. *J Clin Oncol.* 2009;27:1069–1074.

395. **Monk BJ, Mas Lopez L, Zarba JJ, et al.** Phase II, open-label-study of pazopanib or lapatinib monotherapy compared with pazopanib plus lapatinib combination therapy in patients with advanced and recurrent cervical cancer. *J Clin Oncol.* 2010;28:3562–3569.

396. **Mackay HJ, Tinker A, Winquist E, et al.** A phase II study of sunitinib in patients with locally advanced or metastatic cervical carcinoma: NCIC CTG Trial IND.184. *Gynecol Oncol.* 2010;116:163–167.

397. **Santin AD, Sill MW, McMeekin DS, et al.** Phase II trial of cetuximab in the treatment of persistent or recurrent squamous or non-squamous cell carcinoma of the cervix: A Gynecologic Oncology Group study. *Gynecol Oncol.* 2011;122:495–500.

398. **Farley J, Sill MW, Birrer M, et al.** Phase II study of cisplatin plus cetuximab in advanced, recurrent, and previously treated cancers of the cervix and evaluation of epidermal growth factor receptor immunohistochemical expression: A Gynecologic Oncology Group study. *Gynecol Oncol.* 2011;121:303–308.

399. **Kurtz JE, Hardy-Bessards AC, Deslandres M, et al.** Cetuximab, topotecan and cisplatin for the treatment of advanced cervical: A phase II GINECO trial. *Gynecol Oncol.* 2009;113:16–20.

400. **Schilder RJ, Sill MW, Lee YC, et al.** A phase II trial of erlotinib in recurrent squamous cell carcinoma of the cervix: A Gynecologic Oncology Group study. *Int J Gynecol Cancer.* 2009;19:929–933.

401. **Goncalves A, Fabbro M, Lhomme C, et al.** A phase II trial to evaluate gefitinib as second- or third-line treatment in patients with recurring locoregionally advanced or metastatic cervical cancer. *Gynecol Oncol.* 2008;108:42–46.

402. **Monk BJ, Pandite LN.** Survival data from a phase II, open-label study of pazopanib or lapatinib monotherapy in patients with advanced and recurrent cervical cancer. *J Clin Oncol.* 2011;29:4845.

403. **Scambia G, Ferrandina G, Distefano M, et al.** Epidermal growth factor receptor (EGFR) is not related to prognosis of cervical cancer. *Cancer Lett.* 1998;123:135–139.

404. **Kersemaekers AM, Fleuren GJ, Kenter GG, et al.** Oncogene alterations in carcinomas of the uterine cervix: Overexpression of the epidermal growth factor receptor is associated with poor prognosis. *Clin Cancer Res.* 1999;5:577–586.

405. **Del Campo JM, Prat A, Gil-Moreno A, et al.** Update on novel therapeutic agents for cervical cancer. *Gynecol Oncol.* 2008;110:S72–S76.

406. **Fan Z, Baselga J, Masui H, et al.** Antitumor effect of anti-epidermal growth factor receptor monoclonal antibodies plus cis-diamminedichloroplatinum on well established A431 cell xenografts. *Cancer Res.* 1993;53:4637–4642.

407. **Liang K, Ang KK, Milas L, et al.** The epidermal growth factor receptor mediates radioresistance. *Int J Radiat Oncol Biol Phys.* 2003;57:246–254.

408. **Fadare O, Zheng W.** HER2 protein (p185[HER2]) is only rarely overexpressed in cervical cancer. *Int J Gynecol Pathol.* 2004;23:410–411.

409. **Vermorken JB, Avall-Ludqvist E, Pfisterer J, et al.** The Gynecologic Cancer Intergroup (GCIG); History and current status. *Ann Oncol.* 2005;16(suppl. 8):viii32–viii42.

410. **Bacon M, Kitchener H, Stuart G, et al.** Gynecologic Cancer InterGroup and participants of the 4th Ovarian Cancer Consensus Conference. The global impact of the Gynecologic Cancer InterGroup in enhancing clinical trials in ovarian cancer. *Int J Gynecol Cancer.* 2011;21:746–749.

9

Uterine Cancer

Neville F. Hacker
Michael L. Friedlander

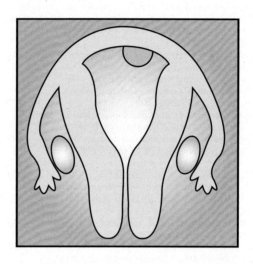

Endometrial carcinoma is the most common malignancy of the female genital tract in developed countries, and the fourth most common cancer in women after breast, lung, and colorectum. Developing countries and Japan have incidence rates four to five times lower than Western industrialized nations, with the lowest rates being in India and South Asia (1).

In the United States, it was anticipated there would, not will be 53,630 new cases and 8,590 deaths from the disease in 2014 (2). **African American women have a 40% lower risk of developing the disease but a 54% greater risk of dying from it,** mainly because of late diagnosis (3).

Two different clinicopathologic subtypes of endometrial cancer are recognized: The estrogen related (Type I, endometrioid), and the nonestrogen related (Type II, nonendometrioid). Each subtype has specific genetic alterations, with endometrioid tumors commonly exhibiting microsatellite instability and mutations in *PTEN, PIK3CA, K-ras,* and *CTNNBI* (β-*catenin*), while nonendometrioid (predominantly serous and clear cell) tumors are characterized by having *p53* mutations and chromosomal instability (4). **Patients with Type II tumors are more likely to be older, nonwhite, multiparous, current smokers, nonobese, and to have had breast cancer treated with *tamoxifen*** (5).

Approximately 80% of newly diagnosed endometrial carcinomas in the Western world are endometrioid in type (4). **Any factor that increases exposure to unopposed estrogen (e.g., estrogen replacement therapy, obesity, anovulatory cycles, estrogen-secreting tumors) increases the risk of these tumors, whereas factors that decrease exposure to estrogens or increase progesterone levels (e.g., oral contraceptives or smoking) tend to be protective** (1). A population-based Finnish study reported that use of continuous estradiol–progestin therapy for 3 years or more decreased the risk of Type I cancers by 76%, whereas sequential estradiol–progestin therapy for at least 5 years increased the risk by 69% if the progestin was added monthly, and by 76% if the progestin was added three monthly (6). **Women with Type I cancers associated with obesity are more likely to die of cardiovascular disease than cancer** (7), **and lifestyle issues need to be addressed when treating these women** (8).

The average age of patients with endometrioid cancer is approximately 63 years, and 70% or so are confined to the corpus at the time of diagnosis. Their 5-year survival is approximately 83% (9). By contrast, the average age of patients with nonendometrioid cancer is 67 years, and at least half have already spread beyond the corpus at the time of diagnosis. Their 5-year survival is approximately 62% for clear cell carcinomas and 53% for serous cancers (9).

Endometrial cancer may occasionally develop after radiation treatment for cervical or other pelvic cancers. Kumar et al. (10) reported 205 radiation-associated cancers and 1,001 sporadic second endometrial cancers in women with a primary cancer of pelvic organs (bladder, rectum, cervix, vulva, or vagina). The cases were identified from the Surveillance, Epidemiology, and End Results (SEER) database between 1973 and 2005. **Lesions in the radiation-associated cohort were more likely to be nonendometrioid histology** (76% vs. 51%; $p < 0.001$), **poorly differentiated** (58% vs. 28%; $p < 0.001$), **and advanced stage** (43% vs. 16%; $p < 0.001$). The 5-year survival for radiation-associated and sporadic endometrial cancers was 27.1% and 57.1%, respectively ($p < 0.001$) (10).

Screening of Asymptomatic Women

The ideal method for outpatient sampling of the endometrium has not yet been devised, and no blood test of sufficient sensitivity and specificity has been developed. Therefore, mass screening of the population is not practical. Screening for endometrial carcinoma or its precursors is justified for certain high-risk people, including those shown in Table 9.1.

Only about 50% of women with endometrial cancer have malignant cells on a Papanicolaou (Pap) smear, but compared with patients who have normal cervical cytology, patients with suspicious or malignant cells are more likely to have deeper myometrial invasion, higher tumor grade, positive peritoneal cytologic findings, and a more advanced stage of disease (11).

The appearance of normal-appearing endometrial cells in cervical smears taken in the second half of the menstrual cycle or in postmenopausal women is controversial. Montz reported endometrial histology from 93 asymptomatic postmenopausal women receiving hormone replacement therapy (HRT) with normal endometrial cells on a Pap smear. Eighteen patients (19%) had abnormalities identified, including seven endometrial polyps, seven cases of simple hyperplasia (one with atypia), three cases of complex hyperplasia (one with atypia), and one endometrial carcinoma (12). A Dutch study of 29,144 asymptomatic postmenopausal women found that **when normal endometrial cells were reported in the cervical smear, the prevalence rate of premalignant uterine disease was significantly higher** (6.5%) as compared to smears without these cells (0.2%), resulting in a relative risk of 40.2 (95% confidence interval [CI] 9.4 to 172.2) (13). **If morphologically abnormal endometrial cells are present, then approximately 25% of women have endometrial carcinoma** (14).

Guidelines from the Bethesda system recommended that benign endometrial cells should be reported in women of age 40 years and older. Beal et al. (15) reported that benign endometrial cells were rarely associated with significant endometrial pathology in asymptomatic premenopausal women and that these women may not need further evaluation. By contrast, Moroney et al. (16) using liquid-based cytology, reported that 2.1% of asymptomatic premenopausal women with benign endometrial cells had significant endometrial pathology.

The unsatisfactory results obtained with cervical cytology are the result of the indirect sampling of the endometrium, and **several commercially available devices have been developed to allow direct sampling (e.g., Pipelle, Gyno Sampler, Vabra aspirator).** A satisfactory endometrial biopsy specimen also may be obtained in the office with a small curette such as a Novak or Kevorkian. All of these office techniques for endometrial sampling cause the patient some discomfort, and in approximately 8% of patients it is not possible to obtain a specimen because of a stenotic os.

A meta-analysis reported that the Pipelle was the best device, with detection rates for endometrial cancer in postmenopausal and premenopausal women of 99.6% and 91%, respectively (17). The sensitivity for the detection of endometrial hyperplasia was 81%. The specificity for all devices was 98%.

Table 9.1 Patients for Whom Screening for Endometrial Cancer is Justified
1. Postmenopausal women on exogenous estrogens without *progestins*
2. Women from families with Lynch syndrome (HNPCC syndrome)
3. Premenopausal women with anovulatory cycles, such as those with polycystic ovarian disease

Table 9.2 Patients in Whom a Diagnosis of Endometrial Cancer Should be Excluded

1. All patients with postmenopausal bleeding

2. Postmenopausal women with a pyometra

3. Asymptomatic postmenopausal women with endometrial cells on a Papanicolaou smear, particularly if they are atypical

4. Perimenopausal patients with intermenstrual bleeding or increasingly heavy periods

5. Premenopausal patients with abnormal uterine bleeding, particularly if there is a history of anovulation

In the 1990s, transvaginal ultrasonography, with or without color flow imaging, was investigated as a screening technique. Mean thickness of the endometrial strip was measured as 3.4 ± 1.2 mm in women with atrophic endometrium, 9.7 ± 2.5 mm in women with hyperplasia, and 18.2 ± 6.2 mm in women with endometrial cancer (18). In a large, multi-institutional study of 1,168 women, all 114 women with endometrial cancer and 95% of the 112 women with endometrial hyperplasia had an endometrial thickness of 5 mm or more (19). **An earlier meta-analysis reported that 4% of endometrial cancers would be missed using transvaginal ultrasonography for the investigation of postmenopausal bleeding, with a false-positive rate as high as 50%** (20), while a more recent meta-analysis suggested the cut-off for endometrial thickness should be 3 mm (21).

Tamoxifen **increases the risk of endometrial cancer twofold to threefold (22) and produces a sonographically unique picture of an irregularly echogenic endometrium that is attributed to cystic glandular dilatation, stromal edema, and edema and hyperplasia of the adjacent myometrium** (23). Routine ultrasonic surveillance of asymptomatic women on *tamoxifen* is not useful because of its low specificity and positive predictive value. Canadian investigators studied 304 women on *tamoxifen* as therapy for breast cancer. Using an endometrial thickness cut-off of 9 mm, the positive predictive value for the detection of endometrial cancer was only 1.4% (24).

Patients taking *tamoxifen* **should be informed of the increased risk of endometrial cancer and told to report any abnormal bleeding or spotting immediately. Any bleeding or spotting must be investigated by biopsy.** A retrospective review of *tamoxifen*-treated women who underwent dilatation and curettage found that uterine cancer was found only in those with vaginal bleeding (23).

Clinical Features

Symptoms

Endometrial carcinoma should be excluded in all patients shown in Table 9.2. **Ninety percent of patients with endometrial cancer will have abnormal vaginal bleeding,** most commonly postmenopausal bleeding, and the bleeding usually occurs early in the course of the disease. The usual causes of postmenopausal bleeding are shown in Table 9.3.

Table 9.3 Etiology of Postmenopausal Bleeding

Factor	Approximate Percentage
Exogenous estrogens	30
Atrophic endometritis/vaginitis	30
Endometrial cancer	15
Endometrial or cervical polyps	10
Endometrial hyperplasia	5
Miscellaneous (e.g., cervical cancer, uterine sarcoma, urethral caruncle, trauma)	10

Reproduced from **Hacker and Moore's**. In: **Hacker, Hobel C, Gambone JC, eds**. *Essentials of Obstetrics and Gynecology*. 5th ed. Philadelphia, PA: Elsevier; 2010:479, with permission.

Intermenstrual bleeding or heavy prolonged bleeding in perimenopausal or anovulatory premenopausal women should arouse suspicion. The diagnosis may be delayed unnecessarily in these women because the bleeding is usually ascribed to "hormonal imbalance."

Occasionally, vaginal bleeding does not occur because of cervical stenosis, particularly in thin, elderly, estrogen-deficient patients. In some patients with cervical stenosis, a hematometra develops, and a small percentage of patients have a purulent vaginal discharge resulting from a pyometra.

Signs

Physical examination commonly reveals an obese, hypertensive, postmenopausal woman, although approximately one-third of patients are not overweight. Abdominal examination is usually unremarkable, except in advanced cases when ascites may be present and hepatic or omental metastases may be palpable. Occasionally, a hematometra appears as a large, smooth midline mass arising from the pelvis.

On pelvic examination, it is important to inspect and palpate the vulva, vagina, and cervix to exclude metastatic spread or other causes of abnormal vaginal bleeding. The uterus may be bulky, but often it is not significantly enlarged. Rectovaginal examination should be performed to evaluate the fallopian tubes, ovaries, and cul-de-sac. Endometrial carcinoma may metastasize to these sites or, alternatively, a coexistent ovarian tumor such as a granulosa cell tumor, thecoma, or epithelial ovarian carcinoma may be noted.

Diagnosis

All patients suspected of having endometrial carcinoma should have an endocervical curettage and an office endometrial biopsy. **A histologically positive endometrial biopsy allows the planning of definitive treatment.** If insufficient tissue is obtained, light bleeding may be ascribed to atrophic endometritis without need for further curettage if the endometrial thickness on transvaginal ultrasound is 4 mm or less (25).

Because there is a false-negative rate of approximately 10%, a negative endometrial biopsy in a patient with heavy bleeding, or with an endometrial thickness greater than 4 mm, must be followed by a fractional curettage under anesthesia. Hysteroscopy is usually performed in conjunction with the curettage, and may identify some small bleeding polyps that would otherwise have been missed. **The development of smaller diameter hysteroscopes has improved patient acceptance, and allowed hysteroscopy to be performed in an outpatient setting without anesthesia** (26). There has been speculation that fluid hysteroscopy may facilitate the abdominal dissemination of malignant cells, but there is no evidence that it has any impact on the disease-free survival (27).

Fractional Curettage

While the patient is under anesthesia, careful bimanual rectovaginal examination is performed, a weighted speculum is placed in the vagina, and the cervix is grasped with a tenaculum. The endocervical canal is curetted before cervical dilatation, and the tissue placed in a specially labeled container. The uterus is sounded, the cervix dilated, and the endometrium systematically curetted. The tissue is placed in a separate container so that the histopathologic status of the endocervix and endometrium can be determined separately.

Preoperative Investigations

Routine preoperative hematology and biochemistry should be performed, and a **chest, pelvic, and abdominal computed tomographic (CT) scan is usually performed**. **It has limited usefulness in determining the depth of myometrial invasion or the presence of nodal disease** (28), but has been the traditional investigation to exclude liver or lung metastases, adnexal masses, or hydronephrosis in high-risk cases. If a fractional curettage has not been performed, an endocervical curettage should be performed to evaluate the endocervix.

Nonroutine tests are sometimes indicated, particularly for more advanced cases or high-risk histologies on curettage. A **colonoscopy** should be performed if there is occult blood in the stool or a recent change in bowel habits because concomitant colon cancer occasionally occurs, particularly if there is a family history of bowel cancer.

A **magnetic resonance imaging (MRI) scan** has been shown to have an 83.3% accuracy (100 of 120 cases) for differentiating deep from superficial myometrial invasion (29) and a positive predictive value of 89.8% for the detection of cervical involvement (30). **MRI may help to differentiate between low- and high-risk patients, which may be useful in triaging cases to a gynecologic oncologist in some areas.**

Positron emission tomography (PET) has an overall diagnostic accuracy of 89.5% for the detection of lymph node metastases in patients with untreated endometrial cancer (31), but it is not considered part of the routine work-up (32). **Elevated CA125 levels** have been demonstrated to correlate with **advanced stage of disease, including positive lymph node status** (33).

Staging

In 1988, the Cancer Committee of the International Federation of Gynecology and Obstetrics (FIGO) replaced the old clinical staging system for endometrial cancer (Table 9.4) **with a surgical staging system** (Table 9.5). This was done in response to the Gynecologic Oncology Group (GOG) staging studies of the 1970s and early 1980s, which demonstrated the high incidence of lymph node metastases in high-risk cases (34,35). **This surgical staging was further refined in 2009** (Table 9.6), after a critical review of its accuracy, reproducibility, and utility, particularly from pathologists (36).

The major differences between the FIGO 1988 and FIGO 2009 staging systems are as follows:

1. **Cancer confined to the endometrium is no longer a separate stage** (i.e., stage IA). All tumors with inner half myometrial invasion are now stage IA.
2. **Only cases with cervical stromal invasion are classified as stage II.** Cervical mucosal involvement, formerly stage IIA, is now merged with stage I.
3. **There is no longer a separate stage** (i.e., stage IIIA) **for patients with positive peritoneal cytology.**
4. **Cases with metastases to lymph nodes are subdivided into stages IIIC1 and IIIC2**, specifying the presence of positive pelvic and para-aortic lymph nodes, respectively.

Two large studies of women with endometrial cancer identified from the SEER database both reported that the 2009 FIGO staging system was highly prognostic (37,38). Distribution by 1988 FIGO surgical stage is shown in Table 9.7.

Table 9.4 1971 FIGO Clinical Staging for Endometrial Carcinoma	
Stage 0	Carcinoma *in situ*
Stage I	The carcinoma is confined to the corpus.
Stage IA	The length of the uterine cavity is 8 cm or less.
Stage IB	The length of the uterine cavity is more than 8 cm.
	Stage I cases should be subgrouped with regard to the histologic grade of the adenocarcinoma as follows:
Grade 1	Highly differentiated adenomatous carcinoma
Grade 2	Moderately differentiated adenomatous carcinoma with partly solid areas
Grade 3	Predominantly solid or entirely undifferentiated carcinoma
Stage II	The carcinoma has involved the corpus and the cervix but has not extended outside the uterus.
Stage III	The carcinoma has extended outside the uterus but not outside the true pelvis.
Stage IV	The carcinoma has extended outside the true pelvis or has obviously involved the mucosa of the bladder or rectum. A bullous edema as such does not permit a case to be allocated to stage IV.
Stage IVA	Spread of the growth to adjacent organs.
Stage IVB	Spread to distant organs.

FIGO, International Federation of Gynecology and Obstetrics.

Table 9.5 1988 FIGO Surgical Staging for Endometrial Carcinoma

Stage IA G123	Tumor limited to endometrium
Stage IB G123	Invasion to less than one-half of the myometrium
Stage IC G123	Invasion to more than one-half of the myometrium
Stage IIA G123	Endocervical glandular involvement only
Stage IIB G123	Cervical stromal invasion
Stage IIIA G123	Tumor invades serosa and/or adnexa, and/or positive peritoneal cytology
Stage IIIB G123	Vaginal metastases
Stage IIIC G123	Metastases to pelvic and/or para-aortic lymph nodes
Stage IVA G123	Tumor invasion of bladder and/or bowel mucosa
Stage IVB G123	Distant metastases including intra-abdominal and/or inguinal lymph nodes

Histopathology—degree of differentiation:

Cases of carcinoma of the corpus should be classified (or graded) according to the degree of histologic differentiation, as follows:

G1 = 5% or less of a nonsquamous or nonmorular solid growth pattern

G2 = 6–50% of a nonsquamous or nonmorular solid growth pattern

G3 = more than 50% of a nonsquamous or nonmorular solid growth pattern

Notes on pathologic grading:

1. Notable nuclear atypia, inappropriate for the architectural grade, raises the grade of a grade 1 or a grade 2 tumor by 1.

2. In serous adenocarcinomas, clear cell adenocarcinomas, and squamous cell carcinomas, nuclear grading takes precedence.

3. Adenocarcinomas with squamous differentiation are graded according to the nuclear grade of the glandular component.

Rules related to staging:

1. Because corpus cancer is now staged surgically, procedures previously used for determination of stages are no longer applicable, such as the findings from fractional dilatation and curettage to differentiate between stage I and stage II.

2. It is appreciated that there may be a small number of patients with corpus cancer who will be treated primarily with radiation therapy. If that is the case, the clinical staging adopted by FIGO in 1971 would still apply, but designation of that staging system should be noted.

3. Ideally, width of the myometrium should be measured along with the width of tumor invasion.

Reproduced from **International Federation of Gynecology and Obstetrics**. Annual report on the results of treatment in gynecologic cancer. *Int J Gynecol Obstet.* 1989;28:189–190, with permission.

Spread Patterns

Endometrial carcinoma spreads by the following routes:

1. Direct extension to adjacent structures
2. Transtubal passage of exfoliated cells
3. Lymphatic dissemination
4. Hematogenous dissemination

Direct Extension

Direct extension is the most common route of spread, and it results in penetration of the myometrium and eventually the serosa of the uterus. The cervix, fallopian tubes, and ultimately the vagina and parametrium may be invaded. Tumors arising in the upper corpus may involve the tube or serosa before involving the cervix, whereas tumors arising from the lower segment of the uterus

Table 9.6 2009 FIGO Surgical Staging for Carcinoma of the Endometrium	
Stage I[a]	Tumor confined to the corpus uteri
IA[a]	No or less than half myometrial invasion
IB[a]	Invasion equal to or more than half of the myometrium
Stage II[a]	Tumor invades cervical stroma, but does not extend beyond the uterus[b]
Stage III[a]	Local and/or regional spread of the tumor
IIIA[a]	Tumor invades the serosa of the corpus uteri and/or adnexae[c]
IIIB[a]	Vaginal and/or parametrial involvement[c]
IIIC[a]	Metastases to pelvic and/or para-aortic lymph nodes[c]
IIIC1[a]	Positive pelvic nodes
IIIC2[a]	Positive para-aortic lymph nodes with or without positive pelvic lymph nodes
Stage IV[a]	Tumor invades bladder and/or bowel mucosa, and/or distant metastases
IVA[a]	Tumor invasion of bladder and/or bowel mucosa
IVB[a]	Distant metastases, including intra-abdominal metastases and/or inguinal lymph nodes

[a]Either Grade 1, Grade 2, or Grade 3.

[b]Endocervical glandular involvement only should be considered as stage I and no longer as stage II.

[c]Positive cytology has to be reported separately without changing the stage.

FIGO Committee on Gynecologic Oncology. Revised FIGO staging for carcinoma of the vulva, cervix, and endometrium. *Int J Gynecol Obst.* 2009;105:103–104.

involve the cervix early. The exact anatomic route by which endometrial cancer involves the cervix has not been clearly defined, but it probably involves a combination of contiguous surface spread, invasion of deep tissue planes, and lymphatic dissemination (39).

Transtubal Dissemination

The presence of malignant cells in peritoneal washings and the development of widespread intra-abdominal metastases in some patients with early-stage endometrial cancer strongly suggest that cells may be exfoliated from the primary tumor and transported to the peritoneal cavity by retrograde flow along the fallopian tubes.

Lymphatic Dissemination

Lymphatic dissemination is clearly responsible for spread to pelvic and para-aortic lymph nodes. **Although lymphatic channels pass directly from the fundus to the para-aortic nodes through the infundibulopelvic ligament, it is rare to find positive para-aortic nodes in the absence of positive pelvic nodes.** It is quite common to find microscopic metastases in both pelvic and para-aortic nodes, suggesting simultaneous spread to pelvic and para-aortic nodes in some patients. This is in contrast to cervical cancer, where para-aortic nodal metastases are virtually always secondary to pelvic nodal metastases.

Table 9.7 Carcinoma of the Endometrium: Distribution by 1988 FIGO Surgical Stage Patients Treated in 1999 to 2001		
Stage	*No.*	*Percent*
I	6,260	71.1
II	1,071	12.1
III	1,190	13.5
IV	280	3.3
Total	8,807	100

Modified from the 26th FIGO Annual Report on the Results of Treatment in Gynecological Cancer (9).

It seems likely that vaginal metastases also result from lymph-vascular spread. They commonly occur in the absence of cervical involvement, excluding direct spread as the mechanism, and may occur despite preoperative sterilization of the uterus with intracavitary radiation, excluding implantation of cells at the time of surgery as the mechanism (40). In a study of 632 patients with stage I endometrial cancer managed with hysterectomy at the Mayo Clinic between 1984 and 1996, Mariani et al. (41) reported that **grade 3 histology and lymphovascular invasion were significant predictors of vaginal relapse,** whereas depth of myometrial invasion was not.

Hematogenous Spread

Hematogenous spread most commonly results in lung metastases; liver, brain, bone, and other sites are involved less commonly.

Prognostic Variables

Although stage of disease is the most significant prognostic variable, a number of factors have been shown to correlate with outcome within the same stage of disease. These prognostic variables are summarized in Table 9.8. Knowledge of them is essential if appropriate treatment programs are to be devised.

Age

Age appears to be an independent prognostic variable. The GOG reported 5-year relative survival rates of 96.3% for 28 patients 40 years of age or younger, 87.3% for 261 patients 51 to 60 years, 78% for 312 patients 61 to 70 years, 70.7% for 119 patients 71 to 80 years, and 53.6% for 23 patients older than 80 ($p = 0.001$) (42). All patients had clinical stage I or occult stage II disease. Using proportional hazards modeling of relative survival time, and taking 45 years of age as the arbitrary reference point, the relative risks for death from disease were as follows: 2 at 55 years, 3.4 at 65 years, and 4.7 at 75 years of age.

A study of 51,471 patients from the SEER database of the National Cancer Institute in the United States demonstrated that patients 40 years and younger had an overall survival advantage compared with women older than 40 years, independent of other clinicopathologic prognosticators (43).

Japanese researchers have reported menopausal status to be an independent prognostic variable for early endometrial cancer but not for patients with advanced disease (44).

Histologic Type

Zaino et al. (45) investigated the prognostic significance of squamous differentiation in 456 patients with typical adenocarcinomas and 175 women with areas of squamous differentiation who had been entered into a GOG clinicopathologic study of stage I and II disease. They reported that the biologic behavior of these tumors reflected the histologic grade and depth of invasion of the

Table 9.8 Prognostic Variables in Endometrial Cancer Other than FIGO Stage
Age
Histologic type
Histologic grade
Nuclear grade
Myometrial invasion
Vascular space invasion
Tumor size
Peritoneal cytology
Hormone receptor status
DNA ploidy and other biologic markers
Type of therapy (surgery vs. radiation)

FIGO, International Federation of Gynecology and Obstetrics.

glandular component. Prognostically valuable information was provided by dividing these tumors into adenoacanthomas and adenosquamous carcinomas, and more information was gained when they were stratified by the histologic grade of the glandular component. **They recommended that the terms *adenoacanthoma* and *adenosquamous carcinoma* be replaced by the simple term *adenocarcinoma with squamous differentiation*** (45).

Serous carcinomas have a poor prognosis, even in the absence of deep myometrial invasion or lymph node metastasis (4,46–49). They disseminate widely, with a particular predilection for recurrence in the upper abdomen. The mechanisms that have been proposed to explain the characteristic intra-abdominal dissemination of these tumors include transtubal spread, vascular-lymphatic invasion, and multifocal disease. Sherman et al. (49) observed that "intraepithelial serous carcinoma" was present in the endocervix in 22% of their cases, in the fallopian tube in 5%, on the surface of the ovary in 10%, and on peritoneal surfaces or omentum in 25%. **Serous elements are often admixed with endometrioid carcinomas, but a serous component of 25% will portend a poor prognosis** (49).

In contrast to the slow, estrogen-driven pathway leading to the biologically more indolent endometrioid carcinoma, a rapid, *p53*-driven pathway appears to lead to the aggressive serous (4,49) and clear cell carcinomas (4).

Clear cell carcinomas represent fewer than 5% of endometrial carcinomas, although clear cell elements are commonly present in serous tumors (49). **Vascular space invasion is more common in these lesions.** In a review of 181 patients with clear cell endometrial carcinoma treated between 1970 and 1992 at the Norwegian Radium Hospital, 5- and 10-year actuarial disease-free survival rates were 43% and 39%, respectively. Two-thirds of the relapses were outside the pelvis, most frequently in the upper abdomen, liver, and lungs (50).

SEER data from 1988 to 2001 were used to compare uterine serous ($n = 1,473$), clear cell ($n = 391$), and grade 3 endometrioid carcinomas ($n = 2,316$) (48). Serous and clear cell carcinomas occurred in older patients, and were diagnosed at a more advanced stage. They represented 10%, 3%, and 15% of endometrial cancer, respectively, but accounted for 39%, 8%, and 27% of cancer deaths.

When serous or clear cell carcinomas are limited to the curettings, with no adverse features in the hysterectomy specimen, prognosis may not be impaired (51).

Squamous cell carcinomas of the endometrium are rare. In a review of the literature, Abeler and Kjorstad (52) estimated that the survival rate for patients with clinical stage I disease was 36%.

Histologic Grade and Myometrial Invasion

There is a strong correlation between histologic grade, myometrial invasion, and prognosis. The GOG reported the surgicopathologic features of 621 patients with stage I endometrial carcinoma (35). The frequency of positive pelvic and para-aortic nodal metastases in relation to histologic grade and depth of myometrial invasion is shown in Tables 9.9 and 9.10. **When grade 1 carcinomas were confined to the inner third of the myometrium, the incidence of positive pelvic nodes was less than 3%, whereas when grade 3 lesions involved the outer third, the incidence**

Table 9.9 Grade, Depth of Invasion, and Pelvic Nodal Metastasis of Endometrial Carcinoma

Depth of Myometrial Invasion	*Histologic Grade*		
	G1 ($n = 180$)	G2 ($n = 288$)	G3 ($n = 153$)
Endometrium only ($n = 86$)	0/44 (0%)	1/31 (3%)	0/11 (0%)
Inner third ($n = 281$)	3/96 (3%)	7/131 (5%)	5/54 (9%)
Middle third ($n = 115$)	0/22 (0%)	6/69 (9%)	1/24 (4%)
Outer third ($n = 139$)	2/18 (11%)	11/57 (19%)	22/64 (34%)

Reproduced from **Creasman WT, Morrow CP, Bundy BN, et al**. Surgical pathologic spread patterns of endometrial cancer: A Gynecologic Oncology Group study. *Cancer*. 1987;60:2035–2041, with permission.

Table 9.10 Grade, Depth of Invasion, and Aortic Nodal Metastasis of Endometrial Carcinoma			
	Histologic Grade		
Depth of Myometrial Invasion	**G1 (*n* = 180)**	**G2 (*n* = 288)**	**G3 (*n* = 153)**
Endometrium only (*n* = 86)	0/44 (0%)	1/31 (3%)	0/11 (0%)
Inner third (*n* = 281)	1/96 (1%)	5/131 (4%)	2/54 (4%)
Middle third (*n* = 115)	1/22 (5%)	0/69 (0%)	0/24 (0%)
Outer third (*n* = 139)	1/18 (6%)	8/57 (14%)	15/64 (23%)

Reproduced from **Creasman WT, Morrow CP, Bundy BN, et al**. Surgical pathologic spread patterns of endometrial cancer: A Gynecologic Oncology Group study. *Cancer.* 1987;60:2035–2041, with permission.

of positive pelvic nodes was 34%. For aortic nodes, the corresponding figures were less than 1% and 23%, respectively.

A combined European-Mayo review of 527 patients with grade 1 endometrioid endometrial cancer revealed 88 patients (16.8%) in whom the background endometrium was atrophic, rather than hyperplastic or proliferative (53). **Atrophic endometrium correlated with older age, lower body mass index, advanced FIGO stage, lymph node metastases, vascular space invasion, and deep myometrial invasion.** The authors concluded that atrophic endometrium was an independent prognostic factor for patients with grade 1 endometrioid carcinoma, and that these tumors may arise through unique carcinogenic pathways (53).

Recurrence at the vaginal vault can usually be prevented by prophylactic vault brachytherapy, and the risk of distant metastases in relation to histologic grade and myometrial invasion is shown in Table 9.11 (54).

Vascular Space Invasion

Vascular space invasion appears to be an independent risk factor for recurrence and death from endometrial carcinoma of all histologic types (42,55–61,62). In a GOG study, vascular space invasion carried a relative risk of death of 1.5 (42).

Abeler et al. (55) reviewed 1,974 cases of endometrial carcinoma from the Norwegian Radium Hospital and reported an 83.5% 5-year survival rate for patients without demonstrable vascular invasion compared with 64.5% for those in whom vascular invasion was present. A Japanese study

Table 9.11 Clinical Stage I Endometrial Carcinoma: Distant Metastases versus Histologic Grade and Myometrial Invasion[a]			
Variable	*Number*	*Metastases*	*Percent*
Histologic grade			
Grade 1	93	2	2.2
Grade 2	88	9	10.2
Grade 3	41	16	39
Myometrial invasion			
None	92	4	4.3
Inner third	80	8	10
Middle third	17	2	11.8
Outer third	33	13	39.4

[a]Gynecologic Oncology Group data.

Reproduced from **DiSaia PJ, Creasman WT, Boronow RC, et al**. Risk factors and recurrent patterns in stage I endometrial cancer. *Am J Obstet Gynecol.* 1985;151:1009–1015, with permission.

reported that lymph-vascular space invasion and the number of positive para-aortic lymph nodes were independent prognostic factors for patients with stage IIIC endometrial cancer (56).

The overall incidence of lymph-vascular invasion in stage I endometrial carcinoma is approximately 15%, although it increases with increasing myometrial invasion and decreasing tumor differentiation. Hanson et al. (58) reported vascular space invasion in 5% of patients with invasion limited to the inner one-third of the myometrium compared with 70% of those with invasion to the outer one-third. Similarly, it was present in 2% of grade 1 carcinomas and 42% of grade 3 lesions.

Lymphovascular space invasion is an independent risk factor for vaginal cuff recurrence (62), distant recurrence (59,62), lymph node metastases (60), and parametrial involvement (61) in patients with early-stage endometrial cancer.

Peritoneal Cytologic Results

The significance of positive peritoneal cytology is controversial (63), and it is no longer part of the FIGO staging system. About half the papers on early-stage endometrial cancer report increased recurrence rates and decreased survival in patients with positive cytology (64–68), while in the other half, no differences were detected (69–74). **Positive washings are most common in patients with grade 3 histology, metastases to the adnexae, deep myometrial invasion, or positive pelvic or para-aortic nodes.**

The GOG study reported by Morrow et al. (66) analyzed 697 patients with information on peritoneal cytology and adequate follow-up. Disease recurred in 25 of 86 patients (29.1%) with positive washings, compared to 64 of 611 patients (10.5%) with negative washings. The authors noted that 17 of the 25 recurrences were outside the peritoneal cavity. **The GOG estimated that the relative risk of death for patients with positive cytologic washings was increased threefold (42).**

In a review of the literature concerning patients with clinical stage I endometrial cancer, Milosevic et al. (64) reported positive peritoneal cytology in 8.3%, 12.1%, and 15.9% of patients with grades 1, 2, and 3 histologic types, respectively. Superficial and deep myometrial invasion were associated with positive washings in 7.6% and 17.2% of the cases, respectively. They concluded that the poor prognosis associated with malignant washings was largely a reflection of other adverse prognostic factors.

Takeshima et al. (70) studied 534 patients with endometrial cancer to assess the prognostic significance of positive peritoneal washings. They concluded that positive washings were not an independent negative prognostic factor, but potentiated other negative prognostic indicators. **They felt that patients with positive peritoneal cytology, in the absence of other adverse prognostic factors, did not warrant upstaging.**

These same researchers placed a tube in the abdomen to allow peritoneal irrigation in 50 patients with early-stage endometrial cancer and positive peritoneal smears detected at surgery (73). Washings were obtained via the tube 7 and 14 days postoperatively. Persistence of positive peritoneal cytology was observed in only 5 of 50 patients (10%), and 4 of these patients had adnexal metastases completely resected. They concluded that **malignant cells found in the peritoneal cavity generally have a low malignant potential** and that **only malignant cells from special cases, such as patients with adnexal metastases, may be capable of independent growth.**

Hormone Receptor Status

Estrogen receptor (ER) and progesterone receptor (PR) levels have been shown to be independent prognostic factors for endometrial cancer; that is, patients whose tumor is positive for one or both receptors have longer survival than patients whose carcinoma lacks the corresponding receptors (75–79). Liao et al. (76) reported that, even for patients with lymph node metastases, the prognosis was significantly improved if the tumor was receptor positive. **PR appears to be a stronger predictor of survival than ER** and, at least for the ER, the absolute level of the receptors may be important: the higher the level, the better the prognosis (79).

Nuclear Grade

Nuclear grade is a significant prognostic indicator (79). Christopherson et al. (80) found **nuclear grading to be a more accurate prognosticator than histologic grade.**

The FIGO grading system takes into account the nuclear grade of the tumor, and "nuclear atypia" inappropriate for the architectural grade raises the grade by 1. There is great variability in the literature regarding the criteria for nuclear grading, and intraobserver and interobserver reproducibility of nuclear grading are poor (81).

Tumor Size

In an analysis of 142 patients with clinical stage I endometrial carcinoma, Schink et al. (82) reported tumor size as an independent prognostic factor. Lymph node metastases occurred in 4% of the patients with tumors no more than 2 cm in diameter, 15% with tumors greater than 2 cm in diameter, and 35% with tumors involving the entire uterine cavity. Japanese researchers used tumor diameter in addition to intraoperative frozen section to identify low-risk cases (83). **None of 55 patients with grade 1 or 2 tumors and less than 50% myometrial invasion had positive nodes if the tumor diameter was 3 cm or less.** Mayo Clinic workers incorporated tumor diameter (2 cm or less vs. greater than 2 cm) into a ***Risk-scoring System*** for prediction of lymphatic dissemination in patients with endometrioid endometrial cancer (84).

DNA Ploidy and Other Biologic Markers

Only about 25% of patients with endometrial carcinomas have aneuploid tumors, but these patients are at significantly increased risk of early recurrence and death from disease (85–87).

In a prospective study of 174 patients, Susini et al. (86) reported a 10-year survival probability of 53.2% for patients with DNA aneuploid tumors, compared to 91% for patients with DNA diploid tumors. By multivariate analysis, DNA aneuploid type was the strongest independent predictor of poor outcome, followed by age and stage. **The GOG estimated the relative risk to be 4.1 for disease-related death for patients with aneuploid tumors** (87).

A number of genetic mutations have been shown to have prognostic significance in endometrial cancer. Greek investigators reported that **loss of *beta-catenin* expression was a strong, independent predictor of a poor prognosis, whereas loss of *PTEN* was associated with a worse prognosis for patients with early-stage disease** (88). The *p53* mutation correlated with increased stage, lymph node metastases, and nonendometrioid histology in univariate analysis but was not an independent prognostic factor in multivariate analysis (88). **Increasing expression of matrix metalloproteinases** (MMPs) (89), **nuclear *Bcl-2* expression** (90), and **Ki-67 expression** (91) also have prognostic significance. The clinical implications of these biologic markers are not yet clear.

Method of Treatment

In contrast to cervical cancer, **patients with endometrial cancer treated with hysterectomy alone or hysterectomy and radiation do significantly better than those treated with radiation alone.** This appears to be related to the inability of radiation therapy effectively to eliminate disease in the myometrium (92,93). Grigsby et al. (92) reported on 116 patients with stage II endometrial carcinoma. Ninety were treated with combined radiation and surgery, whereas 26 received radiation alone. The results of treatment are shown in Table 9.12.

Endometrial Hyperplasia

Classic teaching has been that endometrial hyperplasias represent a continuum of morphologic severity; the most severe form, termed *atypical adenomatous hyperplasia* or *carcinoma in situ,* was considered the immediate precursor of endometrial carcinoma (94). Since the mid-1980s, this continuum concept has been challenged. Independent studies by Kurman et al. (95) and Ferenczy et al. (96) have suggested the following:

1. **Endometrial hyperplasia and endometrial neoplasia are two biologically different diseases.**
2. **The only important distinguishing feature is the presence or absence of cytologic atypia.**

Table 9.12 Clinical Stage II Carcinoma of the Endometrium: Comparison of Treatment Methods

	No. of Patients	Distant Metastases (%)	Pelvic Recurrence (%)	5-Year Survival Rate (%)
Radiation and surgery	90	13.3	8.9	78
Radiation alone	26	11.5	34.6	48

Reproduced from **Grigsby PW, Perez CA, Camel HM, et al**. Stage II carcinoma of the endometrium: Results of therapy and prognostic factors. *Int J Radiat Oncol Biol Phys*. 1985;11:1915–1921, with permission.

Table 9.13 World Health Organization Classification of Endometrial Hyperplasia
Hyperplasia (typical)
Simple hyperplasia without atypia
Complex hyperplasia without atypia (adenomatous without atypia)
Atypical hyperplasia
Simple atypical hyperplasia
Complex atypical hyperplasia (adenomatous with atypia)

Reproduced from **Silverberg SG, Mutter GL, Kurman RJ, et al**. Tumors of the uterine corpus: Epithelial tumors and related lesions. In: *WHO Classification of Tumors: Pathology and Genetics of Tumors of the Breast and Female Genital Organs*. Lyon, France: IARC Press; 2003:221–232.

Ferenczy et al. (96) suggested a two-class classification, with **endometrial hyperplasia** being used for any degree of glandular proliferation devoid of cytologic atypia, and **endometrial intraepithelial neoplasia (EIN) for lesions with cytologic atypia**. Using similar criteria in a long-term follow-up study of 170 patients with endometrial hyperplasia, Kurman et al. (95) reported a 1.6% risk of progression to carcinoma in patients devoid of cytologic atypia, compared with a 23% risk in patients with cytologic atypia. A case-control study was reported among a cohort of 7,947 women diagnosed with endometrial hyperplasia at one prepaid health plan in the United States from 1970 to 2002. **The cumulative 20-year progression risk among women who remained at risk for at least 1 year was less than 5% for women without atypia, and 28% for those with atypical hyperplasia** (97).

The World Health Organization (WHO) still uses a four-class classification of endometrial hyperplasia, as shown in Table 9.13 (98). It is based on morphologic features of the architectural complexity of the glands, and the presence or absence of cytologic and nuclear atypia.

Although the studies of Kurman and Ferenczy are important, **the reproducibility of the diagnosis has been questioned**. In a GOG study, a panel of three expert gynecologic pathologists reviewed outside slides from **306 patients referred with a diagnosis of atypical endometrial hyperplasia**. The majority panel diagnosis was adenocarcinoma in 29%, cycling endometrium in 7%, and non-atypical hyperplasia in 18% of cases (99).

Hysterectomy slides from the same GOG study **were reviewed** by the study pathologists, and 289 hysterectomy specimens were available for review (100). **Concurrent endometrial carcinoma was present in 42.6%** (123 of 289 specimens). Of these, 30.9% (38 of 123 specimens) had myometrial invasion, and 10.6% (13 of 123 specimens) had invasion to the outer half of the myometrium. Even when the study panel consensus diagnosis was less than atypical endometrial hyperplasia, 14 of 74 women (18.9%) still had carcinoma in the hysterectomy specimen.

Diagnosis

Complex atypical endometrial hyperplasia frequently coexists with endometrial carcinoma. Of 824 women with atypical hyperplasia on endometrial biopsy, 48% were found to have endometrial cancer on subsequent hysterectomy (101). If dilatation and curettage were performed, the risk of concurrent endometrial cancer was 30%. Increasing age was strongly correlated with the risk of cancer.

Immunohistochemical staining of complex atypical endometrial hyperplasia for PTEN has been reported to improve the prediction of a coexistent endometrial cancer, and the prediction may be better when *MIB-1* and *p53* expressions are added (102).

Treatment

Most women with endometrial hyperplasia without atypia respond to *progestin* therapy. A pooled analysis of the published literature revealed a 96% regression rate for these patients when treated with the *levonorgestrel* intrauterine device (103).

Patients with atypical endometrial hyperplasia should be advised to have a hysterectomy, but if a decision is made to retain the uterus because of medical comorbidities or fertility considerations, progestins should be tried. Those who do not respond are at a significantly increased risk of progressing to invasive cancer, although individual patient outcomes cannot be predicted (104).

Gunderson et al. (105) reviewed English language studies published from 2004 to 2011 to report oncologic and pregnancy outcomes in women with complex atypical endometrial hyperplasia or grade 1 adenocarcinoma treated with hormone therapy. Forty-five studies with 391 patients were identified, and the median age was 31.7 years. The major therapies were medroxyprogesterone (49%), megestrol acetate (25%), and the *levonorgestrel* intrauterine device (19%). **Overall, 344 women (77.7%) responded to hormonal therapy. After a median follow-up of 39 months, a durable complete response was noted in 53.2%.** The complete response rate was significantly higher for those with hyperplasia than carcinoma (65.8% vs. 48.2%; $p = 0.002$). **The median time to complete response was 6 months (range 1 to 18 months).** Recurrence after an initial response occurred in 23.2% with hyperplasia and 35.4% with carcinoma ($p = 0.03$). During the study period, 41.2% of those with hyperplasia and 34.8% with carcinoma became pregnant ($p = 0.39$), with 117 live births.

The type of *progestin* used does not appear to be important, the optimal dosage has not been investigated, and the regimens advocated are essentially arbitrary (104), because no clinical trials have been conducted (107). High doses of *progestins* are often better tolerated than lower doses. The main side effects are weight gain, edema, thrombophlebitis, and occasionally hypertension and depression. The incidence of venous thromboembolism may be slightly increased.

A suggested scheme of management is outlined in Figure 9.1.

Treatment of Endometrial Cancer

The cornerstone of treatment for endometrial cancer is total hysterectomy and bilateral salpingo-oophorectomy; this operation should be performed in all cases whenever feasible. Many patients require some type of adjuvant radiation therapy to help prevent vaginal vault recurrence and to sterilize disease in lymph nodes.

The surgery has traditionally been via laparotomy, but many of these patients are elderly and have comorbidities such as diabetes, hypertension, and obesity. **Minimally invasive approaches are replacing open laparotomy for most patients with endometrial cancer.** Laparoscopic-assisted vaginal hysterectomy, total laparoscopic hysterectomy, or robotic-assisted laparoscopic hysterectomy have all been compared to open laparotomy in randomized, prospective studies (108–110). These trials mainly focused on patients with Type I tumors, but when managed by expert laparoscopic or robotic surgeons, a high-risk histologic subtype does not seem to be a contraindication in patients with apparent early-stage disease (111).

Although long-term survival data are not yet available, the minimally invasive approach is associated with shorter hospital stay, less postoperative pain, and quicker resumption of normal daily activities. Minimally invasive operations do take longer, and the lymphadenectomy in particular has a steep learning curve; the former has implications for allocation of operating room resources, and the latter for the training of junior surgeons.

Stage I and Stage II Occult

Operative Technique

A recommended treatment plan is shown in Figure 9.2.

The initial approach for all medically fit patients should be total hysterectomy and bilateral salpingo-oophorectomy. Removal of a vaginal cuff is not necessary. The adnexa should be removed because they may be the site of microscopic metastases, and patients with endometrial carcinoma are at increased risk for ovarian cancer. Such tumors sometimes occur concurrently (112). Surgical staging, including lymphadenectomy, should be performed in those patients listed in Table 9.14. The use of minimally invasive surgery is addressed in detail in Chapters 21 and 22, but there will always be a minority of patients for whom an open laparotomy is more appropriate, for example, those with a large volume uterus, an adnexal mass, or extensive adhesions.

The laparotomy is best performed through a lower midline abdominal incision, particularly in the obese patient. This incision allows easy access to the upper abdomen, including the

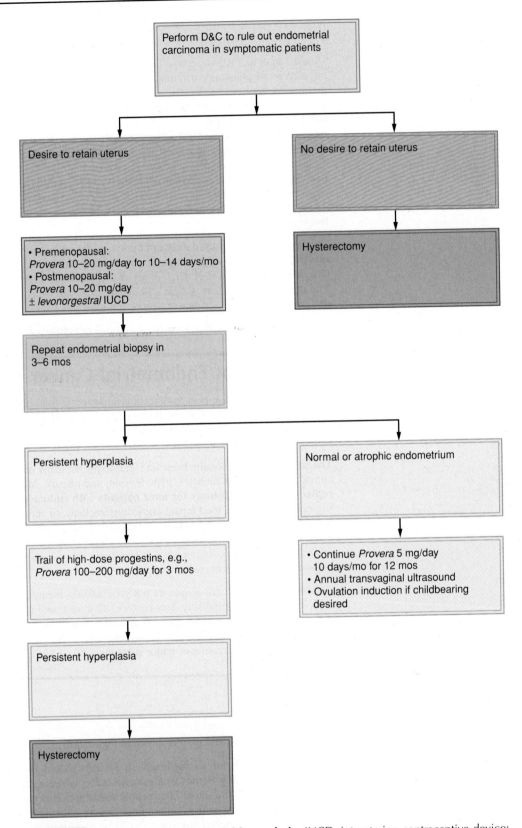

Figure 9.1 Management of endometrial hyperplasia. IUCD, intrauterine contraceptive device; mos, months.

omentum and para-aortic lymph nodes. A Pfannenstiel incision is commonly used for patients with grade 1 or 2 tumors and a normal-sized uterus. **An alternative approach is to use a transverse, muscle-dividing incision (e.g., the Maylard or Cherney),** as discussed in Chapter 20. This incision gives reasonable access to the upper abdomen.

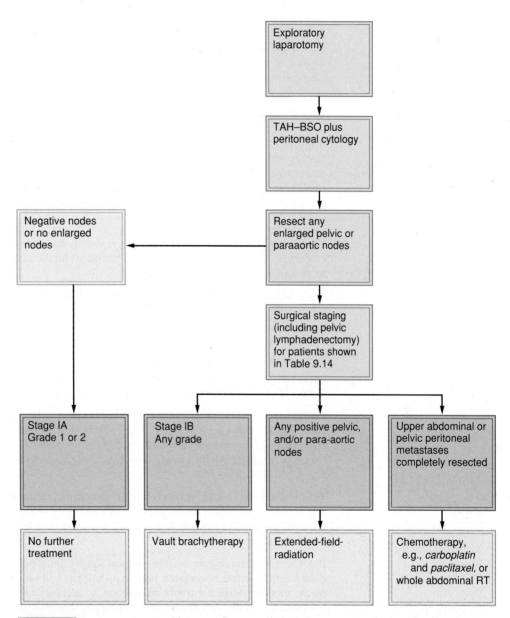

Figure 9.2 **Management of patients with stage I and occult stage II endometrial carcinoma.** TAH, total abdominal hysterectomy; BSO, bilateral salpingo-oophorectomy; RT, radiation therapy.

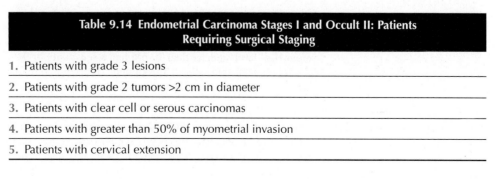

Table 9.14 Endometrial Carcinoma Stages I and Occult II: Patients Requiring Surgical Staging
1. Patients with grade 3 lesions
2. Patients with grade 2 tumors >2 cm in diameter
3. Patients with clear cell or serous carcinomas
4. Patients with greater than 50% of myometrial invasion
5. Patients with cervical extension

After the abdomen is opened, peritoneal washings are taken for cytology, and the abdomen and pelvis are explored, with particular attention to the liver, diaphragm, omentum, and retroperitoneal nodes. Any suspicious lesions are excised or biopsied, and any enlarged lymph nodes removed.

Technique for hysterectomy and bilateral salpingo-oophorectomy. The uterus is grasped with clamps that encompass the round and ovarian ligaments and the fallopian tube. After the round ligaments are divided, the incision is carried anteriorly around the vesicouterine fold of peritoneum, and posteriorly parallel and lateral to the infundibulopelvic ligaments. With a narrow Deaver retractor in the retroperitoneum providing gentle traction cephalad in the direction of the common iliac vessels, the iliac vessels and ureter are displayed. With the retroperitoneum displayed, the pelvic lymph nodes can be visualized and palpated, and any enlarged nodes can be removed and sent for frozen section.

With each ureter under direct vision, the infundibulopelvic ligaments are divided and tied. The bladder is dissected off the front of the cervix, and the uterine vessels are skeletonized and divided at the level of the isthmus. Straight Kocher clamps are used to secure the cardinal and uterosacral ligaments. A circumferential incision is made around the upper vagina, the uterus, tubes, and ovaries are removed, and the vaginal vault is closed. The pelvic peritoneum is not closed, and no drains are placed in the pelvis. The sigmoid colon is placed in the pelvis to help exclude loops of small bowel. A vertical abdominal wound is best closed with a continuous Smead–Jones type of internal retention suture, using a long-acting, absorbable suture such as Maxon or PDS.

Surgical Staging

The decision to undertake surgical staging is usually based on the histopathology from the uterine curettings, the gross findings on opening the uterus on the operating table, and possibly a frozen section of the resected uterus.

A relatively poor correlation has been reported between the grade of cancer on curettings or biopsy and the final grade in the resected uterus, presumably because of a sampling error in the diagnostic procedure. The poorest correlation is for grade 1 tumors, where 20–40% may be upgraded after evaluation of the hysterectomy specimen (113–115).

Our practice is to open the specimen on the operating table to determine the need for surgical staging in patients with grade 1 or 2 tumors (Figs. 9.3 and 9.4). All patients with grade 3 endometrioid, serous, or clear cell carcinomas are surgically staged.

For grade 1 tumors, gross examination fairly accurately predicts depth of myometrial invasion (115,116). A Greek study of 142 patients with apparent early-stage endometrial cancer reported a 93.5% accuracy for estimating depth of myometrial invasion for grade 1 tumors, 80.4% for grade 2, and 58.6% for grade 3. Cervical involvement was correctly determined in 138 of the 142 patients (97.2%) (116).

Tumor diameter should be taken into account when determining the need for surgical staging. Schink et al. (82) reported a 22% incidence of lymph node metastases for grade 2 tumors greater than 2 cm in diameter (7 of 32). None of 19 grade 2 tumors less than 2 cm in diameter had nodal metastases.

If doubt exists regarding the need for surgical staging, intraoperative frozen section can be obtained if sufficient expertise is available, but the pathologist still needs to use gross inspection to decide on the site(s) of deepest myometrial invasion, so accuracy rates of 77% (117) to 96% (118) have been reported. If the final histopathology is worse than was anticipated intraoperatively, the prognosis will not be impaired if external-beam pelvic radiation is given on the basis of histologic grade and depth of myometrial invasion, as long as any enlarged pelvic and/or para-aortic nodes have been resected as part of the standard management for all patients.

Other approaches that have been used to determine depth of myometrial invasion include preoperative MRI (115,119), transvaginal ultrasonography (120), or serum human epididymis protein 4 (HE4) titers (121). A pilot study of 96 patients with endometrioid adenocarcinomas revealed that serum HE4 levels greater than 70 pM had a sensitivity of 94% and a negative predictive value of 97% for distinguishing stage IA from stage IB disease. If these results can be duplicated, this could be a helpful way to triage high-risk patients to a gynecologic oncologist.

Pelvic Lymphadenectomy

No preoperative scan is able to detect micrometastases in lymph nodes, so if accurate surgical staging is to be obtained, full pelvic lymphadenectomy should be performed on all patients who meet the criteria in Table 9.14. Sampling will only lead to inaccurate information (122).

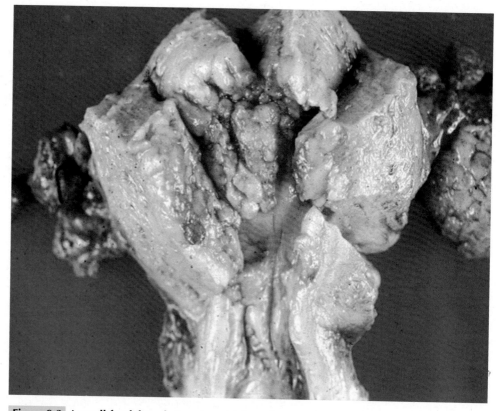

Figure 9.3 **A small fundal grade 1 endometrial carcinoma.** This patient does not require surgical staging.

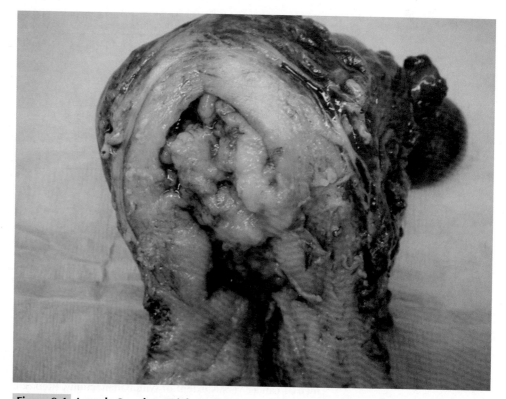

Figure 9.4 **A grade 2 endometrial carcinoma occupying most of the corpus.** A patient such as this should undergo surgical staging.

In an analysis of 11,443 patients registered on the SEER database between 1990 and 2001, Chan et al. (123) reported that the removal of 21 to 25 lymph nodes significantly increased the probability of detecting at least one positive lymph node in endometrioid uterine cancer. Lutman et al. (124) reported that the pelvic lymph node count was an important prognostic variable for patients with FIGO stages I and II endometrial carcinoma and high-risk histology. In an analysis of 5,556 patients with low-risk endometrioid endometrial carcinoma from the SEER database, Chan et al. (125) were unable to find any survival advantage regardless of the extent of the lymphadenectomy (Fig. 9.5).

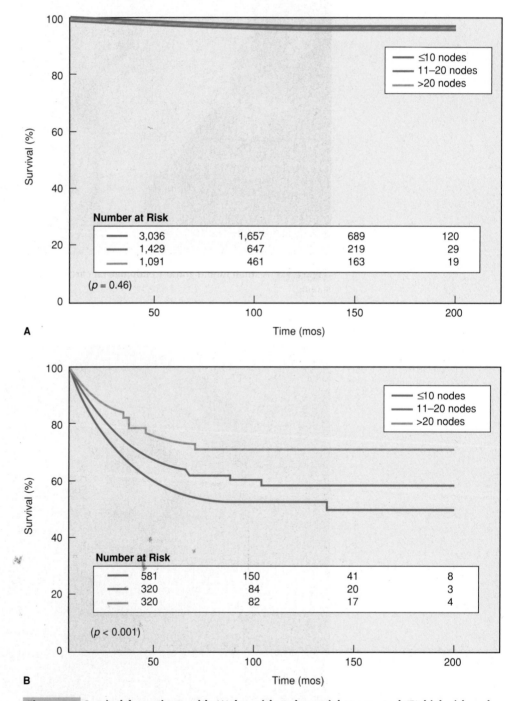

Figure 9.5 Survival for patients with (A) low-risk endometrial cancer and (B) high-risk endometrial cancer versus extent of lymphadenectomy. (Reproduced with permission from **Chan J, Cheung MK, Huh WK, et al**. Therapeutic role of lymph node resection in endometrioid corpus cancer: A study of 12,333 patients. *Cancer.* 2006;107:1823–1828.)

The risk of lymph node metastases in patients with grade 1 or 2 endometrioid tumors which are less than 2 cm diameter, and invading less than 50% of the myometrium, is less than 1%. This cohort represents about 40% of all endometrial cancer patients (126). Performing lymphadenectomy in this low-risk cohort dramatically increases morbidity and cost of care without any discernible benefit (127). Patients with grade 1 or 2 tumors and deep myometrial invasion (intermediate-risk cases), have a 9% risk of positive nodes (128).

The dissection should include removal of common iliac nodes and the fat pad overlying the distal inferior vena cava. If full pelvic lymphadenectomy is considered inadvisable because of the patient's general medical condition, which is uncommon, then resection of any enlarged pelvic nodes should be performed.

Management of Para-aortic Lymph Nodes

Although some authors recommend systematic para-aortic lymphadenectomy on all high-risk patients (129) or in patients with two or more positive pelvic lymph nodes (130), this is major surgery for a group of patients who are usually elderly and obese. **An extensive para-aortic lymphadenectomy significantly increases operating time, blood loss, and postoperative morbidity, particularly lower limb lymphedema.** The latter occurs in about 20% of patients (131).

Lymphedema is a lifelong affliction, which is often complicated by recurrent episodes of cellulitis. To avoid progressive deterioration of the condition, regular massage and use of surgical stockings are essential, and both become progressively more burdensome, particularly for elderly patients. Primary prevention of lymphedema by selective use of pelvic lymphadenectomy, and avoidance of systematic para-aortic lymphadenectomy, is highly desirable.

The GOG data (66) suggested that patients with positive para-aortic nodes were likely to have the following:

1. Grossly positive pelvic nodes,
2. Grossly positive adnexae, or
3. Grade 2 or 3 lesions with outer-third myometrial invasion.

Nomura et al. (132) retrospectively reviewed 841 patients with endometrial cancer who underwent their initial surgery at Keio University Hospital in Japan. In a multivariate analysis, the clinico-pathologic factor most strongly related to para-aortic nodal metastasis was pelvic lymph node metastasis. Among 155 patients who underwent systematic pelvic and para-aortic lymphadenectomy, **96.2% (101 of 105 cases) had negative para-aortic nodes when the pelvic nodes were negative**. When the pelvic nodes were positive, 48% (24 of 50 cases) also had positive para-aortic nodes. These findings are consistent with those from the Mayo Clinic (129).

The author's current surgical approach is to resect any enlarged nodes in all patients, and to perform complete pelvic lymphadenectomy on patients shown in Table 9.14. Complete para-aortic lymphadenectomy is not performed, but any enlarged para-aortic nodes are resected.

Omental Biopsy

In addition to the lymphadenectomy, **an omental biopsy is also performed as part of the surgical staging** because occult omental metastases may occur, particularly in patients with grade 3 tumors or deeply invasive lesions (133). The omentum should be carefully inspected, along with all peritoneal surfaces, and any suspicious lesions excised. If the omentum appears normal, a generous biopsy (e.g., 5 × 5 cm) should be taken.

Sentinel Node Biopsy

Sentinel node identification has been investigated in a number of solid tumors, the hypothesis being that if one or more sentinel nodes are negative, the remainder of the regional nodes will be negative, so complete lymphadenectomy can be avoided (134). Lymphatic mapping is performed by injecting tracers around the tumor and identifying the draining node(s). Usually, a blue dye and a radioactive tracer are used, and the best results are achieved when both techniques are used together. Technetium-99 is the most commonly used radioactive substance because of its short half-life (6 hours).

Three approaches have been used for sentinel node identification in endometrial cancer: (i) injection into the cervix, (ii) injection around the tumor via a hysteroscope, and (iii) injection into the subserosal myometrium at the fundus.

A Korean meta-analysis of 26 studies reported a detection rate of 78% and a sensitivity of 93%. The cervical injection approach was associated with an increase in the detection rate ($p = 0.031$), the hysteroscopic technique with a decrease in the detection rate ($p = 0.045$), and the subserosal injection technique with a decrease in the sensitivity ($p = 0.049$), if they were not combined with another injection technique (135). The authors suggested that the current evidence was not sufficient to establish the true performance of sentinel node biopsy in endometrial cancer.

The hysteroscopic approach seems to represent the only method able to highlight the complete lymphatic drainage of the uterus, as suggested by a higher incidence of positive para-aortic lymph nodes in that cohort (136,137) although Robova et al. (138) from Prague reported that the subserosal technique gave superior detection rates compared to the hysteroscopic approach.

Role of Lymphadenectomy

There are three potential roles for lymphadenectomy:

1. To assign a surgical stage, and provide prognostic information
2. To treat patients with positive nodes
3. To direct adjuvant radiation

The importance of lymphatic spread in endometrial cancer has been appreciated since the publication of the GOG staging studies in the 1980s (34,35). These studies caused the FIGO Cancer Committee to change the staging from a clinical to a surgical system in 1988.

The therapeutic role of lymphadenectomy is less well understood. A large retrospective, cohort study strongly suggested a therapeutic benefit to lymphadenectomy (139), but two subsequent prospective studies have shown no benefit (140,141). Both studies have been strongly criticized (142–144), and neither had a consistent approach to the para-aortic nodes, which are positive in about half the patients with positive pelvic nodes. Any study to validate the therapeutic effect of lymphadenectomy should include both pelvic and para-aortic lymphadenectomy in patients with intermediate or high-risk disease (145).

In the U.K. Medical Research Council's ASTEC study, over 1,400 patients with clinical stage I or II endometrial cancer underwent total abdominal hysterectomy and bilateral salpingo-oophorectomy, and were then randomized to pelvic lymphadenectomy or no lymph node removal (140). **Para-aortic node sampling was not required,** although palpably suspicious nodes could be removed at the surgeon's discretion. Patients with intermediate- or high-risk disease were randomized to receive external pelvic radiation ± brachytherapy, or observation ± brachytherapy, but **the lymph node status was not taken into account in the radiation randomization**. The number of lymph nodes resected was insufficient to show a benefit in at least one-third of patients, (35% of patients had <10 nodes removed), and **43% of patients had low-risk disease, which would have diluted any possible beneficial effect of lymphadenectomy in the high-risk group.** Decision analysis modeling has suggested that **even if the lymphadenectomy had been therapeutic, the study would have been negative because of the poor study design** (143).

In the Italian study, 514 patients with stage I endometrial cancer were randomly assigned to systematic pelvic lymphadenectomy or no lymphadenectomy after undergoing total abdominal hysterectomy and bilateral salpingo-oophorectomy (141). Patients with grade 1 tumors invading the inner half of the myometrium were excluded, and resection of bulky nodes (>1 cm) was allowed in the control arm. Although the quality of the lymphadenectomy was better controlled in this study, failure to address the para-aortic nodes, and to standardize the postoperative adjuvant radiation, make the validity of the conclusions questionable.

The feasibility of using the results of pelvic lymphadenectomy to modify adjuvant radiation therapy has been addressed in several nonrandomized trials and will be discussed under adjuvant radiation. This role is being increasingly accepted.

Vaginal Hysterectomy

In selected patients with marked obesity and medical problems that place them at high risk for abdominal operations, vaginal hysterectomy should be considered.

Japanese researchers reported on 171 patients aged 70 years and older, 128 (75%) of whom were treated with vaginal hysterectomy and 43 of whom underwent abdominal hysterectomy (146). The 10-year disease-specific survival rates were 83% and 84%, respectively ($p = $ ns). **Patients in the vaginal hysterectomy group had significantly shorter operating times, less**

blood loss, and shorter postoperative stays. Severe complications occurred in 5.4% of the vaginal, and 7% of the abdominal procedures. Perioperative mortality was zero after vaginal hysterectomy and 2.3% after abdominal hysterectomy. They concluded that vaginal hysterectomy should be considered the elective approach for the treatment of elderly patients with endometrial cancer.

Adjuvant Radiation

The use of adjuvant radiation is decreasing for patients with endometrial cancer. This reflects the fact that randomized trials and large population-based studies have failed to show a survival benefit in low-risk cases, and concern for the morbidity associated with radiation therapy, including the risk of inducing a second malignancy. Kumar et al. (147) studied 90,502 patients with endometrial cancer identified from the SEER database, 31,643 (34.9%) of whom received radiation therapy. **The overall relative risk of developing a second primary in the radiation-exposed cohort was 1.25 (95% CI 1.20 to 1.29), and increased with latency of exposure, peaking at >10 years, when it was 40% ($p < 0.001$).** The increase in relative risk for individual organs was as follows: Urinary bladder, 124%; vagina, 88%; vulva, 83%; sarcoma, 70%; colon and rectum, 43%.

For high-risk patients, surgical staging has allowed the therapy to be better tailored to the needs of the individual patient. Nevertheless, the indications for adjuvant radiation remain controversial, and there is significant variation in practice by geographic location (148). The options for postoperative management are as follows:

1. Observation
2. Vault brachytherapy
3. External pelvic radiation
4. Extended-field radiation
5. Whole-abdominal radiation

Observation

Patients with FIGO stage IA, grade 1 or 2 tumors have an excellent prognosis, and no adjuvant radiation is necessary for this group. The Danish Endometrial Cancer Group (DEMCA) was the first to report results of a national protocol of observation for the treatment of patients with low-risk endometrial cancer. After total abdominal hysterectomy and bilateral salpingo-oophorectomy, they prospectively followed 641 patients with grade 1 or 2 tumors and no more than 50% myometrial invasion (stage IA) without adjuvant radiation (149). With follow-up of 68 to 92 months, the disease-free survival rate was 93% (596 of 641).

Sorbe et al. (150) reported results of a randomized controlled trial of 645 patients with grade 1 or 2 endometrioid carcinomas confined to the inner half of the myometrium. Vaginal recurrences occurred in 1.2% of patients receiving vault brachytherapy, and 3.1% in the observation group ($p = 0.114$). The overall recurrence rate and survival were similar in the two groups.

A second standardized protocol was instituted by the Danish group in 1998 to 1999 to determine whether postoperative radiation could be omitted in the intermediate-risk group (151). Of 1,166 patients entered onto the study, 232 (19.9%) were intermediate risk, i.e., grade 1 or 2 with >50% myometrial invasion, or grade 3 with <50% myometrial invasion. Bulky nodes could be resected, but pelvic lymphadenectomy was not performed. The cancer-specific 5-year survival for this intermediate-risk group was 87%, and 96% for 99 patients in the low-risk intermediate group (i.e., (a) younger than 50 years with more than two-thirds myometrial invasion and grade 2 or 3 histology, or (b) younger than 70 years with more than two-thirds myometrial invasion or grade 2 or 3). These results were replicated in a retrospective study of 575 surgically staged patients with intermediate-risk endometrial cancer reported from Brisbane, Australia (152).

If patients are treated without adjuvant therapy, they must be followed carefully so that vault recurrences can be diagnosed early, when they are eminently curable (149,153,154). The diagnosis of recurrence is sometimes first suspected when adenocarcinoma cells are seen on a routine vault smear.

Vaginal Brachytherapy

Vaginal brachytherapy significantly reduces the incidence of vault recurrence. With high–dose-rate therapy, treatment can be accomplished as an outpatient, and the morbidity is low. A study from the University of Virginia reported that compared to observation, postoperative brachytherapy improved survival at a cost of $65,900 per survivor (155).

The Postoperative Radiation Therapy in Endometrial Carcinoma-2 (PORTEC-2) study was a prospective, randomized trial designed to determine whether or not vaginal brachytherapy was as effective as pelvic external-beam radiation for patients with high intermediate risk disease (156). The latter was defined as (i) age greater than 60 years and 1988 FIGO stage IC, grade 1 or 2 disease, or stage IB grade 3 disease, and (ii) stage IIA disease, any age (apart from grade 3 with >50% myometrial invasion). No routine lymphadenectomy was performed, although bulky nodes could be removed. The target volume for the external pelvic radiation included the proximal half of the vagina, the dose being 46 Gy in 2 Gy fractions five times per week. Brachytherapy was delivered with a cylinder with the reference isodose covering the proximal half of the vagina. The dose to the vaginal mucosa was 45 to 50 Gy. **Vaginal recurrence rates were 1.8% for brachytherapy versus 1.6% for external-beam therapy ($p = 0.74$),** and although pelvic recurrence rates were somewhat higher in the brachytherapy group (3.8% vs. 0.5%), there were no differences in overall or disease-free survival. **The vaginal brachytherapy had fewer side effects, and the authors considered it should be the treatment of choice for patients with high intermediate risk disease.**

A Swedish randomized trial of external pelvic radiation plus vaginal brachytherapy versus brachytherapy alone for patients with medium-risk endometrial cancer demonstrated that despite a significant locoregional control benefit with combined radiotherapy, no survival benefit occurred. Late toxicity to the bowel and bladder contributed to a significantly decreased quality of life (157).

Several studies have demonstrated low recurrence rates at the vaginal vault and pelvic sidewall when vault brachytherapy is given without external pelvic radiation after lymphadenectomy with negative nodes. Table 9.15 reveals an incidence of vault recurrence of 0.6% and an incidence of pelvic sidewall recurrence of 1.2% following this approach in 1,297 mainly high-risk patients with stage I and occult stage II disease. Data from the Mayo Clinic would suggest that high–dose-rate brachytherapy should also be considered in low-risk cases with extensive vascular space invasion (41).

External Pelvic Radiation

With an increasing number of patients in cancer centers having pelvic lymphadenectomy as part of their primary surgery, the indications for external pelvic radiation are decreasing. **Patients with negative pelvic nodes generally receive vault brachytherapy alone, whereas patients with positive pelvic nodes are better treated with pelvic and para-aortic radiation.** External pelvic

Table 9.15 Vault Brachytherapy for Stage I or Occult Stage II Endometrial Cancer after Pelvic Lymphadenectomy

Author	Number	Dose	Fractions	Follow-up	Recurrence Vault	Recurrence Sidewall
COSA-NZ-UK, 1996 (158)	207	LDR 60 Gy to surface	1	3–10 yrs	2	7
Orr et al., 1997 (159)	310	LDR 60 Gy to surface	1	Up to 10 yrs	0	0
Mohan et al., 1998 (160)	159	LDR 20 Gy at 10 mm HDR 21 Gy	1 3	96 mos median	0	1
Ng et al., 2000 (161)	77	LDR 60 Gy to surface HDR 36 Gy to mucosa	1 6	45 mos median	2[a]	1
Fanning, 2001 (162)	66	LDR 40 Gy at 0.5 cm HDR 21 Gy at 0.5 cm	1 3	4.4 yrs mean	0	0
Seago et al., 2001 (163)	23	HDR 21 Gy at 0.5 cm	3	25 mos median	0	0
Horrowitz et al., 2002 (164)	143	HDR 21 Gy	3	65 mos median	1	2
Jolly et al., 2005 (165)	50	HDR 30 Gy	6	38 mos median	2	1
Solhjem et al., 2005 (166)	100	HDR 21 Gy	3	23 mos median	0	0
Kumar et al., 2010 (167)	162	HDR 25 Gy at 0.5 cm	5	53 mos median	1	3
Total	1,297				8 (0.6%)	15 (1.2%)

[a]Five recurrences in lower 2/3 of vagina.

radiation is a reasonable option for high-risk patients who have not undergone surgical staging, but have a negative pelvic and abdominal CT scan and a normal serum CA125 level.

A European randomized trial (the PORTEC study) of surgery and postoperative external pelvic radiation (46 Gy) versus surgery alone for patients with stage I endometrial cancer was published in 2000 (168). Eligible patients were those with stage IC, grade 1; stage IB or IC, grade 2; or stage IB, grade 3 disease. Patients with serous papillary or clear cell carcinoma were also eligible. Surgery consisted of total abdominal hysterectomy and bilateral salpingo-oophorectomy *without* lymphadenectomy. A total of 715 patients from 19 radiation oncology centers were randomized.

Actuarial 5-year overall survival rates were similar in the two groups: 81% (radiotherapy) and 85% (controls) ($p = 0.31$). Endometrial cancer–related death rates were 9% in the radiotherapy group and 6% in the control group ($p = 0.37$). Treatment-related complications occurred in 25% of the radiotherapy patients and in 6% of the controls ($p = 0.0001$). Grade 3 to 4 complications were seen in eight patients, of which seven were in the radiotherapy group (2%). **Two-year survival after vaginal recurrence was 79%, in contrast to 21% after pelvic recurrence or distant metastases.** Survival after relapse was significantly better ($p = 0.02$) for patients in the control group. After multivariate analysis, **investigators concluded that postoperative radiotherapy was not indicated in patients with stage I endometrial cancer younger than 60 years and in patients with grade 2 tumors with superficial invasion**.

A subsequent 10-year follow-up of the PORTEC trial revealed that the 10-year locoregional relapse rates were 5% after radiation and 14% for controls ($p < 0.0001$), and the 10-year overall survival rates were 66% and 73%, respectively ($p = 0.09$) (169). Endometrial cancer–related death rates were 11% (radiation therapy) and 9% (controls) ($p = 0.47$). **The investigators concluded that radiotherapy was indicated for patients who were unstaged surgically but had high-risk features because of the significant locoregional control benefit.**

The GOG reported results of a randomized study of adjuvant pelvic radiation after complete surgical staging for patients with intermediate-risk endometrial carcinoma in 2004 (170). Eligible patients had 1988 FIGO stages IB, IC, IIA (occult), or IIB (occult) disease and were randomized to receive either no additional therapy or 5,040 cGy of external pelvic radiation therapy. There were 390 eligible patients in the study, and median follow-up was 56 months.

The 2-year progression-free survival rate was significantly higher in the group receiving adjuvant radiation (96% vs. 88%; $p = 0.004$). Overall survival rates were not significantly different because there were more pelvic or vaginal recurrences in the no-treatment arm (17 vs. 3), and these were often effectively treated with second-line therapy.

To clarify the effect of postoperative external-beam pelvic radiotherapy in patients with early endometrial cancer, Johnson and Cornes from the United Kingdom performed **a meta-analysis of data from five randomized trials**. Pelvic lymphadenectomy was performed in only two of the five trials. The authors **concluded that adjuvant external-beam pelvic radiation** should not be used for low- (IA or IB, grade 1) or intermediate-risk (IB, grade 2) cancer, but **was associated with a 10% survival advantage for patients with high-risk (stage IC, grade 3) disease** (171).

There seems to be no reason to give both external and vault radiation postoperatively, because **external pelvic radiation appears to be as effective as vaginal brachytherapy for preventing vault recurrence,** and morbidity will be significantly increased by the combination. Weiss et al. (172) reported no vaginal recurrences among 61 women with stage IC endometrial cancer treated with postoperative pelvic radiation without vaginal brachytherapy.

For patients who have had surgical staging and have negative nodes, small-field pelvic radiation is associated with less short- and long-term morbidity than standard pelvic radiation (173), and may be used as an alternative to vault brachytherapy if the latter is not available.

The authors use external pelvic radiation for unstaged patients with a high-risk histologic type or deep myometrial invasion, as long as their CT scan of the pelvis and abdomen and CA125 level are normal.

Extended-Field Radiation

Surgical staging studies have demonstrated that **approximately 50% of patients with positive pelvic nodes will have positive para-aortic nodes** (132), **but isolated para-aortic nodal metastases in patients with negative pelvic nodes are rare.** They occur in less than 2% of cases (174,175), and virtually all occur in patients with high-grade tumors (176). Para-aortic lymph node metastases have been reported to be associated with an increasing number of pelvic lymph node metastases and with bilateral nodal involvement (177), but a recent study has refuted this claim. Japanese researchers reported 15 patients who had positive pelvic nodes and negative para-aortic nodes after pelvic and para-aortic lymphadenectomy (178). Eleven of the 15 patients (73.3%) had occult para-aortic lymph node metastases on ultrastaging, and the rate of occult para-aortic nodal metastasis was not related to the number of positive pelvic nodes. This suggests that all patients with any positive pelvic nodes should receive extended-field radiation.

Approximately 40% of patients with positive para-aortic nodes may be expected to achieve long-term disease-free survival with extended-field radiation therapy (179), and external-beam radiation is superior to chemotherapy alone for patients with positive nodes (180). Mariani et al. (129) reported that none of 11 patients with positive para-aortic nodes failed in the para-aortic area after adequate lymphadenectomy (defined as removal of five or more para-aortic nodes) and extended-field radiation.

The author's current approach to the para-aortic lymph nodes is to resect any enlarged nodes, perform systematic pelvic lymphadenectomy on all except low-risk cases, and give extended-field radiation to anyone with any positive pelvic nodes or proven positive para-aortic nodes.

Whole-Abdominal Radiation

Whole-abdominal radiation has been used for many years in selected patients with omental, adnexal, or peritoneal metastases that have been completely resected.

In 2005, the GOG reported a nonrandomized study of 180 patients with surgically staged III and IV endometrial cancer treated with whole-abdominal radiation with pelvic, plus or minus a para-aortic boost. The 3-year recurrence-free survival rates were 29% for endometrioid and 27% for serous and clear cell carcinomas, respectively (181). No patient with gross residual disease survived. Severe toxicity included bone marrow depression in 12.6%, gastrointestinal toxicity in 15%, and hepatic toxicity in 2.2% of patients.

The following year, the same group reported a randomized phase III trial of whole-abdominal radiation versus chemotherapy in patients with stage III or IV endometrial carcinoma having a maximum of 2 cm of residual disease postoperatively. There were 396 assessable patients. Radiation dosage was 30 Gy in 20 fractions, with a 15 Gy pelvic boost. Chemotherapy consisted of *doxorubicin* 60 mg/m^2 and *cisplatin* 50 mg/m^2 every 3 weeks for seven cycles, followed by one cycle of *cisplatin* (182).

The study showed a significant improvement in 2-year disease-free survival for the chemotherapy arm, 58% versus 46% ($p < 0.01$), confirming that radiation cannot be given in high enough doses to sterilize gross residual disease in the abdomen. At 60 months, adjusting for stage, 55% of chemotherapy patients were predicted to be alive compared to 42% of patients receiving radiation. Chemotherapy was more toxic and probably contributed to the deaths of eight patients (4%) compared to five (2%) on the radiation arm. In the chemotherapy arm, distant failure was reduced from 18% to 10%, but there was no difference in pelvic or abdominal failure rates in the two arms.

Alvarez Secord et al. (183) from Duke University reported on **356 patients with advanced-stage endometrial cancer**. Postoperatively, whole-abdominal radiation alone was used in 48% ($n = 171$), chemotherapy alone in 29% ($n = 102$), and chemotherapy plus radiation in 23% ($n = 83$) of patients. After adjusting for age, grade, stage, and debulking status, **there was a significant survival benefit for combined therapy compared to either modality used alone**.

A retrospective review of 86 patients from the University of Minnesota with peritoneal spread of endometrial carcinoma reported **a recurrence rate of only 16% for patients with stage IIIA disease after treatment with whole-abdominal radiation** (184). **Six percent of patients required surgical intervention for small-bowel obstruction.**

Martinez et al. (185) reported 10-year survival data on a nonrandomized, **prospective trial of whole-abdominal radiation with a pelvic boost in patients with stages I to III endometrial cancer** who were considered at high risk for intra-abdominopelvic recurrence. There were 132 patients treated between 1981 and 2001, including 89 (68%) with stage III disease and 58 (45%) with serous or clear cell histology. **The 5- and 10-year cause-specific survival for patients with serous or clear cell tumors was 80% and 74%, respectively.** Chronic grade 3 or 4 gastrointestinal toxicity was seen in 14% of patients, and 2% developed grade 3 renal toxicity.

The above **studies suggest an advantage to combining radiation with chemotherapy in patients with advanced-stage endometrial cancer.** The authors use whole-abdominal radiation sparingly because of its bowel toxicity, but consider its use in the circumstances shown in Table 9.16.

Table 9.16 Possible Indications for Whole-abdominal Radiation in Patients with Endometrial Cancer
1. Patients with endometrioid, serous, or clear cell carcinomas and omental, adnexal, or peritoneal metastases that have been completely excised
2. Patients with serous or clear cell carcinomas with positive peritoneal washings

Adjuvant Progestins

Although the role of *progestins* in the management of patients with advanced and recurrent endometrial cancer has been established, they have not been shown to be of value in an adjuvant setting (186–188). In a randomized study of 1,148 patients with clinical stage I or II endometrial cancer at the Norwegian Radium Hospital, death resulting from intercurrent disease, particularly cardiovascular disease, was more common in the *progesterone*-treated group ($p = 0.04$) (187). In 461 high-risk patients, a tendency toward fewer cancer-related deaths and a better disease-free survival rate in the treatment group was observed, but crude survival was unchanged. It was concluded that further studies were needed in high-risk patients but that the evidence suggested that prophylactic *progestin* therapy was not likely to be a cost-effective approach for patients with endometrial cancer unless the patient had a high-risk, receptor-positive tumor.

An Australian, New Zealand, and United Kingdom trial of 1,012 patients with high-risk disease showed more relapses in the control group, but no difference in survival (188). Patients received *medroxyprogesterone acetate* (MPA) 200 mg twice daily for at least 3 years or until recurrence. Steroid receptor status had no influence on outcome in either arm.

Adjuvant Chemotherapy

Endometrioid Carcinoma

The value of adjuvant systemic therapy in patients with high-risk early-stage endometrioid endometrial cancer is still controversial.

Five randomized trials have been conducted that evaluated the efficacy of chemotherapy in the adjuvant setting. The oldest trial (GOG 34), using single-agent *doxorubicin*, did not show any benefit in a study of 192 patients with clinical stage I or II (occult) disease who had one or more risk factors for recurrence after surgical staging (189). Maggi et al. (190) conducted a randomized controlled trial in 345 high-risk endometrial cancer patients comparing five cycles of *cisplatin*, *doxorubicin*, and *cyclophosphamide* with external pelvic radiation. In a multivariate analysis, the investigators reported no difference between therapies in terms of progression-free or overall survival.

A Japanese multicenter randomized trial compared whole-pelvic radiation with three or more cycles of *cyclophosphamide, doxorubicin,* and *cisplatin* (CAP) chemotherapy in 385 evaluable patients with stages IC to IIIC endometrioid adenocarcinoma ("intermediate risk"; 60% stage IC, 15% grade 3) (191). At a median follow-up of 5 years, there were no significant differences in progression-free (pelvic radiation 83.5% vs. CAP 81.8%) or overall survival (85.3% vs. 86.7%). In a subgroup analysis of "high to intermediate risk" cases (stage IC >70 years; stage IC grade 3; stage II or stage IIIA [cytology], $n = 120$), a survival benefit for CAP was suggested (191).

Hogberg et al. (192) presented the results of a European trial of radiation alone *versus* adjuvant chemotherapy before or after radiation in 382 patients with stage I, II, IIIA (positive peritoneal cytology only), or IIIC disease who had high-risk factors for recurrence (one or more of deep myometrial invasion, nondiploid DNA, or serous, clear cell, grade 3, anaplastic histology). Chemotherapy was not standardized and included *doxorubicin* and *platinum* (AP); *paclitaxel, doxorubicin,* and *platinum* (TAP); *paclitaxel* and *platinum* (TP); or *paclitaxel, cisplatin,* and *epirubicin*. The study suggested an improvement in progression-free survival with chemotherapy (7% improvement at 5 years, $p = 0.03$), but survival data were too early to draw any conclusions (192).

Hogberg et al. (193) subsequently reported more mature results, and combined the results with a similar study carried out by the Mario Negri Institute (MaNGO) trials group in Italy (ILIADE-III). The two studies included 540 patients with endometrial cancer (FIGO stages I–III) with no residual tumor, and randomly allocated patients to adjuvant radiotherapy with or without sequential chemotherapy (193). In the combined analysis, there was a significant reduction in risk of relapse in the chemotherapy arm (hazard ratio [HR] 0.63, CI 0.44 to 0.89; $p = 0.009$). Neither trial alone showed any significant difference in overall survival. In the combined analysis, overall survival approached statistical significance (HR 0.69, CI 0.46 to 1.03; $p = 0.07$) and cancer-specific survival (CSS) was significant (HR 0.55, CI 0.35 to 0.88; $p = 0.01$) (193).

A recent **Cochrane analysis** investigated the role of adjuvant chemotherapy in endometrial cancer (194). The authors analyzed the results of five randomized trials of chemotherapy compared to no systemic treatment. Four of these studies included platinum-based chemotherapy and the studies recruited almost 2,200 patients. The authors **concluded that postoperative platinum-based chemotherapy was associated with a small benefit in progression-free and overall survival irrespective of radiotherapy treatment, but the absolute risk reduction was only about 4%** (194).

Increased pelvic relapse rates have been reported when using adjuvant chemotherapy alone in patients with high-risk or advanced-stage disease, and this was noted in the recent Cochrane analysis. The international PORTEC 3 is a phase III randomized trial comparing adjuvant pelvic radiation with concomitant *cisplatin* followed by four cycles of *paclitaxel* and *carboplatin* with standard pelvic radiation in patients with high-risk endometrial cancer. It has recruited over 650 patients, and will close to recruitment in late 2013. It should establish the role, if any, of adjuvant chemotherapy in patients with high-risk endometrial cancer.

Serous and Clear Cell Carcinomas

Although serous carcinomas comprise less than 10% of endometrial cancers, they account for over 50% of all recurrences and disease-related deaths, because of the frequent extrapelvic recurrences and distant metastases. Clear cell cancers comprise 6% of uterine cancers. They share many similarities with clear cell cancers of the ovary and kidney, and are associated with a higher risk of relapse.

The role of adjuvant chemotherapy in patients with these two high-risk histologic subtypes is not known. In the NSGO study reported by Hogberg et al. (192) there did not appear to be any benefit of adjuvant chemotherapy in serous/clear cell carcinomas, but the number of patients was relatively small and the CIs were wide. Similar findings were reported in GOG-122, where the HR for death in the 83 women with serous carcinomas was just over 1, in contrast to the HR of 0.48 favoring chemotherapy for patients with endometrioid cell types (195).

There have been a number of retrospective case series suggesting a possible benefit for adjuvant chemotherapy in women with serous cancers, and a recommendation by the SGO to consider adjuvant chemotherapy in women with clear cell cancers. Einstein et al. (196) reported the results of a pilot study of 84 patients with uterine serous cancers. Postoperatively, they were treated with three cycles of *paclitaxel* (175 mg/m^2) and *carboplatin* (AUC, 6 to 7.5) every 3 weeks, followed by radiotherapy, then an additional three cycles of chemotherapy. The 3-year survival probability for patients with stage I and II disease was 84%, while for patients with stages III and IV disease, it was 50%. They concluded that radiotherapy sandwiched between *carboplatin* and *paclitaxel* was well tolerated, and appeared to be effective in women with completely resected uterine serous cancers.

Although platinum- and taxane-based chemotherapy is commonly used in patients with serous and clear cell carcinomas, there are at present no data from randomized trials to demonstrate benefit. It is hoped that PORTEC 3 will help answer this important clinical question.

Clinical Stage II

When both the cervix and the endometrium are clinically involved with adenocarcinoma, it may be difficult to distinguish between a stage IB adenocarcinoma of the cervix and a stage II endometrial carcinoma. Histopathologic evaluation with hematoxylin and eosin is not helpful in the differentiation of these two conditions, and the diagnosis is usually based on clinical and epidemiologic features. The obese, elderly woman with a bulky uterus is more likely to have endometrial cancer, whereas the younger woman with a bulky cervix and a normal corpus is more likely to have cervical cancer. Immunohistochemical staining for p16 as a surrogate marker for HPV virus will usually differentiate them, cervical cancers being HPV positive.

There are no randomized, prospective studies of treatment for stage II endometrial cancer, but retrospective studies favor primary surgery, including surgical staging, with adjuvant radiation tailored to the surgical findings.

A large retrospective Italian study reported on 203 patients who underwent primary surgery for stage II endometrial cancer (197). Simple hysterectomy was performed in 135 patients (66%) and radical hysterectomy in 68 (34%). Adjuvant radiation was given to 66 of 111 patients (59%) with stage IIA disease and to 67 of 92 patients (73%) with stage IIB. Survival rates were 79% in the simple hysterectomy group and 94% in the radical hysterectomy group at 5 years, and 74% and 94% at 10 years, respectively ($p = 0.05$). Although adjuvant radiation reduced locoregional recurrence, there was no significant difference in survival.

SEER data were used in the United States to determine whether primary treatment with simple or radical hysterectomy, with or without adjuvant radiation, altered disease-related survival for patients with FIGO stage II endometrial cancer (198). Cases diagnosed between 1988 and 1994 were analyzed, and included 555 patients (60%) undergoing simple hysterectomy and 377 patients (40%) undergoing radical hysterectomy. The 5-year cumulative survival rate for patients who received surgery alone was 84.4% with simple hysterectomy and 93% with radical hysterectomy ($p = 0.05$). There was no significant survival difference for adjuvant radiation versus no radiation in either arm. **The researchers concluded that radical hysterectomy was associated with better survival when compared with simple hysterectomy for FIGO stage II corpus adenocarcinoma.**

A multicenter study from the United States evaluated 162 patients with surgical stage II endometrial cancer (199). An extrafascial hysterectomy was performed in 75% of patients and a radical hysterectomy in 25%. At least ten nodes were removed in more than 90% of cases. **A significantly better 5-year disease-free survival was seen in patients undergoing radical hysterectomy (94%) compared with extrafascial hysterectomy (76%)** ($p = 0.05$). **Adjuvant radiation did not improve survival.**

Our current approach to patients with stage II endometrial carcinoma is to perform primary surgery and surgical staging, provided the patient is medically fit.

The surgery is as follows:

1. Modified (Type II) radical hysterectomy
2. Bilateral salpingo-oophorectomy
3. Peritoneal washings for cytologic study
4. Pelvic lymphadenectomy to the midcommon iliac area
5. Resection of grossly enlarged para-aortic nodes
6. Omental biopsy
7. Biopsy of any suspicious peritoneal nodules

Postoperatively, adjuvant radiation is individualized. If lymph nodes are negative, no adjuvant radiation is given. Patients with nodal metastases receive extended-field, external-beam radiation therapy.

Surgical Stage IIIA

Patients with stage IIIA endometrial cancer include those with tumor involving the uterine serosa, and those with disease involving the tubes or ovaries. All macroscopic disease can be removed in these patients. Although there are no definitive randomized studies to guide adjuvant therapy, external pelvic radiation and systemic chemotherapy are appropriate, based on the available data (195,200).

Surgical Stage IIIB

The only study specifically of patients with surgical FIGO stage IIIB endometrial cancer was reported by Nicklin and Petersen in 2000 (201). Isolated vaginal metastases are very uncommon, and only 14 (0.7%) out of 1,940 patients with endometrial cancer treated at the Queensland Centre for Gynaecological Cancer from January 1982 to December 1996 could be identified. None of the 14 patients in the study had pelvic or para-aortic lymph node dissection, so many may have been upstaged to IIIC had this been done. **Survival was similar to patients with stage IIIC disease,** and the authors concluded that a case could be made to abolish this substage and include these patients with those currently classified as having stage IIIC disease.

Surgical Stage IVA

Endometrial cancer extending only into the bladder or rectal mucosa is very uncommon. In the latest FIGO Annual Report, only 49 of 7,990 patients (0.6%) with endometrial cancer had stage IVA disease (5). Treatment must be individualized, but would require some type of modified pelvic exenteration, with or without pelvic radiation and chemotherapy.

Surgical Stage IVB

Stage IVB endometrial carcinoma is uncommon, and the results of therapy are poor. An occasional patient is seen with a well-differentiated adenocarcinoma that has metastasized because of prolonged patient or physician delay or because cervical stenosis has prevented the appearance of abnormal bleeding. Such tumors are usually ER-positive and PR-positive and prolonged survival may occur with *progestin* therapy before or after total abdominal hysterectomy, bilateral salpingo-oophorectomy, and possibly radiation therapy.

In a series of 83 patients reported by Aalders et al. (202) from the Norwegian Radium Hospital, the lung was the main site of extrapelvic spread, with 36% of patients having lung metastases. **Treatment of stage IV disease must be individualized but usually involves a combination of surgery, radiation therapy, and either hormonal therapy or chemotherapy.**

There may be a role for cytoreductive surgery, although data are limited to small, retrospective studies. The largest series, from Baltimore, reported results from 65 patients (203). Optimal cytoreduction, defined as residual tumor up to 1 cm diameter, was accomplished in 36 patients (55.4%), whereas 29 patients (44.6%) underwent suboptimal resection. Median survival was 34 months in the optimal group compared with 11 months in the suboptimal group ($p = 0.0001$). Patients with no macroscopic residual disease had a median survival of 40.6 months. Similar results have been reported from the Netherlands in a smaller series (204).

A major objective of therapy should be to try to achieve local disease control in the pelvis, in order to palliate bleeding, vaginal discharge, pain, and fistula formation.

Hormonal therapy and chemotherapy for patients with advanced and recurrent endometrial cancer is discussed later in the chapter.

Special Clinical Circumstances

Endometrial Cancer Diagnosed after Hysterectomy

This situation is best avoided by the appropriate investigation of any abnormal vaginal bleeding preoperatively, and by routinely opening the excised uterus in the operating room. If unsuspected endometrial cancer is discovered, the adnexae can be removed and appropriate surgical staging performed.

When the diagnosis is made during the postoperative period, the following investigations are recommended:

1. PET scan, or CT scan of the chest, pelvis, and abdomen
2. Serum CA125 measurement

If the CA125 level is elevated or if the PET or CT scan reveals lymphadenopathy or other evidence of metastatic disease, laparotomy is usually indicated.

If all investigations are negative, the authors' approach is as follows:

1. **Grade 1 or 2 endometrioid lesions with less than one-half myometrial invasion: No further treatment,** although laparoscopic prophylactic oophorectomy is advisable because of the risk of subsequent ovarian cancer. This is particularly important if there is any family history of breast, ovarian, or colon cancer (Lynch syndrome).
2. **All other lesions: Further laparotomy with removal of adnexae, surgical staging, and appropriate postoperative radiation.**

Synchronous Primary Tumors in the Endometrium and Ovary

This uncommon circumstance occurs much more commonly in young women (205). A SEER study of 56,986 epithelial ovarian cancers diagnosed between 1973 and 2005 reported synchronous endometrial cancers in less than 3% of cases (206). **In at least half of the cases, both endometrial and ovarian tumors are of the endometrioid type,** and distinguishing between primary and metastatic lesions may be difficult.

Israeli investigators reported that 62% of cases with simultaneous tumors of the endometrium and ovary could be differentiated from metastatic tumors by distinct immunohistochemical expression of ER and PR ($p = 0.0006$), and 32% could be differentiated by distinct immunostaining for *Bcl-2* ($p = 0.03$) (207).

The GOG reported 74 cases, 23 (31%) of which had microscopic spread of tumor in the pelvis or abdomen (112). Sixty-four patients (86%) had endometrioid tumors in both sites, and endometriosis was found in the ovary in 23 patients (31%). Patients with tumor confined to the uterus and ovary had a 10% probability of recurrence within 5 years, compared with a 27% probability for those with metastatic disease ($p = 0.006$). Similarly, patients with no more than grade 1 disease at either site had an 8% probability of recurrence within 5 years, compared with a 22% probability for those with a higher grade in either the ovary or the endometrium ($p = 0.05$).

Treatment should be determined on the premise that each represents a primary lesion, and many cases require surgery alone.

Endometrial Carcinoma in Young Women

Approximately 5% of endometrial cancers occur in women aged 40 years or younger. The majority of women have a history of chronic anovulation and the tumors are usually well differentiated. A minority (10%) occur in association with the Lynch syndrome (hereditary nonpolyposis colorectal cancer [HNPCC] syndrome) in which case there is a more variable histologic spectrum (208). **Adenocarcinomas of the endometrium occasionally develop in very young women (30 years of age or younger), usually in association with the polycystic ovarian syndrome. Approximately 90% of the lesions are well differentiated and limited to the endometrium** (209).

Fertility preservation is often a concern for these young women. An MRI is desirable pretreatment to exclude significant myometrial invasion, and the tumors should have grade 1 histology and be PR-positive.

Several small series have reported **regression of the carcinoma in 70–85% of cases with a variety of *progestins*** (210–216). In a review of 278 patients from 13 series reported by the Royal College of Obstetricians and Gynaecologists, 208 patients (75%) responded to hormonal therapy (217). Sixty-five of the 208 (31%) developed a recurrence, although these patients were often successfully retreated, which is similar to the experience reported from Korea (218). Only 89 of the 278 patients (32%) gave birth to a live infant (217).

A 3-month trial of *megestrol acetate* orally 160 to 320 mg/d or MPA 200 to 500 mg/d is the usual approach, followed by an endometrial biopsy or curettage. Using *megestrol acetate,* Eftekhar et al. reported a complete response in 18 of 21 patients (85%), although 13 of the 18 patients (72%) required the higher dose. The mean treatment duration was 9 months, and pregnancy occurred in five of the responders (27.8%). Three patients (16.6%) recurred, and two (66.6%) responded to further hormonal treatment (215). Taiwanese researchers reported complete remission in eight of nine patients (89%) using a combination of *megestrol acetate* and *tamoxifen* (216). One patient failed to respond but achieved complete remission after a change from *tamoxifen* to a gonadotropin-releasing hormone analog. Four (50%) of the responders later developed recurrent endometrial cancer.

The progesterone-releasing intrauterine devices theoretically should be able to deliver a much higher dose of hormone to the tumor, with better compliance, while decreasing systemic side effects, such as weight gain and venous thromboembolic events. Gallos et al. (219) conducted a systematic review and meta-analysis of oral progestogens versus *levonorgestrel*-releasing intrauterine devices for patients with endometrial hyperplasia. They concluded that although there was a paucity of high-quality evidence to reliably inform clinical practice, there was a higher chance of disease regression with the intrauterine devices. By contrast, **English investigators have raised doubts about the efficacy of the *levonorgestrel* intrauterine system (Mirena) for the treatment of early-stage endometrial cancer, and have suggested that the myometrium may provide a "sanctuary" for these tumors** (220).

A recent study from South Korea reported **the use of photodynamic therapy for fertility preservation in 16 young women with endometrial cancer** (221). Surface photoillumination with red laser light at a wavelength of 630 nm was applied to the endometrial cavity and endocervical canal of the patients 48 hours after a hemoporphyrin derivative-type photosensitizer was injected intravenously. In 11 patients, the photodynamic therapy was used as primary treatment, while in five patients, it was given for recurrence after hormonal therapy. **Complete remission was observed in 12 (75%) of the 16 patients.**

Adequate imaging of the ovaries is important before any decision is made regarding conservative management. In a review of 254 patients with endometrial cancer at the Royal Hospital for

Women in Sydney, synchronous ovarian malignancies were found in 5 of 17 patients (29.4%) younger than 45 years of age, compared with 11 of 237 older patients (4.6%) ($p < 0.001$). Three other younger patients (17.7%) had secondary ovarian involvement (205). In a series of 102 women aged 24 to 45 years who underwent hysterectomy for endometrial cancer in Los Angeles, 26 (25%) were found to have a coexisting epithelial ovarian tumor; 23 were classified as synchronous primaries, and three were metastases (222).

There is no consensus on long-term management for these younger women, although it is reasonable to recommend hysterectomy after childbearing has been completed to avoid the need for ongoing hormonal manipulation and surveillance with transvaginal ultrasonography. Given the significant incidence of ovarian involvement (205,222) and the efficacy of modern hormonal therapy, there seems little justification for ovarian preservation, unless for psychological reasons. Yale researchers reported that bilateral salpingo-oophorectomy at the time of hysterectomy for young patients with stage I endometrial cancer was associated with a significantly better disease-free survival ($p = 0.013$) (223), although two large studies from South Korea reported no increased recurrence rate following ovarian preservation (224,225).

Endometrial Carcinoma and Lynch Syndrome

Lynch syndrome, (also known as HNPCC syndrome), is caused by germline mutations in the DNA mismatch repair genes (specifically *MLH1, MSH2, MSH6,* and *PMS2*). It is inherited as an autosomal dominant, and accounts for 2–5% of all endometrial cancers (226). Zauber et al. (227) reported a presumptive diagnosis of Lynch syndrome in 13% of women with endometrial cancer presenting before the age of 50 years, and in 5% of older women. **Endometrial cancer is the sentinel cancer for Lynch syndrome in about 50% of cases.** A full family history of cancers should be taken in all patients, but over 50% of women with endometrial cancer who are diagnosed with Lynch syndrome will have no relevant family history, so it is not possible to triage patients for testing using family history alone. **Women with Lynch syndrome have a 25–60% risk of developing endometrial cancer, and are ideal candidates for screening and risk-reducing measures, such as oral contraceptives during reproductive years and hysterectomy following childbearing** (226).

Endometrial cancer patients are a rich population in which to screen for Lynch syndrome. Although most women with endometrial cancer present with early-stage disease, identification of the germline mutation allows screening and other preventive strategies for colorectal cancer, which carries a worse prognosis. The most cost-effective screening strategy seems to be immunohistochemistry for the DNA mismatch repair genes on the cancer of all women under the age of 60, followed by single gene sequencing for those women lacking protein expression (228).

An Australian study of 127 women who had a diagnosis of endometrial cancer and who carried a mutation in one of the mismatch repair genes estimated that the 20-year risk of other cancers was as follows: colorectal cancer, 48% (95% CI 35–62%); cancer of the kidney, renal pelvis, or ureter, 11% (95% CI 3–20%); urinary bladder cancer, 9% (95% CI 2–17%); and breast cancer, 11%, (95% CI 4–19%) (229).

Endometrial Carcinoma after Endometrial Ablation

With increasing use of endometrial ablation as an alternative to hysterectomy for some women with dysfunctional uterine bleeding unresponsive to hormonal therapy, there have been several reports of the subsequent development of endometrial cancer.

Valle and Baggish (230) reviewed eight case reports and cautioned about the need for proper patient selection. They recommended that all patients should have a preablation biopsy showing a normal endometrium, and patients with persistent hyperplasia unresponsive to hormonal therapy should be recommended for hysterectomy. They suggested that if endometrial ablation were to be performed in high-risk patients because of medical contraindications to laparotomy, vigorous follow-up, including periodic ultrasonography and endometrial sampling, would be mandatory. Hysteroscopy, with biopsies of the endometrium, should be done for vaginal bleeding.

Follow-Up

Follow-up after management of endometrial cancer should be negotiated with the patient, but the authors' policy is to recommend follow-up, and to alternate visits with the referring gynecologist. An Italian study of 282 patients with recurrent endometrial cancer reported that **patients with an asymptomatic recurrence had a median survival from relapse of 35 months versus 13 months for a symptomatic relapse ($p = 0.0001$).** Among the 165 asymptomatic patients, diagnosis was based on clinical examination alone in 60 patients (36.4%), imaging in 103 (62.4%), and vaginal cytology in two (1.2%) (231).

Visits are scheduled every 3 months for the first year, every 4 months for the second year, and every 6 months until 5 years. **Approximately 10% of recurrences occur beyond 5 years** (232), so patients should be told to report early with any abnormal bleeding or other symptoms.

Women with endometrial cancer have a comparable risk of breast cancer, but a higher risk of colorectal cancer, compared to the general population. **Surveillance provides valuable psychological support, and an opportunity for the initiation of secondary cancer preventative strategies, such as mammography for breast cancer and fecal occult blood testing or colonoscopy for colorectal cancer** (233).

At each visit, a relevant history should be taken, and any suspicious symptoms investigated appropriately. Routine radiologic studies are not performed, but **a vault smear is performed if adjuvant radiation has not been given**. Bristow et al. (234) reported that routine vaginal cytology detected an asymptomatic isolated vault recurrence in only 2 of 377 patients (0.5%), and that it was not cost-effective. Most of their patients had received postoperative radiation and would not benefit from early detection of vault recurrence. Salani et al. (235) reported a 2.6% recurrence rate among 154 patients with FIGO 1988 stage IA disease, all of whom were symptomatic or had clinically apparent disease on speculum examination.

PET or PET/CT imaging has been reported to be helpful in the follow-up of patients with endometrial cancer, and a systematic review and meta-analysis of the literature revealed a **sensitivity of 95.8% (92.2 to 98.1) and specificity of 92.5% (89.3 to 94.9) for detection of recurrent disease** (236). Most of the PET scans were done in patients with clinical, radiologic, or tumor marker suspicion of recurrent disease. The treatment plan was changed in 22–35% of the studied patients.

Recurrent Endometrial Cancer

According to figures reported in the *26th Annual Report on the Results of Treatment in Gynecological Cancer,* approximately 22% of patients treated for endometrial cancer die within 5 years (9). The large series of 379 patients with recurrent disease reported by Aalders et al. (232) from the **Norwegian Radium Hospital** provides some important information, although management protocols have changed somewhat since that report (237). **Local recurrence was found in 50% of the patients, distant metastases in 29%, and simultaneous local and distant metastases in 21%.** The median time from primary treatment to detection of recurrence was 14 months for patients with local recurrence and 19 months for those with distant metastases. **Thirty-four percent of all recurrences were detected within 1 year and 76% within 3 years of primary treatment.** At the time of diagnosis, 32% of all patients were free of symptoms, and the diagnosis was made on routine physical or radiologic examination. For patients with local recurrence, 36% were asymptomatic, 37% had vaginal bleeding, and 16% had pelvic pain.

Isolated Vaginal Recurrence

Isolated vaginal metastases are the most amenable to therapy with curative intent. Before undertaking treatment for an apparent localized recurrence, a PET or CT scan should be obtained to exclude systematic spread.

In the Danish endometrial cancer study in which low-risk patients were followed without radiation, 17 vaginal recurrences were reported, and 15 of these **(88.2%) responded completely to radiation therapy**. By contrast, none of the seven patients with a pelvic recurrence could be cured (149).

A multi-institutional study in the United States identified 69 patients with surgical stage I endometrial cancer who were treated without adjuvant radiation and developed an isolated vaginal recurrence (154). Of these, ten (15%) were diagnosed initially with stage IA disease. Histologically, 22 patients (32%) had grade 1 disease, 26 (38%) grade 2, and 21 (30%) grade 3. **Radiation therapy controlled 81% of these vault recurrences,** although 18% died from a subsequent relapse.

A 5-year disease-free survival of 68% for 50 patients with an isolated vaginal recurrence was reported from St. Louis, with a low rate of complications. Median time to recurrence was 25 months (range 4 to 179 months) (237). On multivariate analysis, age, histologic grade, and size of recurrence were significant predictors of overall survival. All patients who had grade 3 disease were dead by 3.6 years from the time of recurrence.

High–dose-rate brachytherapy, usually combined with external-beam therapy, has been reported in a series of 22 patients from Canada (238). After a median follow-up of 32 months, all patients had locoregional control. One developed a distant metastasis and died from disease.

For bulky lesions (>4 cm diameter), surgical resection before radiation may improve local control. Laparotomy has the advantage of allowing a thorough exploration of the pelvis and abdomen to exclude other metastatic foci.

If the patient has had prior pelvic radiation, exploratory laparotomy with a view to some type of pelvic exenteration, offers the only possibility for cure. A study of 21 patients undergoing pelvic exenteration for recurrent endometrial cancer at Memorial Sloan-Kettering Cancer Center (total exenteration, 14 cases; anterior, 6 cases; and posterior, 1 case) reported a 5-year survival of 40% (239). Five patients (24%) required reoperation in the first 90 days postsurgery.

Systemic Recurrence: Role of Surgery

Surgery—usually combined with radiation, chemotherapy, or hormonal therapy—may play a role in selected patients with recurrent endometrial cancer, particularly if all residual disease can be resected.

A study of 35 patients undergoing salvage cytoreductive surgery at Johns Hopkins Medical Center reported complete cytoreduction in 23 patients (66%) (240). These patients had a median survival of 39 months, compared to 13.5 months for patients with gross residual disease. **On multivariate analysis, salvage surgery and residual disease status were significant and independent predictors of postrecurrence survival.** Similar conclusions were drawn from a smaller series of patients from Memorial Sloan-Kettering Cancer Center (241).

Patients with a long disease-free interval (>2 years) and an isolated recurrence at any site (e.g., lungs, liver, or lymph nodes) should be considered for surgical resection if the patient is medically fit and the surgery is technically feasible.

Role of Hormonal Therapy

Progestational agents have been used successfully as treatment for patients with advanced or recurrent endometrial cancer. Although parenteral administration has been used, oral administration appears to be equally effective. The reported response rates have been variable, but using more rigorous response criteria in multi-institutional studies, the objective response rates are in the range of 15–20%. Features that predict a better response are hormone receptor expression, low-grade histology, and a long disease-free interval.

The GOG randomized 299 patients with advanced or recurrent endometrial cancer to receive either 200 mg/d or 1,000 mg/d of oral MPA (242). Among 145 patients receiving the low-dose regimen, there were 25 complete (17%) and 11 partial (8%) responses, for an overall response rate of 25%. For the 154 patients receiving the high-dose regimen, there were 14 complete (9%) and 10 partial (6%) responses, for an overall response rate of 15%. Median survival durations were 11.1 months and 7 months, respectively, for the low-dose and high-dose regimens.

The GOG concluded that 200 mg/d of MPA was a reasonable initial approach to the treatment of advanced or recurrent endometrial cancer, particularly for patients whose tumors were well differentiated or PR-positive. Patients with poorly differentiated or PR-negative tumors had only an 8–9% response rate (242).

If an objective response is obtained, the progestogen should be continued indefinitely. Some responses may be sustained for several years. Side effects from *progestins* include weight gain, edema, thrombophlebitis, tremor, headache, and hypertension. There is also an increased risk of thromboembolism.

The nonsteroidal antiestrogen *tamoxifen* has been used to treat patients with recurrent endometrial cancer. It is a first-generation selective estrogen response modulator (SERM) and inhibits the binding of estradiol to uterine ER, presumably blocking the proliferative stimulus of circulating estrogens. **Responses are usually seen in patients who have previously responded to *progestins,*** but an occasional response may occur in a patient who is unresponsive to them (243,244). *Tamoxifen* is administered orally at a dose of 20 mg daily or twice daily, and is continued for as long as the disease is responding. In a review of the literature, Moore et al. (245) reported **a pooled response rate of 22% for single-agent** *tamoxifen*.

In postmenopausal women, the principal source of estrogen is through the conversion of androstenedione by aromatase in peripheral adipose tissue. Aromatase is also elevated in endometrial cancer stroma, and locally produced estrogen may act in a paracrine fashion to stimulate cancer growth. **The response rates to aromatase inhibitors in recurrent and metastatic endometrial cancer have been only about 10%, but the majority of patients in the reported studies have had high-grade, hormone receptor–negative cancers,** where the likelihood of response is low (246). Studies are in progress to evaluate aromatase inhibitors in women with well differentiated or hormone receptor–positive tumors.

Role of Cytotoxic Chemotherapy

Cytotoxic therapy for metastatic endometrial cancer is given with palliative intent, and responses are generally of short duration. Many women with endometrial cancer are elderly and have other comorbidities such as obesity, diabetes mellitus, and cardiovascular disease. They may have had pelvic radiation, which can limit bone marrow reserve. All of these factors have to be taken into consideration when making treatment recommendations, but chemotherapy should be considered in patients with a good performance status.

The most active drugs are the *platinum* **agents,** *taxanes,* **and** *anthracyclines.* **Response rates are in the order of 30–60%, with the progression-free survival 5 to 12 months** (247–249).

The response to second-line therapy is generally poor. The best response rates are with a *taxane,* and the GOG reported *paclitaxel* to have a 35% response rate in previously untreated women (250) and a 27% response rate in previously treated patients. In the latter group, the median duration of response was 4.2 months, and the median overall survival was 10.3 months. *Topotecan* has been studied as a second-line agent by the GOG, but the response rate was only 9% (251).

There have been a number of randomized trials of combination versus single-agent chemotherapy, and two systematic reviews of chemotherapy for metastatic endometrial cancer. Both concluded that **combination chemotherapy with** *doxorubicin* **and** *cisplatin* **resulted in higher response rates than** *doxorubicin* **alone** (252,253). The combination was associated with response rates in the order of 40%, with progression-free survivals of 5 to 7 months. The addition of *paclitaxel* to either of the above regimens resulted in a higher response rate (57% vs. 37%) and a small survival advantage. However, the toxicity was excessive, and there were a number of treatment-related deaths (254).

The combination of *carboplatin* **and** *paclitaxel* has been evaluated in a nonrandomized setting, and response rates as high as 67%, with 29% complete responses, have been reported. Toxicity was acceptable, the median progression-free survival was as high as 14 months, and overall survival was approximately 26 months (255,256). **This regimen is commonly used to treat patients with metastatic endometrial cancer.**

The GOG presented the results of a randomized trial comparing *carboplatin* and *paclitaxel* with a three-drug combination of *paclitaxel, doxorubicin,* and *cisplatin* (TAP) at the SGO annual meeting in 2012 (195). There were 1,381 patients treated from 2003 to 2009. The median progression-free survival was 14 months in both trial arms, with a median overall survival of 32 months for *carboplatin and paclitaxel* and 38 months for TAP, respectively (HR, 1.01). The *carboplatin* and *paclitaxel* combination was associated with a more favorable toxicity profile.

Newer targeted treatments are being investigated. In a phase II GOG study of 52 women with recurrent endometrial cancer, *bevacizumab* induced clinical responses in seven patients (13.5%), and 21 patients (40.4%) survived progression free for at least 6 months. Median PFS and overall survival times were 4.2 and 10.5 months, respectively (257).

One of the most active new agents (*temsirolimus*) is directed against the mammalian target of *rapamycin (mTOR).* Oza et al. (258) recently reported the results of a phase II study of *temsirolimus* in patients with advanced endometrial cancer. There was no correlation between molecular markers and clinical outcomes, but the partial response rate was 14%, and 69% of patients had stable disease.

The GOG recently reported a phase II study combining *temsirolimus* with *bevacizumab* in 49 women with metastatic endometrial cancer who had 1 to 2 lines of prior chemotherapy. Although 12 patients (24.5%) had clinical responses (1 complete and 11 partial responses) it was associated with significant toxicity (259).

Table 9.17 Carcinoma of the Corpus Uteri: Patients Treated from 1999 to 2001; Survival Rates by FIGO Surgical Stage (n = 7,990)

Strata	Patients	Overall Survival (%)		
		1-Year	3-Year	5-Year
IA	1,054	98.2	95.3	90.8
IB	2,833	98.7	94.6	91.1
IC	1,426	97.5	89.7	85.4
IIA	430	95.2	89.0	83.3
IIB	543	93.5	80.3	74.2
IIIA	612	89	73.3	66.2
IIIB	80	73.5	56.7	49.9
IIIC	356	89.9	66.3	57.3
IVA	49	63.4	34.4	25.5
IVB	206	59.5	29	20.1

Modified from the 26th FIGO Annual Report on the Results of Treatment in Gynecological Cancer (9).

Table 9.18 Carcinoma of the Corpus Uteri: Patients Treated from 1999 to 2001; Survival Rates for Surgical Stages I and II by Histologic Grade

Grade	Overall 5-Year Survival Rates (%)			
	Stage I		Stage II	
	No.	Percent	No.	Percent
1	2,373	92.9	267	86
2	2,014	89.9	444	82.1
3	708	78.9	208	66

Modified from the 26th FIGO Annual Report on the Results of Treatment in Gynecological Cancer (9).

Table 9.19 Carcinoma of the Corpus Uteri: Patients Treated from 1999 to 2001; Survival Rates in Stage I by Surgical Stage and Grade of Differentiation (n = 5,095)

Strata	Patients	Overall Survival Rates (%)		
		1-Year	3-Year	5-Year
IA G1	627	98.9	97.7	93.4
IB G1	1,113	99.2	94.9	91.6
IC G1	441	98.6	93.9	90.6
IA G2	253	98.8	95	91.3
IB G2	1,305	98.8	96.2	93.4
IC G2	648	98	90.7	86.3
IA G3	107	94.2	83.5	79.5
IB G3	328	97.2	88.1	82
IC G3	273	95.5	80	74.9

Modified from the 26th FIGO Annual Report on the Results of Treatment in Gynecological Cancer (9).

Table 9.20 Carcinoma of the Corpus Uteri: Patients Treated from 1999 to 2001; Survival Rates by Histologic Type (n = 8,033)		
Histologic Type	No.	5-Year Survival Rate (%)
Endometrioid	6,735	83.2
Adenosquamous	338	80.6
Mucinous	80	77
Clear cell	173	62.5
Serous	323	52.6
Squamous	25	68.9

Modified from the 26th FIGO Annual Report on the Results of Treatment in Gynecological Cancer (9).

Uterine serous carcinomas are histologically similar to ovarian serous tumors, but the reported response rate to *cisplatin*-containing combination chemotherapy has been inconsistent, with some studies suggesting a lower response (260). Rodriguez et al. (261) reported a complete response in 3 of 13 (23%) and a partial response in 8 of 13 patients (62%) to various *platinum* combinations, including *cisplatin* and *paclitaxel* in three patients. Median duration of response was 7.5 months (range 1 to 30 months).

Hormone Replacement Therapy (HRT)

Historically, HRT has been withheld after treatment for endometrial cancer, because of the theoretical risk of stimulating occult foci of estrogen-sensitive disease. Patients with stage I disease have a good prognosis, and protection against osteoporosis and quality-of-life issues are important, particularly for younger women.

Studies of the use of HRT have not shown any increased rate of recurrence in users (262–264). A matched control study from California reported 249 patients with surgical stages I, II, and III disease who were treated between 1984 and 1998 (264). Estrogen alone was used in 130 patients (52.2%). They were matched with nonusers for age, stage, postoperative radiation, and concurrent diseases. Estrogen replacement therapy, with or without progestins, did not increase the rate of recurrence and death among endometrial cancer patients, and hormone users had a statistically significant longer disease-free interval than nonusers ($p = 0.006$).

The authors' practice is to offer symptomatic patients daily conjugated estrogens, (*Premarin*), or *tibolone* (*Livial*).

Prognosis

Although individual institutions may report superior results, the most comprehensive survival data are provided in the *Annual Report on the Results of Treatment in Gynecological Cancer*. Survival by 1988 FIGO surgical stage for the years 1999 through 2001 is shown in Table 9.17. Survival by histologic grade is shown in Table 9.18. The significance of histologic grade is highlighted by the fact that **patients with stage II, grade 1 and 2 tumors have a better prognosis than patients with stage I, grade 3 lesions.**

Survival in relation to grade and depth of myometrial invasion for stage I disease is shown in Table 9.19, and the poor prognosis associated with serous and clear cell carcinomas is shown in Table 9.20.

Uterine Sarcoma

Uterine sarcomas are rare mesodermal tumors that account for 3–7% of uterine cancers (265). They are a heterogeneous group of tumors, and individual experience with each lesion is limited. Historically, uterine sarcomas have been classified into **carcinosarcomas, accounting for 40% of cases, leiomyosarcomas (40%), endometrial stromal sarcomas (10–15%), and undifferentiated sarcomas (5–10%)** (266). Although **carcinosarcomas have been reclassified as a metaplastic form of endometrial carcinoma,** they have been included with uterine sarcomas in most retrospective studies, and not included in clinical trials of endometrial carcinomas. Leiomyosarcomas and carcinosarcomas have a higher incidence in African American women in the United States (267). **Most subgroups behave in an aggressive manner** and have a poor prognosis, with high rates of local recurrence and distant metastases (268).

Pelvic radiation has long been believed to predispose to the subsequent development of uterine sarcomas (269), **but Finnish researchers have shown that the use of combined HRT in postmenopausal women for 5 years or longer is also associated with an increased risk.** A nationwide cohort study of all Finnish women 50 years of age or older who had used estradiol–progestin therapy for at least 6 months was performed (270). There were 243,857 estradiol–progestin therapy users identified from the national Medical Reimbursement Registry, and their incidence of uterine stromal and leiomyosarcomas was compared to that of the background population with the aid of the Finnish Cancer Registry. Exposure to estradiol–progestin therapy for less than 5 years was not associated with any significantly increased risk, but the standardized incidence ratio for 5 to 10 years of use was 2 (95% CI 1.4 to 2.9) and for 10 years of use or longer it was 3 (95% CI 1.3 to 5.9) (270).

Zelmanowicz et al. (271) reported that endometrial carcinomas and malignant mixed müllerian tumors have a similar risk factor profile, which is compatible with the hypothesis that the pathogenesis of these two tumors is similar.

Criteria for the histopathologic classification of sarcomas have been changing, and such lesions should be reviewed by an expert gynecologic pathologist. **Much less emphasis is placed on mitotic counts than was previously the case.**

Smooth Muscle Tumors

Leiomyosarcomas, which must be distinguished from cellular leiomyomas and atypical leiomyomas (see Chapter 5), occur most commonly in the 45- to 55-year age group. In the SEER study of 1,396 patients, the median age of the patients was 52 years (273).

Leiomyosarcomas usually arise *de novo* from uterine smooth muscle, although rarely they may arise in a pre-existing leiomyoma. A subset of myomas, with a deletion of a specific portion of chromosome 1, has a specific cellular morphology and a genetic transcription profile similar to those of leiomyosarcomas. Thus **cytogenetics may** help identify these exceptions to the rule, and possibly **allow prediction of malignant progression** (274). A review of 1,432 patients undergoing hysterectomy for presumed fibroids at the University of Southern California revealed leiomyosarcoma in the hysterectomy specimen in 10 patients (0.7%). The incidence increased steadily from the fourth to the seventh decade of life (0.2%, 0.9%, 1.4%, and 1.7%, respectively) (275).

Most leiomyosarcomas are accompanied by pain, a sensation of pressure, abnormal uterine bleeding, or a lower abdominal mass. Rapid enlargement of a fibroid is a possible sign of malignancy. A few patients may have signs of metastatic disease such as a persistent cough, back pain, or ascites. On physical examination, it is impossible to distinguish leiomyosarcomas from large leiomyomas. Pap smears are unrewarding, and uterine curettings are diagnostic for only the 10–20% of tumors that are submucosal (276). Diagnosis usually is not made before surgery.

Uterine smooth muscle tumors of uncertain malignant potential (STUMP) represent a subcategory of uterine smooth muscle tumors, whose clinical behavior is poorly understood. A series of 45 patients was reported from the M. D. Anderson Cancer Center in 2009 (277). Their mean age was 43 years, with a range of 25 to 75 years. **With a mean follow-up of 45 months, three (7.3%) recurrences were seen.** Recurrence rates were similar for patients having a myomectomy or hysterectomy. One of the recurrences was a leiomyosarcoma, but all three patients were alive and disease-free at a mean follow-up of 121 months.

Intravenous leiomyomatosis is a rare, relatively benign uterine smooth muscle tumor in which much of the tumor is present in (and may arise from) veins (278). It may extend as rubbery cords beyond the uterus into the parametrium or occasionally into the vena cava. Some patients may survive for prolonged periods in spite of incomplete resection of diseased tissue. High levels of ER and PR are present in some tumors, and regression may occur after menopause.

Leiomyomatosis peritonealis disseminata is a condition in which numerous nodules of histologically benign smooth muscle are present on peritoneal surfaces (279). It is frequently associated

Table 9.21 FIGO Staging for Leiomyosarcomas (2009)	
Stage	*Definition*
Stage I	Tumor limited to uterus
IA	<5 cm
IB	>5 cm
Stage II	Tumor extends to the pelvis
IIA	Adnexal involvement
IIB	Tumor extends to extrauterine pelvic tissue
Stage III	Tumor invades abdominal tissues (not just protruding into the abdomen)
IIIA	One site
IIIB	More than one site
IIIC	Metastasis to pelvic and/or para-aortic lymph nodes
Stage IV	
IVA	Tumor invades bladder and/or rectum
IVB	Distant metastasis

FIGO Committee on Gynecologic Oncology. FIGO staging for uterine sarcomas. *Int J Gynecol Obstet.* 2009;104:179.

with a term pregnancy or with the use of oral contraceptives, and regression may occur after termination of pregnancy.

Benign metastasizing leiomyoma is a rare disorder characterized by a histologically benign smooth muscle tumor that originates in the uterus and spreads elsewhere, usually to the lungs. Controversy exists regarding whether lung lesions represent metastases of a benign uterine primary tumor or synchronous or metachronous development of an independent lung lesion. Optimal therapy is unclear, but surgical resection and hormonal therapy are generally recommended (280).

Staging

A new FIGO staging system for Uterine Sarcomas was developed in 2009, to reflect the biologic behavior of these tumors (272). The staging for leiomyosarcomas is shown in Table 9.21.

Surgical Treatment

The only treatment of any proven curative value for the frankly malignant leiomyosarcoma is surgical excision. This typically involves total abdominal hysterectomy, bilateral salpingo-oophorectomy, and debulking of any tumor outside the uterus, including any enlarged lymph nodes. In young patients, it is reasonable to preserve the ovaries, particularly if the tumor has arisen in a fibroid (281,282). **Tumor morcellation increases intraperitoneal dissemination,** and adversely affects survival (283,284).

Lissoni et al. (285) reported eight young patients with a diagnosis of leiomyosarcoma after **myomectomy** who were followed conservatively. All were nulliparous, and all had no evidence of disease on ultrasonography, hysteroscopy, chest radiography, and pelvic and abdominal CT scan or MRI. The mean mitotic count of the leiomyosarcomas was 6 per 10 high-power fields (HPF), with a range of 5 to 33. With a median follow-up of 42 months, three live births were recorded, but one patient recurred and died.

For leiomyosarcomas, the GOG study of 59 patients reported positive lymph nodes in only 3.5% of patients, positive washings in only 5.3%, and adnexal involvement in only 3.4% (265). For 71 patients with leiomyosarcoma confined to the uterus or cervix, the Memorial Sloan-Kettering group reported ovarian metastases in two patients (2.8%) and lymph node metastases in none. Three of 37 patients (8.1%) with gross extrauterine disease had positive nodes, and all were clinically suspicious (286). Wu et al. (287) reported no pelvic or para-aortic lymph node involvement in 21 patients who underwent complete surgical staging. **The SEER study reported lymph node metastases in 23 of 348 patients (6.6%) who underwent lymphadenectomy, but performance of a lymphadenectomy was not associated with improved survival** (273), because most lymph node metastases were found in patients with advanced disease.

A possible role for **secondary cytoreduction** for leiomyosarcomas was reported from the Johns Hopkins Medical Center (288). In a recent review of 128 patients with recurrent uterine leiomyosarcoma, researchers reported prolonged survival **in a select group who had a prolonged progression-free survival and an isolated site of recurrent disease amenable to complete resection.** Neither chemotherapy nor radiation therapy was beneficial.

Chemotherapy

The most active drugs include *doxorubicin, ifosfamide, paclitaxel, docetaxel,* and *gemcitabine.* In the GOG trials, leiomyosarcomas had a 25% (7 of 28) overall response rate to ***doxorubicin*** (289), and a 17.2% (6 of 35) partial response rate to ***ifosfamide*** (290). There was only a 3% (1 of 33) partial response rate to ***cisplatin*** (291). For ***paclitaxel,*** there were three complete responses (9%) whereas eight patients (24%) had stable disease for at least two courses of treatment (292).

Because of the propensity for early hematogenous spread, adjuvant chemotherapy after hysterectomy to eliminate micrometastases is an attractive concept. A large study of 1,042 patients with uterine sarcomas recorded in the Cancer Registry of Norway from 1956 to 1992 reported no change in the 5-year survival rate after the introduction of chemotherapy into the treatment protocols (293). However, a prospective study of 25 patients with completely resected stages I–IV leiomyosarcomas from Memorial Sloan-Kettering Cancer Center reported **2-year progression-free survival rates superior to historical controls for adjuvant *docetaxel* and *gemcitabine.*** The latter was given at a dose of 900 mg/m^2 on days 1 and 8, and *docetaxel* 75 mg/m^2 on day 8, every 3 weeks for four cycles (294). A prospective multicenter phase II study of 46 evaluable patients with disease limited to the uterus treated with four cycles of adjuvant *gemcitabine* plus *docetaxel* followed by four cycles of *doxorubicin* reported a 78% progression-free survival at 2 years, and a 57% progression-free survival at 3 years (295). **An international, randomized, phase III trial of observation versus adjuvant chemotherapy is ongoing, with the primary end point being overall survival.**

For patients with metastatic leiomyosarcoma, the GOG has reported objective responses in 15 of 42 patients (35.8%) treated with ***gemcitabine*** plus ***docetaxel***. The complete response rate was 4.8%, and the partial response rate was 31%, with an additional 11 patients (26.2%) having stable disease (296).

The combination of *docetaxel* and *gemcitabine* has also been reported to be active as second-line therapy for patients with metastatic leiomyosarcoma. In a study of 48 patients, 90% of whom had progressed following *doxorubicin*-based chemotherapy, Hensley et al. (297) reported a complete response in three patients (8.8%) and a partial response in 15 patients (44.1%) for an overall response of 53% (95% CI 35–70%). An additional seven patients (20.6%) had stable disease. Fifty percent of patients who were treated previously with *doxorubicin* had a response. The median time to progression was 5.6 months.

Radiation Therapy

Postoperative external-beam pelvic radiation is of no proven benefit in terms of survival, although it has been thought to improve tumor control in the pelvis (298,299). **The recent randomized clinical trial of adjuvant external pelvic radiation versus observation for patients with nonmetastatic leiomyosarcomas revealed no benefit even in terms of local control** (300).

Prognosis

Data on 819 patients with 2009 FIGO stage I leiomyosarcoma were extracted from the SEER database between 1988 and 2005 (301). **The 5-year overall survival rate was 76.6% for patients with stage IA disease and 48.4% for those with stage IB ($p < 0.001$).** Although cervical involvement is not part of the 2009 FIGO staging system, the 5-year overall survival for women with and without cervical involvement was significantly different, 28.5% versus 55.3% ($p = 0.014$). Significant prognostic variables on multivariate analysis were age ($p = 0.007$), tumor size ($p \leq 0.001$), tumor grade ($p < 0.001$), and performance of salpingo-oophorectomy ($p = 0.02$).

Using tissue microarrays of 84 uterine leiomyosarcomas, researchers have been able to identify two different prognostic groups: Good prognosis tumors were <10 cm diameter, with a mitotic index of <20 MF/10 HPF, negative for Ki67 and positive or negative for *Bcl-2* immunostaining. Poor prognosis tumors were ≥10 cm diameter, had a higher mitotic index (≥20 MF/10HPF), and were positive for Ki67 and negative for *Bcl-2* ($p = 0.001$) (282). A recent study of 167 patients with leiomyosarcomas from three Boston institutions also reported that tumor size >10 cm and a mitotic count of 25/10 HPF or greater were independent poor prognostic factors (302).

Summary of Management of Leiomyosarcoma

The only proven benefit for patients with leiomyosarcomas is total abdominal hysterectomy. Ovaries should normally be removed in postmenopausal women. Systematic lymphadenectomy appears to be of no value, but any enlarged nodes should be removed. These patients should be entered onto clinical trials of new therapeutic agents, particularly *docetaxel* and *gemcitabine,* if possible.

Endometrial Stromal Tumor

In the past, endometrial stromal tumors have been divided into three major categories: **Benign endometrial stromal nodules, low-grade endometrial stromal sarcomas, and high-grade endometrial stromal sarcomas. In 2003, the WHO changed the diagnostic criteria.** The term **Endometrial Stromal Sarcoma** was restricted to an invasive endometrial stromal neoplasm with a distinct, uniform histologic appearance and a very good prognosis, whereas the term **Undifferentiated Endometrial Sarcoma** was introduced for a tumor with a more pleomorphic appearance, often with prominent tumor necrosis, and a very poor prognosis (303). Mitotic counts were no longer used to differentiate high-grade from low-grade lesions.

These tumors were staged for the first time by FIGO in 2009, and the staging is shown in Table 9.22.

Table 9.22 FIGO Staging of Endometrial Stromal Sarcomas and Adenosarcomas

Stage	Definition
Stage I	Tumor limited to uterus
IA	Tumor limited to endometrium/endocervix with no myometrial invasion
IB	Less than or equal to half myometrial invasion
IC	More than half myometrial invasion
Stage II	Tumor extends to the pelvis
IIA	Adnexal involvement
IIB	Tumor extends to extrauterine pelvic tissue
Stage III	Tumor invades abdominal tissues (not just protruding into the abdomen)
IIIA	One site
IIIB	>One site
IIIC	Metastasis to pelvic and/or para-aortic lymph nodes
Stage IV	
IVA	Tumor invades bladder and/or rectum
IVB	Distant metastasis

Note: Simultaneous tumors of the uterine corpus and ovary/pelvis in association with ovarian/pelvic endometriosis should be classified as independent primary tumors.

FIGO Committee on Gynecologic Oncology. FIGO staging for uterine sarcomas. *Int J Gynecol Obst.* 2009; 104:179.

Endometrial Stromal Sarcoma (Low Grade)

These tumors constitute 15–25% of uterine sarcomas (304). Most patients are in the age range of 42 to 53 years. More than half the patients are premenopausal, and young women and girls may be affected. Abnormal vaginal bleeding is the most common presenting symptom, and abdominal pain and uterine enlargement may occur (305). **Although they may be intramural, most endometrial stromal sarcomas involve the endometrium, and uterine curettage usually leads to the diagnosis.**

Surgical Treatment

Total abdominal hysterectomy and bilateral salpingo-oophorectomy, with radical cytoreductive surgery for extrauterine involvement, has been the standard recommendation for endometrial stromal sarcomas (306).

Preservation of the ovaries may be an option for premenopausal women with stage I disease. Adnexal metastases were identified in 11 of 87 cases (13%) in the series from Memorial Sloan Kettering, and all were macroscopically apparent (307). A review of 384 patients with low-grade endometrial stromal sarcomas identified from the SEER database between 1988 and 2005 reported that ovarian preservation did not affect the excellent overall survival of these patients (308). By contrast, a Chinese study of 57 patients reported higher recurrence rates in patients having ovarian preservation (309).

There are limited data available on lymph node metastases in endometrial stromal sarcomas, but a literature review of 13 series revealed an incidence of 4.7% (5 of 106) among patients with macroscopic stage I and II disease (310). The authors concluded that retroperitoneal surgery should be limited to resection of bulky nodes. Others have reported that neither lymphadenectomy (309) nor the presence of lymph node metastases (308) had any influence on survival.

Patients with a late recurrence of an endometrial stromal sarcoma may benefit from aggressive cytoreductive surgery to remove all macroscopic disease if possible, including disease in lymph nodes (310).

Hormonal Therapy

Endometrial stromal sarcomas are commonly ER and PR positive (311), **and patients with advanced and recurrent disease respond well to** *progestins* **or aromatase inhibitors such as** *letrozole.* Chu et al. (312) reported eight patients with recurrent endometrial stromal sarcoma who were treated with *progestin* therapy. Complete responses were seen in four patients (50%), and three others (38%) had stable disease. Pink et al. (313) reported 10 patients treated with *letrozole,* and observed eight responses (80%). There are many anecdotal case reports of hormonal therapy, and the responses can be very durable. There are no data to support adjuvant hormonal therapy (312).

Patients with a previous history of low-grade endometrial stromal sarcoma should not receive estrogens or *tamoxifen* (313) because there may be stimulation of growth, although the estrogen and progesterone of normally functioning ovaries does not seem to be a problem (311,312).

Summation of Management for Endometrial Stromal Tumors

Patients with endometrial stromal sarcomas should undergo total abdominal hysterectomy, bilateral salpingo-oophorectomy, and resection of any extrauterine disease. There is no role for systematic retroperitoneal lymphadenectomy. Preservation of ovaries is an option for premenopausal patients with stage I disease. Patients with advanced or recurrent disease respond well to *progestins* or aromatase inhibitors. **Late recurrences are not infrequent, and aggressive secondary cytoreduction to remove all macroscopic disease may result in long-term survival.**

Undifferentiated Uterine Sarcoma

These tumors behave aggressively regardless of the stage at diagnosis. The group at Memorial Sloan Kettering reported 21 patients seen at their institution between January 2000 and March 2011 (314). FIGO 2009 stage distribution was as follows: Seven (33%) had stage I, one (5%) stage II, two (10%) stage III, and 11 (52%) had stage IV. **Although 18 patients underwent resection of all gross disease at primary surgery, 11 (61%) had progression within the abdomen by the time they underwent postoperative imaging.**

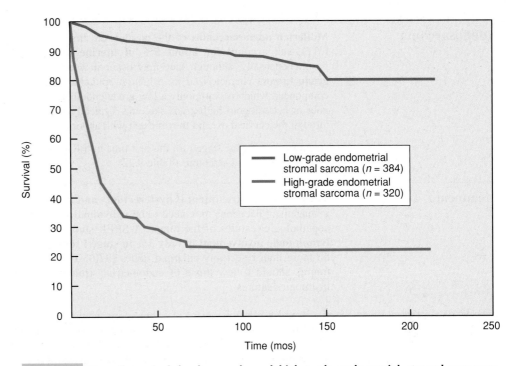

Figure 9.6 Overall survival for low-grade and high-grade endometrial stromal sarcomas. (Reproduced with permission from **Shah JP, Bryant CS, Kumar S, et al**. Lymphadenectomy and ovarian preservation in low-grade endometrial stromal sarcoma. *Obstet Gynecol.* 2008;112: 1102–1108.)

Chemotherapy

Of 13 patients who received first-line chemotherapy for measurable disease, the overall response rate was 62%. Responses were observed with *gemcitabine and docetaxel* (6 of 8) and *doxorubicin*-based regimens (2 of 5) (314).

A report from China suggested that a **combination of *ifosfamide, epirubicin,* and *cisplatin* had activity in patients with undifferentiated endometrial sarcomas** (315).

Radiation Therapy

Radiation therapy may decrease pelvic recurrence without improving survival for patients with endometrial sarcomas.

Summation of Management for Uterine Sarcomas

Management should include total hysterectomy and bilateral salpingo-oophorectomy. The value of lymphadenectomy and debulking of gross extrauterine disease remain unclear (314). Chemotherapy with *gemcitabine and docetaxel* may be used, but responses are short-lived.

Prognosis for Endometrial Stromal Tumors and Endometrial Sarcomas

Endometrial stromal nodules are benign, but can usually only be distinguished from endometrial stromal sarcomas after hysterectomy. For younger women wishing to preserve fertility, a combination of diagnostic imaging and hysteroscopy may be useful in monitoring the growth of the lesion, and local excision has been successful in occasional cases (316).

In a review of 384 patients with **low-grade endometrial stromal sarcomas** and 320 patients with **high-grade lesions** extracted from the SEER database from 1988 to 2005, Shah et al. (308) reported **overall 5-year survival rates of 92% and 25% respectively (*p* < 0.001)** (Fig. 9.6). This study did not have central pathologic review, and pre-WHO 2003 low-grade endometrial stromal sarcomas tended to have more recurrences than the low-grade lesions as currently defined (309).

Adenosarcoma

Müllerian adenosarcomas of the uterus were first described by Clement and Scully in 1974 (317), and **account for about 5% of uterine sarcomas**. They are most commonly seen postmenopausally, although they may occur in young women (318). **They are typically low-grade tumors** characterized by a benign epithelial component and a malignant mesenchymal component, which is commonly a low-grade endometrial stromal sarcoma, but can be a homologous or heterologous high-grade sarcoma. Typically, they are polypoid lesions that may protrude through the cervical os, and they present with abnormal vaginal bleeding (319).

Adenosarcomas were staged for the first time by FIGO in 2009, and the staging is the same as for endometrial stromal sarcomas (Table 9.22).

Treatment

The mainstay of treatment is hysterectomy and bilateral salpingo-oophorectomy, although management decisions may need to be individualized based on the patient's age and the clinicopathologic features of the tumor. A SEER study of 544 patients reported an **incidence of lymph node involvement of only 3% in stage I tumors,** so there seems to be no indication to do more than resect any enlarged nodes (320). The principles of adjuvant therapy for these tumors should follow those of endometrial stromal or uterine sarcomas, depending on the histologic features.

Prognosis

The largest study is the SEER registry report of 544 patients (320). Most cases were confined to the endometrium at diagnosis, although 6% had myometrial invasion into the outer half. The 5-year survival for stage IA uterine adenosarcomas was 84%, compared to 62% for carcinosarcomas. The 5-year survival for stage IB disease was 69%, while it was 63% for stage IC, 69% for stage II, 48% for stage III, and 15% for stage IV. Women over the age of 60 years had a worse prognosis than women under 40.

Carcinosarcoma

Malignant mixed mesodermal tumors (MMMTs) or carcinosarcomas usually occur in an older age group, most patients being postmenopausal (265). They grow rapidly and usually present with postmenopausal bleeding, pelvic pain, or symptoms of metastatic disease. **Most patients have an enlarged uterus, and the tumor protrudes through the cervical os like a polyp in approximately half the patients** (266). Extrauterine disease is found in up to one-third of cases at presentation (266). Uterine curettage usually detects malignant tissue in the uterus, although determination of the exact nature of the tumor may require histologic examination of the entire specimen. **Carcinosarcomas are staged the same as carcinomas.**

There is convincing evidence that most, but not all, uterine carcinosarcomas are monoclonal tumors and really metaplastic carcinomas (321). The behavior of these tumors is similar to that of high-grade endometrioid adenocarcinomas, and they should be managed as such. Metastases are usually from the carcinomatous element, and the sarcomatous element is believed to be derived as a result of dedifferentiation of the carcinomatous component (322). Heterologous differentiation, including rhabdomyosarcomatous differentiation, is not uncommon in MMMTs, and occasionally pure heterologous sarcomas have been reported (323).

Up to 37% of patients with carcinosarcomas have a history of prior pelvic radiation. Such cases tend to occur in younger women, to contain heterologous elements, and to be found at an advanced stage (266).

Surgery

Carcinosarcomas should undergo total hysterectomy, bilateral salpingo-oophorectomy, and surgical staging in the same manner as high-grade endometrial carcinomas. The GOG reported a clinicopathologic study of 301 carcinosarcomas in 1993 (265). Adnexal metastases were present in 12% of patients, lymph node metastases in 18%, and positive peritoneal washings in 21%. No omental biopsies were taken.

A Californian study of 62 patients with carcinosarcoma apparently confined to the uterus reported occult metastases in 38 patients (61%) (324). Adnexal metastases were present in 23% of patients, positive pelvic nodes in 31%, positive para-aortic nodes in 6%, omental involvement in 13%, and positive peritoneal washings in 29%.

Cytoreductive surgery, with the goal of resecting all macroscopic disease, has been reported to be associated with an improvement in overall survival in patients with advanced uterine carcinosarcomas (325).

Chemotherapy

There are a number of active agents, including *cisplatin, carboplatin, anthracyclines, ifosfamide,* and *paclitaxel.* As these are relatively uncommon tumors, the studies have generally been small and patient accrual has been slow. For *cisplatin* (50 mg/m^2 every 3 weeks), the GOG reported a complete response rate of 8% and a partial response rate of 11% among 63 patients with advanced or recurrent disease who had received no previous chemotherapy (291).

Ifosfamide is an active agent for these tumors, the GOG demonstrating nine responses among 28 patients (31.2%) (326). A small improvement in progression-free survival was noted with the addition of *cisplatin* to *ifosfamide* in a phase III GOG trial, but the added toxicity may not justify use of this combination (327).

The GOG evaluated *paclitaxel* in 44 patients with carcinosarcoma of the uterus. Four patients (9.1%) had a complete response, and four (9.1%) had a partial response (328). The GOG subsequently reported the results of a randomized study comparing *ifosfamide* alone versus *ifosfamide* and *paclitaxel* in 179 patients with advanced uterine carcinosarcomas (329). They reported a response rate of 29% with *ifosfamide* alone and 45% with the combination. The odds of response stratified by performance status were 2.21 times greater for the combination arm ($p = 0.017$). The median progression-free and overall survivals for *ifosfamide* compared with *ifosfamide* and *paclitaxel* were 3.6 versus 5.8 months and 8.4 versus 13.5 months, respectively.

A number of phase II trials have reported high response rates to *carboplatin* and *paclitaxel* (54–69%) in patients with advanced carcinosarcomas (330,331). The ongoing GOG 261 phase III noninferiority trial is comparing *ifosfamide* and *paclitaxel* to *carboplatin* and *paclitaxel* in newly diagnosed patients with Stages I–IV carcinosarcomas.

Adjuvant Chemotherapy for Early-Stage Disease

In a prospective phase II study of 65 patients with completely resected clinical stage I or II disease treated with three cycles of adjuvant *ifosfamide* and *cisplatin*, the GOG reported a 54% progression-free and 52% overall survival at 7 years. No postoperative radiation was given, and the authors commented that pelvic relapse remained problematic (332).

Wolfson et al. (333) reported the results of a relatively large randomized clinical trial comparing whole-abdominal radiation with three cycles of *cisplatin, ifosfamide,* and *mesna* (CIM) in 201 patients with stages I to IV uterine carcinosarcomas. The estimated crude probability of recurring within 5 years was 58% for whole-abdominal radiation and 52% for CIM. Adjusting for stage and age, the recurrence rate was 29% lower for patients receiving CIM. They concluded that the results of the trial favored chemotherapy although the differences were small.

Einstein et al. (334) reported a phase II trial of 27 patients with no gross residual disease treated with adjuvant pelvic radiation "sandwiched" between *ifosfamide* alone, or ifosfamide and *cisplatin*. The ifosfamide was given at a dose of 1.2 g/m^2/d × 5 days, and the *cisplatin* at a dose of 20 mg/m^2/d × 5 days, every 3 weeks for three cycles, followed by external pelvic radiation and brachytherapy, then three additional cycles of chemotherapy. They concluded that this treatment was efficacious, but that the addition of *cisplatin* to the regimen added toxicity without improving efficacy.

Radiation

Several nonrandomized studies have suggested that radiotherapy reduces local recurrence (335–337). In a report of 300 patients treated at the M. D. Anderson Hospital between 1954 and 1998, Callister et al. (337) reported that radiotherapy reduced the risk of local recurrence from 48% to 28% and prolonged the time to distant relapse but did not improve overall survival. An EORTC randomized study of stages I and II uterine sarcomas confirmed that external pelvic radiation decreases pelvic relapse but does not improve overall survival for carcinosarcomas (300). There were 91 patients with carcinosarcomas in the study.

The authors' experience suggests that good survival rates can be obtained in patients with carcinosarcomas if they are subjected to surgical staging, targeted postoperative radiation based on the surgical findings, and adjuvant chemotherapy with *cisplatin* and *epirubicin* (338).

Summation of Management of Carcinosarcomas	**Current evidence would suggest that carcinosarcomas of the uterus should undergo full surgical staging and resection of any gross metastatic disease. Postoperative radiation should be tailored to the operative findings. Adjuvant chemotherapy** with *cisplatin* and *epirubicin*, an *ifosfamide*-based combination, or *carboplatin* and *paclitaxel* **may be beneficial** based on small phase II studies, but confirmation requires a randomized phase III trial.
Prognosis	**For 301 MMMTs, the GOG reported a recurrence rate of 53%** (homologous 44%; heterologous 63%) (265). Factors significantly related to progression-free interval by univariate analysis were adnexal spread, lymph node metastases, tumor size, vascular space invasion, depth of myometrial invasion, positive peritoneal washings, histologic grade, and cell type. **On multivariate analysis, the significant prognostic factors were adnexal spread, lymph node metastases, cell type, and cell grade.** Better survivals have been reported in smaller studies following surgical staging, tailored radiation, and adjuvant chemotherapy (338). The role of adjuvant chemotherapy after surgical staging and tailored postoperative radiation must await a randomized trial.

References

1. **Parazzini F, LaVecchia C, Bocciolone L, et al.** The epidemiology of endometrial cancer. *Gynecol Oncol.* 1991;41:1–16.
2. **Siegel R, Ma J, Zou Z, et al.** Cancer statistics, 2014. *CA Cancer J Clin.* 2014;64:9–29.
3. **Madison T, Schottenfeld D, Baker V.** Cancer of the corpus uteri in white and black women in Michigan, 1985–1994: An analysis of trends in incidence and mortality and their relation to histologic subtype and stage. *Cancer.* 1998;83:1546–1554.
4. **Prat J, Gallardo A, Cuatrecasas M, et al.** Endometrial carcinoma: Pathology and genetics. *Pathology.* 2007;39:72–87.
5. **Brinton LA, Felix AS, McMeekin DS, et al.** Etiologic heterogeneity in endometrial cancer: Evidence from a Gynecologic Oncology Group trial. *Gynecol Oncol.* 2013;129:277–284.
6. **Jaakkola S, Lyytinen H, Pukkala E, et al.** Endometrial cancer in postmenopausal women using estradiol-progestin therapy. *Obstet Gynecol.* 2009;114:1197–1204.
7. **Ward KK, Shah NR, Saenz CS, et al.** Cardiovascular disease is the leading cause of death among endometrial cancer patients. *Gynecol Oncol.* 2012;126:176–179.
8. **Von Gruenigen VE, Waggoner SE, Frasure HE, et al.** Lifestyle challenges in endometrial cancer survivorship. *Obstet Gynecol.* 2011; 117:93–100.
9. **Creasman WT, Odicino F, Mausinneuve P, et al.** Carcinoma of the corpus uteri. FIGO Annual Report, Vol 26. *Int J Gynaecol Obstet.* 2006;95(suppl 1):S105–S143.
10. **Kumar S, Shah JP, Bryant CS, et al.** Radiation-associated endometrial cancer. *Obstet Gynecol.* 2009;113:319–325.
11. **DuBeshter B, Warshal DP, Angel C, et al.** Endometrial carcinoma: The relevance of cervical cytology. *Obstet Gynecol.* 1991;77:458–462.
12. **Montz FJ.** Significance of "normal" endometrial cells in cervical cytology from asymptomatic postmenopausal women receiving hormone replacement therapy. *Gynecol Oncol.* 2001;81:33–39.
13. **Siebers AG, Verbeck ALM, Massuger LF, et al.** Normal appearing endometrial cells in cervical smears of asymptomatic postmenopausal women have predictive value of significant endometrial pathology. *Int J Gynecol Cancer.* 2006;16:1069–1074.
14. **Zucker PK, Kasdon EJ, Feldstein ML.** The validity of Pap smear parameters as predictors of endometrial pathology in menopausal women. *Cancer.* 1985;56:2256–2263.
15. **Beal HN, Stone J, Beckman MJ, et al.** Endometrial cells identified in cervical cytology in women >40 years of age: Criteria for appropriate endometrial evaluation. *Am J Obstet Gynecol.* 2007; 196:568.e1–e5; discussion 568.e5–e6.
16. **Moroney JW, Zahn CM, Heaton RB, et al.** Normal endometrial cells in liquid-based cervical cytology specimens in women aged 40 or older. *Gynecol Oncol.* 2007;105:672–676.
17. **Dijkhuizen FPH, Mol BWJ, Brolmann HAM, et al.** The accuracy of endometrial sampling in the diagnosis of patients with endometrial carcinoma and hyperplasia. *Cancer.* 2000;89:1765–1772.
18. **Granberg S, Wikland M, Karlsson B, et al.** Endometrial thickness as measured by endovaginal ultrasonography for identifying endometrial abnormality. *Am J Obstet Gynecol.* 1991;164:47–52.
19. **Karlsson B, Granberg S, Wikland M, et al.** Transvaginal ultrasonography of the endometrium in women with postmenopausal bleeding: A Nordic multicenter study. *Am J Obstet Gynecol.* 1995;172:1488–1494.
20. **Tabor A, Watt HC, Wald NJ.** Endometrial thickness as a test for endometrial cancer in women with postmenopausal vaginal bleeding. *Obstet Gynecol.* 2002;99:663–670.
21. **Timmermans A, Opmeer BC, Khan KS, et al.** Endometrial thickness measurement for detecting endometrial cancer in women with postmenopausal bleeding: A systematic review and meta-analysis. *Obstet Gynecol.* 2010;116:160–167.
22. **Fisher B, Constantino JP, Redmond CK, et al.** Endometrial cancer in tamoxifen-treated breast cancer patients: Findings from the National Surgical Adjuvant Breast and Bowel Project B-14. *J Natl Cancer Inst.* 1994;86:527–537.
23. **Assikis VJ, Neven P, Jordan VC, et al.** A realistic clinical perspective on tamoxifen and endometrial carcinogenesis. *Eur J Cancer.* 1996;32A:1464–1476.
24. **Fung MFK, Reid A, Faught W, et al.** Prospective longitudinal study of ultrasound screening for endometrial abnormalities in women with breast cancer receiving tamoxifen. *Gynecol Oncol.* 2003;91:154–159.
25. **Bakour SH, Khan KS, Gupta JK.** Controlled analysis of factors associated with insufficient sample on outpatient endometrial biopsy. *BJOG.* 2000;10:1312–1314.
26. **Clark TJ, Voit D, Gupta JK, et al.** Accuracy of hysteroscopy in the diagnosis of endometrial cancer and hyperplasia: A systematic quantitative review. *JAMA.* 2002;288:1610–1621.
27. **Obermair O, Geramou M, Gücer F, et al.** Impact of hysteroscopy on disease-free survival in clinically stage I endometrial cancer patients. *Int J Gynecol Cancer.* 2000;10:275–279.
28. **Zerbe MJ, Bristow R, Grumbine FC, et al.** Inability of preoperative computed tomography scans to accurately detect the extent of myometrial invasion and extracorporal spread in endometrial cancer. *Gynecol Oncol.* 2000;78:67–70.
29. **Chung HH, Kang SB, Cho JY, et al.** Accuracy of MR imaging for the prediction of myometrial invasion of endometrial carcinoma. *Gynecol Oncol.* 2007;104:654–659.
30. **Nagar H, Dodds S, McClelland HR, et al.** The diagnostic accuracy of magnetic resonance imaging in detecting cervical involvement in endometrial cancer. *Gynecol Oncol.* 2006;103:431–434.

31. **Chang MC, Chen JH, Laing JA, et al.** 18 F-FDG PET or PET/CT for detection of metastatic lymph nodes in patients with endometrial cancer: A systematic review and meta-analysis. *Eur J Radiol.* 2012;81:3511–3517.

32. **Palma MD, Gregianin M, Fiduccia P, et al.** PET/CT imaging in gynecologic malignancies: A critical overview of its clinical impact and our retrospective single center analysis. *Clin Rev Oncol/Hematol.* 2012;83:84–98.

33. **Jhang H, Chuang L, Visintainer P, et al.** CA125 levels in the preoperative assessment of advanced stage uterine cancer. *Am J Obstet Gynecol.* 2003;188:1195–1197.

34. **Boronow RC, Morrow CP, Creasman WT, et al.** Surgical staging in endometrial cancer: Clinicopathologic findings of a prospective study. *Obstet Gynecol.* 1984;63:825–832.

35. **Creasman WT, Morrow CP, Bundy BN, et al.** Surgical pathologic spread patterns of endometrial cancer. *Cancer.* 1987;60:2035–2041.

36. **Zaino RJ.** FIGO staging of endometrial adenocarcinoma: A critical review and proposal. *Int J Gynecol Pathol.* 2009;28:1–9.

37. **Lewin SN, Herzog TJ, Medel NIB, et al.** Comparative performance of the 2009 International Federation of Gynecology and Obstetrics' staging system for uterine corpus cancer. *Obstet Gynecol.* 2010;116:1141–1149.

38. **Cooke EW, Pappas L, Gaffey DK.** Does the revised International Federation of Gynecology and Obstetrics staging system for endometrial cancer lead to increased discrimination in patient outcomes? *Cancer.* 2011;117:4231–4237.

39. **Bigelow B, Vekshtein V, Demopoulos RI.** Endometrial carcinoma, stage II: Route and extent of spread to the cervix. *Obstet Gynecol.* 1983;62:363–366.

40. **Truskett ID, Constable WC.** Management of carcinoma of the corpus uteri. *Am J Obstet Gynecol.* 1968;101:689–694.

41. **Mariani A, Dowdy SC, Keeney GL, et al.** Predictors of vaginal relapse in stage I endometrial cancer. *Gynecol Oncol.* 2005;97:820–827.

42. **Zaino RJ, Kurman RJ, Diana KL, et al.** Prognostic models to predict outcome for women with endometrial adeno-carcinoma. *Cancer.* 1996;77:1115–1121.

43. **Lee NK, Cheung MK, Shin JY, et al.** Prognostic factors for uterine cancer in reproductive-aged women. *Obstet Gynecol.* 2007;109:655–662.

44. **Nakanishi T, Ishikawa H, Suzuki Y, et al.** Association between menopausal state and prognosis of endometrial cancer. *Int J Gynecol Cancer.* 2001;11:483–487.

45. **Zaino RJ, Kurman R, Herbold D, et al.** The significance of squamous differentiation in endometrial carcinoma. *Cancer.* 1991;68:2293–2302.

46. **Sherman ME, Bitterman P, Rosenshein NB, et al.** Uterine serous carcinoma. *Am J Surg Pathol.* 1992;16:600–610.

47. **Sakuragi N, Hareyama H, Todo Y, et al.** Prognostic significance of serous and clear cell adenocarcinoma in surgically staged endometrial carcinoma. *Acta Obstet Gynecol Scand.* 2000;79:311–316.

48. **Hamilton CA, Cheung MK, Osann K, et al.** Uterine papillary serous and clear cell carcinomas predict for poorer survival compared to grade 3 endometrioid corpus cancers. *Brit J Cancer.* 2006;94:642–646.

49. **Sherman ME, Bur ME, Kurman RJ.** P53 in endometrial carcinoma and its putative precursors: Evidence for diverse pathways for tumorigenesis. *Hum Pathol.* 1995;26:1268–1274.

50. **Abeler VM, Vergote IB, Kjorstad KE, et al.** Clear cell carcinoma of the endometrium. *Cancer.* 1996;78:1740–1747.

51. **Aquino-Parsons C, Lim P, Wong F, et al.** Papillary serous and clear cell carcinoma limited to endometrial curettings in FIGO stage Ia and Ib endometrial adenocarcinoma: Treatment implications. *Gynecol Oncol.* 1998;71:83–86.

52. **Abeler VM, Kjorstad KE.** Endometrial squamous cell carcinoma: Report of three cases and review of the literature. *Gynecol Oncol.* 1990;36:321–326.

53. **Geels YP, Pijnenborg JMA, van den Berg-van Erp SH, et al.** Endometrioid endometrial carcinoma with atrophic endometrium and poor prognosis. *Obstet Gynecol.* 2012;120:1124–1131.

54. **DiSaia PJ, Creasman WT, Boronow RC, et al.** Risk factors and recurrent patterns in stage I endometrial cancer. *Am J Obstet Gynecol.* 1985;151:1009–1015.

55. **Abeler VM, Kjorstad KE, Berle E.** Carcinoma of the endometrium in Norway: A histopathological and prognostic survey of a total population. *Int J Gynecol Cancer.* 1992;2:9–22.

56. **Watari H, Todo Y, Takeda M, et al.** Lymph-vascular space invasion and number of positive paraaortic node groups predict survival in node positive patients with endometrial cancer. *Gynecol Oncol.* 2005;96:651–657.

57. **Simpkins F, Papadia A, Kunos C, et al.** Patterns of recurrence in stage I endometrioid endometrial adenocarcinoma with lymphovascular space invasion. *Int J Gynecol Cancer.* 2013;23:98–103.

58. **Hanson MB, van Nagell JR Jr, Powell DE, et al.** The prognostic significance of lymph-vascular space invasion in stage I endometrial cancer. *Cancer.* 1985;55:1753–1757.

59. **Nofech-Mozes S, Ackerman I, Ghorab Z, et al.** Lymphovascular invasion is a significant predictor for distant recurrence in patients with early-stage endometrial endometrioid adenocarcinoma. *Am J Clin Pathol.* 2008;129:912–917.

60. **Guntupalli SR, Zighelboim I, Kizer NT, et al.** Lymphovascular space invasion is an independent risk factor for nodal disease and poor outcomes in endometrioid endometrial cancer. *Gynecol Oncol.* 2012;124:31–35.

61. **Watanabe Y, Satou T, Natai H, et al.** Evaluation of parametrial spread in endometrial carcinoma. *Obstet Gynecol.* 2010;116:1027–1034.

62. **Weinberg LE, Kunos CA, Zanotti KM.** Lymphovascular space invasion (LVSI) is an isolated poor prognostic factor for recurrence and survival among women with intermediate to high-risk early-stage endometrioid endometrial cancer. *Int J Gynecol Cancer.* 2013;23:1438–1445.

63. **Lurain JR.** The significance of positive peritoneal cytology in endometrial cancer. *Gynecol Oncol.* 1992;46:143–144.

64. **Milosevic MF, Dembo AJ, Thomas GM.** The clinical significance of malignant peritoneal cytology in stage I endometrial carcinoma. *Int J Gynecol Cancer.* 1992;2:225–235.

65. **Garg G, Gao F, Wright JD, et al.** Positive peritoneal cytology is an independent risk-factor in early stage endometrial cancer. *Gynecol Oncol.* 2013;128:77–82.

66. **Morrow CP, Bundy BN, Kurman RJ, et al.** Relationship between surgical-pathologic risk factors and outcome in clinical stage I and II carcinoma of the endometrium: A Gynecologic Oncology Group study. *Gynecol Oncol.* 1991;40:55–65.

67. **Havrilesky LJ, Cragan JM, Calingaert B, et al.** The prognostic significance of positive peritoneal cytology and adnexal/serosal metastasis in stage IIIA endometrial cancer. *Gynecol Oncol.* 2007;104:401–405.

68. **Saga Y, Imai M, Jobo T, et al.** Is peritoneal cytology a prognostic factor of endometrial cancer confined to the uterus? *Gynecol Oncol.* 2006;103:277–280.

69. **Kadar N, Homesley HD, Malfetano JH.** Positive peritoneal cytology is an adverse factor in endometrial carcinoma only if there is other evidence of extrauterine disease. *Gynecol Oncol.* 1992;46:145–149.

70. **Takeshima N, Nishida H, Tabata T, et al.** Positive peritoneal cytology in endometrial cancer: Enhancement of other prognostic indicators. *Gynecol Oncol.* 2001;82:470–473.

71. **Tebeu PM, Popowski Y, Verkooijen HM, et al.** Positive peritoneal cytology in early-stage endometrial cancer does not influence prognosis. *Br J Cancer.* 2004;91:720–724.

72. **Fadare O, Mariappan MR, Hileeto D, et al.** Upstaging based solely on positive peritoneal washings does not affect outcome in endometrial cancer. *Mod Pathol.* 2005;18:673–80.

73. **Hirai Y, Takeshima N, Kato T, et al.** Malignant potential of positive peritoneal cytology in endometrial cancer. *Obstet Gynecol.* 2001;97:725–728.

74. **Kasamatsu T, Onda T, Katsumata N, et al.** Prognostic significance of positive peritoneal cytology in endometrial carcinoma confined to the uterus. *Brit J Cancer.* 2003;88:245–250.

75. **Ehrlich CE, Young PCM, Stehman FB, et al.** Steroid receptors and clinical outcome in patients with adenocarcinoma of the endometrium. *Am J Obstet Gynecol.* 1988;158:796–807.

76. **Liao BS, Twiggs LB, Leung BS, et al.** Cytoplasmic estrogen and progesterone receptors as prognostic parameters in primary endometrial carcinoma. *Obstet Gynecol.* 1986;67:463–467.

77. **Creasman WT, Soper JT, McCarty KS Jr, et al.** Influence of cytoplasmic steroid receptor content on prognosis of early stage endometrial carcinoma. *Am J Obstet Gynecol.* 1985;151:922–932.

78. **Palmer DC, Muir IM, Alexander AI, et al.** The prognostic importance of steroid receptors in endometrial carcinoma. *Obstet Gynecol.* 1988;72:388–393.

79. **Geisinger KR, Homesley HD, Morgan TM, et al.** Endometrial adenocarcinoma: A multiparameter clinicopathologic analysis including DNA profile and the sex steroid hormone receptors. *Cancer.* 1986;58:1518–1525.

80. **Christopherson WM, Connelly PJ, Alberhasky RC.** Carcinoma of the endometrium. V. An analysis of prognosticators in patients with favorable subtypes and stage I disease. *Cancer.* 1983;51:1705–1709.

81. **Nielson AL, Thomsen HK, Nyholm HCJ.** Evaluation of the reproducibility of the revised 1988 International Federation of Gynecology and Obstetrics grading system of endometrial cancers with special emphasis on nuclear grading. *Cancer.* 1991;68:2303–2309.

82. **Schink JC, Lurain JR, Wallemark CB, et al.** Tumor size in endometrial cancer: A prognostic factor for lymph node metastasis. *Obstet Gynecol.* 1987;70:216–219.

83. **Yanazume S, Saito T, Eto T, et al.** Reassessment of the utility of frozen sections in endometrial cancer surgery using tumor diameter as an additional factor. *Am J Obstet Gynecol.* 2011;204:531.e1–e7.

84. **Al Hilli MM, Podratz KC, Dowdy SC, et al.** Risk-scoring system for individualized prediction of lymphatic dissemination in patients with endometrioid endometrial cancer. *Gynecol Oncol.* 2013;131:103–108.

85. **Larson DM, Berg R, Shaw G, et al.** Prognostic significance of DNA ploidy in endometrial cancer. *Gynecol Oncol.* 1999;74:356–360.

86. **Susini T, Amunni G, Molino C, et al.** Ten-year results of a prospective study on the prognostic role of ploidy in endometrial carcinoma. *Cancer.* 2007;109:882–890.

87. **Zaino RJ, Davis ATL, Ohlsson-Wilhelm BM, et al.** DNA content is an independent prognostic indicator in endometrial adenocarcinoma. *Int J Gynecol Pathol.* 1998;17:312–319.

88. **Athanassiadou P, Athanassiades P, Grapsa D, et al.** The prognostic value of *PTEN, p53,* and *beta-catenin* in endometrial carcinoma: A prospective immunocytochemical study. *Int J Gynecol Cancer.* 2007;17:697–704.

89. **Di Nezza LA, Misajon A, Zhang J, et al.** Presence of active gelatinases in endometrial carcinoma and correlation of matrix metalloproteinase expression with increasing tumor grade and invasion. *Cancer.* 2002;94:1466–1475.

90. **Sakuragi N, Ohkouchi T, Hareyama H, et al.** Bcl-2 expression and prognosis of patients with endometrial carcinoma. *Int J Cancer.* 1998;79:153–158.

91. **Salvesen H, Iversen OE, Akslen LA.** Prognostic significance of angiogenesis and Ki-67, *p53,* and p21 expression: A population-based endometrial carcinoma study. *J Clin Oncol.* 1999;17:1382–1390.

92. **Grigsby PW, Perez CA, Camel HM, et al.** Stage II carcinoma of the endometrium: Results of therapy and prognostic factors. *Int J Radiat Oncol Biol Phys.* 1985;11:1915–1923.

93. **Nahhas WA, Whitney CW, Stryker JA, et al.** Stage II endometrial carcinoma. *Gynecol Oncol.* 1980;10:303–311.

94. **Vellios F.** Endometrial hyperplasias, precursors of endometrial carcinoma. *Pathol Annu.* 1972;7:201–229.

95. **Kurman RJ, Kaminski PF, Norris HJ.** The behavior of endometrial hyperplasia: A long-term study of "untreated" hyperplasia in 170 patients. *Cancer.* 1985;56:403–412.

96. **Ferenczy A, Gelfand MM, Tzipris F.** The cytodynamics of endometrial hyperplasia and carcinoma: A review. *Ann Pathol.* 1983;3:189–201.

97. **Lacey JV Jr, Sherman ME, Rush BB, et al.** Absolute risk of endometrial carcinoma during 20-year follow-up among women with endometrial hyperplasia. *J Clin Oncol.* 2010;28:788–792.

98. **Zaino RJ, Kauderer J, Trimble CL, et al.** Reproducibility of the diagnosis of atypical hyperplasia. A GOG study. *Cancer.* 2006;106:804–811.

99. **Trimble CL, Kauderer J, Zaino R, et al.** Concurrent endometrial carcinoma in women with a biopsy diagnosis of atypical endometrial hyperplasia: A GOG study. *Cancer.* 2006;106:812–819.

100. **Silverberg SG, Mutter GL, Kurman RJ, et al.** Tumors of the uterine corpus: Epithelial tumors and related lesions. In: **Tavassoli FA, Stratton MR, eds.** *WHO Classification of Tumors: Pathology and Genetics of Tumors of the Breast and Female Genital Organs.* Lyon: IARC Press; 2003:221–232.

101. **Suh-Burgmann E, Hung YY, Armstrong MA.** Complex atypical endometrial hyperplasia. The risk of unrecognized adenocarcinoma and value of preoperative dilation and curettage. *Obstet Gynecol.* 2009;114:523–529.

102. **Robbe EJM, van Kuijk SMJ, de Boed EM, et al.** Predicting the coexistence of an endometrial adenocarcinoma in the presence of atypical complex hyperplasia. Immunohistochemical analysis of endometrial samples. *Int J Gynecol Cancer.* 2012;22:1264–1272.

103. **Buttini MJ, Jordan SJ, Webb PM.** The effect of the levonorgestrel releasing intrauterine system on endometrial hyperplasia: An Australian study and systematic review. *Aust N Z J Obstet Gynaecol.* 2009;49:316–322.

104. **Semere LG, Ko E, Johnson NR, et al.** Endometrial intraepithelial neoplasia clinical correlates and outcomes. *Obstet Gynecol.* 2011;118:21–28.

105. **Gunderson CC, Fader AN, Carson KA, et al.** Oncologic and reproductive outcomes with progestin therapy in women with endometrial hyperplasia and grade 1 adenocarcinoma: A systematic review. *Gynecol Oncol.* 2012;125:477–482.

106. **Marsden DE, Hacker NF.** The classification, diagnosis and management of endometrial hyperplasia. *Rev Gynecol Pract.* 2003;3:89–97.

107. **Trimble CL, Method M, Leitao M, et al.** Management of endometrial precancers. *Obstet Gynecol.* 2012;120:1160–1175.

108. **Walker JL, Piedmonte MR, Spirtos NM, et al.** Laparoscopy compared with laparotomy for comprehensive surgical staging of uterine cancer: A Gynecologic Oncology Group Study LAP2. *J Clin Oncol.* 2009;27:5331–5336.

109. **Maurits MJE, Bijen CB, Arts HJ, et al.** Safety of laparoscopy versus laparotomy in early-stage endometrial cancer: A randomised trial. *Lancet Oncol.* 2010;11:763–771.

110. **Janda M, Gebski V, Brand A, et al.** Quality of life after total laparoscopic hysterectomy versus total abdominal hysterectomy for stage 1 endometrial cancer (LACE): A randomized trial. *Lancet Oncol.* 2010;11:772–780.

111. **Fader AN, Seamon LG, Escobar PF, et al.** Minimally invasive surgery versus laparotomy in women with high grade endometrial cancer: A multisite study performed at high volume cancer centers. *Gynecol Oncol.* 2012;126:180–185.

112. **Zaino R, Whitney C, Brady MF, et al.** Simultaneously detected endometrial and ovarian carcinomas—a prospective clinicopathologic study of 74 cases: A Gynecologic Oncology Group study. *Gynecol Oncol.* 2001;83:355–362.

113. **Obermair A, Geramou M, Gücer F, et al.** Endometrial cancer: Accuracy of the finding of a well differentiated tumor at dilatation and curettage compared to the findings at subsequent hysterectomy. *Int J Gynecol Cancer.* 1999;9:383–386.

114. **Petersen RW, Quinlivan JA, Casper GR, et al.** Endometrial adenocarcinoma–presenting pathology is a poor guide to surgical management. *Aust N Z J Obstet Gynaecol.* 2000;40:191–194.

115. **Sato S, Itamochi H, Shimada M, et al.** Preoperative and intraoperative assessments of depth of myometrial invasion in endometrial cancer. *Int J Gynecol Cancer.* 2009;19:884–887.

116. **Fotiou S, Vlahos N, Kondi-Pafiti A, et al.** Intraoperative gross assessment of myometrial invasion and cervical involvement in endometrial cancer: Role of tumor grade and size. *Gynecol Oncol.* 2009;112:517–520.

117. **Ugaki H, Kimura T, Miyatake T, et al.** Intraoperative frozen section assessment of myometrial invasion and histology of endometrial cancer using the revised FIGO staging system. *Int J Gynecol Oncol.* 2011;21:1180–1184.

118. **Kumar S, Medeiros F, Dowdy SC, et al.** A prospective assessment of the reliability of frozen section to direct intraoperative decision making in endometrial cancer. *Gynecol Oncol.* 2012;127:525–531.

119. **Cade TJ, Quinn MA, McNally OM, et al.** Predictive value of magnetic resonance imaging in assessing myometrial invasion in endometrial cancer: Is radiological staging sufficient for planning conservative treatment? *Int J Gynecol Oncol.* 2010;20:1166–1169.

120. **Savelli L, Testa AC, Mabrouk M, et al.** A prospective blinded comparison of the accuracy of transvaginal sonography and frozen section in the assessment of myometrial invasion in endometrial cancer. *Gynecol Oncol.* 2012;124:549–552.

121. **Moore RG, Miller CM, Brown AK, et al.** Utility of tumor marker HE4 to predict depth of myometrial invasion in endometrioid adenocarcinoma of the uterus. *Int J Gynecol Cancer.* 2011;21:1185–1190.

122. **Boronow RC.** Endometrial cancer and lymph node sampling: Short on science and common sense, long on cost and hazard. *J Pelvic Surg.* 2001;7:187–190.

123. **Chan JK, Urban R, Cheung MK, et al.** Lymphadenectomy in endometrioid uterine cancer staging. How many nodes are enough? A study of 11,443 patients. *Cancer.* 2007;109:2454–2460.

124. **Lutman CV, Havrilesky LJ, Cragun JM, et al.** Pelvic lymph node count is an important prognostic variable for FIGO stage I and II endometrial carcinoma with high-risk histology. *Gynecol Oncol.* 2006;102:92–97.

125. **Chan JK, Cheung MK, Huh WK, et al.** Therapeutic role of lymph node resection in endometrioid corpus cancer. *Cancer.* 2006;107:1823–1830.

126. **Milan MR, Java J, Walker JL, et al.** Nodal metastasis risk in endometrioid endometrial cancer. *Obstet Gynecol.* 2012;119:286–292.

127. **Dowdy SC, Borah BJ, Bakkum JN, et al.** Prospective assessment of survival, morbidity, and cost associated with lymphadenectomy in low-risk endometrial cancer. *Gynecol Oncol.* 2012;127:5–10.

128. **Kwon JS, Mazgani M, Miller DM, et al.** The significance of surgical staging in intermediate-risk endometrial cancer. *Gynecol Oncol.* 2011;122:50–54.

129. **Mariani A, Dowdy SC, Cliby WA, et al.** Efficacy of systematic lymphadenectomy and adjuvant radiotherapy in node-positive endometrial cancer patients. *Gynecol Oncol.* 2006;10:200–208.

130. **Fujimoto T, Nanjyo H, Nakamura A, et al.** Paraaortic lymphadenectomy may improve disease-related survival in patients with multipositive pelvic lymph node stage IIIC endometrial cancer. *Gynecol Oncol.* 2007;107:253–259.

131. **Ryan M, Stainton C, Slaytor EK, et al.** Aetiology and prevalence of lower limb lymphoedema following treatment for gynaecological cancer. *Aust N Z J Obstet Gynaecol.* 2003;43:148–151.

132. **Nomura H, Aoki D, Suzuki N, et al.** Analysis of clinicopathologic factors predicting paraaortic lymph node metastasis in endometrial cancer. *Int J Gynecol Cancer.* 2006;16:799–804.

133. **Saygili U, Kavaz S, Altunyurt S, et al.** Omentectomy, peritoneal biopsy and appendectomy in patients with clinical stage I endometrial carcinoma. *Int J Gynecol Cancer.* 2001;11:471–474.

134. **Morton DL, Wen DR, Wong JH, et al.** Technical details of intraoperative lymphatic mapping for early stage melanoma. *Arch Surg.* 1992;127:392–399.

135. **Kang S, Yoo HJ, Hwang JH, et al.** Sentinel lymph node biopsy in endometrial cancer: A meta-analysis of 26 studies. *Gynecol Oncol.* 2011;123:522–527.

136. **Perrone AM, Casadio P, Formelli G, et al.** Cervical and hysteroscopic injection for identification of sentinel lymph nodes in endometrial cancer. *Gynecol Oncol.* 2008;111:62–67.

137. **Solima E, Martinelli F, Ditto A, et al.** Diagnostic accuracy of sentinel node in endometrial cancer by using hysteroscopic injection of radiolabeled tracer. *Gynecol Oncol.* 2012;126:419–423.

138. **Robova H, Charvat M, Strnad P, et al.** Lymphatic mapping in endometrial cancer. Comparison of hysteroscopic and subserosal injection and the distribution of sentinel nodes. *Int J Gynecol Cancer.* 2009;19:391–394.

139. **Kilgore LC, Partridge EE, Alvarez RD, et al.** Adenocarcinoma of the endometrium: Survival comparisons of patients with and without pelvic node sampling. *Gynecol Oncol.* 1995;56:29–33.

140. **ASTEC study group, Kitchener H, Swart AM, et al.** Efficacy of systematic pelvic lymphadenectomy in endometrial cancer (MRC ASTEC trial): A randomized study. *Lancet.* 2009;373:125–136.

141. **Benedetti Panici P, Stefano B, Maneschi F, et al.** Systematic pelvic lymphadenectomy vs no lymphadenectomy in early-stage endometrial carcinoma: Randomized clinical trial. *J Natl Cancer Inst.* 2008;100:1707–1716.

142. **Creasman WT, Mutch DE, Herzog TJ.** ASTEC lymphadenectomy and radiation therapy studies: Are conclusions valid? *Gynecol Oncol.* 2010;116:293–294.

143. **Naumann RW.** The role of lymphadenectomy in endometrial cancer: Was the ASTEC trial doomed by design and are we destined to repeat that mistake? *Gynecol Oncol.* 2012;126:5–11.

144. **Seamon LG, Fowler JM, Cohn DE.** Lymphadenectomy for endometrial cancer: The controversy. *Gynecol Oncol.* 2010;117:6–8.

145. **Todo Y, Kato H, Kaneuchi M, et al.** Survival effect of para-aortic lymphadenectomy in endometrial cancer (SEPAL study): A retrospective cohort study. *Lancet.* 2010;375:1165–1172.

146. **Susini T, Massi G, Amunni G, et al.** Vaginal hysterectomy and abdominal hysterectomy for treatment of endometrial cancer in the elderly. *Gynecol Oncol.* 2005;96:362–367.

147. **Kumar S, Shah JP, Bryant CS, et al.** Second neoplasms in survivors of endometrial cancer: Impact of radiation therapy. *Gynecol Oncol.* 2009;113:233–239.

148. **Ko EM, Funk MJ, Clark LH, et al.** Did GOG 99 and PORTEC 1 change clinical practice in the United States. *Gynecol Oncol.* 2013;129:12–17.

149. **Poulsen HK, Jacobsen M, Bertelsen K, et al.** Adjuvant radiation therapy is not necessary in the management of endometrial carcinoma stage I, low-risk cases. *Int J Gynecol Cancer.* 1996;6:38–43.

150. **Sorbe B, Nordstrom B, Maenpaa J, et al.** Intravaginal brachytherapy in FIGO stage I low-risk endometrial cancer: A controlled randomized study. *Int J Gynecol Cancer.* 2009;19:873–878.

151. **Bertelsen K, Ortoft G, Hansen ES.** Survival of Danish patients with endometrial cancer in the intermediate-risk group not given postoperative radiotherapy: The Danish endometrial cancer study (DEMCA). *Int J Gynecol Cancer.* 2011;21:1191–1199.

152. **Obermair A, Cheuk R, Pak SC, et al.** Disease-free survival after vaginal vault brachytherapy versus observation for patients with node-negative intermediate–risk endometrial cancer. *Gynecol Oncol.* 2008;110:280–285.

153. **Ackerman I, Malone S, Thomas G, et al.** Endometrial carcinoma: Relative effectiveness of adjuvant radiation vs therapy reserved for relapse. *Gynecol Oncol.* 1996;60:177–183.

154. **Huh WK, Straughn JM Jr, Mariani A, et al.** Salvage of isolated vaginal recurrences in women with surgical stage I endometrial cancer: A multi-institutional experience. *Int J Gynecol Cancer.* 2007;17:886–889.

155. **Lachance JA, Stukenborg GJ, Schneider BF, et al.** A cost-effective analysis of adjuvant therapies for the treatment of stage I endometrial adenocarcinoma. *Gynecol Oncol.* 2008;108:77–83.

156. **Nout RA, Smit VT, Putter H, et al.** Vaginal brachytherapy versus pelvic external beam radiotherapy for patients with endometrial cancer of high-intermediate risk (PORTEC-2): An open-label, non-inferiority, randomized trial. *Lancet.* 2010;375:816–823.

157. **Sorbe BG, Horvath G, Andersson H, et al.** External pelvic and vaginal irradiation versus vaginal irradiation alone as postoperative therapy in medium-risk endometrial carcinoma: A prospective, randomized study – quality-of-life analysis. *Int J Gynecol Cancer.* 2012;22:1281–1288.

158. **COSA-NZ-UK Endometrial Cancer Study Groups.** Pelvic lymphadenectomy in high-risk endometrial cancer. *Int J Gynecol Cancer.* 1996;6:102–107.

159. **Orr JW, Holimon JL, Orr PF.** Stage I corpus cancer: Is teletherapy necessary. *Am J Obstet Gynecol.* 1997;176:777–789.

160. **Mohan DS, Samuels MA, Selim MA, et al.** Long-term outcomes of therapeutic pelvic lymphadenectomy for stage I endometrial adenocarcinoma. *Gynecol Oncol.* 1998;70:165–171.

161. **Ng TY, Perrin LC, Nicklin JL, et al.** Local recurrence in high-risk node-negative stage I endometrial carcinoma treated with postoperative vaginal vault brachytherapy. *Gynecol Oncol.* 2000;79:490–494.

162. **Fanning J.** Long term survival of intermediate risk endometrial cancer (stage IG3, IC, II) treated with full lymphadenectomy and brachytherapy without teletherapy. *Gynecol Oncol.* 2001;82:371–374.

163. **Seago DP, Raman A, Lele S.** Potential benefit of lymphadenectomy for the treatment of node-negative locally advanced uterine cancers. *Gynecol Oncol.* 2001;83:282–285.

164. **Horowitz NS, Peters WA, Smith MR, et al.** Adjuvant high dose rate vaginal brachytherapy as treatment of stage I and II endometrial cancer. *Obstet Gynecol.* 2002;99:235–240.

165. **Jolly S, Vargas C, Kumar T, et al.** Vaginal brachytherapy alone: An alternative to adjuvant whole pelvis radiation for early stage endometrial cancer. *Gynecol Oncol.* 2005;97:887–892.

166. **Solhjem MC, Petersen IA, Haddock MG.** Vaginal brachytherapy alone is sufficient adjuvant treatment of surgical stage I endometrial cancer. *Int J Radiat Oncol Biol Phys.* 2005;62:1379–1384.

167. **Kumar VJ, Chia YN, Lim YK, et al.** Survival and disease relapse in surgical stage I endometrioid adenocarcinoma of the uterus after adjuvant vaginal vault brachytherapy. *Int J Gynecol Oncol.* 2010; 20:564–569.

168. **Creutzberg CL, van Putten WLJ, Koper PCM, et al.** Surgery and postoperative radiotherapy versus surgery alone for patients with stage I endometrial carcinoma: A multicenter randomized trial. Post Operative Radiation Therapy in Endometrial Carcinoma (PORTEC) Study Group. *Lancet.* 2000;355:1404–1411.

169. **Scholten AN, van Putten WLJ, Beerman H, et al.** Postoperative radiotherapy for stage I endometrial carcinoma: Long term outcome of the randomized PORTEC trial with central pathology review. *Int J Radiat Oncol Biol Phys.* 2005;63:834–838.

170. **Keys HM, Roberts JA, Brunetto VL, et al.** A phase III randomized trial of surgery with or without adjunctive external pelvic radiation therapy in intermediate risk endometrial adenocarcinoma: A Gynecologic Oncology Group study. *Gynecol Oncol.* 2004;92:744–751.

171. **Johnson N, Cornes P.** Survival and recurrent disease after postoperative radiotherapy for early endometrial cancer: Systematic review and meta-analysis. *Brit J Obstet Gynaecol.* 2007;114:1313–1320.

172. **Weiss MF, Connell PP, Waggoner S, et al.** External pelvic radiation therapy in stage IC endometrial carcinoma. *Obstet Gynecol.* 1999; 93:599–602.

173. **De Jong RA, Pras E, Boezen M, et al.** Less gastrointestinal toxicity after adjuvant radiotherapy on a small pelvic field compared to a standard pelvic field in patients with endometrial carcinoma. *Int J Gynecol Cancer.* 2012;22:1177–1186.

174. **Abu-Rustum NR, Gomez JD, Alektiar KM, et al.** The incidence of isolated paraaortic nodal metastasis in surgically staged endometrial cancer patients with negative pelvic lymph nodes. *Gynecol Oncol.* 2009;115:236–238.

175. **Chiang AJ, Yu KJ, Chao KC, et al.** The incidence of isolated paraaortic nodal metastasis in completely staged endometrial cancer patients. *Gynecol Oncol.* 2011;121:122–125.

176. **Abu-Rustum NR, Chi DS, Leitao M, et al.** What is the incidence of isolated paraaortic nodal recurrence in grade I endometrial carcinoma? *Gynecol Oncol.* 2008;111:46–48.

177. **McMeekin DS, Lashbrook D, Gold M, et al.** Nodal distribution and its significance in FIGO stage IIIC endometrial cancer. *Gynecol Oncol.* 2001;82:375–379.

178. **Todo Y, Suzuki Y, Azuma M, et al.** Ultrastaging of paraaortic lymph nodes in stage IIIC1 endometrial cancer: A preliminary report. *Gynecol Oncol.* 2012;127:532–537.

179. **Aalders JG, Thomas G.** Endometrial cancer—revisiting the importance of pelvic and paraaortic lymph nodes. *Gynecol Oncol.* 2007; 104:222–231.

180. **Klopp AH, Jhingran A, Ramondetta L, et al.** Node-positive adenocarcinoma of the endometrium: Outcome and patterns of recurrence with and without external beam irradiation. *Gynecol Oncol.* 2009;115:6–11.

181. **Sutton G, Axelrod JH, Bundy BN, et al.** Whole-abdominal radiotherapy in the adjuvant treatment of patients with stage III and IV endometrial cancer: A Gynecologic Oncology Group Study. *Gynecol Oncol.* 2005;97:755–763.

182. **Randall ME, Filiaci VL, Muss H, et al.** Randomized phase III trial of whole-abdominal irradiation versus doxorubicin and cisplatin chemotherapy in advanced endometrial carcinoma: A Gynecologic Oncology Group Study. *J Clin Oncol.* 2006;24:36–44.

183. **Alvarez Secord A, Havrilesky LJ, Bae-Jump V, et al.** The role of multimodality chemotherapy and radiation in women with advanced stage endometrial cancer. *Gynecol Oncol.* 2007;107:285–291.

184. **Dusenbery KE, Potish RA, Gold DG, et al.** Utility and limitations of abdominal radiotherapy in the management of endometrial carcinomas. *Gynecol Oncol.* 2005;96:635–642.

185. **Martinez AA, Weiner S, Podratz K, et al.** Improved outcome at 10 years for serous papillary/clear cell or high-risk endometrial cancer patients treated by adjuvant high-dose whole-abdominal pelvic irradiation. *Gynecol Oncol.* 2003;90:537–546.

186. **Hirsch M, Lilford RJ, Jarvis GJ.** Adjuvant progestogen therapy for the treatment of endometrial cancer: Review and meta-analysis of published, randomized controlled trials. *Eur J Obstet Gynecol Reprod Biol.* 1996;65:201–207.

187. **Vergote I, Kjorstad K, Abeler V, et al.** A randomized trial of adjuvant progestogen in early endometrial cancer. *Cancer.* 1989;64: 1011–1016.

188. **COSA-NZ-UK Endometrial Cancer Study Groups.** Adjuvant medroxyprogesterone acetate in high-risk endometrial cancer. *Int J Gynecol Cancer.* 1998;8:387–391.

189. **Thigpen T, Vance RB, Balducci L, et al.** Chemotherapy in the management of advanced or recurrent cervical and endometrial carcinoma. *Cancer.* 1981;48(2 supp l):658–665.

190. **Maggi R, Lissoni A, Spina F, et al.** Adjuvant chemotherapy vs radiotherapy in high-risk endometrial carcinoma: Results of a randomized trial. *Br J Cancer.* 2006;95:266–271.

191. **Sasumu N, Sagae S, Udagawa Y, et al.** Randomized phase III trial of pelvic radiotherapy versus cisplatin-based combined chemotherapy in patients with intermediate and high-risk endometrial cancer: A Japanese Gynecologic Oncology Group study. *Gynecol Oncol.* 2008;108:226–233.

192. **Hogberg T, Rosenberg P, Kristensen G, et al.** A randomized phase III study on adjuvant treatment with radiation (RT) ± chemotherapy (CT) in early-stage high-risk endometrial cancer (NSGO-EC-9501/EORTC 55991). *J Clin Oncol.* 2007;25(18 S): 5503.

193. **Hogberg T, Signorelli M, de Oliveira CF, et al.** Sequential adjuvant chemotherapy and radiotherapy in endometrial cancer-results from two randomised studies. *Eur J Cancer.* 2010;13: 2422–2431.

194. **Johnson N, Bryant A, Miles T, et al.** Adjuvant chemotherapy for endometrial cancer after hysterectomy. *Cochrane Database Syst Rev.* 2011;(10):CD003175.

195. **Miller D, Filiaci V, Fleming G, et al.** Late-breaking abstract 1: A randomized phase III noninferiority trial of first-line chemotherapy for metastatic or recurrent endometrial carcinoma: A Gynecologic Oncology Group study. *Gynecol Oncol.* 2012;125:771.

196. **Einstein MH, Frimer M, Kuo DY, et al.** Phase II trial of adjuvant pelvic radiation "sandwiched" between combination paclitaxel and carboplatin in women with uterine papillary serous carcinoma. *Gynecol Oncol.* 2012;124:21–25.

197. **Sartori E, Gadducci A, Landoni F, et al.** Clinical behavior of 203 stage II endometrial cancer cases: The impact of primary surgical approach and of adjuvant radiation therapy. *Int J Gynecol Cancer.* 2001;11:430–437.

198. **Cornelison TL, Trimble EL, Kosary CL.** SEER data, corpus uteri cancer: Treatment trends versus survival for FIGO stage II, 1988–1994. *Gynecol Oncol.* 1999;74:350–355.

199. **Cohn DE, Woeste EM, Cacchio S, et al.** Clinical and pathologic correlates in surgical stage II endometrial carcinoma. *Obstet Gynecol.* 2007;109:1062–1067.

200. **Havrilesky LJ, Secord AV, O'Malley DM, et al.** Multicenter analysis of recurrence and survival in stage IIIA endometrial cancer. *Gynecol Oncol.* 2009;114:279–283.

201. **Nicklin JL, Petersen RW.** Stage 3B adenocarcinoma of the endometrium: A clinicopathologic study. *Gynecol Oncol.* 2000;78:203–207.

202. **Aalders J, Abeler V, Kolstad P.** Stage IV endometrial carcinoma: A clinical and histopathological study of 83 patients. *Gynecol Oncol.* 1984;17:75–84.

203. **Bristow RE, Zerbe MJ, Rosenshein NB, et al.** Stage IVB endometrial carcinoma: The role of cytoreductive surgery and determinants of survival. *Gynecol Oncol.* 2000;78:85–91.

204. **Van Wijk FH, Huikeshoven FJ, Abdulkadir L, et al.** Stage III and IV endometrial cancer: A 20 year review of patients. *Int J Gynecol Cancer.* 2006;16:1648–1655.

205. **Gitsch G, Hanzal E, Jensen D, et al.** Endometrial cancer in premenopausal women 45 years and younger. *Obstet Gynecol.* 1995; 85:504–508.

206. **Williams MG, Bandera EV, Demissie K, et al.** Synchronous primary ovarian and endometrial cancers. *Obstet Gynecol.* 2009;113: 783–789.

207. **Halperin R, Zehavi S, Hadas E, et al.** Simultaneous carcinoma of the endometrium and ovary vs endometrial carcinoma with ovarian metastases: A clinical and immunohistochemical determination. *Int J Gynecol Cancer.* 2003;13:32–37.

208. **Broaddus RR, Lynch HT, Chen LM, et al.** Pathologic features of endometrial carcinoma associated with HNPCC: A comparison with sporadic endometrial carcinoma. *Cancer.* 2006;106:87–94.

209. **Farhi DC, Nosanchuk J, Silberberg SG.** Endometrial adenocarcinoma in women under 25 years of age. *Obstet Gynecol.* 1986;68:741–745.

210. **Gotlieb WH, Beiner ME, Shalmon B, et al.** Outcome of fertility-sparing treatment with *progestins* in young patients with endometrial cancer. *Obstet Gynecol.* 2003;102:718–725.

211. **Wang CB, Wang CJ, Huang HJ, et al.** Fertility-preserving treatment in young patients with endometrial adenocarcinoma. *Cancer.* 2002;94:2192–2198.

212. **Yamazawa K, Hirai M, Fujito A, et al.** Fertility-preserving treatment with *progestin* and pathological criteria to predict responses in young women with endometrial cancer. *Hum Reprod.* 2007;22: 1953–1958.

213. **Niwa K, Tagami K, Lian Z, et al.** Outcome of fertility-preserving treatment in young women with endometrial carcinomas. *BJOG.* 2005;112:317–320.

214. **Oda T, Yoshida M, Kimura M, et al.** Clinicopathologic study of uterine endometrial carcinoma in young women aged 40 years and younger. *Int J Gynecol Cancer.* 2005;15:657–662.

215. **Eftekhar Z, Izadi-Mood N, Yarandi F, et al.** Efficiency of megestrol acetate (Megace) in the treatment of patients with early endometrial adenocarcinoma: Our experiences with 21 patients. *Int J Gynecol Cancer.* 2009;19:249–252.

216. **Hahn HS, Yoon SG, Hong JS, et al.** Conservative treatment with progestin and pregnancy outcomes in endometrial cancer. *Int J Gynecol Cancer.* 2009;19:1068–1073.

217. **Royal College of Obstetricians and Gynaecologists.** Fertility sparing treatments in gynaecological oncology. Scientific Impact Paper No. 35, February 2013.

218. **Park JY, Lee SH, Seong SJ, et al.** Progestin re-treatment in patients with recurrent endometrial adenocarcinoma after successful fertility-sparing management using progestin. *Gynecol Oncol.* 2013;129: 7–11.

219. **Gallos ID, Shehmar M, Thangaratinam S, et al.** Oral progestogens vs levonorgestrel-releasing intrauterine system for endometrial hyperplasia: A systematic review and meta-analysis. *Am J Obstet Gynecol.* 2010;203:547.e1–e10.

220. **Dhar KK, NeedhiRajan T, Koslowski M, et al.** Is levonorgestrel intrauterine system effective for treatment of early endometrial cancer? Report of four cases and review of the literature. *Gynecol Oncol.* 2005;97:924–927.

221. **Choi MC, Jung SG, Park H, et al.** Fertility preservation via photodynamic therapy in young patients with early-stage uterine endometrial cancer. A long-term follow-up study. *Int J Gynecol Cancer.* 2013;23:698–704.

222. **Walsh C, Holschneider C, Hoang Y, et al.** Coexisting ovarian malignancy in young women with endometrial cancer. *Obstet Gynecol.* 2005;106:693–699.

223. **Richter CE, Qian B, Martel M, et al.** Ovarian preservation and staging in reproductive-age endometrial cancer patients. *Gynecol Oncol.* 2009;114:99–104.

224. **Lee TS, Kim JW, Kim TJ, et al.** Ovarian preservation during the surgical treatment of early stage endometrial cancer: A nation-wide study conducted by the Korean Gynecologic Oncology Group. *Gynecol Oncol.* 2009;115:26–31.

225. **Lee TS, Lee JY, Kim JW, et al.** Outcomes of ovarian preservation in a cohort of premenopausal women with early-stage endometrial cancer: A Korean Gynecologic Oncology Group study. *Gynecol Oncol.* 2013;131:289–293.

226. **Modesitt SC.** Missed opportunities for primary endometrial cancer prevention: How to optimize early identification and treatment of high-risk women. *Obstet Gynecol.* 2012;120:989–991.

227. **Zauber NP, Denehy TR, Taylor RR, et al.** Microsatellite instability and DNA methylation of endometrial tumors and clinical features in young women compared with older women. *Int J Gynecol Cancer.* 2010;20:1549–1556.

228. **Resnick K, Straughn JM Jr, Backes F, et al.** Lynch syndrome screening strategies among newly diagnosed endometrial cancer patients. *Obstet Gynecol.* 2009;114:530–536.

229. **Win AK, Lindor NM, Winship I, et al.** Risks of colorectal and other cancers after endometrial cancer for women with Lynch syndrome. *J Natl Cancer Inst.* 2013;105:274–279.

230. **Valle RF, Baggish MS.** Endometrial carcinoma after endometrial ablation: High-risk factors predicting its occurrence. *Am J Obstet Gynecol.* 1998;179:569–572.

231. **Carrara L, Gadducci A, Landoni F, et al.** Could different follow-up modalities play a role in the diagnosis of asymptomatic endometrial cancer relapses: An Italian multicenter retrospective analysis. *Int J Gynecol Cancer.* 2012;22:1013–1019.

232. **Aalders J, Abeler V, Kolstad P.** Recurrent adenocarcinoma of the endometrium: A clinical and histopathological study of 379 patients. *Gynecol Oncol.* 1984;17:85–103.

233. **Kwon JS, Elit L, Saskin R, et al.** Secondary cancer prevention during follow-up for endometrial cancer. *Obstet Gynecol.* 2009;113: 790–795.

234. **Bristow RE, Purinton SC, Santillan A, et al.** Cost effectiveness of routine vaginal cytology for endometrial cancer surveillance. *Gynecol Oncol.* 2006;103:709–713.

235. **Salani R, Nagel CI, Drennen E, et al.** Recurrence patterns and surveillance for patients with early stage endometrial cancer. *Gynecol Oncol.* 2011;123:205–207.

236. **Kadkhodayan S, Shahriari S, Treglia G, et al.** Accuracy of 18-F FDG PET imaging in the follow-up of endometrial cancer patients: Systemic review and meta-analysis of the literature. *Gynecol Oncol.* 2013;128:397–404.

237. **Lin LL, Grigsby PW, Powell MA, et al.** Definitive radiotherapy in the management of isolated vaginal recurrences of endometrial cancer. *Int J Radiat Oncol Biol Phys.* 2005;63:500–504.

238. **Petignat P, Jolicoeur M, Alobaid A, et al.** Salvage treatment with high-dose-rate brachytherapy for isolated vaginal endometrial cancer recurrence. *Gynecol Oncol.* 2006;101:445–449.

239. **Khoury-Collado F, Einstein MH, Bochner BH, et al.** Pelvic exenteration with curative intent for recurrent uterine malignancies. *Gynecol Oncol.* 2012;124:42–47.

240. **Bristow RE, Santillan A, Zahurak ML, et al.** Salvage cytoreductive surgery for recurrent endometrial cancer. *Gynecol Oncol.* 2006;103:281–287.

241. **Awtrey CS, Cadungog MG, Leitao MM, et al.** Surgical resection of recurrent endometrial cancer. *Gynecol Oncol.* 2006;102:480–488.

242. **Thigpen JT, Brady MF, Alvarez RD, et al.** Oral medroxyprogesterone acetate in the treatment of advanced or recurrent endometrial carcinoma: A dose-response study by the Gynecologic Oncology Group. *J Clin Oncol.* 1999;17:1736–1744.

243. **Swenerton KD.** Treatment of advanced endometrial adenocarcinoma with tamoxifen. *Cancer Treat Rep.* 1980;64:805–811.

244. **Bonte J, Ide P, Billiet G, et al.** Tamoxifen as a possible chemotherapeutic agent in endometrial adenocarcinoma. *Gynecol Oncol.* 1981;11:140–161.

245. Moore TD, Phillips PH, Nerenstone SR, et al. Systemic treatment of advanced and recurrent endometrial carcinoma: Current status and future directions. *J Clin Oncol.* 1991;9:1071–1088.

246. Bellone S, Shah HR, Mc Kenney JK, et al. Recurrent endometrial carcinoma regression with the use of the aromatase inhibitor anastrozole. *Am J Obstet Gynecol.* 2008;199:e7–e10.

247. Thigpen JT, Buchsbaum HJ, Mangan C, et al. Phase II trial of Adriamycin in the treatment of advanced or recurrent endometrial carcinoma: A Gynecologic Oncology Group study. *Cancer Treat Rep.* 1979;63:21–27.

248. Thigpen T, Blessing J, Homesley H, et al. Phase III trial of doxorubicin ± cisplatin in advanced or recurrent endometrial carcinoma: A Gynecologic Oncology Group (GOG) Study. *Proc Am Soc Clin Onc.* 1993;12:261(abst).

249. Ball HG, Blessing JA, Lentz SS, et al. A phase II trial of Taxol in advanced or recurrent adenocarcinoma of the endometrium: A Gynecologic Oncology Group study. *Gynecol Oncol.* 1995;56:120(abst).

250. Lincoln S, Blessing JA, Lee RB, et al. Activity of paclitaxel as second-line chemotherapy in endometrial carcinoma: A Gynecologic Oncology Group study. *Gynecol Oncol.* 2003;88:277–281.

251. Miller DS, Blessing JA, Lentz SS, et al. A phase II trial of topotecan in patients with advanced, persistent, or recurrent endometrial carcinoma: A Gynecologic Oncology Group study. *Gynecol Oncol.* 2002;87:247–251.

252. Carey MS, Gawlik C, Fung-Kee-Fung M, et al.; Cancer Care Ontario Practice Guidelines Initiative Gynecology Cancer Disease Site Group. Systematic review of systemic therapy for advanced or recurrent endometrial cancer. *Gynecol Oncol.* 2006;101:158–167.

253. Humber CE, Tierney JF, Symonds RP, et al. Chemotherapy for advanced, recurrent or metastatic endometrial cancer: A systematic review of the Cochrane collaboration. *Ann Oncol.* 2007;18:409–420.

254. Fleming GF, Brunetto VL, Cella D, et al. Phase III trial of doxorubicin plus cisplatin with or without paclitaxel plus filgrastim in advanced endometrial carcinoma: A Gynecologic Oncology Group Study. *J Clin Oncol.* 2004;22:2159–2166.

255. Sorbe B, Andersson H, Boman K, et al. Treatment of primary advanced and recurrent endometrial carcinoma with a combination of carboplatin and paclitaxel—long-term follow-up. *Int J Gynecol Cancer.* 2008;18:803–808.

256. Hoskins PJ, Swenerton KD, Pike JA, et al. Paclitaxel and carboplatin alone or with irradiation, in advanced or recurrent endometrial cancer: A phase II study. *J Clin Oncol.* 2001;19:4048–4053.

257. Aghajanian C, Sill MW, Darcy KM, et al. Phase II trial of bevacizumab in recurrent or persistent endometrial cancer: A Gynecologic Oncology Group study. *J Clin Oncol.* 2011;29:2259–2265.

258. Oza AM, Elit L, Tsao MS, et al. Phase II study of temsirolimus in women with recurrent or metastatic endometrial cancer: A trial of the NCIC Clinical Trials Group. *J Clin Oncol.* 2011;29:3278–3285.

259. Alvarez EA, Brady WE, Walker JL, et al. Phase II trial of combination bevacizumab and temsirolimus in the treatment of recurrent or persistent endometrial carcinoma: A Gynecologic Oncology Group study. *Gynecol Oncol.* 2013;129:22–27.

260. Levenback C, Burke TW, Silva E, et al. Uterine papillary serous carcinoma (UPSC) treated with cisplatin, doxorubicin, and cyclophosphamide (PAC). *Gynecol Oncol.* 1992;46:317–321.

261. Rodriguez M, Abdul-Karim F, Nelson B, et al. *Platinum* based chemotherapy is an active compound in advanced and recurrent papillary serous carcinoma of the endometrium. *Gynecol Oncol.* 1998;68:135(abst).

262. Creasman WT, Henderson D, Hinshaw W, et al. Estrogen replacement therapy in the patient treated for endometrial cancer. *Obstet Gynecol.* 1986;67:326–330.

263. Ayhan A, Taskiran C, Simsek S, et al. Does immediate hormone replacement therapy affect the oncologic outcome in endometrial cancer survivors? *Int J Gynecol Cancer.* 2006;16:805–808.

264. Suriano KA, McHale M, McLaren CE, et al. Estrogen replacement therapy in endometrial cancer patients: A matched control study. *Obstet Gynecol.* 2001;97:555–560.

265. Major FJ, Blessing JA, Silverberg SG, et al. Prognostic factors in early-stage uterine sarcoma. *Cancer.* 1993;71:1702–1709.

266. DÁngelo E, Prat J. Uterine sarcomas: A review. *Gynecol Oncol.* 2010;116:131–139.

267. Brooks SE, Zhan M, Cote T, et al. Surveillance, Epidemiology and End Results analysis of 2677 cases of uterine sarcoma 1989–1999. *Gynecol Oncol.* 2004;93:204–208.

268. Kelly KLJ, Craighead PS. Characteristics and management of uterine sarcoma patients treated at the Tom Baker Cancer Center. *Int J Gynecol Cancer.* 2005;15:132–139.

269. Norris HJ, Taylor HB. Postirradiation sarcomas of the uterus. *Obstet Gynecol.* 1965;26:689–694.

270. Jaakkola S, Lyytinen HK, Pukkala E, et al. Use of estradiol-progestin therapy associates with increased risk for uterine sarcomas. *Gynecol Oncol.* 2011;122:260–263.

271. Zelmanowicz A, Hildesheim A, Sherman ME, et al. Evidence for a common etiology for endometrial carcinomas and malignant mixed müllerian tumors. *Gynecol Oncol.* 1998;69:253–257.

272. FIGO Committee on Gynecologic Oncology. FIGO staging for uterine sarcomas. *Int J Gynecol Obstet.* 2009;104:179.

273. Kapp DS, Shin JY, Chan JK. Prognostic factors and survival in 1396 patients with uterine leiomyosarcomas: Emphasis on impact of lymphadenectomy and oophorectomy. *Cancer.* 2008;112:820–830.

274. Stewart EA, Morton CC. The genetics of uterine leiomyonta: What clinicians need to know. *Obstet Gynecol.* 2006;107:917–921.

275. Leibsohn S, d'Ablaing G, Mishell DR Jr, et al. Leiomyosarcoma in a series of hysterectomies performed for presumed uterine leiomyomas. *Am J Obstet Gynecol.* 1990;162:968–974; discussion 974–976.

276. Dinh TV, Woodruff JD. Leiomyosarcoma of the uterus. *Am J Obstet Gynecol.* 1982;144:817–823.

277. Guntupalli SR, Ramirez PT, Anderson ML, et al. Uterine smooth muscle tumor of uncertain malignant potential. A retrospective analysis. *Gynecol Oncol.* 2009;113:324–326.

278. Norris HJ, Parmley T. Mesenchymal tumors of the uterus. V. Intravenous leiomyomatosis. A clinical and pathologic study of 14 cases. *Cancer.* 1975;36:2164–2178.

279. Goldberg MF, Hurt WG, Frable WJ. Leiomyomatosis peritonealis disseminata. Report of a case and review of the literature. *Obstet Gynecol.* 1977;49:46–52.

280. Wentling GK, Serin BU, Geiger XJ, et al. Benign metastasing leiomyoma responsive to megestrol: A case report and review of the literature. *Int J Gynecol Cancer.* 2005;15:1213–1217.

281. Giuntoli RL 2nd, Metzinger DS, DiMarco CS, et al. Retrospective review of 208 patients with leiomyosarcoma of the uterus: Prognostic indicators, surgical management, and adjuvant therapy. *Gynecol Oncol.* 2003;89:460–469.

282. DÁngelo E, Espinosa I, Ali R, et al. Uterine leiomyosarcomas: Tumor size, mitotic index, and biomarkers Ki67, and Bcl-2 identify two groups with different prognosis. *Gynecol Oncol.* 2011;121:328–333.

283. Park JY, Park SK, Kim DY, et al. The impact of tumor morcellation during surgery on the prognosis of patients with apparently early uterine leiomyosarcoma. *Gynecol Oncol.* 2011;122:255–259.

284. Perri T, Korach J, Sadetzki S, et al. Uterine leiomyosarcoma: Does the primary surgical procedure matter? *Int J Gynecol Cancer.* 2009;19:257–260.

285. Lissoni A, Cormio G, Bonazzi C, et al. Fertility-sparing surgery in uterine leiomyosarcoma. *Gynecol Oncol.* 1998;70:348–350.

286. Barakat R, Leitao M, Sonoda Y, et al. Incidence of lymph node and ovarian metastases in leiomyosarcoma of the uterus. *Gynecol Oncol.* 2003;91:209–212.

287. Wu TI, Chang TC, Hsueh S, et al. Prognostic factors and impact of adjuvant chemotherapy for uterine leiomyosarcoma. *Gynecol Oncol.* 2006;100:166–172.

288. **Giuntoli RL II, Garrett-Mayer E, Bristow RE, et al.** Secondary cytoreduction in the management of recurrent uterine leiomyosarcoma. *Gynecol Oncol.* 2007;106:82–88.

289. **Omura GA, Major FJ, Blessing JA, et al.** A randomized study of Adriamycin with and without dimethyl triazenoimidazole carboxamide in advanced uterine sarcomas. *Cancer.* 1983;52:626–632.

290. **Sutton GP, Blessing JA, Barrett RJ, et al.** Phase II trial of ifosfamide and mesna in leiomyosarcoma of the uterus: A Gynecologic Oncology Group study. *Am J Obstet Gynecol.* 1992;166:556–559.

291. **Thigpen JT, Blessing JA, Beecham J, et al.** Phase II trial of cisplatin as first-line chemotherapy in patients with advanced or recurrent uterine sarcomas: A Gynecologic Oncology Group study. *J Clin Oncol.* 1991;9:1962–1966.

292. **Sutton G, Blessing JA, Ball H.** Phase II trial of paclitaxel in leiomyosarcoma of the uterus: A Gynecologic Oncology Group study. *Gynecol Oncol.* 1999;74:346–349.

293. **Nordal RR, Thoresen SO.** Uterine sarcomas in Norway 1956–1992: Incidence, survival and mortality. *Eur J Cancer.* 1997;33:907–911.

294. **Hensley ML, Ishill N, Soslow R, et al.** Adjuvant gemcitabine plus docetaxel for completely resected stages I-IV high grade uterine leiomyosarcoma: Results of a prospective study. *Gynecol Oncol.* 2009;112:563–567.

295. **Hensley ML, Wathen JK, Maki RG, et al.** Adjuvant therapy for high-grade, uterus-limited leiomyosarcoma: Results of a phase 2 trial (SARC 005). *Cancer.* 2013;119:1555–1561.

296. **Hensley ML, Blessing JA, Mannel R, et al.** Fixed-dose rate gemcitabine plus docetaxel as first-line therapy for metastatic uterine leiomyosarcoma: A Gynecologic Oncology Group (GOG) phase II trial. *Gynecol Oncol.* 2008;109:329–334.

297. **Hensley ML, Blessing JA, DeGeest K, et al.** Fixed-dose rate gemcitabine and docetaxel as second-line therapy for metastatic uterine leiomyosarcoma: A Gynecologic Oncology Group Phase II study. *Gynecol Oncol.* 2008;109:323–328.

298. **Knocke TH, Kucera H, Dotfler D, et al.** Results of post-operative radiotherapy in the treatment of sarcoma of the corpus uteri. *Cancer.* 1998;83:1972–1979.

299. **Mahdavi A, Monk BJ, Ragazzo J, et al.** Pelvic radiation improves local control after hysterectomy for uterine leiomyosarcoma. A 20-year experience. *Int J Gynecol Cancer.* 2009;19:1080–1084.

300. **Reed NS, Mangioni C, Malmström H, et al.** A phase III randomized study to evaluate the role of adjuvant pelvic radiotherapy in the treatment of uterine sarcomas stages I and II: An European Organization for Research and Treatment of Cancer, Gynaecological Cancer Group Study. *Eur J Cancer.* 2008;44:808–818.

301. **Garg G, Shah JP, Liu JR, et al.** Validation of tumor size as staging variable in the revised International Federation of Gynecology and Obstetrics stage I leiomyosarcoma: A population-based study. *Int J Gynecol Cancer.* 2010;20:1201–1206.

302. **Rauh-Hain JA, Oduyebo T, Diver EJ, et al.** Uterine leiomyosarcoma: An updated series. *Int J Gynecol Cancer.* 2013;23:1036–1043.

303. **Tavassoli FA, Devilee P, eds.** *World Health Organization Classification of Tumors. Pathology and Genetics of Tumors of the Breast and Female Organs.* Lyon: IARC Press; 2003.

304. **DeFusco PA, Gaffey TA, Malkasian GD Jr, et al.** Endometrial stromal sarcoma: Review of Mayo Clinic experience, 1945–1980. *Gynecol Oncol.* 1989;35:8–14.

305. **Chang KL, Crabtree GS, Lim-Tan SK, et al.** Primary uterine endometrial stromal neoplasms. *Am J Surg Pathol.* 1990;14:415–438.

306. **Blank SV, Mikuta JJ.** Low grade stromal sarcoma: Confusion and clarification. *Postgraduate Obstet Gynecol.* 2001;21:1–4.

307. **Dos Santos LA, Garg K, Diaz JP, et al.** Incidence of lymph node and adnexal metastasis in endometrial stromal sarcoma. *Gynecol Oncol.* 2011;121:319–322.

308. **Shah JP, Bryant CS, Kumar S, et al.** Lymphadenectomy and ovarian preservation in low-grade endometrial sarcoma. *Obstet Gynecol.* 2008;112:1102–1108.

309. **Feng W, Hua K, Malpica A, et al.** Stages I and II WHO 2003-defined low-grade endometrial stromal sarcoma: How much primary therapy is needed and how little is enough? *Int J Gynecol Cancer.* 2013;23:488–493.

310. **Signorelli M, Fruscio R, Dell'Anna T, et al.** Lymphadenectomy in uterine low-grade endometrial stromal sarcoma. An analysis of 19 cases and a literature review. *Int J Gynecol Cancer.* 2010;20:1363–1366.

311. **Li AJ, Giuntoli RL 2nd, Drake R, et al.** Ovarian preservation in stage I low-grade endometrial stromal sarcomas. *Obstet Gynecol.* 2005;106:1304–1308.

312. **Chu MC, Mor G, Lim C, et al.** Low grade endometrial stromal sarcoma: Hormonal aspects. *Gynecol Oncol.* 2003;90:170–176.

313. **Pink D, Linder T, Mrozek A, et al.** Harm or benefit of hormonal treatment in metastatic low-grade endometrial stromal sarcoma. Simple center experience with 10 cases and review of the literature. *Gynecol Oncol.* 2006;101:464–469.

314. **Tanner EJ, Garg K, Leitao MM Jr, et al.** High grade undifferentiated uterine sarcoma: Surgery, treatment and survival outcomes. *Gynecol Oncol.* 2012;127:27–31.

315. **Li N, Wu LY, Zhang HT, et al.** Treatment options in stage I endometrial stromal sarcoma: A retrospective analysis of 53 cases. *Gynecol Oncol.* 2008;108:306–311.

316. **Schilder JM, Hurd WW, Roth LM, et al.** Hormonal therapy of an endometrioid stromal nodule followed by local excision. *Obstet Gynecol.* 1999;93:805–807.

317. **Clement PB, Scully RE.** Mullerian adenosarcoma of the uterus. A clinicopathologic analysis of 10 cases of a distinctive type of mullerian mixed tumor. *Cancer.* 1974;34:1138–1149.

318. **Abeler VM, Royne O, Thoresen S, et al.** Uterine sarcomas in Norway. A histopathological and prognostic survey of a total population from 1970 to 2000 including 419 patients. *Histopathology.* 2009;54:355–364.

319. **McCluggage WG.** Mullerian adenosarcoma of the female genital tract. *Adv Anat Pathol.* 2010;17:122–129.

320. **Arend R, Bagaria M, Lewin SN, et al.** Long-term outcome and natural history of uterine adenosarcomas. *Gynecol Oncol.* 2010;119:305–308.

321. **McCluggage WG.** Malignant biphasic uterine tumors: Carcinosarcomas or metaplastic carcinoma? *J Clin Pathol.* 2002;55:321–325.

322. **McCluggage WG.** Uterine carcinosarcomas (malignant mixed müllerian tumors) are metaplastic carcinomas. *Int J Gynecol Cancer.* 2002;12:687–690.

323. **Reynolds EA, Logani S, Moller K, et al.** Embryonal rhabdomyosarcoma of the uterus in a post menopausal woman. Case report and review of the literature. *Gynecol Oncol.* 2006;103:736–739.

324. **Yamada SD, Burger RA, Brewster WR, et al.** Pathologic variables and adjuvant therapy as predictors of recurrence and survival for patients with surgically evaluated carcinosarcoma of the uterus. *Cancer.* 2000;88:2782–2786.

325. **Tanner EJ, Leitao MM, Garg K, et al.** The role of cytoreductive surgery for newly diagnosed advanced-stage uterine carcinosarcomas. *Gynecol Oncol.* 2011;123:548–552.

326. **Sutton G, Blessing JA, Rosenshein N, et al.** Phase II trial of ifosfamide and mesna in mixed mesodermal tumors of the uterus (a Gynecologic Oncology Group study). *Am J Obstet Gynecol.* 1989;161:309–312.

327. **Sutton G, Brunetto VL, Kilgore L, et al.** A phase III trial of ifosphamide with or without cisplatin in carcinosarcoma of the uterus: A Gynecologic Oncology Group study. *Gynecol Oncol.* 2000;79:147–153.

328. **Curtin JP, Blessing JA, Soper JT, et al.** Paclitaxel in the treatment of carcinosarcoma of the uterus: A Gynecologic Oncology Group study. *Gynecol Oncol.* 2001;83:268–270.

329. **Homesley HD, Filiaci V, Markman M, et al.** Phase III trial of ifosfamide with or without paclitaxel in advanced uterine carcinosarcoma: A Gynecologic Oncology Group study. *J Clin Oncol.* 2007;25:526–531.

330. **Hoskins PL, Le N, Ellard S, et al.** Carboplatin plus paclitaxel for advanced or recurrent uterine malignant mixed mullerian tumors. The British Columbia Cancer Agency experience. *Gynecol Oncol.* 2008;108:58–62.

331. **Lacour RA, Eusher E, Atkinson EN, et al.** A phase II trial of paclitaxel and carboplatin in women with advanced or recurrent uterine carcinosarcoma. *Int J Gynecol Cancer.* 2011;21:517–522.

332. **Sutton G, Kauderer J, Carson LF, et al.** Adjuvant ifosphamide and cisplatin in patients with completely resected stage I or II carcinosarcomas (mixed mesodermal tumors) of the uterus: A Gynecology Oncology Group study. *Gynecol Oncol.* 2005;96:630–634.

333. **Wolfson AH, Brady MF, Rocereto T, et al.** A Gynecologic Oncology Group randomized phase III trial of whole-abdominal irradiation (WAI) vs cisplatin-ifosfamide and mesna (CIM) as post-surgical therapy in stage I–IV carcinosarcoma (CS) of the uterus. *Gynecol Oncol.* 2007;107:177–185.

334. **Einstein MH, Klobocista M, Hou JY, et al.** Phase II trial of adjuvant pelvic radiation "sandwiched" between ifosfamide or ifosfamide plus cisplatin in women with uterine carcinosarcoma. *Gynecol Oncol.* 2012;124:26–30.

335. **Molpus KL, Redlin-Frazier S, Reed G, et al.** Postoperative pelvic irradiation in early stage uterine mixed müllerian tumors. *Eur J Gynecol Oncol.* 1998;19:541–546.

336. **Sartori E, Bazzorini L, Gadducci A, et al.** Carcinosarcoma of the uterus: A clinicopathological multicenter CTF study. *Gynecol Oncol.* 1997;67:70–75.

337. **Callister M, Ramondetta LM, Jhingran A, et al.** Malignant mixed müllerian tumors of the uterus: Analysis of patterns of failure, prognostic factors and treatment outcomes. *Int J Radiat Oncol Biol Phys.* 2004;58:786–796.

338. **Manolitsas TP, Wain GV, Williams KE, et al.** Multimodality therapy for patients with clinical stage I and II malignant mixed müllerian tumors of the uterus. *Cancer.* 2001;91:1437–1443.

10 Ovarian Cancer–Tumor Markers and Screening

Aleksandra Gentry-Maharaj
Ian Jacobs
Usha Menon

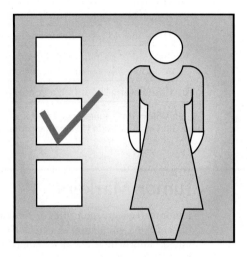

Worldwide, 6,044,000 women are diagnosed with cancer and 3,345,000 die from the disease each year (1). From 1975–2010, the age-standardized incidence rates for cancers in women have increased by 42% (2). The increase has been 6% in women versus 2% in men between 1999 and 2010 (2,3). Gynecologic malignancies account for 12% of these cancers (3,4), with most of this increase occurring in the postmenopausal population.

One of the accepted strategies for combating cancer in the twenty-first century is screening of the asymptomatic population for premalignant conditions and early-stage disease. **Such screening strategies are based on criteria laid down by the World Health Organization (WHO)** (5) (Table 10.1). **Mass screening for cervical cancer fulfills most of these tenets** and organized screening programs in numerous countries have led to a significant reduction in cervical cancer mortality (6). Success is dependent on a number of factors in addition to the effectiveness of the strategy. It includes a recognized need, clear objectives, well-defined target population, detailed screening and management protocols, appropriate infrastructure, quality assurance, and ongoing program evaluation.

Population screening is being investigated for ovarian cancer (7). The disease is usually diagnosed in advanced stages when chances for long-term survival are poor. Effective treatment is available for early-stage disease and there is preliminary evidence from an earlier randomized controlled trial (RCT) that ovarian cancer screening may increase survival (8). Encouraging results have been reported from a single arm ultrasound study using ultrasound, which showed an increased 5-year survival in women who participated in the study compared to women from the same institution who did not (9). However, data from the ovarian arm of the Prostate Lung Colorectal and Ovarian (PLCO) Cancer Screening RCT has shown no impact of screening (using CA125 >35 kU/L and transvaginal scan [TVS]) on mortality from the disease (10). Data from the largest RCT, the United Kingdom Collaborative Trial of Ovarian Cancer Screening (UKC-TOCS), are expected in 2015 (11,12). Encouraging sensitivity, specificity, and positive predictive value (PPV) has been reported in the latter trial for the multimodal strategy, which uses CA125 interpreted using the Risk of Ovarian Cancer (ROC) algorithm (12).

Table 10.1 World Health Organization Criteria for a Screening Program
1. The condition sought should be an important health problem.
2. There should be accepted treatment for patients with recognized disease.
3. Facilities for diagnosis and treatment should be available.
4. There should be a recognizable latent or early symptomatic stage.
5. There should be a suitable test or examination.
6. The test should be acceptable to the population.
7. The natural history of the condition, including development from latent to declared disease, should be adequately understood.
8. There should be an agreed policy on whom to screen.
9. The cost of case finding (including diagnosis and treatment of patients diagnosed) should be economically balanced in relation to possible expenditure on medical care as a whole.
10. Case finding should be a continuing process and not a "once and for all" project.

From **Wilson JMG, Jungner G**. *Principles and practice of screening for disease*. WHO Public Health Paper no. 34. Geneva: World Health Organization, 1968.

Tumor Markers

Tumor markers are molecules or substances produced by or in response to neoplastic proliferation that enter the circulation in detectable amounts. They indicate the likely presence of cancer, or provide information about its behavior. In the context of screening **the value of the marker depends heavily on its sensitivity (proportion of cancers detected by a positive test) and specificity (proportion of those without cancer identified by a negative test)**. An ideal tumor marker would have a 100% sensitivity, specificity, and positive predictive value (PPV). In practice, this is never achieved. **The most limiting factor is *lack of specificity*** because the majority of markers are tumor-associated rather than tumor-specific and are elevated in multiple cancers as well as in benign and physiologic conditions. In most diseases, tumor markers are not diagnostic, but contribute to the differential diagnosis. They may also have an important role to play in screening, determining therapeutic efficacy, detecting recurrence, and predicting prognosis.

A wide variety of macromolecular tumor antigens—including enzymes, hormones, receptors, growth factors, biologic response modifiers, and glycoconjugates—have been investigated as potential tumor markers. Innovative techniques such as mass-spectrometry and next generation sequencing are constantly identifying novel biomarkers that could complement those previously identified by candidate gene or antibody-based techniques.

The number of clinically useful markers is limited, despite significant research and the discovery of a large number of markers. Poor study design leading to inconsistent conclusions has been cited as an important reason (13,14). These design problems relate to all three phases of biomarker discovery and validation; preanalytical (selection of cases and controls, sample processing, and storage), analytical (detection limits and precision of assays), and postanalytical (overfitting and data interpretation to yield "the next promising" marker) (14).

General guidelines on the application and use of tumor markers have been developed by a number of multidisciplinary groups following critical appraisal of available evidence (15–19). **The National Cancer Institute's Early Detection Research Network has suggested five phases for biomarker development: Preclinical exploration, clinical assays and validation, retrospective longitudinal repository studies, prospective screening studies, and clinical randomized trials** for assessing end points of cancer screening. Guidelines covering methodologic issues related to measurement and internal and external quality control have been published. However, systematic reviews such as those conducted by Cochrane Collaboration are lacking in relation to tumor markers. Use of clinical sample sets to identify early detection markers adds further bias. To address this, the use of the PRoBE (prospective-specimen collection, with retrospective-blinded evaluation) design for biomarker discovery and validation has been recommended (20). This approach involves blinded case-control studies nested within a prospective cohort that represents the target population, with biologic specimens and clinical data being collected prior to ascertainment of outcome such as ovarian cancer diagnosis on follow-up.

A variety of imaging modalities have also been explored to identify morphologic character-istics of cancer. In gynecology, real-time ultrasound is most commonly used because it has mini-mal side effects and provides detailed tumor morphology, which can be quantified using a variety of scoring systems. **Detailed characterization of morphology on transvaginal scanning remains an important component of ovarian cancer screening. However as our understanding of the natural history of high-grade serous cancer improves, it is likely that higher resolution imag-ing modalities will be increasingly important.**

Neovascularization associated with malignancy is another marker that has been exploited in screening. Color-flow Doppler to detect altered patterns of blood flow and decreased resistance in the thin-walled new vessels in ovarian cancers has not been successful, but emerging strategies such as targeted microbubbles or autofluorescence, which have been successful in cervical and oral cancer screening, may play a role in ovarian cancer screening in the future.

An important aspect of screening is defining the risk groups. The target population for sporadic ovarian cancer is defined by age (50 years and older) in clinical trials, and for familial ovarian malignancy by family history criteria and the presence of *BRCA1* or *BRCA2* mutations. In the last decade, there has been significant progress in better defining risk based on mutations in moderate risk genes such as *RAD51,* and on alterations in the more common low penetrance genes, together with lifestyle and reproductive factors.

Ovarian and Fallopian Tube Cancer

Ovarian cancer accounts for 4% of cancers occurring in women, with more than 190,000 new cases diagnosed worldwide each year. Incidence rates are highest in the United States and North-ern Europe, and lowest in Africa and Asia, with ovarian cancer accounting for most of the gyne-cologic cancer mortality in the developed world. **Women without a significant family history or known gene mutations have a 1–2% lifetime risk of developing the disease.** Approximately 85% of cases occur after age 50, and 80–85% of cancers are epithelial in origin. High-grade serous tumors are the most common, present at an advanced stage, and have the poorest outcome (21).

Our ability to screen for the disease has been hampered by our lack of knowledge of the molecular and biologic events in ovarian cancer. This has limited the goal of screening to detection of asymp-tomatic, early-stage disease in the absence of a known **precursor lesion** (7). However, this has changed dramatically with descriptive molecular pathology and experimental evidence suggesting that a significant proportion of high-grade serous cancers start as premalignant serous tubal intraepithelial carcinoma (STIC) lesions in the fimbrial end of the fallopian tube (22,23). This has opened up the exploration of novel techniques and biospecimens for detecting these early lesions. While it is likely that detecting these lesions will significantly impact future screening strategies, current evidence does not support screening. **Although the US ovarian cancer screening trial demonstrated no mortality benefit of screening with CA125 cut-off and transvaginal ultra-sound (TVS) (10), the US Preventive Services Task Force is still awaiting the final results of the UK trial (12), which is using an algorithm-based approach (11).**

Biochemical Markers

CA125

CA125 is a 200-kilodalton (kd) glycoprotein recognized by the OC125 murine monoclonal antibody and first described by Bast et al. (24) in 1981. On cloning, it was found to have characteristics of mucin designated as MUC16 (25). It carries two major antigenic domains, clas-sified as A, the domain binding monoclonal antibody OC125; and B, the domain binding mono-clonal antibody M11 (26). The first CA125 immunoassay used the OC125 antibody for both capture and detection (27,28). **The second-generation heterologous CA125 II assay incorpo-rated M11 and OC125 antibodies and is widely used for measuring CA125.** There are a number of CA125 assays available, most of which correlate well with each other and are clinically reliable (29). However, differences in reagent specificities and assay design can lead to variation in the values obtained, and the results may not be interchangeable. **Changes in methodology may require baseline samples to be retested or parallel tested using both assays** (29,30).

This is of particular importance for patients who are undergoing serial monitoring, such as in screening trials.

CA125 is not specific to ovarian cancer and is widely distributed in adult tissues. It is found in structures derived from the coelomic epithelium (such as endocervix, endometrium, and fallopian tube) and in tissues developed from mesothelial cells (such as pleura, pericardium, and peritoneum) (31). It is expressed in the normal adult ovary (32), and has been characterized in epithelial tissues of the colon, pancreas, lung, kidney, prostate, breast, stomach, and gall bladder (27,28).

CA125 levels in body fluids or ovarian cysts do not correlate well with serum levels. Serum concentration is a function of antigen production by the tumor and of other factors that affect its release into the circulation (33,34). The widely adopted cutoff value of 35 kU/L is based upon the distribution of values in healthy subjects, where 99% of 888 men and women were found to have levels below 35 kU/L (35). However, CA125 values can show wide variation, and are influenced by age, race, menstrual cycle, pregnancy, hysterectomy, and a number of benign conditions. In postmenopausal women, CA125 levels tend to be lower than in the general population, and levels below 20 kU/L have been found (36–39). Levels fluctuate during the menstrual cycle and increase during menstruation (27,40). Levels in white women have been found to be higher than in African or Asian women (41). Caffeine intake, hysterectomy, and smoking in some (41) but not all reports (42,43) have been found to be associated with lower levels of CA125 (41).

A number of benign gynecologic conditions such as endometriosis, fibroids, infections, and pelvic inflammatory disease may increase CA125 levels. In pregnancy, peak CA125 values occur in the first trimester and postpartum (27,44–46), with wide fluctuations in levels as high as 300 kU/L being reported at these times; levels return to normal by 10 weeks postpartum (45). Levels of 112 kU/L and 65 kU/L have been found to correspond to the ninety-ninth percentile and the ninety-sixth percentile in the first trimester, respectively (47,48) but ideally different levels need to be defined for different stages of pregnancy and puerperium (49). CA125 may also be elevated by nongynecologic diseases causing any inflammation of the peritoneum, pleura or pericardium, pancreatitis, hepatitis, cirrhosis, ascites, tuberculosis, and other malignancies such as pancreatic, breast, colon, and lung cancer (27,33). The benign and physiologic conditions associated with an elevated CA125 can cause false-positive results when CA125 is used in diagnosis or screening.

Approximately 85% of patients with epithelial ovarian cancer have CA125 levels of greater than 35 kU/L (35,50), with elevated levels found in 50% of patients with stage I disease and more than 90% of patients with stage II to IV disease (27). CA125 levels are less frequently elevated in mucinous and borderline tumors compared to serous tumors (27,51,52). CA125 can be elevated in the preclinical asymptomatic phase of the disease, because raised levels have been found in 25% of 59 stored serum samples collected 5 years before the diagnosis of ovarian cancer (37).

In a prospective ovarian cancer screening study of Swedish women, a specificity of 97% and PPV of 4.6% were achieved using CA125 (30 kU/L) in 4,290 volunteers aged 50 years and older (53). Data from the Shizuoka Cohort Study on Ovarian Cancer Screening (SCSOCS) found that the interval between the first detection of a slightly elevated CA125 level and the diagnosis of disease at surgery was significantly shorter in patients with serous-type ovarian cancer, compared with those with nonserous-type disease (1.4 vs. 3.8 years, $p = 0.011$) (54). Although 47% of nonserous-type ovarian cancers developed in the setting of elevated CA125 levels between 35 and 65 kU/L, 75% of serous ovarian cancers developed when the CA125 levels were normal (<35 kU/L) (54).

In postmenopausal women, an elevated CA125 in the absence of ovarian cancer has been found to be a risk factor for death from other malignant disease (55,56). These findings have implications when screening asymptomatic postmenopausal women.

Improving Sensitivity, Specificity, and Discriminatory Ability

Pelvic Ultrasound as a Second-Line Test

The specificity of screening with CA125 was initially improved by the addition of pelvic ultrasound as a second-line test to assess ovarian volume and morphology. Using multimodal screening incorporating sequential CA125 measurements and pelvic ultrasound, a specificity of 99.9% and PPV of 26.8% for detection of ovarian and fallopian tube cancer were achieved in an RCT of 22,000 postmenopausal women (57,58). With the accumulation of data, ovarian morphology has been used to refine algorithms for the interpretation of ultrasound in postmenopausal women with elevated CA125 levels (59,60). In UKCTOCS, the addition of TVS in the multimodal arm has shown similarly encouraging results (12).

Time-series Algorithms

Developing a more sophisticated approach to replace absolute cutoff levels for the interpretation of CA125 levels has been a key step in strategy development. Detailed analysis of more than 50,000 serum CA125 levels involving 22,000 volunteers followed for a median of 8.6 years in the study by Jacobs et al. (8,58) revealed that **elevated CA125 levels in women without ovarian cancer were static or decreased with time, whereas levels associated with malignancy tended to rise. This finding has been incorporated into a computerized algorithm that uses an individual's age-specific incidence of ovarian cancer and CA125 profile to estimate her Risk of Ovarian Cancer (ROC)** (61–63). The closer the CA125 profile to the CA125 behavior of known cases of ovarian cancer, the greater the ROC. The final result is presented as the individual's estimated risk of having ovarian cancer with a ROC of 2% implying a risk of 1 in 50. **The ROC algorithm increases the sensitivity of CA125 compared with a single cutoff value, because women with normal but rising levels are identified as being at increased risk. At the same time, specificity is improved because women with static but elevated levels are classified as low risk. Based on the risk categories** (low-, intermediate-, and elevated-risk) women can be triaged to repeat CA125 alone, or CA125 and TVS. An abnormal TVS, or a high (1 in 5) risk based on CA125 levels leads to gynecologic assessment with a view to surgery. For a target specificity of 98%, the ROC calculation achieved a sensitivity of 86% for preclinical detection of ovarian cancer (61).

This approach first showed encouraging performance characteristics when evaluated prospectively in a pilot RCT in the mid-1990s (64). On prevalence screening in the ongoing UKCTOCS (12,65), the ROC has achieved encouragingly high sensitivity (89%), specificity (99%), and PPV (40%) in the prevalence screening (12), which has persisted during incidence screening (66,67). Similarly high specificity and PPV were reported in a single arm ovarian cancer screening study of 4,051 postmenopausal US women who underwent up to 9 screens (68).

The ROC algorithm is being evaluated prospectively in pilot ovarian cancer screening trials in high-risk women under the auspices of the Cancer Genetics Network (CGN) (69) and Gynecology Oncology Group (GOG) (70) in the United States, and in the United Kingdom Familial Ovarian Cancer Screening Study (UKFOCSS) (71). Preliminary data from UKFOCSS (Phase II) where women have been screened 4-monthly have indicated high (67–100%) sensitivity for ovarian and tubal cancer. There were no interval cancers diagnosed, and the only cancers not detected on screening were occult cancers picked up at risk reducing surgery. Although only 42% of incident screen-detected ovarian/fallopian tube cancers were Stages I and II, 92% were completely cytoreduced (71).

Preliminary data from UKCTOCS have indicated that serial CA125 monitoring using the ROC algorithm is able to detect ovarian cancer at tumor sizes that are too small to be detected by transvaginal ultrasound. Independent retrospective data from the PLCO trial suggest that CA125 velocity in the women with cancer (19.749 kU/L/month) is more than 500 times that (0.035 kU/L/month) of those who do not have cancer, indicating that CA125 velocity and time-series algorithms are significant predictors of ovarian cancer (72).

The **parametric empirical Bayes (PEB) longitudinal screening algorithm** has been described. When evaluated in the PLCO samples, it was found to detect ovarian cancer earlier than the single threshold rule (73). The recent focus has been on developing algorithms incorporating multiple markers. Serial sample sets from trial biobanks such as PLCO and UKCTOCS are crucial to this effort.

Other Markers

Accurate discrimination between benign and malignant masses is essential to avoid unnecessary operations in women with benign lesions, and to plan suitable surgery by appropriately trained gynecologic oncologists in tertiary care centers for those with cancer (74–76). Both prospective and retrospective data show that CA125 can be used as an adjunct in distinguishing benign from malignant masses, particularly in postmenopausal women (77–80). Using an upper limit of 35 kU/L, a sensitivity of 78%, specificity of 95%, and PPV of 82% can be achieved for ovarian cancer. The addition of human epididymis protein 4 (HE4) may add to this in premenopausal women, because it is elevated in ovarian cancer and less frequently elevated in benign conditions, especially endometriosis, which is commonly found in younger women (81). It is commercially available as **Risk of Ovarian Malignancy Algorithm (ROMA),** a test that combines HE4, CA125 II, and menopausal status. A systematic review by Ferraro et al. (82) looking at the performance of HE4 and CA125 in identification of ovarian cancer in women with suspected gynecologic disease has concluded that HE4 is superior to CA125. In addition, HE4 may improve sensitivity (83). Immunohistochemical data suggest that both HE4 and mesothelin may be discriminatory in CA125-negative cancers (84). Analysis of a panel of nine markers—CA125, SMRP, HE4, CA72–4, activin, inhibin, osteopontin, epidermal growth factor, and ERBB2 (HER2)—found that the addition of HE4 to CA125 without the use of ultrasound increased sensitivity to 76.4% at a specificity of 90% and 81% at a specificity of 90% (85).

The option of using a combination or panel of markers rather than a single biomarker to improve screening performance has been explored. Of the many hundreds of serum markers that have been investigated, only a few have been validated for clinical use (86–89). Limited sensitivities and specificities further constrain their use for screening purposes. The majority of studies trying to identify markers complementary to CA125 have focused on clinical sample sets that were collected from symptomatic patients at the time of diagnosis, and controls recruited in hospital settings. They are therefore not representative of the population undergoing screening. Over the past few years, preclinical samples have become increasingly available from the biobanks of the large screening trials. Nested case-control studies within the PLCO cohort using the PRoBE design (20) have reported that within 6 months of diagnosis, serum CA125 remained the single-best biomarker for ovarian cancer (sensitivity of 86%, 95% CI 0.76 to 0.97) with HE4 the second best, with a sensitivity of 73% (95% CI 0.60 to 0.86).

The repeated validation of CA125 as the best single biomarker for ovarian cancer has led to efforts to further characterize CA125 in order to improve the performance characteristics. A cancer-specific glycoform of CA125 (O-glycosylated CA125) has been able to discriminate between invasive and benign ovarian neoplasms in women with CA125 elevations in the range of 30 to 500 kilounit/L, with a specificity of 60% at a sensitivity of 90% (90).

Modeling has been undertaken to define the requirements of a screening test that would be able to detect the tumor earlier than is currently possible. A model, which incorporates ovarian tumor growth and CA125 shedding data, has suggested that **a tumor may grow unnoticed for over 10.1 years and reach a volume of 25 mm^3 before becoming detectable by current blood assays**. The specificity and detection limit of biomarker assays would need to improve 100-fold in order to enable detection within this first decade of tumor growth (91). Brown and Palmer (92) reached similar conclusions using published data from occult serous cancers found following prophylactic salpingo-oophorectomy in BRCA mutation carriers. They showed that serous cancers spend, on average, greater than 4 years *in situ,* stage I or II, and possibly a further 1 year as stage III or IV, before they present clinically. **The tumors are less than 1 cm during this occult period, only increasing to 3 cm when they progress to stage III or IV** (93). An annual screen would need to detect tumors 1.3 cm in diameter to detect half the tumors in stage I and II, and tumors of 0.5 cm diameter to achieve a 50% reduction in serous ovarian cancer mortality. **The goal in detecting high-grade serous ovarian cancer may need to be in detection of low volume rather than early-stage disease.**

New High-Throughput Approaches

Proteomics is the study of the expression, structure, and function of all proteins as a function of state, time, age, and environment (94). Although the initial euphoria related to ovarian cancer proteomic profiles and markers has been significantly moderated by a number of reports pointing out potential issues such as cross-platform reliability, reproducibility, sample processing, and analytical sensitivity of minute samples (95–99), significant progress has been made in the last decade in use of proteomic technologies to identify peptides or individual markers that relate to cancer risk (100,101). A combination of mass spectra generated by these new technologies and artificial intelligence–based informatic algorithms is being used to discover small sets of key protein markers that can discriminate normal from ovarian cancer patients (102) and can then be validated using more conventional assays. Recent refinements in these technologies have meant that fine mapping of a number of markers is feasible in a much shorter space of time (97,103). Advances in bioinformatics are leading to the development of sophisticated algorithms to analyze the large volume of preprocessed mass-spectrometric data and identify the most informative "common" peaks, but these approaches still need further refinement (96,98).

Recent studies using proteomic technology have confirmed that CA125 remains the best single marker for nonmucinous ovarian cancer, but 60 autoantibodies specific to ovarian cancer and independent of CA125 levels have also been discovered (104). Other identified proteomic markers such as C-reactive protein (105) are proteins and peptides that are produced as part of the host response to inflammation and are unlikely to be of clinical utility. It is likely that markers discovered through proteomic profiling will be important in the future. Well-designed, large prospective, multicenter clinical trials are required to validate and standardize this technology (99,106).

Metabolomics refers to the rapid, high-throughput characterization, and quantification of small-molecule metabolites, which are the end products of cellular regulatory processes. Preliminary data suggest that metabolomics is a promising automated approach, in addition to functional genomics and proteomics, for analyses of molecular changes in malignant tumors. In a preliminary study of 66 invasive ovarian carcinomas and 9 borderline ovarian tumors, a gas chromatography/time-of-flight mass spectrometry (GC-TOF MS) was able to detect 291 metabolites, of which 114 were already annotated compounds. A model built on these data could distinguish 88% of the borderline tumors from the carcinomas (107).

Epigenetic mechanisms have been shown to be extremely important in the initiation and progression of human cancer (108). Freely circulating hypermethylated tumor-derived DNA has been shown to be present in serum or plasma of patients with cancer (109,110). However, before the clinical utility of circulating epigenetic markers can be determined, a number of issues related to standardization of methodology, type of assay, reproducibility, efficacy, and comparison with other markers need to be addressed (111). In a clinical case-control series, a DNA methylation signature was found to distinguish patients from healthy controls (112). More promising, a multiplex methylation-specific PCR assay of seven candidate genes that analyzes the methylation status of cell-free serum DNA was shown to have superior sensitivity (85.3% vs. 56.1%) and specificity (90.5% vs. 64.15%) compared with CA125 alone in detecting early-stage ovarian cancer (113).

miRNAs are generally stable and can be detected in serum and plasma. Initial tissue based studies identified some miRNA that were upregulated and others that were downregulated when profiling ovarian cancers and normal ovaries (114–116). DNA released from dead cancer cells varies in size, whereas DNA released from nondiseased cells undergoing apoptosis is uniformly truncated (117). **Circulating tumor DNA may serve as a surrogate marker for active, fast-growing invasive tumors** (111). **Cell-free DNA has been suggested as a potential marker, as it reflects the release of both normal and tumor-derived DNA into the circulation through cellular necrosis and apoptosis.** In a study of 164 women with invasive epithelial ovarian carcinoma, 49 with benign ovarian neoplasms and 75 age-matched controls, elevated preoperative total plasma cell-free DNA levels were observed. Women with levels >22,000 GE/mL had decreased survival ($p < 0.001$), and a 2.83-fold increased risk of death from ovarian cancer ($p < .001$) (118).

Cancer Specific Biomarkers and Novel Biospecimens

Mutations in cancer-related genes *TP53, EGFR, BRAF* and *KRAS* are some of the early molecular genetic events in ovarian cancer. New technologies, such as BEAMing, are able to detect small amounts of mutant alleles in cell-free body fluids, which can be quantified with unprecedented sensitivity (119). Forshew et al. (120) recently identified mutations in *TP53* at allelic frequencies of 2–65%, in plasma from patients with advanced ovarian cancer who had high levels of circulating tumor DNA (ctDNA).

Kinde et al. (121) recently reported a sensitive massively parallel sequencing method to detect mutations in a panel of 12 genes. Applying this method to 14 liquid cytology cervical samples from women with ovarian cancer who had mutations, they were able to identify the expected tumor-specific mutations. **These results suggest that tumor DNA can be detected in a proportion of patients with ovarian cancer in a standard liquid-based cervical cytology specimen** (121). Salivary transcriptomes have also been evaluated as possible ovarian cancer markers (122).

Morphologic Markers

Real-time ultrasonic screening is aimed at detecting the earliest possible architectural changes in the ovary that accompany carcinogenesis. The transvaginal route is preferred because its better resolution leads to a more accurate assessment of ovarian and endometrial morphology, and it does not require a full bladder. However ultrasound has a subjective element (123), and therefore there is a need for accreditation and quality assurance in large multicentre screening. Encouragingly, postmenopausal women undergoing screening find TVS acceptable (124).

Both ovarian volume and morphology have been assessed, with cutoffs for volume ranging from 10–20 mL, depending on menopausal status (125). The persistence of abnormalities on repeat scanning 4 to 6 weeks after initial detection helps to reduce false-positive rates and increase PPV (126). Even when ovarian lesions appear to be complex, solid, or bilateral, many may resolve, as demonstrated by serial ultrasonography in the University of Kentucky Ovarian Cancer Screening Program (127). The lack of physiologic changes in ovarian volume in postmenopausal women further decreases the number of false positives in this group.

Even in older women, there is a high prevalence of benign ovarian lesions. In an ultrasonic and histopathologic autopsy study of 52 consecutive postmenopausal women who died from causes other than gynecologic or intraperitoneal cancer, 56% were found to have a histologically confirmed benign adnexal lesion of 50 mm in diameter (128). Ultrasonography used in this manner can therefore lead to the detection of many benign ovarian tumors, which results in unnecessary surgery in healthy, asymptomatic women.

As data accumulate with long-term follow-up of the participants of the early screening trials, it has been possible to further define the risk of ovarian cancer associated with various ultrasonic morphologic findings. **Unilocular ovarian cysts less than 10 cm in diameter are found in 18% of asymptomatic postmenopausal women aged over 50 years and are associated with an extremely low risk of malignancy** (129). In contrast, complex ovarian cysts with wall abnormalities or solid areas are associated with a significant risk of malignancy (126,129). Restricting the definition of abnormality to such complex ovarian morphology helps increase the specificity and PPV of ultrasonic screening (60).

To further decrease the number of false positives, some screening protocols use a weighted scoring system or morphologic index based on ovarian volume, outline, presence of papillary projections, and cyst complexity (i.e., number of locules, wall structure, thickness of septae, and echogenicity of fluid). There is no standardized index as yet (130–135). Others use subjective assessment of the gray-scale images. Based on gross anatomic changes at the time of surgery, papillary projections have the highest and simple cysts and septal thickness the lowest correlation with a diagnosis of ovarian malignancy (136). The University of Kentucky group has developed a serial morphologic index, which increased with time in the cancers, whereas it either decreased or remained stable in those with benign tumors, akin to the change in CA125 with time. The addition of this index in a serial-performing algorithm may increase specificity in screening by reducing the false positives (137). Newer modalities, such as pattern-recognition computer models and artificial neural networks (138–141), may increase the reproducibility of results and improve ultrasonic performance.

In the differential diagnosis of benign from malignant disease, a number of strategies have been explored to reduce the false-positive rate and facilitate discrimination between benign and malignant ovarian lesions. **Subjective evaluation using gray scale and Doppler (pattern recognition) by an experienced examiner has been reported to be better than mathematical logistic regression models** (141) **or CA125 alone** (142). In a systematic review of risk scores available to triage pelvic masses, the **Risk of Malignancy Index (RMI)** has been found to be the best predictor of malignancy and the model of choice (143). **The RMI combines serum CA125 values with ultrasound detected ovarian morphology and menopausal status** (144). The pooled sensitivity for an RMI cutoff of 200 was 78% at 87% specificity (143). Ultrasonic assessment for an **"ovarian crescent sign"** in women with an RMI above 200 has been shown to improve accuracy (145).

The sensitivity of RMI for early-stage disease is low when CA125 levels are normal and scan findings a poor discriminator. Nevertheless, in the premobile computing era, the ease of applying the RMI has gained widespread clinical use. The International Ovarian Tumor Analysis (IOTA) group reported a logistic regression model incorporating 12 variables, which was superior to CA125 alone (146,147) and equivalent to RMI even when the ultrasonic scanning was performed by operators with varied training (148). A systematic review looking at various imaging modalities has suggested that 3D ultrasonography has a higher sensitivity and specificity when compared to 2D ultrasonography, and **of the more sophisticated imaging modalities, magnetic resonance imaging performed the best** (149). Formal evidence of their effectiveness in reducing surgical intervention in screening trials is awaited.

Increasingly, conservative management is the norm for adnexal cysts judged to be benign at transvaginal ultrasonic examination when they are detected either incidentally (150) or in screening trials in postmenopausal women. Follow-up of such women in ongoing randomized screening trials will be important in validating such strategies.

Development of new imaging diagnostic approaches is expected to significantly advance detection of ovarian cancer. One such approach explores use of light-induced intrinsic tissue fluorescence or autofluorescence, which is lost in cancerous/precancerous epithelial tissue and has been successfully used in cervical and oral cancer screening. In a preliminary study using ex vivo reflectance and autofluorescent optical imaging of fallopian tubes removed at surgery, McAlpine et al. (151) demonstrated encouraging sensitivity (73–100%), specificity (83–92%), PPV (50–78%), and NPV (91–100%) for detection of STIC lesions. Its use in screening will require improvement of the predictive ability, and its incorporation into endoscopy to allow *in vivo* real-time imaging of the fallopian tube lumen. Other modalities being explored in mouse models include laparoscopic nonlinear microscopy (152).

Vascular Markers

Neovascularization is an obligate early event in tumor growth and neoplasia (153). Fast-growing tumors contain many new vessels that have less smooth muscle in their walls and therefore provide less resistance to blood flow when compared with vessels within benign ovarian tumors. **Color-flow Doppler imaging uses these altered blood-flow patterns as markers to differentiate malignant from physiologic and benign lesions.** It has been used as a first-line screening test in combination with transvaginal ultrasound (154,155) and as a second-line test following an abnormal ultrasound (156,157) in both general and high-risk population screening.

The early promise of Doppler to differentiate between malignant and benign ovarian masses and therefore improve the specificity of ultrasound (154,155) was not confirmed in subsequent studies (135,158,159). Although it was demonstrated that the mean pulsatility index of vessels supplying ovarian cancers was lower than that of vessels supplying benign ovarian tumors, the overlap in vascular resistance between these two groups prevented reliable separation of malignant from benign disease. It was thought that lack of blood flow in an ovarian tumor, as detected by color Doppler, may preclude cancer (159), but this was not substantiated, as 6% of ovarian tumors without blood flow were malignant in the Kentucky screening trial (135). Even when Doppler examinations were simplified and limited to the expression of internal color flow, gray-scale sonography was still a more sensitive indicator of malignancy than Doppler sonography (160). The effectiveness of a screening strategy that incorporates Doppler evaluation of ovarian masses in addition to gray-scale sonography is yet to be established. Although UKCTOCS is collecting Doppler data on abnormal adnexal masses detected on ultrasonic screening, these data are not part of the screening algorithm (12).

For differential diagnosis of women presenting with pelvic masses, color Doppler flow indices and tumor morphology, as assessed by gray-scale imaging, have been incorporated into a logistic regression model (146), which has been prospectively validated in a multicenter study (147). Pattern-recognition models using a combination of gray-scale and color Doppler ultrasound have been found to be better than CA125 alone in differential diagnosis (142). Some studies have shown that three-dimensional power Doppler examinations may be more accurate than two-dimensional Doppler examinations (161,162), although this remains controversial (163). Data have demonstrated the superior performance of color flow Doppler compared to 2D scanning to analyze blood flow to suspicious areas or masses (149).

Contrast-enhanced transvaginal ultrasound with microbubbles that are small enough to pass through capillaries can detect abnormal flow found in areas of neovascularization (164). The higher resolution of such techniques may allow detection of low-volume tumors in future screening strategies. A more powerful use of contrast-enhanced ultrasonic imaging is by targeting tumor angiogenesis at the molecular level. Ultrasonographic microbubbles may be targeted with one of several antibodies. As the tumors grow, there is a change in the relative uptake of each targeted microbubble, suggesting that such noninvasive molecular profiling of tumor angiogenesis could be useful as a diagnostic tool (165).

Target Populations

Two distinct populations are at increased risk for ovarian cancer: the general population and a high-risk population.

General Population

Most ovarian cancers are sporadic, and occur in the general population. More than 90% of sporadic cancers occur in women older than 50 years, so screening studies in the general population usually target this group. Some of the **other known risk factors** in the general population such **as oral contraceptive use, parity, and hysterectomy** have the potential for determining risk. Over the past few years, as a result of a massive international effort of **the Ovarian Cancer Association Consortium (OCAC), genome-wide association studies (GWAS) have identified eight susceptibility loci for serous epithelial ovarian cancer** (166–170). By themselves, these loci confer increased risk of magnitude less than 1.5-fold. However, a multiplicative effect of gene–gene and gene–environment interaction may allow better risk prediction (171), similar to the "polygenic" approach of combining multiple, low-penetrance susceptibility alleles to refine breast cancer risk stratification (172). The implementation of such a screening strategy will depend on organizational, ethical, legal, and social factors, in addition to usefulness and cost-effectiveness (173).

High-Risk Population

Hereditary syndromes account for approximately 5–10% of ovarian cancers. Female relatives of affected members from ovarian, breast, breast and ovarian, or Lynch syndrome (LS) families who have a greater than 10% lifetime risk of developing ovarian cancer are considered to be high risk. Much of this risk results from mutations arising in the *BRCA1, BRCA2,* and mismatch repair (*MMR*) genes. A recent meta-analysis has indicated that **the average cumulative risk by age 70 for ovarian cancer is 40% (35–46%) in *BRCA1* mutation carriers and 18% (13–23%) in *BRCA2* mutation carriers** (174). A genome-wide association study (GWAS) of BRCA1 carriers has identified **two novel ovarian cancer risk modifier loci, 17q21.31 and 4q32.3.** The first is associated with both *BRCA1* and *BRCA2,* while the latter has only a *BRCA1*-specific association. **The risk of ovarian cancer can now be recalculated based on these known ovarian cancer risk-modifying loci. It could be 28% or lower (in the 5% of *BRCA1* carriers at the lowest risk), or 63% or higher (in the 5% at the highest risk)** (175). These recent findings have important implications for risk prediction and clinical management for BRCA1 carriers. **MMR gene-mutation carriers have a lifetime risk of ovarian cancer of approximately 10–12%** (176).

Current Ovarian Cancer Screening Trials

Two distinct screening strategies have emerged, one based on ultrasound and the other on measurement of serum CA125, with ultrasound as the second-line test (multimodal screening) (12,68,125,177–188). Overall, the data from large prospective studies in the general population (Table 10.2) suggest that sequential multimodal screening has superior specificity and PPV. However, ultrasonography as a first-line test may offer greater sensitivity for early-stage disease.

Trials in the General Population

The RCTs in the general population aim to assess the impact of screening on ovarian cancer mortality. **In the UKCTOCS trial, 202,638 postmenopausal women aged 50 to 74 have been randomized in a 2:1:1 fashion to either control or annual screening with transvaginal ultrasound (ultrasound group) or CA125 interpreted using the ROC algorithm followed by TVS as a second-line test (multimodal group).** Apart from ovarian cancer mortality, the trial also addresses the issues of compliance, health economics, and the physical and psychological morbidity of screening. Both strategies have had encouraging sensitivity for primary invasive epithelial ovarian and fallopian tube cancers (89.5% and 75%, respectively) on the prevalence (initial) screen. The multimodal strategy had a significantly higher PPV (35.1% vs. 2.8%), resulting in lower rates of repeat testing and surgery, likely reflecting the higher detection rates of benign adnexal masses and borderline tumors in the ultrasound group (12). **The superior sensitivity (87.7% vs. 67.6%) and PPV (22.3% vs. 4.4%) of the multimodal compared to the ultrasound strategy was confirmed on incidence screening** (66,67). Screening in UKCTOCS was completed in December 2011, with the results of the mortality impact of screening awaited in 2015.

Multimodal screening is currently ongoing in the single-arm prospective study of 4,051 low-risk postmenopausal US women aged 50 and older in the MD Anderson study (68). During 11 years of screening, the ROC algorithm had picked up 4 of the 10 women with ovarian cancer, all of whom had "early-stage, high-grade" disease, with no interval cancers reported. This study has provided independent validation of the UK findings.

The PLCO Cancer Screening Trial enrolled 78,237 women aged 55 to 74 at 10 screening centers in the United States, with balanced randomization to intervention and control arms. The women underwent annual screening with both serum CA125 (interpreted using a 35 kU/L cutoff) and transvaginal ultrasound for 3 years followed by CA125 alone for a further 2 years. In the trial,

Table 10.2 Prospective Ovarian Cancer Screening Studies in the General Population

Study	Population	Screening Strategy	No. Screened	No. of Invasive Epithelial Ovarian Cancers Detected[a]	No. of Positive Screens	No. of Operations per Cancer Detected
CA125 Alone						
Einhorn et al. 1992 (53)	Age ≥40 yrs	Serum CA125	5,550	6 2 stage I	175[b]	29[b]
Multimodal Approach: CA125 (Level 1 Screen), then USS (Level 2 Screen)						
Menon et al. 2005 (64)	Age ≥50 yrs Postmenopausal	Serum CA125 ROCA, TVS if ROC ↑	6,532	3 (1) 2 stage I	16	3
Menon et al. 2009 (12)	Postmenopausal ≥50–74	Serum CA125 ROCA, TVS if ROC ↑	50,078	34 16 Stage I/II	97	3
Jacobs et al. 2012 (66)	Postmenopausal ≥50–74	Serum CA125 ROCA, TVS if ROC ↑	189,058 women screen-years	93 (includes borderline)	357	4
Jacobs et al. 1993 (57)	Age ≥45 yrs (median 56) Postmenopausal	Serum CA125 TAS, if CA125 ↑	22,000	11 4 stage I	41	3.7
Jacobs et al. 1999 (8)	Age ≥45 yrs (median 56) Postmenopausal	RCT Serum CA125 TAS/TVS, if CA125 ↑	10,958 3 annual screens	6 3 stage I	29	4.8
Grover et al. 1995 (184)	Age ≥40 yrs (median 51) or with family history (3%)	Serum CA125 TAS/TVS, if CA125 ↑	2,550	1 0 stage I	16	16
Adonakis et al. 1996 (180)	Age ≥45 yrs (mean 58)	Serum CA125 TVS, if CA125 ↑	2,000	1 (1) 1 stage I	15	15
USS-Only Approach: USS (Level 1 Screen), then Repeat USS (Level 2 Screen)						
De Priest et al. 1997 (182)	Age ≥50 yrs and postmenopausal or ≥30 with FH	TVS Annual screens Mean 4 screens per woman	6,470	6 5 stage I	90	18
Menon et al. 2009 (12)	Postmenopausal ≥50–74	TVS (annual) First scan	48,215	24 12 Stage I/II	845	35
Menon et al. 2012 (67)	Postmenopausal ≥50–74	TVS (annual) Incidence screening	176,659 women screen-years	72 (includes borderline)	769	11
van Nagell et al. 2000 (125) van Nagell et al. 2007 (177)	Postmenopausal >50 and >25 with FH of ovarian cancer	TVS (annual) CA125 and CDI if TVS persistent positive	14,469 25,312	11 (3) 1 PC 29 (10) 14 stage 1	180 364	16.3 12.5
Sato et al. 2000 (222)	Part of general screening program	TVS TVS + markers at level 2	51,550	22 17 stage I	324	14.7
Hayashi et al. 1999 (185)	Age ≥50 yrs	TVS	23,451	3 (3)	258	[c]

(Continued)

Table 10.2 Prospective Ovarian Cancer Screening Studies in the General Population (*Continued*)

Study	Population	Screening Strategy	No. Screened	No. of Invasive Epithelial Ovarian Cancers Detected[a]	No. of Positive Screens	No. of Operations per Cancer Detected
Tabor et al. 1994 (188)	Aged 46–65 yrs	TVS	435	0	9	—
Campbell et al. 1989 (181)	Age ≥45 yrs (mean 53) or with family history (4%)	TAS 3 screens at 18-monthly intervals	5,479	2 (3) 2 stage I	326	163
Millo et al. 1989 (187)	Age ≥45 yrs or postmenopausal (mean 54)	USS (mode not specified)	500	0	11	—
Goswamy et al. 1983 (183)	Age 39–78 Postmenopausal	TAS	1,084	1 1 stage I		
USS and CDI (Level 1 Screen)						
Kurjak et al. 1995 (186)	Aged 40–71 yrs (mean 45)	TVS and CDI	5,013	4 4 stage I	38	9.5
Vuento et al. 1995 (155)	Aged 56–61 yrs (mean 59)	TVS and CDI	1,364	(1)	5	—
USS (Level 1) and Other Tests (Level 2 Screen)						
Parkes et al. 1994 (157)	Aged 50–64 yrs	TVS then CDI if TVS positive	2,953	1 1 stage I	15[d]	15
Holbert et al. 1994 (223)	Postmenopausal aged 30–89 yrs	TVS then CA125 if TVS positive	478	1 1 stage I	33[e]	33
USS and CA125						
Buys et al. 2005 (178)	Postmenopausal aged 55–74 yrs	TVS and CA125 (annual)	28,816	18 (9) 2 stage 1 1 PC	1,706[b] (570: Surgery)	28.5
Kobayashi et al. 2007 (179)	Postmenopausal >50 yrs	TVS and CA125 (annual)	41,688	27	4,744[b] (305: Surgery)	11.3

[a]Primary invasive epithelial ovarian cancers. The borderline and granulosa tumors detected are shown in parentheses.

[b]Not all of these women underwent surgical investigation because the study design involved intensive surveillance rather than surgical intervention.

[c]Only 95 women consented to surgery, and there are no follow-up details on the remaining.

[d]86 women had abnormal USS before CDI.

[e]Only 11 of these women underwent surgery.

TVS, transvaginal ultrasound; ROC, risk of ovarian cancer; TAS, transabdominal ultrasound; RCT, randomized controlled trial; FH, family history; CDI, color Doppler imaging; USS, ultrasound; PC, peritoneal cancer; mos, months.

all positive screening tests and abnormal findings were evaluated and managed by the participants' physicians, with no prescribed study protocol (178). The results of the prevalence screen in 28,816 screened women reported 29 neoplasms, of which 20 were invasive and 9 borderline. Of all screened women, 4.7% had an abnormal scan and 1.4% an abnormal CA125. The PPV for invasive cancer was 3.7%, 1%, and 23.5% for abnormal CA125, TVS, and both CA125 and TVS, respectively (178). The trial has reported on the impact of screening on mortality. At a median follow-up of 12.4 years (25th–75th percentile 10.9 to 13), there were 118 and 100 deaths in the screening and control arm, respectively, with a mortality rate ratio of 1.18 (95% CI 0.91 to 1.54) (10). The validity of these findings has been questioned in view of the lengthy follow-up after end of screening, with 40.6% of the ovarian cancers being diagnosed after screening had been completed, and lack of a protocol driven screening and treatment (189). Crucially, a single threshold rule was used to interpret CA125. The trial reported a high (15%) complication rate in women undergoing surgery for false-positive findings (10). **Based on these findings, USPSTF reaffirmed their previous recommendation that screening for ovarian cancer should not be undertaken in the general population** (11). Despite this, a survey of US physicians showed that one in three physicians believed that ovarian cancer screening was effective and were likely to offer it to the women (190).

The Japanese Shizuoka Cohort Study of Ovarian Cancer Screening RCT, using an annual ultrasound and absolute CA125-based strategy in 82,487 low-risk postmenopausal women, did not find a statistically significant difference in the number of screen-detected ovarian cancers between the study ($n = 27$) **and the control arm** ($n = 32$). Eight additional interval cancers occurred in the screened arm. Early-stage disease (stage I) was more likely to be detected in the screened women (63%) compared to the control group (38%), although this did not reach statistical significance ($p = 0.2285$). Ovarian cancer detection rates of 0.31 per 1,000 at prevalent screen and 0.38 to 0.74 per 1,000 at subsequent screens were found (179). The mortality impact has not been reported as yet.

The only single-arm study of ovarian cancer screening, **the Kentucky Screening Study,** of 25,327 women has shown encouraging performance of an ultrasound-only strategy, with a larger proportion of cancers detected at an early stage (82%) (177). The study also reported significantly higher 5-year survival rates for women diagnosed with primary invasive epithelial ovarian cancer (screen positives and interval cancers) in the screening study (74.8% ± 6.6%) compared to women treated at the same institution during the same period who were not study participants (53.7% ± 2.3%) (mean follow-up of 5.8 years) (9). However the groups were not comparable, because of the "lead time effect" of screening. Furthermore, study participation would have been associated with a significant "healthy volunteer effect." In both PLCO and UKCTOCS, all-cause mortality in the control arm was less than half that expected as a result of a "healthy volunteer effect" (191,192).

Trials in a High-Risk Population

In women with strong evidence of a hereditary predisposition, screening from the age of 35 is frequently advocated. However the efficacy of such surveillance is yet to be determined. Data suggest that if undertaken, more frequent screening than annual is essential in this population (71). **Screening premenopausal women can be problematic because of the frequency of both physiologic (e.g., menstrual cycle variations) and benign (e.g., endometriosis, ovarian cysts) conditions that can give rise to false-positive abnormalities on both ultrasound and CA125.** Hence, criteria for the interpretation of the screening tests need to be more stringent than those for postmenopausal women in the general population.

To date, 26 studies have reported on screening for familial ovarian cancer (Table 10.3). Most studies have used a combination of absolute CA125 levels and ultrasound. Criteria for the interpretation of the test results vary, and screening protocols are not always clearly reported (69,125,193–200). In addition, **multifocal peritoneal cancer is probably a phenotypic variant of familial ovarian cancer** (195,201), **and neither CA125 nor ultrasound is reliable in detecting early-stage disease**.

Annual screening with CA125 using a cutoff and TVS **does not seem to be effective** (197,198). This has been confirmed by the results of Phase I (2002 to 2008) of the UKFOCSS, where 3,563 women underwent annual screening with serum CA125 and TVS. The study reported encouraging sensitivity for the detection of incident ovarian/fallopian tube cancers within a year of the last annual screen (81.3–87.5% depending on whether occult cancers were classified as interval cancers or true positives). Only 30.8% of the cancers detected by screening were Stage I and II. **Advanced-stage disease (stage IIIC and IV) was more likely in those that did not adhere to annual screening compared to those that did (85.7% vs. 26.1%; $p = 0.009$).**

Phase II of UKFOCSS and those undertaken under the auspices of the CGN (69) and GOG (70) **in the United States** have therefore adopted a more **frequent 3- to 4-month approach to screening using the ROC algorithm**. In all three trials, screening is now complete and the results are expected soon, with the scope for meta-analysis in the future. In the United States trials, screening is based on 3-monthly serum CA125 levels, which are interpreted using the ROC algorithm. In the United States-based CGN trial involving 2,343 high-risk women, 38 women underwent surgery following 6,284 screens. Five ovarian cancers were detected: two prevalent (one early, one late stage) and three incident (three early) cases, resulting in a PPV of 13%. Three further occult cancers were detected at risk-reducing salpingo-oophorectomy, and one woman developed an interval (late-stage) cancer (202). The preliminary results of Phase II of UKFOCSS (4-monthly serum CA125 interpreted using the ROC algorithm and annual TVS) have suggested that high (67–100%)

					No. of Invasive	

Table 10.3 Prospective Ovarian Cancer Screening Studies in Women with a Family History of Ovarian or Breast Cancer or a Personal History of Breast Cancer

Study	Population	Screening Protocol	No. Screened (Premenopausal %)	No. Referred for Diagnostic Tests[a] (%)	No. of Invasive EOC Detected (Borderline Tumors)	Cancers in Screen-Negative Women
Bourne et al. 1994 (193)	Aged >17 (mean 47) FH Ov cancer	TVS then CDI	1,502 (60)	62 (3.8)	4 (3) 2 stage I	2: PC (2–8 mos) 4: EOC (24–44 mos)
Weiner et al. 1993 (208)	PH Br cancer	TVS and CDI	600	12 (3)	3 1 stage I	Not stated
Muto et al. 1993 (209)	Aged >25 FH Ov cancer	TVS and CA125	384 (85.4)	15 (3.9)	0	Not stated
Schwartz et al. 1995 (210)	Aged. >30 FH Ov cancer	TVS and CDI and CA125	247	1 (0.4)	0	Not stated
Belinson et al. 1995 (211)	Aged >23 (mean 43) FH Ov cancer	TVS and CDI and CA125	137	2 (1.5)	1	Not stated
Menkiszak et al. 1998 (212)	Aged >20 FH Br, Ov cancer	TVS and CA125 (every 6 mos)	124	Not available	1 (3)	Not available
Karlan et al. 1993 (213) Karlan et al. 1999 (195)	Aged >35 FH Ov, Br, Endo, Colon cancer PH Br cancer	TVS and CDI and CA125 (every 6 mos until 1995, then annually)	597[b] (75) 1,261	10 (1.7) Not stated	0 (1) 1 EOC, 3 PC (2) 1 stage I	Not stated 4 PC (5, 6, 15, 16 mos)
Dorum et al. 1996 (214)	Aged >25 (mean 43)	TVS and CA125	180[b]	16 (8.9)	4 (3)[b]	2[c]
Dorum et al. 1999 (194)	Strict criteria for FH Br, Ov cancer		803	Not stated	16 (4)	Not stated
Van Nagell et al. 2000 (125)	FH Ov cancer	TVS and CDI and CA125	3,299	Not stated	3 EOC (1) 2 stage I	2 (12, 14 mos)
Scheuer et al. 2002 (215)	Aged >35 BRCA1, BRCA2 mutation carriers	TVS and CA125 (every 6 mos)	62	22 (35.5) 10 had surgery	5 4 EOC, 1 PC 3 stage I	0[d]
Laframboise et al. 2002 (216)	Age >22 (mean 47) Strict criteria for FH Br, Ov cancer	TVS and CA125 (every 6 mos)	311	9 (3)	1	Not stated
Liede et al. 2002 (217)	Mean age 47 Jewish FH Br, Ov cancer	TVS and CA125 (every 6 mos)	290	Not stated	1 EOC 2 PC 1 stage I	Not stated
Tailor et al. 2003 (199)	Age >17 (mean 47) FH Ov cancer	TVS and CDI	2,500 (65)	104 (3)	6 EOC (4) 4 stage I	2 PC (20–40 mos) 7 EOC (9–46 mos)

Table 10.3 Prospective Ovarian Cancer Screening Studies in Women with a Family History of Ovarian or Breast Cancer or a Personal History of Breast Cancer (*Continued*)

Study	Population	Screening Protocol	No. Screened (Premenopausal %)	No. Referred for Diagnostic Tests[a] (%)	No. of Invasive EOC Detected (Borderline Tumors)	Cancers in Screen-Negative Women
Fries et al. 2004 (218)	Age >28 (mean 53) FH Br, Ov cancer	TVS and CA125 (every 6 mos)	53	3 (6)	0	Not stated
Stirling et al. 2005 (198)	Strict criteria for FH Br, Ov cancer	TVS and CA125 (annually)	1,110	39 (4)	9 EOC (1) 2 stage I	3 (2, 4, 12 mos)
Vasen et al. 2005 (200)	*BRCA1, BRCA2* carriers, relatives	TVS and CA125 (annually)	138	Not stated	5	1 (11 mos)
Meeuwissen et al. 2005 (219)	Age >18 (mean 42) Strict criteria for FH Br, Ov cancer	TVS and CA125 (annually)	383	20 (5)	0	0
Oei et al. 2006 (220)	Age >20 (mean 40) Strict criteria for FH Br, Ov cancer	TVS and CA125 (annually)	512	24 (4.7)	1 EOC	0
Garenstrom et al. 2006 (196)	Age >27 (mean 45) Strict criteria for FH Br, Ov cancer	TVS and CA125 (annually)	269	26 (9.6)	3 EOC (1) 2 PC 1 stage I	2 (8, 10 mos)
Bosse et al. 2006 (221)	Median 40–45 Strict criteria for FH Br, Ov cancer 85 *BRCA* carriers	TVS and CA125 (every 6 mos)	676 (77)	10 (1.5)	1 EOC Stage I	0
Hermsen et al. 2007 (197)	>35 *BRCA1, BRCA2* mutation carriers	TVS and CA125 (annually)	888	25 (4)	10 EOC 1 stage II	5 (3–10 mos)
Skates et al. 2007 (202)	Strict criteria for FH Br, Ov cancer	TVS and CA125 (every 3 mos) ROC Algorithm	2,343	38	2 EOC (2) 1 PC 1 stage I	1
Rosenthal et al. 2013 (71)	Strict criteria for FH Ov cancer or *BRCA1, BRCA2* mutation carriers	TVS and CA125 (every 4 mos) ROC Algorithm	4,531	18	18 EOC 6 stage I	0

[a]Following positive secondary screens.

[b]Not included in total because there are more recent updates on the trial.

[c]Further 13 women underwent oophorectomy for breast cancer; two had ovarian cancer not detected by TVS.

[d]Two women who opted for oophorectomy with normal scans and CA125 had stage I ovarian cancer.

FH, family history; Ov, ovarian; TVS, transvaginal ultrasound; CDI, color Doppler imaging; EOC, epithelial ovarian cancer; PH, personal history; Br, breast; Endo, endometrial; ROC, risk of ovarian cancer; PC, peritoneal cancer; mos, months.

sensitivity for ovarian and fallopian tube cancer could be achieved using this strategy, with no interval cancers reported. Only 42% of incident screen-detected ovarian/fallopian tube cancers were Stage I and II. Most notably, 92% of the screen-detected cancers were completely cytoreduced compared to 62% on Phase I ($p = 0.16$) (71).

Women in the high-risk population who request screening should be counseled about the current lack of evidence for the efficacy of both CA125 and ultrasonic screening, and the associated false-positive rates. Some will still opt for screening. They should be counseled that **the recommendation in high-risk women is risk-reducing salpingo-oophorectomy after completion of their families** (203–205) **and that at present, screening cannot be considered an effective alternative** (71).

One of the established strategies for combating cancer in the twenty-first century is screening the asymptomatic population for premalignant conditions and early-stage disease. **The effectiveness of ovarian cancer screening in the general population using a cutoff to interpret CA125 has not shown a mortality benefit. The results of the UK trial using the time-series algorithm ROC algorithm to interpret CA125 are awaited. Screening outside the context of research trials is not recommended.**

References

1. **IARC.** Estimated Incidence, Mortality and Prevalence Worldwide in 2008;All Cancers (excluding non-melanoma skin cancer) 2008. Available from: http://globocan.iarc.fr/factsheet.asp, Accessed October 20, 2013

2. **CRUK.** Cancer incidence for all cancers combined 2013. Available from: http://www.cancerresearchuk.org/cancer-info/cancerstats/incidence/all-cancers-combined/, Accessed October 11, 2013

3. **CRUK.** Cancer incidence statistics 2013. Available from: http://www.cancerresearchuk.org/cancer-info/cancerstats/incidence/, Accessed October 11, 2013

4. **Siegel R, Ma J, Zou Z, et al.** Cancer statistics, 2014. *CA Cancer J Clin.* 2014;64:9–29.

5. **Wilson JMG, Jungner G.** Principles and practice of screening for disease. WHO Public Health Paper no. 34. Geneva: World Health Organization, 1968.

6. **Castle PE.** Gynecological cancer: More evidence supporting human papillomavirus testing. *Nat rev Clin Oncol.* 2012;9(3):131–132.

7. **Gentry-Maharaj A, Menon U.** Screening for ovarian cancer in the general population. *Best Pract Res Clin Obstet Gynaecol.* 2012;26(2): 243–256.

8. **Jacobs IJ, Skates SJ, MacDonald N, et al.** Screening for ovarian cancer: A pilot randomised controlled trial. *Lancet.* 1999;353(9160): 1207–1210.

9. **van Nagell JR, Jr., Miller RW, DeSimone CP, et al.** Long-term survival of women with epithelial ovarian cancer detected by ultrasonographic screening. *Obstet Gynecol.* 2011;118(6):1212–1221.

10. **Buys SS, Partridge E, Black A, et al.** Effect of screening on ovarian cancer mortality: The Prostate, Lung, Colorectal and Ovarian (PLCO) Cancer Screening Randomized Controlled Trial. *JAMA.* 2011; 305(22):2295–2303.

11. **Moyer VA; U.S. Preventive Services Task Force.** Screening for ovarian cancer: U.S. Preventive Services Task Force reaffirmation recommendation statement. *Ann Inter Med.* 2012;157(12):900–904.

12. **Menon U, Gentry-Maharaj A, Hallett R, et al.** Sensitivity and specificity of multimodal and ultrasound screening for ovarian cancer, and stage distribution of detected cancers: Results of the prevalence screen of the UK Collaborative Trial of Ovarian Cancer Screening (UKCTOCS). *Lancet Oncol.* 2009;10(4):327–340.

13. **Jacobs I, Menon U.** The sine qua non of discovering novel biomarkers for early detection of ovarian cancer: Carefully selected preclinical samples. *Cancer Prev Res (Phila).* 2011;4(3):299–302.

14. **Diamandis EP.** Cancer biomarkers: Can we turn recent failures into success? *J Nat Cancer Inst.* 2010;102(19):1462–1467.

15. **Duffy MJ, Bonfrer JM, Kulpa J, et al.** CA125 in ovarian cancer: European Group on Tumor Markers guidelines for clinical use. *Int J Gynecol Cancer.* 2005;15(5):679–691.

16. **Sturgeon C.** Practice guidelines for tumor marker use in the clinic. *Clin Chem.* 2002;48(8):1151–1159.

17. **Aebi S, Castiglione M, Group EGW.** Epithelial ovarian carcinoma: ESMO clinical recommendations for diagnosis, treatment and follow-up. *Ann Oncol.* 2008;19(suppl 2):ii14–ii16.

18. **Duffy MJ.** Evidence for the clinical use of tumour markers. *Ann Clin Biochem.* 2004;41(Pt 5):370–375.

19. **Sturgeon CM, Lai LC, Duffy MJ.** Serum tumour markers: How to order and interpret them. *BMJ.* 2009;339:b3527.

20. **Pepe MS, Feng Z, Janes H, et al.** Pivotal evaluation of the accuracy of a biomarker used for classification or prediction: Standards for study design. *J Natl Cancer Inst.* 2008;100(20):1432–1438.

21. **Seidman JD, Horkayne-Szakaly I, Haiba M, et al.** The histologic type and stage distribution of ovarian carcinomas of surface epithelial origin. *Int J Gynecol Pathol.* 2004;23(1):41–44.

22. **Crum CP, Drapkin R, Miron A, et al.** The distal fallopian tube: A new model for pelvic serous carcinogenesis. *Curr Opin Obstet and Gynecol.* 2007;19(1):3–9.

23. **Crum CP, McKeon FD, Xian W.** The oviduct and ovarian cancer: Causality, clinical implications, and "targeted prevention". *Clin Obstet Gynecol.* 2012;55(1):24–35.

24. **Bast RC, Jr., Feeney M, Lazarus H, et al.** Reactivity of a monoclonal antibody with human ovarian carcinoma. *J Clin Invest.* 1981; 68(5):1331–1337.

25. **Yin BW, Lloyd KO.** Molecular cloning of the CA125 ovarian cancer antigen: Identification as a new mucin, MUC16. *J Biol Chem.* 2001; 276(29):27371–27375.

26. **Nustad K, Bast RC, Jr., Brien TJ, et al.** Specificity and affinity of 26 monoclonal antibodies against the CA 125 antigen: First report from the ISOBM TD-1 workshop. International Society for Oncodevelopmental Biology and Medicine. *Tumour Biol.* 1996;17(4): 196–219.

27. **Jacobs I, Bast RC, Jr.** The CA 125 tumour-associated antigen: A review of the literature. *Hum Reprod.* 1989;4(1):1–12.

28. **Bast RC, Jr., Xu FJ, Yu YH, et al.** CA 125: The past and the future. *Int J Biol Markers.* 1998;13(4):179–187.

29. **Davelaar EM, van Kamp GJ, Verstraeten RA, et al.** Comparison of seven immunoassays for the quantification of CA 125 antigen in serum. *Clin Chem.* 1998;44(7):1417–1422.

30. **Mongia SK, Rawlins ML, Owen WE, et al.** Performance characteristics of seven automated CA 125 assays. *Am J Clin Pathol.* 2006;125(6):921–927.

31. **Kabawat SE, Bast RC, Jr., Bhan AK, et al.** Tissue distribution of a coelomic-epithelium-related antigen recognized by the monoclonal antibody OC125. *Int J Gynecol Pathol.* 1983;2(3):275–285.

32. **Nouwen EJ, Hendrix PG, Dauwe S, et al.** Tumor markers in the human ovary and its neoplasms. A comparative immunohistochemical study. *Am J Pathol.* 1987;126(2):230–242.

33. **Tuxen MK, Soletormos G, Dombernowsky P.** Tumor markers in the management of patients with ovarian cancer. *Cancer Treat Rev.* 1995;21(3):215–245.

34. **Fleuren GJ, Nap M, Aalders JG, et al.** Explanation of the limited correlation between tumor CA 125 content and serum CA 125 antigen levels in patients with ovarian tumors. *Cancer.* 1987;60(10):2437–2442.

35. **Bast RC, Jr., Klug TL, St John E, et al.** A radioimmunoassay using a monoclonal antibody to monitor the course of epithelial ovarian cancer. *N Engl J Med.* 1983;309(15):883–887.

36. **Bon GG, Kenemans P, Verstraeten R, et al.** Serum tumor marker immunoassays in gynecologic oncology: Establishment of reference values. *Am J Obstet Gynecol.* 1996;174(1 Pt 1):107–114.

37. **Zurawski VR Jr, Orjaseter H, Andersen A, et al.** Elevated serum CA 125 levels prior to diagnosis of ovarian neoplasia: Relevance for early detection of ovarian cancer. *Int J Cancer.* 1988;42(5):677–680.

38. **Alagoz T, Buller RE, Berman M, et al.** What is a normal CA125 level? *Gynecol Oncol.* 1994;53(1):93–97.

39. **Bonfrer JM, Korse CM, Verstraeten RA, et al.** Clinical evaluation of the Byk LIA-mat CA125 II assay: Discussion of a reference value. *Clin Chem.* 1997;43(3):491–497.

40. **Grover S, Koh H, Weideman P, et al.** The effect of the menstrual cycle on serum CA 125 levels: A population study. *Am J Obstet Gynecol.* 1992;167(5):1379–1381.

41. **Pauler DK, Menon U, McIntosh M, et al.** Factors influencing serum CA125II levels in healthy postmenopausal women. *Cancer epidemiol, Biomarkers Prev.* 2001;10(5):489–493.

42. **Green PJ, Ballas SK, Westkaemper P, et al.** CA 19–9 and CA 125 levels in the sera of normal blood donors in relation to smoking history. *J Natl Cancer Inst.* 1986;77(2):337–341.

43. **Tuxen MK, Soletormos G, Petersen PH, et al.** Assessment of biological variation and analytical imprecision of CA 125, CEA, and TPA in relation to monitoring of ovarian cancer. *Gynecol Oncol.* 1999;74(1):12–22.

44. **Gocze PM, Szabo DG, Than GN, et al.** Occurrence of CA 125 and CA 19–9 tumor-associated antigens in sera of patients with gynecologic, trophoblastic, and colorectal tumors. *Gynecol Obstet Invest.* 1988;25(4):268–272.

45. **Spitzer M, Kaushal N, Benjamin F.** Maternal CA-125 levels in pregnancy and the puerperium. *J Reprod Med.* 1998;43(4):387–392.

46. **Urbancsek J, Hauzman EE, Lagarde AR, et al.** Serum CA-125 levels in the second week after embryo transfer predict clinical pregnancy. *Fertil Steril.* 2005;83(5):1414–1421.

47. **El-Shawarby SA, Henderson AF, Mossa MA.** Ovarian cysts during pregnancy: Dilemmas in diagnosis and management. *J Obstet Gynaecol.* 2005;25(7):669–675.

48. **Sarandakou A, Protonotariou E, Rizos D.** Tumor markers in biological fluids associated with pregnancy. *Crit Rev Clin Lab Sci.* 2007;44(2):151–178.

49. **Aslam N, Ong C, Woelfer B, et al.** Serum CA125 at 11–14 weeks of gestation in women with morphologically normal ovaries. *BJOG.* 2000;107(5):689–690.

50. **Canney PA, Moore M, Wilkinson PM, et al.** Ovarian cancer antigen CA125: A prospective clinical assessment of its role as a tumour marker. *Br J Cancer.* 1984;50(6):765–769.

51. **Tamakoshi K, Kikkawa F, Shibata K, et al.** Clinical value of CA125, CA19-9, CEA, CA72-4, and TPA in borderline ovarian tumor. *Gynecol Oncol.* 1996;62(1):67–72.

52. **Vergote IB, Bormer OP, Abeler VM.** Evaluation of serum CA 125 levels in the monitoring of ovarian cancer. *Am J Obstet Gynecol.* 1987;157(1):88–92.

53. **Einhorn N, Sjovall K, Knapp RC, et al.** Prospective evaluation of serum CA 125 levels for early detection of ovarian cancer. *Obstet Gynecol.* 1992;80(1):14–18.

54. **Kobayashi H, Ooi H, Yamada Y, et al.** Serum CA125 level before the development of ovarian cancer. *Int J Gynaecol Obstet.* 2007;99(2):95–99.

55. **Jeyarajah AR, Ind TE, MacDonald N, et al.** Increased mortality in postmenopausal women with serum CA125 elevation. *Gynecol Oncol.* 1999;73(2):242–246.

56. **Sjovall K, Nilsson B, Einhorn N.** The significance of serum CA 125 elevation in malignant and nonmalignant diseases. *Gynecol Oncol.* 2002;85(1):175–178.

57. **Jacobs I, Davies AP, Bridges J, et al.** Prevalence screening for ovarian cancer in postmenopausal women by CA 125 measurement and ultrasonography. *BMJ.* 1993;306(6884):1030–1034.

58. **Jacobs IJ, Skates S, Davies AP, et al.** Risk of diagnosis of ovarian cancer after raised serum CA 125 concentration: A prospective cohort study. *BMJ.* 1996;313(7069):1355–1358.

59. **Menon U, Talaat A, Jeyarajah AR, et al.** Ultrasound assessment of ovarian cancer risk in postmenopausal women with CA125 elevation. *Br J Cancer.* 1999;80(10):1644–1647.

60. **Menon U, Talaat A, Rosenthal AN, et al.** Performance of ultrasound as a second line test to serum CA125 in ovarian cancer screening. *BJOG.* 2000;107(2):165–169.

61. **Skates SJ, Menon U, MacDonald N, et al.** Calculation of the risk of ovarian cancer from serial CA-125 values for preclinical detection in postmenopausal women. *J Clin Oncol.* 2003;21(10 Suppl):206s–210s.

62. **Skates SJ, Xu FJ, Yu YH, et al.** Toward an optimal algorithm for ovarian cancer screening with longitudinal tumor markers. *Cancer.* 1995;76(10 suppl):2004–2010.

63. **Skates SJ, Pauler DK, Jacobs IJ.** Screening based on risk of cancer calculation from Bayesian hierarchical change point and mixture models of longitudinal markers. *J Am Stat Assoc.* 2001(96):429–435.

64. **Menon U, Skates SJ, Lewis S, et al.** Prospective study using the risk of ovarian cancer algorithm to screen for ovarian cancer. *J Clin Oncol.* 2005;23(31):7919–7926.

65. **Menon U, Gentry-Maharaj A, Ryan A, et al.** Recruitment to multicentre trials–lessons from UKCTOCS: Descriptive study. *BMJ.* 2008;337:a2079.

66. **Jacobs I, Ryan, A, Skates S, et al.** Performance characteristics of multimodal screening with serum CA125 in the United Kingdom Collaborative Trial of Ovarian Cancer Screening (UKCTOCS). NCRI; Liverpool: 2012.

67. **Menon U, Ryan A, Campbell S, et al.** Performance characteristics of ultrasound screening in the United Kingdom Collaborative Trial of Ovarian Cancer Screening (UKCTOCS). NCRI; Liverpool: 2012.

68. **Lu KH, Skates S, Hernandez MA, et al.** A 2-stage ovarian cancer screening strategy using the Risk of Ovarian Cancer Algorithm (ROCA) identifies early-stage incident cancers and demonstrates high positive predictive value. *Cancer.* 2013;119(19):3454–3461.

69. **Skates SJ, Mai P, Horick NK, et al.** Large prospective study of ovarian cancer screening in high-risk women: CA125 cut-point defined by menopausal status. *Cancer Prev Res.* 2011;4(9):1401–1408.

70. **Greene MH, Piedmonte M, Alberts D, et al.** A prospective study of risk-reducing salpingo-oophorectomy and longitudinal CA-125 screening among women at increased genetic risk of ovarian cancer: Design and baseline characteristics: A Gynecologic Oncology Group study. *Cancer Epidemiol, Biomarkers Prev.* 2008;17(3):594–604.

71. **Rosenthal AN, Fraser L, Manchanda R, et al.** Results of annual screening in phase I of the United Kingdom familial ovarian cancer screening study highlight the need for strict adherence to screening schedule. *J Clin Oncol.* 2013;31(1):49–57.

72. **Xu JL, Commins J, Partridge E, et al.** Longitudinal evaluation of CA-125 velocity and prediction of ovarian cancer. *Gynecol Oncol.* 2012;125(1):70–74.

73. **Drescher CW, Shah C, Thorpe J, et al.** Longitudinal screening algorithm that incorporates change over time in CA125 levels identifies ovarian cancer earlier than a single-threshold rule. *J Clin Oncol.* 2013;31(3):387–392.

74. **Engelen MJ, Kos HE, Willemse PH, et al.** Surgery by consultant gynecologic oncologists improves survival in patients with ovarian carcinoma. *Cancer.* 2006;106(3):589–598.

75. **Giede KC, Kieser K, Dodge J, et al.** Who should operate on patients with ovarian cancer? An evidence-based review. *Gynecol Oncol.* 2005;99(2):447–461.

76. **Paulsen T, Kjaerheim K, Kaern J, et al.** Improved short-term survival for advanced ovarian, tubal, and peritoneal cancer patients operated at teaching hospitals. *Int J Gynecol Cancer.* 2006;16 (suppl 1):11–17.

77. **Finkler NJ.** Clinical utility of CA 125 in preoperative diagnosis of patients with pelvic masses. *Eur J Obstet, Gynecol Reprod Biol.* 1993;49(1–2):105–107.

78. **Jacobs IJ, Rivera H, Oram DH, et al.** Differential diagnosis of ovarian cancer with tumour markers CA 125, CA 15–3 and TAG 72.3. *Br J Obstet Gynaecol.* 1993;100(12):1120–1124.

79. **Mogensen O, Mogensen B, Jakobsen A.** Tumour-associated trypsin inhibitor (TATI) and cancer antigen 125 (CA 125) in mucinous ovarian tumours. *Br J Cancer.* 1990;61(2):327–329.

80. **Schutter EM, Kenemans P, Sohn C, et al.** Diagnostic value of pelvic examination, ultrasound, and serum CA 125 in postmenopausal women with a pelvic mass. An international multicenter study. *Cancer.* 1994;74(4):1398–1406.

81. **Moore RG, Miller MC, Steinhoff MM, et al.** Serum HE4 levels are less frequently elevated than CA125 in women with benign gynecologic disorders. *Am J Obstet Gynecol.* 2012;206(4):351e1–351e8.

82. **Ferraro S, Braga F, Lanzoni M, et al.** Serum human epididymis protein 4 vs carbohydrate antigen 125 for ovarian cancer diagnosis: A systematic review. *J Clin Pathol.* 2013;66(4):273–281.

83. **Zhu CS, Pinsky PF, Cramer DW, et al.** A framework for evaluating biomarkers for early detection: Validation of biomarker panels for ovarian cancer. *Cancer Prev Res(Phila).* 2011;4(3):375–383.

84. **Rosen DG, Wang L, Atkinson JN, et al.** Potential markers that complement expression of CA125 in epithelial ovarian cancer. *Gynecol Oncol.* 2005;99(2):267–277.

85. **Woolas RP, Conaway MR, Xu F, et al.** Combinations of multiple serum markers are superior to individual assays for discriminating malignant from benign pelvic masses. *Gynecol Oncol.* 1995;59(1):111–116.

86. **Cramer DW, Bast RC, Jr., Berg CD, et al.** Ovarian cancer biomarker performance in prostate, lung, colorectal, and ovarian cancer screening trial specimens. *Cancer Prev Res(Phila).* 2011;4(3):365–374.

87. **Anderson GL, McIntosh M, Wu L, et al.** Assessing lead time of selected ovarian cancer biomarkers: A nested case-control study. *J Natl Cancer Inst.* 2010;102(1):26–38.

88. **Moore LE, Pfeiffer RM, Zhang Z, et al.** Proteomic biomarkers in combination with CA 125 for detection of epithelial ovarian cancer using prediagnostic serum samples from the Prostate, Lung, Colorectal, and Ovarian (PLCO) Cancer Screening Trial. *Cancer.* 2012;118(1):91–100.

89. **Timms JF, Menon U, Devetyarov D, et al.** Early detection of ovarian cancer in samples pre-diagnosis using CA125 and MALDI-MS peaks. *Cancer Genomics Proteomics.* 2011;8(6):289–305.

90. **Chen K, Gentry-Maharaj A, Burnell M, et al.** Microarray Glycoprofiling of CA125 improves differential diagnosis of ovarian cancer. *J Proteome Res.* 2013;12(3):1408–1418.

91. **Hori SS, Gambhir SS.** Mathematical model identifies blood biomarker-based early cancer detection strategies and limitations. *Sci Transl Med.* 2011;3(109):109ra16.

92. **Brown PO, Palmer C.** The preclinical natural history of serous ovarian cancer: Defining the target for early detection. *PLoS Med.* 2009;6(7):e1000114.

93. **Hori SS, Gambhir SS.** Mathematical model identifies blood biomarker-based early cancer detection strategies and limitations. *Sci Transl Med.* 2011;3(109):109ra16.

94. **Reynolds T.** For proteomics research, a new race has begun. *J Natl Cancer Inst.* 2002;94(8):552–554.

95. **Timms JF, Arslan-Low E, Gentry-Maharaj A, et al.** Preanalytic influence of sample handling on SELDI-TOF serum protein profiles. *Clin Chem.* 2007;53(4):645–656.

96. **Fushiki T, Fujisawa H, Eguchi S.** Identification of biomarkers from mass spectrometry data using a "common" peak approach. *BMC Bioinformatics.* 2006;7:358.

97. **Skates SJ, Horick NK, Moy JM, et al.** Pooling of case specimens to create standard serum sets for screening cancer biomarkers. *Cancer Epidemiol Biomarkers and Prev.* 2007;16(2):334–341.

98. **Bast RC, Jr., Badgwell D, Lu Z, et al.** New tumor markers: CA125 and beyond. *Int J Gynecol Cancer.* 2005;15(suppl 3):274–281.

99. **van der Merwe DE, Oikonomopoulou K, Marshall J, et al.** Mass spectrometry: Uncovering the cancer proteome for diagnostics. *Adv Cancer Res.* 2007;96:23–50.

100. **Baak JP, Path FR, Hermsen MA, et al.** Genomics and proteomics in cancer. *Eur J Cancer.* 2003;39(9):1199–1215.

101. **Mills GB, Bast RC Jr., Srivastava S.** Future for ovarian cancer screening: Novel markers from emerging technologies of transcriptional profiling and proteomics. *J Natl Cancer Inst.* 2001;93(19):1437–1439.

102. **Plebani M.** Proteomics: The next revolution in laboratory medicine? *Clin Chim Acta.* 2005;357(2):113–122.

103. **Zhang Y, Fonslow BR, Shan B, et al.** Protein analysis by shotgun/bottom-up proteomics. *Chem Rev.* 2013;113(4):2343–2394.

104. **Karabudak AA, Hafner J, Shetty V, et al.** Autoantibody biomarkers identified by proteomics methods distinguish ovarian cancer from non-ovarian cancer with various CA-125 levels. *J Cancer Res Clin Oncol.* 2013;139(10):1757–1770.

105. **Shield-Artin KL, Bailey MJ, Oliva K, et al.** Identification of ovarian cancer-associated proteins in symptomatic women: A novel method for semi-quantitative plasma proteomics. *Proteomics Clin Appl.* 2012;6(3–4):170–181.

106. **Sturgeon CM, Duffy MJ, Stenman UH, et al.** National Academy of Clinical Biochemistry laboratory medicine practice guidelines for use of tumor markers in testicular, prostate, colorectal, breast, and ovarian cancers. *Clin Chem.* 2008;54(12):e11–e79.

107. **Denkert C, Budczies J, Kind T, et al.** Mass spectrometry-based metabolic profiling reveals different metabolite patterns in invasive ovarian carcinomas and ovarian borderline tumors. *Cancer Res.* 2006;66(22):10795–10804.

108. **Jones PA, Baylin SB.** The fundamental role of epigenetic events in cancer. *Nat Rev Genet.* 2002;3(6):415–428.

109. **Jen J, Wu L, Sidransky D.** An overview on the isolation and analysis of circulating tumor DNA in plasma and serum. *Ann N Y Acad Sci.* 2000;906:8–12.

110. **Laird PW.** The power and the promise of DNA methylation markers. *Nat Rev Cancer.* 2003;3(4):253–266.

111. **Widschwendter M, Menon U.** Circulating methylated DNA: A new generation of tumor markers. *Clin Cancer Res.* 2006;12(24):7205–7208.

112. **Teschendorff AE, Menon U, Gentry-Maharaj A, et al.** An epigenetic signature in peripheral blood predicts active ovarian cancer. *PLoS One.* 2009;4(12):e8274.

113. **Zhang Q, Hu G, Yang Q, et al.** A multiplex methylation-specific PCR assay for the detection of early-stage ovarian cancer using cell-free serum DNA. *Gynecol Oncol.* 2013;130(1):132–139.

114. **Iorio MV, Visone R, Di Leva G, et al.** MicroRNA signatures in human ovarian cancer. *Cancer Res.* 2007;67(18):8699–8707.

115. **Taylor DD, Gercel-Taylor C.** MicroRNA signatures of tumor-derived exosomes as diagnostic biomarkers of ovarian cancer. *Gynecol Oncol.* 2008;110(1):13–21.

116. **Resnick KE, Alder H, Hagan JP, et al.** The detection of differentially expressed microRNAs from the serum of ovarian cancer patients using a novel real-time PCR platform. *Gynecol Oncol.* 2009;112(1):55–59.

117. **Giacona MB, Ruben GC, Iczkowski KA, et al.** Cell-free DNA in human blood plasma: Length measurements in patients with pancreatic cancer and healthy controls. *Pancreas.* 1998;17(1):89–97.

118. **Kamat AA, Baldwin M, Urbauer D, et al.** Plasma cell-free DNA in ovarian cancer: An independent prognostic biomarker. *Cancer.* 2010;116(8):1918–1925.

119. **Li M, Diehl F, Dressman D, et al.** BEAMing up for detection and quantification of rare sequence variants. *Nat Methods.* 2006;3(2):95–97.

120. **Forshew T, Murtaza M, Parkinson C, et al.** Noninvasive identification and monitoring of cancer mutations by targeted deep sequencing of plasma DNA. *Sci Transl Med.* 2012;4(136):136ra68.

121. **Kinde I, Bettegowda C, Wang Y, et al.** Evaluation of DNA from the Papanicolaou test to detect ovarian and endometrial cancers. *Sci Transl Med.* 2013;5(167):167ra4.

122. **Lee YH, Kim JH, Zhou H, et al.** Salivary transcriptomic biomarkers for detection of ovarian cancer: For serous papillary adenocarcinoma. *J Mole Med (Berl).* 2012;90(4):427–434.

123. **Sladkevicius P, Valentin L.** Intra- and interobserver agreement when describing adnexal masses using the International Ovarian Tumor Analysis terms and definitions: A study on three-dimensional ultrasound volumes. *Ultrasound Obstet Gynecol.* 2013;41(3):318–327.

124. **Gentry-Maharaj A, Sharma A, Burnell M, et al.** Acceptance of transvaginal sonography by postmenopausal women participating in the United Kingdom Collaborative Trial of Ovarian Cancer Screening. *Ultrasound Obstet Gynecol.* 2013;41(1):73–79.

125. **van Nagell JR, Jr., DePriest PD, Reedy MB, et al.** The efficacy of transvaginal sonographic screening in asymptomatic women at risk for ovarian cancer. *Gynecol Oncol.* 2000;77(3):350–356.

126. **Bailey CL, Ueland FR, Land GL, et al.** The malignant potential of small cystic ovarian tumors in women over 50 years of age. *Gynecol Oncol.* 1998;69(1):3–7.

127. **Pavlik EJ, Ueland FR, Miller RW, et al.** Frequency and disposition of ovarian abnormalities followed with serial transvaginal ultrasonography. *Obstet Gynecol.* 2013;122(2 Pt 1):210–217.

128. **Valentin L, Skoog L, Epstein E.** Frequency and type of adnexal lesions in autopsy material from postmenopausal women: Ultrasound study with histological correlation. *Ultrasound Obstet Gynecol.* 2003;22(3):284–289.

129. **Modesitt SC, Pavlik EJ, Ueland FR, et al.** Risk of malignancy in unilocular ovarian cystic tumors less than 10 centimeters in diameter. *Obstet Gynecol.* 2003;102(3):594–599.

130. **Ferrazzi E, Zanetta G, Dordoni D, et al.** Transvaginal ultrasonographic characterization of ovarian masses: Comparison of five scoring systems in a multicenter study. *Ultrasound Obstet Gynecol.* 1997;10(3):192–197.

131. **Lerner JP, Timor-Tritsch IE, Federman A, et al.** Transvaginal ultrasonographic characterization of ovarian masses with an improved, weighted scoring system. *Am J Obstet Gynecol.* 1994;170(1 Pt 1):81–85.

132. **Mol BW, Boll D, De Kanter M, et al.** Distinguishing the benign and malignant adnexal mass: An external validation of prognostic models. *Gynecol Oncol.* 2001;80(2):162–167.

133. **Sassone AM, Timor-Tritsch IE, Artner A, et al.** Transvaginal sonographic characterization of ovarian disease: Evaluation of a new scoring system to predict ovarian malignancy. *Obstet Gynecol.* 1991;78(1):70–76.

134. **Timmerman D, Bourne TH, Tailor A, et al.** A comparison of methods for preoperative discrimination between malignant and benign adnexal masses: The development of a new logistic regression model. *Am J Obstet Gynecol.* 1999;181(1):57–65.

135. **Ueland FR, DePriest PD, Pavlik EJ, et al.** Preoperative differentiation of malignant from benign ovarian tumors: The efficacy of morphology indexing and Doppler flow sonography. *Gynecol Oncol.* 2003;91(1):46–50.

136. **Granberg S, Wikland M, Jansson I.** Macroscopic characterization of ovarian tumors and the relation to the histological diagnosis: Criteria to be used for ultrasound evaluation. *Gynecol Oncol.* 1989;35(2):139–144.

137. **Elder JW, Pavlik EJ, Long A, et al., Ueland FR.** Serial ultrasonographic evaluation of ovarian abnormalities with a morphology index. *Gynecologic Oncology.* 2014 Jul 25.

138. **Clayton RD, Snowden S, Weston MJ, et al.** Neural networks in the diagnosis of malignant ovarian tumours. *Br J Obstet Gynaecol.* 1999;106(10):1078–1082.

139. **Tailor A, Jurkovic D, Bourne TH, et al.** Sonographic prediction of malignancy in adnexal masses using an artificial neural network. *Br J Obstet Gynaecol.* 1999;106(1):21–30.

140. **Timmerman D, Verrelst H, Bourne TH, et al.** Artificial neural network models for the preoperative discrimination between malignant and benign adnexal masses. *Ultrasound Obstet Gynecol.* 1999;13(1):17–25.

141. **Valentin L, Hagen B, Tingulstad S, et al.** Comparison of 'pattern recognition' and logistic regression models for discrimination between benign and malignant pelvic masses: A prospective cross validation. *Ultrasound Obstet Gynecol.* 2001;18(4):357–365.

142. **Van Calster B, Timmerman D, Bourne T, et al.** Discrimination between benign and malignant adnexal masses by specialist ultrasound examination versus serum CA-125. *J Natl Cancer Inst.* 2007;99(22):1706–1714.

143. **Geomini P, Kruitwagen R, Bremer GL, et al.** The accuracy of risk scores in predicting ovarian malignancy: A systematic review. *Obstet Gynecol.* 2009;113(2 Pt 1):384–394.

144. **Jacobs I, Oram D, Fairbanks J, et al.** A risk of malignancy index incorporating CA 125, ultrasound and menopausal status for the accurate preoperative diagnosis of ovarian cancer. *Br J Obstet Gynaecol.* 1990;97(10):922–929.

145. **Yazbek J, Aslam N, Tailor A, et al.** A comparative study of the risk of malignancy index and the ovarian crescent sign for the diagnosis of invasive ovarian cancer. *Ultrasound Obstet Gynecol.* 2006;28(3):320–324.

146. **Timmerman D, Testa AC, Bourne T, et al.** Logistic regression model to distinguish between the benign and malignant adnexal mass before surgery: A multicenter study by the International Ovarian Tumor Analysis Group. *J clin Oncol.* 2005;23(34):8794–801.

147. **Timmerman D, Van Calster B, Jurkovic D, et al.** Inclusion of CA-125 does not improve mathematical models developed to distinguish between benign and malignant adnexal tumors. *J Clin Oncol.* 2007;25(27):4194–4200.

148. **Sayasneh A, Wynants L, Preisler J, et al.** Multicentre external validation of IOTA prediction models and RMI by operators with varied training. *Br J Cancer.* 2013;108(12):2448–2454.

149. **Dodge JE, Covens AL, Lacchetti C, et al.** Preoperative identification of a suspicious adnexal mass: A systematic review and meta-analysis. *Gynecol Oncol.* 2012;126(1):157–166.

150. **Valentin L, Akrawi D.** The natural history of adnexal cysts incidentally detected at transvaginal ultrasound examination in postmenopausal women. *Ultrasound Obstet Gynecol.* 2002;20(2):174–180.

151. **McAlpine JN, El Hallani S, Lam SF, et al.** Autofluorescence imaging can identify preinvasive or clinically occult lesions in fallopian tube epithelium: A promising step towards screening and early detection. *Gynecol Oncol.* 2011;120(3):385–392.

152. **Williams RM, Flesken-Nikitin A, Ellenson LH, et al.** Strategies for high-resolution imaging of epithelial ovarian cancer by laparoscopic nonlinear microscopy. *Transl Oncol.* 2010;3(3):181–194.

153. **Folkman J, Watson K, Ingber D, et al.** Induction of angiogenesis during the transition from hyperplasia to neoplasia. *Nature.* 1989;339(6219):58–61.

154. **Kurjak A, Shalan H, Kupesic S, et al.** An attempt to screen asymptomatic women for ovarian and endometrial cancer with transvaginal color and pulsed Doppler sonography. *J Ultrasound Med.* 1994;13(4):295–301.

155. **Vuento MH, Pirhonen JP, Makinen JI, et al.** Evaluation of ovarian findings in asymptomatic postmenopausal women with color Doppler ultrasound. *Cancer.* 1995;76(7):1214–1218.

156. **Bourne TH, Campbell S, Reynolds KM, et al.** Screening for early familial ovarian cancer with transvaginal ultrasonography and colour blood flow imaging. *BMJ.* 1993;306(6884):1025–1029.

157. **Parkes CA, Smith D, Wald NJ, et al.** Feasibility study of a randomised trial of ovarian cancer screening among the general population. *J Med Screen.* 1994;1(4):209–214.

158. **Brown DL, Frates MC, Laing FC, et al.** Ovarian masses: Can benign and malignant lesions be differentiated with color and pulsed Doppler US? *Radiology.* 1994;190(2):333–336.

159. **Timor-Tritsch LE, Lerner JP, Monteagudo A, et al.** Transvaginal ultrasonographic characterization of ovarian masses by means of color flow-directed Doppler measurements and a morphologic scoring system. *Am J Obstet Gynecol.* 1993;168(3 Pt 1):909–913.

160. **Valentin L.** Pattern recognition of pelvic masses by gray-scale ultrasound imaging: The contribution of Doppler ultrasound. *Ultrasound Obstet Gynecol.* 1999;14(5):338–347.

161. **Cohen LS, Escobar PF, Scharm C, et al.** Three-dimensional power Doppler ultrasound improves the diagnostic accuracy for ovarian cancer prediction. *Gynecol Oncol.* 2001;82(1):40–48.

162. **Kurjak A, Kupesic S, Sparac V, et al.** The detection of stage I ovarian cancer by three-dimensional sonography and power Doppler. *Gynecol Oncol.* 2003;90(2):258–264.

163. **Guerriero S, Alcazar JL, Ajossa S, et al.** Comparison of conventional color Doppler imaging and power doppler imaging for the diagnosis of ovarian cancer: Results of a European study. *Gynecol Oncol.* 2001;83(2):299–304.

164. **Fleischer AC, Lyshchik A, Andreotti RF, et al.** Advances in sonographic detection of ovarian cancer: Depiction of tumor neovascularity with microbubbles. *Am J Roentgenol.* 2010;194(2):343–348.

165. **Deshpande N, Ren Y, Foygel K, et al.** Tumor angiogenic marker expression levels during tumor growth: Longitudinal assessment with molecularly targeted microbubbles and US imaging. *Radiology.* 2011;258(3):804–811.

166. **Song H, Ramus SJ, Tyrer J, et al.** A genome-wide association study identifies a new ovarian cancer susceptibility locus on 9p22.2. *Nat Genet.* 2009;41(9):996–1000.

167. **Pharoah PD, Tsai YY, Ramus SJ, et al.** GWAS meta-analysis and replication identifies three new susceptibility loci for ovarian cancer. *Nat Genet.* 2013;45(4):362–370, 370e1–370e2.

168. **Permuth-Wey J, Lawrenson K, Shen HC, et al.** Identification and molecular characterization of a new ovarian cancer susceptibility locus at 17q21.31. *Nat Comm.* 2013;4:1627.

169. **Bojesen SE, Pooley KA, Johnatty SE, et al.** Multiple independent variants at the TERT locus are associated with telomere length and risks of breast and ovarian cancer. *Nat Genet.* 2013;45(4):371–384, 384e1–384e2.

170. **Goode EL, Chenevix-Trench G, Song H, et al.** A genome-wide association study identifies susceptibility loci for ovarian cancer at 2q31 and 8q24. *Nat Genet.* 2010;42(10):874–879.

171. **Pearce CL, Rossing MA, Lee AW, et al.** Combined and interactive effects of environmental and GWAS-identified risk factors in ovarian cancer. *Cancer Epidemiol Biomarkers Prev.* 2013;22(5):880–890.

172. **Pharoah PD, Antoniou AC, Easton DF, et al.** Polygenes, risk prediction, and targeted prevention of breast cancer. *N Engl J Med.* 2008;358(26):2796–2803.

173. **Burton H, Chowdhury S, Dent T, et al.** Public health implications from COGS and potential for risk stratification and screening. *Nat Genet.* 2013;45(4):349–351.

174. **Chen S, Parmigiani G.** Meta-analysis of BRCA1 and BRCA2 penetrance. *J Clin Oncol.* 2007;25(11):1329–1333.

175. **Couch FJ, Wang X, McGuffog L, et al.** Genome-wide association study in BRCA1 mutation carriers identifies novel loci associated with breast and ovarian cancer risk. *PLoS Genet.* 2013;9(3):e1003212.

176. **Aarnio M, Sankila R, Pukkala E, et al.** Cancer risk in mutation carriers of DNA-mismatch-repair genes. *Int J Cancer.* 1999;81(2):214–218.

177. **van Nagell JR, Jr., DePriest PD, Ueland FR, et al.** Ovarian cancer screening with annual transvaginal sonography: Findings of 25,000 women screened. *Cancer.* 2007;109(9):1887–1896.

178. **Buys SS, Partridge E, Greene MH, et al.** Ovarian cancer screening in the Prostate, Lung, Colorectal and Ovarian (PLCO) cancer screening trial: Findings from the initial screen of a randomized trial. *Am J Obstet Gynecol.* 2005;193(5):1630–1639.

179. **Kobayashi H, Yamada Y, Sado T, et al.** A randomized study of screening for ovarian cancer: A multicenter study in Japan. *Int J Gynecol Cancer.* 2008;18(3):414–420.

180. **Adonakis GL, Paraskevaidis E, Tsiga S, et al.** A combined approach for the early detection of ovarian cancer in asymptomatic women. *Eur J Obstet, Gynecol Reprod Biol.* 1996;65(2):221–225.

181. **Campbell S, Bhan V, Royston P, et al.** Transabdominal ultrasound screening for early ovarian cancer. *BMJ.* 1989;299(6712):1363–1367.

182. **DePriest PD, Gallion HH, Pavlik EJ, et al.** Transvaginal sonography as a screening method for the detection of early ovarian cancer. *Gynecol Oncol.* 1997;65(3):408–414.

183. **Goswamy RK, Campbell S, Whitehead MI.** Screening for ovarian cancer. *Clin Obstet Gynaecol.* 1983;10(3):621–643.

184. **Grover S, Quinn MA, Weideman P, et al.** Screening for ovarian cancer using serum CA125 and vaginal examination: Report on 2550 females. *Int J Gynecol Cancer.* 1995;5(4):291–295.

185. **Hayashi H, Yaginuma Y, Kitamura S, et al.** Bilateral oophorectomy in asymptomatic women over 50 years old selected by ovarian cancer screening. *Gynecol Obstet Invest.* 1999;47(1):58–64.

186. **Kurjak A, Kupesic S.** Transvaginal color Doppler and pelvic tumor vascularity: Lessons learned and future challenges. *Ultrasound Obstet and Gynecol.* 1995;6(2):145–159.

187. **Millo R, Facca MC, Alberico S.** Sonographic evaluation of ovarian volume in postmenopausal women: A screening test for ovarian cancer? *Clin Exp Obstet Gynecol.* 1989;16(2–3):72–78.

188. **Tabor A, Jensen FR, Bock JE, et al.** Feasibility study of a randomised trial of ovarian cancer screening. *J Med Screen.* 1994;1(4):215–219.

189. **Menon U, Gentry-Maharaj A, Jacobs I.** Ovarian cancer screening and mortality. *JAMA.* 2011;306(14):1544; author reply -1544-1545.

190. **Baldwin LM, Trivers KF, Matthews B, et al.** Vignette-based study of ovarian cancer screening: Do U.S. physicians report adhering to evidence-based recommendations? *Ann Inter Med.* 2012;156(3):182–194.

191. **Burnell M, Gentry-Maharaj A, et al.** Impact on mortality and cancer incidence rates of using random invitation from population registers for recruitment to trials. *Trials.* 2011;12:61.

192. **Pinsky PF, Miller A, Kramer BS, et al.** Evidence of a healthy volunteer effect in the prostate, lung, colorectal, and ovarian cancer screening trial. *Am J Epidemiol.* 2007;165(8):874–881.

193. **Bourne TH, Campbell S, Reynolds K, et al.** The potential role of serum CA 125 in an ultrasound-based screening program for familial ovarian cancer. *Gynecol Oncol.* 1994;52(3):379–385.

194. **Dorum A, Heimdal K, Lovslett K, et al.** Prospectively detected cancer in familial breast/ovarian cancer screening. *Acta Obstet Gynecol Scand.* 1999;78(10):906–911.

195. **Karlan BY, Baldwin RL, Lopez-Luevanos E, et al.** Peritoneal serous papillary carcinoma, a phenotypic variant of familial ovarian cancer: Implications for ovarian cancer screening. *Am J Obstet Gynecol.* 1999;180(4):917–928.

196. **Gaarenstroom KN, van der Hiel B, Tollenaar RA, et al.** Efficacy of screening women at high risk of hereditary ovarian cancer: Results of an 11-year cohort study. *Int J Gynecol Cancer.* 2006;16 (suppl 1):54–59.

197. **Hermsen BB, Olivier RI, Verheijen RH, et al.** No efficacy of annual gynaecological screening in BRCA1/2 mutation carriers; an observational follow-up study. *Br J Cancer.* 2007;96(9):1335–1342.

198. **Stirling D, Evans DG, Pichert G, et al.** Screening for familial ovarian cancer: Failure of current protocols to detect ovarian cancer at an early stage according to the international Federation of gynecology and obstetrics system. *J Clin Oncol.* 2005;23(24):5588–5596.

199. **Tailor A, Bourne TH, Campbell S, et al.** Results from an ultrasound-based familial ovarian cancer screening clinic: A 10-year observational study. *Ultrasound Obstet Gynecol.* 2003;21(4):378–385.

200. **Vasen HF, Tesfay E, Boonstra H, et al.** Early detection of breast and ovarian cancer in families with BRCA mutations. *Eur J Cancer.* 2005;41(4):549–554.

201. **Schorge JO, Muto MG, Welch WR, et al.** Molecular evidence for multifocal papillary serous carcinoma of the peritoneum in patients with germline BRCA1 mutations. *J Natl Cancer Inst.* 1998;90(11):841–845.

202. **Skates SJ, Drescher CW, Isaacs C, et al.** A prospective multi-centre ovarian cancer screening study in women at increased risk. *J Clin Oncol.* American Society of Clinical Oncology; Chicago, IL. 2007; 25(18S):5510.

203. **Finch A, Beiner M, Lubinski J, et al.** Salpingo-oophorectomy and the risk of ovarian, fallopian tube, and peritoneal cancers in women with a BRCA1 or BRCA2 Mutation. *JAMA.* 2006;296(2):185–192.

204. **Kauff ND, Barakat RR.** Risk-reducing salpingo-oophorectomy in patients with germline mutations in BRCA1 or BRCA2. *J Clin Oncol.* 2007;25(20):2921–2927.

205. **Kauff ND, Satagopan JM, Robson ME, et al.** Risk-reducing salpingo-oophorectomy in women with a BRCA1 or BRCA2 mutation. *N Engl J Med.* 2002;346(21):1609–1615.

206. **Anderson CK, Wallace S, Guiahi M, et al.** Risk-reducing salpingectomy as preventative strategy for pelvic serous cancer. *Int J Gynecol Cancer.* 2013;23(3):417–421.

207. **Kamran MW, Vaughan D, Crosby D, et al.** Opportunistic and interventional salpingectomy in women at risk: A strategy for preventing pelvic serous cancer (PSC). *Eur J Obstet, Gynecol Reprod Biol.* 2013;170(1):251–254.

208. **Weiner Z, Beck D, Shteiner M, et al.** Screening for ovarian cancer in women with breast cancer with transvaginal sonography and color flow imaging. *J Ultrasound Med.* 1993;12(7):387–393.

209. **Muto MG, Cramer DW, Brown DL, et al.** Screening for ovarian cancer: The preliminary experience of a familial ovarian cancer center. *Gynecol Oncol.* 1993;51(1):12–20.

210. **Schwartz PE, Chambers JT, Taylor KJ.** Early detection and screening for ovarian cancer. *J Cell Biochem Suppl.* 1995;23:233–237.

211. **Belinson JL, Okin C, Casey G, et al.** The familial ovarian cancer registry: Progress report. *Clev Clin J Med.* 1995;62(2):129–134.

212. **Menkiszak J, Jakubowska A, Gronwald J, et al.** [Hereditary ovarian cancer: Summary of 5 years of experience]. *Ginekol Pol.* 1998;69(5):283–287.

213. **Karlan BY, Raffel LJ, Crvenkovic G, et al.** A multidisciplinary approach to the early detection of ovarian carcinoma: Rationale,

protocol design, and early results. *Am J Obstet Gynecol.* 1993;169(3): 494–501.

214. **Dorum A, Kristensen GB, Abeler VM, et al.** Early detection of familial ovarian cancer. *Eur J Cancer.* 1996;32A(10):1645–1651.

215. **Scheuer L, Kauff N, Robson M, et al.** Outcome of preventive surgery and screening for breast and ovarian cancer in BRCA mutation carriers. *J Clin Oncol.* 2002;20(5):1260–1268.

216. **Laframboise S, Nedelcu R, Murphy J, et al.** Use of CA-125 and ultrasound in high-risk women. *Int J Gynecol Cancer.* 2002;12(1): 86–91.

217. **Liede A, Karlan BY, Baldwin RL, et al.** Cancer incidence in a population of Jewish women at risk of ovarian cancer. *J Clin Oncol.* 2002;20(6):1570–1577.

218. **Fries MH, Hailey BJ, Flanagan J, et al.** Outcome of five years of accelerated surveillance in patients at high risk for inherited breast/ovarian cancer: Report of a phase II trial. *Mil Med.* 2004;169(6): 411–416.

219. **Meeuwissen PA, Seynaeve C, Brekelmans CT, et al.** Outcome of surveillance and prophylactic salpingo-oophorectomy in asymptomatic women at high risk for ovarian cancer. *Gynecol Oncol.* 2005; 97(2):476–482.

220. **Oei AL, Massuger LF, Bulten J, et al.** Surveillance of women at high risk for hereditary ovarian cancer is inefficient. *Br J Cancer.* 2006; 94(6):814–819.

221. **Bosse K, Rhiem K, Wappenschmidt B, et al.** Screening for ovarian cancer by transvaginal ultrasound and serum CA125 measurement in women with a familial predisposition: A prospective cohort study. *Gynecol Oncol.* 2006;103(3):1077–1082.

222. **Sato S, Yokoyama Y, Sakamoto T, et al.** Usefulness of mass screening for ovarian carcinoma using transvaginal ultrasonography. *Cancer.* 2000;89(3):582–588.

223. **Holbert TR.** Screening transvaginal ultrasonography of postmenopausal women in a private office setting. *Am J Obstet Gynecol.* 1994; 170(6):1699–1703; discussion 1703–1704.

11 Epithelial Ovarian, Fallopian Tube, and Peritoneal Cancer

Jonathan S. Berek
Michael L. Friedlander
Neville F. Hacker

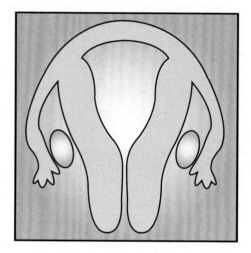

Epithelial ovarian cancer has the highest fatality-to-case ratio of all the gynecologic malignancies, because more than two-thirds of patients have advanced disease at diagnosis (1,2). It presents a major surgical challenge, requires intensive and often complex therapies, and is extremely demanding of the patient's psychological and physical energy. **High-grade serous carcinomas, which are the most common, are now believed to be related etiologically to fallopian tube and peritoneal cancer and most appear to arise from the fimbria of the fallopian tube** (3–11).

There are nearly 22,000 new cases of ovarian cancer annually in the United States, and more than 14,000 women can be expected to succumb to their illness (1). It is the fifth most common cancer in women in the United States after cancers of the lung, breast, colon, and uterus. It accounts for 4% of all female cancers and 31% of cancers of the female genital tract. Ovarian cancer is the fourth most common cause of death from malignancy in women (1). **A woman's risk at birth of having ovarian cancer some time in her lifetime is nearly 1.4%, and the risk of dying from ovarian cancer is almost 1%** (2). The number of new cases per 10,000 women per year was 12.5 in 2010 (2).

There is a trend toward improved survival for ovarian cancer (1,2). Based on Surveillance, Epidemiology, and End Results (SEER) data in the United States, the 5-year survival for all stages combined increased from 33.6% in 1975 to 44.2% in 2003 to 2009 (2). Using statistical models for analysis, rates for new ovarian cancer cases have been falling on average 1% per year over the last 10 years. Death rates have been falling on average 1.6% per year over the same period. The numbers of new cases, deaths, and 5-year relative survival trends are presented in Figure 11.1. The death rate decreased 22% from 10 per 100,000 women per year in 1976 to 7.8 per 100,000 per women per year in 2010 (2). Ovarian cancer rates are highest in women aged 55 to 64 years (median age 63 years), and deaths are highest in people aged 75 to 84 years (median age 71 years) (2). The percentage of new ovarian cancer cases by age group and the percentage of deaths by age group are presented in Figure 11.2.

Classification

Approximately 90% of ovarian cancers are derived from cells of the coelomic epithelium or *modified mesothelium* (3). The cells are a product of the primitive mesoderm, which can undergo

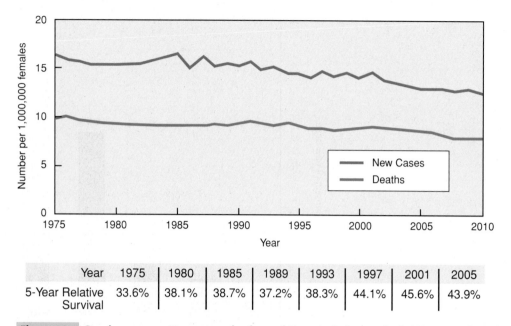

Year	1975	1980	1985	1989	1993	1997	2001	2005
5-Year Relative Survival	33.6%	38.1%	38.7%	37.2%	38.3%	44.1%	45.6%	43.9%

Figure 11.1 **Ovarian cancer: New cases, deaths, and 5-year relative survival.** SEER 9 Incidence and U.S. Mortality 1975–2010, all races, females. Rates are age adjusted. SEER Cancer Statistics Factsheets: Ovary Cancer. National Cancer Institute. Bethesda, MD. http://seer.cancer.gov/statfacts/html/ovary.html

metaplasia. Neoplastic transformation can occur when the cells are genetically predisposed to oncogenesis or exposed to an oncogenic agent.

Epithelial ovarian cancers are thought to arise either from the fimbriated end of the fallopian tube or from a single layer of cells that covers the ovary or lines cysts immediately beneath the ovarian surface. These latter cells are generally quiescent, but proliferate following ovulation to repair the defect created by rupture of a follicle.

There are at least two different molecular pathways that lead to the development of ovarian cancers, and these develop into tumors that have quite distinct biologic behaviors and probably different cells of origin (4). **There are those tumors (so-called type I tumors) that arise from ovarian surface epithelium and müllerian inclusions,** either from endosalpingiosis or invagination of the ovarian surface epithelium during repair of ovulation or implantation of cells from endometrium. This process typically **involves a relatively slow and multistep pathway and accounts for many early-stage cancers** such as endometrioid, clear cell, mucinous, and low-grade serous cancers. In contrast, **the more common high-grade serous cancers (type II) have a phenotype that resembles the fallopian tube mucosa, and they commonly have *p53* mutations.** These tumors **appear to develop rapidly,** and are almost always at an advanced stage at presentation. Many appear to arise in the fallopian tube (4).

Pathology

Invasive Cancer

Approximately 75–80% of epithelial cancers are of the serous histologic type, with the majority being high-grade cancers. Less common subtypes are mucinous (10%), endometrioid (10%), clear cell, Brenner, and undifferentiated carcinomas (3). Each tumor type has a histologic pattern that recapitulates the epithelial features of a section of the lower genital tract. For example, the serous pattern has an appearance similar to that of the glandular epithelium lining the fallopian tube, and **it is now appreciated that many high-grade serous epithelial cancers originate in fimbriae of the distal fallopian tubal epithelium** (5–11). High-grade serous cancers commonly involve both the ovaries and tubes and it can be difficult to ascertain the site of origin (7–11). **Mucinous tumors** resemble the endocervical glands, and the **endometrioid tumors** resemble the endometrium. More specific details of the histopathology are discussed in Chapter 5.

There is increasing evidence to demonstrate that many high-grade serous ovarian cancers arise in the fallopian tube (7–11), a situation that may have been obscured by an overly rigid

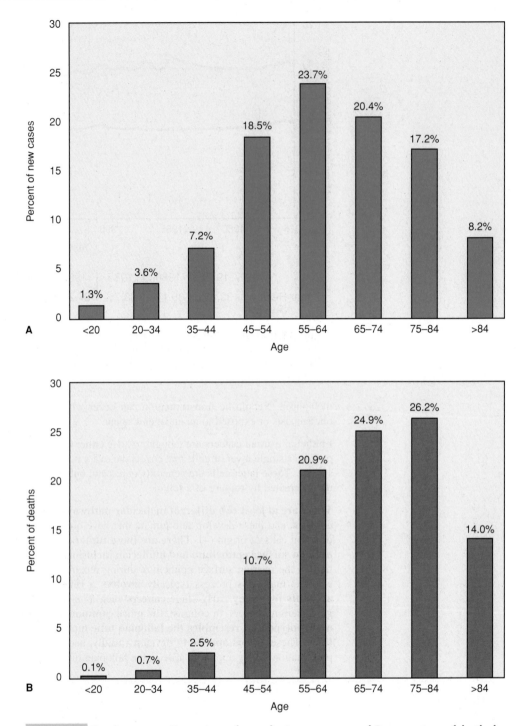

Figure 11.2 Ovarian cancer: Percentage of cases by A: age group, and B: percentage of deaths by age group. U.S. 2006–2010, all races, females. SEER Cancer Statistics Factsheets: Ovary Cancer. National Cancer Institute. Bethesda, MD. http://seer.cancer.gov/statfacts/html/ovary.html

WHO definition of fallopian tube cancer. Molecular and genetic evidence supports this etiology, as well as the finding of carcinoma in situ in the tubal epithelium that appears to be the precursor of high-grade serous carcinomas (4).

It is now believed that most high-grade serous cancers of the ovary , fallopian tube carcinomas, and peritoneal carcinomas should be regarded as a single disease entity. Although a substantial proportion of cancers appear to arise in the fimbriated end of the fallopian tube,

this site cannot account for all of these cancers, and a proportion is thought to be derived from components of the secondary müllerian system (12).

In histologic features and clinical behavior, fallopian tube carcinoma is the same as ovarian cancer; thus, the management is the same. Almost all fallopian tube cancers are of "epithelial" origin, most frequently of serous histology. Rarely, sarcomas have also been reported. The fallopian tubes are frequently involved secondarily from other primary sites, most often the ovaries, endometrium, gastrointestinal tract, or breast (1). They may be secondarily involved in peritoneal cancer.

Peritoneal serous carcinomas are identical pathologically to serous cancers arising in the fallopian tube or ovary and have the same biologic behavior as well as response to chemotherapy. They are thought to arise from müllerian remnants in the coelomic epithelium or alternatively to arise in the fimbria of the fallopian tube. In most cases there may be microscopic or small macroscopic cancer on the surface of the ovary and extensive disease in the upper abdomen, particularly in the omentum. Peritoneal carcinoma also explains how "ovarian cancer" can arise in a patient whose ovaries were surgically removed many years earlier, although in some patients this may be due to the fallopian tubes not being removed or due to an ovarian remnant (13–15).

Based on these data, patients with epithelial ovarian, fallopian tube, and peritoneal cancer are now staged by the same International Federation of Gynecology and Obstetrics (FIGO) system, and evaluated and treated in the same manner. The discussion that follows regarding ovarian cancer includes patients with fallopian tube and peritoneal cancer.

Borderline Tumors

An important group of tumors to distinguish is the tumors of low malignant potential, also called the **borderline tumors** (16–19). Borderline tumors are usually confined to the ovary at diagnosis, occur predominantly in premenopausal women, and are associated with a very good prognosis. **They are diagnosed most frequently between the ages of 30 and 50 years,** while invasive carcinomas occur more commonly between the ages of 50 and 70 years (3). **Although uncommon, peritoneal implants may occur** and may be either noninvasive or invasive. Invasive implants are associated with a higher likelihood of progression, which can lead to intestinal obstruction and death (17–19).

Clinical Features

As noted above, **the peak incidence of invasive epithelial ovarian cancer is ages 55 to 64 years with a median of age 63 years** (2,3,20) (Fig. 11.2). The age-specific incidence of this disease rises precipitously from 20 to 80 years of age and subsequently declines (21). By contrast, the average patient age of those with borderline tumors is approximately 46 years (3,12). Eighty percent to 90% of ovarian cancers, including borderline forms, occur after the age of 40 years.

The chance that a primary epithelial tumor will be of borderline or invasive malignancy in a patient younger than age 40 years is approximately 1 in 10, but after that age, it rises to 1 in 3 (3). Less than 1% of epithelial ovarian cancers occur before the age of 20, two-thirds of ovarian malignancies in such patients being germ cell tumors (3,21). **Approximately 30% of ovarian neoplasms in postmenopausal women are malignant, whereas only about 7% of ovarian epithelial tumors in premenopausal patients are frankly malignant** (3).

Epidemiology

Ovarian cancer has been associated with low parity and infertility (22). Although there has been a variety of epidemiologic variables correlated with ovarian cancer—such as increased risk with talc use, galactose consumption, and decreased risk with tubal ligation and the oral contraceptive pill usage (see Chapter 6)—none has been so strongly correlated as prior reproductive history and duration of the reproductive career (22–24). **Early menarche and late menopause increase the risk of ovarian cancer** (23). These factors and the relationship of parity and infertility to the risk of ovarian cancer have led to the hypothesis that suppression of ovulation may be an important factor. Theoretically, the surface epithelium undergoes repetitive disruption and repair. It is thought that this process might lead to a higher probability of spontaneous mutations that can unmask germ line mutations or otherwise lead to the oncogenic phenotype (see Chapter 1).

In a cohort study of more than 1.1 million Norwegian women, a positive association was found between body mass index (BMI), height, and risk of ovarian cancer, particularly of the endometrioid type in women younger than 60 years (25). Women who had a very high BMI and were clinically obese in adolescence and childhood had a relative risk of 1.56 of developing ovarian cancer compared with women with a medium BMI.

There has been considerable controversy as to whether fertility-enhancing drugs increase the risk of ovarian cancer. In a meta-analysis of eight case-control studies (26), there were 5,207 women with cancer compared with 7,705 controls. The relative risk (RR) of fertility drug exposure for ovarian cancer was 0.97—that is, the use of the drugs was not associated with an increased risk. However, in the same cohort, nulliparity (compared with multiparity greater than 4) carried a RR of 2.42, and infertility per se for 5 years or longer (compared with shorter than 1 year) carried a RR of 2.7. These results support the hypothesis that the higher risk in these women is related to infertility, independent of fertility drug use.

Most case-control and cohort studies have failed to link hormone replacement therapy to an increased risk of epithelial ovarian cancer (27). A large cohort study has reopened controversy regarding this issue (28). Among 44,241 postmenopausal women in the Breast Cancer Detection Demonstration Project, 329 developed ovarian cancer. Women who had received estrogen replacement therapy only for more than 10 years without progestin were at increased risk. By 20 years, the relative risk was 3.2-fold.

The incidence of ovarian cancer varies in different geographic locations throughout the world. Western countries, including the United States and the United Kingdom, have an incidence of ovarian cancer that is three to seven times greater than in Japan, where epithelial ovarian tumors are considered rare (3). In Asia, the incidence of germ cell tumors of the ovary appears to be somewhat higher than in the West. Japanese immigrants to the United States exhibit a significant increase in the incidence of epithelial ovarian cancer, the rate eventually approaching that of white US women. The incidence of epithelial tumors is about 1.5 times greater in whites than in blacks (1).

Prevention

As parity is inversely related to the risk of ovarian cancer, having at least one child is protective of the disease, with a risk reduction of 0.3 to 0.4. The oral contraceptive reduces the risk of epithelial ovarian cancer (22). Women who use the oral contraceptive for 5 or more years reduce their relative risk to 0.5—that is, there is a 50% reduction in the likelihood of developing ovarian cancer. Women who have had two children and have used the oral contraceptive for 5 or more years have a relative risk of ovarian cancer as low as 0.3, or a 70% reduction (29). Therefore, the oral contraceptive pill is the only documented method of chemoprevention for ovarian cancer, and it should be recommended to women for this purpose. When counseling patients regarding birth control options, this important benefit of the oral contraceptive should be emphasized. This is also important for women with a strong family history of ovarian cancer.

Fenretinide, a retinoid, was thought to be a chemoprophylactic agent for ovarian cancer (30). However, in a prospective, randomized, placebo-controlled trial, there was no difference in the incidence or survival from ovarian cancer after 5 years (31). The Gynecology Oncology Group (GOG) initiated a confirmatory trial, but it was closed because of poor accrual.

As many high-grade serous epithelial tumors arise in the fallopian tube and because there is a higher rate of tubal carcinoma in women with BRCA1 and BRCA2 mutations, it is essential that risk-reducing prophylactic surgery includes the removal of both ovaries and both fallopian tubes. The performance of a prophylactic salpingo-oophorectomy will significantly reduce, but not eliminate, the risk of ovarian and fallopian tube cancer (14,15) because the entire peritoneum is potentially at risk and serous cancers may arise in the secondary müllerian system (19). The ovaries provide protection from cardiovascular disease and osteoporosis, so prophylactic bilateral salpingo-oophorectomy should not be routinely performed in premenopausal women at low risk for ovarian cancer.

Screening

There is no proven effective method of screening for ovarian cancer (see Chapter 10). Routine annual pelvic examinations are not considered to be an effective method of screening (32), and given the false positive results for both CA125 and transvaginal ultrasonography, particularly in premenopausal women, these tests are not cost-effective and have not been

found to detect ovarian cancer at an early stage. Recent advances in transvaginal ultrasonography (33–39) have been reported by some groups to have a very high (>95%) sensitivity for the detection of early-stage ovarian cancer, although this test alone might result in up to 15 unnecessary laparotomies for every ovarian cancer detected (40). Transvaginal color-flow Doppler to assess the vascularity of the ovarian vessels may be a useful adjunct to ultrasonography (34–36).

In the future, new markers or technologies may improve the specificity of screening, but proof of this will require large prospective studies (37–47). **Even screening in women at higher risk of ovarian cancer because of a strong family history or known *BRCA* mutation has not been found to be effective. These women should be advised to have risk reducing bilateral salpingo-oophorectomy.**

CA125 screening has previously been thought to allow the earlier diagnosis of epithelial ovarian cancer (40–47). However, screening trials have not found a lower incidence of stage I tumors in women at population risk. For example, in the **Prostate, Lung, Colon, Ovarian (PLCO) Screening Trial,** which included an annual CA125 and transvaginal ultrasound, the stage distributions were similar to the study group, with stage III and IV cancers comprising the majority of cases in both the screened group (77%) and usual care group (78%).

CA125 has been cloned, and although the function of the molecule is unclear, the elucidation of the *MUC16* gene and its control may enhance the understanding of this important marker in ovarian cancer (48–50). Binding of *MUC16* to mesothelin appears to mediate cell adhesion and facilitates peritoneal metastasis in animal models (51–53). Data suggest that the specificity of CA125 is improved when the CA125 levels are followed over time (47–57). The risk of ovarian cancer (ROC) algorithm might help to improve the efficacy of screening (57), although this was not confirmed even with every 4-month CA125 levels in the UKFOCSS trial (58).

A number of novel markers for ovarian cancer have been identified in recent years, including mesothelin, a 110-kd fragment of EGFR (sEGFR), and **HE4** (59–65). **Multiplex assays** can measure more than 50 biomarkers with a few hundred microliters of serum (66), and using this technology, a combination of CA125, HE4, sEGFR, and soluble vCAM-1 has distinguished 90% of stage I ovarian cancer patients from 98% of healthy controls. The use of surface-enhanced laser desorption and ionization (SELDI) with subsequent resolution by mass spectroscopy has demonstrated a pattern of low molecular weight moieties that has been reported to distinguish sera from ovarian cancer patients from those of healthy individuals (67); however, methodologic issues have been raised regarding these data (68,69).

Genetic Risk for Epithelial Ovarian Cancer

Hereditary Ovarian Cancer

The risk of ovarian cancer is higher than that of the general population in women with a family history of breast or ovarian cancer as well as in families with Lynch syndrome (70–86). Although **most epithelial ovarian cancer is sporadic, at least 10–14% of patients have a germ line mutation in *BRCA1* or *BRCA2*** (73,85,86). Further discussion of germ line mutations and their biology is presented in Chapter 1.

BRCA1 and *BRCA2*

Most hereditary ovarian cancer results from mutations in the *BRCA1* gene, which is located on chromosome 17 (72), **with a smaller proportion associated with mutations in *BRCA2*, which is located on chromosome 13** (47). Although these appear to be responsible for most hereditary ovarian cancers, it is likely that there are other, as yet undiscovered, genes that also predispose to ovarian or breast cancer or both (81).

In the past, it had been thought that there were two distinct syndromes associated with a genetic risk: site-specific hereditary ovarian cancer and hereditary breast or ovarian cancer syndrome. It is now accepted that these groups represent a continuum of mutations of *BRCA1* and *BRCA2*, with different degrees of penetrance within a given family (49,57). There are other less common genetic causes of ovarian cancer, and **there is a higher risk of ovarian and endometrial cancer in women with the Lynch syndrome, which was also known as the *hereditary nonpolyposis colorectal cancer syndrome* (HNPCC syndrome)** (82).

The mutations are autosomal dominant, and thus a complete family history and pedigree analysis, including both maternal and paternal sides of the family, must be evaluated (76). There are numerous distinct mutations that have been identified on each of these genes, and the mutations may have different degrees of penetrance, which may explain the preponderance of either breast cancer, ovarian cancer, or both, in any given family. **A combined analysis of 22 studies unselected for family history has found that women who have a germ line mutation in the *BRCA1* gene have a lifetime risk of ovarian cancer of 39% (18–54%), and the risk has been calculated to be 11% (2.4–19%) for women with a *BRCA2* mutation (73,74,80). In this study, women with a *BRCA1* or *BRCA2* mutation had a risk of breast cancer of 65% and 45%, respectively** (87). These figures are somewhat lower than the estimates based on multiple case families, which may be enriched for mutations of higher risk. A large consortium found genetic risk modifiers on 4q32.2 and 17q21.31 that significantly increased the risk of developing ovarian cancer in *BRCA1*-mutation carriers, which may explain the variable risks that have been reported (88).

Hereditary ovarian cancers, in particular, *BRCA1*-associated ovarian cancers, generally occur in women approximately 10 years younger than those with nonhereditary tumors (73,84). As the median age of epithelial ovarian cancer is 62 to 63 years, a woman with a first- or second-degree relative who had early onset ovarian cancer may have a higher probability of having a *BRCA* 1 or *BRCA* 2 mutation. For example, a recent Australian population based study found that 22.2% of women diagnosed before age 50 years carried a *BRCA* mutation, compared with 12.1% of those older than 50 years. **There was no potentially significant family history in 44% (95% CI, 35.8–52.2%) of mutation-positive women, which underscores the importance of offering mutation testing to all women with ovarian cancer under the age of 70 irrespective of family history** (89).

Women with *BRCA* mutations are also at increased risk of breast cancer. The breast cancers typically occur at a young age and may be bilateral. There is a higher incidence of triple-negative breast cancers in women with *BRCA1* mutations.

Founder Effect

There is a higher carrier rate of *BRCA1* and *BRCA2* mutations in women of Ashkenazi Jewish descent, Icelandic women, and in other ethnic groups (78,79,81). There are three specific founder mutations that are carried by the Ashkenazi population: 185delAG and 5382insC on *BRCA1*, and 6174delT on *BRCA2*. **The carrier rate of at least one of these mutations for a patient of Ashkenazi Jewish descent is 1 in 40 or 2.5%, which is considerably higher than the general Caucasian population.** The increased risk is a result of the *founder effect*—that is, a higher rate of mutations that have occurred within a specific population group within a defined geographic area.

Pedigree Analysis

The risk of ovarian cancer depends on the number of first- or second-degree relatives with a history of epithelial ovarian carcinoma or breast cancer, and on the age of onset. The degree of risk is difficult to determine precisely unless a full pedigree analysis is performed, and all patients should be referred to a familial cancer service for genetic counseling.

Risch et al. (85) reported that **the hereditary proportion of invasive ovarian tumors was approximately 13%, and was as high as 18% in the large subgroup of women with high-grade serous ovarian cancers.** This was independent of family history. Similar findings have been reported in a smaller study from Poland (86), and confirmed in a large prospective Australian study (89). **These findings have major implications for genetic testing, and argue for consideration of *BRCA* genetic testing in all patients with high-grade serous cancers irrespective of the pedigree and family history. Recent Australian guidelines recommend genetic testing for all women diagnosed with nonmucinous ovarian cancer under the age of 70.**

Lynch Syndrome

Lynch syndrome is defined as a hereditary predisposition to colorectal cancer and a wide range of other malignancies (e.g., endometrial, ovarian, and gastric cancer) as a result of a germ line mismatch repair (MMR) genetic mutation (82). The mutations that have been associated with this syndrome are *MSH2, MSH6, MLH1, PMS1*, and *PMS2*. **The risk of endometrial cancer equals or exceeds that of colorectal cancer in women with Lynch Syndrome. The**

diagnosis of gynecologic cancer precedes that of colorectal cancer in over half the cases, making gynecologic cancer a "sentinel cancer" for Lynch syndrome.

The lifetime risk of ovarian cancer in women with Lynch Syndrome has been estimated at approximately 6–12%. The mean age at diagnosis is 42.7 to 49.5 years. There is a higher risk of endometrioid and clear cell subtypes, and the majority of cases are stages I or II at diagnosis. It is important to take a full family history in all patients, but family history alone cannot be relied on to identify cases (90).

Management of Women at High Risk for Ovarian Cancer

The management of a woman with a strong family history of epithelial ovarian cancer must be individualized and will depend on her age, her reproductive plans, and the estimated level of risk. A thorough pedigree analysis is important. A geneticist should evaluate the family pedigree for at least three generations. Decisions about management are best made after careful study of the pedigree and, whenever possible, verification of the histologic diagnosis of the family members' ovarian cancer as well as the age of onset and other tumors in the family.

The value of testing for *BRCA1* and *BRCA2* has been clearly established, and guidelines for testing now exist (76,83,84). The American Society of Clinical Oncologists has provided guidelines that emphasize careful evaluation by geneticists, careful maintenance of medical records, and a clear understanding of how to counsel and manage these patients. There remain concerns of the impact on insurability, how the results will be interpreted, and how the information will be used within a specific family—for example, to counsel children.

Although there are some conflicting data, the outcomes of women with breast cancer and with germ line mutations in *BRCA1* or *BRCA2* are comparable to women with sporadic tumors (75,91,92). **Women with breast cancer who carry these mutations are at a greatly increased risk of ovarian cancer, as well as of a second breast cancer. The lifetime risk of ovarian cancer is 54% for women who have a *BRCA1* mutation and 23% for those with a *BRCA2* mutation; for the two groups together, there is an 82% lifetime risk of breast cancer** (84).

Although recommended by the National Institutes of Health Consensus Conference on Ovarian Cancer (93), **the value of screening with transvaginal ultrasonography and CA125 has not been established in women at high risk. The findings of two prospective studies of annual transvaginal ultrasonography and CA125 screening** in 888 *BRCA1* and *BRCA2* mutation carriers in the Netherlands and 279 mutation carriers in the United Kingdom are not encouraging, and **suggest a very limited benefit, if any, of screening even in high-risk women** (94,95). Despite annual gynecologic screening, Hermsen et al. (94) reported that a high proportion of ovarian cancers in *BRCA1* and *BRCA2* carriers were interval cancers, and the majority of all cancers diagnosed were at an advanced stage. Similar findings were reported by Woodward (95). **Therefore, it is unlikely that annual screening will reduce mortality from ovarian cancer in *BRCA1* and *BRCA2* mutation carriers** (94,96).

This important question has also been addressed in GOG 199, a study of screening with annual transvaginal ultrasonography and CA125 ROCA compared to prophylactic bilateral salpingo-oophorectomy. Study accrual was completed in November 2006, with 2,605 participants enrolled: 1,030 (40%) in the surgical cohort and 1,575 (60%) in the screening cohort (97). Five years of prospective follow-up ended in November 2011 (see Chapter 10).

Data derived from a multi-institutional consortium of genetic screening centers has suggested that the use of the oral contraceptive pill is associated with a lower risk of ovarian cancer in women who have a *BRCA1* or *BRCA2* mutation (98). In women who had taken the oral contraceptive pill for five or more years, the relative risk of ovarian cancer was 0.4, or a 60% reduction in incidence. Another study failed to confirm this finding (99). Tubal ligation may also decrease the risk of ovarian cancer in patients with a *BRCA1* but not *BRCA2* mutation in one study, but the protective effect is not nearly as strong as risk-reducing bilateral salpingo-oophorectomy (100).

The value of prophylactic risk-reducing bilateral salpingo-oophorectomy in these patients has been well documented (101–106). Occult ovarian/fallopian tube cancers detected at the time of risk-reducing bilateral salpingo-oophorectomy have been reported in many studies with wide variability in reported prevalence ranging from 2.3–23%. This may reflect selection bias as well as inadequate pathologic review of the fallopian tubes and ovaries (102). Domchek et al. (102) estimated the prevalence of occult cancers in a prospective cohort of 647 *BRCA1/2* mutation carriers from 18 centers (PROSE consortium) who underwent risk-reducing bilateral salpingo-**oophorectomy** between

2001 and 2008. An occult cancer was detected in 16 of 647 women (2.5%). Thirty-eight percent of women had stage I cancer versus none of the women in the PROSE database diagnosed with ovarian cancer outside of screening. Ovarian and fallopian tube tissues removed at major genetic referral centers were significantly more likely to have been examined completely by pathologists compared to specimens obtained at nonreferral centers (75% vs. 30%, $p < 0.001$), and the authors commented that an unacceptably high proportion of pathologic examinations did not adequately examine ovaries and fallopian tubes obtained at risk-reducing bilateral salpingo-oophorectomy (RRSO) (102).

The performance of a prophylactic salpingo-oophorectomy reduces the risk of BRCA-related gynecologic cancer by 96% (104). There remains a small risk of subsequently developing a peritoneal carcinoma, a tumor that may also have a higher predisposition in women who have mutations in the *BRCA1* and *BRCA2* genes. In these series, the risk of developing peritoneal carcinoma was 0.8% and 1%, respectively (102,103). **Prophylactic salpingo-oophorectomy in premenopausal women reduced the risk of developing subsequent breast cancer by 50–80%** (102,103).

The role of hysterectomy is more controversial. Although most studies show no increase in the rate of uterine and cervical tumors, there are some isolated reports of an increased risk of papillary serous tumors of the endometrium (107). **Women on *tamoxifen* are at higher risk for benign endometrial lesions (e.g., polyps) and have a twofold higher risk of endometrial cancer.** In selected patients who have completed childbearing, the performance of a prophylactic hysterectomy in conjunction with salpingo-oophorectomy may be considered on an individual basis.

Grann et al. (108) reported the application of Markov modeling—that is, quality-adjusted survival estimate analysis—in a simulated cohort of 30-year-old women who tested positive for *BRCA1* or *BRCA2* mutations. The analysis predicted that **a 30-year-old woman could prolong her survival beyond that associated with surveillance alone by 1.8 years with *tamoxifen*, 2.6 years with prophylactic salpingo-oophorectomy, 4.6 years with both *tamoxifen* and prophylactic salpingo-oophorectomy, 3.5 years with prophylactic mastectomy, and 4.9 years with both prophylactic surgeries.** Quality-adjusted life expectancy was estimated to be prolonged by 2.8 years for *tamoxifen*, 4.4 years with prophylactic salpingo-oophorectomy, 6.3 years for *tamoxifen* and prophylactic salpingo-oophorectomy, 2.6 years with mastectomy, and 2.6 years with both operations. This has been supported by a study of women with *BRCA1* and *BRCA2* mutations which found that risk-reducing mastectomy was associated with a lower risk of breast cancer, risk-reducing bilateral salpingo-oophorectomy was associated with a lower risk of ovarian cancer, and that there was an improvement in all-cause mortality, breast cancer-specific mortality as well as ovarian cancer-specific mortality (109).

The survival of women who have a *BRCA1* or *BRCA2* mutation and develop ovarian cancer is longer than that for those who do not have a mutation. In one study, the median survival for mutation carriers was 53.4 months compared with 37.8 months for those with sporadic ovarian cancer from the same institution (110). These findings have recently been confirmed in a population-based study from Israel in which Chetrit et al. (111) reported that among Ashkenazi women with ovarian cancer, those with *BRCA1* and *BRCA2* mutations had an improved long-term survival (38% vs. 24% at 5 years). This may result from distinct clinical behavior or from a better response to chemotherapy.

Recommendations

Current recommendations are that all women under the age of 70 with a nonmucinous epithelial ovarian, fallopian tube, or peritoneal cancer should undergo testing for *BRCA*1 to *BRCA*2 (112). The recommendations for management of women at high risk for ovarian cancers are summarized below (83,84,93,98–108):

1. Women who appear to be at high risk for ovarian and or breast cancer should undergo genetic counseling; if there is a probability of 10% or greater of having a *BRCA* mutation, they should be offered genetic testing for *BRCA1* and *BRCA2*.

2. Women who wish to preserve their reproductive capability or delay prophylactic surgery should undergo periodic screening by transvaginal ultrasonography every 6 months, although the efficacy of this approach has not been established.

3. Oral contraceptives should be recommended to young women before a planned family.

4. Women who do not wish to maintain their fertility or who have completed their family should be recommended to undergo prophylactic bilateral salpingo-oophorectomy. The majority of *BRCA1*-related ovarian cancers occur in women

after the age of 40, and *BRCA2* **ovarian cancers are more likely in postmenopausal women. The risk of ovarian cancer under the age of 40 is very low.** The potential risk should be clearly documented and preferably established by *BRCA1* and *BRCA2* testing. These women should be counseled that this operation does not offer absolute protection, because peritoneal carcinomas may occasionally occur (102,103). A prophylactic hysterectomy is acceptable, and the option should be discussed with these patients.

5. **In women who have a strong family history of breast or ovarian cancer, annual mammographic and magnetic resonance imaging (MRI) screening should be performed commencing at age 30 years, or younger if there are family members with documented very early onset breast cancer.**

6. **Women with a documented Lynch syndrome should be counseled about prophylactic hysterectomy and oophorectomy after childbearing, in view of the risk of both endometrial and ovarian cancer.** Although there are no definitive studies to support screening, endometrial sampling and transvaginal ultrasound of the ovaries may be considered from ages 30 to 35. **Colonoscopy is recommended every 1 to 2 years starting from age 20 to 25 or 10 years younger than the youngest person diagnosed in the family** (82,90,113).

Symptoms

The majority of women with epithelial ovarian cancer have vague and nonspecific pelvic, abdominal, and menstrual symptoms (114–118). Goff et al. (119) recently developed an ovarian cancer symptom index and reported that symptoms associated with ovarian cancer were pelvic or abdominal pain, urinary frequency or urgency, increased abdominal size or bloating, and difficulty eating or feeling full. These symptoms were particularly suspicious when they were present for less than 1 year and lasted longer than 12 days a month. The index had a sensitivity of 56.7% for the diagnosis of early ovarian cancer and 79.5% for advanced-stage disease.

A study from the Royal Hospital for Women in Sydney compared 100 patients with early-stage epithelial ovarian cancer with 100 patients with advanced-stage disease. **Ninety percent of women with early disease and 100% with advanced disease reported at least one symptom.** With early disease, abdominal pain was reported by 51% and abdominal swelling by 32%. With advanced disease, abdominal swelling was reported by 62% and abdominal pain by 40%. **Seventy percent of patients with early disease and 69% of those with advanced disease reported symptoms of less than 3 months duration.** Patients with tumors less than 5 cm in diameter were three times more likely to have advanced disease. Patients with grade 1 tumors were 40 times more likely to have early-stage disease when compared to patients with grade 3 tumors (120). **These findings were confirmed in a population-based study from Australia in which there did not appear to be a significant difference in the duration of symptoms or the nature of symptoms in patients with early as opposed to advanced-stage disease** (121). These two studies reinforce the concept that early- and late-stage ovarian cancer are biologically different entities, and argue against the widely held misconception that ovarian cancer is diagnosed at an early stage because the symptoms are recognized earlier than in patients with more advanced disease (96,120–122).

Of historical interest is the so-called "classic triad" of symptoms and signs associated with fallopian tube cancer: watery vaginal discharge (*hydrops tubae profluens*)**,** pelvic pain, and a pelvic mass. This triad is noted in fewer than 15% of patients (123).

Signs

The most important sign is the presence of a pelvic mass on physical examination. A solid, irregular, fixed pelvic mass is highly suggestive of an ovarian malignancy. If, in addition, an upper abdominal mass or ascites is present, then the diagnosis of ovarian cancer is almost certain. Because the patient usually reports abdominal symptoms, she may not be subjected to a pelvic examination, and the presence of a tumor may be missed. Pleural effusions commonly occur in association with ascites, and very occasionally in the absence of ascites in patients with advanced disease.

Diagnosis

The diagnosis of an ovarian cancer requires histologic examination of a resected ovary. The preoperative evaluation of the patient with an adnexal mass is outlined in Figure 11.3.

Ultrasonographic signs of malignancy include an adnexal pelvic mass with areas of complexity such as irregular borders; multiple echogenic patterns within the mass; and dense, multiple, irregular

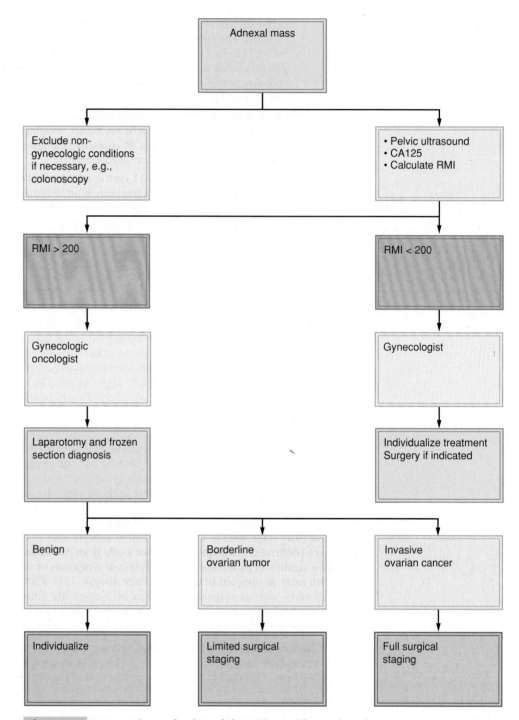

Figure 11.3 **Preoperative evaluation of the patient with an adnexal mass.** RMI, Risk of Malignancy Index.

septae. Bilateral tumors are more likely to be malignant, although the individual characteristics of the lesions are of greater significance. **Transvaginal ultrasonography may have a somewhat better resolution than transabdominal ultrasonography for adnexal neoplasms** (33,37–39), and Doppler color-flow imaging may enhance the specificity (34–36).

The size of the lesion is of importance. If a complex cystic mass is more than 8 to 10 cm in diameter, the probability is high that the lesion is neoplastic, unless the patient has been taking *clomiphene citrate* or other agents to induce ovulation (115). **In the premenopausal patient, a period of observation is reasonable, provided it is not clinically suspicious** (i.e., it is mobile, mostly cystic, unilateral, and of regular contour). Generally, an interval of no more than 2 months should be allowed for observation. If the lesion is not neoplastic, it should remain stable or regress. If a mass increases in size or complexity, it must be presumed to be neoplastic and removed surgically.

In postmenopausal women with unilocular cysts measuring 8 to 10 cm or less and normal serial CA125 levels, expectant management is acceptable, and this approach may decrease the number of surgical interventions (124–126). **Premenopausal patients whose lesions are clinically suspicious (i.e., large, predominantly solid, relatively fixed, or irregularly shaped) should undergo laparotomy, as should postmenopausal patients with complex adnexal masses of any size.**

Before the planned exploration, the patient should undergo routine hematologic and biochemical assessments. A preoperative evaluation in a patient older than 40 years should include a radiograph of the chest. An abdominal and pelvic computed tomographic (CT) or MRI scan is of limited value in patients with a definite pelvic mass (127–131). Patients with ascites and no pelvic mass should have a CT or MRI scan to look particularly for liver or pancreatic tumors (128). The value of positron emission tomography (PET) scans is being evaluated but may contribute to the specificity of the CT scan findings (130,131).

The preoperative evaluation should exclude other primary cancers metastatic to the ovary. A **colonoscopy** is indicated in selected patients with symptoms and signs suspicious for colon cancer. This would include any patient who has evidence of frank or occult blood in the stool or a recent history of diarrhea or constipation. A **gastroscopy** is indicated if there are upper gastrointestinal symptoms such as nausea, vomiting, or hematemesis (132). **Bilateral mammography** is indicated if there is any breast mass, and **patients who have irregular menses or postmenopausal bleeding should have an endometrial biopsy and an endocervical curettage** to exclude the presence of endometrial or endocervical cancer metastatic to the ovary.

Differential Diagnosis

Ovarian epithelial cancers must be differentiated from benign neoplasms and functional cysts of the ovaries (40,133,134). A variety of benign conditions of the reproductive tract—such as pelvic inflammatory disease, endometriosis, and pedunculated uterine leiomyomata—can simulate ovarian cancer. Nongynecologic causes of a pelvic tumor, such as an inflammatory or neoplastic colonic mass must be excluded (115). A pelvic kidney can simulate ovarian cancer.

The **risk of malignancy index** (RMI), first described by Jacobs in 1990, is one method of differentiating between benign and malignant masses (133). Utilization of this index may facilitate better triage of suspicious pelvic masses to gynecologic oncologists. **The RMI incorporates the menopausal status, an ultrasonic score, and the serum CA125 level.**

In an analysis of 204 consecutive patients with an ovarian mass seen at the Royal Hospital for Women in Sydney, an RMI of <200 correctly identified 83 of 108 (77%) benign ovarian masses (133). **An RMI of >200 correctly identified 11 of 19 (58%) borderline ovarian tumors and 70 of 77 (91%) invasive ovarian cancers.** An RMI of >200 had a sensitivity of 84%, specificity of 77%, positive predictive value of 76%, and a negative predictive value of 85% for the detection of both borderline and invasive ovarian tumors (133).

Patterns of Spread

Ovarian epithelial cancers spread primarily by exfoliation of cells into the peritoneal cavity, but also by lymphatic and hematogenous dissemination.

Transcoelomic   **The most common mode of dissemination is by exfoliation of cells that implant on the peritoneal surfaces.** The cells tend to follow the circulatory path of the peritoneal fluid, which moves with the forces of respiration from the pelvis, up the paracolic gutters, especially on the right, along the intestinal mesenteries, to the right hemidiaphragm. Therefore, metastases are typically seen on the posterior cul-de-sac, paracolic gutters, right hemidiaphragm, liver capsule, the peritoneal surfaces of the intestines and their mesenteries, and the omentum. **The disease seldom invades the intestinal lumen** but progressively agglutinates loops of bowel, leading to a functional intestinal obstruction. This condition is known as **carcinomatous ileus**.

Lymphatic   **Lymphatic dissemination to the pelvic and para-aortic lymph nodes is common, particularly in advanced-stage disease** (135–138). Spreading through the lymphatic channels of the diaphragm and through the retroperitoneal lymph nodes can lead to dissemination above the diaphragm, especially to the supraclavicular lymph nodes (135).

475

Burghardt et al. (137) performed systematic pelvic and para-aortic lymphadenectomy on 123 patients and reported that 78% of patients with stage III disease had metastases to the pelvic lymph nodes. In another series (138), the rate of positive para-aortic lymph nodes was 18% in stage I, 20% in stage II, 42% in stage III, and 67% in stage IV.

Hematogenous   **Hematogenous dissemination at the time of diagnosis is uncommon,** with spread to vital organ parenchyma, such as the lungs and liver, in only some 2–3% of patients. Most patients presenting with disease above the diaphragm have a right pleural effusion. Systemic metastases are seen more frequently in patients who have survived for some years. Dauplat et al. (139) from UCLA reported that **distant metastasis consistent with stage IV disease ultimately occurred in 38% of the patients whose disease was originally intraperitoneal.** Sites of hematogenous spread and their median survivals were as follows.

- Parenchymal lung metastasis in 7.1%, median survival 9 months
- Subcutaneous nodules in 3.5%, 12 months
- Malignant pericardial effusion in 2.4%, 2.3 months
- Central nervous system in 2%, 1.3 months
- Bone metastases in 1.6%, 4 months

Significant risk factors for distant metastases were malignant ascites, peritoneal carcinomatosis, large metastatic disease within the abdomen, and retroperitoneal lymph node involvement at the time of initial surgery.

Prognosis

The outcome of patients after treatment can be evaluated in the context of prognostic factors, which can be grouped into pathologic and clinical factors.

Pathologic Factors

The morphologic and histologic pattern, including the architecture and grade of the lesion, are important prognostic variables (140–145). **In general, stage for stage, histologic type is not of prognostic significance, with the exception of clear cell and mucinous carcinomas,** which are associated with a worse prognosis than the other histologic types when diagnosed at an advanced stage (143,144,146–148). Traditionally, stage I clear cell cancers have been thought also to have a high risk of recurrence, but more recent data have challenged this belief and Stage IA clear cell cancers appear to have a good prognosis, and probably do not benefit from adjuvant chemotherapy (148,149).

Histologic grade, as determined either by the pattern of differentiation or by the extent of cellular anaplasia and the proportion of undifferentiated cells, seems to be of prognostic significance (144,150). However, studies of the reproducibility of ovarian cancer grading have shown a high degree of intraobserver and interobserver variation (145). **Because there is significant heterogeneity of tumors and observational bias, the value of histologic grade as an independent prognostic factor has not been clearly established.**

Clinical Factors

In addition to FIGO stage, the extent of residual disease after primary surgery, the volume of ascites, patient age, and performance status are all independent prognostic variables (149,151–165). Among patients with stage I disease, Dembo et al. (152) showed, in a multivariate analysis, that tumor grade and "dense adherence" to the pelvic peritoneum had a significant adverse impact on prognosis, whereas intraoperative tumor spillage or rupture did not. A subsequent study by Sjövall et al. (153) confirmed these findings. A multivariate analysis of these and several other studies was performed by Vergote et al. (155), who reported that poor prognostic variables for early-stage disease were the tumor grade, capsular penetrance, surfaces excrescences, and malignant ascites, but not iatrogenic rupture. More recent studies have supported these findings and reported that **the most important prognostic factors in patients with early-stage ovarian cancer include substage, grade, age, positive cytology, dense adherence, capsular rupture, and histologic subtype** (156).

FIGO reported a statistically significant improvement in survival for all stages from 29.8% for the interval 1976 to 1978 to 49.7% for the interval 1999 to 2001 (157). The 5-year survival

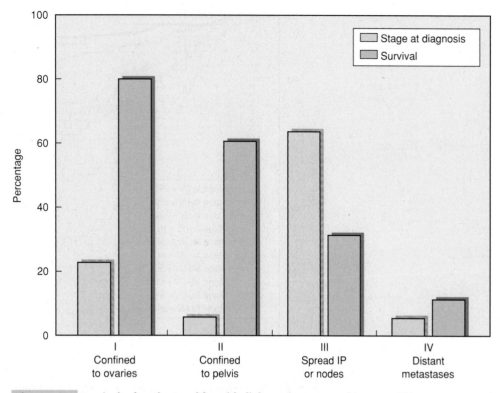

Figure 11.4 Survival of patients with epithelial ovarian cancer by stage. The percentage of patients diagnosed at a particular stage (green bars) is shown next to the 5-year survival by stage (blue bars). Data from **Heintz APM, Odicino F, Maisonneuve P, et al.** Carcinoma of the ovary. 26th Annual Report on the Results of Treatment in Gynaecological Cancer. *Int J Gynaecol Obstet.* 2006;95(suppl 1):S161–S192, with permission.

rate for carefully staged patients with stage IA disease is about 90%, while it is 70–80% for stage IC. The 5-year survival for stage II disease is about 70%, 45–50% or stage IIIA, 40% for stage IIIB, 30–35% for stage IIIC, and 15–20% for stage IV (157). The percentage of patients by stage at the time of diagnosis is shown next to the 5-year survival by stage in Figure 11.4, and the survival by substage is presented in Figure 11.5. **The 5-year survival of patients with stage III disease and microscopic residual after cytoreductive surgery is 63.5%, compared with 32.9% for those with optimal residual disease, and 25% for those with suboptimal residual disease.** Patients whose Karnofsky's index (KI) is low (76) have a significantly shorter survival than those with a KI > 70 (158). For stages I and II disease, the 5-year survival rate for grade 1 cancer is about 90%, compared with approximately 80% for grade 2 and 70–75% for grade 3 (Fig. 11.6). For patients with stages III and IV disease, the 5-year survivals for grades 1, 2, and 3 are about 60%, 30%, and 25%, respectively (157,159) (Fig. 11.7). **Survival of patients with borderline tumors is excellent, with stage I lesions having a 98% 10-year survival** (16,18,63). When all stages of borderline tumors are included, the 5-year survival rate is 87% (157).

Initial Surgery for Ovarian Cancer

Staging

Ovarian epithelial malignancies are staged according to the FIGO system, and the staging system of 2013 is presented in Table 11.1. The TNM staging is correlated with the FIGO stage in Figure 11.8. **The 2014 FIGO staging for ovarian, fallopian tube and peritoneal cancers are now grouped into a single staging system (160). The FIGO staging is based on findings at surgical exploration.** A preoperative evaluation should exclude the presence of extraperitoneal metastases.

Surgical staging should be performed because subsequent treatment will be determined by the stage of disease. In patients in whom exploratory laparotomy does not reveal any macroscopic evidence of disease beyond the ovaries, a careful search for microscopic spread must be undertaken.

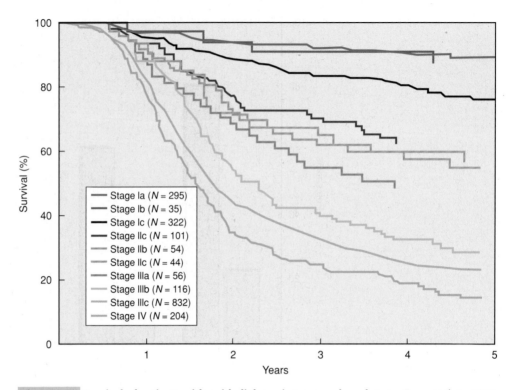

Figure 11.5 Survival of patients with epithelial ovarian cancer by substage. From **Heintz APM, Odicino F, Maisonneuve P, et al.** Carcinoma of the ovary. 26th Annual Report on the Results of Treatment in Gynaecological Cancer. *Int J Gynaecol Obstet.* 2006;95(suppl 1):S161–S192, with permission.

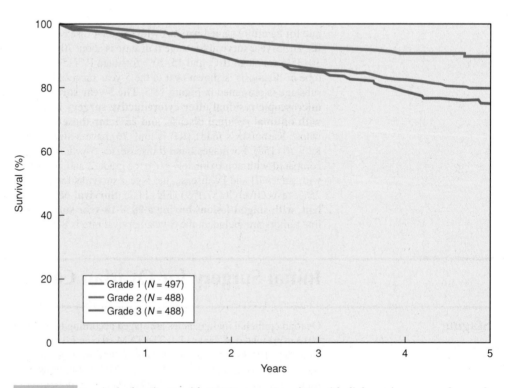

Figure 11.6 Survival of patients with FIGO stages I and II epithelial ovarian cancer by grade of the tumor. From **Heintz APM, Odicino F, Maisonneuve P, et al.** Carcinoma of the ovary. 26th Annual Report on the Results of Treatment in Gynaecological Cancer. *Int J Gynaecol Obstet.* 2006;95(suppl 1):S161–S192, with permission.

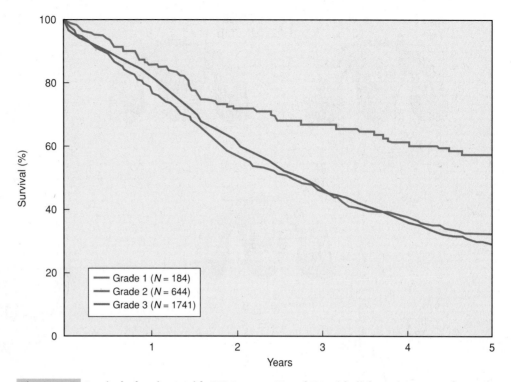

Figure 11.7 **Survival of patients with FIGO stages III and IV epithelial ovarian cancer by grade of the tumor.** From **Heintz APM, Odicino F, Maisonneuve P, et al.** Carcinoma of the ovary. 26th Annual Report on the Results of Treatment in Gynaecological Cancer. *Int J Gynaecol Obstet.* 2006;95(suppl 1):S161–S192, with permission.

In earlier series in which patients did not undergo careful surgical staging, the overall 5-year survival for patients with apparent stage I epithelial ovarian cancer was only approximately 60% (166). Since then, survival rates of 90–100% have been reported for patients who have been surgically staged and found to have disease confined to one or both ovaries (166–170).

Technique for Surgical Staging

In patients whose preoperative evaluation suggests a probable ovarian malignancy, a midline or paramedian abdominal incision is recommended to allow adequate access to the upper abdomen. When a malignancy is unexpectedly discovered in a patient who has a lower transverse incision, the rectus muscles can be either divided or detached from the symphysis pubis to allow better access to the upper abdomen (see Chapter 20). If this is not sufficient, the incision can be extended on one side to create a "J" incision.

The ovarian tumor should be removed intact, if possible, and a frozen histologic section obtained. If ovarian malignancy is confirmed and the tumor is apparently confined to the ovaries or the pelvis, thorough surgical staging should be carried out. This involves the following steps:

1. **Any free fluid, especially in the pelvic cul-de-sac, should be submitted for cytologic evaluation.**

2. **If no free fluid is present, peritoneal "washings" should be performed by instilling and recovering 50 to 100 dL of saline from the pelvic cul-de-sac, each paracolic gutter, and from beneath each hemidiaphragm.** Obtaining the specimens from under the diaphragms can be facilitated with the use of a red rubber catheter attached to the end of a bulb syringe.

3. **A systematic exploration of all the intra-abdominal surfaces and viscera is performed.** This should proceed in a clockwise fashion from the cecum cephalad along the paracolic gutter and the ascending colon to the right kidney, the liver and gallbladder, the right hemidiaphragm, the entrance to the lesser sac at the para-aortic area, across the transverse colon to the left hemidiaphragm, and down the left gutter and the descending colon to the rectosigmoid colon. The small intestine and its mesentery from the ligament of Treitz to the cecum should be inspected.

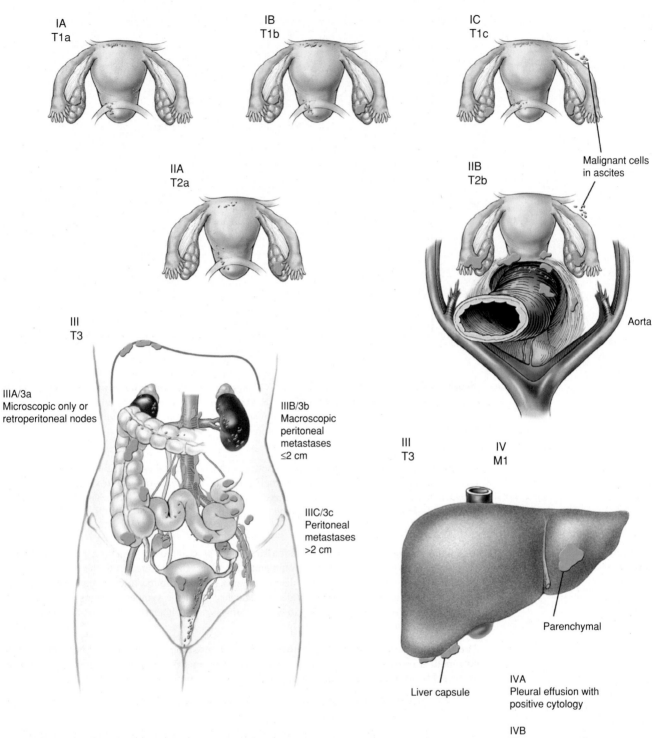

Figure 11.8 Staging ovarian cancer (FIGO and TNM). Updated and redrawn from **Heintz APM, Odicino F, Maisonneuve P, et al.** Carcinoma of the ovary. 26th Annual Report on the Results of Treatment in Gynaecological Cancer. *Int J Gynaecol Obstet.* 2006;95(suppl 1):S161–S192, with permission.

Table 11.1 FIGO Staging Cancer of the Ovary, Fallopian Tube, and Peritoneum (2014)

FIGO		TNM
Ov	**Primary tumor, ovary**	**Tov**
FT	**Primary tumor, fallopian tube**	**Tft**
P	**Primary tumor, peritoneum**	**Tp**
X	**Primary tumor cannot be assessed**	**Tx**
Designate histologic type:		
High-Grade Serous (HGS), Endometrioid (E), Clear Cell (CC), Mucinous (M), Low-Grade Serous (LG), Other or cannot be classified (O); Germ Cell (GC), Sex-Cord Stromal Cell Tumor (SC)		
Stage I	**Tumor confined to ovaries or fallopian tube(s)**	**T1**
IA	Tumor limited to one ovary (capsule intact) or fallopian tube	**T1a**
	No tumor on ovarian or fallopian tube surface	
	No malignant cells in the ascites or peritoneal washings	
IB	Tumor limited to both ovaries (capsules intact) or fallopian tubes	**T1b**
	No tumor on ovarian or fallopian tube surface	
	No malignant cells in the ascites or peritoneal washings	
IC	Tumor limited to one or both ovaries or fallopian tubes, with any of the following:	**T1c**
IC1	Surgical spill intraoperatively	
IC2	Capsule ruptured before surgery or tumor on ovarian or fallopian tube surface	
IC3	Malignant cells in the ascites or peritoneal washings	
Stage II	**Tumor involves one or both ovaries or fallopian tubes with pelvic extension (below pelvic brim) or peritoneal cancer (Tp)**	**T2**
IIA	Extension and/or implants on the uterus and/or fallopian tubes/and/or ovaries	**T2a**
IIB	Extension to other pelvic intraperitoneal tissues	**T2b**
Stage III	**Tumor involves one or both ovaries, fallopian tubes, or peritoneal cancer, with cytologically or histologically confirmed spread to the peritoneum outside the pelvis and/or metastasis to the retroperitoneal lymph nodes**	**T3**
IIIA	Metastasis to the retroperitoneal lymph nodes with or without microscopic peritoneal involvement beyond the pelvis	**T1, T2, T3aN1**
IIIA1	Positive retroperitoneal lymph nodes only (cytologically or histologically proven)	
IIIA1(i)	Metastasis ≤10 mm in greatest dimension	
IIIA1(ii)	Metastasis >10 mm in greatest dimension	
IIIA2	Microscopic extrapelvic (above the pelvic brim) peritoneal involvement with or without positive retroperitoneal lymph nodes	**T3a/T3aN1**
IIIB	Macroscopic peritoneal metastases beyond the pelvic brim ≤2 cms in greatest dimension, with or without metastasis to the retroperitoneal lymph nodes	**T3b/T3bN1**
IIIC	Macroscopic peritoneal metastases beyond the pelvic brim >2 cms in greatest dimension, with or without metastases to the retroperitoneal nodes (Note 1)	**T3c/T3cN1**
Stage IV	**Distant metastasis excluding peritoneal metastases**	**Any T, Any N, M1**
IVA	Pleural effusion with positive cytology	
IVB	Metastases to extra-abdominal organs (including inguinal lymph nodes and lymph nodes outside of abdominal cavity)	
Note 1: Includes extension of tumor to capsule of liver and spleen without parenchymal involvement of either organ		
Note 2: Parenchymal metastases are stage IVB		

(Continued)

Table 11.1 FIGO Staging Cancer of the Ovary, Fallopian Tube, and Peritoneum (2014) (*Continued*)

Carcinoma of the ovary–fallopian tube–peritoneum—Stage grouping

FIGO			UICC
(Designate primary: Tov, Tft, Tp, or Tx)			
Stage	T	N	M
IA	T1a	N0	M0
IB	T1b	N0	M0
IC	T1c	N0	M0
IIA	T2a	N0	M0
IIB	T2b	N0	M0
IIC	T2c	N0	M0
IIIA	T3a	N0	M0
	T3a	N1	M0
IIIB	T3b	N0	M0
	T3b	N1	M0
IIIC	T3c	N0–1	M0
	T3c	N1	M0
IV	Any T	Any N	M1

Regional Nodes (N)

Nx	Regional lymph nodes cannot be assessed
N0	No regional lymph node metastasis
N1	Regional lymph node metastasis

Distant Metastasis (M)

Mx	Distant metastasis cannot be assessed
M0	No distant metastasis
M1	Distant metastasis (excluding peritoneal metastasis)

Notes:

1. The primary site—that is, ovary, fallopian tube, or peritoneum—should be designated where possible. In some cases, it may not be possible to clearly delineate the primary site, and these should be listed as "undesignated."
2. The histologic type should be recorded.
3. The staging includes a revision of the stage III patients and allotment to stage IIIA1 is based on spread to the retroperitoneal lymph nodes without intraperitoneal dissemination, because an analysis of these patients indicates that their survival is significantly better than those who have intraperitoneal dissemination.
4. Involvement of retroperitoneal lymph nodes must be proven cytologically or histologically.
5. Extension of tumor from omentum to spleen or liver (stage IIIC) should be differentiated from isolated parenchymal splenic or liver metastases (stage IVB).

*FIGO Committee on Gynecologic Oncology.** Pratt J on behalf of FIGO committee. Staging classification for cancer of ovary, fallopian tube and peritoneum. *Internat J Gynaecol Obstet* 2014;124(1):1–5 (160).

4. **Any suspicious areas or adhesions on the peritoneal surfaces should be biopsied.** If there is no evidence of disease, multiple intraperitoneal biopsies should be performed. The peritoneum of the pelvic cul-de-sac, both paracolic gutters, the peritoneum over the bladder, and the intestinal mesenteries should be biopsied.

5. **The diaphragm should be sampled either by biopsy or by scraping with a tongue depressor and making a cytologic smear** (171). Biopsies of any irregularities on the surface of the diaphragm can be facilitated by use of the laparoscope and the associated biopsy instrument.

6. **The omentum should be resected from the transverse colon, a procedure called an *infracolic omentectomy.*** The procedure is initiated on the underside of the greater omentum,

where the peritoneum is incised just a few millimeters away from the transverse colon. The branches of the gastroepiploic vessels are clamped, ligated, and divided, along with all the small branching vessels that feed the infracolic omentum. If the gastrocolic ligament is palpably normal, it does not need to be resected.

7. **The retroperitoneal spaces should be dissected and explored to evaluate the pelvic lymph nodes.** The pelvic retroperitoneal dissection is performed by incising the peritoneum over the psoas muscles. This may be done on the ipsilateral side only for unilateral tumors. Any enlarged lymph nodes should be resected and submitted for frozen section. If no metastases are present, a formal pelvic lymphadenectomy should be performed.

8. **The para-aortic area should be explored.** A vertical incision should be made cephalad in the paracolic gutter and an oblique incision across the posterior parietal peritoneum from the right iliac fossa to the ligament of Treitz. The right colon can then be mobilized and the para-aortic lymph nodes exposed. Any enlarged nodes should be removed and at least the nodes caudal to the inferior mesenteric artery resected (172).

Results

As many as three in ten patients whose tumor appears confined to the pelvis will have occult metastatic disease in the upper abdomen or the retroperitoneal lymph nodes. At surgical staging, metastases in apparent low-stage epithelial ovarian cancer have been reported in the diaphragm in approximately 7% of patients, in para-aortic lymph nodes in 15%, pelvic nodes in 6%, omentum in 9%, and peritoneal cytology in 26% (135,166–169).

The importance of careful initial surgical staging is emphasized by the findings of a cooperative national study (166) in which 100 patients with apparent Stages I and II disease, who were referred for subsequent therapy, underwent surgical staging. In this series, 28% of the patients initially thought to have stage I disease were "upstaged," as were 43% of those thought to have stage II. A total of 31% of the patients were upstaged as a result of additional surgery, and 77% were reclassified as having stage III disease. **Histologic grade was a significant predictor of occult metastasis;** 16% of the patients with grade 1 lesions were upstaged, compared to 34% with grade 2 and 46% with grade 3.

After a comprehensive staging laparotomy, only a minority of women will have local disease (FIGO stage I). Of the 21,650 women diagnosed yearly with epithelial ovarian cancer in the United States, only about 4,000 have disease confined to the ovaries (1,173). The prognosis for these patients depends on the clinical–pathologic features, as outlined below. Because of this emphasis on the importance of surgical staging, the rate of lymph node sampling has increased in the United States, with a study showing that for women with stages I and II disease, the percentage having lymph nodes sampled increased from 38% to 59% from 1991 to 1996 (174).

Early-Stage Ovarian Cancer

The primary treatment for stage I epithelial ovarian cancer is surgical—that is, a total abdominal hysterectomy, bilateral salpingo-oophorectomy, and surgical staging (166,175). In certain circumstances, a unilateral oophorectomy may be permitted, as discussed below. Based on the prognostic variables outlined above (135,141,152–161,163,164,175), early-stage epithelial ovarian cancer can be subdivided into low-risk and high-risk disease (Table 11.2).

Table 11.2 Prognostic Variables in Early-Stage Epithelial Ovarian Cancer	
Low-Risk	*High-Risk*
Low-grade	High-grade
Intact capsule	Tumor growth through capsule
No surface excrescences	Surface excrescences
No ascites	Ascites
Negative peritoneal cytologic findings	Malignant cells in fluid
Unruptured or intraoperative rupture	Preoperative rupture
No dense adherence	Dense adherence
Diploid tumor	Aneuploid tumor

Borderline Tumors

The principal treatment of borderline ovarian tumors is surgical resection of the primary tumor (4,176–183). There are no data to suggest that either adjuvant chemotherapy or radiation therapy improves survival (184–186). After a frozen section has determined that the histology is borderline, premenopausal patients who desire preservation of ovarian function may be managed with a "conservative" operation—that is, a unilateral oophorectomy (4,177,179). In a study of patients who underwent unilateral ovarian cystectomy only for apparent stage I borderline serous tumors, Lim-Tan et al. (178) found that this conservative operation was also safe, only 8% of the patients having recurrences 2 to 18 years later, all with curable disease confined to the ovaries. Recurrence was associated with "positive margins" of the removed ovarian cyst.

In a retrospective series of 339 patients by Zanetta et al. (182), seven (2%) progressed to invasive carcinoma, five serous, and two mucinous tumors. **Although the recurrence rate after fertility-sparing surgery was 18.5% versus 4.6% after nonfertility-sparing surgery, all but one woman with recurrence of borderline tumor or progression to carcinoma was cured.** The disease-free survival was 99.6% for patients with stage I disease, 95.8% for stage II, and 89% for stage III. Thus, hormonal function and fertility can be maintained in the majority of patients with borderline tumors. In patients in whom an oophorectomy or cystectomy has been performed and a borderline tumor is later documented in the permanent pathology, no additional staging surgery is necessary, but the patient should be monitored with transvaginal ultrasonography.

Fertility Preservation in Early-Stage Ovarian Cancer

In patients who have undergone a thorough staging laparotomy and in whom there is no evidence of spread beyond the ovary, the uterus and contralateral ovary can be retained in women who wish to preserve fertility (187–194). **In several studies, women with stages IA–IC have undergone fertility-sparing surgery, and there have been no recurrences in women whose disease was grade 1 or 2** (189–194). **Women with grade 3 or higher-stage disease have had a significantly higher recurrence rate and lower survival.** Women who have undergone fertility-sparing surgery for low-stage, low-grade epithelial ovarian cancer should be followed carefully with routine transvaginal ultrasonography and determination of serum CA125 levels. Generally, the other ovary and the uterus should be removed at the completion of childbearing (see treatment section below).

Advanced-Stage Ovarian Cancer

The surgical management of all patients with advanced-stage disease is approached in a similar manner, with modifications made for the overall status and general health of the patient. A treatment scheme is outlined in Figure 11.9.

If the patient is medically stable, she should undergo an initial exploratory procedure with removal of as much disease as possible (195–215). **The operation to remove the primary tumor as well as the associated metastatic disease is referred to as** *debulking* or *cytoreductive surgery.* Most patients subsequently receive combination intravenous chemotherapy with an empiric number of cycles, six to eight. In some patients with completely resected disease, intra-peritoneal chemotherapy may be considered. In selected patients who are not candidates for initial cytoreductive surgery, neoadjuvant chemotherapy may be given for a few cycles before surgery, as discussed below. Second-look laparotomy has not been shown to improve outcomes and is best limited to investigational protocols (216).

The preoperative assessment of resectability is limited. Using a cutoff of 500 International Unit, CA125 levels have been suggested as a means of predicting the probability of an optimal resection (206,209), but others have shown that these determinations have low predictive value (210). **CT and MRI scans have been used to try to predict suboptimal resection** (215,217–220). In a series from the Mayo Clinic (215), the presence of diffuse peritoneal thickening and ascites on CT scan was associated with a 32% optimal debulking rate, as opposed 71% in the group that did not have these findings, with a positive predictive value of 68%. **However, in a larger multi-institutional validation study, the accuracy of CT in predicting suboptimal cytoreduction dropped to as low as 34% in some cohorts** (218). CT–PET also has limited positive predictive value (219,220).

Vergote and colleagues from Belgium reported the use of open laparoscopy in 173 patients with a pelvic mass, an omental "cake," or large volume ascites to exclude other primary tumors and to determine resectability. Seventy-one of the patients (41%) developed a port site metastasis (221). **In our experience, it is almost always possible to remove the primary**

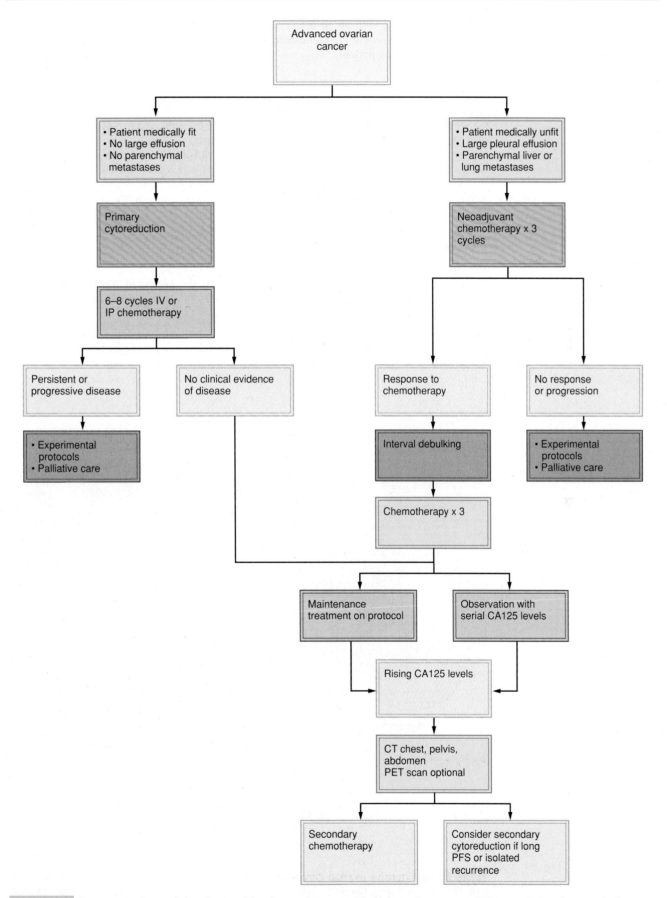

Figure 11.9 **Treatment scheme for patients with advanced-stage epithelial ovarian cancer.** PFS, progression-free survival.

tumor (if necessary, with an *en bloc* resection of the rectosigmoid colon) and the omental cake, so the major reason for recommending neoadjuvant chemotherapy is to improve the medical fitness of the patient.

Cytoreductive Surgery

Patients with advanced-stage epithelial ovarian cancer documented at initial exploratory laparotomy should undergo cytoreductive surgery (195–215). The operation typically includes the performance of a total abdominal hysterectomy and bilateral salpingo-oophorectomy, along with a complete omentectomy and resection of any metastatic lesions from the peritoneal surfaces or from the intestines. The pelvic tumor often directly involves the rectosigmoid colon, the terminal ileum, and the cecum (Fig. 11.10). In a minority of patients, most or all of the disease is confined to the pelvic viscera and the omentum so that removal of these organs will result in extirpation of all gross tumors, a situation that is associated with a reasonable chance of prolonged progression-free survival (PFS).

Theoretic Rationale

The rationale for cytoreductive surgery relates to general theoretic considerations (203,222,223): **(i) the physiologic benefits of tumor excision and (ii) the improved tumor perfusion and increased growth fraction,** both of which increase the likelihood of response to chemotherapy or radiation therapy.

Physiologic Benefits   Ascites may be sometimes reasonably well controlled after removal of the primary tumor and a large omental cake. Also, removal of the omental cake often alleviates the nausea and early satiety that many patients experience. Removal of intestinal metastases may

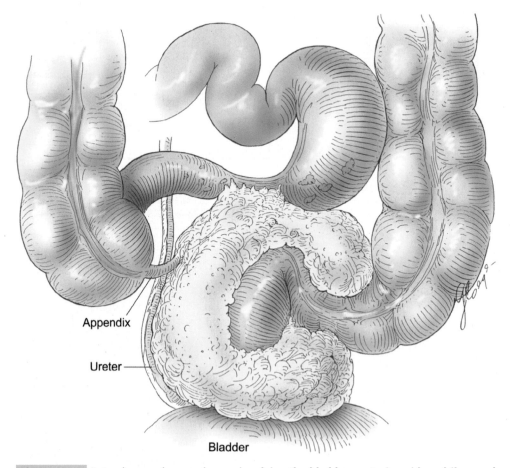

Appendix

Ureter

Bladder

Figure 11.10 Extensive ovarian carcinoma involving the bladder, rectosigmoid, and ileocecal area. From **Heintz APM, Berek JS.** Cytoreductive surgery for ovarian carcinoma. In: **Piver MS, ed.** *Ovarian Malignancies.* Edinburgh: Churchill Livingstone; 1987:134, with permission.

restore adequate intestinal function and lead to an improvement in the overall nutritional status of the patient, thereby facilitating the patient's ability to tolerate subsequent chemotherapy.

Tumor Perfusion and Cellular Kinetics   **A large, bulky tumor may contain areas that are poorly vascularized, and such areas will be exposed to suboptimal concentrations of chemotherapeutic agents.** Similarly, these areas will be poorly oxygenated, so radiation therapy, which requires adequate oxygenation to achieve maximal cell kill, will be less effective. Thus, surgical removal of bulky tumors may eliminate areas that are most likely to be relatively resistant to treatment.

In addition, larger tumor masses tend to be composed of a higher proportion of cells that are either nondividing or in the "resting" phase (i.e., G_0 cells), which are essentially resistant to the therapy. A low growth fraction is characteristic of bulky tumor masses, and cytoreductive surgery can result in smaller residual masses with a relatively higher growth fraction.

The fractional cell kill hypothesis of Skipper (222) postulates that a constant proportion of the tumor cells are destroyed with each treatment. This theory suggests that a given dose of a drug will kill a constant fraction of cells as long as the growth fraction and phenotype are the same. Therefore, a treatment that reduces a population of tumor cells from 10^9 to 10^4 cells also would reduce a population of 10^5 cells to a single cell. If the absolute number of tumor cells is lower at the initiation of treatment, then fewer cycles of therapy should be necessary to eradicate the cancer, provided that the cells are not inherently resistant to the therapy.

The larger the initial tumor burden, the longer the necessary exposure to the drug and, therefore, the greater the chance of developing acquired drug resistance. However, because the spontaneous mutation rate of tumors is an inherent property of the malignancy, the likelihood of developing phenotypic drug resistance also increases as the size of the tumor increases. **The chance of developing a clone of cells resistant to a specific agent is related to both the tumor size and its mutation frequency** (222,223). One of the inherent problems with cytoreductive surgery for large tumor masses is that phenotypic drug resistance may have already developed before any surgical intervention.

Goals of Cytoreductive Surgery

The principal goal of cytoreductive surgery is the removal of all of the primary cancer and, if possible, all metastatic disease. If resection of all metastases is not feasible, the goal should be to reduce the tumor burden by resection of all individual tumor nodules to an "optimal" status.

Griffiths (195) initially proposed that all metastatic nodules should be reduced to ≤1.5 cm in maximum diameter, and showed that survival was significantly longer in such patients. Subsequently, Hacker and Berek (197,200–203) showed that patients whose largest residual lesions were ≤5 mm had a superior survival, and this was substantiated by Hoskins et al. (199) presenting the data of the GOG. The median survival of patients in this category was 40 months, compared with 18 months for patients whose lesions were ≤1.5 cm and 6 months for patients with nodules >1.5 cm (Fig. 11.11). **Patients whose disease has been completely resected have the best prognosis, and approximately 60% of patients in this category will be free of disease at 5 years** (Fig. 11.12). **The goal of "complete resection to no residual disease" is the most optimal postoperative status** (204).

The value of complete cytoreduction was substantiated by du Bois et al. in a retrospective review of 3,126 patients with stages IIB–IV epithelial ovarian cancer who had been entered on three randomized prospective clinical trials, AGO-OVAR 3, 5, and 7 (205). In this analysis, 1,046 patients (33.3%) underwent complete resection of their disease to "no residual disease," 975 (31.3%) had their disease resected to 1 to 10 mm maximum tumor diameter, and 1,105 (35.4%) had >10 mm maximum diameter residual disease. **Progression-free and overall survivals were significantly prolonged in the completely resected group by multivariate analysis** ($p < 0.0001$).

In a study from the Mayo Clinic (206), the relative impact of disease status, patient status, and the aggressiveness of the surgeon on the resectability of disease were analyzed. Surgery by an "aggressive surgeon," presence of carcinomatosis, and ASA score were independently associated with optimal resection to <1 cm maximum residual disease.

The resectability of the metastatic tumor is usually determined by the location of the disease. Optimal cytoreduction is difficult to achieve in the presence of extensive disease on the diaphragm,

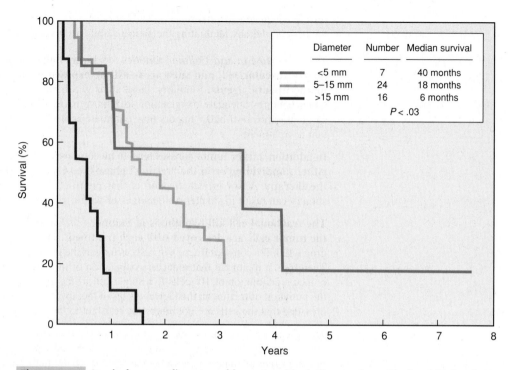

Figure 11.11 Survival versus diameter of largest residual disease. From **Hacker NF, Berek JS, Lagasse LD, et al.** Primary cytoreductive surgery for epithelial ovarian cancer. *Obstet Gynecol.* 1983; 61:413–420, with permission from the American College of Obstetricians and Gynecologists.

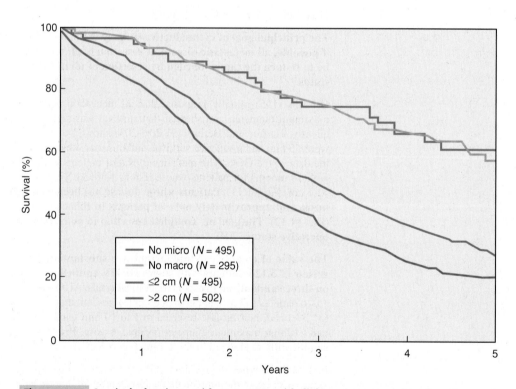

Figure 11.12 Survival of patients with stage IIIC epithelial ovarian cancer based on the maximum size of the residual tumor after exploratory laparotomy and tumor resection. From **Heintz APM, Odicino F, Maisonneuve P, et al.** Carcinoma of the ovary. 26th Annual Report on the Results of Treatment in Gynaecological Cancer. *Int J Gynaecol Obstet.* 2006;95(suppl 1):S161–S192, with permission.

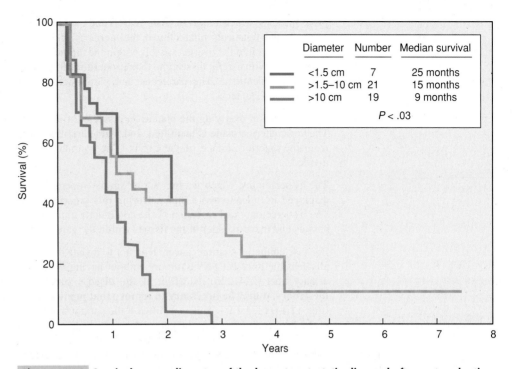

Figure 11.13 **Survival versus diameter of the largest metastatic disease before cytoreduction.** From **Hacker NF, Berek JS, Lagasse LD, et al.** Primary cytoreductive surgery for epithelial ovarian cancer. *Obstet Gynecol.* 1983;61:413–420, with permission from the American College of Obstetricians and Gynecologists.

in the parenchyma of the liver, along the base of the small-bowel mesentery, in the lesser omentum, or in the porta hepatis (211).

The ability of cytoreductive surgery to influence survival is limited by the extent of metastases before cytoreduction, possibly because of the higher likelihood of phenotypically resistant clones of cells in larger metastatic masses (197,200). Patients whose metastatic tumor is very large (i.e., >10 cm) have a shorter survival than those with smaller areas of metastatic disease (134) (Fig. 11.13) regardless of the residual disease. Even with residual lesions <5 mm diameter, extensive carcinomatosis, the presence of ascites, and poor tumor grade are poor prognostic factors (200–203,211).

Exploration

The supine position on the operating table may be sufficient for most patients. However, for those with extensive pelvic disease for whom a low resection of the colon may be necessary, the low lithotomy position should be used. Debulking operations should be performed through a vertical incision in order to gain adequate access to the upper abdomen.

After the peritoneal cavity has been opened, ascitic fluid, if present, should be evacuated. In some centers, fluid is submitted routinely for appropriate in vitro studies, particularly the clonogenic assay. In cases of massive ascites, careful attention must be given to hemodynamic monitoring, especially in patients with borderline cardiovascular function.

A thorough inspection and palpation of the peritoneal cavity and retroperitoneum should be carried out to assess the extent of the primary tumor and the metastatic disease. All abdominal viscera must be palpated to exclude the possibility that the ovarian disease is metastatic, particularly from the stomach, colon, or pancreas. **If optimal status is not considered achievable, extensive bowel and urologic resections are not indicated except to overcome a bowel obstruction. However, removal of the primary tumor and omental cake is usually both feasible and desirable.**

Pelvic Tumor Resection

The essential principle of removal of the pelvic tumor is to use the retroperitoneal approach (202,203). To accomplish this, the retroperitoneum is entered laterally, along the surface of the psoas muscles, which avoids the iliac vessels and the ureters. The procedure is initiated by division of the round ligaments bilaterally if the uterus is present. The peritoneal incision is extended cephalad, lateral to the ovarian vessels within the *infundibulopelvic ligaments* and caudally toward the bladder. With careful dissection, the retroperitoneal space is explored, and the ureter and pelvic vessels are identified. The pararectal and paravesicle spaces are identified and developed as described in Chapter 8.

The peritoneum overlying the bladder is dissected to connect the peritoneal incisions anteriorly. The vesicouterine plane is identified, and, with careful sharp dissection, the bladder is mobilized from the anterior surface of the cervix. The ovarian vessels are isolated, doubly ligated, and divided.

The hysterectomy, which is often not a "simple" operation, is performed. The ureters need to be displayed in order to avoid injury. During this procedure, the uterine vessels can be identified. The hysterectomy and resection of the contiguous tumor are completed by ligation of the uterine vessels and the remainder of the tissues within the cardinal ligaments.

Because epithelial ovarian cancers tend not to invade the lumina of the colon or bladder, it is usually feasible to resect pelvic tumors without having to resect portions of the lower colon or the urinary tract (224–226). However, **if the disease surrounds the rectosigmoid colon and its mesentery, it may be necessary to remove that portion of the colon to clear the pelvic disease** (Fig. 11.14) (224,225). This is justified if the patient will be left with "optimal" disease at the end of the cytoreduction. After the pararectal space has been identified in such patients, the proximal site of colonic involvement is identified, the colon and its mesentery are divided, and the rectosigmoid is removed along with the uterus *en bloc*. A reanastomosis of the colon is performed, as described in Chapter 20.

It is rarely necessary to resect portions of the lower urinary tract (226). Occasionally, resection of a small portion of the bladder may be required. If so, a cystotomy should be performed to

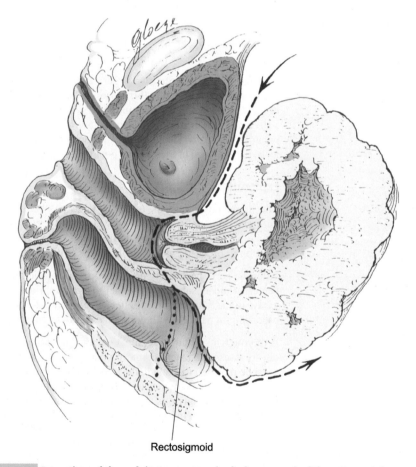

Rectosigmoid

Figure 11.14 Resection of the pelvic tumor may include removal of the uterus, tubes, and ovaries, as well as portions of the lower intestinal tract. The *arrows* represent the plane of resection.

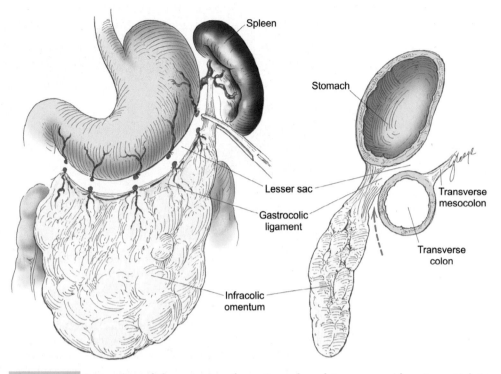

Figure 11.15 **Separation of the omentum from stomach and transverse colon.** From **Heintz APM, Berek JS.** Cytoreductive surgery for ovarian carcinoma. In: **Piver MS, ed.** *Ovarian Malignancies*. Edinburgh: Churchill Livingstone; 1987:134, with permission.

assist in resection of the disease. Rarely, partial ureteric resection may be necessary, followed by primary reanastomosis (ureteroureterostomy), ureteroneocystostomy, or transureteroureterostomy, as described in Chapter 20.

Omentectomy

Advanced epithelial ovarian cancer often completely replaces the omentum, forming an omental cake. This disease may be adherent to the parietal peritoneum of the anterior abdominal wall, making entry into the abdominal cavity difficult. After freeing the omentum from any adhesions to parietal peritoneum, adherent loops of small intestine are freed by sharp dissection. The omentum is then lifted and pulled gently in the cranial direction, exposing the attachment of the infracolic omentum to the transverse colon. The peritoneum is incised to open the appropriate plane, which is developed by sharp dissection along the serosa of the transverse colon. Small vessels are ligated with hemoclips. The omentum is then separated from the greater curvature of the stomach by ligation of the right and left gastroepiploic arteries and ligation of the short gastric arteries (Fig. 11.15).

The disease in the gastrocolic ligament can extend to the hilum of the spleen and splenic flexure of the colon on the left and to the capsule of the liver and the hepatic flexure of the colon on the right. Usually, the disease does not invade the parenchyma of the liver or spleen, and a plane can be found between the tumor and these organs. However, **it will occasionally be necessary to perform splenectomy to remove all the omental disease** (212,226–229) (Fig. 11.16). Diaphragmatic stripping and diaphragmatic resection have been used to optimally resect upper abdominal disease in selected cases (212).

Intestinal Resection

The disease may involve focal areas of the small or large intestine, and resection should be performed if it would permit the removal of all or most of the abdominal metastases. Apart from the rectosigmoid colon, the most frequent sites of intestinal metastasis are the terminal ileum, the cecum, and the transverse colon. Resection of one or more of these segments of bowel may be necessary (224–229).

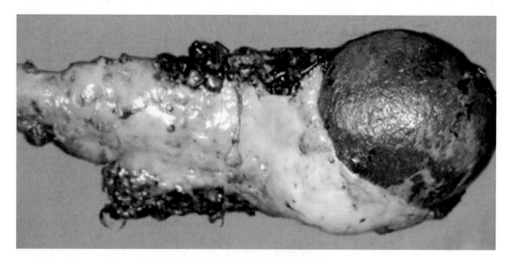

Figure 11.16 Omental "cake" densely adherent to the spleen.

Resection of Other Metastases

A discussion of extended upper abdominal resection for debulking operations is presented in Chapter 20. Other large masses of tumor that are located on the parietal peritoneum should be removed, particularly if they are isolated masses, and their removal would permit optimal cytore-duction. The use of the Cavitron Ultrasonic Surgical Aspirator (CUSA), the argon beam laser, and the loop electrosurgical device may help facilitate resection of small tumor nodules, especially those on flat surfaces (230–232).

Resection of Pelvic and Para-aortic Lymph Nodes

The performance of a pelvic and para-aortic lymphadenectomy in patients with stage IIIC–IV disease has been reported to prolong survival (138), but an international randomized study failed to confirm this (233). **Patients who were optimally cytoreduced in the peritoneal cavity were randomized between systematic pelvic and para-aortic lymphadenectomy versus resection of bulky nodes only.** There were 216 evaluable patients in the systematic lymphadenectomy arm and 211 in the nodal debulking arm of the study. Patients in each group were well matched for clinical characteristics such as stage of disease, grade of tumor, and residual disease status. Although there was a 6-month improvement in PFS, **there was no difference in 5-year overall survival** (48.5% vs. 47%, respectively; 95% confidence interval [CI]—8.4–10.6%).

Du Bois et al. (234) analyzed the three phase III German trials (AGO-OVAR 3, 5, 7) to retrospec-tively determine the role of lymphadenectomy. In this analysis, 3,336 patients were evaluated, of whom 1,059 (32%) had no macroscopic residual intraperitoneal disease. Retroperitoneal lymph-adenectomy was performed in 757 of the 1,059 patients (72%), and there was a significant survival advantage for the group having the lymphadenectomy (66% vs. 55%; $p = 0.003$). No advantage could be demonstrated if there was any macroscopic residual disease. There may have been a selection bias in the patients having the lymphadenectomy, and resolution of this issue will require a further randomized controlled trial.

Feasibility and Outcome

An analysis of the retrospective data available suggests that these operations are feasible in 70–90% of patients when performed by gynecologic oncologists (201,203,206,209,212). Major morbidity is in the range of 5% and operative mortality in the range of 1% (178,183). Intestinal resection in these patients does not appear to increase the overall morbidity of the operation (200,202,206,235). Patients with stage IV disease can also benefit from optimal cytoreduction (207,236,237).

In a meta-analysis of 81 studies of women who had undergone cytoreductive surgery for advanced ovarian cancer, Bristow et al. (236) documented that the greater the percentage of tumor reduction, the longer the survival. Each 10% increase in cytoreduction equated to a 5.5% increase in median survival. Women whose cytoreduction was greater than 75% of their tumor burden had a median survival of 33.9 months compared with 22.7 months for women whose tumors were cytoreduced to less than 75% ($p < 0.001$).

Interval Cytoreductive Surgery	**A prospective randomized study of "interval" cytoreductive surgery was reported by the European Organization for the Research and Treatment of Cancer (EORTC) in 1995.** Interval surgery was performed after three cycles of platinum-combination chemotherapy in patients whose primary attempt at cytoreduction was suboptimal. Patients in the surgical arm of the study demonstrated a survival benefit when compared with those who did not undergo interval debulking (238). In a 10-year follow-up analysis, the risk of mortality was reduced by more than 40% in the group that was randomized to the debulking arm of the study (239). A prospective phase III study of interval cytoreductive surgery conducted by the GOG (240) failed to confirm these findings: The median survival of the 216 women who underwent interval cytoreduction was 32 months, compared with 33 months for the 209 women who did not undergo cytoreduction. This analysis reflected the fact that all patients had initially been operated on by a gynecologic oncologist, so they had already undergone a maximal attempt at tumor resection (241).

Several investigators suggested that neoadjuvant chemotherapy followed by an interval cytoreduction might be appropriate in women whose performance status was poor (242–245). In 2010, Vergote et al. (246) reported the results of **a randomized EORTC-NCIC (National Cancer Institute of Canada) study of primary debulking surgery (PDS) versus three cycles of neoadjuvant chemotherapy followed by interval debulking surgery in 670 patients with Stages IIIC–IV epithelial ovarian, fallopian tube, and peritoneal cancer.** All the patients were reported to have had extensive stage IIIC or IV disease. Just over 60% had metastatic lesions that were larger than 10 cm in diameter, and 74.5% had lesions larger than 5 cm. Patients were randomly assigned either to PDS followed by at least six courses of platinum-based chemotherapy or to three courses of neoadjuvant platinum-based chemotherapy followed by interval debulking surgery in all patients with a response or stable disease, followed by at least three further courses of platinum-based chemotherapy. The primary end point of the study was overall survival. The group undergoing PDS was considered to be the standard-treatment group. The median overall survival was 29 months in the primary-surgery group and 30 months in the neoadjuvant chemotherapy group. **The median PFS in both groups was 12 months suggesting that the study included a relatively poor prognostic subset of patients. There was lower morbidity and mortality reported in the group that received neoadjuvant chemotherapy.** Postoperative death (defined as death within 28 days after surgery) occurred in 2.5% of patients in the primary-surgery group and in 0.7% of patients in the neoadjuvant chemotherapy group. Grade 3 or 4 hemorrhage occurred in 7.4% of patients after primary debulking and in 4.1% after interval debulking, infection in 8.1% and 1.7%, respectively, and venous complications in 2.6% and 0%, respectively.

Complete tumor resection was the strongest independent predictor of overall survival in both groups. The results of this study have been widely debated and the findings criticized by a number of authors (247–250). In an analysis of this study, Du Bois et al. noted that the patients recruited to this study had a poorer performance status than those in most upfront randomized trials, and that the complete resection rates varied considerably from country to country and were considered to be low (247). In the PDS group, only about 20% of patients were completely cytoreduced to no residual disease, which is much lower than what would be expected in experienced centers. Indeed, there were very different optimal debulking rates reported in different countries, ranging from 62% in Belgium to 3.9% in the Netherlands suggesting very variable surgical expertise. **The median OS was only 30 months, which is considerably less than the 60+ months expected with optimal cytoreduction followed by chemotherapy, suggesting that the study included a poor performance status cohort of patients with very advanced disease.**

There have been two other randomized trials of neoadjuvant chemotherapy that have completed enrollment. The first study is the chemotherapy or upfront surgery (CHORUS) trial, which had a similar design to the EORTC trial and was conducted in the United Kingdom. It was reported at ASCO in 2013 (251). The CHORUS study had very similar findings to the EORTC study. They randomized 552 patients to receive either neoadjuvant chemotherapy followed by interval debulking and then three additional cycles, or to have PDS followed by six cycles of platinum-based chemotherapy. The optimal debulking rate was only 16% in the PDS group, compared to 40% following neoadjuvant chemotherapy. The median duration of surgery was only 120 minutes in both groups, which is clearly not long enough for aggressive debulking surgery. There was a 5.6% postoperative mortality rate in the PDS group, which is much higher than expected and may reflect patient selection. The median PFS was approximately 11 months in both groups and the median survival similar at 2 years. The Japanese GOG (JGOG) is also conducting a trial comparing PDS followed by eight cycles of chemotherapy to four cycles of neoadjuvant chemotherapy followed by surgery and four more cycles of chemotherapy, and the results of this study are pending.

There remain very divergent views regarding the place of neoadjuvant chemotherapy. A survey of SGO members found the 82% felt there was not enough evidence to justify the use of neoadjuvant chemotherapy (252). In contrast, 70% of ESGO members felt there was sufficient evidence to recommend neoadjuvant chemotherapy.

Based on the above considerations, the performance of a debulking operation as early as possible in the course of the patient's treatment should be considered the standard of care (253). Neoadjuvant chemotherapy followed by interval debulking should be reserved for patients with a poor performance and nutritional status, as these patients will usually have decreased postoperative morbidity if given chemotherapy prior to their planned debulking operation. These are usually patients with large volume ascites or pleural effusions.

Surgical Experience and Outcome	**Wright and colleagues studied 28,651 women who underwent surgery for ovarian cancer in the United States from 1998 to 2007, using data from The Nationwide Inpatient Sample (250). They reported that the operative complication rate increased with age**—from 17.1% in women under age 50 years, to 29.7% in women 70 to 79 years of age and 31.5% in women 80 years and older. The occurrence of two perioperative complications and initiation of chemotherapy longer than 12 weeks after the primary surgery were associated with lower survival rates.

In addition, there is evidence that the survival of women with advanced ovarian cancer is improved when the surgeon is specifically trained to perform cytoreductive surgery (254) and when there is centralization of care (255). **Whenever feasible, patients with advanced ovarian malignancy should be referred to a subspecialty unit for primary surgery, and every effort should be made to attain as complete a cytoreduction as possible.**

Treatment with Chemotherapy and Radiation

Early-Stage Low-risk Ovarian Cancer	In 1984, Guthrie et al. (175) studied the outcome of 656 patients with early-stage epithelial ovarian cancer. No untreated patients who had stage IA, grade 1 cancer died of their disease so adjuvant therapy was not necessary. Furthermore, in 1990 the GOG reported the results of a prospective, randomized trial of observation versus *melphalan* for patients with stages IA and IB, grades 1 and 2 disease. **Five-year survival for each group was 94% and 96%, respectively, confirming that no further adjuvant treatment was needed for such patients** (256).
Early-Stage High-risk Ovarian Cancer	In patients with high-risk features—for example, poorly differentiated carcinoma or with capsular involvement or evidence of malignant cells either in ascitic fluid or in peritoneal washings—additional therapy is indicated. Treatment options include adjuvant chemotherapy, whole-abdominal radiation, or pelvic radiation plus chemotherapy in selected subsets (177–202,216). These adjuvant treatment options are summarized below.
Chemotherapy	**Chemotherapy for patients with early-stage high-risk epithelial ovarian cancer can be either single agent *carboplatin* or platinum/taxane combination chemotherapy** (256–264). Historically, *cisplatin* or *cyclophosphamide* or both (PC) were used to treat patients with stage I disease (265–276). In a GOG trial of three cycles of *cisplatin* and *cyclophosphamide* versus intraperitoneal ^{32}P in patients with stages IB and IC disease, the PFS of women receiving the platinum-based chemotherapy was 31% higher than that of those receiving the radiocolloid (267). Similar results were reported from a multicenter trial performed in Italy by the Gruppo Italiano Collaborativo Oncologica Ginecologica for PFS, although there was no overall survival advantage (275). *Carboplatin* **can be substituted for** *cisplatin* **in these patients because it is much better tolerated, has fewer side effects, and has similar efficacy** (276).

Two large, parallel, randomized phase III clinical trials have been conducted in women with early-stage disease: The **International Collaborative Ovarian Neoplasm Trial 1 (ICON1)** and the **Adjuvant Chemotherapy Trial in Ovarian Neoplasia (ACTION)** (276,277).

In the ICON1 trial, 477 patients from 84 centers in Europe were entered. Patients of all stages were eligible for the trial if, in the opinion of the investigator, it was unclear whether adjuvant therapy would be of benefit. Most patients were said to have stages I and IIA disease, but optimal **surgical staging was not required,** so it is likely that a number of these women really had stage III disease. Adjuvant platinum-based chemotherapy was given to 241 patients, and no adjuvant chemotherapy was given to 236 patients. **The 5-year survival was 73% in the group that received adjuvant chemotherapy compared with 62% in the control group** (hazard ratio [HR] = 0.65, $p = 0.01$) (277).

In the ACTION trial, 440 patients from 40 European centers were randomized; 224 patients received adjuvant platinum-based chemotherapy, and 224 patients did not (276). Patients with stages I and IIA grades 2 and 3 were eligible. Only **one-third of the total group was optimally staged** (151 patients). **In the observation arm, optimal staging was associated with a better survival** (HR = 2.31, $p = 0.03$); **in the nonoptimally staged patients, adjuvant chemotherapy was associated with an improved survival** (HR = 1.78, $p = 0.009$). **In optimally staged patients, no benefit of adjuvant chemotherapy was seen** (Fig. 11.17). Therefore, in the ACTION trial, the benefit from adjuvant chemotherapy was limited to the patients with suboptimal staging, suggesting that patients might only benefit if they had a higher likelihood of occult microscopic dissemination.

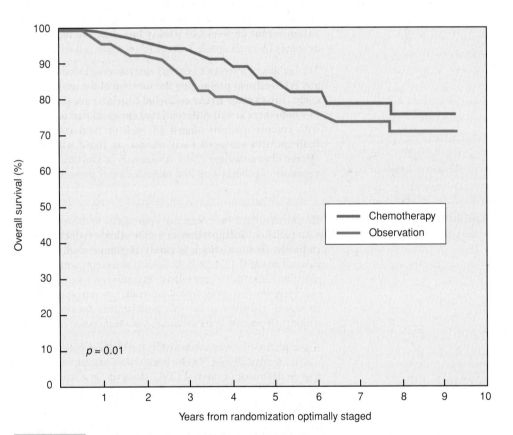

Figure 11.17 **Overall survival in patients with optimally staged early-stage ovarian cancer** (ACTION Trial). Adjuvant chemotherapy patients (*n* = 224 patients) (*purple line*) were those patients who received immediate adjuvant chemotherapy versus Observation patients (*n* = 224) (*blue line*) were those patients who were observed until adjuvant chemotherapy was indicated. The hazard ratio is 1.45 (95% CI = 0.93 to 2.27, $p = 0.01$ using log-rank test). Five-year survivals were 85% for the adjuvant chemotherapy group versus 78% for those who did not receive adjuvant chemotherapy. Reproduced with permission from **Trimbos JB, Vergote I, Bolis G, et al.** Impact of adjuvant chemotherapy and surgical staging in early-stage ovarian carcinoma: European Organisation for Research and Treatment of Cancer-Adjuvant Chemotherapy in Ovarian Neoplasm Trial. *J Natl Cancer Inst.* 2003;95:113–125.

When the data from the two trials were combined and analyzed (278), a total of 465 patients were randomized to receive platinum-based adjuvant chemotherapy and 460 to observation until disease progression. After a median follow-up of more than 4 years, the overall survival was 82% in the chemotherapy arm and 74% in the observation arm (HR = 0.67, p = 0.001). Recurrence-free survival was also better in the chemotherapy arm: 76% versus 65% (HR = 0.64, p = 0.001). The results of this analysis must be interpreted with caution because most of the patients did not undergo thorough surgical staging, but the findings suggest that platinum-based chemotherapy should be given to patients who have not been optimally staged or who have high-risk pathologic features.

The GOG reported the results of a randomized study of three cycles versus six cycles of *carboplatin* and *paclitaxel* in 457 patients with early-stage ovarian cancer (232). An unexpectedly large number of patients (126, or approximately 28%) had incomplete or inadequately documented surgical staging. The recurrence rate was 24% lower (HR = 0.76, CI = 0.5–1.13, p = 0.18) for six versus three cycles, but this was not statistically significant. The estimated probability of recurrence at 5 years was 20.1% for six cycles and 25.4% for three cycles. They concluded that three cycles of adjuvant *carboplatin* and *paclitaxel* was a reasonable option for women with high-risk early-stage ovarian cancer. In a subset analysis of this study, patients with high-grade serous cancers had a lower risk of recurrence with six cycles of chemotherapy compared with three cycles (HR = 0.33, CI = 0.14 to 0.77; p = 0.04) while this was not the case for the nonserous tumors. Further studies are needed to confirm these findings (279).

The current ongoing GOG trial includes patients with high-risk stages I and II disease, and offers three cycles of *carboplatin* and *paclitaxel* followed by a randomization to either observation versus 26 weeks of weekly low-dose (40 mg/m^2) *paclitaxel.* High-risk stage I is defined as stages IA or IB, grade 3, stage IC, or clear cell carcinomas.

The authors of a recent Cochrane analysis concluded that "adjuvant platinum-based chemotherapy is effective in prolonging the survival of the majority of patients who are assessed as having early (FIGO stage I/IIA) epithelial ovarian cancer. However, it may be withheld from women in whom there is well-differentiated encapsulated unilateral disease (stage IA, grade 1) or those with comprehensively staged IB, well or moderately differentiated (grade 1 to 2) disease." Patients with unstaged early disease or those with poorly differentiated tumors should be offered chemotherapy (280). A summary of randomized phase III trials reported since 1995 for the treatment of patients with low-stage disease is presented in Table 11.3 (241,246,254,256,260).

Radiation Therapy

Historically, there have been two approaches to the treatment of low-stage epithelial ovarian cancer with radiation: Intraperitoneal radiocolloids (which is no longer used), and whole-abdominal radiation therapy, which is rarely recommended. In one retrospective study of ^{32}P, the 5-year survival was 85% (256,267). In a series of patients with stage I disease treated with whole-abdominal radiation (261), the 5-year relapse-free survival rate was 78%, but many of these patients had high-risk variables (e.g., poor histologic grade). A retrospective examination of early trials using whole abdominal radiation as the sole postoperative treatment in ovarian cancer has suggested that the majority of patients in these studies who were cured had the nonserous subtypes (268).

A prospective trial was conducted by the GOG of patients with stage IB, grade 3, stage IC, or stage II with no residual disease. Twelve cycles of *melphalan* were compared with intraperitoneal ^{32}P, and there was no difference in survival (256). However, in a multicenter Italian trial (271), a randomized comparison of six cycles of *cisplatin* as a single agent versus ^{32}P showed an 84% disease-free survival with *cisplatin* and 61% with ^{32}P (p < 0.01). Furthermore, the GOG protocol that randomized *cisplatin* and *cyclophosphamide* versus ^{32}P showed that the platinum-based chemotherapy was superior (267). Therefore, although ^{32}P produces results similar to single-agent *melphalan*, platinum-based chemotherapy is preferable, and melphalan and ^{32}P are of historical interest only (Table 11.3).

There has been a resurgence of interest in the role of whole abdominal radiation following the recent report of a population-based study from British Columbia that suggested that whole abdominal radiation provided a survival benefit when added to chemotherapy, particularly in low-stage, nonserous cancers (269). This study retrospectively examined the outcomes for 703 patients with stages I or II ovarian cancer, of whom 351 had radiotherapy based on physician choice (270). Surgery consisted of abdominal hysterectomy, bilateral salpingo-oophorectomy, omentectomy, washings, and removal of suspicion nodes. Patients were treated with three cycles of platinum based chemotherapy alone, or followed by pelvic and whole abdominal

Table 11.3 Randomized Trials in Stage I Epithelial Ovarian Cancer (Since 1995)

Study	Patients (Author)	Stages	Treatment	Best Arm
Italian Cooperative (271)	47 (Bolis et al., 1995)	Stage I low risk	Observation vs. *cisplatin* × 6	No difference
Italian Cooperative (271)	104 (Bolis et al., 1995)	Stage I high risk	^{32}P vs. *cisplatin* × 6	*Cisplatin* 79% vs. 69% 5-yr survival
GOG 7601 (256)	81 (Young et al., 2003)	Stage I low risk	Observation vs. *melphalan*	No difference
GOG 7602 (256)	141 (Young et al., 2003)	Stage I high risk, II	^{32}P vs. *melphalan*	No difference
GOG 95 (267)	205 (Young et al., 2003)	Stage I high risk, II	*Cisplatin* 75 mg/m^2; *cyclophosphamide* 750 mg/m^2 vs. ^{32}P	*Cisplatin, cyclophosphamide* 77% vs. 66% 5-yr survival
Scandinavian Cooperative (274)	134 (Tropé et al., 2003)	Stage I high risk	*Carboplatin* AUC × vs. observation	No difference
ICON1 (277)	477 (Trimbos et al., 2003)	Most stage I and II, optimal staging not required	Platinum-based vs. observation	73% (chemotherapy) vs. 62% (observation) 5-yr survival
ACTION (276)	448 (Trimbos et al., 2003)	Stage I high risk, IIA, one-third staged	Platinum-based vs. observation	Improved survival in optimally staged patients only
ICON1–ACTION (278)	925 (Trimbos et al., 2003)	Combined analysis		82% (chemotherapy) vs. 72% (observation) 5-yr survival
GOG 157 (281)	421 (Bell et al., 2006)	Stage I high risk/II	*Paclitaxel* 175 mg/m^2; *carboplatin* AUC 7.5 3 vs. six cycles	Three cycles equivalent to six cycles of chemotherapy
GOG 175	Accruing	Stage I high risk/II	*Paclitaxel* 175 mg/m^2; *carboplatin* AUC 6 followed by observation vs. *paclitaxel* 40 mg/m^2 weekly × 26 wks	

GOG, Gynecologic Oncology Group; AUC, area under the curve.

radiation at a dose of 22.5 Gy to the pelvis in 10 fractions and 22.5 Gy in 22 fractions to the whole abdomen. An additional three cycles of chemotherapy were administered to patients who were not offered, or who declined, radiotherapy. **There was a 40% reduction in disease-specific mortality and a 43% reduction in overall mortality in patients with clear cell, endometrioid, and mucinous cancers.** Patients with serous cancers did not appear to benefit from the adjuvant irradiation. This finding is biologically plausible, given that nonserous tumors are more likely to be confined to the pelvis in contrast to high-grade serous cancers, which disseminate early throughout the peritoneal cavity.

The same group later reported **a separate analysis of 241 patients with stage I or II clear cell ovarian cancer** (270). They found that adjuvant irradiation was associated with improved disease-free survival, and it reduced pelvic relapse rates from 76–62%. Abdominal recurrence occurred in 42% with chemotherapy and only 13% with whole-abdominal and pelvic irradiation. **The 5-year disease-free survival was 25% with chemotherapy and 81% with irradiation.** They found that patients with stage IA/B and IC disease with rupture only did not appear to benefit from additional radiation as they had a relatively good prognosis (5- and 10-year disease-free survival rates were 92% and 71%, respectively). **Radiotherapy appeared to be of particular benefit for patients with stage IC based on positive cytology or surface involvement, and those with stage II disease.** These patients had a 20% improved disease-free survival at 5 years (relative risk, 0.5). Regarding morbidity, **45% of patients had long-term, mild/moderate diarrhea and cramping** (Radiation Therapy Oncology Group grades 1 and 2), but grade 3 and 4 late-radiation toxicities were uncommon (grade 3 in 3% and grade 4 in 1% of patients). In view of these data, **there has been renewed interest in the role of radiotherapy in early-stage ovarian cancer.** The group from British Columbia is currently treating selected patients with early-stage ovarian cancer with a pelvic field alone after three cycles of *carboplatin* and *paclitaxel*, as most recurrences were in the pelvis.

Recommendation for Adjuvant Treatment of Early-Stage Ovarian Cancer

Low-risk Early-Stage Disease

No adjuvant chemotherapy is recommended for these patients.

High-risk Early-Stage Disease

1. Patients with high-risk stage I epithelial ovarian cancer should be given adjuvant chemotherapy. The type depends on the patient's overall health and the presence of medical comorbidities.

2. Treatment with *carboplatin* and *paclitaxel* chemotherapy for three to six cycles is used in most patients, although single-agent *carboplatin* may be preferable for women with significant medical comorbidities.

3. Consideration should also be given to the addition of pelvic radiation in selected patients with clear cell and endometrioid cancers at risk for local recurrence.

Advanced-Stage Ovarian Cancer

Chemotherapy

Platinum- and taxane-based combination chemotherapy is the standard of care for women with advanced-stage epithelial ovarian cancer (279–307). After the introduction of *cisplatin* in the latter half of the 1970s, platinum-based combination chemotherapy has become the most frequently used treatment regimen in the United States (290). *Paclitaxel* was made available in the 1980s, and was incorporated into ovarian combination chemotherapy in the 1990s (279–290). Comparative trials of *paclitaxel, cisplatin,* and *carboplatin* are summarized below (Table 11.4).

Cisplatin Combination Chemotherapy

Combination chemotherapy has been shown to be superior to single-agent therapy in most studies of initial chemotherapy in patients with advanced epithelial ovarian cancer (290–304). After *cisplatin* became available for the treatment of ovarian cancer, a prospective study conducted in England showed that *cisplatin* was better than an *alkylating agent, cyclophosphamide,* as a single agent (295). Concurrently, *cisplatin* was tested in a variety of different combinations, and the platinum-containing regimens were superior (296). A meta-analysis compared outcomes for patients given *cisplatin*-containing combination chemotherapy with those for patients not receiving *cisplatin* (293). The *cisplatin* group had a slight survival advantage from 2 to 5 years, but this difference disappeared by 8 years.

Most studies using the PC (*cisplatin* and *cyclophosphamide*) or PAC (*cisplatin, doxorubicin, and cyclophosphamide*) regimen have reported similar survival rates (297–302). The GOG's randomized prospective comparison of equitoxic doses of PAC versus PC showed no benefit to the inclusion of *doxorubicin* in the combination (298). Although a meta-analysis of the combined data from four trials showed a 7% survival advantage at 6 years for those patients treated with the *doxorubicin*-containing regimen (302), the survival curves converged at 8 years.

Paclitaxel

The next major advance was the incorporation of *paclitaxel* into the chemotherapeutic regimens. A series of randomized, prospective clinical trials with *paclitaxel*-containing arms have defined the current recommended treatment protocol in advanced epithelial ovarian cancer (290–292,306). These studies are listed in Table 11.4.

***Paclitaxel* was shown to have an overall response rate of 36% in phase II trials in previously treated patients** (286), which was a higher rate than was seen for *cisplatin* when it was first tested (282–290).

Reporting the GOG data (Protocol 111), McGuire et al. (290) showed that **the combination of *cisplatin* (75 mg/m^2) and *paclitaxel* (135 mg/m^2) was superior to *cisplatin* (75 mg/m^2) and *cyclophosphamide* (600 mg/m^2), each given for six cycles.** In suboptimally resected patients, the *paclitaxel*-containing arm produced a 36% reduction in mortality. These data were verified in a trial conducted jointly by the EORTC, the Nordic Ovarian Cancer Study Group (NOCOVA), and NCIC, in which patients with both optimal and suboptimal diseases were treated (291). In this

Table 11.4 First-Line Intravenous Chemotherapy with Platinum and Taxane: Randomized Trials Involving in Patients with Advanced-Stage Epithelial Ovarian Cancer

Group Protocol	Ref.	Year	Author	Status	Drugs/Doses/(hrs)[a]	Best
GOG 111	(290)	1996	McQuire et al.	Subopt	*Paclitaxel* 135 (3 hrs) & *cisplatin* 75 vs. *cyclophosphamide* 750 & *cisplatin* 75	*Paclitaxel, cisplatin*
OV 10 EORTC, NOCOVA, NCIC	(291)	1998	Piccart et al.	Opt, subopt	*Paclitaxel* 175 & *cisplatin* 75 vs. *cyclophosphamide* 750 & *cisplatin* 75	*Paclitaxel, cisplatin*
SCOT-ROC	(307)	1999	Vasey et al.	Opt, subopt	*Docetaxel & cisplatin* vs. *paclitaxel & cisplatin*	*Docetaxel, carboplatin*
GOG 132	(292)	2000	Muggia et al.	Subopt	*Cisplatin* 100 vs. *paclitaxel* 200 (24 hrs) vs. *cisplatin* 75 & *paclitaxel* 135 (24 hrs)	*Paclitaxel, cisplatin*
ICON 3	(308)	2002	ICON3 collaborators	Opt, subopt	*Carboplatin & paclitaxel* vs. *carboplatin* vs. *cisplatin & cyclophosphamide & doxorubicin*	*Carboplatin*
GOG 158	(306)	2003	Ozols et al.	Opt	*Carboplatin* 7.5 & *paclitaxel* 175 (3 hrs) vs. *cisplatin* 75 & *paclitaxel* 135 (24 hrs)	*Paclitaxel, carboplatin*
GOG 182, ICON 5	(309)	2004	Bookman et al.	Opt, subopt	*Paclitaxel & carboplatin* × 8 vs. *paclitaxel & carboplatin & gemcitabine* × 8 vs. *paclitaxel & carboplatin & liposomal doxorubicin* × 8 vs. *carboplatin & topotecan* × 4 followed by *paclitaxel & carboplatin* × 4 vs. *carboplatin & gemcitabine* × 4 followed by *paclitaxel & carboplatin* × 4	*Carboplatin[a], paclitaxel*
GOG 218	(311)	2011	Burger et al.	III–IV (suboptimal)	*Carboplatin* AUC 6 q 3 weeks × 6 + *paclitaxel* 175/m^2 over 3 hrs q 3 weeks + either 1 of 3 arms: (arm 1) *bevacizumab* 15 mg/kg × 2–6 followed by placebo cycles 7–22 vs. (arm 2) *bevacizumab* 15 mg/kg × 2–6 followed by *bevacizumab* cycles 7–22 vs. (arm 3) placebo cycles 2–22	*Bevacizumab* (arm 2)
ICON 7	(312)	2011	Perren et al.	Ic–IV	*Carboplatin* AUC 5–6 Q 3 weeks × 6 + *paclitaxel* 175/m^2 over 3 hrs q 3 weeks + either: (arm 1) *bevacizumab* 7.5 mg/kg with chemoRx followed by 12 more q 3 weeks vs. (arm 2) no *bevacizumab*	*Bevacizumab* (arm 1)
JGOG	(310)	2013	Katsumata et al.	II–IV	*Carboplatin* AUC 6 Q 3 weeks × 6–9 + *Paclitaxel* 180/m^2 over 3 hrs q × 3 weeks vs. *carboplatin* AUC 6 q 3 weeks × 6–9 & *Paclitaxel* 80/m^2 q week	Dose-dense using *paclitaxel* q week

[a]*Carboplatin* doses in area under the curve; others in mg/m^2.

GOG, Gynecologic Oncology Group; subopt, suboptimal; OV 10, Ovarian Protocol; EORTC, European Organization for the Research and Treatment of Cancer; NOCOVA, Nordic Ovarian Cancer Study Group; NCIC, National Cancer Institute of Canada; opt, optimal; SCOT-ROC, Scottish Gynaecological Cancer Trials Group; ICON, International Collaborative Ovarian Neoplasm Group; AUC, area under the curve (Calvert formula); JGOG, Japanese Gynecologic Oncology Group.

study, the *paclitaxel*-containing arm produced a significant improvement in both progression-free and overall survival in both groups. **Based on these two studies, *paclitaxel* should be included in the primary treatment of all women with advanced-stage epithelial ovarian cancer, unless precluded by toxicity or significant medical comorbidities.**

A three-arm comparison of *paclitaxel* (T) versus *cisplatin* (P) versus PT in suboptimal stage III and IV patients (protocol 132) showed equivalency in the three groups, but crossover from one drug to the other was permitted (292). The study essentially showed that the combination regimen was better tolerated than the sequential administration of the agents in suboptimally resected patients.

Carboplatin

The second-generation platinum analog, *carboplatin*, was introduced and developed to have less toxicity than its parent compound, *cisplatin*. **Fewer gastrointestinal side effects, especially nausea and vomiting, were observed with *carboplatin*, and there was significantly less nephrotoxicity, neurotoxicity, and ototoxicity** (303–306,313). However, *carboplatin* is associated with a higher degree of myelosuppression than *cisplatin*.

The initial studies showed that *carboplatin* and *cisplatin* had approximately a 4:1 equivalency ratio. Thus, a standard single-agent dose of approximately 400 mg/m^2 *carboplatin* was used in most phase II trials, but dosing is no longer based on surface area. **The optimal way to dose *carboplatin* is by using the area under the curve (AUC) and the glomerular filtration rate according to the Calvert formula** (305), as discussed in Chapter 3. **The target AUC is 5 to 6 for previously untreated patients.** A platelet nadir of approximately 50,000 dL is a suitable target (305).

Carboplatin and *Paclitaxel*

Two randomized, prospective clinical studies have compared the combination of *paclitaxel* and *carboplatin* with *paclitaxel* and *cisplatin* (306,313) (Table 11.4). **In both studies, the efficacy and survival were similar, but the toxicity was more acceptable for the *carboplatin*-containing regimen.**

In the first trial, GOG Protocol 158, the randomization was *carboplatin* AUC 7.5 and *paclitaxel* 175 mg/m^2 over 3 hours, versus *cisplatin* 75 mg/m^2 and *paclitaxel* 135 mg/m^2 over 24 hours (306). The PFS of the *carboplatin*-containing arm was 20.7 months, versus 19.4 months for the control arm. The overall survival was 57.4 months for the *carboplatin* arm versus 48.7 months for control arm. The relative risk of progression for the *carboplatin* plus *paclitaxel* group was 0.88, and the RR of death was 0.84. **The gastrointestinal and neurotoxicity of the *carboplatin* arm were appreciably lower than in the *cisplatin* arm.**

A similar result was obtained in a large randomized trial in Germany (313) in which the dose of *carboplatin* was AUC = 6, and *paclitaxel* dosage was 185 mg/m^2 over 3 hours, compared with the same dose of *paclitaxel* and *cisplatin* 75 mg/m^2. The overall survival was 44.1 months for the *carboplatin*-containing arm versus 43.3 months for the control arm. **Thus, the preferred regimen in patients with advanced-stage disease is the *paclitaxel* plus *carboplatin* combination.**

The International Collaborative Ovarian Neoplasm 3 (ICON3) trial studied 2,074 women with all stages of ovarian cancer, including 20% who had stage I or II disease (308). The combination of *carboplatin* plus *paclitaxel* was compared with two *nonpaclitaxel* regimens, *carboplatin* alone **(70%), or *cyclophosphamide*, *doxorubicin*, and *cisplatin* (CAP) (30%). The regimens were chosen before randomization, and were based on the clinical preference of the treating physician.** One-third of patients who received *carboplatin* or CAP subsequently received second-line *paclitaxel*, and this additional chemotherapy was often given before clinical progression. With a median follow-up of 51 months, the *carboplatin* plus *paclitaxel* and the control groups had a similar progression-free (0.93) and overall survival (0.98). **The median survival for the *paclitaxel* plus *carboplatin* and control groups was 36.1 and 35.4 months, respectively.** The median duration of PFS was 17.3 and 16.1 months, respectively. **The researchers concluded that single-agent *carboplatin* and CAP were as effective as *paclitaxel* and *carboplatin* for first-line chemotherapy.** Because *carboplatin* as a single agent had a lower toxicity than the other regimens and the median survival was similar in a prior trial that had compared *carboplatin* and CAP as first-line treatment (314), **the researchers suggested that *carboplatin* alone should be the preferred therapy.**

The design of this study limits drawing any definitive conclusions. Patients with FIGO stages I to IV ovarian cancer were included, the extent of primary surgery was variable, and the majority (85%) of patients who relapsed after single-agent *carboplatin* subsequently

received *paclitaxel.* The investigators suggested that one explanation for the favorable outcome with *carboplatin* alone was that 30% of patients had dose escalation based on their nadir counts not falling significantly, although this was not protocol driven. They then commenced a study comparing standard AUC dosing of *carboplatin* with dose escalation based on nadir counts to try and confirm this hypothesis. However, they recently reported that dose escalation did not result in an improvement in PFS or OS compared with flat dosing, which illustrates the importance of randomized clinical trials in informing clinical practice (315). **The findings of the ICON 3 study have not altered the standard of care.**

Carboplatin and *Docetaxel*

Docetaxel **has a different toxicity profile to** *paclitaxel* **and appears to be equivalent to** *paclitaxel* **when combined with** *carboplatin.* The Scottish Gynaecological Cancer Trials Group (SCOT-ROC) study randomly assigned 1,077 women with stages IC to IV epithelial ovarian cancer to *carboplatin* with either *paclitaxel* or *docetaxel* (307). **The efficacy of** *docetaxel* **was similar to** *paclitaxel:* The median PFS was 15.1 months versus 15.4 months, and **the** *docetaxel* **group had less extremity weakness, sensory peripheral neuropathy, arthralgias, and myalgias** than the *paclitaxel* group. However, **the** *docetaxel* **plus** *carboplatin* **regimen was associated with significantly more myelosuppression and febrile neutropenia** (11% compared to 2%). *Docetaxel* is not commonly used, but is a reasonable substitute for *paclitaxel* in patients who are at greater risk of neuropathy or who have an allergic reaction to *paclitaxel.*

Five-Arm Trial

A large intergroup, international trial (GOG 182/SWOG 182/ICON5/ANZGOG) compared the standard **combination of** *carboplatin* **and** *paclitaxel* **with these drugs in combination with** *gemcitabine,* *topotecan,* **or** *liposomal doxorubicin* **in sequential doublets or triplets** (315). This was the largest randomized trial ever conducted in women with advanced ovarian cancer, and recruited more than 4,000 patients. **There were no differences between any of the arms in terms of progression-free or median survival,** although there were differences in the side effects experienced in the different arms. **The authors concluded that the combination of** *carboplatin* **and** *paclitaxel* **should remain the standard of care.** A summary of these trials is presented in Table 11.4.

Dose Intensification with Intravenous Chemotherapy	The issue of dose intensification of *cisplatin* was examined in a prospective trial conducted by the GOG (317). In this study, **243 patients with suboptimal ovarian cancer were randomized to receive 50 mg/m^2 or 100 mg/m^2 *cisplatin* plus 500 mg/m^2 *cyclophosphamide*. There were no differences in the response rates in patients with measurable disease,** and the overall survival times were identical. There was greater toxicity associated with the high-dose regimen. A Scottish group reported that patients who received 100 mg/m^2 *cisplatin* plus 750 mg/m^2 *cyclophosphamide* had a significantly longer median survival compared with those receiving 50 mg/m^2 *cisplatin* plus the same dose of *cyclophosphamide* (318). The overall median survival time was 114 weeks in the high-dose group and 69 weeks in the low-dose group ($p = 0.0008$), but this difference disappeared with longer follow-up (319). **Therefore, the doubling of the dose of *cisplatin* does not improve the survival of patients with advanced ovarian cancer.**

Dose escalations of *paclitaxel* and *carboplatin* require granulocyte colony-stimulating factor (G-CSF) because of the combined myelosuppressive effects, but there is no evidence to support a role for a more intensive course of either agent (288,320).

Intraperitoneal Chemotherapy	A randomized, prospective trial in 546 evaluable patients of intraperitoneal (IP) *cisplatin* versus intravenous (IV) *cisplatin* (100 mg/m^2), each given with 750 mg/m^2 *cyclophosphamide,* was performed jointly by the Southwest Oncology Group (SWOG) and the GOG in patients with advanced ovarian cancer following optimal cytoreduction (residual nodules <2 cm diameter) (321). **The IP *cisplatin* arm had a longer overall median survival than the IV arm, 49 versus 41 months** ($p = 0.03$). **In the patients with minimal residual disease (<0.5 cm maximum residual diameter), who would be expected to derive the most benefit, there was no difference between the two treatments, 51 versus 46 months** ($p = 0.08$) (Table 11.5).

In a follow-up trial of 532 patients (GOG Protocol 114), the dose-intense arm was initiated by giving a moderately high dose of *carboplatin* (dose AUC = 9) for two induction cycles, followed by IP *cisplatin* 100 mg/m^2 and IV *paclitaxel* 135 mg/m^2 over 24 hours versus IV *cisplatin* 75 mg/m^2

Table 11.5 Randomized Trials of IV Versus IP Chemotherapy in Patients with Advanced Epithelial Ovarian Cancer

Group Protocol	Ref.	Year	Author	Status	Drugs/Doses/(hrs)	Best Arm
GOG 104	(321)	1996	Alberts et al.	Optimal	IP cisplatin & IV cyclophosphamide vs. IV cisplatin & cyclophosphamide	IP cisplatin & IV cyclophosphamide 49 vs. 41 mos (p = 0.03)
GOG 114	(322)	2001	Markman et al.	Optimal	IV carboplatin AUC = 9 IP cisplatin 100 mg & IV paclitaxel 135 mg (24 hrs) vs. IV cisplatin 75 & IV paclitaxel 135 mg (24 hrs)	IP cisplatin & IV carboplatin & IV paclitaxel[b] 52.9 vs. 47.6 mos (p = 0.056)
GOG 172	(323)	2006	Armstrong et al.	Optimal	IV paclitaxel 135 mg (24 hrs) & IP cisplatin 100 mg on day 2 & IP paclitaxel 60 mg on day 8 vs. IV paclitaxel 135 mg (24 hrs) & IV cisplatin 75 mg	IP cisplatin, IV paclitaxel, & IP paclitaxel 65.6 vs. 49.7 mos (p = 0.03)

[a]Median survival longer in IP arm, not in minimal residual (<0.5 mm) group.

[b]Progression-free survival longer in IP arm, no difference in overall survival.

AUC, area under the curve; all mg doses are mg/m^2.

and IV *paclitaxel* 135 mg/m^2 (322). In the dose-intense arm, progression-free median survival was 27.6 months compared with 22.5 months for the control arm ($p = 0.02$). However, there was no difference in overall survival (59.9 months versus 47.6 months, $p = 0.056$). Thus, **it is unclear if dose intensification with IP *cisplatin* has a long-term impact on the survival of these patients.** A phase II trial of IV *paclitaxel* plus intraperitoneal *cisplatin* and *paclitaxel* was well tolerated and associated with a 2-year survival of 91% (324).

A randomized prospective GOG study compared IP *cisplatin* and *paclitaxel* with IV *cisplatin* and *paclitaxel* (323). Patients with stage III ovarian or peritoneal carcinoma with residual masses ≤ 1 cm were randomly assigned to receive IV *paclitaxel* 135 mg/m^2 over 24 hours followed by either IV *cisplatin* 75 mg/m^2 on day 2 (IV therapy group) or IP *cisplatin* 100 mg/m^2 on day 2 and IP *paclitaxel* 60 mg/m^2 on day 8 (IP therapy group). Treatment was given every 3 weeks for six cycles. Four hundred and twenty-nine patients were randomly assigned, and 415 were eligible. **The median PFS was 23.8 months in the IP arm versus 18.3 months in the IV arm ($p = 0.05$). The median overall survival was 65.6 months in the IP group and 49.7 months in the IV group ($p = 0.03$)** (Fig. 11.18). Ninety percent of patients in the IV arm received the six planned cycles of therapy, whereas **only 42% of patients received the assigned 6 cycles of IP therapy, with the remainder switching to IV therapy.** The reasons for discontinuation were primarily for catheter-related problems, but there were also significantly more side effects in the IP group, with more patients experiencing severe fatigue, pain, hematologic toxicity, nausea, and vomiting as well as metabolic and neurotoxicity. It is likely that with more training, appropriate dose modifications, and better antiemetics, the toxicity can be reduced (325).

The results of this study, together with the previous studies, led to an NCI clinical announcement recommending that women with optimally debulked stage III ovarian cancer should be considered for IP chemotherapy. There has been a Cochrane Review as well as a separate meta-analysis, and both concluded that IP chemotherapy was associated with better outcomes than intravenous chemotherapy (326,327).

The meta-analysis included six randomized trials with a total of 1,716 ovarian cancer patients. The pooled HR for PFS of IP *cisplatin* as compared to IV treatment regimens was 0.792 (95% CI: 0.688 to 0.912, $p = 0.001$), and the pooled hazard ratio for overall survival was 0.799 (95% CI: 0.702 to 0.910, $p = 0.0007$). **The authors concluded that these findings strongly supported the incorporation of an IP *cisplatin* regimen in the first-line treatment of patients with stage III optimally debulked ovarian cancer** (326).

In the **Cochrane review, the conclusion was that IP chemotherapy was associated with an increased overall and PFS in patients with optimally debulked stage III ovarian cancer.** However, **they also commented on the potential for catheter-related complications and increased toxicity with IP therapy,** and concluded that the optimal dose, timing, and mechanism of administration should be addressed in the next phase of clinical trials (327). Most of the current clinical

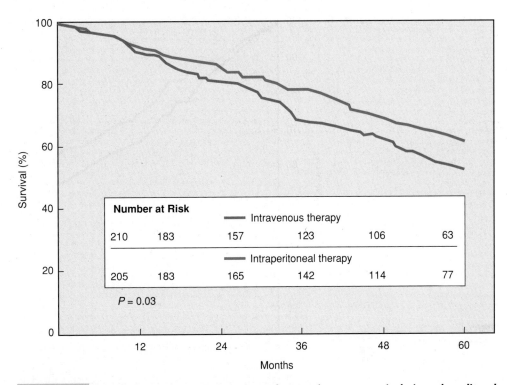

Figure 11.18 Overall survival after intraperitoneal versus intravenous *cisplatin* and *paclitaxel* chemotherapy. From **Armstrong DK, Bundy B, Wenzel L, et al.** Intraperitoneal *cisplatin* and *paclitaxel* in ovarian cancer. *N Eng J Med.* 2006;354:34–43.

trials have reduced the dose of *cisplatin* to 75 mg/m² to try to reduce toxicity, and there are also studies of IP *carboplatin*.

Tewari et al. recently presented the results of IP chemotherapy in 876 patients treated on GOG clinical trials 114 and 172, who have more than 10 years of follow-up (328). The median survival was 61.8 months for IP therapy compared with 51.4 months for IV therapy ($p = 0.048$). There was a significantly decreased risk of death associated with IP therapy (adjusted hazard ratio, 0.83). Significant predictors of improved survival after IP therapy included: younger age, better performance status, nonclear cell/mucinous histology, low-grade histology, and microscopic residual disease. Patients with microscopic and gross residual disease had a survival advantage with IP therapy. There was also an association with the number of cycles administered. Five-year overall survival in patients who completed five or six cycles of IP therapy was 59%, compared to 18% in those who completed one or two cycles (18%), and 33% for those who received three or four cycles.

The role of IP chemotherapy remains contentious, with some researchers arguing that the trials to date have been flawed (329). It has been suggested that the IP protocols are just a more complicated way of administering dose-dense chemotherapy, and that the results are very similar to the Japanese GOG IV dose-dense regimen (330). In addition, concerns have been raised about the technical difficulties and increased toxicity of IP therapy (331).

Neoadjuvant Chemotherapy

Neoadjuvant chemotherapy is a viable approach for the limited number of patients felt to be optimally unresectable by an experienced ovarian cancer surgical team, that is, in selected patients who are at high risk for operative morbidity or mortality (241–252). As discussed above, primary cytoreductive surgery should be considered the standard of care for most patients. There may be a role for neoadjuvant chemotherapy in selected patients with stage IIIC or stage IV ovarian cancer with large-volume disease with extensive ascites and large pleural effusions as well as in patients who have a poor performance status and are therefore at high operative risk because of medical comorbidities (253).

Dose-Dense Chemotherapy

There is preclinical evidence as well as clinical evidence to suggest that dose-dense, dose-fractionated chemotherapy with *carboplatin* and *paclitaxel* may be more active than the same treatments

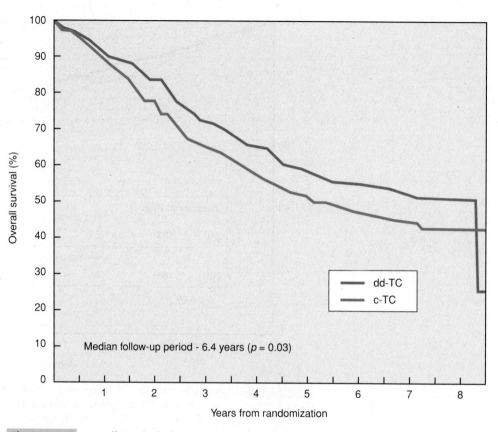

Figure 11.19 Overall survival after dose-dense chemotherapy: the Japanese GOG Study. Katsumata N, Yasuda M, Isonishi S, et al. Long-term results of dose-dense *paclitaxel* and *carboplatin* versus conventional *paclitaxel* and *carboplatin* for treatment of advanced epithelial ovarian, fallopian tube, or primary peritoneal cancer (JGOG 3016): A randomised, controlled, open-label trial. *Lancet Oncol.* 2013;14(10):1020–1026, with permission.

given every 3 weeks. There are a number of explanations for this, including an antiangiogenic effect of weekly metronomic *paclitaxel*, as well as decreasing the accelerated repopulation of cancer cells between cycles, and reducing the acquisition of drug resistance (332,333).

A phase III study by the JGOG randomized 637 women with FIGO stages II to IV ovarian cancer to receive either weekly *paclitaxel* at a dose of 80 mg/m² in combination with three-weekly *carboplatin* (AUC 6) or three-weekly dosing of both drugs (*carboplatin* AUC 6 and *paclitaxel* 180 mg/m²) (310,330). After a median follow-up of 29 months, they reported that the median PFS was 17.2 months in the standard three-weekly *paclitaxel* arm, compared to 28 months in the weekly *paclitaxel* arm (HR 0.71; 95% CI 0.58–0.88, p = 0.0015) and the 3-year OS (at 42 months follow-up) was 65.1% and 72.1%, respectively (HR 0.75; 95% CI 0.57 to 0.98, p = 0.03) (Fig. 11.19). The median PFS in patients with residual disease at least 1 cm was 17.6 months in the dose-dense arm compared to 12.1 months in the conventional arm. The median progression survival in the patients with residual disease <1 cm was not statistically different between the two arms. The median overall survival in the patients with residual disease at least 1 cm was better in the dose-dense arm compared to the conventional arm (51.2 months vs. 33.5 months).

They concluded that dose-dense treatment offered better survival than conventional treatment, and was a potential new standard of care for first-line chemotherapy for patients with advanced epithelial ovarian cancer. The improvements in PFS and overall survival exceed any benefits previously seen in any phase III trial in ovarian cancer. It is unclear whether these benefits relate to pharmacogenomic or pharmacodynamic differences in the Japanese population. **This and other studies have suggested that Asian patients with ovarian cancer have a significantly better survival than do Caucasian patients** (334). A GOG Phase III study of patients with advanced-stage ovarian cancer (Protocol 218) revealed that the overall survival was significantly higher in Asian patients when adjusted for age, stage, residual disease, performance status, and histology (335).

It is essential that the JGOG study be confirmed in a predominantly Caucasian population of patients. An Italian trial (MITO-7; NCT00660842) investigated a different schedule of weekly *carboplatin* (AUC 2 mg/mL/min) plus weekly *paclitaxel* (60 mg/m^2) compared with *carboplatin* (AUC 6 mg/mL/min, administered every 3 weeks) and *paclitaxel* (175 mg/m^2). The weekly regimen did not significantly improve PFS compared with the conventional regimen (18.8 months vs. 16.5 months; $p = 0.18$), but was associated with better quality of life and fewer toxic effects (336). **Other ongoing studies, including the ICON 8 trial (NCT01654146) and the GOG 262 trial (NCT01167712) are assessing dose-dense chemotherapy,** and will help address the role of dose-dense chemotherapy in a Caucasian population.

The GOG 262 study has recently been presented (337), and its findings underscore the importance of the ICON 8 trial, which is currently recruiting. The design of GOG 262 was similar to the JGOG 3016 trial, the main difference being that patients could be also treated with IV *bevacizumab* 15 mg/kg every 3 weeks in both arms. The decision to receive *bevacizumab* was dependent on the treating doctors and patient wishes. The vast majority of patients (84%) received *bevacizumab* until progression. The population of patients included a high proportion with gross residual disease (63%) and 13% of patients received neoadjuvant chemotherapy. Only 24% had microscopic residual disease. The median PFS was the same in both arms and was just over 14 months. Only 112 patients did not have *bevacizumab,* with approximately equal numbers in both arms and interestingly, the median PFS was 14.2 months with dose-dense *paclitaxel* and only 10.3 months with three-weekly scheduling of *paclitaxel.* This was a subset analysis and it is difficult to draw definitive conclusions. ICON 8 trial is an effort to replicate the JGOG study in non-Asian women. If the Japanese results can be confirmed, it would be a major advance in ovarian cancer treatment.

Chemotherapy and Molecular Targeted Therapies	**Inhibition of angiogenesis with drugs such as *bevacizumab* has demonstrated activity and benefit in women with recurrent ovarian cancer.** In view of this, there have been two large randomized trials investigating the impact, if any, of the addition of *bevacizumab* to standard *carboplatin* and *paclitaxel* in patients with advanced ovarian cancer. There is evidence in other tumor types such as breast, colon, and lung cancer that the addition of *bevacizumab* to chemotherapy increases response rates and PFS and also overall survival in some studies (338–340).

Two large Phase III studies, (GOG 218 and ICON 7) have investigated the role of *bevacizumab* in the first-line setting. The GOG 218 trial was a three-arm randomized study that recruited 1,873 patients with stage III to IV ovarian, fallopian tube, and peritoneal cancer (311). Patients with stage III disease were required to have macroscopic residual disease. The patients were randomly assigned to one of the following: (i) a control group, who received 6 cycles of *carboplatin* and *paclitaxel* chemotherapy with concurrent placebo in cycles 2 through 6, followed by placebo alone every 3 weeks for a total of 22 cycles; (ii) a group who received standard chemotherapy for 6 cycles in combination with *bevacizumab* (15 mg/kg) in cycles 2 through 6, followed by placebo alone for a total of 22 cycles; and (iii) a group who received standard chemotherapy for 6 cycles with *bevacizumab* in cycles 2 through 6, followed by the continuation of *bevacizumab* alone, for a total of 22 cycles. **At a median follow-up of 17.4 months, the hazard of progression or death was the same in the *bevacizumab* with chemotherapy group compared with the control group (hazard ratio [HR], 0.908; $p = 0.16$), and significantly lower in the *bevacizumab* with chemotherapy and maintenance group (HR, 0.717; $p < 0.001$).** In an analysis of PFS, in which patients with an elevated CA-125 were censored, the median PFS was 12 months in the control group but 18 months in the *bevacizumab* maintenance group (HR, 0.645; $p < 0.001$). This was confirmed in a recent analysis on independent radiologic review of all patients in GOG 218. To date there does not appear to be any significant difference in OS, and this may be due to many patients receiving multiple subsequent regimens at relapse, including crossover to *bevacizumab* or other anti-VEGF agents that could potentially influence overall survival.

The ICON7 trial had a similar design and enrolled 1,528 patients with high-risk (clear cell or grade 3 tumors) (341). Patients with stages I and II ovarian, fallopian tube, or peritoneal cancer, as well as stages III and IV were included. They were randomized to six cycles of chemotherapy alone or six cycles of chemotherapy plus *bevacizumab* (7.5 mg/kg), followed by 12 cycles of maintenance *bevacizumab* every 3 weeks. With a median follow-up of 19.4 months, the median PFS was 17.3 months in the control group and 19 months in the *bevacizumab* group (HR, 0.81; $p = 0.004$). The improvement in PFS with *bevacizumab* was maintained with a median follow-up of 28 months. An exploratory OS analysis showed a significant improvement in survival in the high-risk subgroups (stage III with >1 cm residual and stage IV [HR, 0.64; $p = 0.002$]). This was confirmed in a recently presented update of the survival data, which showed that there was a 4-month improvement in median survival from 35 to 39 months in the high-risk subgroup (342). However, **there was no survival advantage found between the two arms in ICON7, suggesting that patients who are optimally cytoreduced may not gain a significant benefit from the addition of** *bevacizumab.* In contrast to GOG 218, in the ICON7 trial, only 3% of the patients in the control group received postprogression antiangiogenic therapy, which could explain the difference in survival observed between the high-risk subgroup in ICON7 and GOG 218. *Bevacizumab* **was associated with an increase in toxicity,** which included bleeding (mainly grade 1 mucocutaneous bleeding), grade 2 or higher hypertension (18% with *bevacizumab* vs. 2% with standard therapy), grade 3 or higher thromboembolic events (7% with *bevacizumab* vs. 3% with standard therapy), and gastrointestinal perforations (occurring in 10 patients in the *bevacizumab* group vs. 3 patients in the standard-therapy group).

In contrast to the GOG 218 study, the ICON7 study enrolled patients with advanced-stage cancer with no visible residual disease, as well as patients with high-risk early-stage disease (342). In the ICON7 study, a lower dose of *bevacizumab* was used (7.5 mg/kg vs. 15 mg/kg in GOG 218) for a shorter maintenance period (12 cycles, vs. 16 cycles). **In both studies, PFS curves converged a few months after bevacizumab was discontinued, suggesting that antiangiogenic treatment may delay, but not prevent, disease progression. This raises the issue of the advisability of patients with high-risk disease continuing treatment indefinitely.** This is currently being investigated, but has significant cost-benefit implications.

There are still no good biologic markers to identify which patients are most likely to benefit from the incorporation of *bevacizumab* **into the first-line setting. The optimal dose is also unclear.**

Maintenance of Complete Clinical Response to First-Line Chemotherapy

Because as many as 80% of women with advanced ovarian cancer who have had a complete response to first-line chemotherapy will ultimately relapse, **several trials of maintenance therapy have been conducted in an attempt to prolong PFS, and possibly improve overall survival.**

Paclitaxel

In a study conducted by the GOG and SWOG, 277 women with advanced ovarian cancer who had a complete clinical response to first-line chemotherapy were randomized to receive 3 or 12 cycles of additional single-agent *paclitaxel* (175 or 135 mg/m^2 every 28 days) (343). Patients were excluded if they had developed grade 2 or 3 neurotoxicity during their initial chemotherapy. Because of cumulative toxicity, the mean number of actual cycles of *paclitaxel* received by the group assigned to receive 12 cycles was 9. The treatment-related grade 2 to 3 neuropathy was more common with longer treatment, 24% versus 14% of patients, respectively. **The study was closed after a median follow-up of only 8.5 months, and an interim analysis showed a significant 7-month prolongation in median PFS (28 vs. 21 months) with 9 versus 3 months of consolidation** *paclitaxel.* **However, there was no difference in median overall survival.** The absolute difference in PFS of 7 months was less than the difference in treatment duration of 9 months between the two arms. The rate of disease progression increased significantly after maintenance therapy was discontinued. **It is unlikely that a survival benefit will be seen with longer follow-up, because patients assigned to three cycles were given the option of receiving an additional nine courses of** *paclitaxel* **after the study was discontinued** (344).

GOG 212 is a three-arm study in which patients are randomized to observation, *paclitaxel* **or** *polyglutamated paclitaxel* **for 12 months.** The study has recently completed accrual and will help answer the question regarding the role of maintenance chemotherapy.

Topotecan

Four additional courses of *topotecan* were administered to patients following six cycles of *carboplatin* and *paclitaxel* in two randomized trials, one conducted in Italy (312) and the other in Germany (345). In the larger trial conducted in Germany, 1,059 evaluable patients were randomly assigned to six cycles of *paclitaxel* (175 mg/m^2 over 3 hours) and *carboplatin* (AUC 5) with (537 patients) or without (522 patients) four additional cycles of *topotecan* (1.25 mg/m^2 IV 1 to 5 days every 3 weeks) (312). In the Italian trial, 273 women were randomly assigned to receive four additional cycles (137 patients) of *topotecan* at a dose of 1 mg/m^2 on days 1 to 5 every 3 weeks or no further chemotherapy

(136 patients) (312). **There were no significant differences in either progression-free or overall survival in patients who received four to six cycles of maintenance** *topotecan.*

Cochrane Meta-analysis

There has been a recent Cochrane meta-analysis of all maintenance chemotherapy studies. It concluded that there was no evidence to suggest that maintenance chemotherapy was more effective than observation alone (346). However, as noted above, the data regarding *bevacizumab* and other VEGF-R modulators for maintenance therapy are encouraging.

Toxicity of Platinum and *Paclitaxel*

There are a number of adverse effects associated with the *paclitaxel* **and** *carboplatin* **combination and they include alopecia, nausea and vomiting, fatigue, myelosuppression, and neurotoxicity.** Shorter infusions of *paclitaxel 175 mg/m²* (e.g., over 3 hours) tend to reduce the likelihood of bone marrow depression when combining the drug with *carboplatin* (288), although in practice myelosuppression is not usually a problem and febrile neutropenia is very uncommon. The appropriate dosing of *carboplatin* is discussed in Chapter 3. **Neurotoxicity is the major toxicity when** *paclitaxel* **is combined with** *cisplatin.* This can be reduced by using a lower dose of *paclitaxel* administered over a longer period of time (e.g., 135 mg/m² over 24 hours), but this is much more inconvenient than the 3-hour infusion with *carboplatin,* and is not commonly used (347).

The renal and gastrointestinal toxicities of *carboplatin* **are modest compared with** *cisplatin;* thus, patients do not require prehydration, and outpatient administration is standard practice. *Carboplatin* does tend to have more bone marrow toxicity than *cisplatin.* **Growth factors such as G-CSF have facilitated the administration of drug combinations that have neutropenia as a dose-limiting toxicity,** although they are not commonly required with *carboplatin* and *paclitaxel.* The use of growth factors is discussed more fully in Chapter 3.

Cisplatin combination chemotherapy is given every 3 to 4 weeks by intravenous infusion over 1 to 1.5 hours. *Cisplatin* **requires appropriate pre- and posthydration as well as antiemetics, and can be administered on either an inpatient or outpatient basis, depending on the dose used and the patient's performance status.** The principal toxicities of this regimen are renal, gastrointestinal, hematologic, and neurologic. The renal and neurologic toxicities generally limit the duration of treatment to six cycles.

The acute and delayed gastrointestinal toxicity of *cisplatin* **(i.e., nausea and vomiting) can be minimized with appropriate antiemetics, including a 5HT3 antagonist, together with** *dexamethasone* **and** *aprepitant,* **an NK1 receptor blocker.** All three published guidelines recommend this approach to prevent acute nausea and vomiting, and they also recommend *dexamethasone* and *aprepitant* to reduce delayed nausea and vomiting (348–350). For example, the ASCO guidelines recommend a 5HT3 antagonist (e.g., *ondansetron* 8 mg IV, *palonsetron* 0.25 mg, or one other 5HT3 antagonist) as well as *dexamethasone* 12 mg orally and *aprepitant* 125 mg orally prior to *cisplatin,* followed by *dexamethasone* 8 mg daily from days 2 to 4, and *aprepitant* 80 mg orally on days 2 and 3, as appropriate antiemetic cover (350).

Radiation Therapy

An alternative to first-line combination chemotherapy for selected patients with metastatic ovarian cancer is whole-abdominal radiation. This approach has not been used in the United States, but it has been standard treatment in some institutions in Canada for patients with no residual macroscopic tumor in the upper abdomen (260). It has been compared with oral *chlorambucil* and appears to be superior (260), but it has not been tested against combination chemotherapy. A trial of three cycles of high-dose *cisplatin* and *cyclophosphamide* "induction" chemotherapy followed by whole-abdominal radiation therapy to "consolidate" the initial response has been reported (351). No apparent benefit could be shown by adding whole-abdominal radiation after chemotherapy in patients with optimal disease. **There has been renewed interest in the potential role of radiation in selected subsets of patients with clear cell and endometrioid cancer,** as discussed above.

Hormonal Therapy

There is no evidence that hormonal therapy alone is appropriate primary therapy for advanced ovarian cancer (352), although it may have a role in selected women with recurrent disease (see discussion below).

Immunotherapy

There are some data using biologic and immunotherapy in ovarian cancer, and a full discussion of immunotherapy is presented in Chapter 2.

In a trial of *gamma interferon* (γ*-interferon*) **with** *cisplatin* **and** *cyclophosphamide*, there appeared to be a benefit from the addition of the *interferon* (353). **A trial of** *carboplatin* **and** *paclitaxel* **with or without** γ*-interferon* concluded that there were more adverse events with γ*-interferon* and no survival benefits in women with advanced ovarian cancer (354).

Trials of monoclonal antibodies directed toward ovarian cancer-associated antigens have been conducted (355–361). Women who were in clinical remission following platinum and *taxane* chemotherapy were studied in a randomized, prospective trial of maintenance **OvaRex,** a monoclonal antibody directed toward CA125. No PFS benefit was seen (357,358). Studies with monoclonal antibodies directed against human milk fat globulin (HMFG) tumor-associated antigens for consolidation have shown no survival benefit (359), although there was an improved control of intraperitoneal disease, which was offset by increased extraperitoneal disease (360).

Treatment Assessment

Many patients who undergo optimal cytoreductive surgery and subsequent chemotherapy will have no evidence of disease at the completion of treatment. The *second-look operation* was previously considered to be standard practice, but is now seldom performed (362–370).

Tumor Markers

Elevated CA125 levels are useful in predicting the presence of disease, but normal levels are an insensitive determinant of the absence of disease. In a prospective study by Berek et al. (371), the positive predictive value was shown to be 100%—that is, if the level of CA125 was >35 unit/dL, disease was always detectable in patients at second-look laparotomy. The predictive value of a negative test was only 56%—that is, if the level was <35 unit/dL, disease was present in 44% of the patients. **A review of the literature suggests that an elevated CA125 level predicts persistent disease at second-look in 97% of the cases** (42).

Serum CA125 levels can be used during chemotherapy to follow those patients whose level was elevated at the initiation of treatment (42,371). The change in level generally correlates with response. **Rising levels on treatment almost invariably indicate treatment failure. A retrospective study determined that a doubling of the CA125 level from its nadir in those patients with a persistently elevated level accurately predicted disease progression** (372).

The Gynecologic Cancer Intergroup (GCIG) developed a standard definition for CA125 level progression, which is now widely used in clinical trials. **Patients with elevated CA125 levels pretreatment who normalize their levels must demonstrate CA125 levels greater than or equal to twice the upper limit of normal on two occasions at least 1 week apart. Patients with elevated CA125 levels pretreatment, which never normalize, must show evidence of CA125 levels greater than or equal to twice the nadir value on two occasions at least 1 week apart** (373).

A trial of 527 patients, randomized to early treatment of relapse based on CA 125 level progression versus delaying treatment until the development of symptoms showed no survival benefits from early treatment (374). In view of this many centers, particularly in the United Kingdom and parts of Europe do not routinely follow up patients with CA125 levels after first-line chemotherapy, but base investigations and treatment decisions on symptoms and signs of recurrence (375).

Radiologic Assessment

In patients with stages I to III epithelial ovarian cancer, radiologic investigations, with the exception of CT-PET scans, have generally been of limited value in determining the presence of small volume disease. Ascites can be readily detected, but **even quite large omental metastases can be missed on CT scan** (128,376–381). The false-negative rate of a CT scan is approximately 45% (376).

Positron-emission tomography, with or without CT imaging, may help in the detection of relapse, but there appears to be a higher false-positive rate with PET compared with CT (129–131). A review concluded that PET had a sensitivity of 90% and a specificity of 85% for the detection of recurrent ovarian cancer, and that it appeared to be particularly useful for the diagnosis of recurrent disease when CA125 levels were rising and conventional imaging was inconclusive or negative (129). Technologic advances have led to a combined ^{18}fluorodeoxyglucose (^{18}FDG)-PET–CT machine that provides contemporaneous ^{18}FDG-PET and CT images. **The role of ^{18}FDG-PET–CT for the detection of recurrent ovarian cancer is promising,** and may be especially useful for the selection of patients with late recurrent disease who may benefit from secondary cytoreductive surgery (378–383). **MRI can be used as an alternative to CT in patients with allergies to the contrast medium** (131).

Second-Look Operations

A second-look operation was historically performed in patients who had no clinical evidence of disease after completion of first line chemotherapy. Approximately 30% of patients with no evidence of macroscopic disease will have microscopic metastases (362). **Second-look laparotomy has not been shown to influence patient survival, although the information obtained is of prognostic significance** (363–366,369,370). **The likelihood that a patient will have a recurrence after a negative second-look laparotomy ranges from 30–60% at 5 years** (366–369). The majority of recurrences after a negative second-look laparotomy are in patients with poorly differentiated cancers (369). Patients whose tumors are initially stages I or II have negative second-look laparotomy rates of 85–95% and 70–80%, respectively. In patients with optimally resected stage III disease treated with the platinum and *paclitaxel* regimen, the negative second-look rate is approximately 45–50% (272).

Secondary Therapy

Secondary Cytoreduction

Secondary cytoreduction is defined as an attempt to resect or optimally debulk selected patients with recurrent disease following first-line chemotherapy (384). Patients with platinum-refractory or platinum-resistant disease are not suitable candidates for secondary cytoreduction, but selected patients with platinum-sensitive recurrent ovarian cancer may benefit if all macroscopic residual disease can be resected. **There have been many retrospective studies as well as literature reviews that have shown a survival advantage for secondary cytoreduction for selected patients in whom all macroscopic disease could be resected** (385–397). The patients who appear to have the greatest benefit are those with localized late recurrence, absence of ascites, complete cytoreduction, and potentially platinum-sensitive recurrent disease.

The role of secondary surgery is being studied in a large randomized controlled trial led by the AGO in Europe. At the present time, **it should be considered in patients with platinum-sensitive recurrent ovarian cancer who have had a disease-free interval of at least 12 months, and where it is anticipated that all macroscopic disease can be resected** (386,388,389,395–397).

Chemotherapy for Recurrent Ovarian Cancer

The majority of women who relapse will be offered further chemotherapy with the likelihood of benefit related in part to the initial response and the duration of response. **The goals of treatment include improving disease-related symptoms, maintaining or improving quality of life, delaying time to progression, and possibly prolonging survival, particularly in women with platinum-sensitive recurrences.**

Many active chemotherapeutic agents (platinum, *paclitaxel, topotecan, liposomal doxorubicin, docetaxel, gemcitabine,* and *etoposide*) as well as targeted agents (*bevacizumab, cediranib, AMG386*) are available, and the choice of treatment is based on factors including likelihood of benefit, potential toxicity, and patient convenience (398,399). **Women who relapse later than 6 months after primary chemotherapy are classified as platinum-sensitive** and usually receive further platinum-based chemotherapy, with response rates ranging from 27–65% and a median survival of 12 to 24 months (400,401). **Patients who relapse within 6 months of completing first-line chemotherapy are classified as *platinum-resistant,*** and have a median survival of 6 to 9 months and a 10–30% response rate to chemotherapy. **Patients who progress while on treatment are classified as having *platinum-refractory disease.*** Objective response rates to chemotherapy in patients with platinum-refractory ovarian cancer are generally less than 10% (399).

Patients with platinum-refractory and platinum-resistant ovarian cancer are commonly treated with chemotherapy and may have a number of lines of therapy depending on response,

Table 11.6 Chemotherapy for Advanced Epithelial Ovarian Cancer: Recommended Regimens				
Drugs	*Dose*	*Administration (hr)*	*Interval*	*No. of Treatments*
Standard Regimens				
Carboplatin	AUC = 5–6	3	Every 3 wks	6–8 cycles
Paclitaxel	175 mg/m^2			
Carboplatin	AUC = 5–6	3	Every 3 wks	6 cycles
Paclitaxel	80 mg/m^2		Every week	18 weeks
Carboplatin	AUC = 5	3	Every week	6 cycles
Docetaxel	75 mg/m^2		Every 3 wks	
Cisplatin	75 mg/m^2	3	Every 3 wks	6 cycles
Paclitaxel	135 mg/m^2	24		
Carboplatin (single agent)^a	AUC 5	3	Every 3 wks	6 cycles, as tolerated

^{a}In patients who are elderly, frail, or poor performance status.

AUC, area under the curve dose by Calvert formula (305).

performance status, patient request, and doctor recommendations. A study comparing *topotecan* with *liposomal doxorubicin* demonstrated the **low response rates and poor prognosis for women with platinum-resistant ovarian cancer** (402). In a subset analysis of platinum-resistant patients, the median time to progression ranged from 9.1 to 13.6 weeks for *topotecan* and *liposomal doxorubicin*, respectively. The median survival was 35.6 weeks for *pegylated liposomal doxorubicin* (PLD) and 41.3 weeks for *topotecan* ($p = 0.455$). Objective response rates were recorded in 6.5% of patients who received *topotecan* and in 12.3% of those who received PLD ($p = 0.118$). Symptom control and quality-of-life issues were not specifically addressed.

The potential adverse effects associated with chemotherapy should not be underestimated. The three most commonly used drugs are *paclitaxel, topotecan,* and *liposomal doxorubicin.* The reported adverse effects associated with ***paclitaxel*** are **alopecia** in 62–100% of patients, **neurotoxicity** (any grade) in 5–42%, and **severe leukopenia** in 4–24%. *Topotecan* is associated with **myelosuppression** in 49–76% of patients, which is significantly greater than with *liposomal doxorubicin* or *paclitaxel.* *Liposomal doxorubicin* is associated with **palmar–plantar erythrodysesthesia** of any grade in more than 50% of patients, and it is severe in 23%. In addition, severe stomatitis has been reported in as many as 10% of patients (399). A large international study to evaluate the impact of chemotherapy on quality of life and symptom improvement in patients with platinum-resistant or platinum-refractory ovarian cancer is currently underway.

The most important prognostic factors are response to first-line chemotherapy and the treatment-free interval (401–488) (Tables 11.6 and 11.7).

Platinum-Sensitive Disease

In general, randomized trials have shown that response rates, median PFS, and overall survival rates are superior for platinum-based combination chemotherapy compared to single-agent platinum chemotherapy. The use of combination platinum plus *paclitaxel* chemotherapy versus single-agent platinum has been tested in two multinational randomized phase III trials (407) **and a randomized phase II study** (408). In a report (407) of the ICON4 and AGO-OVAR-2.2 trials, 802 women with platinum-sensitive ovarian cancer who relapsed after being treatment free for at least 6 to 12 months were randomized to platinum-based chemotherapy (72% *carboplatin*, or *cisplatin* alone; 17% CAP; 4% *carboplatin* plus *cisplatin;* and 3% *cisplatin* plus *doxorubicin*) or *paclitaxel* plus platinum-based chemotherapy (80% *paclitaxel* plus *carboplatin*; 10% *paclitaxel* plus *cisplatin*; 5% *paclitaxel* plus both *carboplatin* and *cisplatin*; and 4% *paclitaxel* alone). The AGO-OVAR-2.2 trial did not accrue its planned number of patients. **In both trials, a significant proportion of the patients had not received *paclitaxel* initially. Combining the trials for analysis, there was a significant survival advantage for the *paclitaxel*-containing therapy** (HR = 0.82), with a median follow-up of 42 months. **The absolute 2-year survival advantage was 7% (57% vs. 50%), and there was a 5-month improvement in median survival (29 vs. 24 months).** PFS was better with the *paclitaxel* regimen (HR = 0.76); there was a 10% difference in 1-year PFS (50% vs. 40%) and a 3-month prolongation in median PFS

(13 vs. 10 months). The toxicities were comparable, except there was a significantly higher incidence of neurologic toxicity and alopecia in the *paclitaxel* group, whereas myelosuppression was significantly greater with the non–*paclitaxel*-containing regimens.

Two randomized trials have compared *carboplatin* alone to *carboplatin* and *gemcitabine* or *liposomal doxorubicin* (463,464). There was a higher response rate with the combination therapy and a longer PFS, but the studies were not powered to look at overall survival. **In the GCIG study comparing *carboplatin* and *gemcitabine* with *carboplatin* alone, the response rate was 47.2% for the combination and 30.9% for *carboplatin*, with the PFSs being 8.6 and 5.8 months, respectively** (463). A SWOG study of *carboplatin* versus *carboplatin* and *liposomal doxorubicin* was closed early because of poor accrual, but with 61 patients recruited, the response rate was 67% for the combination and 32% for *carboplatin*. The PFS was 12 months versus 8 months; intriguingly, the overall survival was 26 months compared to 18 months ($p = 0.02$) (467). A phase II study from France confirmed the high response rate of 67% with *carboplatin* and *liposomal doxorubicin* in patients with platinum-sensitive recurrent ovarian cancer (464).

A large GCIG study (CALYPSO) comparing *carboplatin* and *liposomal doxorubicin* (CD) with *carboplatin* and *paclitaxel* (CP) recruited almost 1,000 patients, and has been recently reported (467). With a median follow-up of 22 months, PFS for the CD arm was statistically superior to the CP arm (hazard ratio, 0.821; 95% CI, 0.72 to 0.94; $p = 0.005$); median PFS was 11.3 versus 9.4 months, respectively. Overall severe nonhematologic toxicity (36.8% vs. 28.4%; $p < 0.01$) leading to early discontinuation (15% vs. 6%; $p < 0.001$) occurred more frequently in the CP arm. More frequent grade 2 or greater alopecia (83.6% vs. 7%), hypersensitivity reactions (18.8% vs. 5.6%), and sensory neuropathy (26.9% vs. 4.9%) were observed in the CP arm; more hand–foot syndrome (grade 2 to 3, 12% vs. 2.2%), nausea (35.2% vs. 24.2%), and mucositis (grade 2 to 3, 13.9% vs. 7%) in the CD arm. **This trial demonstrated superiority in PFS and better therapeutic index of *carboplatin* and *liposomal doxorubicin* compared to *carboplatin* and *paclitaxel*, and this regimen is now widely used.**

Non-Platinum Chemotherapy in Platinum-Sensitive Recurrent Ovarian Cancer

Some researchers have hypothesized that treating patients with non-platinum drugs to prolong the *platinum-free interval* will allow the tumor to again become more platinum-sensitive over time (466). However, **there are no data to support the hypothesis that the interposition of a non-platinum agent will result in an increase in platinum-sensitivity because of a longer interval since the last platinum treatment.**

Non-platinum regimens have been investigated as second-line therapy (468,469), including a large Phase III trial of *trabectedin* plus *liposomal doxorubicin* compared to *liposomal doxorubicin* alone (470). This trial included patients with platinum-resistant as well as platinum-sensitive recurrent disease. In patients with "platinum-sensitive" recurrence, response rates were higher for the combination of *trabectedin* plus *liposomal doxorubicin* (35% vs. 23%) and the median PFS was 9.2 versus 7.5 months, respectively (hazard ratio, 0.73; 95% CI, 0.56 to 0.95; $p = 0.0170$) (470). The authors did not report on the response rates to subsequent platinum based chemotherapy in patients with either platinum-sensitive or platinum-resistant disease and whether there was any apparent increase likelihood or response to platinum as a result of increasing the platinum free interval.

Platinum-Resistant and Refractory Disease

In platinum-refractory patients—defined as those progressing on treatment—the response rates to second-line chemotherapy are less than 10% (Table 11.7). The management of women who are platinum-resistant (i.e., progressing within 6 months of completion of chemotherapy) is complex and these patients should be offered clinical trials if available. However, **the Aurelia trial recently demonstrated the added benefit of *bevacizumab* to chemotherapy, and this is likely to change the standard of care** (486).

All randomized trials of combination versus single-agent chemotherapy in resistant/refractory ovarian cancer have failed to show superiority of combination chemotherapy over single-agent treatment (463,464). **There are a variety of potentially active single agents, the most frequently used being *paclitaxel*, *docetaxel*, *topotecan*, *liposomal doxorubicin*, *gemcitabine*, *ifosfamide*, *trabectedin* oral *etoposide*, *tamoxifen*, and *bevacizumab*** (441–456,468,469).

Almost 200 patients with platinum-resistant ovarian cancer were randomized to receive either *gemcitabine* or *liposomal doxorubicin*. In the *gemcitabine* and *liposomal doxorubicin* groups, median PFSs were 3.6 versus 3.1 months, median overall survivals were 12.7 versus 13.5 months, and overall response rates were 6.1% versus 8.3%, respectively. In the subset of patients with measurable disease,

Table 11.7 Key Randomized Trials in Platinum-Resistant Ovarian Cancer					
Trials (Reference)	*N (Patients)*	*RR (%)*	*PFS (months)*	*OS (months)*	*Comments*
Topotecan vs.	124	6.5	3.1	9.5	No significant difference
PLD	130	12.3	2.1	8.2	
Gordon et al., 2001 (435)					
Gemcitabine vs.	99	6.1	3.6	12	No significant difference
PLD	96	8.3	3.1	13	
Mutch et al., 2007 (476)					
Topotecan vs.	57	19.3	4.2	11.2	*P* = 0.04 PFS
Treosulfan	57	7	2.2	7.3	OS—no difference
Meier et al., 2009 (475)					
PLD or Topotecan vs.	229	10.9	4.3	13.5	3rd line therapy
Canfosfamide	232	4.3	2.3	8.5	*Canfosfamide* inferior
Vergote et al., 2009 (478)					
PLD vs.	117	12.2	3.7	NR	No difference seen
PLD/trabectedin	115	13.4	4	No difference in 2 arms	in platinum-resistant
Monk et al., 2010 (470)					
PLD vs.	417	7.9	3.7	12.7	Not significant
Patupilone	412	15.5	3.7	13.2	
Columbo et al., 2012 (474)					
TRINOVA 1 Trial	919	30	5.4	17.3	PFS *p* < 0.001
weekly *paclitaxel*		38	7.2	19	OS—not significant
± *trebananib*					
Monk et al., 2013 (487)					
PRECEDENT Trial	53	12	2.7	NR	CA125 RR
PLD ± *vintafolide*	109	18	5	No difference in 2 arms	38% vs. 19%
Naumann et al., 2013 (477)					PFS *p* = 0.03
Paclitaxel + placebo vs.	36	43	5.3	12.3	No benefit of *saracatinib*
Paclitaxel + *saracatinib*	71	21	4.7	10.1	PFS and OS greatest if
McNeish et al., 2014 (481)					taxane-free interval >6 mo
AURELIA Trial	182	12	3.4	13.3	PFS *p* = 0.001
PLD/topotecan/	179	31	6.7	16.6	OS *p* = 0.17
weekly *paclitaxel*					
± *bevacizumab*					
Pujade-Lauraine et al.,					
2014 (486)					

PLD, pegylated liposomal doxorubicin; PFS, progression-free survival; OS, overall survival; RR, response rate; NR, not reported.

overall response rates were 9.2% versus 11.7%, respectively. None of the efficacy end points showed a statistically significant difference between treatment groups. The *liposomal doxorubicin* group experienced significantly more hand–foot syndrome and mucositis, whereas the *gemcitabine* group experienced significantly more constipation, nausea and vomiting, fatigue, and neutropenia (473).

These findings are similar to the results of a large randomized phase III trial comparing *patupilone* to *liposomal doxorubicin* in 829 patients with platinum-refractory/resistant ovarian cancer (474). *Patupilone* has been reported to have a 16% overall response rate in patients with platinum-refractory and platinum-resistant recurrent ovarian cancer. The primary end point of the study was overall survival. There was no difference in patient outcomes between the two treatments. The median PFS was 3.7 months in both arms, and the overall survival was 13.2 months in the *patupilone* arm and 12.7 months in the *liposomal doxorubicin* arm; 20% of patients in the experimental arm discontinued treatment because of toxicity. Frequently observed adverse events of all grades were common and included diarrhea (85%) and peripheral neuropathy (39%) in the *patupilone* arm and stomatitis/mucositis (43%) and hand–foot syndrome (41.8%) in the *liposomal doxorubicin* arm. The majority of patients in this trial had platinum resistant, not platinum-refractory disease. Furthermore, almost all had a WHO performance status of 0 or 1, so this selected population is not necessarily representative of the large number of women with platinum-resistant/refractory ovarian cancer. **The results highlight the poor prognosis of these patients, and underscore the importance of symptom benefit and quality-of-life considerations.** Arguably, **these should be the primary aim of chemotherapy, and should be used as coprimary end points, along with traditional end points such as PFS and OS in clinical trials.**

Taxanes

Single-agent *paclitaxel* **has shown objective responses in 20–30% of patients in phase II trials of women with platinum-resistant ovarian cancer** (409–414). The main toxicities have been asthenia and peripheral neuropathy. **Weekly** *paclitaxel* **is more active than three-weekly dosing and is also associated with less toxicity.** In a study of 53 women with platinum-resistant ovarian cancer, weekly *paclitaxel* (80 mg/m^2 over 1 hour) had an objective response of 25% in patients with measurable disease, and 27% of patients without measurable disease had a 75% decline in serum CA125 levels (412).

Docetaxel **also has some activity in these patients** (415–417). The GOG studied 60 women with platinum-resistant ovarian or primary peritoneal cancer (417). Although there was a 22% objective response rate, the median response duration was only 2.5 months, and therapy was complicated by severe neutropenia in three-quarters of the patients.

Topotecan

Topotecan **is an active second-line treatment for patients with platinum-sensitive and platinum-resistant disease** (418–433). In a study of 139 women receiving *topotecan* 1.5 mg/m^2 daily for 5 days, response rates were 19% and 13% in patients with platinum-sensitive and platinum-resistant disease, respectively (418). **The predominant toxicity of** *topotecan* **is hematologic, especially neutropenia.** With the 5-day dosing schedule, 70–80% of patients have severe neutropenia, and 25% have febrile neutropenia, with or without infection (418,423). In some studies, regimens of 5 days produce better response rates than regimens of shorter duration (418–428), but in others, reducing the dose to 1 mg/m^2/d for 3 days is associated with similar response rates but lower toxicity (429,430). In a study of 31 patients, one-half of whom were platinum refractory (431), *topotecan* 2 mg/m^2/d for 3 days every 21 days had a 32% response rate. Continuous infusion *topotecan* (0.4 mg/m^2/d for 14 to 21 days) had a 27–35% objective response rate in platinum-refractory patients (424,455). **Weekly** *topotecan* **administered at a dose of 4 mg/m^2/wk for 3 weeks with a week off every month produced a response rate similar to the 5-day regimen with considerably less toxicity. Therefore, this is now considered the regimen of choice for this agent** (433).

Liposomal Doxorubicin

Liposomal doxorubicin (*Doxil* in the United States and *Caelyx* in Europe) has activity in platinum- and *taxane*-refractory disease (402,435,438). **Its predominant severe toxicity is the** *hand–foot syndrome,* **also known as** *palmar–plantar erythrodysesthesia* **or** *acral erythema,* **which is observed in 20% of patients who receive 50 mg/m^2 every 4 weeks** (435). *Liposomal doxorubicin* does not cause neurologic toxicity or alopecia. It is administered every 4 weeks, which makes it convenient, and it is relatively well tolerated at the lower dose of 40 mg/m^2, which is widely used. In a study of 89 patients with platinum-refractory disease, including 82 *paclitaxel*-resistant patients, *liposomal doxorubicin* (50 mg/m^2 every 3 weeks) produced a response in 17% (one complete and 14 partial responses) (435). In another study, an objective response rate of 26% was reported, although there were no responses in women who progressed during first-line therapy (434).

There have been two randomized trials comparing *liposomal doxorubicin* **with either** *topotecan* **or** *paclitaxel*. In a study of 237 women who relapsed after receiving one platinum-containing regimen, 117 of whom (49.4%) had platinum-refractory disease, *liposomal doxorubicin* 50 mg/m^2 over 1 hour every 4 weeks **was compared with** *topotecan* 1.5 mg/m^2/d for 5 days every 3 weeks (402,435). **The two treatments had a similar overall response rate** (20% vs. 17%), **time to progression** (22 vs. 20 weeks), **and median overall survival** (66 vs. 56 weeks). The myelotoxicity was significantly lower in the *liposomal doxorubicin*–treated patients. **In a second study comparing** *liposomal doxorubicin* **with single-agent** *paclitaxel* **in 214 platinum-treated patients who had not received prior** *taxanes* (436), **the overall response rates for** *liposomal doxorubicin* **and** *paclitaxel* **were 18% and 22%, respectively, and median survivals were 46 and 56 weeks, respectively.** Neither was significantly different. In practice, most patients are treated with a starting dose of 40 mg/m^2 of *liposomal doxorubicin* every 4 weeks because of the need to commonly dose reduce when 50 mg/m^2 is initially used.

Gemcitabine

Gemcitabine is a nucleoside analogue of cytidine and has been reported to have response rates of 10–20% in patients who have platinum-resistant disease and 6% in those with platinum-refractory disease (439–443). **The principal toxicities are myelosuppression and gastrointestinal.**

Oral *Etoposide*

The most common toxicities with oral *etoposide* are myelosuppression and gastrointestinal. Grade 4 neutropenia is observed in approximately one-fourth of patients, and 10–15% have severe nausea and vomiting (444–446). Although an initial study of intravenous *etoposide* reported an objective response rate of only 8% among 24 patients (444), a subsequent study of oral *etoposide* given for a prolonged period (50 mg/m^2 daily for 21 days every 4 weeks) had a 27% response rate in 41 women with platinum-resistant disease, three of whom had durable complete responses (445). In 25 patients with platinum- and *taxane*-resistant disease, eight objective responses (32%) were reported. **Oral *etoposide* should be considered in patients with *paclitaxel*- and platinum-resistant disease.**

Hormonal Therapy

Although response rates have been generally low with hormonal therapy, there is evidence that a subset of patients with recurrent or metastatic ovarian cancer do benefit (452–461).

Tamoxifen has been reported to have activity in some patients with recurrent ovarian cancer, with a reported response rate of 17% in heavily pretreated patients (452). A Cochrane review of *tamoxifen* in ovarian cancer reported an average response rate of 9.6%, ranging from 0–56% in different phase II studies (454). The meta-analysis was based on phase II trials only, and the authors concluded that there was only limited evidence for activity of *tamoxifen* in patients with recurrent ovarian cancer.

More recently, **there has been a randomized phase III trial comparing *tamoxifen* with *thalidomide* in patients with recurrent ovarian cancer** with GCIG CA125 progression. This study was closed prematurely after **an interim analysis showed similar PFS, but shorter overall survival in the *thalidomide* arm (median survival 24 months vs. 33.2 months in *tamoxifen* arm),** as well as more toxicity in the *thalidomide* arm.

The gonadotropin-agonist *leuprolide acetate (Lupron)* has produced a response rate of 10% in one series (457). Aromatase inhibitors (e.g., *letrozole, anastrozole,* and *exemestane*), which have been shown to be more active than *tamoxifen* in postmenopausal women with breast cancer, **are being investigated in relapsed ovarian cancer (460).** Patients with tumors that highly express ER or PR may have the best responses to hormonal treatment. This is categorized by the Allred score, which uses the percentage of cells that stain by immunohistochemistry for ER and stratifies a breast cancer patient's ER status into cancers that are likely to respond to hormone therapy with *tamoxifen* or *letrozole*. An association between the Allred score and CA125 response to *letrozole* has been observed in preselected patients with ER-positive recurrent ovarian cancer. The response rate was 0% in the lowest ER score group, 12% in the middle score group, and 33% in the highest score group. Higher ER expression has also been associated with a greater CA125 response in unselected patients with relapsed ovarian cancer (460). However, this has not been a consistent finding. One major advantage of this class of agent is the relatively low toxicity compared to chemotherapy (462).

Targeted Therapies

A new era of cancer treatment is being entered in which knowledge of molecular pathways within normal and malignant cells has led to the development of molecular targeted therapies (a full discussion is presented in Chapter 2).

The best success to date in ovarian cancer has been achieved by targeting angiogenesis, in particular VEGF, which has been found to play a major role in the biology of epithelial ovarian cancer (482). The VEGF family includes VEGF-A, VEGF-B, VEGF-C, VEGF-D, VEGF-E, and placental growth factor, with VEGF-A being the major mediator of angiogenesis. These proteins interact with VEGF tyrosine kinase receptors to initiate a cascade of downstream signaling pathways leading to the formation of new blood vessels, and an increase in the permeability of existing blood vessels. **There are two main approaches to the inhibition of the VEGF pathway: inhibition of the VEGF ligand with antibodies such as *bevacizumab*, and inhibition of the VEGF-R with tyrosine kinase inhibitors such as *pazopanib* or *cediranib*.** Therapies that specifically target the VEGF ligand inhibit only the proangiogenic VEGF pathway. In contrast, tyrosine kinase inhibitors that target the receptor have a wider range of inhibitory effects, and also have "off target" effects, which explain the different side effect profiles.

Bevacizumab **is the first targeted agent to show significant single-agent activity in ovarian cancer.** It is a humanized monoclonal antibody that targets angiogenesis by binding to VEGF-A, thereby blocking the interaction of VEGF with its receptor. There have been a number of phase II studies reporting the **use of** *bevacizumab* **in patients with platinum-sensitive and platinum-resistant ovarian cancer, with response rates ranging from 16–22%** in both platinum-sensitive and platinum-refractory patients (479,480). **About 40% of patients had stabile disease for at least 6 months.**

A study of 70 patients with recurrent ovarian cancer using low-dose metronomic chemotherapy with 50 mg of *cyclophosphamide* daily and *bevacizumab* 10 mg/kg intravenously every 2 weeks showed significant activity (483). The primary end point was PFS at 6 months. **The probability of being alive and progression free at 6 months was 56%.** A partial response was achieved in 17 patients (24%). Median times to progression and survival were 7.2 and 16.9 months, respectively. The **side effects** of *bevacizumab* **include hypertension, fatigue, proteinuria, and gastrointestinal perforation or fistula.** Uncommonly, vascular thrombosis and CNS ischemia, pulmonary hypertension, bleeding, and wound healing complications may occur. The most common side effect is hypertension. This is grade 3 in 7% of patients and is usually readily treatable, whereas the most concerning side effect is bowel perforation. The study by Cannistra was stopped after recruiting 44 patients because of an **11% incidence of bowel perforation** (479).

It has been suggested that bowel perforation can be avoided by careful screening of patients. Simpkins et al. (484) limited *bevacizumab* to patients without clinical symptoms of bowel obstruction, evidence of rectosigmoid involvement on pelvic examination, or bowel involvement on CT scan. Their study included 25 patients with platinum-resistant ovarian cancer, and all had been heavily pretreated. They observed a response rate of 28% and had no bowel perforations or any other grade 3 or 4 toxicity (484).

The role of *bevacizumab* has been investigated in a number of randomized trials. The first-line studies have been reviewed above, and the studies in recurrent ovarian cancer are discussed below.

OCEANS is a randomized trial of bevacizumab in 484 women with platinum-sensitive recurrent ovarian cancer (485). Patients with recurrence ≥6 months after first-line platinum-based therapy and measurable disease were randomly assigned to *carboplatin* and *gemcitabine* plus either *bevacizumab* or placebo for six to 10 cycles. *Bevacizumab* or placebo was then continued until disease progression. The primary end point was PFS by RECIST. The PFS for the *bevacizumab* arm was superior to that for the placebo arm (hazard ratio [HR], 0.484; 95% CI, 0.388 to 0.605; $p < 0.0001$). **The median PFS was 12.4 months in the** *bevacizumab* **arm compared to 8.4 months in the placebo arm.** The objective response rate (78.5% vs. 57.4%; $p < 0.0001$) and duration of response (10.4 vs. 7.4 months; HR, 0.534; 95% CI, 0.408 to 0.698) were also significantly improved with the addition of *bevacizumab*. Quality of life was not assessed but there were no new or unexpected toxicities observed. There are no data regarding the impact on overall survival. **The findings of this study support the role of** *bevacizumab* **in selected patients with platinum-sensitive recurrent ovarian cancer.**

AURELIA is a randomized study in which women with platinum-resistant recurrent ovarian cancer received either the standard of care (e.g., *pegylated doxorubicin* **monthly,** *topotecan* **weekly, or** *paclitaxel* **weekly) or these agents combined with** *bevacizumab* **(15 mg/kg q3wks)** (486). Women at high risk for GI perforations were excluded from participation and patients could not have had more than 3 lines of prior chemotherapy. **The women in the experimental arm had a substantially longer PFS (6.7 months vs. 3.4 months,** HR 0.48; $p < 0.001$**) and a higher overall response rate** (30.9% vs. 12.6%; $p < 0.001$). There was no difference in the overall survival between the groups with or without *bevacizumab* but there was a planned crossover, so that patients who had not received *bevacizumab* initially could receive it at relapse. **In a subgroup analysis, there was a highly significant overall survival benefit in the weekly** *paclitaxel* **group. The median survival for weekly** *paclitaxel* **alone was approximately 13 months and when** *bevacizumab* **was added to** *paclitaxel***, the median survival was 22 months. This study supports the addition of** *bevacizumab* **to chemotherapy in selected patients with platinum-resistant ovarian cancer, and in particular suggests that** *bevacizumab* **should be combined with weekly** *paclitaxel***.**

Trebananib (AMG386) is an angiopoietin antagonist that targets Tie1 and 2 receptors and blocks angiogenesis. **The TRINOVA-1 study was a large randomized trial with 919 patients who had either platinum-resistant disease or partially platinum-sensitive recurrence, who all received weekly** *paclitaxel.* **The patients and were randomized to a placebo or** *trebananib* (487). The primary end point was PFS and the authors recently reported that **there was a significant prolongation of PFS from 5.4 to 7.2 months for the** *trebananib* **arm**. (HR of 0.66) *Trebananib*, which is given weekly intravenously, does not cause hypertension or bowel perforation, but can cause edema and ascites.

The ICON6 study (488) **was run by the Medical Research Council in the United Kingdom and had a similar study design and patient population to the OCEANS trial. However, instead of *bevacizumab* they used *cediranib*, which is an oral tyrosine kinase inhibitor, which targets vascular endothelial growth factors 1, 2, and 3.** The aim of the study was to determine whether *cediranib* added to chemotherapy, either concurrently or sequentially, would provide benefit. The study planned to enrol 2,000 patients, but the pharmaceutical company sponsoring the trial decided to discontinue the development of the drug because of negative results in other diseases. The study was closed after 480 enrolled patients. Using a restrictive-means analysis, **there was a 3- to 4-month benefit in PFS, a hazard ratio of 0.57, and approximately a 3-month benefit in overall survival, which appeared to be due to the maintenance *cediranib* study.** This is a very important observation, and the first evidence to suggest that maintenance therapy with the antiangiogenesis inhibitor is associated with an overall survival benefit.

VEGF-Trap **functions as a soluble decoy receptor, soaking up a ligand before it can interact with its receptor.** It is currently being evaluated in phase II trials in patients with recurrent ovarian cancer, either as a single agent or in combination with chemotherapy (489). **A randomized phase II study, of intravenous *aflibercept* at 2 different doses (2 mg/kg or 4 mg/kg) in patients with recurrent, platinum-resistant ovarian, peritoneal, or fallopian tube cancer who developed disease progression after receiving *topotecan* and/or *PLD* has recently been reported. The authors reported the results in 215 evaluable patients, which were disappointing** and including 1 responder among 106 patients (0.9%) in the 2-mg/kg cohort, and 5 responders among 109 patients (4.6%) in the 4-mg/kg cohort, which did not meet the primary end point for response (490).

A recent study of *aflibercept* 4 mg/kg every 2 weeks compared to placebo in patients with platinum-resistant/platinum-refractory cancer and ascites found that the time to repeat paracentesis was significantly longer with *aflibercept* than with placebo (55.1 vs. 23.3 days $p = 0.0019$), but there was significant toxicity with the *aflibercept*, which restricted its use in this setting (489). Coleman et al. (491) reported that **the combination of *aflibercept* (6 mg/kg) and *docetaxel* (75 mg/m^2) had significant activity (54% RR) in a phase I-II trial** that included patients with platinum-sensitive as well as recurrent disease, and this requires confirmation.

Dose-Intense Second-Line Chemotherapy

In patients with minimal residual (≤5 mm) or microscopic disease confined to the peritoneal cavity, intraperitoneal chemotherapy or immunotherapy has been used (493–509). Cytotoxic chemotherapeutic agents such as *cisplatin, paclitaxel, 5-fluorouracil (5-FU), etoposide* (VP-16), and *mitoxantrone,* have been used as single agents in patients with persistent epithelial ovarian cancer (493–501), and complete responses have been seen in patients who have started their treatment with minimal residual disease. The surgically documented response rates reported with this approach have been 20–40% for carefully selected patients, with a complete response rate of 10–20%. Although it has been suggested that this approach may produce a significant improvement in survival (503), there are no prospective phase III data to demonstrate this.

Of historical interest is intraperitoneal immunotherapy with *alpha interferon (α-interferon), γ-interferon,* tumor necrosis factor, and *interleukin 2,* which were shown to have some activity in patients with minimal residual disease (502–510) (see Chapter 2). The response rate for the intraperitoneal cytokines, *α-interferon* and *γ-interferon,* was the same as that for the cytotoxic agents: Approximately 28–50% (502–505). The combination of *cisplatin* and *α-interferon* has produced a surgically documented 50% complete response rate, which was greater than that produced by the single agent alone (504). However, because *interferons* are not FDA approved for use in ovarian cancer, they are no longer used.

Second-line intraperitoneal treatment is not suitable for most patients, because they often have extensive intraperitoneal adhesions or extraperitoneal disease. Therefore, second-line intraperitoneal chemotherapy and immunotherapy should be considered experimental (see Chapter 2).

High-Dose Chemotherapy and Autologous Bone Marrow Transplantation

The use of high-dose chemotherapy and either autologous bone marrow transplantation or peripheral stem cell protection has been tested in patients with advanced ovarian cancer (511–514). **In one trial of high-dose *carboplatin* with autologous bone marrow transplantation, 7 of the 11 patients with extensive refractory disease had an objective response.** The maximum tolerated dose of high-dose *carboplatin* was 2 g/m^2 (511).

A phase III randomized trial of 57 patients treated with high-dose chemotherapy (*cyclophosphamide* 6,000 mg/m^2 and *carboplatin* 1,600 mg/m^2) with peripheral blood stem cell support

as consolidation versus 53 patients treated with conventional dose maintenance (*cyclophosphamide* 600 mg/m^2 and *carboplatin* 300 mg/m^2) has been reported (512). Only 43 of the 57 women (75%) completed the high-dose therapy, while 48 of 53 (92%) completed the standard dose regimen. There was no statistically significant difference in progression-free or overall survival between the two groups of patients.

A European study of high-dose chemotherapy was a negative study (514). One hundred and forty-nine patients with untreated ovarian cancer were randomly assigned after debulking surgery to receive standard combination chemotherapy or sequential high-dose treatment with two cycles of *cyclophosphamide* and *paclitaxel* followed by three cycles of high-dose *carboplatin* and *paclitaxel* with stem cell support. High-dose *melphalan* was added to the final cycle. After a median follow-up of 38 months, the PFS was 20.5 months in the standard arm and 29.6 months in the high-dose arm. The median overall survival was 62.8 months in the standard arm and 54.4 months in the high-dose arm. This is the first randomized trial comparing sequential high-dose with standard-dose chemotherapy in first-line treatment of patients with advanced ovarian cancer, and no statistically significant difference in progression-free or overall survival was observed. The investigators concluded that high-dose chemotherapy does not appear to be superior to conventional-dose chemotherapy.

Whole-Abdominal Radiation

Whole-abdominal radiation given as a second-line treatment has been shown to be potentially effective in a small subset of patients with microscopic disease, but it is associated with a relatively high morbidity. The principal problem associated with this approach is the development of acute and chronic intestinal morbidity. As many as 30% of patients treated with this approach develop intestinal obstruction, and this may necessitate potentially morbid exploratory surgery (510). Because there are many new chemotherapeutic agents available for the treatment of relapsed ovarian cancer, most centers have stopped using second-line whole-abdominal radiation therapy.

Intestinal Obstruction

Patients with epithelial ovarian cancer often develop intestinal obstruction, either at the time of initial diagnosis or, more frequently, in association with recurrent disease (515–526). Obstruction may be related to a mechanical blockage or to carcinomatous ileus. Correction of the intestinal blockage can be accomplished in most patients whose obstruction appears at the time of initial diagnosis. However, the decision to perform an exploratory procedure to palliate intestinal obstruction in patients with recurrent disease is more difficult. In patients whose life expectancy is very short (e.g., shorter than 2 months), surgical relief of the obstruction is not indicated (518). In those whose projected life span is longer, features that predict a reasonable likelihood of success include young age, good nutritional status, and the absence of rapidly accumulating ascites.

For most patients with recurrent ovarian cancer who present with intestinal obstruction, initial management should include radiographic documentation of the obstruction, hydration, correction of any electrolyte disturbances, and possibly parenteral alimentation (516,518). In many patients, the obstruction may be alleviated by this conservative approach. A preoperative upper gastrointestinal series and a barium enema will define possible sites of obstruction.

If exploratory surgery is deemed appropriate, the type of operation to be performed will depend on (i) the site and (ii) the number of obstructions. Multiple sites of obstruction are not uncommon in patients with recurrent epithelial ovarian cancer. More than one-half of the patients have a small-bowel obstruction, one-third have a colonic obstruction, and one-sixth have both (516–518). If the obstruction is principally contained in one area of the bowel (e.g., the terminal ileum), this area can either be resected or bypassed, depending on what can be accomplished safely. Intestinal bypass is generally less morbid than resection, and in patients with progressive cancer, the survival time after these two operations is the same (522,524). If multiple obstructions are present, resection of several segments of intestine is usually not indicated, and intestinal bypass or colostomy should usually be performed. A gastrostomy may occasionally be useful in this circumstance (525), and this can usually be placed percutaneously (526).

Surgery for bowel obstruction in patients with ovarian cancer carries an operative mortality of approximately 10% and a major complication rate of about 30% (517–519). The need for multiple reanastomoses and preceding radiation therapy increases the morbidity, which consists primarily of sepsis and enterocutaneous fistulae. The median survival ranges from 3 to 12 months, although approximately 20% of such patients survive longer than 12 months (518). Further discussion of the palliative care of intestinal obstruction in these patients is presented in Chapter 25.

References

1. **Siegel R, Ma J, Zou Z, et al.** Cancer statistics. 2014. *CA Cancer J Clin.* 2014;64:9–29.
2. **SEER Cancer Statistics Factsheets.** *Ovary Cancer.* National Cancer Institute. Bethesda, MD. http://seer.cancer.gov/statfacts/html/ovary.html
3. **Scully RE, Young RH, Clement PB.** Tumors of the ovary, maldeveloped gonads, fallopian tube, and broad ligament. In: *Atlas of Tumor Pathology.* 3rd Series, Fascicle 23. Washington, DC: Armed Forces Institute of Pathology; 1998:1–168.
4. **Kurman RJ, Shih IeM.** Pathogenesis of ovarian cancer: Lessons from morphology and molecular biology and their clinical implications. *Int J Gynecol Pathol.* 2008;27:151–160.
5. **Crum CP, Drapkin R, Miron A, et al.** The distal fallopian tube: A new model for pelvic serous carcinogenesis. *Curr Opin Obstet Gynecol.* 2007;19:3–9.
6. **Berek JS, Crum C, Friedlander MF.** Cancer of the ovary, fallopian tube, and peritoneum. *Int J Gynaecol Obstet.* 2012;119(suppl 2); S118–S129.
7. **Kindelberger DW, Lee Y, Miron A, et al.** Intraepithelial carcinoma of the fimbria and pelvic serous carcinoma: Evidence for a causal relationship. *Am J Surg Pathol.* 2007;31:161–169.
8. **Callahan MJ, Crum CP, Medeiros F, et al.** Primary fallopian tube malignancies in *BRCA*-positive women undergoing surgery for ovarian cancer risk reduction. *J Clin Oncol.* 2007;25:3985–3990.
9. **Carlson JW, Miron A, Jarboe EA, et al.** Serous tubal intraepithelial carcinoma: Its potential role in primary peritoneal serous carcinoma and serous cancer prevention. *J Clin Oncol.* 2008;26:4160–4165.
10. **Levanon K, Crum C, Drapkin R.** New insights into the pathogenesis of serous ovarian cancer and its clinical impact. *J Clin Oncol.* 2008; 26:5284–5293.
11. **Erickson BK, Conner MG, Landen CN.** The role of the fallopian tube in the origin of ovarian cancer. *Am J Obstet Gynecol.* 2013;209: 409–414. http://dx.doi.org/10.1016/j.acog.2013.04.019
12. **Dubeau L.** The cell of origin of ovarian epithelial tumours. *Lancet Oncol.* 2008;9:1191–1197.
13. **Fowler JM, Nieberg RK, Schooler TA, et al.** Peritoneal adenocarcinoma (serous) of müllerian type: A subgroup of women presenting with peritoneal carcinomatosis. *Int J Gynecol Cancer.* 1994;4: 43–51.
14. **Tobacman JK, Greene MH, Tucker MA, et al.** Intra-abdominal carcinomatosis after prophylactic oophorectomy in ovarian cancer-prone families. *Lancet.* 1982;2:795–797.
15. **Piver MS, Jishi MF, Tsukada Y, et al.** Primary peritoneal carcinoma after prophylactic oophorectomy in women with a family history of ovarian cancer: A report of the Gilda Radner Familial Ovarian Cancer Registry. *Cancer.* 1993;71:2751–2755.
16. **Barnhill DR, Kurman RJ, Brady MF, et al.** Preliminary analysis of the behavior of stage I ovarian serous tumors of low malignant potential: A Gynecologic Oncology Group study. *J Clin Oncol.* 1995;13: 2752–2756.
17. **Seidman JD, Kurman RJ.** Subclassification of serous borderline tumors of the ovary into benign and malignant types: A clinicopathologic study of 65 advanced stage cases. *Am J Surg Pathol.* 1996;20: 1331–1345.
18. **Seidman JD, Kurman RJ.** Pathology of ovarian carcinoma. *Hematol Oncol Clin North Am.* 2003;17:909–925.
19. **Bell DA, Weinstock MA, Scully RE.** Peritoneal implants of ovarian serous borderline tumors: Histologic features and prognosis. *Cancer.* 1988;62:2212–2222.
20. **Heintz APM, Odicino F, Maisonneuve P, et al.** Carcinoma of the ovary. *Int J Gynecol Obstet.* 2003;83(suppl 1):135–166.
21. **Koonings PP, Campbell K, Mishell DR Jr, et al.** Relative frequency of primary ovarian neoplasms: A 10-year review. *Obstet Gynecol.* 1989;74:921–926.
22. **Negri E, Franceschi S, Tzonou A, et al.** Pooled analysis of three European case-control studies of epithelial ovarian cancer: I. Reproductive factors and risk of epithelial ovarian cancer. *Int J Cancer.* 1991;49:50–56.
23. **Franceschi S, La Vecchia C, Booth M, et al.** Pooled analysis of three European case-control studies of epithelial ovarian cancer: II. Age at menarche and menopause. *Int J Cancer.* 1991;49:57–60.
24. **Moorman PG, Havrilesky LJ, Gierisch JM, et al.** Oral contraceptives and risk of ovarian cancer and breast cancer among high-risk women: A systematic review and meta-analysis. *J Clin Oncol.* 2013; 31:4188–4198.
25. **Engeland A, Tretli S, Bjorge T.** Height, body mass index, and ovarian cancer: A follow-up of 1.1 million Norwegian women. *J Natl Cancer Inst.* 2003;95:1244–1248.
26. **Ness RB, Cramer DW, Goodman MT, et al.** Infertility, fertility drugs, and ovarian cancer: A pooled analysis of case-control studies. *Am J Epidemiol.* 2002;155:217–224.
27. **Sit AS, Modugno F, Weissfeld JL, et al.** Hormone replacement therapy and formulations and risk of epithelial ovarian carcinoma. *Gynecol Oncol.* 2002;86:118–123.
28. **Lacey JV Jr, Mink PJ, Lubin JH, et al.** Menopausal hormone replacement therapy and risk of ovarian cancer. *J Am Med Assoc.* 2002;288:334–341.
29. **Franceschi S, Parazzini F, Negri E, et al.** Pooled analysis of three European case-control studies of epithelial ovarian cancer: III. Oral contraceptive use. *Int J Cancer.* 1991;49:61–65.
30. **De Palo G, Vceronesi U, Camerini T, et al.** Can fenretinide protect women against ovarian cancer? *J Natl Cancer Inst.* 1995;87:146–147.
31. **De Palo G, Mariani L, Camerini T, et al.** Effect of fenretinide on ovarian carcinoma occurrence. *Gynecol Oncol.* 2002;86:24–27.
32. **Rulin MC, Preston AL.** Adnexal masses in postmenopausal women. *Obstet Gynecol.* 1987;70:578–581.
33. **van Nagell JR Jr, DePriest PD, Reedy MB, et al.** The efficacy of transvaginal sonographic screening in asymptomatic women at risk for ovarian cancer. *Gynecol Oncol.* 2000;77:350–356.
34. **Ueland FR, DePriest PD, Pavlik EJ, et al.** Preoperative differentiation of malignant from benign ovarian tumors: The efficacy of morphology indexing and Doppler flow sonography. *Gynecol Oncol.* 2003;91:46–50.
35. **Cohen LS, Escobar PF, Scharm C, et al.** Three-dimensional power Doppler ultrasound improves the diagnostic accuracy for ovarian cancer prediction. *Gynecol Oncol.* 2001;82:40–48.
36. **Kurjak A, Kupesic S, Sparac V, et al.** The detection of stage I ovarian cancer by three-dimensional sonography and power Doppler. *Gynecol Oncol.* 2003;90:258–264.
37. **Campbell S, Royston P, Bhan V, et al.** Novel screening strategies for early ovarian cancer by transabdominal ultrasonography. *Br J Obstet Gynaecol.* 1990;97:304–311.
38. **van Nagell JR Jr, Higgins RV, Donaldson ES, et al.** Transvaginal sonography as a screening method for ovarian cancer: A report of the first 1000 cases screened. *Cancer.* 1990;65:573–577.
39. **van Nagell JR Jr, Gallion HH, Pavlik EJ, et al.** Ovarian cancer screening. *Cancer.* 1995;76:2086–2091.
40. **Jacobs I, Oram D, Fairbanks J, et al.** A risk of malignancy index incorporating CA125, ultrasound and menopausal status for the accurate preoperative diagnosis of ovarian cancer. *Br J Obstet Gynaecol.* 1990;97:922–929.
41. **Jacobs I, Davies AP, Bridges J, et al.** Prevalence screening for ovarian cancer in postmenopausal women by CA125 measurements and ultrasonography. *BMJ.* 1993;306:1030–1034.
42. **Rustin GJS, van der Burg MEL, et al.** Tumor markers. *Ann Oncol.* 1993;4:71–77.
43. **Jacobs IJ, Skates S, Davies AP, et al.** Risk of diagnosis of ovarian cancer after raised serum CA125 concentration: A prospective cohort study. *BMJ.* 1996;313:1355–1358.
44. **Einhorn N, Sjövall K, Knapp RC, et al.** A prospective evaluation of serum CA125 levels for early detection of ovarian cancer. *Obstet Gynecol.* 1992;80:14–18.
45. **Jacobs IJ, Oram DH, Bast RC Jr.** Strategies for improving the specificity of screening for ovarian cancer with tumor-associated antigens CA125, CA15-3, and TAG 72.3. *Obstet Gynecol.* 1992;80: 396–399.
46. **Berek JS, Bast RC Jr.** Ovarian cancer screening: The use of serial complementary tumor markers to improve sensitivity and specificity for early detection. *Cancer.* 1995;76:2092–2096.
47. **Skates SJ, Xu FJ, Yu YH, et al.** Towards an optimal algorithm for ovarian cancer screening with longitudinal tumour markers. *Cancer.* 1995;76:2004–2010.

48. **Yin BW, Lloyd KO.** Molecular cloning of the CA125 ovarian cancer antigen: Identification of a new mucin, MUC16. *J Biol Chem.* 2001; 27:371–375.

49. **Lloyd KO, Yin BW, Kudryashov V.** Isolation and characterization of ovarian cancer antigen CA125 using a new monoclonal antibody (VK-8): Identification as a mucin-type molecule. *Int J Cancer.* 1997;71:842–850.

50. **O'Brien TJ, Beard JB, Underwood LJ, et al.** The CA125 gene: An extracellular superstructure dominated by repeat sequences. *Tumour Biol.* 2001;22:345–347.

51. **Gubbels JA, Belisle J, Onda M, et al.** Mesothelin-MUC16 binding is a high affinity, N-glycan dependent interaction that facilitates peritoneal metastasis of ovarian tumors. *Mol Cancer.* 2006;5:50.

52. **Maeda T, Inoue M, Koshiba S, et al.** Solution structure of the SEA domain from the murine homologue of ovarian cancer antigen CA125 (MUC16). *J Biol Chem.* 2004;279:13174–13182.

53. **Rump A, Morikawa Y, Tanaka M, et al.** Binding of ovarian cancer antigen CA125/MUC16 to mesothelin mediates cell adhesion. *J Biol Chem.* 2004;279:9190–9198.

54. **Jacobs IJ, Skates SJ, MacDonald N, et al.** Screening for ovarian cancer: A pilot randomised controlled trial. *Lancet.* 1999;353:1207–1210.

55. **Bourne TH, Campbell S, Reynolds KM, et al.** Screening for early familial ovarian cancer with transvaginal ultrasonography and colour blood flow imaging. *BMJ.* 1993;306:1025–1029.

56. **European Randomised Trial of Ovarian Cancer Screening (protocol).** Department of Environmental and Preventive Medicine, Wolfson Institute of Preventive Medicine, Barts and The London, Queen Mary's School of Medicine and Dentistry, London, United Kingdom, 1999.

57. **Skates SJ, Menon U, MacDonald N, et al.** Calculation of the risk of ovarian cancer from serial CA-125 values for preclinical detection in postmenopausal women. *J Clin Oncol.* 2003;21(suppl 10):206–210.

58. **Rosenthal AN, Fraser L, Manchanda R, et al.** Final results of 4-monthly screening in the UK Familial Ovarian Cancer Screening Study (UKFOCSS Phase 2). *J Clin Oncol.* 2013;Abstract 5507 ASCO Annual Meeting.

59. **Scholler N, Fu N, Yang Y, et al.** Soluble member(s) of the mesothelin/megakaryocyte potentiating factor family are detectable in sera from patients with ovarian carcinoma. *Proc Natl Acad Sci U S A.* 1999;96:11531–11536.

60. **Baron AT, Lafky JM, Boardman CH, et al.** Serum sErbB1 and epidermal growth factor levels as tumor biomarkers in women with stage III or IV epithelial ovarian cancer. *Cancer Epidemiol Biomarkers.* 1999;8:129–137.

61. **Schummer M, Ng WV, Bumgarner RE, et al.** Comparative hybridization of an array of 21500 ovarian cDNAs for the discovery of genes overexpressed in ovarian carcinomas. *Gene.* 1999;238:375–385.

62. **Mok SC, Chao J, Skates S, et al.** Prostasin, a potential serum marker for ovarian cancer: Identification through microarray technology. *J Natl Cancer Inst.* 2001;93:1458–1464.

63. **Kim JH, Skates SJ, Uede T, et al.** Osteopontin as a potential diagnostic for ovarian cancer. *JAMA.* 2002;282:1671–1679.

64. **Diamandis EP, Yousef GM, Soosaipillai AR, et al.** Human kallikrein 6 (zyme/protease M/neurosin): A new serum biomarker of ovarian carcinoma. *Clin Biochem.* 2000;33:579–583.

65. **Luo LY, Bunting P, Scorilas A, et al.** Human kallikrein 10: A novel tumor marker for ovarian carcinoma? *Clin Chim Acta.* 2001;306:111–118.

66. **Gorelik E, Landsittel DP, Morangonni AM, et al.** Multiplexed immunobead-based cytokine profiling for early detection of ovarian cancer. *Epidemiol Biomarkers Prev.* 2005;14:981–987.

67. **Petricoin EF, Ardekani AM, Hitt BA, et al.** Use of proteomic patterns in serum to identify ovarian cancer. *Lancet.* 2002;359:572–577.

68. **Baggerly KA, Morris JS, Coombes KR.** Reproducibility of SELDI-TOF protein patterns in serum: Comparing datasets from different experiments. *Bioinformatics.* 2004;20:777–785.

69. **Zhang Z, Bast RC Jr, Yu Y, et al.** Three biomarkers identified from serum proteomic analysis for the detection of early stage ovarian cancer. *Cancer Res.* 2004;64:5882–5890.

70. **Mok CH, Tsao SW, Knapp RC, et al.** Unifocal origin of advanced human epithelial ovarian cancers. *Cancer Res.* 1992;52:5119–5122.

71. **Muto MG, Welch WR, Mok SC, et al.** Evidence for a multifocal origin of papillary serous carcinoma of the peritoneum. *Cancer Res.* 1995;55:490–492.

72. **Easton DF, Ford D, Bishop DT.** Breast and ovarian cancer incidence in *BRCA1*-mutation carriers. Breast Cancer Linkage Consortium. *Am J Hum Genet.* 1995;56:265–271.

73. **Whittemore AS, Gong G, Itnyre J.** Prevalence and contribution of *BRCA1* mutations in breast cancer and ovarian cancer: Results from three U.S. population-based case-control studies of ovarian cancer. *Am J Hum Genet.* 1997;60:496–504.

74. **Frank TS, Manley SA, Olopade OI, et al.** Sequence analysis of *BRCA1* and *BRCA2:* Correlation of mutations with family history and ovarian cancer risk. *J Clin Oncol.* 1998;16:2417–2425.

75. **Johannsson OT, Ranstam J, Borg A, et al.** Survival of *BRCA1* breast and ovarian cancer patients: A population-based study from southern Sweden. *J Clin Oncol.* 1998;16:397–404.

76. **Burke W, Daly M, Garber J, et al.** Recommendations for follow-up care of individuals with an inherited predisposition to cancer. II. *BRCA1* and *BRCA2.* Cancer Genetics Studies Consortium. *JAMA.* 1997;277:997–1003.

77. **Berchuck A, Cirisano F, Lancaster JM, et al.** Role of *BRCA1* mutation screening in the management of familial ovarian cancer. *Am J Obstet Gynecol.* 1996;175:738–746.

78. **Struewing JP, Hartge P, Wacholder S, et al.** The risk of cancer associated with specific mutations of *BRCA1* and *BRCA2* among Ashkenazi Jews. *N Engl J Med.* 1997;336:1401–1408.

79. **Beller U, Halle D, Catane R, et al.** High frequency of *BRCA1* and *BRCA2* germline mutations in Ashkenazi Jewish ovarian cancer patients, regardless of family history. *Gynecol Oncol.* 1997;67:123–126.

80. **Lerman C, Narod S, Schulman K, et al.** *BRCA1* testing in families with hereditary breast-ovarian cancer: A prospective study of patient decision making and outcomes. *JAMA.* 1996;275:1885–1892.

81. **Ponder B.** Genetic testing for cancer risk. *Science.* 1997;278:1050–1058.

82. **Lynch HT, Cavalieri RJ, Lynch JF, et al.** Gynecologic cancer clues to Lynch syndrome II diagnosis: A family report. *Gynecol Oncol.* 1992;44:198–203.

83. **American Society of Clinical Oncology.** Statement of the American Society of Clinical Oncology: Genetic testing for cancer susceptibility. *J Clin Oncol.* 1996;14:1730–1736.

84. **King MC, Marks JH, Mandell JB, New York Breast Cancer Study Group.** Breast and ovarian cancer risks due to inherited mutations in *BRCA1* and *BRCA2. Science.* 2003;302:643–646.

85. **Risch HA, McLaughlin JR, Cole DE, et al.** Population *BRCA1* and *BRCA2* mutation frequencies and cancer penetrances: A kin-cohort study in Ontario, Canada. *J Natl Cancer Inst.* 2006;98:1694–1706.

86. **Brozek I, Ochman K, Debniak J, et al.** High frequency of *BRCA1/2* germline mutations in consecutive ovarian cancer patients in Poland. *Gynecol Oncol.* 2008;108:433–437.

87. **Antoniou A, Pharoah PD, Narod S, et al.** Average risks of breast and ovarian cancer associated with BRCA1 or BRCA2 mutations detected in case Series unselected for family history: A combined analysis of 22 studies. *Am J Hum Genet.* 2003;72(5):1117–1130.

88. **Couch FJ, Wang X, McGuffog L, et al.** Genome-wide association study in BRCA1 mutation carriers identifies novel loci associated with breast and ovarian cancer risk. *PLoS Genet.* 2013;9(3):e1003212.

89. **Alsop K, Fereday S, Meldrum C, et al.** *BRCA* Mutation Frequency and Patterns of Treatment Response in *BRCA* Mutation–Positive Women With Ovarian Cancer: A Report From the Australian Ovarian Cancer Study Group. *J Clin Oncol.* 2012;20;30(21):2654–2663.

90. **Crispens MA.** Endometrial and ovarian cancer in lynch syndrome. *Clin Colon Rectal Surg.* 2012;25(2):97–102.

91. **Huzarski T, Byrski T, Gronwald J, et al.** Ten-Year Survival in Patients With BRCA1-Negative and BRCA1-Positive Breast Cancer. *J Clin Oncol.* 2013;31(26):3191–3196.

92. **Goodwin PJ, Phillips KA, West DW, et al.** Breast cancer prognosis in BRCA1 and BRCA2 mutation carriers: An International Prospective Breast Cancer Family Registry population-based cohort study. *J Clin Oncol.* 2012;30(1):19–26.

93. **Moyer VA; U.S. Preventive Services Task Force.** Screening for ovarian cancer: U.S. Preventive Services Task Force reaffirmation recommendation statement. *Ann Intern Med.* 2012;157(12):900–904.

94. **Hermsen BB, Olivier RI, Verheijen RH, et al.** No efficacy of annual gynaecological screening in BRCA1/2 mutation carriers; an observational follow-up study. *Br J Cancer.* 2007;96:1335–1342.

95. **Woodward ER, Sleightholme HV, Considine AM, et al.** Annual surveillance by CA125 and transvaginal ultrasound for ovarian

cancer in both high-risk and population risk women is ineffective. *BJOG.* 2007;114:1500–1509.

96. **Hogg R, Friedlander M.** Biology of epithelial ovarian cancer: Implications for screening women at high genetic risk. *J Clin Oncol.* 2004;22:1315–1327.

97. **Greene MH, Piedmonte M, Alberts D, et al.** Prospective study of risk-reducing salpingo-oophorectomy and longitudinal CA-125 screening among women at increased genetic risk of ovarian cancer: Design and baseline characteristics: A Gynecologic Oncology Group study. *Cancer Epidemiol Biomarkers Prev.* 2008;17: 594–604.

98. **Narod SA, Risch H, Moslehi R, et al.** Oral contraceptives and the risk of hereditary ovarian cancer. Hereditary Ovarian Cancer Clinical Study Group. *N Engl J Med.* 1998;339:424–428.

99. **Modan B, Hartge P, Hirsh-Yechezkel G, et al.** Parity, oral contraceptives, and the risk of ovarian cancer among carriers and noncarriers of a *BRCA1* or *BRCA2* mutation. *N Engl J Med.* 2001;345: 235–240.

100. **Narod SA, Sun P, Ghadirian P, et al.** Tubal ligation and risk of ovarian cancer in carriers of *BRCA1* or *BRCA2* mutations: A case-control study. *Lancet.* 2001;357:1467–1470.

101. **Averette HE, Nguyen HN.** The role of prophylactic oophorectomy in cancer prevention. *Gynecol Oncol.* 1994;55:S38–S41.

102. **Domchek SM, Friebel TM, Garber JE, et al.** Occult ovarian cancers identified at risk-reducing salpingo-oophorectomy in a prospective cohort of *BRCA1/2* mutation carriers. *Breast Cancer Res Treat.* 2010;124(1):195–203

103. **Rebbeck TR, Lynch HT, Neuhausen SL, et al.** Prophylactic oophorectomy in carriers of *BRCA1* or *BRCA2* mutations. *N Engl J Med.* 2002;346:1616–1622.

104. **Haber D.** Prophylactic oophorectomy to reduce the risk of ovarian and breast cancer in carriers of *BRCA* mutations. *N Engl J Med.* 2002; 346:1660–1661.

105. **Rebbeck TR, Levin AM, Eisen A, et al.** Breast cancer risk after bilateral prophylactic oophorectomy in *BRCA1* mutation carriers. *J Natl Cancer Inst.* 1999;91:1475–1479.

106. **Schrag D, Kuntz KM, Garber JE, et al.** Decision analysis-effects of prophylactic mastectomy and oophorectomy on life expectancy among women with *BRCA1* and *BRCA2* mutations. *N Engl J Med.* 1997;336:1465–1471. [erratum, *N Engl J Med* 1997; 337:434].

107. **Lavie O, Hornreich G, Ben-Arie A.** BRCA germline mutations in Jewish women with uterine papillary carcinoma. *Gynecol Oncol.* 2004;92:521–524.

108. **Grann VR, Jacobson JS, Thomason D, et al.** Effect of prevention strategies on survival and quality-adjusted survival of women with *BRCA1/2* mutations: An updated decision analysis. *J Clin Oncol.* 2002;20:2520–2529.

109. **Domchek SM, Friebel TM, Singer CF, et al.** Association of risk-reducing surgery in BRCA1 or BRCA2 mutation carriers with cancer risk and mortality. *JAMA.* 2010;304(9):967–975.

110. **Ben David Y, Chetrit A, Hirsh-Yechezkel G, et al.** Effect of *BRCA* mutations on the length of survival in epithelial ovarian tumors. *J Clin Oncol.* 2002;20:463–466.

111. **Chetrit A, Hirsh-Yechezkel G, Ben-David Y, et al.** Effect of *BRCA1/2* mutations on long-term survival of patients with invasive ovarian cancer: The national Israeli study of ovarian cancer. *J Clin Oncol.* 2008;26:20–25.

112. **Genetic Testing for Heritable Mutations in the BRCA1 and BRCA2 Genes EVIQ Guidelines Cancer Institute NSW November 2013** https://www.eviq.org.au

113. **Schmeler KM, Lynch HT, Chen LM et al.** Prophylactic surgery to reduce the risk of gynecologic cancers in the Lynch syndrome. *N Engl J Med.* 2006;19:354(3):261–269

114. **Chen LM, Berek JS.** Ovarian and fallopian tubes. In: **Haskell CM, ed.** *Cancer Treatment.* 5th ed. Philadelphia, PA: WB Saunders; 2000: 900–932.

115. **Berek JS, Bast RC.** *Ovarian Cancer.* In: **Kufe DW, Pollock RE, Weichselbaum RR, et al.** *Cancer Medicine.* 6th ed. Hamilton, ON: BC Decker 2004:1831–1861.

116. **Goff BA, Masndel L, Muntz HG, et al.** Ovarian carcinoma diagnosis. *Cancer.* 2000;89:2068–2075.

117. **Olson SH, Mignone L, Nakraseive C, et al.** Symptoms of ovarian cancer. *Obstet Gynecol* 2001;98:212–217.

118. **Vine MF, Calingaert B, Berchuck A, et al.** Characterization of prediagnostic symptoms among primary epithelial ovarian cancer cases and controls. *Gynecol Oncol.* 2003;90:75–82.

119. **Goff BA, Mandel LS, Drescher CW, et al.** Development of an ovarian cancer symptom index: Possibilities for earlier detection. *Cancer.* 2007;109:221–227.

120. **Lataifeh I, Marsden DE, Robertson G, et al.** Presenting symptoms of epithelial ovarian cancer. *Aust NZ J Obstet Gynaecol.* 2005;45:211–214.

121. **Olsen CM, Cnossen J, Green AC, et al.** Comparison of symptoms and presentation of women with benign, low malignant potential and invasive ovarian tumors. *Eur J Gynaecol Oncol.* 2007;28:376–380.

122. **Barber HK, Grober EA.** The PMPO syndrome (postmenopausal palpable ovary syndrome). *Obstet Gynecol.* 1971;138:921–923.

123. **Baekelandt M, Nesbakken A, Kristensen GB, et al.** Carcinoma of the fallopian tube. *Cancer.* 2000;89:2076–2084.

124. **Nardo LG, Kroon ND, Reginald PW.** Persistent unilocular ovarian cysts in a general population of postmenopausal women: Is there a place for expectant management? *Obstet Gynecol.* 2003;102: 589–593.

125. **Modesitt SC, Pavlik EJ, Ueland FR, et al.** Risk of malignancy in unilocular ovarian cystic tumors less than 10 centimeters in diameter. *Obstet Gynecol.* 2003;102:594–599.

126. **Roman LD.** Small cystic pelvic masses in older women: Is surgical removal necessary? *Gynecol Oncol.* 1998;69:1–2.

127. **Bristow RE, Duska LR, Lambrou NC, et al.** A model for predicting surgical outcome in patients with advanced ovarian carcinoma using computed tomography. *Cancer.* 2000;89:1532–1540.

128. **Togashi K.** Ovarian cancer: The clinical role of US, CT, and MRI. *Eur Radiol.* 2003;13(suppl 4):S87–S104.

129. **Makhija S, Howden N, Edwards R, et al.** Positron emission tomography/computed tomography imaging for the detection of recurrent ovarian and fallopian tube carcinoma: A retrospective review. *Gynecol Oncol.* 2002;85:53–58.

130. **Kurokawa T, Yoshida Y, Kawahara K, et al.** Whole-body PET with FDG is useful for following up an ovarian cancer patient with only rising CA-125 levels within the normal range. *Ann Nucl Med.* 2002;16:491–493.

131. **Jung SE, Lee JM, Rha SE, et al.** CT and MR imaging of ovarian tumors with emphasis on differential diagnosis. *Radiographics.* 2002;22:1305–1325.

132. **Hacker NF, Berek JS, Lagasse LD.** Gastrointestinal operations in gynecologic oncology. In: **Knapp RE, Berkowitz RS, eds.** *Gynecologic Oncology.* 2nd ed. New York: McGraw-Hill; 1993:361–375.

133. **Chia YN, Marsden DE, Robertson G, et al.** Triage of ovarian masses. *Aust NZ J Obstet Gynaecol.* 2008;48:322–328.

134. **Malkasian GD, Knapp RC, Lavin PT, et al.** Preoperative evaluation of serum CA125 levels in premenopausal and postmenopausal patients with pelvic masses: Discrimination of benign from malignant disease. *Am J Obstet Gynecol.* 1988;159:341–346.

135. **Plentl AM, Friedman EA.** *Lymphatic System of the Female Genitalia.* Philadelphia: WB Saunders, 1971.

136. **Chen SS, Lee L.** Incidence of paraaortic and pelvic lymph node metastasis in epithelial ovarian cancer. *Gynecol Oncol.* 1983;16: 95–100.

137. **Burghardt E, Pickel H, Lahousen M, et al.** Pelvic lymphadenectomy in operative treatment of ovarian cancer. *Am J Obstet Gynecol.* 1986;155:315–319.

138. **Scarabelli C, Gallo A, Zarrelli A, et al.** Systematic pelvic and para-aortic lymphadenectomy during cytoreductive surgery in advanced ovarian cancer: Potential benefit on survival. *Gynecol Oncol.* 1995;56:328–337.

139. **Dauplat J, Hacker NF, Neiberg RK, et al.** Distant metastasis in epithelial ovarian carcinoma. *Cancer.* 1987;60:1561–1566.

140. **Krag KJ, Canellos GP, Griffiths CT, et al.** Predictive factors for long term survival in patients with advanced ovarian cancer. *Gynecol Oncol.* 1989;34:88–93.

141. **Haapasalo H, Collan Y, Atkin NB.** Major prognostic factors in ovarian carcinomas. *Int J Gynecol Cancer.* 1991;1:155–162.

142. **Haapasalo H, Collan Y, Seppa A, et al.** Prognostic value of ovarian carcinoma grading methods: A method comparison study. *Histopathology.* 1990;16:1–7.

143. **Silverberg SG.** Prognostic significance of pathologic features of ovarian carcinoma. *Curr Top Pathol.* 1989;78:85–109.

144. **Ludescher C, Weger AR, Lindholm J, et al.** Prognostic significance of tumor cell morphometry, histopathology, and clinical parameters in advanced ovarian carcinoma. *Int J Gynecol Pathol.* 1990;9:343–351.

145. **Henson DE.** The histologic grading of neoplasms. *Arch Pathol Lab Med.* 1988;112:1091–1096.

146. **Takada T, Iwase H, Iitsuka C, et al.** Adjuvant chemotherapy for stage I clear cell carcinoma of the ovary: An analysis of fully staged patients. *Int J Gynecol Cancer.* 2012;22(4):573–578

147. **Takano M, Sugiyama T, Yaegashi N, et al.** Less impact of adjuvant chemotherapy for stage I clear cell carcinoma of the ovary: A retrospective Japan Clear Cell Carcinoma Study. *Int J Gynecol Cancer.* 2010;20(9):1506–1510.

148. **Mizuno M, Kajiyama H, Shibata K, et al.** Adjuvant chemotherapy for stage 1 ovarian clear cell carcinoma: Is it necessary for stage IA? *Int J Gynecol Cancer.* 2012;22(7):1143–1149.

149. **Berek JS, Martinez-Maza O.** Molecular and biological factors in the pathogenesis of ovarian cancer. *J Reprod Med.* 1994;39:241–248.

150. **Baak JP, Chan KK, Stolk JG, et al.** Prognostic factors in borderline and invasive ovarian tumours of the common epithelial type. *Pathol Res Pract.* 1987;182:755–774.

151. **Berek JS, Martinez-Maza O, Hamilton T, et al.** Molecular and biological factors in the pathogenesis of ovarian cancer. *Ann Oncol.* 1993;4:S3–S16.

152. **Dembo AJ, Davy M, Stenwig AE, et al.** Prognostic factors in patients with stage I epithelial ovarian cancer. *Obstet Gynecol.* 1990; 75:263–273.

153. **Sjövall K, Nilsson B, Einhorn N.** Different types of rupture of the tumour capsule and the impact on survival in early ovarian cancer. *Int J Gynecol Cancer.* 1994;4:333–336.

154. **Sevelda P, Dittich C, Salzer H.** Prognostic value of the rupture of the capsule in stage I epithelial ovarian carcinoma. *Gynecol Oncol.* 1989;35:321–322.

155. **Vergote I, De Brabanter J, Fyles A, et al.** Prognostic importance of degree of differentiation and cyst rupture in stage I invasive epithelial ovarian cancer. *Lancet.* 2001;357:176–182.

156. **Tognon G, Carnazza M, Ragnoli M, et al.** Prognostic factors in early-stage ovarian cancer. *Ecancermedicalscience.* 2013;7:325.

157. **Heintz APM, Odicino F, Maisonneuve P, et al.** Carcinoma of the ovary. 26th Annual Report on the Results of Treatment in Gynaecological Cancer. *Int J Gynaecol Obstet.* 2006;95(suppl 1):S161–S192.

158. **Voest EE, van Houwelingen JC, Neijt JP.** A meta-analysis of prognostic factors in advanced ovarian cancer with median survival and overall survival measured with log (relative risk) as main objectives. *Eur J Cancer Clin Oncol.* 1989;25:711–720.

159. **Fader AN, Java J, Ueda S, et al.** Survival in women with grade 1 serous ovarian carcinoma. *Obstet Gynecol.* 2013;122:225–232.

160. **FIGO Committee on gynecologic oncology.** Pratt J on behalf of FIGO committee. Staging classification for cancer of ovary, fallopian tube and peritoneum. *Int J Gynaecol Obstet.* 2014;124(1):1–5.

161. **van Houwelingen JC, ten Bokkel Huinink WW, van der Burg ATM, et al.** Predictability of the survival of patients with ovarian cancer. *J Clin Oncol.* 1989;7:769–773.

162. **Berek JS, Bertelsen K, du Bois A, et al.** Advanced epithelial ovarian cancer: 1998 consensus statement. *Ann Oncol.* 1999;10(suppl 1):87–92.

163. **Sharp F, Blackett AD, Berek JS, et al.** Conclusions and recommendations from the Helene Harris Memorial Trust sixth biennial international forum on ovarian cancer. *Int J Gynecol Cancer.* 1997;7:416–424.

164. **Balkwill F, Bast RC, Berek JS, et al.** Current research and treatment for epithelial ovarian cancer: A position paper from the Helene Harris Memorial Trust. *Eur J Cancer.* 2003;39:1818–1827.

165. **Omura GA, Brady MF, Homesley HD, et al.** Long-term follow-up and prognostic factor analysis in advanced ovarian carcinoma: The Gynecologic Oncology Group experience. *J Clin Oncol.* 1991;9:1138–1150.

166. **Young RC, Decker DG, Wharton JT, et al.** Staging laparotomy in early ovarian cancer. *JAMA.* 1983;250:3072–3076.

167. **Yoshimura S, Scully RE, Bell DA, et al.** Correlation of ascitic fluid cytology with histologic findings before and after treatment of ovarian cancer. *Am J Obstet Gynecol.* 1984;148:716–721.

168. **Benedetti-Panici P, Greggi S, Maneschi F, et al.** Anatomical and pathological study of retroperitoneal nodes in epithelial ovarian cancer. *Gynecol Oncol.* 1993;51:150–154.

169. **Zanetta G, Rota S, Chiari S, et al.** The accuracy of staging: An important prognostic determinator in stage I ovarian carcinoma. *Ann Oncol.* 1998;9:1097–1101.

170. **Schueler JA, Cornelisse CJ, Hermans J, et al.** Prognostic factors in well-differentiated early-stage epithelial ovarian cancer. *Cancer.* 1993;71:787–795.

171. **Eltabbakh GH, Mount SL.** Comparison of diaphragmatic wash and scrape specimens in staging of women with ovarian cancer. *Gynecol Oncol.* 2001;81:461–465.

172. **Benedetti-Panici P, Scambia G, Baiocchi G, et al.** Technique and feasibility of radical para-aortic and pelvic lymphadenectomy for gynecologic malignancies: A prospective study. *Int J Gynecol Cancer.* 1991;1:133–140.

173. **Green JA.** Early ovarian cancer—time for a rethink on stage? *Gynecol Oncol.* 2003;90:235–237.

174. **Harlan LC, Clegg LX, Trimble EL.** Trends in surgery and chemotherapy for women diagnosed with ovarian cancer in the United States. *J Clin Oncol.* 2003;21:3488–3494.

175. **Guthrie D, Davy MLJ, Phillips PR.** Study of 656 patients with "early" ovarian cancer. *Gynecol Oncol.* 1984;17:363–369.

176. **Gershenson DM.** Clinical management potential tumours of low malignancy. *Best Pract Res Clin Obstet Gynaecol.* 2002;16:513–527.

177. **Kurman RJ, Trimble CL.** The behavior of serous tumors of low malignant potential: Are they ever malignant? *Int J Gynecol Pathol.* 1993;12:120–127.

178. **Lim-Tan SK, Cajigas HE, Scully RE.** Ovarian cystectomy for serous borderline tumors: A follow-up study of 35 cases. *Obstet Gynecol.* 1988;72:775–781.

179. **Rose PG, Rubin RB, Nelson BE, et al.** Accuracy of frozen section (intraoperative consultation) diagnosis of ovarian tumors. *Am J Obstet Gynecol.* 1994;171:823–826.

180. **Tropé C, Kaern J, Vergote IB, et al.** Are borderline tumors of the ovary overtreated both surgically and systemically? A review of four prospective randomized trials including 253 patients with borderline tumors. *Gynecol Oncol.* 1993;51:236–243.

181. **Kaern J, Tropé CG, Abeler VM.** A retrospective study of 370 borderline tumors of the ovary treated at the Norwegian Radium Hospital from 1979 to 1982: A review of clinicopathologic features and treatment modalities. *Cancer.* 1993;71:1810–1820.

182. **Zanetta G, Rota S, Chiari S, et al.** Behavior of borderline tumors with particular interest to persistence, recurrence, and progression to invasive carcinoma: A prospective study. *J Clin Oncol.* 2001;19:2658–2664.

183. **Trimble CL, Korsary C, Trimble EL.** Long-term survival and patterns of care in women with ovarian tumors of low malignant potential. *Gynecol Oncol.* 2002;86:34–37.

184. **Sutton GP, Bundy GN, Omura GA, et al.** Stage III ovarian tumors of low malignant potential treated with cisplatin combination therapy: A Gynecologic Oncology Group study. *Gynecol Oncol.* 1991;41:230–233.

185. **Barakat RR, Benjamin IB, Lewis JL Jr, et al.** Platinum-based chemotherapy for advanced-stage serous ovarian tumors of low malignant potential. *Gynecol Oncol.* 1995;59:390–393.

186. **Ronnett BM, Kurman RJ, Shmookler BM, et al.** Pseudomyxoma peritonei in women: A clinicopathologic analysis of 30 cases with emphasis on site of origin, prognosis, and relationship to ovarian mucinous tumors of low malignant potential. *Hum Pathol.* 1995;26:509–524.

187. **Gershenson DM.** Fertility-sparing surgery for malignancies in women. *J Natl Cancer Inst Monogr.* 2005;34:43–47.

188. **Park JY, Kim DY, Suh DS, et al.** Outcomes of fertility-sparing surgery for invasive epithelial ovarian cancer: Oncologic safety and reproductive outcomes. *Gynecol Oncol.* 2008;110:345–353.

189. **Schlaerth AC, Chi DS, Poynor EA, et al.** Long-term survival after fertility-sparing surgery for epithelial ovarian cancer. *Int J Gynecol Cancer.* 2009;19:1199–1204.

190. **Satoh T, Hatae M, Watanabe Y, et al.** Outcomes of fertility-sparing surgery for stage I epithelial ovarian cancer: A proposal for patient selection. *J Clin Oncol.* 2010;28:1727–1732.

191. **Kajiyama H, Shibata K, Suzuki S, et al.** Fertility-sparing surgery in young women with invasive epithelial ovarian cancer. *Eur J Surg Oncol.* 2010;36:404–408.

192. **Kajiyama H, Shibata K, Mizuno M, et al.** Fertility-sparing surgery in young women with mucinous adenocarcinoma of the ovary. *Gynecol Oncol.* 2011;122:334–338.

193. Fruscio R, Corso S, Ceppi L, et al. Conservative management of early-stage epithelial ovarian cancer: Results of a large retrospective series. *Ann Oncol.* 2013;24(1):138–144..

194. Nam JH, Park JY. Fertility-sparing surgery for young women with early-stage epithelial ovarian cancer. *Gynecol Obstet Invest.* 2013; 76:14–24.

195. Griffiths CT. Surgical resection of tumor bulk in the primary treatment of ovarian carcinoma. *J Natl Cancer Inst Monogr.* 1975;42: 101–104.

196. Heintz APM, Berek JS. Cytoreductive surgery in ovarian cancer. In: Piver MS, ed. *Ovarian Cancer.* Edinburgh: Churchill Livingstone, 1987:129–143.

197. Hacker NF, Berek JS, Lagasse LD, et al. Primary cytoreductive surgery for epithelial ovarian cancer. *Obstet Gynecol.* 1983;61:413–420.

198. Hoskins WJ, Bundy BN, Thigpen JT, et al. The influence of cytoreductive surgery on recurrence-free interval and survival in small volume stage III epithelial ovarian cancer: A Gynecologic Oncology Group study. *Gynecol Oncol.* 1992;47:159–166.

199. Hoskins WJ, McGuire WP, Brady MF, et al. The effect of diameter of largest residual disease on survival after primary cytoreductive surgery in patients with suboptimal residual epithelial ovarian carcinoma. *Am J Obstet Gynecol.* 1994;170:974–979.

200. Farias-Eisner R, Teng F, Oliveira M, et al. The influence of tumor grade, distribution and extent of carcinomatosis in minimal residual epithelial ovarian cancer after optimal primary cytoreductive surgery. *Gynecol Oncol.* 1994;55:108–110.

201. Berek JS. Complete debulking of advanced ovarian cancer. *Cancer J.* 1996;2:134–135.

202. Farias-Eisner R, Kim YB, Berek JS. Surgical management of ovarian cancer. *Semin Surg Oncol.* 1994;10:268–275.

203. Hacker NF. Cytoreduction for advanced ovarian cancer in perspective. *Int J Gynecol Cancer.* 1996;6:159–160.

204. Eisenkop SM, Friedman RL, Wang H-J. Complete cytoreductive surgery is feasible and maximizes survival in patients with advanced epithelial ovarian cancer: A prospective study. *Gynecol Oncol.* 1998; 69:103–108.

205. Du Bois A, Reuss A, Pujade-Lauraine E, et al. Role of surgical outcome as prognostic factor in advanced epithelial ovarian cancer: A combined exploratory analysis of 3 prospectively randomized phase 3 multicenter trials. *Cancer.* 2009;115:1234–1244.

206. Aletti GO, Gostout BS, Podratz KC, et al. Ovarian cancer surgical resectability: Relative impact of disease, patient status, and surgeon. *Gynecol Oncol.* 2006;100:33–37.

207. Bristow R, Montz FJ, Lagasse LD, et al. Survival impact of surgical cytoreduction in stage IV epithelial ovarian cancer. *Gynecol Oncol.* 1999;72:278–287.

208. Hunter RW, Alexander NDE, Soutter WP. Meta-analysis of surgery in advanced ovarian carcinoma: Is maximum cytoreductive surgery an independent determinant of prognosis? *Am J Obstet Gynecol.* 1992;166:504–511.

209. Eisenkop SM, Spirtos NM, Friedman RL, et al. Relative influences of tumor volume before surgery and the cytoreductive outcome on survival for patients with advanced ovarian cancer: A prospective study. *Gynecol Oncol.* 2003;90:390–396.

210. Brockbank EC, Ind TE, Barton DP, et al. Preoperative predictors of suboptimal primary surgical cytoreduction in women with clinical evidence of advanced primary epithelial ovarian cancer. *Int J Gynecol Cancer.* 2004;14:42–50.

211. Crawford SC, Vasey PA, Paul J, et al. Does aggressive surgery only benefit patients with less advanced ovarian cancer? Results from an international comparison within the SCOTROC-1 Trial. *J Clin Oncol.* 2005;23:8802–8811.

212. Eisenkop SM, Spirtos NM, Lin WC. Splenectomy in the context of primary cytoreductive operations for advanced ovarian cancer. *Gynecol Oncol.* 2006;100:344–348.

213. de Jong D, Eijkemans MJ, Lie Fong S, et al. Preoperative predictors for residual tumor after surgery in patients with ovarian carcinoma. *Oncology.* 2007;72:293–301.

214. Memarzadeh S, Lee SB, Berek JS, et al. CA125 levels are a weak predictor of optimal cytoreductive surgery in patients with advanced epithelial ovarian cancer. *Int J Gynecol Cancer.* 2003;13:120–124.

215. Dowdy SC, Mullany SA, Brandt KR, et al. The utility of computed tomography scans in predicting suboptimal cytoreductive surgery in women with advanced ovarian cancer. *Cancer.* 2004;101:346–352.

216. Greer BE, Bundy BN, Ozols RF, et al. Implications of second-look laparotomy in the context of optimally resected stage III ovarian cancer: A non-randomized comparison using an explanatory analysis: A Gynecologic Oncology Group study. *Gynecol Oncol.* 2005; 99:71–79.

217. Oayyum A, Coakley FV, Westphalen AC, et al. Role of CT and MR imaging in predicting optimal cytoreduction of newly diagnosed primary epithelial ovarian cancer. *Gynecol Oncol.* 2005;96:301–306.

218. Axtell AE, Lee MH, Bristow RE, et al. Multi-institutional reciprocal validation study of computed tomography predictors of suboptimal primary cytoreduction in patients with advanced ovarian cancer. *J Clin Oncol.* 2007;25:384–389.

219. Risum S, Høgdall C, Loft A, et al. Prediction of suboptimal primary ovarian cancer with combined positron emission tomography/computed tomography: A prospective study. *Gynecol Oncol.* 2008; 108:265–270.

220. Hynninen J, Auranen A, Carpen O, et al. FDG PET/CT in staging of advanced epithelial ovarian cancer: Frequency of supradiaphragmatic lymph node metastasis challenges the traditional pattern of disease spread. *Gynecol Oncol.* 2012;126:64–68.

221. Vergote I, Marquette S, Amant F, et al. Port-site metastases after open laparoscopy: A study in 173 patients with advanced ovarian cancer. *Int J Gynecol Cancer.* 2005;15:776–779.

222. Skipper HE. Adjuvant chemotherapy. *Cancer.* 1978;41:936–940.

223. Goldie JH, Coldman AJ. A mathematic model for relating the drug sensitivity of tumors to their spontaneous mutation rate. *Cancer Treat Rep.* 1979;63:1727–1733.

224. Berek JS, Hacker NF, Lagasse LD. Rectosigmoid colectomy and reanastomosis to facilitate resection of primary and recurrent gynecologic cancer. *Obstet Gynecol.* 1984;64:715–720.

225. Bridges JE, Leung Y, Hammond IG, et al. En bloc resection of epithelial ovarian tumors with concomitant rectosigmoid colectomy: The KEMH experience. *Int J Gynecol Cancer.* 1993;3: 199–202.

226. Berek JS, Hacker NF, Lagasse LD, et al. Lower urinary tract resection as part of cytoreductive surgery for ovarian cancer. *Gynecol Oncol.* 1982;13:87–92.

227. Heintz AM, Hacker NF, Berek JS, et al. Cytoreductive surgery in ovarian carcinoma: Feasibility and morbidity. *Obstet Gynecol.* 1986; 67:783–788.

228. Montz FJ, Schlaerth J, Berek JS. Resection of diaphragmatic peritoneum and muscle: Role in cytoreductive surgery for ovarian carcinoma. *Gynecol Oncol.* 1989;35:338–340.

229. Nicklin JL, Copeland LJ, O'Toole RV, et al. Splenectomy as part of cytoreductive surgery for ovarian carcinoma. *Gynecol Oncol.* 1995;58:244–247.

230. Brand E, Pearlman N. Electrosurgical debulking of ovarian cancer: A new technique using the argon beam coagulator. *Gynecol Oncol.* 1990;39:115–118.

231. Deppe G, Malviya VK, Boike G, et al. Use of Cavitron surgical aspirator for debulking of diaphragmatic metastases in patients with advanced carcinoma of the ovaries. *Surg Gynecol Obstet.* 1989; 168:455–456.

232. Fanning J, Hilgers R. Loop electrosurgical excision procedure for intensified cytoreduction of ovarian cancer. *Gynecol Oncol.* 1995; 57:188–190.

233. Panici PB, Maggioni A, Hacker NF, et al. Systematic aortic and pelvic lymphadenectomy versus resection of bulky nodes only in optimally debulked advanced ovarian cancer: A randomized clinical trial. *J Nat Cancer Inst.* 2005;97:560–566.

234. du Bois A, Reuss A, Harter A, et al. The role of lymphadenectomy in advanced epithelial ovarian cancer in patients with macroscopically complete resection of intraperitoneal disease. *Int J Gyn Cancer.* 2006;16(suppl 3):601.

235. Venesmaa P, Ylikorkala O. Morbidity and mortality associated with primary and repeat operations for ovarian cancer. *Obstet Gynecol.* 1992;79:168–172.

236. Bristow RE, Tomacruz RS, Armstrong DK, et al. Survival effect of maximal cytoreductive surgery for advanced ovarian carcinoma during the platinum era: A meta-analysis. *J Clin Oncol.* 2002; 20:1248–1259.

237. Naik R, Nordin A, Cross PA, et al. Optimal cytoreductive surgery is an independent prognostic indicator in stage IV epithelial ovarian cancer with hepatic metastases. *Gynecol Oncol.* 2000;78:171–175.

238. van der Burg MEL, van Lent M, Buyse M, et al. The effect of debulking surgery after induction chemotherapy on the prognosis in advanced epithelial ovarian cancer. *N Engl J Med.* 1995;332: 629–634.

239. van der Burg MEL, Vergote I. The role of interval debulking surgery in ovarian cancer. *Curr Oncol Rep.* 2003;5:473–481.

240. Rose PG, Nerenstone S, Brady MF, et al. Secondary surgical cytoreduction for advanced ovarian carcinoma. *N Engl J Med.* 2004;351: 2544–2546.

241. Berek JS. Interval debulking of ovarian cancer—an interim measure. *N Engl J Med.* 1995;332:675–677.

242. Schwartz PE, Rutherford TJ, Chambers JT, et al. Neoadjuvant chemotherapy for advanced ovarian cancer: long-term survival. *Gynecol Oncol.* 1999;72:93–99.

243. Shibata K, Kikkawa F, Mika M, et al. Neoadjuvant chemotherapy for FIGO stage III or IV ovarian cancer: Survival benefit and prognostic factors. *Int J Gynecol Cancer.* 2003;13:587–592.

244. Chan YM, Ng TY, Ngan HY, et al. Quality of life in women treated with neoadjuvant chemotherapy for advanced ovarian cancer: A prospective longitudinal study. *Gynecol Oncol.* 2003;88:9–16.

245. Bristow RE, Eisenhauer EL, Santillan A, et al. Delaying the primary surgical effort for advanced ovarian cancer: A systematic review of neoadjuvant chemotherapy and interval cytoreduction. *Gynecol Oncol.* 2007;104:480–490.

246. Vergote I, Tropé CG, Amant F, et al. Neoadjuvant chemotherapy or primary surgery in stage IIIC or IV ovarian cancer. *N Engl J Med.* 2010;363:943–953.

247. Du Bois A, Marth C, Pfisterer J, et al. Neoadjuvant chemotherapy cannot be regarded as adequate routine therapy strategy of advanced ovarian cancer. *Int J Gynecol Cancer.* 2012;22:182–185.

248. Aletti CD, Eisenhauer EL, Santillan A, et al. Identification of patient groups at highest risk from traditional approach to ovarian cancer treatment. *Gynecol Oncol.* 2011;120:23–28.

249. Wright JD, Lewin SN, Deutsch I, et al. Defining the limits of radical cytoreductive surgery for ovarian cancer. *Gynecol Oncol.* 2011; 123:467–473.

250. Wright JD, Herzog TJ, Neugut AI, et al. Effect of radical cytoreductive surgery on omission and delay of chemotherapy for advanced-stage ovarian cancer. *Obstet Gynecol.* 2012;120:871–881.

251. Kehoe S, Hook J, Nankivell M, et al. Chemotherapy or upfront surgery for newly diagnosed ovarian cancer: Results from the MRC CHORUS trial. *J Clin Oncol.* 2013 ASCO Meeting Abstracts;31:15.

252. Dewdney SB, Rimel BJ, Reinhart AJ, et al. The role of neoadjuvant chemotherapy in the management of patients with advanced stage ovarian cancer: Survey results from members of the Society of Gynecologic Oncologists. *Gynecol Oncol.* 2010;119:18–21.

253. Hacker NF. State of the art of surgery in advanced epithelial ovarian cancer. *Ann Oncol.* 2013;24(suppl 10):x27–x32.

254. Junor EJ, Hole DJ, McNulty L, et al. Specialist gynecologists and survival outcome in ovarian cancer: A Scottish National Study of 1966 patients. *Br J Obstet Gynaecol.* 1999;106:1130–1136.

255. Tingulstad S, Skjeldestad FE, Hagen B. The effect of centralization of primary surgery on survival in ovarian cancer patients. *Obstet Gynecol.* 2003;102:499–505.

256. Young RC, Walton LA, Ellenberg SS, et al. Adjuvant therapy in stage I and stage II epithelial ovarian cancer: Results of two prospective randomized trials. *N Engl J Med.* 1990;322:1021–1027.

257. Hreshchyshyn MM, Park RC, Blessing JA, et al. The role of adjuvant therapy in stage I ovarian cancer. *Am J Obstet Gynecol.* 1980; 138:139–145.

258. Greene MH, Boice JD, Greer BE, et al. Acute nonlymphocytic leukemia after therapy with *alkylating agents* for ovarian cancer: A study of the five randomized clinical trials. *N Engl J Med.* 1982; 307:1416–1421.

259. Travis LB, Holowaty EJ, Bergfeldt K, et al. Risk of leukemia after platinum-based chemotherapy for ovarian cancer. *N Engl J Med.* 1999;340:351–357.

260. Thomas GM. Radiotherapy in early ovarian cancer. *Gynecol Oncol.* 1994;55:S73–S79.

261. Sell A, Bertelsen K, Andersen JE, et al. Randomized study of whole-abdomen irradiation versus pelvic irradiation plus cyclophosphamide in treatment of early ovarian cancer. *Gynecol Oncol.* 1990; 37:367–373.

262. Berek JS. Adjuvant therapy for early-stage ovarian cancer. *N Engl J Med.* 1990;322:1076–1078.

263. Ahmed FY, Wiltshaw E, Hern RP, et al. Natural history and prognosis of untreated stage I epithelial ovarian carcinoma. *J Clin Oncol.* 1996;14:2968–2975.

264. Finn CB, Luesley DM, Buxton EJ, et al. Is stage I epithelial ovarian cancer overtreated both surgically and systemically? Results of a five-year cancer registry review. *Br J Obstet Gynaecol.* 1992;99: 54–58.

265. Vergote I, Vergote-De Vos LN, Abeler V, et al. Randomized trial comparing cisplatin with radioactive phosphorus or whole abdominal irradiation as adjuvant treatment of ovarian cancer. *Cancer.* 1992; 69:741–749.

266. Rubin SC, Wong GY, Curtin JP, et al. Platinum based chemotherapy of high risk stage I epithelial ovarian cancer following comprehensive surgical staging. *Obstet Gynecol.* 1993;82:143–147.

267. Young RC, Brady MF, Nieberg RK, et al. Adjuvant treatment for early ovarian cancer: A randomized phase III trial of intraperitoneal 32P or intravenous cyclophosphamide and cisplatin: A Gynecologic Oncology Group study. *J Clin Oncol.* 2003;21:4350–4355.

268. Thomas G. Revisiting the role of radiation treatment for non-serous subtypes of epithelial ovarian cancer. *Am Soc Clin Oncol Educ Book.* 2013;2013:205–208.

269. Swenerton KD, Santos JL, Gilks CB, et al. Histotype predicts the curative potential of radiotherapy: The example of ovarian cancers. *Ann Oncol.* 2011;22:341–347.

270. Hoskins PJ, Le N, Gilks B, et al. Low-stage ovarian clear cell carcinoma: Population-based outcomes in British Columbia, Canada, with evidence for a survival benefit as a result of irradiation. *J Clin Oncol.* 2012;30:1656–1662.

271. Bolis G, Colombo N, Pecorelli S, et al. Adjuvant treatment for early epithelial ovarian cancer: Results of two randomized clinical trials comparing cisplatin to no further treatment or chromic phosphate (32P). *Ann Oncol.* 1995;6:887–893.

272. Colombo N, Maggioni A, Bocciolone L, et al. Multimodality therapy of early-stage (FIGO I-II) ovarian cancer: Review of surgical management and postoperative adjuvant treatment. *Int J Gynecol Cancer.* 1996;6:13–17.

273. Vermorken JB, Pecorelli S. Clinical trials in patients with epithelial ovarian cancer: Past, present and future. *Eur J Surg Oncol.* 1996;22: 455–466.

274. Tropé C, Kaern J, Hogberg T, et al. Randomized study on adjuvant chemotherapy in stage I high-risk ovarian cancer with evaluation of DNA-ploidy as prognostic instrument. *Ann Oncol.* 200;11:281–288.

275. Gadducci A, Sartori E, Maggino T, et al. Analysis of failure in patients with stage I ovarian cancer: An Italian multicenter study. *Int J Gynecol Cancer.* 1997;7:445–450.

276. Trimbos JB, Vergote I, Bolis G, et al. Impact of adjuvant chemotherapy and surgical staging in early-stage ovarian carcinoma: European Organisation for Research and Treatment of Cancer-Adjuvant Chemotherapy in Ovarian Neoplasm Trial. *J Natl Cancer Inst.* 2003; 95:113–125.

277. Trimbos JB1, Parmar M, Vergote I, et al.; International Collaborative Ovarian Neoplasm (ICON1) Collaborators. International collaborative ovarian neoplasm trial 1: A randomized trial of adjuvant chemotherapy in women with early-stage ovarian cancer. *J Natl Cancer Inst.* 2003;95:125–132.

278. Trimbos JB, Parmar M, Vergote I, et al. International Collaborative Ovarian Neoplasm Trial 1 and Adjuvant Chemotherapy in Ovarian Neoplasm Trial: Two parallel randomized phase III trials of adjuvant chemotherapy in patients with early-stage ovarian carcinoma. *J Natl Cancer Inst.* 2003;95:105–112.

279. Chan JK, Tian C, Fleming GF, et al. The potential benefit of 6 vs. 3 cycles of chemotherapy in subsets of women with early-stage high-risk epithelial ovarian cancer: An exploratory analysis of a Gynecologic Oncology Group study. *Gynecol Oncol.* 2010;116(3):301–306.

280. Winter-Roach BA, Kitchener HC, Lawrie TA. Adjuvant (postsurgery) chemotherapy for early stage epithelial ovarian cancer. *Cochrane Database Syst Rev.* 2012;14:3.

281. Bell J, Brady MF, Young RC, et al.; Gynecologic Oncology Group. Randomized phase III trial of three versus six cycles of adjuvant carboplatin and paclitaxel in early stage epithelial ovarian carcinoma: A Gynecologic Oncology Group study. *Gynecol Oncol.* 2006; 102:432–439.

282. **McGuire WP, Rowinsky EK, Rosensheim NE, et al.** Taxol: A unique antineoplastic agent with significant activity in advanced ovarian epithelial neoplasms. *Ann Intern Med.* 1989;111:273–279.

283. **Rowinsky EK, Cazenave LA, Donehower RC.** Taxol: A novel investigational antimicrotubule agent. *J Natl Cancer Inst.* 1990;82: 1247–1259.

284. **Sarosy G, Kohn E, Stone DA, et al.** Phase I study of Taxol and granulocyte colony-stimulating factor in patients with refractory ovarian cancer. *J Clin Oncol.* 1992;10:1165–1170.

285. **Einzig AI, Wiernik PH, Sasloff J, et al.** Phase II study and long-term follow-up of patients treated with *Taxol* for advanced ovarian adenocarcinoma. *J Clin Oncol.* 1992;10:1748–1753.

286. **Trimble EL, Adams JD, Vena D, et al.** Paclitaxel for platinum-refractory ovarian cancer: Results from the first 1000 patients registered to National Cancer Institute Treatment Referral Center 9103. *J Clin Oncol.* 1993;11:2405–2410.

287. **Thigpen JT, Blessing JA, Ball H, et al.** Phase II trial of paclitaxel in patients with progressive ovarian carcinoma after platinum-based chemotherapy: A Gynecologic Oncology Group study. *J Clin Oncol.* 1994;12:1748–1753.

288. **Eisenhauer EA, ten Bokkel Huinink WW, Swenerton KD, et al.** European-Canadian randomized trial of paclitaxel in relapsed ovarian cancer: High-dose versus low-dose and long versus short infusion. *J Clin Oncol.* 1994;12:2654–2666.

289. **Bookman MA, McGuire WP, Kilpatrick D, et al.** Carboplatin and paclitaxel in ovarian cancer: A phase I study of the Gynecologic Oncology Group. *J Clin Oncol.* 1996;14:1895–1902.

290. **McGuire WP, Hoskins WJ, Brady MF, et al.** Cyclophosphamide and cisplatin compared with paclitaxel and cisplatin in patients with stage III and stage IV ovarian cancer. *N Engl J Med.* 1996;334: 1–6.

291. **Piccart MJ, Bertelsen K, Stuart G, et al.** Long-term follow-up confirms a survival advantage of the paclitaxel-cisplatin regimen over the cyclophosphamide-cisplatin combination in advanced ovarian cancer. *Int J Gynecol Cancer.* 2003;13(suppl 2):144–148.

292. **Muggia FM, Braly PS, Brady MF, et al.** Phase III randomized study of cisplatin versus paclitaxel versus cisplatin and paclitaxel in patients with suboptimal stage III or IV ovarian cancer: A gynecologic oncology group study. *J Clin Oncol.* 2000;18:106–115.

293. **Advanced Ovarian Cancer Trialists Group.** Chemotherapy in advanced ovarian cancer: An overview of randomized clinical trials. *BMJ.* 1991;303:884–891.

294. **Young RC, Chabner BA, Hubbard SP, et al.** Advanced ovarian adenocarcinoma: A prospective clinical trial of melphalan (L-PAM) versus combination chemotherapy. *N Engl J Med.* 1978;299: 1261–1266.

295. **Lambert HE, Berry RI.** High dose cisplatin compared with high dose cyclophosphamide in the management of advanced epithelial ovarian cancer (FIGO Stages III and IV): Report from the North Thames Cooperative Group. *BMJ.* 1985;290:889–893.

296. **Neijt JP, ten Bokkel Huinink WW, van der Burg ME, et al.** Randomized trial comparing two combination chemotherapy regions (Hexa-CAF vs. CHAP-5) in advanced ovarian carcinoma. *Lancet.* 1984;2:594–600.

297. **Neijt JP, ten Bokkel Huinink WW, van der Burg MEL, et al.** Randomized trial comparing two combination chemotherapy regimens (CHAP-5 versus CP) in advanced ovarian carcinoma: A randomized trial of the Netherlands joint study group for ovarian cancer. *J Clin Oncol.* 1987;5:1157–1168.

298. **Omura G, Bundy B, Berek JS, et al.** Randomized trial of cyclophosphamide plus cisplatin with or without doxorubicin in ovarian carcinoma: A Gynecologic Oncology Group study. *J Clin Oncol.* 1989;7:457–465.

299. **Bertelsen K, Jakobsen A, Andersen JE, et al.** A randomized study of cyclophosphamide and cisplatin with or without doxorubicin in advanced ovarian cancer. *Gynecol Oncol.* 1987;28:161–169.

300. **Conte PF, Bruzzone M, Chiara S, et al.** A randomized trial comparing cisplatin plus cyclophosphamide versus cisplatin, doxorubicin and cyclophosphamide in advanced ovarian cancer. *J Clin Oncol.* 1986;4:965–971.

301. **Gruppo Interegionale Cooperativo Oncologico Ginecologia.** Randomized comparison of cisplatin with cyclophosphamide/cisplatin with cyclophosphamide/doxorubicin/cisplatin in advanced ovarian cancer. *Lancet.* 1987;2:353–359.

302. **Ovarian Cancer Meta-Analysis Project.** Cyclophosphamide plus cisplatin versus cyclophosphamide, doxorubicin, and cisplatin chemotherapy of ovarian carcinoma: A meta-analysis. *J Clin Oncol.* 1991; 9:1668–1674.

303. **Swenerton K, Jeffrey J, Stuart G, et al.** Cisplatin-cyclophosphamide versus carboplatin-cyclophosphamide in advanced ovarian cancer: A randomized phase III study of the National Cancer Institute of Canada Clinical Trials Group. *J Clin Oncol.* 1992;10:718–726.

304. **Alberts DS, Green S, Hannigan EV, et al.** Improved therapeutic index of carboplatin plus cyclophosphamide versus cisplatin plus cyclophosphamide: Final report by the Southwest Oncology Group of a phase III randomized trial in stages III (suboptimal) and IV ovarian cancer. *J Clin Oncol.* 1992;10:706–717.

305. **Calvert AH, Newell DR, Gumbrell LA, et al.** Carboplatin dosage: Prospective evaluation of a simple formula based on renal function. *J Clin Oncol.* 1989;7:1748–1756.

306. **Ozols RF, Bundy BN, Greer B, et al.** Phase III trial of carboplatin and paclitaxel compared with cisplatin and paclitaxel in patients with optimally resected stage III ovarian cancer: A Gynecologic Oncology Group study. *J Clin Oncol.* 2003;21:3194–3200.

307. **Vasey PA, Paul J, Birt A, et al.** Docetaxel and cisplatin in combination as first-line chemotherapy for advanced epithelial ovarian cancer. Scottish Gynaecological Cancer Trials Group. *J Clin Oncol.* 1999;17: 2069–2080.

308. **The International Collaborative Ovarian Neoplasm (ICON) Group.** Paclitaxel plus carboplatin versus standard chemotherapy with either single agent carboplatin or cyclophosphamide, doxorubicin, and cisplatin in women with ovarian cancer: The ICON3 randomised trial. *Lancet.* 2002;360:505–515.

309. **Bookman MA, Brady MF, McGuire WP, et al.** Evaluation of new platinum-based treatment regimens in advanced-stage ovarian cancer: A Phase III Trial of the Gynecologic Cancer Intergroup. *J Clin Oncol.* 2009;27:1419–1425.

310. **Katsumata N, Yasuda M, Isonishi S, et al.** Long-term results of dose-dense paclitaxel and carboplatin versus conventional paclitaxel and carboplatin for treatment of advanced epithelial ovarian, fallopian tube, or primary peritoneal cancer (JGOG 3016): A randomised, controlled, open-label trial. *Lancet Oncol.* 2013;14(10):1020–1026.

311. **Burger RA, Brady MF, Bookman MA, et al.; Gynecologic Oncology Group.** Incorporation of bevacizumab in the primary treatment of ovarian cancer. *N Engl J Med.* 2011;365(26):2473–2483.

312. **De Placido S, Scambia G, DiVagno G, et al.** Topotecan compared with no therapy after response to surgery and carboplatin/paclitaxel in patients with ovarian cancer: Multicenter Italian trials in ovarian cancer (MITO-1) randomized study. *J Clin Oncol.* 2004;22:2635–2642.

313. **du Bois A, Lück HJ, Meier W, et al.** A randomized clinical trial of cisplatin/paclitaxel versus carboplatin/paclitaxel as first-line treatment of ovarian cancer. *J Natl Cancer Inst.* 2003;95:1320–1330.

314. **ICON Collaborators.** International Collaborative Ovarian Neoplasm Study 2 (ICON2): Randomised trial of single-agent carboplatin against three-drug combination of CAP (cyclophosphamide, doxorubicin, and cisplatin) in women with ovarian cancer. *Lancet.* 1998;352:1571–1576.

315. **Banerjee S, Rustin G, Paul J, et al.** A multicenter, randomized trial of flat dosing versus intrapatient dose escalation of single-agent carboplatin as first-line chemotherapy for advanced ovarian cancer: An SGCTG (SCOTROC 4) and ANZGOG study on behalf of GCIG. *Ann Oncol.* 2013 Mar;24(3):679–687.

316. **Copeland LJ, Bookman M, Trimble E; Gynecologic Oncology Group Protocol GOG 182–ICON5.** Clinical trials of newer regimens for treating ovarian cancer: The rationale for Gynecologic Oncology Group Protocol GOG 182-ICON5. *Gynecol Oncol.* 2003;90:S1–S7.

317. **McGuire WP, Hoskins WJ, Brady MS, et al.** An assessment of dose-intensive therapy in suboptimally debulked ovarian cancer: A Gynecologic Oncology Group study. *J Clin Oncol.* 1995;13: 1589–1599.

318. **Kaye SB, Lewis CR, Paul J, et al.** Randomized study of two doses of cisplatin with cyclophosphamide in epithelial ovarian cancer. *Lancet.* 1992;340:329–333.

319. **Kaye SB, Paul J, Cassidy J, Lewis CR, et al.** Mature results of a randomized trial of two doses of cisplatin for the treatment of ovarian cancer. *J Clin Oncol.* 1996;14:2113–2119.

320. **Reed E, Janik J, Bookman MA, et al.** High-dose carboplatin and recombinant granulocyte-macrophage colony-stimulating factor in

advanced-stage recurrent ovarian cancer. *J Clin Oncol.* 1993;11: 2118–2126.

321. **Alberts DS, Liu PY, Hannigan EV, et al.** Intraperitoneal cisplatin plus intravenous cyclophosphamide versus intravenous cisplatin plus intravenous cyclophosphamide for stage III ovarian cancer. *N Engl J Med.* 1996;335:1950–1955.

322. **Markman M, Bundy BN, Alberts DS, et al.** Phase III trial of standard-dose intravenous cisplatin plus paclitaxel versus moderately high-dose intravenous carboplatin followed by intraperitoneal paclitaxel and intraperitoneal cisplatin in small-volume stage III ovarian cancer: An intergroup study of the Gynecologic Oncology Group, Southwestern Oncology Group, and the Eastern Cooperative Oncology Group. *J Clin Oncol.* 2001;19:1001–1007.

323. **Armstrong DK, Bundy B, Wenzel L, et al.** Intraperitoneal cisplatin and paclitaxel in ovarian cancer. *N Eng J Med.* 2006:354:34–43.

324. **Rothenburg ML, Liu PY, Braly PS, et al.** Combined intraperitoneal and intravenous chemotherapy for women with optimally debulked ovarian cancer: Results from an intergroup phase II trial. *J Clin Oncol.* 2003;21:1313–1319.

325. **Alberts DS, Markman M, Armstrong D, et al.** Intraperitoneal therapy for stage III ovarian cancer: A therapy whose time has come! *J Clin Oncol.* 2002;20:3944–3946.

326. **Hess LM, Benham-Hutchins M, Herzog TJ, et al.** A meta-analysis of the efficacy of intraperitoneal cisplatin for the front-line treatment of ovarian cancer. *Int J Gynecol Cancer.* 2007;17:561–570.

327. **Jaaback K, Johnson N.** Intraperitoneal chemotherapy for the initial management of primary epithelial ovarian cancer. *Cochrane Database Syst Rev* 2006, 25(1):CD005340. DOI: 10.1002/14651858. CD005340.pub2.

328. **Tewari D, Java J, Salani R, et al.** Long-term survival advantage of intraperitoneal chemotherapy treatment in advanced ovarian cancer: An analysis of a Gynecologic Oncology Group ancillary data study (GOG#114/172, abstract). Presented at: 2013 Society of Gynecologic Oncology Annual Meeting on Women's Cancer; March 9–12, 2013; Los Angeles, CA. Abstract 6.

329. **Friedlander M.** Optimally debulked stage III ovarian cancer: Intraperitoneal or intravenous chemotherapy? *Int J Gynecol Cancer.* 2010;20(11 Suppl 2):S20–S23.

330. **Katsumata N, Yasuda M, Takahashi F, et al.** Dose-dense paclitaxel once a week in combination with carboplatin every 3 weeks for advanced ovarian cancer: A phase 3, open-label, randomised controlled trial. *Lancet.* 2009;17;374(9698):1331–1338.

331. **Gore M, du Bois A, Vergote I.** Intraperitoneal chemotherapy in ovarian cancer remains experimental. *J Clin Oncol.* 2006;24: 4528–4530.

332. **Chang CL, Hsu YT, Wu CC, et al.** Dose-dense chemotherapy improves mechanisms of antitumor immune response. *Cancer Res.* 2013;73(1):119–127.

333. **Pinato DJ, Graham J, Gabra H, et al.** Evolving concepts in the management of drug resistant ovarian cancer: Dose dense chemotherapy and the reversal of clinical platinum resistance. *Cancer Treat Rev.* 2013;39(2):153–160.

334. **Fuh K, Shin J, Blansit K, et al.** The treatment and survival differences of Asians versus whites with epithelial ovarian cancer. SGO Annual Meeting. 2013; abstract 53.

335. **duPont NC, Brady MF, Burger RA, et al.** Prognostic significance of ethnicity and age in advanced stage ovarian cancer: An analysis of GOG 218. SGO Annual Meeting. 2013; abstract 54.

336. **Pignata S, Scambia G, Lauria R, et al.** A randomized multicenter phase III study comparing weekly versus every 3 weeks carboplatin (C) plus paclitaxel (P) in patients with advanced ovarian cancer (AOC): Multicenter Italian Trials in Ovarian Cancer (MITO-7)— European Network of Gynaecological Oncological Trial Groups (ENGOT-ov-10) and Gynecologic Cancer Intergroup (GCIG) trial. *Proc Am Soc Clin Oncol.* (2013);31(suppl): abstr LBA5501.

337. **Chan J, Brady M, Penson R, et al.** Phase III trial of every-3-weeks paclitaxel vs. dose dense weekly paclitaxel with carboplatin +/− bevacizumab in epithelial ovarian, peritoneal, fallopian tube cancer: GOG 262 (NCT01167712). European Society of Gynecological Oncology, Liverpool, England, UK, Oct 2013.

338. **Cohen MH, Gootenberg J, Keegan P, et al.** FDA drug approval summary: Bevacizumab (Avastin) plus carboplatin and paclitaxel as first-line treatment of advanced/metastatic recurrent nonsquamous non-small cell lung cancer. *Oncologist.* 2007;12:713–718.

339. **Miller K, Wang M, Gralow J, et al.** Paclitaxel plus bevacizumab versus paclitaxel alone for metastatic breast cancer. *N Engl J Med.* 2007;357:2666–2676.

340. **Hurwitz H, Fehrenbacher L, Novotny W, et al.** Bevacizumab plus irinotecan, fluorouracil, and leucovorin for metastatic colorectal cancer. *N Engl J Med.* 2004;350:2335–2342.

341. **Perren TJ, Swart AM, Pfisterer J, et al.** A phase 3 trial of bevacizumab in ovarian cancer. *N Engl J Med.* 2011;365(26):2484–2496.

342. **Oza A, Perren TJ, Swart AM, et al.** ICON7: Final overall survival results in the GCIG phase III randomized trial of bevacizumab in women with newly diagnosed ovarian cancer. *Eur J Cancer* 2013;49(3): Abstract 6.

343. **Markman M, Liu PY, Wilczynski S, et al.** Southwest Oncology Group and Gynecologic Oncology Group. Phase III randomized trial of 12 versus 3 months of maintenance paclitaxel in patients with advanced ovarian cancer after complete response to platinum and paclitaxel-based chemotherapy: A Southwest Oncology Group and Gynecologic Oncology Group trial. *J Clin Oncol.* 2003;21:2460–2465.

344. **Ozols RF.** Maintenance therapy in advanced ovarian cancer: Progression-free survival and clinical benefit. *J Clin Oncol.* 2003;21: 2451–2453.

345. **Pfisterer J, Weber B, Reuss A, et al.** Randomized phase III trial of topotecan following carboplatin and paclitaxel in first-line treatment of advanced ovarian cancer: A gynecologic cancer intergroup trial of the AGO-OVAR and GINECO. *J Natl Cancer Inst.* 2006;98:1024– 1045.

346. **Mei L1, Chen ML, Wei DM, et al.** Maintenance chemotherapy for ovarian cancer (Review). *Cochrane Database Syst Rev.* 2013;6: CD007414.

347. **Piccart MJ, Floquet A, Scarfone G, et al.** Intraperitoneal cisplatin versus no further treatment: 8-year results of EORTC 55875, a randomized phase III study in ovarian cancer patients with a pathologically complete remission after platinum-based intravenous chemotherapy. *Int J Gynecol Cancer.* 2003;13(suppl 2):196–203.

348. **Jordan K, Sippel C, Schmoll HJ.** Guidelines for antiemetic treatment of chemotherapy-induced nausea and vomiting: Past, present, and future recommendations. *Oncologist.* 2007;12:1143–1150.

349. **Herrstedt J.** Antiemetics: An update and the MASCC guidelines applied in clinical practice. *Nat Clin Pract Oncol.* 2008;1:32–43.

350. **Kris MG, Hesketh PJ, Somerfield MR, et al.** American Society of Clinical Oncology guideline for antiemetics in oncology: Update 2006. *J Clin Oncol.* 2006;24:2932–2947.

351. **Rothenberg ML, Ozols RF, Glatstein E, et al.** Dose-intensive induction therapy with cyclophosphamide, cisplatin and consolidative abdominal radiation in advanced stage epithelial cancer. *J Clin Oncol.* 1992;10:727–734.

352. **Rendina GM, Donadio C, Giovannini M.** Steroid receptors and progestinic therapy in ovarian endometrioid carcinoma. *Eur J Gynaecol Oncol.* 1982;3:241–246.

353. **Windbichler G, Hausmaninger H, Stummvoll W, et al.** Interferon-gamma in the first-line therapy of ovarian cancer: A randomized phase III trial. *Br J Cancer.* 2000;82:1138–1144.

354. **Alberts DS, Marth C, Alvarez RD, et al.** GRACES Clinical Trial Consortium. Randomized phase 3 trial of interferon gamma-1b plus standard carboplatin/paclitaxel versus carboplatin/paclitaxel alone for first-line treatment of advanced ovarian and primary peritoneal carcinomas: Results from a prospectively designed analysis of progression-free survival. *Gynecol Oncol.* 2008;109:174–181.

355. **Berek JS, Schultes BC, Nicodemus CF.** Biologic and immunologic therapies for ovarian cancer. *J Clin Oncol.* 2003;21:168S–174S.

356. **Berek JS, Dorigo O, Schultes BC, et al.** Immunological therapy for ovarian cancer. *Gynecol Oncol.* 2003;88:S105–S109.

357. **Berek JS, Taylor PT, Gordon A, et al.** Randomized placebo-controlled study of oregovomab for consolidation of clinical remission in patients with advanced ovarian cancer. *J Clin Oncol* 2004;22: 3507–3516.

358. **Berek JS, Taylor P, McGuire W, et al.** Oregovamab maintenance therapy in advanced stage ovarian cancer: No impact on relapse-free survival. *J Clin Oncol.* 2008;26:1–8.

359. **Verheijen RH, Massuger LF, Benigno BB, et al.** Phase III trial of intraperitoneal therapy with yttrium-90-labeled HMFG1 murine monoclonal antibody in patients with epithelial ovarian cancer after a surgically defined complete remission. *J Clin Oncol.* 2006;24: 571–578.

360. Oei AL, Verheijen RH, Seiden MV, et al. Decreased intraperitoneal disease recurrence in epithelial ovarian cancer patients receiving intraperitoneal consolidation treatment with yttrium-90-labeled murine HMFG1 without improvement in overall survival. *Int J Cancer.* 2007;120:2710–2714.

361. Bookman MA, Darcy KM, Clarke-Pearson D, et al. Evaluation of monoclonal humanized anti-HER2 antibody, trastuzumab, in patients with recurrent or refractory ovarian or primary peritoneal carcinoma with overexpression of HER2: A phase II trial of the Gynecologic Oncology Group. *J Clin Oncol.* 2003;21:283–290.

362. Berek JS, Hacker NF, Lagasse LD, et al. Second-look laparotomy in stage III epithelial ovarian cancer: Clinical variables associated with disease status. *Obstet Gynecol.* 1984;64:207–212.

363. Schwartz PE, Smith JP. Second-look operation in ovarian cancer. *Am J Obstet Gynecol.* 1980;138:1124–1130.

364. Rubin SC, Jones WB, Curtin JP, et al. Second-look laparotomy in stage I ovarian cancer following comprehensive surgical staging. *Obstet Gynecol.* 1993;82:139–142.

365. Podratz KC, Cliby WA. Second-look surgery in the management of epithelial ovarian carcinoma. *Gynecol Oncol.* 1994;55:S128–S133.

366. Bolis G, Villa A, Guarnerio P, et al. Survival of women with advanced ovarian cancer and complete pathologic response at second-look laparotomy. *Cancer.* 1996;77:128–131.

367. Friedman JB, Weiss NS. Second thoughts about second-look laparotomy in advanced ovarian cancer. *N Engl J Med.* 1990;322:1079–1082.

368. Berek JS. Second-look versus second-nature. *Gynecol Oncol.* 1992; 44:1–2.

369. Rubin SC, Hoskins WJ, Saigo PE, et al. Prognostic factors for recurrence following negative second-look laparotomy in ovarian cancer patients treated with platinum-based chemotherapy. *Gynecol Oncol.* 1991;42:137–141.

370. Dowdy SC, Constantinou CL, Hartmann LC, et al. Long-term follow-up of women with ovarian cancer after positive second-look laparotomy. *Gynecol Oncol.* 2003;91:563–568.

371. Berek JS, Knapp RC, Malkasian GD, et al. CA125 serum levels correlated with second-look operations among ovarian cancer patients. *Obstet Gynecol.* 1986;67:685–698.

372. Rustin GJ, Marples M, Nelstrop AE, et al. Use of CA125 to define progression of ovarian cancer in patients with persistently elevated levels. *J Clin Oncol.* 2001;19:4054–4057.

373. Rustin GJ, Timmers P, Nelstrop A, et al. Comparison of CA-125 and standard definitions of progression of ovarian cancer in the intergroup trial of cisplatin and paclitaxel versus cisplatin and cyclophosphamide. *J Clin Oncol.* 2006;24:45–51.

374. Rustin GJ, van der Burg ME; On behalf of MRC and EORTC collaborators. A randomized trial in ovarian cancer (OC) of early treatment of relapse based on CA125 level alone versus delayed treatment based on conventional clinical indicators (MRC OV05/EORTC 55955 trials). *J Clin Oncol.* 2009;27:18S(abst1).

375. Rustin GJ. Follow-up with CA125 after primary therapy of advanced ovarian cancer has major implications for treatment outcome and trial performances and should not be routinely performed. *Ann Oncol.* 2011;22(suppl 8):viii45–viii48.

376. De Rosa V, Mangioni di Stefano ML, Brunetti A, et al. Computed tomography and second-look surgery in ovarian cancer patients: Correlation, actual role and limitations of CT scan. *Eur J Gynaecol Oncol.* 1995;16:123–129.

377. Lund B, Jacobson K, Rasch L, et al. Correlation of abdominal ultrasound and computed tomography scans with second- or third-look laparotomy in patients with ovarian carcinoma. *Gynecol Oncol.* 1990;37:279–283.

378. Gadducci A, Cosio S, Zola P, et al. Diagnostic accuracy of FDG PET in the follow-up of platinum-sensitive epithelial ovarian carcinoma. *Eur J Nucl Med Mol Imaging.* 2007;34:1396–1405.

379. Kim CK, Park BK, Choi JY, et al. Detection of recurrent ovarian cancer at MRI: Comparison with integrated PET/CT. *J Comput Assist Tomogr.* 2007;31:868–875.

380. Lenhard SM, Burges A, Johnson TRC, et al. Predictive value of PET-CT imaging versus AGO-scoring in patients planned for cytoreductive surgery in recurrent ovarian cancer. *European J Obstet Gynecol Reprod Biol.* 2008;140:263–268.

381. Ebina Y, Watari H, Kaneuchi M, et al. Impact of FDG PET in optimizing patient selection for cytoreductive surgery in recurrent ovarian cancer. *Eur J Nucl Med Mol Imaging.* 2014;41(3):446–451.

382. Bristow RE, del Carmen MG, Pannu HK, et al. Clinically occult recurrent ovarian cancer: A patient selection for secondary cytoreductive surgery using combined PET/CT. *Gynecol Oncol.* 2003;90: 519–528.

383. Bristow RE, Giuntoli RL 2nd, Pannu HK, et al. Combined PET/CT for detecting recurrent ovarian cancer limited to the retroperitoneal nodes. *Gynecol Oncol.* 2005;99:294–300.

384. Berek JS, Hacker NF, Lagasse LD, et al. Survival of patients following secondary cytoreductive surgery in ovarian cancer. *Obstet Gynecol.* 1983;61:189–193.

385. Hoskins WJ, Rubin SC, Dulaney E, et al. Influence of secondary cytoreduction at the time of second-look laparotomy on the survival of patients with epithelial ovarian carcinoma. *Gynecol Oncol.* 1989; 34:365–371.

386. Jänicke F, Hölscher M, Kuhn W, et al. Radical surgical procedure improves survival time in patients with recurrent ovarian cancer. *Cancer.* 1992;70:2129–2136.

387. Rubin SC, Benjamin I, Berek JS. Secondary cytoreductive surgery. In: Gershenson D, McGuire W, eds. *Ovarian Cancer: Controversies in Management.* New York, NY: Churchill Livingstone; 1998:101–113.

388. Tay EH, Grant PT, Gebski V, et al. Secondary cytoreductive surgery for recurrent epithelial ovarian cancer. *Obstet Gynecol.* 2002; 100:1359–1360.

389. Salani R, Santillan A, Zahurak ML, et al. Secondary cytoreductive surgery for localized recurrent epithelial ovarian cancer: Analysis of prognostic factors and survival outcome. *Cancer.* 2007;109:685–691.

390. Rose PG. Surgery for recurrent ovarian cancer. *Semin Oncol.* 2000; 27:17–23.

391. Munkarah A, Levenback C, Wolf JK, et al. Secondary cytoreductive surgery for localized intra-abdominal recurrences in epithelial ovarian cancer. *Gynecol Oncol.* 2001;81:237–241.

392. Segna RA, Dottino PR, Mandeli JP, et al. Secondary cytoreduction for ovarian cancer following cisplatin therapy. *J Clin Oncol.* 1993;11:434–439.

393. Eisenkop SM, Friedman RL, Spirtos NM. The role of secondary cytoreductive surgery in the treatment of patients with recurrent epithelial ovarian carcinoma. *Cancer.* 2000;88:144–153.

394. Scarabelli C, Gallo A, Carbone A. Secondary cytoreductive surgery for patients with recurrent epithelial ovarian cancer. *Gynecol Oncol.* 2001;83:504–512.

395. Chi DS, McCaughty K, Diaz JP, et al. Guidelines and selection criteria for secondary cytoreductive surgery in patients with recurrent, platinum-sensitive epithelial ovarian carcinoma. *Cancer.* 2006; 106:1933–1939.

396. Harter P, du Bois A, Hahmann M, et al. Surgery in recurrent ovarian cancer: The Arbeitsgemeinschaft Gynaekologische Onkologie (AGO) DESKTOP OVAR Trial. *Ann Surg Oncol.* 2006;13: 1702–1710.

397. Al Rawahi T, Lopes AD, Bristow RE, et al. Surgical cytoreduction for recurrent epithelial ovarian cancer. *Cochrane Database Syst Rev.* 2013;2:CD008765.

398. Herzog TJ, Pothuri B. Ovarian cancer: A focus on management of recurrent disease. *Nat Clin Pract Oncol.* 2006;3:604–611.

399. Fung-Kee-Fung M, Oliver T, Elit L, et al. Optimal chemotherapy treatment for women with recurrent ovarian cancer. *Curr Oncol.* 2007;14:195–207.

400. Blackledge G, Lawton F, Redman C, et al. Response of patients in phase II studies of chemotherapy in ovarian cancer: Implications for patient treatment and the design of phase II trials. *Br J Cancer.* 1989; 59:650–653.

401. Markman M, Rothman R, Hakes T, et al. Second-line platinum chemotherapy in patients with ovarian cancer previously treated with cisplatin. *J Clin Oncol.* 1991;9:389–393.

402. Gordon AN, Fleagle JJ, Guthrie D, et al. Recurrent epithelial ovarian carcinoma: A randomized phase III study of pegylated liposomal doxorubicin versus topotecan. *J Clin Oncol.* 2001;19:3312–3322.

403. Gershenson DM, Kavanagh JJ, Copeland LJ, et al. Retreatment of patients with recurrent epithelial ovarian cancer with cisplatin-based chemotherapy. *Obstet Gynecol.* 1989;73:798–802.

404. Ozols RF, Ostchega Y, Curt G, et al. High dose carboplatin in refractory ovarian cancer patients. *J Clin Oncol.* 1987;5:197–201.

405. Gore ME, Fryatt I, Wiltshaw E, et al. Treatment of relapsed carcinoma of the ovary with cisplatin or carboplatin following initial treatment with these compounds. *Gynecol Oncol.* 1990;36:207–211.

406. **Eisenhauer EA, Vermorken JB, van Glabbeke M.** Predictors of response to subsequent chemotherapy in platinum pretreated ovarian cancer: A multivariate analysis of 704 patients. *Ann Oncol.* 1997; 8:963–968.

407. **Parmar MK, Ledermann JA, Colombo N, et al.** Paclitaxel plus platinum-based chemotherapy versus conventional platinum-based chemotherapy in women with relapsed ovarian cancer: The ICON4/AGO-OVAR-2.2 trial. *Lancet.* 2003;361:2099–2106.

408. **Gonzalez-Martin AJ, Calvo E, Bover I, et al.** Randomized phase II study of carboplatin versus paclitaxel and carboplatin in platinum-sensitive recurrent advanced ovarian carcinoma: A GEICO (Grupo Espanol de Investigacion en Cancer de Ovario) study. *Ann Oncol.* 2005;16:749–755.

409. **Greco FA, Hainsworth JD.** One-hour paclitaxel infusion schedules: A phase I/II comparative trial. *Semin Oncol.* 1995;22:118–123.

410. **Chang AY, Boros L, Garrow G, et al.** Paclitaxel by 3-hour infusion followed by 96-hour infusion on failure in patients with refractory malignant disease. *Semin Oncol.* 1995;22:124–127.

411. **Kohn EC, Sarosy G, Bicher A, et al.** Dose-intense Taxol: High response rate in patients with platinum-resistant recurrent ovarian cancer. *J Natl Cancer Inst.* 1994;86:1748–1753.

412. **Omura GA, Brady MF, Look KY, et al.** Phase III trial of paclitaxel at two dose levels, the higher dose accompanied by filgrastim at two dose levels in platinum-pretreated epithelial ovarian cancer: An intergroup study. *J Clin Oncol.* 2003;21:2843–2848.

413. **Markman M, Hall J, Spitz D, Weiner S, et al.** Phase II trial of weekly single-agent paclitaxel in platinum/paclitaxel-refractory ovarian cancer. *J Clin Oncol.* 2002;20:2365–2369.

414. **Ghamande S, Lele S, Marchetti D, et al.** Weekly paclitaxel in patients with recurrent or persistent advanced ovarian cancer. *Int J Gynecol Cancer.* 2003;13:142–147.

415. **Piccart MJ, Gore M, ten Bokkel Huinink W, et al.** Docetaxel: An active new drug for treatment of advanced epithelial ovarian cancer. *J Natl Cancer Inst.* 1995;87:676–681.

416. **Francis P, Schneider J, Hann L, et al.** Phase II trial of docetaxel in patients with platinum-refractory advanced ovarian cancer. *J Clin Oncol.* 1994;12:2301–2308.

417. **Rose PG, Blessing, JA, Ball HG, et al.** A phase II study of docetaxel in paclitaxel-resistant ovarian and peritoneal carcinoma: A Gynecologic Oncology Group study. *Gynecol Oncol.* 2003;88:130–135.

418. **Bookman MA, Malstrom H, Bolis G, et al.** Topotecan for the treatment of advanced epithelial ovarian cancer: An open-label phase II study in patients treated after prior chemotherapy that contained cisplatin or carboplatin and paclitaxel. *J Clin Oncol.* 1998;16:3345–3352.

419. **ten Bokkel Huinink W, Gore M, Carmichael J, et al.** Topotecan versus paclitaxel for the treatment of recurrent epithelial ovarian cancer. *J Clin Oncol.* 1997;15: 2183–2193.

420. **ten Bokkel Huinink W, Lane SR, Ross GA; for the International Topotecan Study Group.** Long-term survival in a phase III, randomised study of topotecan versus paclitaxel in advanced epithelial ovarian carcinoma. *Ann Oncol.* 2004;15:100–103.

421. **Hoskins P, Eisenhauer E, Beare S, et al.** Randomized phase II study of two schedules of topotecan in previously treated patients with ovarian cancer: A National Cancer Institute of Canada Clinical Trials Group study. *J Clin Oncol.* 1998;16:2233–2237.

422. **Markman M, Blessing JA, Alvarez RD, et al.** Phase II evaluation of 24-h continuous infusion topotecan in recurrent, potentially platinum-sensitive ovarian cancer: A Gynecologic Oncology Group study. *Gynecol Oncol.* 2000;77:112–115.

423. **Kudelka AP, Tresukosol D, Edwards CL, et al.** Phase II study of intravenous topotecan as a 5-day infusion for refractory epithelial ovarian carcinoma. *J Clin Oncol.* 1996;14:1552–1557.

424. **Hochster H, Wadler S, Runowicz C, et al.** Activity and pharmacodynamics of 21-day topotecan infusion in patients with ovarian cancer previously treated with platinum-based chemotherapy. New York Gynecologic Oncology Group. *J Clin Oncol.* 1999;17:2553–2561.

425. **Elkas JC, Holschneider CH, Katz B, et al.** The use of continuous infusion topotecan in persistent and recurrent ovarian cancer. *Int J Gynecol Cancer.* 2003;13:138–141.

426. **Markman M, Kennedy A, Webster K, et al.** Phase 2 evaluation of topotecan administered on a 3-day schedule in the treatment of platinum- and paclitaxel-refractory ovarian cancer. *Gynecol Oncol.* 2000;79:116–119.

427. **Clarke-Pearson DL, Van Le L, Iveson T, et al.** Oral topotecan as single-agent second-line chemotherapy in patients with advanced ovarian cancer. *J Clin Oncol.* 2001;19:3967–3975.

428. **McGuire WP, Blessing JA, Bookman MA, et al.** Topotecan has substantial antitumor activity as first-line salvage therapy in platinum-sensitive epithelial ovarian carcinoma: A Gynecologic Oncology Group Study. *J Clin Oncol.* 2000;18:1062–1067.

429. **Rodriguez M, Rose PG.** Improved therapeutic index of lower dose topotecan chemotherapy in recurrent ovarian cancer. *Gynecol Oncol.* 2001;83:257–262.

430. **Gronlund B, Hansen HH, Hogdall C, et al.** Efficacy of low-dose topotecan in second-line treatment for patients with epithelial ovarian carcinoma. *Cancer.* 2002;95:1656–1662.

431. **Brown JV, Peters WA, Rettenmaier MA, et al.** Three-consecutive-day topotecan is an active regimen for recurrent epithelial ovarian cancer. *Gynecol Oncol.* 2003;88:136–140.

432. **Gore M, Oza A, Rustin G, et al.** A randomised trial of oral versus intravenous topotecan in patients with relapsed epithelial ovarian cancer. *Eur J Cancer.* 2002;38:57–63.

433. **Homesley HD, Hall DJ, Martin DA, et al.** A dose-escalating study of weekly bolus topotecan in previously treated ovarian cancer patients. *Gynecol Oncol.* 2001;83:394–399.

434. **Muggia F, Hainsworth J, Jeffers S, et al.** Phase II study of liposomal doxorubicin in refractory ovarian cancer: Antitumor activity and toxicity modification by liposomal encapsulation. *J Clin Oncol.* 1997; 15:987–993.

435. **Gordon AN, Tonda M, Sun S, et al.** Long-term survival advantage for women treated with pegylated liposomal doxorubicin compared with topotecan in a phase 3 randomized study of recurrent and refractory epithelial ovarian cancer. *Gynecol Oncol.* 2004;95(1):1–8.

436. **Smith DH, Adams JR, Johnston SR, et al.** A comparative economic analysis of pegylated liposomal doxorubicin versus topotecan in ovarian cancer in the USA and UK. *Ann Oncol.* 2002;13:1590–1597.

437. **Gold MA, Walker JL, Berek JS, et al.** Amifostine pretreatment for protection against topotecan-induced hematologic toxicity: Results of a multicenter phase III trial in patients with advanced gynecologic malignancies. *Gynecol Oncol.* 2003;90:325–330.

438. **Gore M, ten Bokkel Huinink W, Carmichael J, et al.** Clinical evidence for topotecan-paclitaxel non-cross-resistance in ovarian cancer. *J Clin Oncol.* 2001;19:1893–1900.

439. **Shapiro JD, Millward MJ, Rischin D, et al.** Activity of gemcitabine in patients with advanced ovarian cancer: Responses seen following platinum and paclitaxel. *Gynecol Oncol.* 1996;63:89–93.

440. **Papadimitriou CA, Fountzilas G, Aravantinos G, et al.** Second-line chemotherapy with gemcitabine and carboplatin in paclitaxel-pretreated, platinum-sensitive ovarian cancer patients: A Hellenic Cooperative Oncology Group Study. *Gynecol Oncol.* 2004;92: 152–159.

441. **Look KY, Bookman MA, Schol J, et al.** Phase I feasibility trial of carboplatin, paclitaxel, and gemcitabine in patients with previously untreated epithelial ovarian or primary peritoneal cancer: A Gynecologic Oncology Group study. *Gynecol Oncol.* 2004;92:93–100.

442. **Belpomme D, Krakowski I, Beauduin M, et al.** Gemcitabine combined with cisplatin as first-line treatment in patients with advanced ovarian cancer: A phase I study. *Gynecol Oncol.* 2003;91:32–38.

443. **Markman M, Webster K, Zanotti K, et al.** Phase 2 trial of single-agent gemcitabine in platinum-paclitaxel refractory ovarian cancer. *Gynecol Oncol.* 2003;90:593–596.

444. **Slayton RE, Creasman WT, Petty W, et al.** Phase II trial of VP-16–213 in the treatment of advanced squamous cell carcinoma of the cervix and adenocarcinoma of the ovary: A Gynecologic Oncology Group Study. *Cancer Treat Rep.* 1979;63:2089–2092.

445. **Hoskins PJ, Swenerton KD.** Oral etoposide is active against platinum-resistant epithelial ovarian cancer. *J Clin Oncol.* 1994;12:60–63.

446. **Rose PG, Blessing JA, Mayer AR, et al.** Prolonged oral etoposide as second-line therapy for platinum-resistant and platinum-sensitive ovarian carcinoma: A Gynecologic Oncology Group study. *J Clin Oncol.* 1998;16:405–410.

447. **Manetta A, MacNeill C, Lyter JA, et al.** Hexamethylmelamine as a second-line agent in ovarian cancer. *Gynecol Oncol.* 1990;36:93–96.

448. **Moore DH, Valea F, Crumpler LS, et al.** Hexamethylmelamine (altretamine) as second-line therapy for epithelial ovarian carcinoma. *Gynecol Oncol.* 1993;51:109–112.

449. **Vasey PA, McMahon L, Paul J, et al.** A phase II trial of capecitabine (Xeloda) in recurrent ovarian cancer. *Br J Cancer.* 2003;89:1843–1848.

450. **Look KY, Muss HB, Blessing JA, et al.** A phase II trial of 5-fluorouracil and high-dose leucovorin in recurrent epithelial ovarian carcinoma: A Gynecologic Oncology group study. *Am J Clin Oncol.* 1995;18:19–22.

451. **Sorensen P, Pfeiffer P, Bertelsen K.** A phase II trial of ifosfamide/mesna as salvage therapy in patients with ovarian cancer refractory to or relapsing after prior platinum-containing chemotherapy. *Gynecol Oncol.* 1995;56:75–78.

452. **Perez-Gracia JL, Carrasco EM.** Tamoxifen therapy for ovarian cancer in the adjuvant and advanced settings: Systematic review of the literature and implications for future research. *Gynecol Oncol.* 2002;84:201–209.

453. **Ansink AC, Williams CJ.** The role of tamoxifen in the management of ovarian cancer. *Gynecol Oncol.* 2002;86:390.

454. **Williams CJ.** Tamoxifen for relapse of ovarian cancer. *Cochrane Database Syst Rev.* 2001;(1). Art. No.: CD001034. DOI: 10.1002/14651858.CD001034.

455. **Hatch KD, Beecham JB, Blessing JA, et al.** Responsiveness of patients with advanced ovarian carcinoma to tamoxifen: A Gynecologic Oncology Group study of second-line therapy in 105 patients. *Cancer.* 1991;68:269–271.

456. **Van der Velden J, Gitsch G, Wain GV, et al.** Tamoxifen in patients with advanced epithelial ovarian cancer. *Int J Gynecol Cancer.* 1995;5:301–305.

457. **Miller DS, Brady MF, Barrett RJ.** A phase II trial of leuprolide acetate in patients with advanced epithelial ovarian cancer. *J Clin Oncol.* 1992;15:125–128.

458. **Lopez A, Tessadrelli A, Kudelka AP, et al.** Combination therapy with leuprolide acetate and tamoxifen in refractory ovarian cancer. *Int J Gynecol Cancer.* 1996;6:15–619.

459. **Smith IE, Dowsett M.** Aromatase inhibitors in breast cancer. *N Engl J Med.* 2003;348:2431–2442.

460. **Smyth JF, Gourley C, Walker G, et al.** Antiestrogen therapy is active in selected ovarian cancer cases: The use of letrozole in estrogen receptor–positive patients. *Clin Cancer Res.* 2007;13(12):3617–3622.

461. **Williams C SI, Bryant A.** Tamoxifen for relapse of ovarian cancer. *Cochrane Database Syst rev.* 2010;17(3):CD001034.

462. **Le T, Leis A, Pahwa P, et al.** Quality of life evaluations in patients with ovarian cancer during chemotherapy treatment. *Gynecol Oncol.* 2004;92:839–844.

463. **Pfisterer J, Plante M, Vergote I, et al.; for AGO-OVAR; NCIC CTG; EORTC GCG.** Gemcitabine plus carboplatin compared with carboplatin in patients with platinum-sensitive recurrent ovarian cancer: An intergroup trial of the AGO-OVAR, the NCIC CTG, and the EORTC GCG. *J Clin Oncol.* 2006;24:4699–4707.

464. **Alberts DS, Liu PY, Wilczynski SP, et al.** Randomized trial of pegylated liposomal doxorubicin (PLD) plus carboplatin versus carboplatin in platinum-sensitive (PS) patients with recurrent epithelial ovarian or peritoneal carcinoma after failure of initial platinum-based chemotherapy (Southwest Oncology Group Protocol S0200). *Gynecol Oncol.* 2008;108:90–94.

465. **Weber B, Lortholary A, Mayer F, et al.** Pegylated liposomal doxorubicin and carboplatin in late-relapsing ovarian cancer: A GINECO group phase II trial. *Anticancer Res.* 2009;29(10):4195–4200.

466. **Chuang YT, Chang CL.** Extending platinum-free interval in partially platinum-sensitive recurrent ovarian cancer by a non-platinum regimen: Its possible clinical significance. *Taiwan J Obstet Gynecol.* 2012;51(3):336–341.

467. **Pujade-Lauraine E, Wagner U, Aavall-Lundqvist E, et al.** Pegylated liposomal doxorubicin and carboplatin compared with paclitaxel and carboplatin for patients with platinum-sensitive ovarian cancer in late relapse. *J Clin Oncol.* 2010;28(20):3323–3329.

468. **Sessa C, De Braud F, Perotti A, et al.** Trabectedin for women with ovarian carcinoma after treatment with platinum and taxanes fails. *J Clin Oncol.* 2005;23(9):1867–1874.

469. **Krasner CN, McMeekin DS, Chan S, et al.** Phase II study of trabectedin single agent in patients with recurrent ovarian cancer previously treated with platinum-based regimens. *Br J Cancer.* 2007;97:1618–1624.

470. **Monk BJ, Herzog TJ, Kaye SB, et al.** Trabectedin plus pegylated liposomal doxorubicin in recurrent ovarian cancer. *J Clin Oncol.* 2010;28(19):3107–3114.

471. **Ferrero JM, Weber B, Geay JF, et al.** Second-line chemotherapy with pegylated liposomal doxorubicin and carboplatin is highly effective in patients with advanced ovarian cancer in late relapse: A GINECO phase II trial. *Ann Oncol.* 2007;18:263–268.

472. **van der Burg ME, van der Gaast A, Vergote I, et al.** What is the role of dose-dense therapy? *Int J Gynecol Cancer.* 2005;15(suppl 3):233–240.

473. **Mutch DG, Orlando M, Goss T, et al.** Randomized phase III trial of gemcitabine compared with pegylated liposomal doxorubicin in patients with platinum-resistant ovarian cancer. *J Clin Oncol.* 2007;25:2811–2818.

474. **Colombo N, Kutarska E, Dimopoulos M, et al.** Randomized, open-label, phase III study comparing patupilone (EPO906) with pegylated liposomal doxorubicin in platinum-refractory or resistant patients with recurrent epithelial ovarian, primary fallopian tube, or primary peritoneal cancer. *J Clin Oncol.* 2012;30:3841–3847.

475. **Meier W, du Bois A, Reuss A, et al.** Topotecan versus treosulfan, an alkylating agent, in patients with epithelial ovarian cancer and relapse within 12 months following 1st-line platinum/paclitaxel chemotherapy. A prospectively randomized phase III trial by the Arbeitsgemeinschaft Gynaekologische Onkologie Ovarian Cancer Study Group (AGO-OVAR). *Gynecol Oncol.* 2009;114(2):199–205.

476. **Mutch DG, Orlando M, Goss T, et al.** Randomized phase III trial of gemcitabine compared with pegylated liposomal doxorubicin in patients with platinum-resistant ovarian cancer. *J Clin Oncol.* 2007;25(19):2811–2818.

477. **Naumann RW, Coleman RL, Burger RA, et al.** PRECEDENT: a randomized phase II trial comparing vintafolide (EC145) and pegylated liposomal doxorubicin (PLD) in combination versus PLD alone in patients with platinum-resistant ovarian cancer. *J Clin Oncol.* 2013;31(35):4400–4406.

478. **Vergote I, Finkler N, del Campo J, et al.** ASSIST-1 Study Group. Phase 3 randomised study of canfosfamide (Telcyta, TLK286) versus pegylated liposomal doxorubicin or topotecan as third-line therapy in patients with platinum-refractory or -resistant ovarian cancer. *Eur J Cancer.* 2009;45(13):2324–2332.

479. **Cannistra SA, Matulonis UA, Penson RT, et al.** Phase II study of *bevacizumab* in patients with platinum-resistant ovarian cancer or peritoneal serous cancer. *J Clin Oncol.* 2007;25:5180–5186.

480. **Burger RA, Sill MW, Monk BJ, et al.** Phase II trial of bevacizumab in persistent or recurrent epithelial ovarian cancer or primary peritoneal cancer: A Gynecologic Oncology Group Study. *J Clin Oncol.* 2007;25:5165–5171.

481. **McNeish IA, Ledermann JA, Webber L, et al.** A randomised placebo-controlled trial of weekly paclitaxel and saracatinib (AZD0530) in platinum-resistant ovarian, fallopian tube or primary peritoneal cancer. *Ann Oncol.* 2014 Jul 28. [Epub ahead of print]

482. **Martin L, Schilder R.** Novel approaches in advancing the treatment of epithelial ovarian cancer: The role of angiogenesis inhibition. *J Clin Oncol.* 2007;25:2894–2901.

483. **Garcia AA, Hirte H, Fleming G, et al.** Phase II clinical trial of *bevacizumab* and low-dose metronomic oral cyclophosphamide in recurrent ovarian cancer: A trial of the California, Chicago, and Princess Margaret Hospital phase II consortia. *J Clin Oncol.* 2008;26:76–82.

484. **Simpkins F, Belinson JL, Rose PG.** Avoiding bevacizumab related gastrointestinal toxicity for recurrent ovarian cancer by careful patient screening. *Gynecol Oncol.* 2007;107:118–123.

485. **Aghajanian C, Blank SV, Goff BA, et al.** OCEANS: A randomized, double-blind, placebo-controlled phase III trial of chemotherapy with or without bevacizumab in patients with platinum-sensitive recurrent epithelial ovarian, primary peritoneal, or fallopian tube cancer. *J Clin Oncol.* 2012;30(17):2039–2045.

486. **Pujade-Lauraine E, Hilpert F, Weber B, et al.** Bevacizumab combined with chemotherapy for platinum-resistant recurrent ovarian cancer: The AURELIA open-label randomized phase III trial. *J Clin Oncol.* 2014;32(13):1302–1308.

487. **Monk BJ, Poveda A, Vergote I, et al.** A phase III, randomized, double-blind trial of weekly paclitaxel plus the angiopoietin 1 and 2 inhibitor, trebananib, or placebo in women with recurrent ovarian cancer: TRINOVA-1. *European Cancer Congress.* Abstract 41. Presented October 1, 2013.TRINOVA-1 Trial. ECCO abstract.

488. Ledermann JA, Perren T, Raja FA, et al. ICON6: A randomised three-arm, three stage, double-blind, placebo-controlled multi-centre Gynaecologic Cancer InterGroup (GCIG) phase III trial. *European Cancer Congress.* 2013 (ECCO 17-ESMO 38-ESTRO 32). ECCO Meeting Abstract.

489. Tew WP, Colombo N, Ray-Coquard I, et al. Intravenous aflibercept in patients with platinum-resistant, advanced ovarian cancer: results of a randomized, double-blind, phase 2, parallel-arm study. *Cancer.* 2014;120(3):335–343.

490. Gotlieb WH, Amant F, Advani S, et al. Intravenous aflibercept for treatment of recurrent symptomatic malignant ascites in patients with advanced ovarian cancer: A phase 2, randomised, double-blind, placebo-controlled study. *Lancet Oncol.* 2012;13(2):154–162.

491. Coleman RL, Duska LR, Ramirez PT, et al. Phase 1–2 study of docetaxel plus aflibercept in patients with recurrent ovarian, primary peritoneal, or fallopian tube cancer. *Lancet Oncol.* 2011;12(12):1109–1117.

492. Ma WW, Jimeno A. Strategies for suppressing angiogenesis in gynecological cancers. *Drugs Today (Barc).* 2007;43:259–273.

493. Hacker NF, Berek JS, Pretorius G, et al. Intraperitoneal cisplatinum as salvage therapy in persistent epithelial ovarian cancer. *Obstet Gynecol.* 1987;70:759–764.

494. Braly PS, Berek JS, Blessing JA, et al. Intraperitoneal administration of cisplatin and 5-fluorouracil in residual ovarian cancer: A phase II Gynecologic Oncology Group trial. *Gynecol Oncol.* 1995;34:143–147.

495. Francis P, Rowinsky E, Schneider J, et al. Phase I feasibility study and pharmacologic study of weekly intraperitoneal Taxol: A Gynecologic Oncology Group study. *J Clin Oncol* 1995;13:2961–2967.

496. Feun LG, Blessing JA, Major FJ, et al. A phase II study of intraperitoneal cisplatin and thiotepa in residual ovarian carcinoma: A Gynecologic Oncology Group study. *Gynecol Oncol.* 1998;71:410–415.

497. Markman M, Blessing JA, Major F, et al. Salvage intraperitoneal therapy of ovarian cancer employing cisplatin and etoposide: A Gynecologic Oncology Group study. *Gynecol Oncol.* 1993;50:191–195.

498. Kirmani S, Lucas WE, Kim S, et al. A phase II trial of intraperitoneal cisplatin and etoposide as salvage treatment for minimal residual ovarian carcinoma. *J Clin Oncol.* 1991;9:649–657.

499. Markman M, Hakes T, Reichman B, et al. Phase II trial of weekly or biweekly intraperitoneal mitoxantrone in epithelial ovarian cancer. *J Clin Oncol.* 1991;9:978–982.

500. Markman M, Rowinsky E, Hakes T, et al. Phase I trial of intraperitoneal Taxol: A Gynecologic Oncology Group study. *J Clin Oncol.* 1992;10:1485–1491.

501. Howell SB, Zimm S, Markman M, et al. Long-term survival of advanced refractory ovarian carcinoma patients with small-volume disease treated with intraperitoneal chemotherapy. *J Clin Oncol.* 1987;5:1607–1612.

502. Berek JS, Hacker NF, Lichtenstein A, et al. Intraperitoneal recombinant alpha2 interferon for salvage epithelial ovarian cancer immunotherapy in stage III: A Gynecologic Oncology Group study. *Cancer Res.* 1985;45:4447–4453.

503. Willemse PHB, De Vries EGE, Mulder NH, et al. Intraperitoneal human recombinant interferon alpha-2b in minimal residual ovarian cancer. *Eur J Cancer.* 1990;26:353–358.

504. Nardi M, Cognetti F, Pollera F, et al. Intraperitoneal alpha-2-interferon alternating with cisplatin as salvage therapy for minimal residual disease ovarian cancer: A phase II study. *J Clin Oncol.* 1990;6:1036–1041.

505. Markman M, Berek JS, Blessing JA, et al. Characteristics of patients with small-volume residual ovarian cancer unresponsive to cisplatin-based IP chemotherapy: Lessons learned from a Gynecologic Oncology Group phase II trial of IP cisplatin and recombinant α-interferon. *Gynecol Oncol.* 1992;45:3–8.

506. Berek JS, Markman M, Blessing JA, et al. Intraperitoneal α-interferon alternating with cisplatin in residual ovarian cancer: A phase II Gynecologic Oncology Group study. *Gynecol Oncol.* 1999;74:48–52.

507. Berek JS, Markman M, Stonebraker B, et al. Intraperitoneal α-interferon in residual ovarian cancer: A phase II Gynecologic Oncology Group study. *Gynecol Oncol.* 1999;75:10–14.

508. Bezwoda WR, Golombick T, Dansey R, et al. Treatment of malignant ascites due to recurrent/refractory ovarian cancer: the use of interferon-alpha or interferon-alpha plus chemotherapy. *In vivo* and *in vitro* observations. *Eur J Cancer.* 1991;27:1423–1429.

509. Pujade-Lauraine E, Guastella JP, Colombo N, et al. Intraperitoneal administration of interferon gamma: An efficient adjuvant to chemotherapy of ovarian cancers. Apropos of a European study of 108 patients. *Bull Cancer.* 1993;80:163–170.

510. Steis RG, Urba WJ, Vandermolen LA, et al. Intraperitoneal lymphokine-activated killer cell and interleukin 2 therapy for malignancies limited to the peritoneal cavity. *J Clin Oncol.* 1990;10:1618–1629.

511. Broun ER, Belinson JL, Berek JS, et al. Salvage therapy for recurrent and refractory ovarian cancer with high-dose chemotherapy and autologous bone marrow support: A Gynecologic Oncology Group pilot study. *Gynecol Oncol.* 1994;54:142–146.

512. Stiff P, Bayer R, Camarda M, et al. A phase II trial of high-dose mitoxantrone, carboplatin and cyclophosphamide with autologous bone marrow rescue for recurrent epithelial ovarian carcinoma: Analysis of risk factors for clinical outcome. *Gynecol Oncol.* 1995;57:278–285.

513. Cure H, Battista C, Guastalla JP, et al. Phase III randomized trial of high-dose chemotherapy (HDC) and peripheral blood stem cell (PBSC) support as consolidation in patients with advanced ovarian cancer: 5-year follow-up of a GINECO/FNCLCC/SFGM-TC Study. *Proc Am Soc Clin Oncol.* 2004;23(abst 5006).

514. Möbus V, Wandt H, Frickhofen N, et al. Phase III trial of high-dose sequential chemotherapy with peripheral blood stem cell support compared with standard dose chemotherapy for first-line treatment of advanced ovarian cancer: Intergroup trial of the AGO-Ovar/AIO and EBMT. *J Clin Oncol.* 2007;25:4187–4193.

515. Hacker NF, Berek JS, Burnison CM, et al. Whole abdominal radiation as salvage therapy for epithelial ovarian cancer. *Obstet Gynecol.* 1985;65:60–65.

516. Ripamonti C, Easson AM, Gerdes H. Management of malignant bowel obstruction. *Eur J Cancer.* 2008;44:1105–1115.

517. Feuer DJ, Broadley KE, Shepherd JH, et al. Surgery for the resolution of symptoms in malignant bowel obstruction in advanced gynaecological and gastrointestinal cancer (Cochrane Review). *Cochrane Database Syst Rev* 2000;(4):Art. No.: CD002764. DOI: 10.1002/14651858.CD002764.

518. Ripamonti C, Bruera E. Palliative management of malignant bowel obstruction. *Int J Gynecol Cancer.* 2002;12:135–143.

519. DeBernardo R. Surgical management of malignant bowel obstruction: Strategies toward palliation of patients with advanced cancer. *Curr Oncol Rep.* 2009;11:287–292.

520. Soriano A, Davis MP. Malignant bowel obstruction: Individualized treatment near the end of life. *Cleveland Clinic J Med.* 2011;78:197–206.

521. Coukos G, Rubin SC. Surgical management of epithelial ovarian cancer. *Oncol Spectr.* 2001;2:350–361.

522. Pothuri B, Vaidya A, Aghajanian C, et al. Palliative surgery for bowel obstruction in recurrent ovarian cancer: An updated series. *Gynecol Oncol.* 2003;89:306–313.

523. Tamussino KF, Lim PC, Webb MJ, et al. Gastrointestinal surgery in patients with ovarian cancer. *Gynecol Oncol.* 2001;80:79–84.

524. Winter WE, McBroom JW, Carlson JW, et al. The utility of gastrojejunostomy in secondary cytoreduction and palliation of proximal intestinal obstruction in recurrent ovarian cancer. *Gynecol Oncol.* 2003;91:261–264.

525. Jolicoeur L, Faught W. Managing bowel obstruction in ovarian cancer using a percutaneous endoscopic gastrostomy (PEG) tube. *Can Oncol Nurs J.* 2003;13:212–219.

526. Campagnutta E, Cannizzaro R, Gallo A, et al. Palliative treatment of upper intestinal obstruction by gynecologic malignancy: The usefulness of percutaneous endoscopic gastrostomy. *Gynecol Oncol.* 1996;62:103–105.

12 Germ Cell and Nonepithelial Ovarian Cancer

Jonathan S. Berek
Michael L. Friedlander
Neville F. Hacker

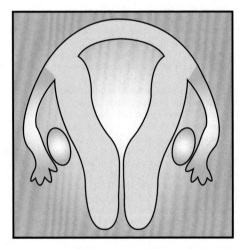

Compared with epithelial ovarian cancers, nonepithelial ovarian tumors are uncommon. They include malignancies of germ cell origin, sex-cord–stromal cell origin, metastatic carcinomas to the ovary, and a variety of extremely rare ovarian cancers, for example, sarcomas and lipoid cell tumors.

Nonepithelial malignancies of the ovary account for approximately 10% of all ovarian cancers (1,2). Although there are many similarities in the presentation, evaluation, and management of these patients, these tumors also have unique features that require a special approach (1–5).

Germ Cell Malignancies

Germ cell tumors are derived from the primordial germ cells of the ovary and occur with only about one-tenth the incidence of malignant germ cell tumors of the testis. Although they can arise in extragonadal sites such as the mediastinum and the retroperitoneum, the majority of germ cell tumors arise in the gonad from undifferentiated germ cells. The variation in the site of these cancers is explained by the embryonic migration of the germ cells from the caudal part of the yolk sac to the dorsal mesentery before their incorporation into the sex cords of the developing gonads (1,2).

Germ cell tumors are a model of a curable cancer. The management of patients with ovarian germ cell tumors has largely been extrapolated from the much greater experience of treating males with the more common testicular germ cell tumors. There have been many randomized trials for testicular germ cell tumors, which have provided a strong evidence base for treatment decision making (6,7). The outcome of patients with testicular germ cell tumors is better in experienced centers, and it is reasonable to suggest the same will be true for the less common ovarian counterparts. The cure rate is high, and attention is now being directed at reducing toxicity without compromising survival. There are still a small number of patients who die from the disease, and studies are in progress to try to improve the outcome for this high-risk, poor-prognostic subset (6,7).

In one of the largest reported series, which included 113 patients with advanced ovarian germ cell tumors treated with *cisplatin*-based chemotherapy, Murugaesu et al. (8) reported that **stage and**

Table 12.1 Histologic Typing of Ovarian Germ Cell Tumors	
I. Primitive Germ Cell Tumors	*III. Monodermal Teratoma and Somatic-Type Tumors Associated with Dermoid Cysts*
Dysgerminoma	Thyroid tumor
Yolk sac tumor	Struma ovarii
Embryonal carcinoma	Benign
Polyembryoma	Malignant
Nongestational choriocarcinoma	Carcinoid
Mixed germ cell tumor	Neuroectodermal tumor
II. Biphasic or Triphasic Teratoma	Carcinoma
Immature teratoma	Melanocytic
Mature teratoma	Sarcoma
Solid	Sebaceous tumor
Cystic	Pituitary-type tumor
Dermoid cyst	Others
Fetiform teratoma (homunculus)	

Adapted from **Tavassoli FA, Devilee P, eds**. World Health Organization classification of tumours. *Pathology and Genetics of Tumours of the Breast and Female Organs.* Lyon, France: IARC Press; 2003.

elevated tumor markers were independent poor prognostic indicators. These findings are important because they identify similar prognostic factors for ovarian and testicular germ cell tumors, and are in accordance with the clinical observation that testicular and ovarian germ cell tumors behave similarly. This is relevant for the management of patients with ovarian germ cell tumors because it may help to identify a poor prognostic subset of patients who require more intensive treatment (8).

Classification

A histologic classification of ovarian germ cell tumors is presented in Table 12.1 (1,9). **Both α-fetoprotein (AFP) and human chorionic gonadotropin (hCG) are secreted by some germ cell malignancies.** An elevated AFP and β-hCG can be clinically useful in the differential diagnosis of patients with a pelvic mass, and in monitoring patients after surgery. **Placental alkaline phosphatase (PLAP) and lactate dehydrogenase (LDH) are elevated in up to 95% of patients with dysgerminomas,** and serial monitoring of serum LDH levels may be useful for monitoring the disease. PLAP is more useful as an immunohistochemical marker than as a serum marker. The classification of germ cell tumors is based both on histologic features and immunohistochemical expression of tumor markers (Fig. 12.1) (10,15).

In this scheme, **embryonal carcinoma,** which is composed of undifferentiated cells that **synthesize both hCG and AFP,** is the progenitor of several other germ cell tumors (4,10). More differentiated germ cell tumors—such as the **endodermal sinus tumor (EST), which secretes AFP, and choriocarcinoma, which secretes hCG—are derived from the extraembryonic tissues; immature teratomas are derived from the embryonic cells** and do not secrete hCG, but may be associated with an elevated AFP. Elevated hCG levels are seen in 3% of dysgerminomas and the level is typically less than 100 International Unit. AFP is never elevated in pure dysgerminomas (1).

Epidemiology

Although 20–25% of all benign and malignant ovarian neoplasms are of germ cell origin, they account for only about 5% of all malignant ovarian neoplasms (1). In Asian and black societies where epithelial ovarian cancers are much less common, they may account for as many as 15% of ovarian cancers. **In the first two decades of life, almost 70% of ovarian tumors are of germ cell origin, and one-third of these are malignant** (1,2). Germ cell tumors account for two-thirds of the ovarian malignancies in this age group. Germ cell cancers also are seen in the third decade, but thereafter they become quite rare.

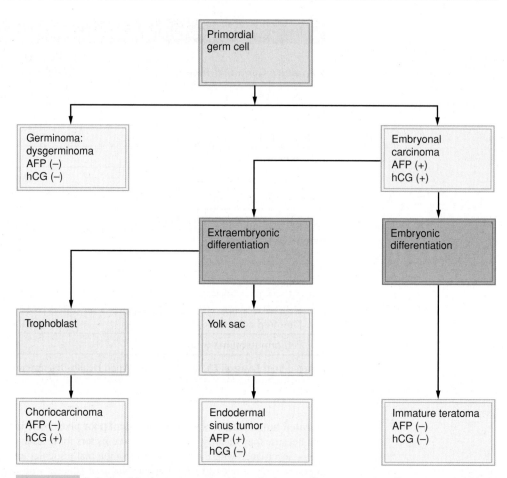

Figure 12.1 Relationship between examples of pure malignant germ cell tumors and their secreted marker substances.

Clinical Features

Symptoms

In contrast to the relatively slow-growing epithelial ovarian tumors, germ cell malignancies grow rapidly, and often are characterized by subacute pelvic pain related to capsular distention, hemorrhage, or necrosis. The rapidly enlarging pelvic mass may produce pressure symptoms on the bladder or rectum, and menstrual irregularities also may occur in menarchal patients. Some young patients may misinterpret the symptoms as those of pregnancy, and this can lead to a delay in diagnosis. Acute symptoms associated with torsion or rupture can develop. These symptoms may be confused with acute appendicitis. In more advanced cases, ascites may develop, and the patient may present with abdominal distention (3).

Signs

In patients with a palpable adnexal mass, the evaluation can proceed as outlined in Chapter 11. Some patients with germ cell tumors will be premenarchal. If the lesions are principally solid, or a combination of solid and cystic on an ultrasonographic evaluation, a neoplasm is probable and a malignancy is possible (Fig. 12.2). The remainder of the physical examination should search for signs of ascites, pleural effusion, and organomegaly.

Diagnosis

Adnexal masses measuring 2 cm or more in premenarchal girls or complex masses 8 cm or more in premenopausal patients will usually require surgical exploration (Fig. 12.3). In young patients, preoperative blood tests should include serum hCG, AFP, LDH and CA125 levels, a complete blood count, and liver function tests. A radiograph of the chest is important because germ cell tumors can metastasize to the lungs or mediastinum. **A karyotype should ideally be obtained preoperatively on all premenarchal girls because of the propensity of these tumors to arise**

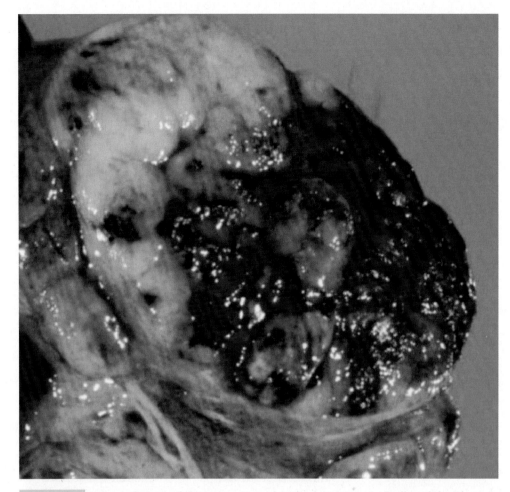

Figure 12.2 Dysgerminoma of the ovary. Note that the lesion is principally solid with some cystic areas and necrosis. (From **Berek JS, Longacre TA, Friedlander M.** Ovarian, fallopian tube and peritoneal cancer. In: **Berek JS, ed.** *Berek & Novak's Gynecology.* 15th ed. Philadelphia, PA: Lippincott Williams & Wilkins; 2012.)

in dysgenetic gonads, but this may not be practical (3,11). A preoperative computed tomographic (CT) scan or magnetic resonance imaging (MRI) may document the presence and extent of retroperitoneal lymphadenopathy or liver metastases, but unless there is very extensive metastatic disease, is unlikely to influence the decision to operate on the patient initially. If postmenarchal patients have predominantly cystic lesions up to 8 cm in diameter, they may undergo observation or a trial of hormonal suppression for two cycles (12).

Dysgerminoma

Dysgerminomas are the most common malignant germ cell tumor, accounting for approximately 30–40% of all ovarian cancers of germ cell origin (2,10). They represent only 1–3% of all ovarian cancers, but represent as many as 5–10% of ovarian cancers in patients younger than 20 years of age. Seventy-five percent of dysgerminomas occur between the ages of 10 and 30 years, 5% occur before the age of 10 years and they rarely occur after age 50 (1,4). They typically occur in young women and 20–30% of ovarian malignancies associated with pregnancy are dysgerminomas.

Approximately 5% of dysgerminomas occur in phenotypic females with abnormal gonads (1,11). Dysgerminomas can be associated with patients who have pure gonadal dysgenesis (46XY, bilateral streak gonads), mixed gonadal dysgenesis (45X/46XY, unilateral streak gonad, contralateral testis), and the androgen insensitivity syndrome (46XY, testicular feminization). Therefore, in premenarchal patients with a pelvic mass, the karyotype should be determined, particularly if a dysgerminoma is considered as the likely diagnosis (Fig. 12.4).

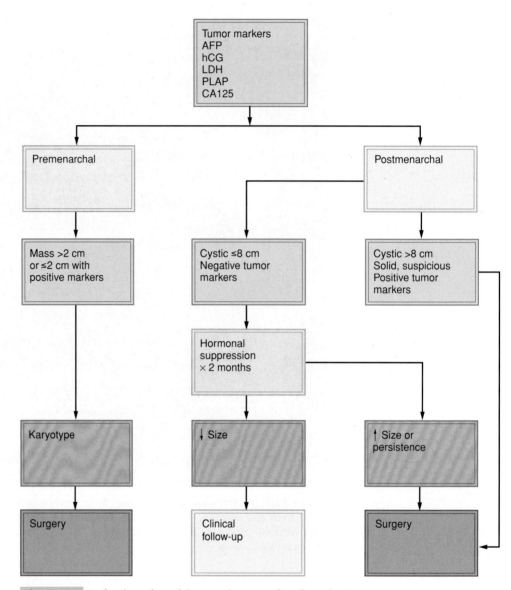

Figure 12.3 Evaluation of a pelvic mass in young female patients.

In most patients with gonadal dysgenesis, dysgerminomas arise in a gonadoblastoma, which is a benign ovarian tumor composed of germ cells and sex-cord stroma. If gonadoblastomas are left *in situ* in patients with gonadal dysgenesis, more than 50% will subsequently develop ovarian malignancies (13).

Approximately 65% of dysgerminomas are stage I at diagnosis (1,3,5,14,16,18–20). **Eighty-five to ninety percent of stage I** tumors are confined to one ovary, while 10–15% are bilateral. All other germ cell tumors are rarely bilateral.

In patients whose contralateral ovary has been preserved, a dysgerminoma can develop in 5–10% of them over the next 2 years (1). This figure includes patients who have not received systemic chemotherapy, as well as patients with gonadal dysgenesis.

In the 25% of patients who present with metastatic disease, the tumor most commonly spreads via the lymphatics, particularly to the higher para-aortic nodes (18). They can also spread hematogenously, or by direct extension through the capsule of the ovary with exfoliation and dissemination of cells throughout the peritoneal surfaces. Metastases to the contralateral ovary may be present when there is no other evidence of spread. An uncommon site of metastatic disease is bone, and when metastasis to this site occurs, the metastases are seen typically in the lower vertebrae. Metastases to the lungs, liver, and brain are rare and seen most often in patients with

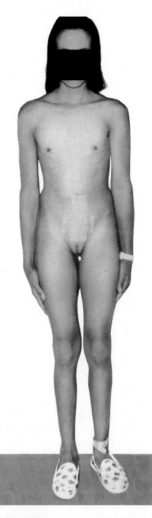

Figure 12.4 A 16-year-old girl with 46XY gonadal dysgenesis, showing lack of secondary sexual features, who developed dysgerminoma.

long-standing or recurrent disease. Metastasis to the mediastinum and supraclavicular lymph nodes is also usually a late manifestation of disease (14,16).

Treatment

The treatment of patients with early dysgerminoma is primarily surgical, including resection of the primary lesion and limited surgical staging–washings, omental biopsy, careful palpation of all peritoneal surfaces and retroperitoneal nodes, and biopsy of anything suspicious. Chemotherapy is administered to patients with metastatic disease. Because the disease principally affects young women, **special consideration must be given to the preservation of fertility** (17,18). A comparison of outcomes based on treatment at the Norwegian Radium Hospital clearly demonstrates the superiority of chemotherapy over radiation. Survival was better and morbidity was lower in the group treated with chemotherapy (17). An algorithm for the management of ovarian dysgerminoma is presented in Figure 12.5.

Surgery

The minimum operation for ovarian dysgerminoma is unilateral oophorectomy (19,21). If there is a desire to preserve fertility, as is usually the case, the contralateral ovary, fallopian tube, and uterus should be left *in situ* even in the presence of metastatic disease, because of the sensitivity of the tumor to chemotherapy. If fertility preservation is not required, it may be appropriate to perform a total abdominal hysterectomy and bilateral salpingo-oophorectomy in patients with advanced disease (5), although this will be appropriate in only a very small minority of patients. **In patients whose karyotype contains a Y chromosome, both ovaries should be**

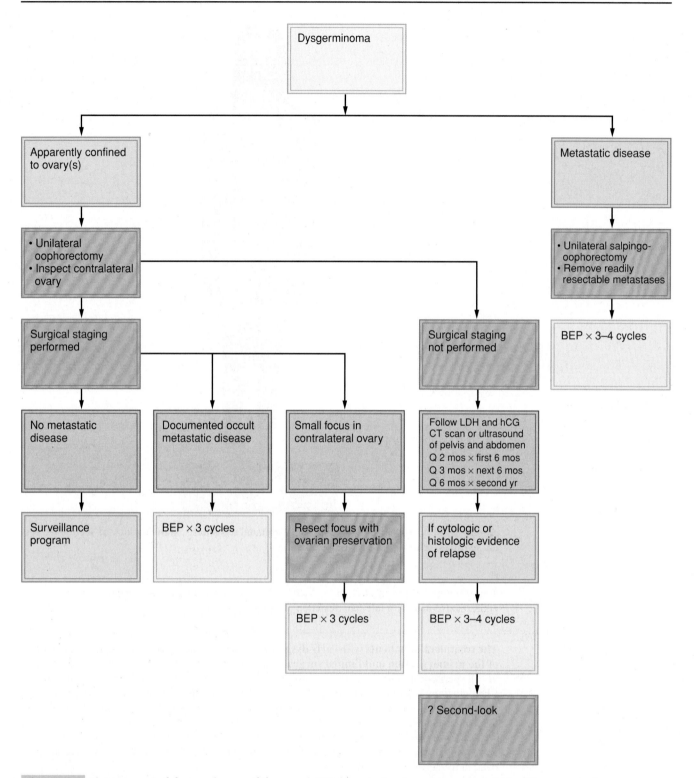

Figure 12.5 **Management of dysgerminoma of the ovary.** BEP, *bleomycin, etoposide,* and *cisplatin;* CT, computed tomogram.

removed, although the uterus may be left *in situ* for possible future embryo transfer. Cytoreductive surgery is of unproven value, but bulky disease that can be readily resected (e.g., an omental cake) should be removed at the initial operation. **It is important not to undertake surgery that is potentially morbid and may delay the initiation of chemotherapy.**

In patients in whom the dysgerminoma appears on inspection to be confined to the ovary, a careful staging operation should be undertaken to determine the presence of any occult

metastatic disease. These tumors often metastasize to the para-aortic nodes around the renal vessels. Peritoneal washings should be taken for cytology, and a thorough exploration made of all peritoneal surfaces and retroperitoneal lymph nodes, with biopsy or resection of any noted abnormalities. The contralateral ovary should be carefully inspected because dysgerminoma is the only germ cell tumor that tends to be bilateral, and not all of the bilateral lesions have obvious ovarian enlargement. Therefore careful inspection and palpation of the contralateral ovary and excisional biopsy of any suspicious lesion are desirable (5,19–21). If a small contralateral tumor is found, it may be possible to resect it and preserve some normal ovary.

Many patients with a dysgerminoma will have a tumor that is apparently confined to one ovary and will be referred after unilateral salpingo-oophorectomy without surgical staging. The options for such patients are (i) repeat laparotomy for surgical staging, (ii) regular pelvic and abdominal CT scans, or (iii) adjuvant chemotherapy (18). Because most dysgerminomas are confined to the ovary at presentation and are rapidly growing tumors, the author's preference is to offer regular and close surveillance to such patients (23,24) (Fig. 12.1).

Radiation

Loss of fertility and second malignancies are important late effects of radiation therapy, so it is no longer used for primary treatment (17). Radiation can be used selectively to treat recurrent disease (5,17,20). Dysgerminomas are very sensitive to radiation therapy, and doses of 2,500 to 3,500 cGy may be curative; however, it is uncommonly used because these tumors are very sensitive to platinum-based chemotherapy, and have a high likelihood of cure.

Chemotherapy

Chemotherapy is regarded as the treatment of choice (21,22,25–32,34). The obvious advantage is the preservation of fertility in most patients, and the reduced risk of second malignancies compared with radiation (21,35–39).

The most frequently used chemotherapeutic regimen is BEP (*bleomycin, etoposide,*** and ***cisplatin***). In the past, VBP (***vinblastine, bleomycin,*** and ***cisplatin***), and VAC (***vincristine, actinomycin,*** and ***cyclophosphamide***) were commonly used but are now rarely used** (21,22,25–28) (Table 12.2).

The Gynecologic Oncology Group (GOG) studied three cycles of EC: *Etoposide* (120 mg/m^2 intravenously on days 1, 2, and 3 every 4 weeks) and *carboplatin* (400 mg/m^2 intravenously on day 1 every 4 weeks) in 39 patients with completely resected ovarian dysgerminoma, stages IB, IC, II, or III (31). The results were excellent, and GOG reported a sustained disease-free remission rate of 100%.

For patients with advanced, incompletely resected germ cell tumors, the GOG studied *cisplatin-*based chemotherapy on two consecutive protocols (25). In the first study, patients received four cycles of *vinblastine* (12 mg/m^2 every 3 weeks), *bleomycin* (20 unit/m^2 intravenously every week for 12 weeks), and *cisplatin* (20 mg/m^2/d intravenously for 5 days every 3 weeks). Patients with persistent or progressive disease at second-look laparotomy were treated with six cycles of VAC. In the second trial, patients received three cycles of BEP initially, followed by consolidation with VAC, which was later discontinued in patients with dysgerminomas (25). VAC does not appear to improve the outcome following the BEP regimen and is no longer used.

Table 12.2 Combination Chemotherapy for Germ Cell Tumors of the Ovary	
Regimen and Drugs	*Dose and Schedule*[a]
BEP	
Bleomycin	30,000 International Units weekly for a total of 12 wks
Etoposide	100 mg/m^2/d × 5 d every 3 wks
Cisplatin	20 mg/m^2/d × 5 d every 3 wks

[a]**Loehrer PJ, Johnson D, Elson P, et al.** Importance of *bleomycin* in favorable-prognosis disseminated germ cell tumors: An Eastern Cooperative Oncology Group trial. *J Clin Oncol.* 1995;13:470–476.

A total of 20 evaluable patients with stages III and IV dysgerminoma were treated in these two protocols, and 19 were alive and free of disease after 6 to 68 months (median = 26 months). Fourteen of these patients had a second-look laparotomy, and all findings were negative. A study at MD Anderson Hospital (28) used BEP in 14 patients with residual disease, and all patients were free of disease with long-term follow-up. In another series of 26 patients with pure ovarian dysgerminomas who received BEP chemotherapy, 54% of whom had stage IIIC or IV disease, 25 (96%) remained continuously disease free following three to six cycles of therapy (34).

These results indicate that patients with an advanced-stage, incompletely resected dysgerminoma have an excellent prognosis when treated with *cisplatin*-**based combination chemotherapy (32–38). The optimal regimen is three to four cycles of BEP based on the data from testis cancers (33,39,40)** with the number of cycles depending on the extent of disease and the presence or absence of visceral metastases. If *bleomycin* is contraindicated or omitted because of lung toxicity, consideration should be given to four cycles of *cisplatin* and *etoposide* rather than three cycles of BEP.

There is no need to perform a second-look laparotomy in patients with dysgerminomas (41–43). The role of surgery to resect residual masses following chemotherapy for dysgerminomas is not clear, as the vast majority of these patients will only have necrotic tissue and nonviable tumor. In general, these patients should be closely monitored with scans and tumor markers. **A positron emission tomography (PET–CT) scan should be considered in patients who have bulky residual masses larger than 3 cm more than 4 weeks after chemotherapy.** A positive PET–CT scan appears to be a sensitive predictor of residual seminoma in males in these circumstances, (44) with residual disease being evident in 30–50% of patients. If the PET–CT is positive or if there is a suggestion of progressive disease on scans, ideally there should be histologic confirmation of residual disease before embarking on salvage therapy (45).

Recurrent Disease

Although recurrences are uncommon, 75% will occur within the first year after initial treatment (1–4), with **the most common sites being the peritoneal cavity and the retroperitoneal lymph nodes.** These patients should be treated with either chemotherapy or radiation, depending on the location of disease and the primary treatment. Patients with recurrent disease who have had no therapy other than surgery should be treated with chemotherapy. If previous chemotherapy with BEP has been given, an alternative regimen such as **TIP (***paclitaxel, ifosfamide,*** and ***cisplatin***),** a commonly used salvage regimen in testicular germ cell tumors (46), may be tried.

These treatment decisions should be made in a multidisciplinary setting with the input of physicians experienced in the management of patients with germ cell tumors. **Consideration may be given to the use of high-dose chemotherapy with peripheral stem cell support in selected patients.** A number of high-dose regimens have been used in phase II studies, and the choice depends on the previous chemotherapy, the time to recurrence, and the residual toxicity from the previous therapy (47,48). It is unclear whether high-dose chemotherapy is superior to conventional dose chemotherapy as first-line salvage therapy for patients with relapsed disease. The only randomized trial, conducted by the European Group for Blood and Marrow Transplantation (EBMT)-IT-94, did not demonstrate superiority for three cycles of VIP or *vinblastine-ifosfamide-cisplatin* (VeIP) followed by high-dose chemotherapy compared with four cycles of conventional dose chemotherapy. An international randomized trial (TIGER) plans to randomize 390 patients with recurrent germ cell tumors to four cycles of conventional dose *cisplatin*-based chemotherapy with TIP, compared with two cycles of *paclitaxel-ifosfamide* followed by three cycles of high-dose *carboplatin* and *etoposide* with autologous stem-cell support (TI-CE) (48).

Radiation therapy may be considered in selected patients with dysgerminomas with a localized recurrence, but this has the major disadvantage of causing loss of fertility if pelvic and abdominal radiation is required, and may also compromise the ability to deliver further chemotherapy if unsuccessful (17).

Pregnancy

Because dysgerminomas tend to occur in young patients, they may coexist with pregnancy. When a stage IA cancer is found, the tumor can be removed intact and the pregnancy continued. In patients with more advanced disease, continuation of the pregnancy will depend on gestational age. **Chemotherapy can be given in the second and third trimesters in the same dosages as** given for the nonpregnant patient without apparent detriment to the fetus (35,49). Relatively few patients have been treated with BEP during pregnancy and some fetal malformations and complications have been reported, underscoring the importance of ensuring that only patients who definitely require chemotherapy during pregnancy should be treated (50).

Prognosis

In patients with stage IA dysgerminoma, unilateral oophorectomy alone results in a 5-year disease-free survival rate of greater than 95% (5,20). The features that have been associated with a higher tendency to recurrence include tumors larger than 10 to 15 cm in diameter, age younger than 20 years, and microscopic features that include numerous mitoses, anaplasia, and a medullary pattern (1,10).

Kumar et al. abstracted data on malignant ovarian germ cell tumors from the Surveillance, Epidemiology, and End Results (SEER) program from 1988 through 2004 (51). There were a total of 1,296 patients with dysgerminomas, immature teratomas, or mixed germ cell tumors, 613 (47.3%) of whom had lymphadenectomies. Lymph node metastases were present in 28% of dysgerminomas, 8% of immature teratomas, and 16% of mixed germ cell tumors ($p < 0.05$). **The 5-year survival for patients with negative nodes was 95.7% compared to 82.8% for patients with positive nodes ($p < 0.001$).** The same group updated the results recently and reported on 1,083 patients with ovarian germ cell tumors who had surgery and who were believed to have disease clinically confined to the ovary (52). This included 590 (54.5%) who had no lymphadenectomy and 493 (45.5%) who had a lymphadenectomy. Of the latter, 52 (10.5%) were upstaged to FIGO stage IIIC due to nodal metastases. The 5-year survival was 96.9% for patients who did not have a lymphadenectomy, 97.7% for those who did, and 93.4% for patients who were found to have stage IIIC disease after lymphadenectomy. These survivals were not statistically different, and underscore the excellent prognosis for patients with dysgerminomas (22,25–32,34–38).

Immature Teratomas

Immature teratomas typically contain immature neuroepithelium and may be pure immature teratomas or occur in combination with other germ cell tumors as mixed germ cell tumors. The pure immature teratoma accounts for fewer than 1% of all ovarian cancers, but it is the second most common germ cell malignancy and represents 10–20% of all ovarian malignancies seen in women younger than 20 years of age (1). Approximately 50% of pure immature teratomas of the ovary occur between the ages of 10 and 20 years, and they rarely occur in postmenopausal women.

Semi-quantification of the amount of neuroepithelium correlates with survival in ovarian immature teratomas and is the basis for the grading of these tumors (53–55). **Those with less than one lower-power field (4) of immature neuroepithelium on the slide with the greatest amount of immature neuroepithelium (grade 1) have a survival of at least 95%, whereas greater amounts of immature neuroepithelium (grades 2 and 3) appear to have a lower overall survival (approximately 85%)** (55). This may not apply to immature teratomas of the ovary in children, because they appear to have a very good outcome with surgery alone, regardless of the degree of immaturity. These findings are from an era when not all patients would have received platinum-based chemotherapy (56,57).

Some pathologists have recommended a two-tiered grading system, suggesting that immature teratomas be categorized as either low grade or high grade because of the significant inter- and intraobserver difficulty with a three-grade system (55). This is the authors' current practice.

Immature ovarian teratomas may be associated with gliomatosis peritonei, which has a favorable prognosis if composed of completely mature tissues. Recent reports have suggested that these glial "implants" are not tumor derived, but represent teratoma-induced metaplasia of pluripotential müllerian stem cells in the peritoneum (56,58,59). The researchers have exploited a unique characteristic of ovarian teratomas. The latter typically contain a duplicated set of maternal chromosomes, and are therefore homozygous at polymorphic microsatellite loci, while DNA from matched normal tissue contains genetic material of both maternal and paternal origin, so exhibits heterozygosity at many of these same polymorphic microsatellite loci.

Malignant transformation of a mature teratoma is a rare event. Squamous cell carcinoma is the most frequent subtype of malignancy, but adenocarcinomas, primary melanomas, and carcinoids may also rarely occur (see below) (30). The risk is reported to be between 0.5% and 2% of teratomas, and usually occurs in postmenopausal patients.

Diagnosis

The preoperative evaluation and differential diagnosis are the same as for patients with other germ cell tumors. Some of these tumors will contain calcifications similar to mature teratomas, and this can be detected by a radiograph of the abdomen or by ultrasonography. Rarely, they are associated with the production of steroid hormones and can be accompanied by sexual pseudoprecocity (4). **AFP may be elevated in some patients with a pure immature teratoma but hCG is not elevated.**

Treatment

Surgery

In a premenopausal patient where the tumor appears confined to a single ovary, unilateral oophorectomy and limited surgical staging should be performed. In the rare postmenopausal patient with an immature teratoma, a total abdominal hysterectomy and bilateral salpingo-oophorectomy may be performed. Contralateral involvement is rare, and routine resection or wedge biopsy of the contralateral ovary is unnecessary (2). Any suspicious lesions on the peritoneal surfaces should be sampled and submitted for histologic evaluation. **The most frequent site of dissemination is the peritoneum and, much less commonly, the retroperitoneal lymph nodes.** Blood-borne metastases to organ parenchyma such as the lungs, liver, or brain are uncommon. When present, they are usually seen in patients with late or recurrent disease and most often in tumors that are high grade (4).

It is unclear whether debulking of metastases improves the response to combination chemotherapy (60,61). Cure ultimately depends on the ability to deliver chemotherapy promptly. **Any surgical resection that may be potentially morbid and therefore delay chemotherapy should be resisted, although surgical resection of any residual disease should be considered at the completion of chemotherapy.**

Chemotherapy

Patients with stage IA, grade 1 tumors have an excellent prognosis, and no adjuvant therapy is required. In patients with high-grade, stage IA immature teratomas, adjuvant chemotherapy has commonly been given, although this has been questioned, as excellent results have been also reported with close surveillance and treating only patients who have a recurrence (17,18,26–28,42,57,62–76).

The most frequently used combination chemotherapeutic regimen in the past was VAC (70–72), but a GOG study reported a relapse-free survival rate in patients with incompletely resected disease of only 75% (72). The approach over the last 20 years has been to incorporate *cisplatin* into the primary treatment of these tumors, and most of the experience has been with the VBP in the past and BEP more recently (65).

The GOG prospectively evaluated three courses of BEP therapy in patients with completely resected stage I, II, and III ovarian germ cell tumors (30). Overall, the toxicity was acceptable, and **91 of 93 patients (97.8%) with nondysgerminomatous tumors were clinically free of disease.** In nonrandomized studies, the BEP regimen is superior to the VAC regimen in the treatment of completely resected nondysgerminomatous germ cell tumors of the ovary. Some patients can progress rapidly postoperatively, and, in general, treatment should be initiated as soon as possible after surgery, preferably within 7 to 10 days, in those patients who require chemotherapy.

The switch from VBP to BEP has been prompted by the experience in patients with testicular cancer, where the replacement of *vinblastine* with *etoposide* has been associated with a better therapeutic index (i.e., equivalent efficacy and lower morbidity), with less neurologic and gastrointestinal toxicity, and improved outcomes (65,66). Furthermore, the use of *bleomycin* appears to be important in this group of patients. In a randomized study of three cycles of *etoposide* plus *cisplatin* with or without *bleomycin* (EP vs. BEP) in 166 patients with germ cell tumors of the testes, **the BEP regimen had a relapse-free survival rate of 84% compared with 69% for the EP regimen ($p = 0.03$)** (40).

Cisplatin **is superior to** *carboplatin* **in metastatic germ cell tumors of the testis.** One hundred and ninety-two patients with good prognosis germ cell tumors of the testes were entered into a study of four cycles of *etoposide* plus *cisplatin* (EP) versus four cycles of *etoposide* plus *carboplatin* (EC). There were three relapses with the EP regimen versus seven with the EC regimen (41). A German group randomized patients to (i) a BEP regimen of three cycles at standard doses given days 1 to 5 versus (ii) a CEB regimen of *carboplatin* (target AUC of 5 [mg/dL × min] on day 1), *etoposide* 120 mg/m^2 on days 1 to 3, and *bleomycin* 30 mg on days 1, 8, and 15 (77). Four cycles of CEB were given, with the omission of *bleomycin* in the fourth cycle so that the cumulative doses of *etoposide* and *bleomycin* in the two treatment arms were comparable. Fifty-four patients were entered on the trial; 29 were treated with BEP and 25 with CEB chemotherapy. More patients treated with CEB relapsed after therapy (32% vs. 13%). Four patients (16%) treated with CEB died of disease progression in contrast to one patient (3%) after BEP therapy. The trial was terminated early after an interim analysis. **The inferiority of carboplatin was confirmed in a larger randomized trial** reported by Horwich et al. (78). In view of these results, **BEP is the preferred treatment regimen** (65,79–81). **The 3-day schedule has been found to be equivalent to a 5-day schedule for BEP chemotherapy.** A cycle of BEP consisted of *etoposide* 500 mg/m^2, administered at either 100 mg/m^2 days 1 through 5 or 165 mg/m^2 days 1 through 3, *cisplatin* 100 mg/m^2, administered at either 20 mg/m^2 days 1 through 5 or 50 mg/m^2 days 1 and 2. *Bleomycin* 30,000 International Unit is administered on days 1, 8, and 15 during cycles 1 through 3.

Recurrent Disease

The principles and approach are identical to the management of recurrent dysgerminoma, as discussed above.

Second-look Laparotomy

Second-look operation for ovarian germ cell tumors (43,44) is not indicated in patients who have received adjuvant chemotherapy (i.e., stage IA, grades 2 and 3). However, **surgery should be considered in patients with metastatic immature teratomas who have residual disease at the completion of chemotherapy** because they may have residual mature teratoma and are at risk of *growing teratoma syndrome,* a rare complication of immature teratomas (90–92). Furthermore, cancers can arise at a later date in residual mature teratoma, and it is important to resect any residual mass and exclude persistent disease, as further chemotherapy may be indicated.

The principles of surgery are based on the much larger experience of surgery in males with residual masses following chemotherapy for germ cell tumors with a component of immature teratoma (93). Mathew et al. (94) reported their experience of laparotomy in assessing the nature of postchemotherapy residual masses in ovarian germ cell tumors. Sixty-eight patients completed combination chemotherapy with *cisplatin* regimens, of whom 35 had radiologic evidence of residual masses. Twenty-nine of these 35 patients underwent laparotomy, and 10 patients (34.5%) had viable tumor, including seven cases (24.2%) of immature teratoma. Nineteen patients (65.5) had no evidence of malignancy, including three (10.3%) cases showing mature teratoma, and 16 (55.2%) showing necrosis or fibrosis only. **None of the patients with a dysgerminoma or embryonal carcinoma and a radiologic residual mass of less than 5 cm had viable tumor present, whereas all patients with primary tumors containing a component of teratoma had residual tumor,** strengthening the case for surgery in patients with metastatic immature teratoma and any residual mass (94,95).

Prognosis

The most important prognostic feature of the immature teratoma is the grade of the lesion (1,53). In addition, the stage of disease and the extent of tumor at the initiation of treatment also have an impact on prognosis (4). Overall, the 5-year survival rate for patients with all stages of pure immature teratomas is 70–80%, and it is 90–95% for patients with surgical stage I tumors (42,53,62).

The degree or grade of immaturity generally predicts the metastatic potential and prognosis. The 5-year survival rates have been reported to be 82%, 62%, and 30% for patients with grades 1, 2, and 3, respectively (53) but many of these patients were treated in an era before optimal chemotherapy was available, and these figures do not match current experience and more recently published data (67). For example, Lai et al. (96) reported on the long-term outcome of 84 patients with ovarian germ cell tumors, including 29 immature teratomas, and the 5-year survival was 97.4%.

Occasionally, these tumors are associated with mature or low-grade glial elements that have implanted throughout the peritoneum. Such patients have a favorable long-term survival (4). **Mature glial elements can grow and mimic malignant disease and may need to be resected to relieve pressure on surrounding structures.**

Endodermal Sinus Tumor

Endodermal sinus tumors (ESTs) have also been referred to as *yolk sac carcinomas* because they are derived from the primitive yolk sac (1). They are the third most frequent malignant germ cell tumor of the ovary.

ESTs have a median age of 18 years at diagnosis (1–3,97,98). Approximately one-third of the patients are premenarchal at presentation. Abdominal or pelvic pain occurs in approximately 75% of patients, whereas an asymptomatic pelvic mass is documented in 10% of patients (3).

Most ESTs secrete AFP and rarely may also elaborate detectable alpha-1-antitrypsin (AAT). There is a good correlation between the extent of disease and the level of AFP, although discordance also has been observed. The serum level of AFP is useful in monitoring the patient's response to treatment, as well as in follow-up (97–104).

Treatment

Surgery

The treatment of an EST consists of surgical exploration, unilateral salpingo-oophorectomy, a frozen section for diagnosis, and limited surgical staging. A hysterectomy and contralateral salpingo-oophorectomy should not be done (4,100,101). Conservative surgery and adjuvant chemotherapy allow fertility preservation as with other germ cell tumors (21). In patients with metastatic disease, all gross disease should be resected if possible. At surgery, the tumors tend to be solid and large, ranging in size from 7 to 28 cm (median = 15 cm) in the GOG series. **Bilaterality is not seen in EST,** and the other ovary is involved with metastatic disease only when there are other metastases in the peritoneal cavity. Most patients have early-stage disease: 71% stage I, 6% stage II, and 23% stage III (101,105).

Chemotherapy

All patients with ESTs should be treated with chemotherapy shortly after recovering from surgery. Prior to the routine use of combination chemotherapy, the 2-year survival rate was approximately 25%. After the introduction of the VAC regimen, the survival rate improved to 60–70%, which highlights the chemosensitivity of the majority of these tumors (71,72). **All patients should be treated with a *cisplatin*-based regimen such as BEP, which is considered the standard of care.** The chance of cure now approaches 100% for patients with early-stage disease, and is at least 75% for patients with more advanced-stage disease (101).

The optimal number of treatment cycles has not been established in ovarian germ cell tumors, but it is reasonable to extrapolate from the much larger experience in testicular germ cell tumors where three cycles of BEP is considered optimal for good prognosis, low-risk patients and four cycles for patients with intermediate to high-risk tumors (7). In patients for whom *bleomycin* is omitted or discontinued because of toxicity, four cycles of *cisplatin* and *etoposide* are recommended. **An alternative approach is to use VIP (*etoposide*, *ifosfamide*, and *cisplatin*) in patients with more advanced disease in whom *bleomycin* is contraindicated.** Four cycles of VIP are equivalent to four cycles of BEP, but it is more myelotoxic and requires growth-factor support (6,7,108). These patients should only be treated by clinicians experienced in the management of germ cell tumors as the outcomes of patients in inexperienced hands are compromised.

Neoadjuvant chemotherapy followed by fertility-sparing surgery may also be a reasonable option for patients with advanced ovarian germ cell tumors not suitable for optimal cytoreduction, as shown in a recent study of 21 patients from India (109).

A number of years ago, the group from the Charing Cross Hospital in London developed the **POMB-ACE** (*cisplatin, vincristine, methotrexate, bleomycin, actinomycin D, cyclophosphamide, etoposide*) **regimen for high-risk germ cell tumors of any histologic type** (104) (Table 12.3). Their results appear to be superior to BEP in patients with poor prognostic features, but this has not been confirmed in randomized controlled trials. **This protocol introduces seven drugs into the initial management, which is intended to reduce the chances of developing drug resistance, which may be particularly relevant for patients with large volume metastatic disease.** The authors have used the POMB-ACE regimen as primary therapy for selected patients with liver or brain metastases, and this regimen is still used at Charing Cross.

The POMB schedule is only moderately myelosuppressive, so the intervals between each course can be kept to a maximum of 14 days (usually 9 to 11 days), thereby minimizing the time for tumor regrowth. When *bleomycin* is given by a 48-hour infusion, pulmonary toxicity is reduced (108). **With a maximum of 9 years of follow-up, the Charing Cross group has seen no long-term side effects in patients treated with POMB-ACE.** Children have developed normally, menstruation has been physiologic, and several women have completed normal pregnancies. There are

Table 12.3 POMB-ACE Chemotherapy for Germ Cell Tumors of the Ovary	
POMB	
Day 1	*Vincristine* 1 mg/m^2 intravenously; *methotrexate* 300 mg/m^2 as a 12-hr infusion
Day 2	*Bleomycin* 15 mg as a 24-hr infusion: Folinic acid rescue started at 24 hr after the start of *methotrexate* in a dose of 15 mg every 12 hr for 4 doses
Day 3	*Bleomycin* infusion 15 mg by 24-hr infusion
Day 4	*Cisplatin* 120 mg/m^2 as a 12-hr infusion, given together with hydration and 3-g magnesium sulfate supplementation
ACE	
Days 1–5	*Etoposide* (VP-16–213) 100 mg/m^2, days 1–5
Day 3, 4, 5	*Actinomycin* D 0.5 mg intravenously, days 3, 4, and 5
Day 5	*Cyclophosphamide* 500 mg/m^2 intravenously, day 5
OMB	
Day 1	*Vincristine* 1 mg/m^2 intravenously; *methotrexate* 300 mg/m^2 as a 12-hr infusion
Day 2	*Bleomycin* 15 mg by 24-hr infusion; folinic acid rescue started at 24 hr after start of *methotrexate* in a dose of 15 mg every 12 hr for 4 doses
Day 3	*Bleomycin* 15 mg by 24-hr infusion

The sequence of treatment schedules is two courses of POMB followed by ACE. POMB is then alternated with ACE until patients are in biochemical remission as measured by human chorionic gonadotropin and α-fetoprotein, and placental alkaline phosphatase and lactate dehydrogenase. The usual number of courses of POMB is three to five. After biochemical remission, patients alternate ACE with OMB until remission has been maintained for approximately 12 weeks. The interval between courses of treatment is kept to the minimum (usually 9 to 11 days). If delays are caused by myelosuppression after courses of ACE, then the first 2 days of *etoposide* are omitted from subsequent courses of ACE.

Reproduced from **Newlands ES, Southall PJ, Paradinas FJ, et al.** Management of ovarian germ cell tumors. In: **Williams CJ, Krikorian JG, Green MR, et al., eds.** *Textbook of uncommon cancer.* New York, NY: John Wiley & Sons; 1988:37–53, with permission.

a number of groups investigating different regimens to treat patients with testicular germ cell tumors who fall into the intermediate or high-risk prognostic subsets, and these regimens include accelerated BEP every 2 weeks.

Second-look Laparotomy   A second-look operation is not required in patients with EST whose AFP values return to normal and remain normal (102,103). There have been reported cases in which the AFP measurement has returned to normal in spite of persistent measurable disease; some of these cases have been mixed germ cell tumors and in patients with residual masses, surgery may be required (103).

Rare Germ Cell Tumors of the Ovary

Embryonal Carcinoma   Embryonal carcinoma of the ovary is an extremely rare tumor that is distinguished from a choriocarcinoma of the ovary by the absence of syncytiotrophoblastic and cytotrophoblastic cells. **The patients are very young,** their ages ranging between 4 and 28 years (median = 14 years) in two series (105). Older patients have been reported (106). **Embryonal carcinomas may secrete estrogens,** with the patient exhibiting symptoms and signs of precocious pseudopuberty or irregular bleeding (1). The presentation is otherwise similar to that of the EST. The primary lesions tend to be large, and approximately two-thirds are confined to one ovary at the time of presentation. **These lesions frequently secrete AFP and hCG,** which are useful for following the response to subsequent therapy (102).

The treatment of embryonal carcinomas is the same as that for ESTs (27,76,107).

Choriocarcinoma of the Ovary

Pure nongestational choriocarcinoma of the ovary is an extremely rare tumor. Histologically, it has the same appearance as gestational choriocarcinoma metastatic to the ovaries (110). **The majority of patients with this cancer are younger than 20 years. The presence of hCG can be useful in monitoring the patient's response to treatment.** In the presence of high hCG levels, **isosexual precocity** has been seen, occurring in approximately 50% of patients whose tumors appear before menarche (111,112).

There are only a few limited reports on the use of chemotherapy for these nongestational choriocarcinomas, but complete responses have been reported to the MAC regimen (*methotrexate, actinomycin D, and cyclophosphamide*) as described for gestational trophoblastic disease (110). These tumors are so rare that no good data are available, but the options also include the BEP or POMB-ACE regimens. The prognosis for ovarian choriocarcinomas has been poor. The majority of patients have metastases to organ parenchyma at the time of initial diagnosis, and they should be managed as high-risk germ cell tumors.

Polyembryoma

Polyembryoma of the ovary is another extremely rare tumor, which is composed of "embryoid bodies." This tumor replicates the structures of early embryonic differentiation (i.e., the three somatic layers: Endoderm, mesoderm, and ectoderm) (1,10). They occur in very young, premenarchal girls with signs of pseudopuberty, and AFP and hCG levels are elevated. **Women with polyembryomas confined to one ovary may be followed with serial tumor markers and diagnostic-imaging techniques to avoid cytotoxic chemotherapy. In patients who require chemotherapy, the BEP regimen is appropriate** (71).

Mixed Germ Cell Tumors

Mixed germ cell malignancies of the ovary contain two or more elements of the tumors described above. In one series (107), **the most common component of a mixed germ cell tumor was dysgerminoma, which occurred in 80%,** followed by EST in 70%, immature teratoma in 53%, choriocarcinoma in 20%, and embryonal carcinoma in 16%. **The most frequent combination was a dysgerminoma and an EST.** The mixed germ cell tumors may secrete either AFP or hCG—or both or neither—depending on the components.

These tumors should be managed with combination chemotherapy, preferably BEP. The serum marker, if positive initially, may become negative during chemotherapy, but this may reflect regression of only a particular component of the mixed lesion. Therefore, **a second-look laparotomy may be indicated if there is residual disease following chemotherapy, particularly if there was an immature teratomatous component in the original tumor.**

The most important prognostic features are the size of the primary tumor and the relative percentage of its most malignant component (107). In stage IA lesions smaller than 10 cm, survival is 100%. Tumors composed of less than one-third EST, choriocarcinoma, or grade 3 immature teratoma also have an excellent prognosis, but it is possibly less favorable when these components comprise the majority of the tumor.

Surveillance for Stage I Ovarian Germ Cell Tumors

Surveillance is a common approach to the management of young men with apparent stage I testicular germ cell tumors. There is a large body of evidence to support this approach, as well as guidelines on what constitutes appropriate surveillance (6,7). **Although as many as 20–30% of patients will relapse, almost all will be cured with salvage chemotherapy with BEP,** and the potential adverse effects of chemotherapy can be avoided in most patients.

Although this is a very common approach in young men, **it has not been widely adopted in females with ovarian germ cell tumors. However, some data are now available to support surveillance in selected patients whose disease is confined to the ovary.** Cushing et al. reported a study of 44 pediatric patients with completely resected ovarian immature teratomas who were followed carefully for recurrence of disease with appropriate diagnostic imaging and serum tumor markers (113). Thirty-one patients (70.5%) had pure ovarian immature teratomas with a tumor grade of 1 ($n = 17$), 2 ($n = 12$), or 3 ($n = 2$). Thirteen patients (29.5%) had an ovarian immature teratoma plus microscopic foci of yolk sac tumor. The 4-year event-free and overall survival for the ovarian immature teratoma group and for the ovarian immature teratoma plus yolk sac tumor group was 97.7% (95% confidence interval, 84.9–99.7%) and 100%, respectively. The only yolk sac tumor relapse occurred in a child with ovarian immature teratoma and yolk sac tumor who was then treated and salvaged with chemotherapy (113).

The Charing Cross Group initially reported a prospective study of 24 patients with stage IA ovarian germ cell tumors who were also enrolled in a surveillance program. The group consisted of nine patients (37.5%) with dysgerminoma, nine (37.5%) with pure immature teratoma, and six (25%) with ESTs (with or without immature teratoma). Treatment consisted of surgical resection without adjuvant chemotherapy, followed by a surveillance program of clinical, serologic, and radiologic review. A second-look operation was performed, and **all but one patient were alive and in remission after a median follow-up of 6.8 years.** The 5-year overall survival was 95%, and the 5-year disease-free survival was 68%. Eight patients required chemotherapy for recurrent disease or a second primary germ cell tumor. This included three patients with a grade II immature teratoma, three patients with a dysgerminoma, and two patients with dysgerminoma who developed a contralateral dysgerminoma 4.5 and 5.2 years after their first tumor. All but one, who died of a pulmonary embolus, was successfully salvaged with chemotherapy (114).

The same group updated its experience and reported on the safety of the ongoing surveillance program of all stage IA female germ cell tumors (24). Thirty-seven patients (median age 26, range 14 to 48 years) with stage I disease were referred to Mount Vernon and Charing Cross Hospitals between 1981 and 2003. Patients underwent surgery and staging followed by intense surveillance, which included regular tumor markers and imaging. The median period of follow-up was 6 years. **Relapse rates for stage IA nondysgerminomatous tumors and dysgerminomas were 8 of 22 (36%) and 2 of 9 (22%), respectively.** In addition, one patient with mature teratoma and glial implants also relapsed. Ten of these 11 patients (91%) were successfully cured with platinum-based chemotherapy. Only one patient died from chemoresistant disease. **All relapses occurred within 13 months of initial surgery.** The overall disease-specific survival of malignant ovarian germ cell tumors was 94%.

More than 50% of patients who underwent fertility-sparing surgery went on to have successful pregnancies. They concluded that surveillance of all stage IA ovarian germ cell tumors was safe and feasible, and that the outcome was comparable with testicular tumors. They questioned the need for potentially toxic adjuvant chemotherapy in all patients with nondysgerminomas who have greater than 90% chance of being salvaged with chemotherapy if they relapse.

This strategy is appealing and is supported by a larger pediatric literature, but there is much less experience in adults. It deserves further study, but this will require international collaboration. **If a surveillance program is to be instigated, it is essential that the protocols used by the Charing Cross group are closely adhered to and that patients understand that the data for adults are limited.**

The surveillance policy is very strict and includes a **CT scan of chest, abdomen, and pelvis** after surgery, if not done preoperatively. At 12 weeks following surgery, a repeat MRI/CT of the abdomen and pelvis or a second-look laparoscopy should be performed if there has been inadequate initial staging. If all of these are negative, MRI/CT imaging should be repeated at 12 months. Patients are reviewed monthly in year one, every 2 months in year two, every 3 months in year three, and so on until year five, after which they are seen every 6 months for another 5 years. **A pelvic ultrasound and chest x-ray should be done on alternate visits. Tumor markers** including AFP, β-hCG, CA125, and LDH measurements should be done every 2 weeks for 6 months, and then monthly for 6 months, every other month in year two, every third month in year three, and so on until year five when they are repeated every 6 months for 5 years (24,114).

Late Effects of Treatment of Malignant Germ Cell Tumors of the Ovary

Although there are substantial data regarding late effects of *cisplatin*-based therapy in men with testicular cancer, much less information is available for women with ovarian germ cell tumors. **The toxicity of BEP chemotherapy** has been well documented in men and includes **significant pulmonary toxicity** in 5% of patients, with fatal lung toxicity in 1%; **acute myeloid leukemia or myelodysplastic syndrome** in 0.2–1% of patients; **neuropathy** in 20–30%; **Raynaud phenomenon** in 20%; **tinnitus** in 24%; and **high-tone hearing loss** in as many as 70% of patients. In addition, late effects occur on **gonadal function,** there is an increased risk of **hypertension and cardiovascular disease,** and some degree of **renal impairment** occurs in 30% of patients (115,116). These side effects underscore the importance of limiting BEP to three cycles for low-risk and to four cycles for high-risk patients, and emphasize the need for these patients to be referred to major referral centers (95,117).

Gonadal Function

An important cause of infertility in patients with ovarian germ cell tumors is unnecessary bilateral salpingo-oophorectomy and hysterectomy. **Although temporary ovarian dysfunction or failure** is common with platinum-based chemotherapy, most women will resume normal ovarian function, and childbearing is usually preserved (11,20,21,35–39). In one representative series of 47 patients treated with combination chemotherapy for germ cell malignancies, 91.5% of patients resumed normal menstrual function, and there were 14 healthy live births and no birth defects (21). **Factors such as older age at initiation of chemotherapy, greater cumulative drug dose, and longer duration of therapy all have adverse effects on future gonadal function** (36,95,117,119,120).

A large study of reproductive and sexual function after platinum-based chemotherapy in ovarian germ cell tumor survivors was recently reported by the GOG, and 132 survivors were included in the study. Surprisingly, only 71 (53.8%) had fertility-sparing surgery; of these, 87.3% were still having regular menstrual periods. Twenty-four survivors had 37 offspring after cancer treatment (80,118).

Secondary Malignancies

An important cause of late morbidity and mortality in patients receiving chemotherapy for germ cell tumors is the development of secondary tumors (95). *Etoposide* **in particular has been implicated in the development of treatment-related leukemias.**

The chance of developing treatment-related leukemia following *etoposide* **is dose related.** The incidence of leukemia is approximately 0.4–0.5% (representing a 30-fold increased likelihood) in patients receiving a cumulative *etoposide* dose of less than 2,000 mg/m^2 (121) compared with as much as 5% (representing a 336-fold increased likelihood) in those receiving more than 2,000 mg/m^2 (122). In a typical three- or four-cycle course of BEP, patients receive a cumulative *etoposide* dose of 1,500 or 2,000 mg/m^2, respectively.

Despite the risk of secondary leukemia, risk–benefit analyses have concluded that *etoposide*-**containing chemotherapy regimens are beneficial in advanced germ cell tumors;** one case of treatment-induced leukemia would be expected for every 20 additionally cured patients who receive BEP as compared with PVB (*cisplatin, vinblastine,* and *bleomycin*). The risk–benefit balance for patients with low-risk disease, or for high-dose *etoposide* in the salvage setting, is less clear (122).

Sex-Cord–Stromal Tumors

Sex-cord–stromal tumors of the ovary account for approximately 5–8% of all ovarian malignancies (1–4,123–128). They are derived from the sex cords and the ovarian stroma or mesenchyme, and are usually composed of various combinations of elements, including the "female" cells (i.e., granulosa and theca cells) and "male" cells (i.e., Sertoli and Leydig cells), as well as morphologically indifferent cells. A classification of this group of tumors is presented in Table 12.4 (9,129).

Granulosa–Stromal-Cell Tumors

Granulosa–stromal-cell tumors include granulosa cell tumors, thecomas, and fibromas. The granulosa cell tumor is a low-grade malignancy. Thecomas and fibromas are benign but rarely may have morphologic features of malignancy and then may be referred to as *fibrosarcomas* (131).

Granulosa cell tumors, which may secrete estrogen, are seen in women of all ages, and are classified as either Adult Granulosa Cell tumors or Juvenile. Five percent of cases are found in prepubertal girls; the others are distributed throughout the reproductive and postmenopausal years (127,128,130,132). They are bilateral in only 2% of patients.

Of the rare prepubertal lesions, 75% are associated with sexual pseudoprecocity because of the estrogen secretion (128). In the reproductive age group, most patients have menstrual irregularities or secondary amenorrhea. In postmenopausal women, abnormal uterine bleeding is frequently the presenting symptom. **Endometrial cancer occurs in association with granulosa cell tumors in at least 5% of cases, and 25–50% are associated with endometrial hyperplasia** (1,125,127,128,130). **Rarely, granulosa cell tumors may produce androgens and cause virilization.**

The other symptoms and signs of granulosa cell tumors are nonspecific and the same as most ovarian malignancies. **Ascites is present in approximately 10% of cases,** and rarely a pleural

Table 12.4 Classification of Sex Cord-Stromal and Steroid Cell Tumors of the Ovary

I. Sex cord-stromal cell tumors
   A. **Granulosa cell tumor group**
      1. Adult-type granulosa cell tumor
      2. Juvenile-type granulosa cell tumor
   B. **Theca–fibroma group**
      1. Thecoma
         a. Typical
         b. Luteinized (partly luteinized theca cell tumor)
         c. Calcified
      2. Fibroma
      3. Cellular fibroma (cellular fibrous tumor of low malignant potential)
      4. Fibrosarcoma
      5. Stromal tumor with minor sex cord elements
      6. Sclerosing stromal tumor
      7. Signet-ring stromal tumor
      8. Unclassified (fibrothecoma)
II. Sertoli-stromal cell tumors
   A. **Sertoli–Leydig cell tumor group (androblastoma)**
      1. Well differentiated
      2. Intermediate differentiation
         Variant with heterologous elements
      3. Poorly differentiated (sarcomatoid)
         Variant with heterologous elements
      4. Retiform
         Variant with heterologous elements
   B. **Sertoli cell tumor**
   C. **Stromal-Leydig cell tumor**
III. Sex cord-stromal cell tumors of mixed or unclassified cell type
   A. **Sex cord tumor with annular tubules**
   B. **Gynandroblastoma (specify components)**
   C. **Sex cord-stromal tumor, unclassified**
IV. Steroid cell tumors
   A. **Stromal luteoma**
      1. Leydig cell tumor group
         a. Hilus cell tumor
         b. Leydig cell tumor, nonhilar type
         c. Leydig cell tumor, not otherwise specified
      2. Steroid cell tumor, not otherwise specified
         a. Well differentiated
         b. Malignant

Modified with permission from the WHO histological classification of tumors of the ovary; **Tavassoli FA, Devilee P, eds.** *Pathology and Genetics of Tumours of the Breast and Female Genital Tract.* Lyon: IARC Press, 2003; **Roth LM.** Recent advances in the pathology and classification of ovarian sex cord-stromal tumors. *Int J Gynecol Pathol.* 2006;25:199–215.

effusion (127,128). Granulosa tumors tend to be hemorrhagic; occasionally they rupture and produce a hemoperitoneum.

Granulosa cell tumors are usually stage I at diagnosis but may recur 5 to 30 years after initial diagnosis (126). The tumors may also spread hematogenously, and metastases can develop in the lungs, liver, and brain years later. Malignant thecomas are extremely rare, and their presentation, management, and outcome are similar to those of the granulosa cell tumors (131,132).

A somatic missense point mutation in the gene encoding the forkhead box protein L2 (*FOXL2*) has been found to be present in all adult-type granulosa cell tumors of the ovary. *FOXL2* 402 CG leads to a gain or change of function and is believed to be a driver mutation for adult granulosa cell tumors. There is an effort to see if it can be targeted (133–135).

Diagnosis

Inhibin is secreted by granulosa cell tumors and is a useful tumor marker for diagnosis and surveillance (136–140). It is a polypeptide hormone secreted primarily by granulosa cells and is an inhibiter of pituitary FSH secretion. **Inhibin decreases to nondetectable levels after menopause.** However, certain ovarian cancers (mucinous epithelial ovarian carcinomas and granulosa cell tumors) produce inhibin, which may predate clinical recurrence (141–143). An elevated serum inhibin level in a premenopausal woman presenting with amenorrhea and infertility is suggestive of a granulosa cell tumor.

In the past, inhibin assays could not distinguish between the two inhibin subunits, inhibin A and B, and total inhibin has been measured. However, there are now specific immunoassays for inhibin A and B. **Inhibin B is the predominant form of inhibin secreted by granulosa cell tumors and has been reported to reflect disease status more accurately than inhibin A. Measurement of serum inhibin B concentrations rather than total inhibin or inhibin A may be better for the follow-up of granulosa cell tumors** (139,144).

Antimüllerian hormone (AMH), also called Müllerian inhibitory substance (MIS), is produced by granulosa cells, and is emerging as a potential marker for these tumors (140). An elevated AMH level appears to have high specificity. The test is commercially available, and its role in the management of granulosa cell tumors is being investigated (145). An elevated estradiol level is not a sensitive marker of this disease (142).

The histologic diagnosis can be facilitated by staining for markers of ovarian granulosa cell tumors (e.g., inhibin, CD99, and AMH) (136,137). Antibodies against inhibin appear to be the most useful, but they are not specific (133). In one report, positive staining for inhibin was present in 94% of granulosa cell tumors and in 10–20% of ovarian endometrioid tumors and metastatic carcinomas to the ovary (140). The latter demonstrated significantly weaker staining. Molecular testing for a mutation in *FOXL2* is now available to help with the diagnosis if it is in doubt (134,135).

Treatment

The treatment of granulosa cell tumors depends on the age of the patient and the extent of disease. **For most patients, surgery alone is sufficient primary therapy,** with radiation and chemotherapy reserved for the treatment of recurrent or metastatic disease (127,128,130,132).

Surgery

Because granulosa cell tumors are bilateral in approximately 2% of patients, a unilateral salpingo-oophorectomy is appropriate therapy for stage IA tumors in children or in women of reproductive age (124). At the time of laparotomy, if a granulosa cell tumor is identified by frozen section, then a limited staging operation is performed, including an assessment of the contralateral ovary (146–149). As with germ cell malignancies, staging is limited to washings, omental biopsy, careful palpation of the peritoneal surfaces and retroperitoneal nodes, and biopsy of any suspicious lesions. If the opposite ovary appears enlarged, it should be biopsied. If there is metastatic disease, an effort should be made to resect all disease because these tumors are typically slow growing and do not respond well to chemotherapy. **In perimenopausal and postmenopausal women for whom ovarian preservation is not important, a hysterectomy and bilateral salpingo-oophorectomy should be performed. In premenopausal patients in whom the uterus is left *in situ*, a dilation and curettage of the uterus should be performed because of the possibility of a coexistent adenocarcinoma of the endometrium** (127).

Radiation

There is no evidence to support the use of adjuvant radiation therapy for granulosa cell tumors, although pelvic radiation may help to palliate isolated pelvic recurrences (127). Radiation can induce clinical responses and occasional long-term remission in patients with persistent or recurrent granulosa cell tumors, particularly if the disease is surgically cytoreduced (143,150,151). In one review of 34 patients treated at one center for more than 40 years, 14 (41.2%) were treated with measurable disease (150). Three (21%) were alive without progression for 10 to 21 years following treatment.

Chemotherapy

There is no evidence that adjuvant chemotherapy in patients with stage I disease will prevent recurrence.

Patients with metastatic granulosa cell tumors have been treated with a variety of different antineoplastic drugs over the years. There has been no one consistently effective regimen, although complete responses have been reported anecdotally in patients treated with the single agents *cyclophosphamide* and *melphalan,* as well as the combinations VAC, PAC (*cisplatin, doxorubicin, cyclophosphamide*), PVB, and BEP (4,124,152–163). More recently, *carboplatin* and *paclitaxel* (143) as well as *bevacizumab* (164) have shown benefit.

The rarity of these tumors has made it impossible to conduct well-designed randomized studies for patients with stages II to IV disease. **In retrospective series, postoperative chemotherapy has been associated with a prolonged progression-free interval in women with stage III or IV disease** (154), but an overall survival benefit has not been shown (155). Despite the absence of data supporting a survival benefit, some experts recommend postoperative chemotherapy for women with completely resected stage II to IV disease, because of the high risk of disease progression and the potential for long-term survival after platinum-based chemotherapy (143,156–159). Acceptable options include **BEP, EP, PAC, and** *carboplatin* **and** *paclitaxel* (143).

For patients with suboptimally cytoreduced disease, combinations of BEP have produced overall response rates of 58–83% (156,160). In one study, 14 of 38 patients (37%) with advanced disease undergoing second-look laparotomy following four courses of BEP had negative findings (156). With a median follow-up of 3 years, 11 of 16 patients (69%) with primary advanced disease and 21of 41 patients (51%) with recurrent disease were progression free. This regimen was associated with severe toxicity and two *bleomycin*-related deaths. *Carboplatin* **and** *etoposide* (161), **PVB** (127,162), and **PAC** (152,163) have also been reported to have relatively high response rates.

There is a need to develop less toxic and equally active regimens for this older group of patients. *Paclitaxel* **is an active agent, and the combination of platinum with a** *taxane* **has been reported to have a response rate of 60%,** which makes it a more attractive alternative (165–167).

Recurrent Disease

The median time to relapse is approximately 4 to 6 years after initial diagnosis (124,126,147,159). There is no standard approach to the management of relapsed disease. A common site of recurrence is the pelvis, although the upper abdomen may also be involved. Further surgery can be effective if the tumor is localized, but diffuse intra-abdominal disease is difficult to treat. Chemotherapy or radiation may be useful in selected patients.

Approximately 30% of these tumors are estrogen receptor-positive and 100% are progesterone receptor-positive on immunostaining (168,169). The use of hormonal agents such as progestins or luteinizing hormone-releasing hormone (LHRH) agonists has been suggested, but there are limited available data (142). LHRH agonists have been reported to have a 50% response rate in 13 patients from small clinical series and case reports (169–171), whereas four of five patients (80%) were reported to respond to a progestational agent (172). Freeman recently reported two patients with recurrent adult granulosa cell tumors who had received multiple treatment modalities, including chemotherapy, and had previously progressed on *leuprolide*. Both patients were treated with *anastrozole*. Inhibin B levels normalized, as did clinical findings. Both were maintained on treatment for 14 and 18 months, respectively (173).

The numbers are too small to draw any conclusions, and it is likely that there has been significant publication bias, with more reports of responses to treatment (174).

Prognosis

The prognosis for granulosa cell tumor of the ovary depends on the surgical stage of disease (126,128,143,175–178). **Most granulosa cell tumors are indolent and are confined to one ovary at diagnosis;** the cure rate for stage I disease is 75–92% (128,149,159,178). However, late recurrences are not uncommon (124,126,128). In one report of 37 women with stage I disease, survival rates at 5, 10, and 20 years were 94%, 82%, and 62%, respectively. The survival rates for stages II to IV at 5 and 10 years were 55% and 34%, respectively (143).

In adult tumors, cellular atypia, mitotic rate, and the absence of Call-Exner bodies are the only significant pathologic predictors of early recurrence (158). Neither an abnormal tumor karyotype nor *p53* overexpression appears to be prognostic (179). The DNA ploidy of the tumors has been correlated with survival. Holland et al. (153) reported DNA aneuploidy in 13 of 37 patients (35%) with primary granulosa cell tumors. **The presence of residual disease was found to be the most important predictor of progression-free survival, but DNA ploidy was an**

independent prognostic factor. Patients with no residual disease and DNA diploid tumors had a 10-year progression-free survival of 96%.

Juvenile Granulosa Cell Tumors

Juvenile granulosa cell tumors of the ovary are rare and make up less than 5% of ovarian tumors in childhood and adolescence (161). Approximately 90% are diagnosed in stage I and have a favorable prognosis. **The juvenile subtype behaves less aggressively than the adult type.** Advanced-stage tumors have been successfully treated with platinum-based combination chemotherapy (e.g., BEP) (143).

Sertoli–Leydig Tumors

Sertoli–Leydig tumors occur most frequently in the third and fourth decades, with 75% of the lesions seen in women younger than 40 years. They account for less than 0.2% of ovarian cancers (1). **Sertoli–Leydig cell tumors are most frequently low-grade malignancies,** although poorly differentiated tumors may behave more aggressively.

The tumors typically produce androgens, and clinical virilization is noted in 70–85% of patients (180,181). **Signs of virilization include oligomenorrhea followed by amenorrhea, breast atrophy, acne, hirsutism, clitoromegaly, a deepening voice, and a receding hairline** (Fig. 12.6). Measurement of plasma androgens may reveal elevated testosterone and androstenedione, with normal or slightly elevated dehydroepiandrosterone sulfate (1). Rarely, the Sertoli–Leydig tumor can be associated with manifestations of estrogenization (i.e., isosexual precocity, irregular or postmenopausal bleeding) (181).

Treatment

Because these low-grade tumors are bilateral in less than 1% of cases, the usual treatment is unilateral salpingo-oophorectomy and evaluation of the contralateral ovary in patients who are in their reproductive years (181). In older patients, hysterectomy and bilateral salpingo-oophorectomy are appropriate.

There are limited data regarding the utility of chemotherapy in patients with persistent disease, but responses in patients with measurable disease have been reported with *cisplatin* in combination

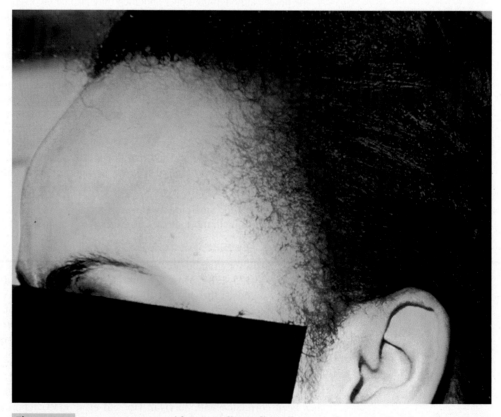

Figure 12.6 A young woman with a Sertoli–Leydig cell tumor demonstrating frontal and temporal baldness.

with *doxorubicin* or *ifosfamide* or both (181) as well as the regimens mentioned above for granulosa cell tumors. Because of their rarity, most series have included them with granulosa cell tumors (157). Pelvic radiation can also be used for recurrent pelvic tumor but with limited responses.

Prognosis

The 5-year survival rate is 70–90%, and recurrences thereafter are uncommon (1,2,181). The majority of fatalities occur with poorly differentiated lesions.

Uncommon Ovarian Cancers

There are several varieties of malignant ovarian tumors, which together constitute only 0.1% of ovarian malignancies. These lesions include lipoid (or lipid) cell tumors, primary ovarian sarcomas, and small cell ovarian carcinomas.

Lipoid Cell Tumors

Lipoid cell tumors are thought to arise in adrenal cortical rests that reside in the vicinity of the ovary. More than 100 cases have been reported, and bilaterality has been noted in only a few (1). **Most are associated with virilization and occasionally with obesity, hypertension, and glucose intolerance,** reflecting glucocorticoid secretion. Rare cases of estrogen secretion and isosexual precocity have been reported.

The majority of these have a benign or low-grade behavior, but approximately 20% develop metastatic lesions in the peritoneal cavity, or rarely at distant sites. The primary treatment is surgical, and there are no data regarding radiation or chemotherapy for this disease.

Sarcomas

Malignant mixed mesodermal sarcomas of the ovary are usually heterologous, and 80% occur in postmenopausal women (182–188). The lesions are biologically aggressive, and their presentation is similar to that of most epithelial ovarian malignancies.

Such patients should be treated by cytoreductive surgery and postoperative platinum-containing combination chemotherapy (187,188). Silasi et al. (189) reported their experience with 22 patients from Yale, all but two of whom presented with advanced-stage disease. The median survival for the entire cohort was 38 months. The median survival was 46 months for 18 optimally debulked (<1 cm) patients and 27 months for four suboptimally debulked (>1 cm) patients. **After optimal cytoreduction, six patients were treated with *cisplatin* and *ifosfamide*; they had a median progression-free interval of 13 months and a median survival of 51 months.** The combination of *carboplatin* and *paclitaxel* was administered to four patients following optimal cytoreduction; their median progression-free interval was 6 months, and median survival was 38 months. The difference in survival between the *cisplatin* and *ifosfamide* group and the *carboplatin* and *paclitaxel* group was not statistically significant ($p = 0.48$). **First-line *cisplatin* and *ifosfamide* or *carboplatin* and *paclitaxel* can achieve survival rates comparable to those observed in epithelial ovarian cancer.**

Leiser et al. (190) reported the **Memorial Sloan-Kettering experience with *platinum* and *paclitaxel*** in 30 patients with carcinosarcomas of the ovary. Twelve patients (40%) had a complete response, seven (23%) a partial response, two (7%) stable disease, and nine (30%) progression of disease. The median time to progression for responders was 12 months; with a median follow-up of 23 months, the median overall survival was 43 months for survivors. **The 3- and 5-year survival rates were 53% and 30%, respectively.**

Small Cell Carcinomas

This rare tumor occurs at an average age of 24 years (range 2 to 46 years) (191). The tumors are all bilateral. **Approximately two-thirds of the tumors are accompanied by paraneoplastic hypercalcemia.** This tumor accounts for one-half of all of the cases of hypercalcemia associated with ovarian tumors. Approximately 50% of the tumors have spread beyond the ovaries at the time of diagnosis (1,2).

Management consists of surgery followed by platinum-based chemotherapy. Radiation therapy may be considered in selected patients. In addition to the primary treatment of the disease, **control of the hypercalcemia may require aggressive hydration, loop diuretics, and the use of bisphosphonates.**

In a collaborative Gynecologic Cancer Intergroup study, data were collected for 17 patients treated in Australia, Canada, and Europe (192). The median follow-up was 13 months for all patients and 35.5 months for surviving patients. Ten patients (58.8%) had FIGO stage I tumors, six (35.3%) stage III, and in one patient, stage was unknown. All underwent surgical resection and adjuvant platinum-based chemotherapy. Seven received adjuvant pelvic, whole-abdominal or extended-field radiation. The median survival for stage I tumors was not reached, whereas it was 6 months for stage III tumors. **For the ten patients with stage I tumors, six also received adjuvant radiotherapy, with five alive and disease-free;** four received no adjuvant radiotherapy, with one alive and disease-free. **Of the seven patients with stage III or unknown tumor stage, all but one have died.** The only long-term survivor was treated with platinum-based chemotherapy (BEP) followed by para-aortic and pelvic radiotherapy. Recurrences were most frequent in the pelvis and the abdomen. **Patients receiving salvage treatment with chemotherapy and radiotherapy did poorly.**

Although the optimal approach to management is not known, in view of these findings, the authors **advocate a multimodality treatment approach, including surgical resection of gross disease, chemotherapy with** *carboplatin* **and** *paclitaxel* **or** *cisplatin* **and** *etoposide,* **and the addition of various fields of pelvic radiotherapy either sequentially or concurrently.** Others have advocated high-dose chemotherapy with stem cell support and have reported a number of long-term survivors (193,194).

Metastatic Tumors

Approximately 5–6% of ovarian tumors are metastatic from other organs, most frequently from the female genital tract, the breast, or the gastrointestinal tract (195–212). The metastases may occur from direct extension of another pelvic neoplasm, by hematogenous spread, by lymphatic spread, or from transcoelomic dissemination, with surface implantation of tumors that spread in the peritoneal cavity.

Gynecologic Primary

Nonovarian cancers of the genital tract can spread by direct extension or metastasize to the ovaries (1). Under some circumstances, it is difficult to know whether the tumor originates in the fallopian tube or in the ovary when both are involved, especially because many serous carcinomas that were thought to be primary ovarian malignancies are now believed to actually arise in the fallopian tube (213) (see Chapter 11). Cervical cancer spreads to the ovary only in rare cases (<1%), and most of these are at an advanced clinical stage or are adenocarcinomas. **Although adenocarcinoma of the endometrium can spread and implant directly onto the surface of the ovaries in as many as 5% of cases, two synchronous primary tumors probably occur with greater frequency.** In these cases, an endometrioid carcinoma of the ovary is usually associated with the adenocarcinoma of the endometrium (214).

Nongynecologic Primary

The frequency of metastatic breast carcinoma to the ovaries varies according to the method of determination, but is relatively common, particularly in patients with estrogen receptor positive metastatic breast cancer. In autopsy data of women who die of metastatic breast cancer, the ovaries are involved in 24% of cases, and 80% of the involvement is bilateral (195–201). Similarly, when ovaries are removed as treatment for metastatic breast cancer in premenopausal women, approximately 20–30% of patients have evidence of ovarian metastases, 60% bilaterally. The involvement of ovaries in early-stage breast cancer is considerably lower, but precise figures are not available. In almost all cases, ovarian involvement is occult but in some patients, a pelvic mass is discovered after other metastatic disease becomes apparent.

Krukenberg Tumor

Krukenberg tumors account for 30–40% of metastatic cancers to the ovaries, and are characterized by mucin-filled, signet-ring cells in the ovarian stroma (205,206). **The primary tumor is most frequently the stomach** (Fig. 12.7) but less common primaries include the colon, breast, or biliary tract. Rarely, the cervix or the bladder may be the primary site. Krukenberg tumors can account for approximately 2% of ovarian cancers, and they are usually bilateral. The tumors are usually not discovered until the primary disease is advanced, and therefore most patients die of their disease within a year. **In some cases, a primary tumor is never found.**

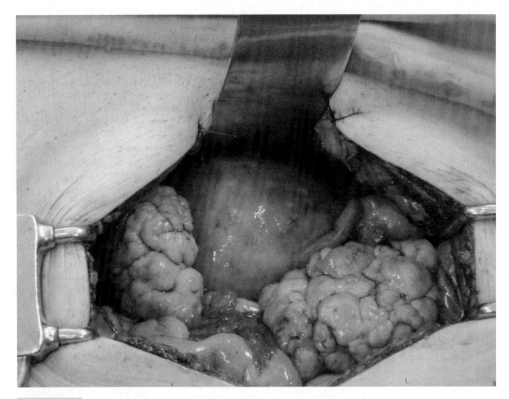

Figure 12.7 Bilateral Krukenberg tumors from a primary stomach cancer.

Other Gastrointestinal Tumors

In other cases of metastasis from the gastrointestinal tract to the ovary, the tumor does not have the classic histologic appearance of a Krukenberg tumor; most of these are from the colon and, less commonly, the small intestine. One to two percent of women with intestinal carcinomas will develop metastases to the ovaries during the course of their disease (197,202–204,207,208). **Before exploration for an adnexal tumor in a woman more than 40 years of age, a colonoscopy or gastroscopy should be performed to exclude a primary gastrointestinal carcinoma with metastases to the ovaries if there are any gastrointestinal symptoms.**

Metastatic colon cancer can mimic a mucinous cystadenocarcinoma of the ovary histologically, and the histologic distinction between the two can be difficult (207–211). Tumors that arise in the appendix may also be associated with ovarian metastasis and have frequently been confused with primary ovarian malignancies, especially when associated with pseudomyxoma peritonei (207,211) (see Chapters 5 and 11). When the ovaries are involved with metastasis, a bilateral salpingo-oophorectomy should be performed at the time of surgery for colon cancer (202,212).

Melanoma

Rare cases of malignant melanoma metastatic to the ovaries have been reported (215), and **must be distinguished from the rare case of a melanoma arising in an ovarian teratoma** (216). In cases of metastatic disease, the melanomas are usually widely disseminated. Removal would be warranted for palliation of abdominal or pelvic pain, bleeding, or torsion.

Carcinoid

Metastatic carcinoid tumors represent fewer than 2% of metastatic lesions to the ovaries (217). Conversely, only some 2% of primary carcinoids have evidence of ovarian metastasis, and **only 40% of these patients have the carcinoid syndrome at the time of discovery of the metastatic carcinoid** (218). In perimenopausal and postmenopausal women explored for an intestinal carcinoid, it is reasonable to remove the ovaries to prevent subsequent ovarian metastasis. Furthermore, the discovery of an ovarian carcinoid should prompt a careful search for a primary intestinal lesion.

Lymphoma and Leukemia

Lymphomas and leukemia can involve the ovary. When they do, the involvement is usually bilateral (219–222). Approximately 5% of patients with Hodgkin disease will have lymphomatous involvement of the ovaries, but this occurs typically with advanced-stage disease. **With Burkitt lymphoma, ovarian involvement is very common.** Other types of lymphoma involve the ovaries much less frequently, and leukemic infiltration of the ovaries is uncommon.

Sometimes the ovaries can be the only apparent sites of involvement of the abdominal or pelvic viscera with a lymphoma—in this circumstance, a careful surgical exploration may be necessary. An intraoperative consultation with a hematologist–oncologist should be obtained to determine the need for such procedures if frozen section of a solid ovarian mass reveals a lymphoma. **In general, most lymphomas no longer require extensive surgical staging,** although enlarged lymph nodes should generally be biopsied. In some cases of Hodgkin disease, a more extensive evaluation may be necessary. Treatment involves that of the lymphoma or leukemia in general. **Removal of a large ovarian mass may improve patient comfort and facilitate a response to subsequent radiation or chemotherapy** (221).

References

1. **Scully RE, Young RH, Clement RB.** Tumors of the ovary, maldeveloped gonads, fallopian tube, and broad ligament. In: *Atlas of Tumor Pathology:* 3rd series, Fascicle 23. Washington, DC: Armed Forces Institute of Pathology; 1998:169–498.

2. **Chen LM, Berek JS.** Ovarian and fallopian tubes. In: **Haskell CM, ed.** *Cancer Treatment.* 5th ed. Philadelphia, PA: WB Saunders; 2000: 900–932.

3. **Imai A, Furui T, Tamaya T.** Gynecologic tumors and symptoms in childhood and adolescence: 10-years' experience. *Int J Gynaecol Obstet.* 1994;45:227–234.

4. **Gershenson DM.** Management of early ovarian cancer: Germ cell and sex-cord stromal tumors. *Gynecol Oncol.* 1994;55:S62–S72.

5. **Gershenson DM.** Update on malignant ovarian germ cell tumors. *Cancer.* 1993;71:1581–1590.

6. **Krege S, Beyer J, Souchon R, et al.** European consensus conference on diagnosis and treatment of germ cell cancer: A report of the second meeting of the European Germ Cell Cancer Consensus group (EGCCCG): Part I. *Eur Urol.* 2008;53:478–496.

7. **Krege S, Beyer J, Souchon R, et al.** European consensus conference on diagnosis and treatment of germ cell cancer: A report of the second meeting of the European Germ Cell Cancer Consensus Group (EGCCCG): Part II. *Eur Urol.* 2008 Mar;53:497–513.

8. **Murugaesu N, Schmid P, Dancey G, et al.** Malignant ovarian germ cell tumors: Identification of novel prognostic markers and long-term outcome after multimodality treatment. *J Clin Oncol.* 2006;24: 4862–4866.

9. **Tavassoli FA, Devilee P, eds.** *Pathology and Genetics of Tumours of the Breast and Female Genital Tract.* Lyon: IARC Press, 2003.

10. **Kurman RJ, Scardino PT, McIntire KR, et al.** Malignant germ cell tumors of the ovary and testis: An immunohistologic study of 69 cases. *Ann Clin Lab Sci.* 1979;9:462–466.

11. **Obata NH, Nakashima N, Kawai M, et al.** Gonadoblastoma with dysgerminoma in one ovary and gonadoblastoma with dysgerminoma and yolk sac tumor in the contralateral ovary in a girl with 46XX karyotype. *Gynecol Oncol.* 1995;58:124–128.

12. **Spanos WJ.** Preoperative hormonal therapy of cystic adnexal masses. *Am J Obstet Gynecol.* 1973;116:551–556.

13. **Bremer GL, Land JA, Tiebosch A, et al.** Five different histologic subtypes of germ cell malignancies in an XY female. *Gynecol Oncol.* 1993;50:247–248.

14. **Mayordomo JI, Paz-Ares L, Rivera F, et al.** Ovarian and extragonadal malignant germ-cell tumors in females: A single-institution experience with 43 patients. *Ann Oncol.* 1994;5:225–231.

15. **Rabban JT, Zaloudek CJ.** A practical approach to immunohistochemical diagnosis of ovarian germ cell tumours and sex cord-stromal tumours. *Histopathology.* 2013;62:71–88.

16. **Piura B, Dgani R, Zalel Y, et al.** Malignant germ cell tumors of the ovary: A study of 20 cases. *J Surg Oncol* 1995;59:155–161.

17. **Solheim O, Kaern J, Trope CG, et al.** Malignant ovarian germ cell tumors: Presentation, survival and second cancer in a population based Norwegian cohort (1953–2009). *Gynecol Oncol.* 2013;131(2): 330–335.

18. **Lu KH, Gershenson DM.** Update on the management of ovarian germ cell tumors. *J Reprod Med.* 2005;50:417–425.

19. **Gordon A, Lipton D, Woodruff JD.** Dysgerminoma: A review of 158 cases from the Emil Novak Ovarian Tumor Registry. *Obstet Gynecol.* 1981;58:497–504.

20. **Thomas GM, Dembo AJ, Hacker NF, et al.** Current therapy for dysgerminoma of the ovary. *Obstet Gynecol* 1987;70:268–275.

21. **Low JJ, Perrin LC, Crandon AJ, et al.** Conservative surgery to preserve ovarian function in patients with malignant ovarian germ cell tumors: A review of 74 cases. *Cancer.* 2000;89:391–398.

22. **Williams SD, Birch R, Einhorn LH, et al.** Treatment of disseminated germ cell tumors with cisplatin, bleomycin and either vinblastine or etoposide. *N Engl J Med.* 1987;316:1435–1440.

23. **Mangili G, Sigismondi C, Lorusso D, et al.** Is surgical restaging indicated in apparent stage IA pure ovarian dysgerminoma? The MITO group retrospective experience. *Gynecol Oncol.* 2011;121: 280–284.

24. **Patterson DM, Murugaesu N, Holden L, et al.** A review of the close surveillance policy for stage I female germ cell tumors of the ovary and other sites. *Int J Gynecol Cancer.* 2008;18(1):43–50. PMID:17466047.

25. **Williams SD, Blessing JA, Hatch K, et al.** Chemotherapy of advanced ovarian dysgerminoma: Trials of the Gynecologic Oncology Group. *J Clin Oncol.* 1991;9:1950–1955.

26. **Williams SD, Blessing JA, Moore DH, et al.** Cisplatin, vinblastine, and bleomycin in advanced and recurrent ovarian germ-cell tumors. *Ann Intern Med.* 1989;111:22–27.

27. **Williams SD, Blessing JA, Liao S, et al.** Adjuvant therapy of ovarian germ cell tumors with cisplatin, etoposide, and bleomycin: A trial of the Gynecologic Oncology Group. *J Clin Oncol.* 1994;12:701–706.

28. **Gershenson DM, Morris M, Cangir A, et al.** Treatment of malignant germ cell tumors of the ovary with bleomycin, etoposide, and cisplatin. *J Clin Oncol.* 1990;8:715–720.

29. **Bekaii-Saab T, Einhorn LH, Williams SD.** Late relapse of ovarian dysgerminoma: Case report and literature review. *Gynecol Oncol.* 1999;72:111–112.

30. **Kurtz JE, Jaeck D, Maloisel F, et al.** Combined modality treatment for malignant transformation of a benign ovarian teratoma. *Gynecol Oncol.* 1999;73:319–321.

31. **Williams SD.** Ovarian germ cell tumors: An update. *Semin Oncol.* 1998;25:407–413.

32. **Pawinski A, Favalli G, Ploch E, et al.** PVB chemotherapy in patients with recurrent or advanced dysgerminoma: A phase II study of the EORTC Gynaecological Cancer Cooperative Group. *Clin Oncol (R Coll Radiol).* 1998;10:301–305.

33. **Rogers PC, Olson TA, Cullen JW, et al.** Treatment of children and adolescents with stage II testicular and stages I and II ovarian

malignant germ cell tumors: A Pediatric Intergroup Study–Pediatric Oncology Group 9048 and Children's Cancer Group 8891. *J Clin Oncol.* 2004; 22:3563–3569.

34. **Brewer M, Gershenson DM, Herzog CE, et al.** Outcome and reproductive function after chemotherapy for ovarian dysgerminoma. *J Clin Oncol.* 1999;17:2670–2675.

35. **Gershenson DM.** Menstrual and reproductive function after treatment with combination chemotherapy for malignant ovarian germ cell tumors. *J Clin Oncol.* 1988;6:270–275.

36. **Kanazawa K, Suzuki T, Sakumoto K.** Treatment of malignant ovarian germ cell tumors with preservation of fertility: Reproductive performance after persistent remission. *Am J Clin Oncol.* 2000;23: 244–248.

37. **El-Lamie IK, Shehata NA, Abou-Loz SK, et al.** Conservative surgical management of malignant ovarian germ cell tumors: The experience of the Gynecologic Oncology Unit at Ain Shams University. *Eur J Gynaecol Oncol.* 2000;21:605–609.

38. **Tangir J, Zelterman D, Ma W, et al.** Reproductive function after conservative surgery and chemotherapy for malignant germ cell tumors of the ovary. *Obstet Gynecol.* 2003;101:251–257.

39. **Loehrer PJ, Johnson D, Elson P, et al.** Importance of bleomycin in favorable-prognosis disseminated germ cell tumors: An Eastern Cooperative Oncology Group trial. *J Clin Oncol.* 1995;13:470–476.

40. **Bajorin DF, Sarosdy MF, Pfister GD, et al.** Randomized trial of etoposide and cisplatin versus etoposide and carboplatin in patients with good-risk germ cell tumors: A multi-institutional study. *J Clin Oncol.* 1993;11:598–606.

41. **Schwartz PE, Chambers SK, Chambers JT, et al.** Ovarian germ cell malignancies: The Yale University experience. *Gynecol Oncol.* 1992;45:26–31.

42. **Williams SD, Blessing JA, DiSaia PJ, et al.** Second-look laparotomy in ovarian germ cell tumors. *Gynecol Oncol.* 1994;52:287–291.

43. **Culine S, Lhomme C, Michel G, et al.** Is there a role for second-look laparotomy in the management of malignant germ cell tumors of the ovary? Experience at Institute Gustave Roussy. *J Surg Oncol.* 1996;62:40–45.

44. **De Santis M, Bokemeyer C, Becherer A, et al.** Predictive impact of 2–18fluoro-2-deoxy-D-glucose positron emission tomography for residual postchemotherapy masses in patients with bulky seminoma. *J Clin Oncol.* 2001;19:3740–3744.

45. **Siekiera J, Małkowski B, Jóźwicki W, et al.** Can we rely on PET in the follow-up of advanced seminoma patients? *Urol Int.* 2012;88(4): 405–409

46. **Motzer RJ, Sheinfeld J, Mazumdar M, et al.** Paclitaxel, ifosfamide, and cisplatin second-line therapy for patients with relapsed testicular germ cell cancer. *J Clin Oncol.* 2000;18:2413–2418.

47. **Pico JL, Rosti G, Kramar A, et al.** A randomised trial of high-dose chemotherapy in the salvage treatment of patients failing first-line platinum chemotherapy for advanced germ cell tumours. *Ann Oncol.* 2005;16:1152–1159.

48. **Feldman D, Huddart R, Hall E, et al.** Is high dose therapy superior to conventional dose therapy as initial treatment for relapsed germ cell tumors? The TIGER trial. *J Cancer.* 2011;2:374–377.

49. **Han JY, Nava-Ocampo AA, Kim TJ, et al.** Pregnancy outcome after prenatal exposure to bleomycin, etoposide and cisplatin for malignant ovarian germ cell tumors: Report of 2 cases. *Reprod Toxicol.* 2005;19(4):557–561.

50. **Elit L, Bocking A, Kenyon C, et al.** An endodermal sinus tumor diagnosed in pregnancy: Case report and review of the literature. *Gynecol Oncol.* 1999;72:123–127

51. **Kumar S, Shah JP, Bryant CS, et al.** The prevalence and prognostic impact of lymph node metastasis in malignant germ cell tumors of the ovary. *Gynecol Oncol.* 2008;110:125–132.

52. **Mahdi H, Swensen RE, Hanna R, et al.** Prognostic impact of lymphadenectomy in clinically early stage malignant germ cell tumour of the ovary. *Br J Cancer.* 2011;105(4):493–497.

53. **O'Conner DM, Norris HJ.** The influence of grade on the outcome of stage I ovarian immature (malignant) teratomas and the reproducibility of grading. *Int J Gynecol Pathol.* 1994;13:283–289.

54. **Norris HJ, Zirkin HJ, Benson WL.** Immature (malignant) teratoma of the ovary: A clinical and pathologic study of 58 cases. *Cancer.* 1976;37:2359–2372.

55. **Ulbright TM.** Germ cell tumors of the gonads: A selective review emphasizing problems in differential diagnosis, newly appreciated,

and controversial issues. A review. *Mod Pathol.* 2005;18(suppl 2): S61–S79.

56. **Heifetz SA, Cushing B, Giller R, et al.** Immature teratomas in children: Pathologic considerations: A report from the combined Pediatric Oncology Group/Children's Cancer Group. *Am J Surg Pathol.* 1998;22:1115–1124.

57. **Marina NM, Cushing B, Giller R, et al.** Complete surgical excision is effective treatment for children with immature teratomas with or without malignant elements: A Pediatric Oncology Group/Children's Cancer Group Intergroup Study. *J Clin Oncol.* 1999;17:2137–2143.

58. **Ferguson AW, Katabuchi H, Ronnett BM, et al.** Glial implants in gliomatosis peritonei arise from normal tissue, not from the associated teratoma. *Am J Pathol.* 2001;159:51–55.

59. **Best DH, Butz GM, Moller K, et al.** Molecular analysis of an immature ovarian teratoma with gliomatosis peritonei and recurrence suggests genetic independence of multiple tumors. *Int J Oncol.* 2004;25:17–25.

60. **Dimopoulos MA, Papadopoulou M, Andreopoulou E, et al.** Favorable outcome of ovarian germ cell malignancies treated with cisplatin or carboplatin-based chemotherapy: A Hellenic Cooperative Oncology Group study. *Gynecol Oncol.* 1998;70:70–74.

61. **Bafna UD, Umadevi K, Kumaran C, et al.** Germ cell tumors of the ovary: Is there a role for aggressive cytoreductive surgery for non-dysgerminomatous tumors? *Int J Gynecol Cancer.* 2001;11:300–304.

62. **De Palo G, Zambetli M, Pilotti S, et al.** Non-dysgerminomatous tumors of the ovary treated with cisplatin, vinblastine, and bleomycin: Long-term results. *Gynecol Oncol.* 1992;47:239–246.

63. **Culine S, Kattan J, Lhomme C, et al.** A phase II study of high-dose cisplatin, vinblastine, bleomycin, and etoposide (PVeBV regimen) in malignant non-dysgerminomatous germ-cell tumors of the ovary. *Gynecol Oncol.* 1994;54:47–53.

64. **Mann JR, Raafat F, Robinson K, et al.** The United Kingdom Children's Cancer Study Group's second germ cell tumor study: Carboplatin, etoposide, and bleomycin are effective treatment for children with malignant extracranial germ cell tumors, with acceptable toxicity. *J Clin Oncol.* 2000;18:3809–3818.

65. **Cushing B, Giller R, Cullen JW, et al.** Randomized comparison of combination chemotherapy with etoposide, bleomycin, and either high-dose or standard-dose cisplatin in children and adolescents with high-risk malignant germ cell tumors: A pediatric intergroup study–Pediatric Oncology Group 9049 and Children's Cancer Group 8882. *J Clin Oncol.* 2004;22:2691–2700.

66. **Lopes LF, Macedo CR, Pontes EM, et al.** Cisplatin and etoposide in childhood germ cell tumor: Brazilian pediatric oncology society protocol GCT-91. *J Clin Oncol.* 2009;27:1297–1303.

67. **Mangili G, Scarfone G, Gadducci A, et al.** Is adjuvant chemotherapy indicated in stage I pure immature ovarian teratoma (IT)? A multicentre Italian trial in ovarian cancer (MITO-9). *Gynecol Oncol.* 2010;119:48–52.

68. **Segelov E, Campbell J, Ng M, et al.** Cisplatin-based chemotherapy for ovarian germ cell malignancies: The Australian experience. *J Clin Oncol.* 1994;12:378–384.

69. **Bonazzi C, Peccatori F, Colombo N, et al.** Pure ovarian immature teratoma, a unique and curable disease: 10 years' experience of 32 prospectively treated patients. *Obstet Gynecol.* 1994;84:598–604.

70. **Cangir A, Smith J, van Eys J.** Improved prognosis in children with ovarian cancers following modified VAC (vincristine sulfate, dactinomycin, and cyclophosphamide) chemotherapy. *Cancer.* 1978;42: 1234–1238.

71. **Chapman DC, Grover R, Schwartz PE.** Conservative management of an ovarian polyembryoma. *Obstet Gynecol.* 1994;83:879–882.

72. **Slayton RE, Park RC, Silverberg SC, et al.** Vincristine, dactinomycin, and cyclophosphamide in the treatment of malignant germ cell tumors of the ovary: A Gynecologic Oncology Group study (a final report). *Cancer.* 1985;56:243–248.

73. **Creasman WJ, Soper JT.** Assessment of the contemporary management of germ cell malignancies of the ovary. *Am J Obstet Gynecol.* 1985;153:828–834.

74. **Taylor MH, DePetrillo AD, Turner AR.** Vinblastine, bleomycin, and cisplatin in malignant germ cell tumors of the ovary. *Cancer.* 1985;56:1341–1349.

75. **Culine S, Lhomme C, Kattan J, et al.** Cisplatin-based chemotherapy in the management of germ cell tumors of the ovary: The Institute Gustave Roussy experience. *Gynecol Oncol.* 1997;64:160–165.

76. **Williams SD, Wong LC, Ngan HYS.** Management of ovarian germ cell tumors. In: Gershenson DM, McGuire WP, eds. *Ovarian Cancer.* New York, NY: Churchill-Livingstone; 1998:399–415.

77. **Bokemeyer C, Köhrmann O, Tischler J, et al.** Schmoll HJA randomized trial of cisplatin, etoposide, and bleomycin (PEB) versus carboplatin, etoposide, and bleomycin (CEB) for patients with "good-risk" metastatic non-seminomatous germ cell tumors. *Ann Oncol.* 1996;7:1015–1021.

78. **Horwich A, Sleijfer DT, Fosså SD, et al.** Randomized trial of bleomycin, etoposide, and cisplatin compared with bleomycin, etoposide, and carboplatin in good-prognosis metastatic nonseminomatous germ cell cancer: A Multiinstitutional Medical Research Council/ European Organization for Research and Treatment of Cancer Trial. *J Clin Oncol.* 1997;15:1844–1852.

79. **de Wit R, Roberts JT, Wilkinson PM, et al.** Equivalence of three or four cycles of bleomycin, etoposide, and cisplatin chemotherapy and of a 3- or 5-day schedule in good-prognosis germ cell cancer: A randomized study of the European Organization for Research and Treatment of Cancer Genitourinary Tract Cancer Cooperative Group and the Medical Research Council. *J. Clin Oncol.* 2001;19(6):1629–1640. PMID:11250991.

80. **Abdul Razak AR, Li L, Bryant A, et al.** Chemotherapy for malignant germ cell ovarian cancer in adult patients with early stage, advanced and recurrent disease. *Cochrane Database Syst Rev.* 2011;(3):CD007584. doi:10.1002/14651858.CD007584.pub2.

81. **Fizazi K, Pagliaro LC, Flechon A, et al.** A phase III trial of personalized chemotherapy based on serum tumor marker decline in poor-prognosis germ cell tumors: Results of GETUG 13. 2013 ASCO Annual Meeting. Abstract LBA4500.

82. **Pectasides D, Pectasides M, Farmakis D, et al.** Gemcitabine and oxaliplatin (GEMOX) in patients with cisplatin-refractory germ cell tumors: A phase II study. *Ann Oncol.* 2004;15(3):493–497. PMID: 14998855.

83. **Einhorn LH, Brames MJ, Juliar B, et al.** Phase II study of paclitaxel plus gemcitabine salvage chemotherapy for germ cell tumors after progression following high-dose chemotherapy with tandem transplant. *J Clin Oncol.* 2007;25(5):513–516. PMID:17290059.

84. **Theodore C, Chevreau C, Yataqhene Y, et al.** A phase II multi-center study of oxaliplatin in combination with paclitaxel in poor prognosis patients who failed cisplatin-based chemotherapy for germ-cell tumors. *Ann Oncol.* 2008;9(8):1465–1469. PMID:18385203.

85. **Shiraishi T, Nakamura T, Mikami K, et al.** Salvage chemotherapy with paclitaxel and gemcitabine plus nedaplatin (TGN) as part of multidisciplinary therapy in patients with heavily pretreated cisplatin-refractory germ cell tumors. *Int J Clin Oncol.* 2009;14(5):436–441. PMID:19856053.

86. **Li J, Yang W, Wu X.** Prognostic factors and role of salvage surgery in chemorefractory ovarian germ cell malignancies: A study in Chinese patients. *Gynecol Oncol.* 2007;105:769–775.

87. **Rezk Y, Sheinfeld J, Chi DS.** Prolonged survival following salvage surgery for chemorefractory ovarian immature teratoma: A case report and review of the literature. *Gynecol Oncol.* 2005;96:883.

88. **Einhorn LH, Williams SD, Chamness A, et al.** High-dose chemotherapy and stem-cell rescue for metastatic germ-cell tumors. *N Engl J Med.* 2007;357(4):340–348. PMID:17652649.

89. **Voigt W, Kegel T, Maher G, et al.** Bevacizumab plus high-dose ifosfamide, etoposide and carboplatin (HD-ICE) as third-line salvage chemotherapy induced an unexpected dramatic response in highly platinum refractory germ-cell cancer. *Ann. Oncol.* 2006; 17(3):531–533. PMID:16234294.

90. **Hariprasad R, Kumar L, Janga D, et al.** Growing teratoma syndrome of ovary. *Int J Clin Oncol.* 2008;13:83–87.

91. **Tangjitgamol S, Manusirivithaya S, Leelahakorn S, et al.** The growing teratoma syndrome: A case report and a review of the literature. *Int J Gynecol Cancer.* 2006;16(suppl 1):384–390.

92. **Mego M, Reckova M, Sycova-Mila Z, et al.** Bevacizumab in a growing teratoma syndrome. Case report. *Ann. Oncol.* 2007;18(5):962–963. PMID:17434900.

93. **Carver BS, Shayegan B, Serio A, et al.** Long-term clinical outcome after postchemotherapy retroperitoneal lymph node dissection in men with residual teratoma. *J Clin Oncol.* 2007;25:1033–1037.

94. **Mathew GK, Singh SS, Swaminathan RG, et al.** Laparotomy for post chemotherapy residue in ovarian germ cell tumors. *J Postgrad Med.* 2006;52:262–265.

95. **Billmire D, Vinocur C, Rescorla F, et al.** Outcome and staging evaluation in malignant germ cell tumors of the ovary in children and adolescents: An intergroup study. *J Pediatr Surg.* 2004;39(3):424–429. PMID:15017564.

96. **Lai CH, Chang TC, Hsueh S, et al.** Outcome and prognostic factors in ovarian germ cell malignancies. *Gynecol Oncol.* 2005;96:784–791.

97. **Talerman A.** Germ cell tumors of the ovary. *Curr Opin Obstet Gynecol.* 1997;9:44–47.

98. **Kleiman GM, Young RH, Scully RE.** Primary neuroectodermal tumors of the ovary: A report of 25 cases. *Am J Surg Pathol.* 1993; 17:764–778.

99. **Sasaki H, Furusata M, Teshima S, et al.** Prognostic significance of histopathological subtypes in stage I pure yolk sac tumour of the ovary. *Br J Cancer.* 1994;69:529–536.

100. **Fujita M, Inoue M, Tanizawa O, et al.** Retrospective review of 41 patients with endodermal sinus tumor of the ovary. *Int J Gynecol Cancer.* 1993;3:329–335.

101. **de La Motte Rouge T, Pautier P, et al.** Prognostic factors in women treated for ovarian yolk sac tumour: A retrospective analysis of 84 cases. *Eur. J. Cancer.* 2011. PMID:20851596.

102. **Kawai M, Kano T, Kikkawa F, et al.** Seven tumor markers in benign and malignant germ cell tumors of the ovary. *Gynecol Oncol.* 1992;45:248–253.

103. **Abu-Rustum NR, Aghajanian C.** Management of malignant germ cell tumors of the ovary. *Semin Oncol.* 1998;25:235–242.

104. **Newlands ES, Southall PJ, Paradinas FJ, et al.** Management of ovarian germ cell tumours. In: **Williams CJ, Krikorian JG, Green MR, et al., eds.** *Textbook of Uncommon Cancer.* New York, NY: John Wiley & Sons; 1988:37–53.

105. **Ueda G, Abe Y, Yoshida M, et al.** Embryonal carcinoma of the ovary: A six-year survival. *Gynecol Oncol.* 1990;31:287–292.

106. **Kammerer-Doak D, Baurick K, Black W, et al.** Endodermal sinus tumor and embryonal carcinoma of the ovary in a 53-year-old woman. *Gynecol Oncol.* 1996;63:133–137.

107. **Tay SK, Tan LK.** Experience of a 2-day BEP regimen in postsurgical adjuvant chemotherapy of ovarian germ cell tumors. *Int J Gynecol Cancer.* 2000;10:13–18.

108. **Haugnes HS, Aass N, Fosså SD, et al.** Pulmonary function in long-term survivors of testicular cancer. *J Clin Oncol.* 2009;27:2779–2786.

109. **Talukdar S, Kumar S, Bhatla N, et al.** Neo-adjuvant chemotherapy in the treatment of advanced malignant germ cell tumors of ovary. *Gynecol Oncol.* 2014;132(1):28–32. pii: S0090–8258(13)01254–7.

110. **Simosek T, Trak B, Thnoc M, et al.** Primary pure choriocarcinoma of the ovary in reproductive ages: A case report. *Eur J Gynaecol Oncol.* 1998;19:284–286.

111. **Oliva E, Andrada E, Pezzica E, et al.** Ovarian carcinomas with choriocarcinomatous differentiation. *Cancer.* 1993;72:2441–2446.

112. **Kong B, Tian YJ, Zhu WW, et al.** A pure nongestational ovarian choriocarcinoma in a 10-year-old girl: Case report and literature review. *J Obstet Gynaecol Res.* 2009;35(3):574–578. PMID: 19527404.

113. **Cushing B, Giller R, Ablin A, et al.** Surgical resection alone is effective treatment for ovarian immature teratoma in children and adolescents: A report of the Pediatric Oncology Group and the Children's Cancer Group. *Am J Obstet Gynecol.* 1999;181:353–358.

114. **Dark GG, Bower M, Newlands ES, et al.** Surveillance policy for stage I ovarian germ cell tumors. *J Clin Oncol.* 1997;15:620–624.

115. **Efstathiou E, Logothetis CJ.** Review of late complications of treatment and late relapse in testicular cancer. *J Natl Compr Canc Netw.* 2006;4:1059–1070.

116. **Chaudhary UB, Haldas JR.** Long-term complications of chemotherapy for germ cell tumours. *Drugs.* 2003;63:1565–1577.

117. **Matei D, Miller AM, Monahan P, et al.** Chronic physical effects and health care utilization in long-term ovarian germ cell tumor survivors: A Gynecologic Oncology Group study. *J Clin Oncol.* 2009; 27:4142–4149.

118. **Gershenson DM, Miller AM, Champion VL, et al.** Reproductive and sexual function after platinum-based chemotherapy in long-term ovarian germ cell tumor survivors: A Gynecologic Oncology Group Study. *J Clin Oncol.* 2007;25:2792–2797.

119. **Zhang R, Sun YC, Zhang GY, et al.** Treatment of malignant germ cell tumors and preservation of fertility. *Eur J Gynaecol Oncol.* 2012; 33:489–492.

120. **Monahan PO, Champion VL, Zhao Q, et al.** Case-control comparison of quality of life in long-term ovarian germ cell tumor survivors: A gynecologic oncology group study. *J Psychosoc Oncol.* 2008; 26(3):19–42. PMID:19042263.

121. **Schneider DT, Hilgenfeld E, Schwabe D, et al.** Acute myelogenous leukemia after treatment for malignant germ cell tumors in children. *J Clin Oncol.* 1999;17:3226–3233.

122. **Kollmannsberger C, Beyer J, Droz JP, et al.** Secondary leukemia following high cumulative doses of etoposide in patients treated for advanced germ cell tumors. *J Clin Oncol.* 1998;16:3386–3391.

123. **Young RE, Scully RE.** Ovarian sex cord-stromal tumors: Problems in differential diagnosis. *Ann Pathol.* 1988;23:237–296.

124. **Miller BE, Barron BA, Wan JY, et al.** Prognostic factors in adult granulosa cell tumor of the ovary. *Cancer.* 1997;79:1951–1955.

125. **Boyce EA, Costaggini I, Vitonis A, et al.** The epidemiology of ovarian granulosa cell tumors: A case-control study. *Gynecol Oncol.* 2009;115:221–225.

126. **Malmström H, Högberg T, Risberg B, et al.** Granulosa cell tumors of the ovary: Prognostic factors and outcome. *Gynecol Oncol.* 1994; 52:50–55.

127. **Segal R, DePetrillo AD, Thomas G.** Clinical review of adult granulosa cell tumors of the ovary. *Gynecol Oncol.* 1995;56:338–344.

128. **Cronje HS, Niemand I, Barn, RH, et al.** Review of the granulosa–theca cell tumors from the Emil Novak ovarian tumor registry. *Am J Obstet Gynecol.* 1999;180:323–328.

129. **Roth LM.** Recent advances in the pathology and classification of ovarian sex cord-stromal tumors. *Internat J Gynecol Pathol.* 2006: 25:199–215.

130. **Aboud E.** A review of granulosa cell tumours and thecomas of the ovary. *Arch Gynecol Obstet.* 1997;259:161–165.

131. **Chechia A, Attia L, Temime RB, et al.** Incidence, clinical analysis, and management of ovarian fibromas and fibrothecomas. *Am J Obstet Gynecol.* 2008;199:473.e1–e4.

132. **Young R, Clement PB, Scully RE.** The ovary. In: Sternberg SS, ed. *Diagnostic Surgical Pathology.* New York, NY: Raven Press, 1989: 1687.

133. **Zhao C, Vinh TN, McManus K, et al.** Identification of the most sensitive and robust immunohistochemical markers in different categories of ovarian sex cord-stromal tumors. *Am J Surg Pathol.* 2009; 33:354–366.

134. **Shah SP, Köbel M, Senz J, et al.** Mutation of FOXL2 in granulosa-cell tumors of the ovary. *N Engl J Med.* 2009;360:2719–2729.

135. **Köbel M, Gilks CB, Huntsman DG.** Adult-type granulosa cell tumors and FOXL2 mutation. *Cancer Res.* 2009;69:9160–9162.

136. **Lappohn RE, Burger HG, Bouma J, et al.** Inhibin as a marker for granulosa-cell tumors. *N Engl J Med.* 1989;321:790–793.

137. **Hildebrandt RH, Rouse RV, Longacre TA.** Value of inhibin in the identification of granulosa cell tumors of the ovary. *Hum Pathol.* 1997;28:1387–1395.

138. **Richi M, Howard LN, Bratthauae GL, et al.** Use of monoclonal antibody against human inhibin as a marker for sex-cord-stromal tumors of the ovary. *Am J Surg Pathol.* 1997;21:583–589.

139. **Mom CH, Engelen MJ, Willemse PH, et al.** Granulosa cell tumors of the ovary: The clinical value of serum inhibin A and B levels in a large single center cohort. *Gynecol Oncol.* 2007;105: 365–372.

140. **Matias-Guiu X, Pons C, Prat J.** Müllerian inhibiting substance, alpha-inhibin, and CD99 expression in sex cord-stromal tumors and endometrioid ovarian carcinomas resembling sex cord-stromal tumors. *Hum Pathol.* 1998;29:840–845.

141. **McCluggage WG.** Recent advances in immunohistochemistry in the diagnosis of ovarian neoplasms. *J Clin Pathol.* 2000;53:327–334.

142. **Rey RA, Lhomme C, Marcillac I, et al.** Antimüllerian hormone as a serum marker of granulosa cell tumors of the ovary: Comparative study with serum alpha-inhibin and estradiol. *Am J Obstet Gynecol.* 1996;174:958–965.

143. **Schumer ST, Cannistra SA.** Granulosa cell tumor of the ovary. *J Clin Oncol.* 2003;21:1180–1189.

144. **Chang HL, Pahlavan N, Halpern EF, et al.** Serum Müllerian Inhibiting Substance/anti-Müllerian hormone levels in patients with adult granulosa cell tumors directly correlate with aggregate tumor mass as determined by pathology or radiology. *Gynecol Oncol.* 2009;114: 57–60.

145. **Geerts I, Vergote I, Neven P, et al.** The role of inhibins B and anti-müllerian hormone for diagnosis and follow-up of granulosa cell tumors. *Int J Gynecol Cancer.* 2009;19(5):847–855.

146. **Kommoss S, Gilks CB, Penzel R, et al.** A current perspective on the pathological assessment of FOXL2 in adult-type granulosa cell tumours of the ovary. *Histopathology.* 2014;64(3):380–388.

147. **Brown J, Sood AK, Deavers MT, et al.** Patterns of metastasis in sex cord-stromal tumors of the ovary: Can routine staging lymphadenectomy be omitted? *Gynecol Oncol.* 2009;113:86–90.

148. **Abu-Rustum NR, Restivo A, Ivy J, et al.** Retroperitoneal nodal metastasis in primary and recurrent granulosa cell tumors of the ovary. *Gynecol Oncol.* 2006;103:31–34.

149. **National Comprehensive Cancer Network (NCCN) guidelines.** Available at: www.nccn.org (Accessed on May 15, 2013).

150. **Wolf JK, Mullen J, Eifel PJ, et al.** Radiation treatment of advanced or recurrent granulosa cell tumor of the ovary. *Gynecol Oncol.* 1999;73:35–41.

151. **Savage P, Constenla D, Fisher C, et al.** Granulosa cell tumours of the ovary: Demographics, survival and the management of advanced disease. *Clin Oncol (R Coll Radiol).* 1998;10:242–245.

152. **Gershenson DM, Copeland IA, Kavanagh JJ, et al.** Treatment of metastatic stromal tumors of the ovary with cisplatin, doxorubicin, and cyclophosphamide. *Obstet Gynecol.* 1987;5:765–769.

153. **Holland DR, Le Riche J, Swenerton KD, et al.** Flow cytometric assessment of DNA ploidy is a useful prognostic factor for patients with granulosa cell ovarian tumors. *Int J Gynecol Cancer.* 1991;1: 227–232.

154. **Uygun K, Aydiner A, Saip P, et al.** Clinical parameters and treatment results in recurrent granulosa cell tumor of the ovary. *Gynecol Oncol.* 2003;88:400–403.

155. **Al-Badawi IA, Brasher PM, Ghatage P, et al.** Postoperative chemotherapy in advanced ovarian granulosa cell tumors. *Int J Gynecol Cancer.* 2002;12:119–123.

156. **Homesley HD, Bundy BN, Hurteau JA, et al.** Bleomycin, etoposide, and cisplatin combination therapy of ovarian granulosa cell tumors and other stromal malignancies: A Gynecologic Oncology Group study. *Gynecol Oncol.* 1999;72:131–137.

157. **Colombo N, Sessa C, Landoni F, et al.** Cisplatin, vinblastine, and bleomycin combination chemotherapy in metastatic granulosa cell tumor of the ovary. *Obstet Gynecol.* 1986;67:265–268.

158. **Zambetti M, Escobedo A, Pilotti S, et al.** Cis-platinum/vinblastine/bleomycin combination chemotherapy in advanced or recurrent granulosa cell tumors of the ovary. *Gynecol Oncol.* 1990;36:317–320.

159. **Lauszus FF, Petersen, AC, Greisen J, et al.** Granulosa cell tumor of the ovary: A population-based study of 37 women with stage I disease. *Gynecol Oncol.* 2001;81:456–460.

160. **Gershenson DM, Morris M, Burke TW, et al.** Treatment of poor-prognosis sex cord-stromal tumors of the ovary with the combination of bleomycin, etoposide, and cisplatin. *Obstet Gynecol.* 1996;87: 527–531.

161. **Powell JL, Otis CN.** Management of advanced juvenile granulosa cell tumor of the ovary. *Gynecol Oncol.* 1997;64:282–284.

162. **Pecorelli S, Wagenaar HC, Vergote IB, et al.** Cisplatin (P), vinblastine (V), and bleomycin (B) combination chemotherapy in recurrent or advanced granulosa(-theca) cell tumours of the ovary. An EORTC Gynaecological Cancer Cooperative Group study. *Eur J Cancer.* 1999;35:1331–1337.

163. **Muntz HG, Goff AF, Fuller AF Jr.** Recurrent ovarian granulosa cell tumor: Role of combination chemotherapy with report of a long-term response to a cyclophosphamide, doxorubicin, and cisplatin regimen. *Eur J Gynaecol Oncol.* 1990;11:263–268.

164. **Tao X, Sood AK, Deavers MT, et al.** Anti-angiogenesis therapy with bevacizumab for patients with ovarian granulosa cell tumors. *Gynecol Oncol.* 2009;114(3):431–436.

165. **Tresukosol D, Kudelka AP, Edwards CL, et al.** Recurrent ovarian granulosa cell tumor: A case report of a dramatic response to *Taxol.* *Int J Gynecol Cancer.* 1995;5:156–159.

166. **Brown J, Shvartsman HS, Deavers MT, et al.** The activity of taxanes in the treatment of sex cord-stromal ovarian tumors. *J Clin Oncol.* 2004; 22:3517.

167. **Brown J, Shvartsman HS, Deavers MT, et al.** The activity of taxanes compared with bleomycin, etoposide, and cisplatin in the treatment of sex cord-stromal ovarian tumors. *Gynecol Oncol.* 2005; 97:489–496.

168. **Hardy RD, Bell JG, Nicely CJ, et al.** Hormonal treatment of a recurrent granulosa cell tumor of the ovary: Case report and review of the literature. *Gynecol Oncol.* 2005;96:865–869.

169. **Emons G, Schally AV.** The use of luteinizing hormone releasing hormone agonists and antagonists in gynaecological cancers. *Hum Reprod.* 1994;9:1364–1379.

170. **Martikainen H, Penttinen J, Huhtaniemi I, et al.** Gonadotropin-releasing hormone agonist analog therapy effective in ovarian granulosa cell malignancy. *Gynecol Oncol.* 1989;35:406–408.

171. **Fishman A, Kudelka AP, Tresukosol D, et al.** Leuprolide acetate for treating refractory or persistent ovarian granulosa cell tumor. *J Reprod Med.* 1996;41:393–396.

172. **Briasoulis E, Karavasilis V, Pavlidis N.** Megestrol activity in recurrent adult type granulosa cell tumour of the ovary. *Ann Oncol.* 1997; 8:811–812.

173. **Freeman SA, Modesitt SC.** Anastrozole therapy in recurrent ovarian adult granulosa cell tumors: A report of 2 cases. *Gynecol Oncol.* 2006;103:755–758.

174. **Sommeijer DW, Sjoquist KM, Friedlander M.** Hormonal treatment in recurrent and metastatic gynaecological cancers: A review of the current literature. *Curr Oncol Rep.* 2013;15(6):541–548.

175. **Lee YK, Park NH, Kim JW, et al.** Characteristics of recurrence in adult-type granulosa cell tumor. *Int J Gynecol Cancer.* 2008;18: 642–647.

176. **Zhang M, Cheung MK, Shin JY, et al.** Prognostic factors responsible for survival in sex cord stromal tumors of the ovary–an analysis of 376 women. *Gynecol Oncol.* 2007;104:396–400.

177. **Chan JK, Zhang M, Kaleb V, et al.** Prognostic factors responsible for survival in sex cord stromal tumors of the ovary–a multivariate analysis. *Gynecol Oncol.* 2005;96:204.

178. **Auranen A, Sundström J, Ijäs J, et al.** Prognostic factors of ovarian granulosa cell tumor: A study of 35 patients and review of the literature. *Int J Gynecol Cancer.* 2007;17:1011–1018.

179. **Ala-Fossi SL, Maenpaa J, Aine R, et al.** Prognostic significance of *p53* expression in ovarian granulosa cell tumors. *Gynecol Oncol.* 1997;66:475–479.

180. **Roth LM, Anderson MC, Govan AD, et al.** Sertoli-Leydig cell tumors: A clinicopathologic study of 34 cases. *Cancer.* 1981;48: 187–197.

181. **Tomlinson MW, Treadwell MC, Deppe G.** Platinum based chemotherapy to treat recurrent Sertoli-Leydig cell ovarian carcinoma during pregnancy. *Eur J Gynaecol Oncol.* 1997;18:44–46.

182. **Le T, Krepart GV, Lotocki RJ, et al.** Malignant mixed mesodermal ovarian tumor treatment and prognosis: A 20-year experience. *Gynecol Oncol.* 1997;65:237–240.

183. **Piura B, Rabinovich A, Yanai-Inbar I, et al.** Primary sarcoma of the ovary: Report of five cases and review of the literature. *Eur J Gynaecol Oncol.* 1998;19:257–261.

184. **Topuz E, Eralp Y, Aydiner A, et al.** The role of chemotherapy in malignant mixed müllerian tumors of the female genital tract. *Eur J Gynaecol Oncol.* 2001;22:469–472.

185. **van Rijswijk RE, Tognon G, Burger CW, et al.** The effect of chemotherapy on the different components of advanced carcinosarcomas (malignant mixed mesodermal tumors) of the female genital tract. *Int J Gynecol Cancer.* 1994;4:52–60.

186. **Berek JS, Hacker NF.** Sarcomas of the female genital tract. In: **Eilber FR, Morton DL, Sondak VK, et al., eds.** *The soft tissue sarcomas.* Orlando, FL: Grune & Stratton; 1987:229–238.

187. **Barakat RR, Rubin SC, Wong G, et al.** Mixed mesodermal tumor of the ovary: Analysis of prognostic factors in 31 cases. *Obstet Gynecol.* 1992;80:660–664.

188. **Fowler JM, Nathan L, Nieberg RK, et al.** Mixed mesodermal sarcoma of the ovary in a young patient. *Eur J Obstet Gynecol Reprod Biol.* 1996;65:249–253.

189. **Silasi DA, Illuzzi JL, Kelly MG, et al.** Carcinosarcoma of the ovary. *Int J Gynecol Cancer.* 2008;18:22–29.

190. **Leiser AL, Chi DS, Ishill NM, et al.** Carcinosarcoma of the ovary treated with platinum and taxane: The Memorial Sloan-Kettering Cancer Center experience. *Gynecol Oncol.* 2007;105:657–661.

191. **Young RH, Oliva E, Scully RE.** Small cell sarcoma of the ovary, hypercalcemic type: A clinicopathological analysis of 150 cases. *Am J Surg Pathol.* 1994;18:1102–1116.

192. **Harrison ML, Hoskins P, du Bois A, et al.** Small cell of the ovary, hypercalcemic type—analysis of combined experience and recommendation for management. A GCIG study. *Gynecol Oncol.* 2006; 100:233–238.

193. **Pautier P, Ribrag V, Duvillard P, et al.** Results of a prospective dose-intensive regimen in 27 patients with small cell carcinoma of the ovary of the hypercalcemic type. *Ann Oncol.* 2007;18:1985–1989.

194. **Nelsen LL, Muirhead DM, Bell MC.** Ovarian small cell carcinoma, hypercalcemic type exhibiting a response to high-dose chemotherapy. *S D Med.* 2010;63(11):375–377.

195. **Petru E, Pickel H, Heydarfadai M, et al.** Non-genital cancers metastatic to the ovary. *Gynecol Oncol.* 1992;44:83–86.

196. **Demopoulos RI, Touger L, Dubin N.** Secondary ovarian carcinoma: A clinical and pathological evaluation. *Int J Gynecol Pathol.* 1987;6:166–175.

197. **Young RH, Scully RE.** Metastatic tumors in the ovary: A problem-oriented approach and review of the recent literature. *Semin Diagn Pathol.* 1991;8:250–276.

198. **Moore RG, Chung M, Granai CO, et al.** Incidence of metastasis to the ovaries from nongenital tract tumors. *Gynecol Oncol.* 2004;93: 87–91.

199. **Ayhan A, Tuncer ZS, Bukulmez O.** Malignant tumors metastatic to the ovaries. *J Surg Oncol.* 1995;60:268–276.

200. **Curtin JP, Barakat RR, Hoskins WJ.** Ovarian disease in women with breast cancer. *Obstet Gynecol.* 1994;84:449–452.

201. **Yada-Hashimoto N, Yamamoto T, Kamiura S, et al.** Metastatic ovarian tumors: A review of 64 cases. *Gynecol Oncol.* 2003;89: 314–317.

202. **Ayhan A, Guvenal T, Salman MC, et al.** The role of cytoreductive surgery in nongenital cancers metastatic to the ovaries. *Gynecol Oncol.* 2005;98:235–241. [PubMed]

203. **Khunamornpong S, Suprasert P, Chiangmai WN, et al.** Metastatic tumors to the ovaries: A study of 170 cases in northern Thailand. *Int J Gynecol Cancer.* 2006;16(Suppl 1):132–138. [PubMed]

204. **Antila R, Jalkanen J, Heikinheimo O.** Comparison of secondary and primary ovarian malignancies reveals differences in their pre- and perioperative characteristics. *Gynecol Oncol.* 2006;101:97–101. [PubMed]

205. **Kim HK, Heo DS, Bang YJ, et al.** Prognostic factors of Krukenberg's tumor. *Gynecol Oncol.* 2001;82:105–109.

206. **Yakushiji M, Tazaki T, Nishimura H, et al.** Krukenberg tumors of the ovary: A clinicopathologic analysis of 112 cases. *Nihon Sanka Fujinka Gakkai Zasshi.* 1987;39:479–485.

207. **Misdraji J, Yantiss RK, Graeme-Cook FM, et al.** Appendiceal mucinous neoplasms: A clinicopathologic analysis of 107 cases. *Am J Surg Pathol.* 2003;27:1089–1103.

208. **Chou YY, Jeng YM, Kao HL, et al.** Differentiation of ovarian mucinous carcinoma and metastatic colorectal adenocarcinoma by immunostaining with beta-catenin. *Histopathology.* 2003;43:151–156.

209. **Seidman JD, Kurman RJ, Ronnett BM.** Primary and metastatic mucinous adenocarcinomas in the ovaries: Incidence in routine practice with a new approach to improve intraoperative diagnosis. *Am J Surg Pathol.* 2003;27:985–993.

210. **Lee KR, Young RH.** The distinction between primary and metastatic mucinous carcinomas of the ovary: Gross and histologic findings in 50 cases. *Am J Surg Pathol.* 2003;27:281–292.

211. **McBroom JW, Parker MF, Krivak TC, et al.** Primary appendiceal malignancy mimicking advanced stage ovarian carcinoma: A case series. *Gynecol Oncol.* 2000;78:388–390.

212. **Schofield A, Pitt J, Biring G, et al.** Oophorectomy in primary colorectal cancer. *Ann R Coll Surg Engl.* 2001;83:81–84.

213. **Levanon K, Crum C, Drapkin R.** New insights into the pathogenesis of serous ovarian cancer and its clinical impact. *J Clin Oncol.* 2008;26:5284–5293.

214. **Ayhan A, Guvenal T, Coskun F, et al.** Survival and prognostic factors in patients with synchronous ovarian and endometrial cancers and endometrial cancers metastatic to the ovaries. *Eur J Gynaecol Oncol.* 2003;24:171–174.

215. **Young RH, Scully RE.** Malignant melanoma metastatic to the ovary: A clinicopathologic analysis of 20 cases. *Am J Surg Pathol.* 1991;15:849–860.

216. **Davis GL.** Malignant melanoma arising in mature ovarian cystic teratoma (dermoid cyst): Report of two cases and literature analysis. *Int J Gynecol Pathol.* 1996;15:356–362.

217. **Motoyama T, Katayama Y, Watanabe H, et al.** Functioning ovarian carcinoids induce severe constipation. *Cancer.* 1991;70:513–518.

218. **Robbins ML, Sunshine TJ.** Metastatic carcinoid diagnosed at laparoscopic excision of pelvic endometriosis. *J Am Assoc Gynecol Laparosc.* 2000;7:251–253.

219. **Fox H, Langley FA, Govan AD, et al.** Malignant lymphoma presenting as an ovarian tumour: A clinicopathological analysis of 34 cases. *BJOG.* 1988;95:386–390.

220. **Monterroso V, Jaffe ES, Merino MJ, et al.** Malignant lymphomas involving the ovary: A clinicopathologic analysis of 39 cases. *Am J Surg Pathol.* 1993;17:154–170.

221. **Azizoglu C, Altinok G, Uner A, et al.** Ovarian lymphomas: A clinicopathological analysis of 10 cases. *Arch Gynecol Obstet.* 2001;265: 91–93.

222. **Sakurai N, Tateoka K, Taguchi J, et al.** Primary precursor B-cell lymphoblastic lymphoma of the ovary: Case report and review of the literature. *Int J Gynecol Pathol.* 2008;27:412–417. [PubMed]

13 Vulvar Cancer

Neville F. Hacker
Patricia J. Eifel

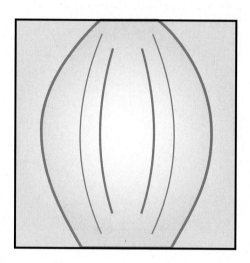

Vulvar cancer represents about 5% of malignancies of the female genital tract and 0.6% of female cancers. There were estimated to be 4,850 new cases of vulvar cancer diagnosed in the United States in 2014 and 1,030 deaths (1). Squamous cell carcinomas account for 85–90% of cases, whereas basal cell carcinomas, melanomas, invasive Paget's disease, Bartholin gland carcinomas, and sarcomas are much less common.

Vulvar cancer is predominantly a disease of older women. In spite of the vulva being an external organ, delayed diagnosis has been typical of this disease.

There has been a significant increase in the incidence of vulvar intraepithelial neoplasia (VIN) in recent decades (2–5), and this has been attributed to changing sexual behavior, human papillomavirus (HPV) infection, and cigarette smoking (6). Judson et al. (2) reviewed 13,176 *in situ* and invasive vulvar carcinomas from the **Surveillance Epidemiology and End Results program (SEER) database** over a 28-year period (1973 to 2000); 57% of the cases were *in situ.* **There was a 411% increase in the incidence of *in situ* carcinoma from 1973 to 2000, while the incidence of invasive carcinoma increased 20% during the same period.** The incidence of *in situ* disease increased until the age of 40 to 49 years, and then decreased, whereas the invasive cancer risk increased with age, and increased more rapidly after age 50. Similar trends have been reported from Denmark, although the increased incidence of invasive vulvar cancer was limited there to women under the age of 60 years (5).

Hampl et al. (3) from Dusseldorf reported that the fraction of vulvar cancers diagnosed in women under the age of 50 years increased from 11% in the 1980s to 41% in the 10 years up to 2007 in their single institution study. Population based SEER data from the United States have shown no comparable increase in incidence. From 1980 to 1989, 15% of 2,271 invasive vulvar cancers occurred in women under the age of 50 years, compared to 18.8% of 5,227 vulvar cancers from 2000 to 2005 (7).

Approximately 40% of vulvar cancers are HPV positive, and about 85% of HPV-positive invasive vulvar cancers are attributable to HPV-16 (8). Prophylactic HPV vaccines have the potential to decrease the incidence of invasive vulvar cancer by about one-third overall (8), and to be even more effective in younger women.

In the early part of the 20th century, patients commonly presented with advanced disease, and surgical techniques were poorly developed; thus, the 5-year survival rate for vulvar cancer was 20–25% (9,10). Basset (11), in France, was the first to suggest an *en bloc* dissection

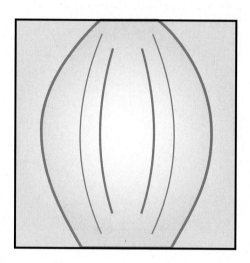

560

of the vulva, groin, and iliac lymph nodes, although he performed the operation only on cadavers. **Taussig (12), in the United States, and Way (13), in Great Britain, pioneered the radical *en bloc* dissection for vulvar cancer, and reported 5-year survival rates of 60–70%.** Postoperative morbidity was high after these procedures, with wound breakdown, infection, and prolonged hospitalization the norm. For patients with disease involving the anus, rectum, or proximal urethra, pelvic exenteration was often combined with radical vulvectomy.

Since approximately 1980, there has been a paradigm shift in the approach to vulvar cancer (14,15). The most significant advances have included the following:

1. **Individualization of treatment** for all patients with invasive disease (16,17).
2. **Vulvar conservation** for patients with unifocal tumors and an otherwise normal vulva (16–20).
3. **Omission of the groin dissection for patients with T_1 tumors and no more than 1 mm of stromal invasion** (16,17).
4. **Elimination of routine pelvic lymphadenectomy** (21–25).
5. **The use of separate groin incisions** for the groin dissection to improve wound healing (26).
6. **Omission of the contralateral groin dissection** in patients with lateral T_1 lesions and negative ipsilateral nodes (16,17,23).
7. **The use of preoperative radiation therapy or definitive radiation therapy** to obviate the need for exenteration in selected patients with advanced disease (27–30).
8. **The use of postoperative radiation to decrease the incidence of groin recurrence and improve survival of patients with multiple positive groin nodes** (25).
9. **Resection of bulky positive groin and pelvic nodes** without complete node dissection to decrease the risk of lymphedema prior to pelvic and groin radiation (31).
10. **The use of sentinel node biopsy** to obviate the need for complete groin dissection in carefully selected patients with early vulvar cancer (32).

This paradigm shift in the management philosophy of vulvar cancer has been well exemplified in retrospective reviews of the experience at the University of Miami (33) and the Mayo Clinic (34). Both centers reported a trend toward a more conservative approach, and both reported decreased postoperative morbidity, without compromised survival.

Etiology of Invasive Squamous Cell Carcinoma

VIN has traditionally been considered to be a premalignant condition, and to be one disease, but **in 2004, the International Society for the Study of Vulvovaginal Disease officially divided VIN into two types: (i) usual type VIN, which is related to HPV infection, and (ii) differentiated VIN, which is unrelated to HPV infection** (Table 13.1) (35). **The term VIN 1 is no longer used, and VIN 2 and VIN 3 are simply called VIN.**

The older classification of VIN 1, 2, and 3 was based on the degree of histologic abnormality, but there is no evidence that the VIN 1 to 3 morphologic spectrum reflects a biologic continuum, or that VIN 1 is a cancer precursor (35).

Table 13.1 Squamous Vulvar Intraepithelial Neoplasia (VIN). 2004 ISSVD Terminology

VIN, usual type
a. **VIN, warty type**
b. **VIN, basaloid type**
c. **VIN, mixed (warty/basaloid) type**
VIN, differentiated type

ISSVD, International Society for the Study of Vulvar Disease.

Reproduced with permission from ISSVD Vulvar Oncology Sub-committee. *J Reprod Med.* 2005;50: 807–810.

It is now generally accepted that there are two different etiologic types of vulvar cancer (36,37). **One type is seen mainly in younger patients, is related to HPV infection and smoking, and is commonly associated with basaloid or warty VIN (36–38). The more common type is seen mainly in elderly patients, is unrelated to smoking or HPV infection, and concurrent VIN is uncommon. There is, however, a high incidence of dystrophic lesions, including lichen sclerosus and squamous hyperplasia, adjacent to the tumor (39–41). If VIN is present, it is of the differentiated type** (42–44).

Using data on 2,685 patients with invasive vulvar cancer from the National Cancer Institute's Surveillance Epidemiology and End Results program (SEER), Sturgeon et al. (45) reported **the increased risk of a subsequent cancer to be 1.3-fold. Most of the second cancers were related to smoking** (i.e., cancers of the lung, buccal cavity, pharynx, nasal cavity, or larynx) **or to infection with human papillomavirus** (e.g., cervix, vagina, or anus).

In a study designed to investigate the malignant potential of the vulvar premalignant conditions, Eva et al. (44) identified 580 women from Birmingham, England, who had vulvar biopsies showing VIN, lichen sclerosus, or squamous hyperplasia over a 5-year period. These women were studied for the presence of a synchronous or metachronous vulvar cancer. The authors reported that **differentiated VIN had a higher risk of malignancy (85.7%) than usual VIN (25.8%), lichen sclerosus (27.7%) or squamous hyperplasia (31.7%).**

Dutch workers retrieved all patients with a primary diagnosis of VIN from the Nationwide Netherlands Database between 1992 and 2005 (43). They reported that the incidence of both usual and differentiated VIN increased during the study period, while the incidence of vulvar squamous cell carcinoma remained stable. In this prospective study, they found the malignant potential of these premalignant conditions to be much lower—5.7% for usual VIN, 32% for differentiated VIN, and 2–6% for lichen sclerosus (43). However, **Jones et al. (46) reported a series of 405 cases of VIN 2–3 seen between 1962 and 2003 in Auckland, New Zealand. Progression to malignant disease occurred between 1.1 and 7.3 years (mean 3.9 years) in 10 of 16 untreated patients (62.5%), but in only 17 treated women (3.8%).**

Patients with lichen sclerosus and concomitant hyperplasia may be at particular risk for malignant transformation. Rodke et al. (47) reported the development of vulvar carcinoma in 3 of 18 such cases (17%), postulating that the areas of hyperplasia were superimposed on a background of lichen sclerosus because of chronic irritation and trauma.

Carli et al. (48) from the Vulvar Clinic at the University of Florence, Italy, reported an association with lichen sclerosus in 32% of their cases of vulvar cancer that were not HPV related. They felt that the existence of accessory conditions necessary to promote the progression from lichen sclerosus to cancer remained to be established. **Scurry believes lichen sclerosus contributes to a vicious cycle of itching and scratching, which leads to superimposed lichen simplex chronicus, squamous cell hyperplasia, and ultimately carcinoma (40).**

The management of VIN is discussed in Chapter 7.

Paget's Disease of the Vulva

The original description of Paget's disease was of a breast lesion (Sir James Paget, 1874), in which the appearance of the nipple heralded an underlying carcinoma. **Extramammary Paget's Disease is a rare neoplasm of the skin, which is estimated to account for 1–6% of all cases of Paget's disease. It** predominantly affects women over 60 years of age (49) and **the vulva accounts for up to 60% of cases** (50).

Paget's disease of the vulva has been the subject of two recent classifications, and that proposed by **Wilkinson and Brown** (51) in 2002 is shown in Table 13.2. In this classification, **Type 1 Paget's disease is of primary cutaneous origin,** and is divided into Type 1a, primary intraepithelial neoplasia; Type 1b, intraepithelial neoplasia with underlying invasion; and Type 1c, a manifestation of an underlying adenocarcinoma of a skin appendage or of vulvar glandular origin. **Type 2 Paget's disease is of noncutaneous origin, such as the rectum, bladder, or upper genital tract.**

In the Kurman classification, Type 2 Paget's disease is a manifestation of an associated primary cancer or a rectal adenocarcinoma, and Type 3 is a manifestation of a urothelial neoplasm (52).

Table 13.2 Classification of Paget's Disease of the Vulva
1. *Primary Paget's disease of the vulva:*
a. **Intraepithelial Paget's disease**
b. **Intraepithelial Paget's disease with stromal invasion**
c. **As a manifestation of an underlying adenocarcinoma of a skin appendage or subcutaneous vulvar gland**
2. *Secondary Paget's disease of the vulva:*
a. **Secondary to an anorectal adenocarcinoma**
b. **Secondary to an urothelial carcinoma**
c. **As a manifestation of another noncutaneous adenocarcinoma (e.g., endocervical, endometrial, ovarian)**

Modified from **Wilkinson RJ and Brown H**. *Human Pathology.* 2002;33:S49–S54.

Type 1 Paget's Disease

In a review of Type 1 cases from the English literature, Niikura et al. (53) reported on 565 cases, including their own series of 22 cases. There were 425 patients (75%) with Type 1a disease; 89 (16%) with Type 1b; and 51 (9%) with Type 1c.

MacLean et al. (54) reported that 6 of 76 patients (8%) on a British registry had an underlying carcinoma (Type 1b), and 14 patients (18.4%) had a systemic cancer. The primary was in the breast in six; bladder in three; and colorectum, cervix, uterus, and ovary in one each. One patient had a melanoma. Only four of these tumors were synchronous cancers. Niikura et al. (53) determined that if only synchronous neoplasms or those occurring within 12 months of the diagnosis were considered, only 8% of patients (44 of 534) with primary Paget's disease had a nonvulvar malignancy.

Fanning et al. (49) reported on a combined series of 100 patients with Paget's disease of the vulva. Their median age was 70 years. There was a 12% prevalence of invasive vulvar Paget's disease, and a 4% prevalence of associated vulvar adenocarcinoma. Thirty-four percent of patients experienced a recurrence at a median of 3 years.

Clinical Features

The disease predominantly affects postmenopausal white women, and the presenting symptoms are usually pruritus and vulvar soreness. **The lesion has an eczematoid appearance macroscopically and usually begins on the hair-bearing portions of the vulva** (Fig. 13.1). It may extend to involve the mons pubis, thighs, and buttocks. Extension to involve the mucosa of the rectum, vagina, or urinary tract also has been described (55). The more extensive lesions are usually raised and velvety in appearance and may weep persistently.

Investigations

All patients with Paget's disease of the vulva should be screened for any associated malignancy. These investigations should include mammography, computed tomography (CT) scan of the pelvis and abdomen, transvaginal ultrasonography, and cervical cytology. If the lesions involve the anus, colonoscopy should be undertaken, while if the urethra is involved, cystoscopy is indicated.

Treatment

The mainstay of treatment is wide superficial resection of the gross disease (56,57). **Underlying adenocarcinomas usually are clinically apparent, but this is not invariable. Paget cells may invade the underlying dermis, which should be removed for adequate histologic evaluation.** For this reason, laser therapy is unsatisfactory for primary Paget's disease. The surgical defect can usually be closed primarily, but sometimes a split thickness skin graft may be required to cover an extensive defect.

Unlike squamous cell carcinoma *in situ*, in which the histologic extent of disease usually correlates reasonably with the macroscopic lesion, Paget's disease usually extends well beyond the gross lesion, resulting in frequent positive surgical margins. The group at Memorial Sloan-Kettering Cancer Center reported positive margins in 20 of 28 patients (71%) (56). Of the 20 patients with

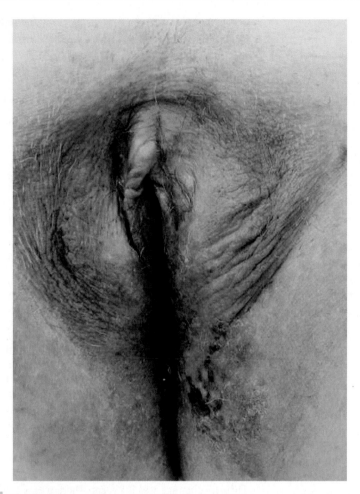

Figure 13.1 Paget's disease of the vulva. Note the weeping, eczematoid appearance, particularly posteriorly on the left, where there is early extension onto the inner thigh.

microscopically positive margins, 14 (70%) developed recurrent disease, while of the 8 patients with negative margins, 3 (38%) developed a recurrence.

Although surgical margins may be checked with frozen sections, these can be misleading (58), **and resection of the entire gross lesion with margins of at least 1 cm will control symptoms and exclude invasive disease.**

The role of **radiotherapy** for vulvar Paget's disease has been reviewed by Brown et al. (59). It **may be most useful when the disease involves the anus or urethra,** and surgery would involve diversion and stoma formation.

Another alternative approach that has been used for primary management is photodynamic therapy. An Italian study reported 32 patients who were treated with three cycles of aminolevulinic acid methyl-esther photodynamic therapy (M-ALA PDT) (60). Three patients (9.4%) had a complete resolution of symptoms and 25 (78.1%) had a partial resolution. The authors felt that **M-ALA PDT was able to control large and multiple lesions regardless of the area involved,** and that it preserved cosmetic and functional anatomy. However, the treatment is not curative. **All patients recurred, and one progressed to invasive disease.**

In general, recurrent lesions should be treated by further surgical resection, although laser therapy may occasionally be useful, particularly for perianal disease. **Topical Imiquimod cream (5%) has been used successfully for patients with recurrent Paget's disease of the vulva** (61). There is no consensus on dosage or duration of use, and it has been prescribed 3 to 7 times a week, for 6 to 24 weeks.

Invasive Paget's Disease   **If an underlying invasive carcinoma is present, it should be treated in the same manner as a squamous vulvar cancer.** This may require radical vulvectomy and at least an ipsilateral inguinofemoral lymphadenectomy. From their literature review, Niikura et al. (53) reported positive nodes in 30% of patients (23 of 70) with Types 1b or 1c Paget's disease of the vulva.

Lymph node metastases have been reported in patients with very superficially invasive tumors. Fine et al. reported a patient who had invasion no greater than 1 mm over a maximum length of 10 mm at her primary operation. Three weeks later, she was noted to have a palpable groin node, and at groin dissection, six positive groin nodes were resected from each groin (53). Ewing et al. (62) reported a positive sentinel node in a patient whose excised Paget's disease had scattered foci of superficial dermal invasion to a maximum depth of 0.7 mm.

Minimally invasive Paget's disease is rare, and in both the above cases, the surgical margins were positive for intraepithelial disease. **It would seem prudent to at least monitor the groins carefully, preferably with ultrasound, if the nodes are not dissected in a patient with superficially invasive Paget's disease.**

Prognosis

A study of 1,439 patients with invasive extramammary Paget's disease, identified from the SEER database from 1973 to 2007, reported that most (80.4%) had localized disease, 17.1% had locoregional spread, and 2.5% had distant disease (63). The 5-year disease-specific survival was 94.9% for patients with localized disease, 84.9% for those with locoregional spread, and 52.5% for those with distant metastases.

The disease is characterized by local recurrences over many years (54–56). Recurrent lesions are usually *in situ*, although 5 of 76 patients (6.7%) in the British registry showed progression to invasive disease between 1 and 21 years after the initial diagnosis (54). Investigators at the Norwegian Radium Hospital reported that nondiploid tumors had an increased risk of recurrence regardless of surgical radicality (64).

Invasive Vulvar Cancer

Squamous Cell Carcinoma

Squamous cell carcinoma of the vulva is predominantly a disease of postmenopausal women, with a mean age at diagnosis of approximately 65 years.

Clinical Features

Most patients present with a vulvar lump or mass, although there is often a long history of pruritus, usually associated with a vulvar dystrophy (Fig. 13.2). Less common presenting symptoms include vulvar bleeding, discharge, dysuria, or occasionally a large metastatic mass in the groin. On physical examination, the lesion is usually raised and may be fleshy, ulcerated, leukoplakic, or warty in appearance (Fig. 13.3). Warty lesions are often initially misdiagnosed as condylomata acuminata.

Most squamous carcinomas of the vulva occur on the labia majora, but the labia minora, clitoris, and perineum also may be primary sites. A study from one University Hospital in Germany reported a recent change in location of the tumor, with 37% of cases occurring between the clitoris and urethra in the 10 years up to 2007, compared to 19% in the 1980s ($p < 0.05$) (3). Approximately 10% of the cases are too extensive to determine a site of origin, and approximately **5% of the cases are multifocal.**

As part of the clinical assessment, the groin lymph nodes should be palpated, a Papanicolaou smear taken from the cervix, and **colposcopy of the cervix and vagina performed because of the common association with other squamous intraepithelial neoplasms of the lower genital tract.**

Diagnosis

Diagnosis requires a wedge or a Keyes biopsy specimen, which usually can be taken in the office under local anesthesia. The biopsy must include some underlying dermis and connective tissue so that the pathologist can adequately evaluate the depth of stromal invasion. It is preferable to leave the primary lesion *in situ* to allow the treating surgeon to fashion adequate surgical margins.

Routes of Spread

Vulvar cancer spreads by the following routes:

1. **Direct extension,** to involve adjacent structures such as the vagina, urethra, and anus.
2. **Lymphatic embolization** to regional lymph nodes.
3. **Hematogenous spread** to distant sites, including the lungs, liver, and bone.

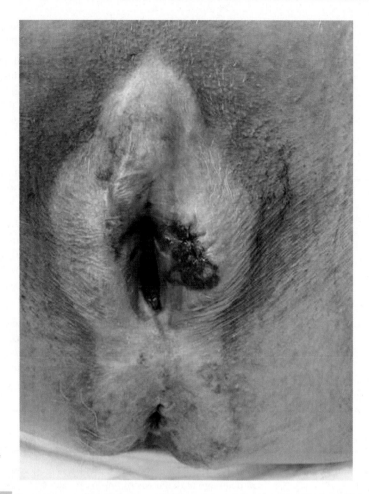

Figure 13.2 Squamous cell carcinoma of the vulva arising in a patient with long-standing lichen sclerosus. Note the butterfly distribution of the lichen sclerosus and the early invasive cancer on the left.

Lymphatic metastases may occur early in the disease. Initially, spread is usually to the inguinal lymph nodes, which are located between Camper's fascia and the fascia lata. From these superficial groin nodes, the disease spreads to the femoral nodes, which are located medial to the femoral vein (Fig. 13.4). Cloquet's node, situated beneath the inguinal ligament, is the most cephalad of the femoral node group. **Metastases to the femoral nodes without involvement of the inguinal nodes have been reported** (65–67). In addition, Gordinier et al. (68) reported groin recurrence in 9 of 104 patients (8.7%) treated by superficial inguinal lymphadenectomy at the M. D. Anderson Cancer Center. The median number of lymph nodes removed per groin was 7, and the median time to recurrence was 22 months.

From the inguinofemoral nodes, the cancer spreads to the pelvic nodes, particularly the external iliac group. **Although direct lymphatic pathways from the clitoris and Bartholin gland to the pelvic nodes have been described, these channels seem to be of minimal clinical significance** (21,69).

Since 1980, the overall incidence of lymph node metastases is reported to be approximately 30% (Table 13.3) (21–23,70–75). The incidence in relation to clinical stage of disease is shown in Table 13.4 (22,71,76), and in relation to depth of invasion in Table 13.5 (16,17,77–84). Data on 446 patients with primary vulvar cancer from the Mayo Clinic revealed that the incidence of lymph node metastases in relation to tumor size was as follows: 1 cm or less, 7%; 1.1 to 2 cm, 22.2%; 2.1 to 3 cm, 26.9%; and 3.1 to 5 cm, 34.1% (73).

Metastases to pelvic nodes are uncommon, the overall reported frequency being approximately 9%. About 20% of patients with positive groin nodes have positive pelvic nodes (85). Pelvic nodal metastases are rare in the absence of clinically suspicious (N_2) groin nodes (22), three or more positive groin nodes (21,22,70,73) and a tumor with invasion >4 mm (73).

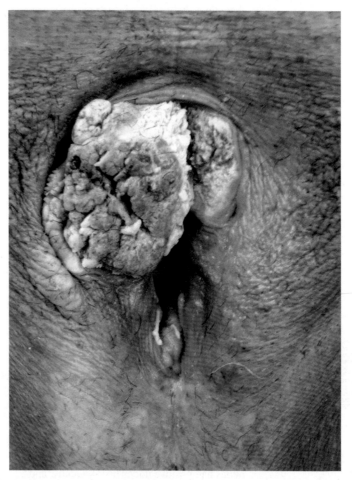

Figure 13.3 Exophytic squamous cell carcinoma involving the clitoris and right anterior labia.

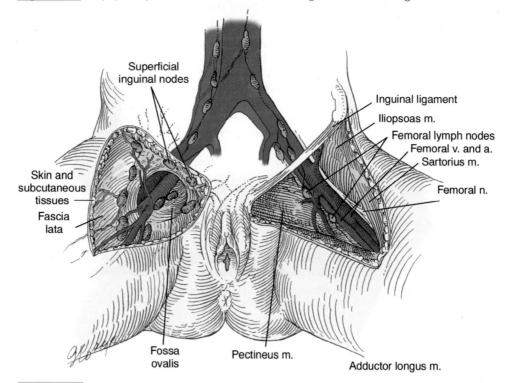

Figure 13.4 **Inguinal-femoral lymph nodes.** (Reproduced from **Hacker NF.** Vulvar cancer. In: **Hacker NF, Moore JG**. *Essentials of Obstetrics and Gynecology.* 5th ed. Philadelphia, PA: Elsevier Saunders; 2008, with permission.)

Table 13.3 Incidence of Lymph Node Metastases in Operable Vulvar Cancer			
Author	*No. of Cases*	*Positive Nodes*	*Percent*
Curry et al., 1980 (21)	191	57	29.8
Iversen et al., 1980 (70)	268	86	32.1
Hacker et al., 1983 (22)	113	31	27.4
Monaghan and Hammond, 1984 (23)	134	37	27.6
Rouzier et al., 2002 (71)	180	54	30
Raspagliesi et al., 2006 (72)	389	110	28.3
Bosquet et al., 2007 (73)	320	108	33.8
Ghebre et al., 2011 (74)	140	37	26.4
Tabbaa et al., 2012 (75)	468	139	29.7
Total	**2,203**	**659**	**29.9**

Hematogenous spread usually occurs late in the course of vulvar cancer and is rare in the absence of lymph node metastases. Hematogenous spread is uncommon in patients with one or two positive groin nodes, but is more common in patients with three or more positive nodes (22).

Staging

A clinical staging system based on the TNM classification was adopted by the International Federation of Gynecology and Obstetrics (FIGO) in 1969 (Table 13.6) (86). The staging was based on a clinical evaluation of the primary tumor and regional lymph nodes and a limited search for distant metastases.

Clinical evaluation of the groin lymph nodes is inaccurate. Bosquet et al. (73) reported that pooled data from six institutions showed that 19.5% of patients (88 of 451) with clinically negative nodes had positive nodes histologically, and 21.8% of patients (53 of 243) with clinically positive nodes had negative nodes histologically. The Gynecologic Oncology Group (GOG) data revealed that compared with surgical staging of vulvar cancer, the percentage of error in clinical staging increased from 18% for stage I disease to 44% for stage IV disease (87).

These factors led the Cancer Committee of FIGO to introduce a surgical staging for vulvar cancer in 1988. Stage I was subdivided in 1994 (Table 13.7). Although this system took the histologic status of the nodes into account, it had four major problems (88). **The first was that patients with negative lymph nodes have a very good prognosis, regardless of the size of the primary tumor.** Data from the Royal Hospital for Women in Sydney revealed a 96.4% 5-year survival for 121 patients with Stages I or II disease (89). **The second was that stage III represented a heterogeneous group of patients prognostically,** because it included patients with and without positive lymph nodes. The GOG analysis of 588 patients reported that survival for patients with stage III disease ranged from 34–100% (87). Rouzier et al. (90) reported a cohort of 895 patients with FIGO Stage III vulvar cancer who had been registered with the SEER database from 1988 through 2004. The 5-year overall survival for patients with regional metastatic nodal disease (39%) was significantly worse than that of patients with locally advanced tumors but negative nodes (62%, $p < 0.0001$). **The third problem was that the number of positive nodes and the**

Table 13.4 Incidence of Lymph Node Metastases in Relation to Clinical Stage of Disease			
Stage	*No. of Cases*	*Positive Nodes*	*Percent*
I	140	15	10.7
II	145	38	26.2
III	137	88	64.2
IV	18	16	88.9

Data compiled from **Green, 1978** (76); **Iversen et al., 1980** (70); and **Hacker et al., 1983** (22).

Table 13.5 Nodal Status in T_1 Squamous Cell Carcinoma of the Vulva versus Depth of Stromal Invasion

Depth of Invasion	No.	Positive Nodes	Nodes
<1 mm	163	0	0
1.1–2 mm	145	11	7.6
2.1–3 mm	131	11	8.4
3.1–5 mm	101	27	26.7
>5 mm	38	13	34.2
Total	578	62	10.7

Data compiled from **Parker et al., 1975** (77); **Magrina et al., 1979** (78); **Iversen et al., 1981** (16); **Wilkinson et al., 1982** (79); **Hoffman et al., 1983** (80); **Hacker et al., 1984** (17); **Boice et al., 1984** (81); **Ross and Ehrmann, 1987** (82); **Rowley et al., 1988** (83); **Struyk et al., 1989** (84).

Table 13.6 FIGO Clinical Staging of Carcinoma of the Vulva (1969)

FIGO Stage	TNM	Clinical Findings
Stage 0		Carcinoma *in situ* (e.g., VIN 3, noninvasive Paget disease)
Stage I	$T_1N_0M_0$ $T_1N_1M_0$	Tumor confined to the vulva, 2 cm or less in largest diameter, and no suspect groin nodes
Stage II	$T_2N_0M_0$ $T_2N_1M_0$	Tumor confined to the vulva more than 2 cm in diameter, and no suspect groin nodes
Stage III	$T_3N_0M_0$ $T_3N_1M_0$ $T_3N_2M_0$ $T_1N_2M_0$ $T_2N_2M_0$	Tumor of any size with: 1. Adjacent spread to the urethra and/or the vagina, the perineum, and the anus, and/or 2. Clinically suspect lymph nodes in either groin
Stage IV	$T_xN_3M_0$ $T_4N_0M_0$ $T_4N_1M_0$ $T_4N_2M_0$ $T_xN_xM_{1a}$ $T_xN_xM_{1b}$	Tumor of any size: 1. Infiltrating the bladder mucosa, or the rectal mucosa, or both, including the upper part of the urethral mucosa, and/or 2. Fixed to the bone, and/or 3. Other distant metastases

TNM Classification

T:	Primary Tumor	N:	Regional Lymph Nodes
T_1	Tumor confined to the vulva, ≤2 cm in largest diameter	N_0	No nodes palpable
T_2	Tumor confined to the vulva, >2 cm in diameter	N_1	Nodes palpable in either groin, not enlarged, mobile (not clinically suspect for neoplasm)
T_3	Tumor of any size with adjacent spread to the urethra and/or vagina and/or perineum and/or anus	N_2	Nodes palpable in either or both groins, enlarged, firm and mobile (clinically suspect for neoplasm)
T_4	Tumor of any size infiltrating the bladder mucosa and/or the rectal mucosa, or including the upper part of the urethral mucosa and/or fixed to the bone	N_3	Fixed or ulcerated nodes

		M:	Distant Metastases
		M_0	No clinical metastases
		M_1	Palpable deep pelvic lymph nodes
		M_{1b}	Other distant metastases

FIGO, International Federation of Gynecology and Obstetrics; VIN, vulvar intraepithelial neoplasia; x, any T or N category.

Table 13.7 FIGO Surgical Staging for Vulvar Cancer (1994)

FIGO Stage	TNM	Clinical/Pathologic Findings
Stage 0	T_{is}	Carcinoma *in situ*, intraepithelial carcinoma
Stage I	$T_1N_0M_0$	Tumor ≤2 cm in greatest diameter, confined to the vulva or perineum; nodes are negative
IA	$T_1N_0M_0$	As above with stromal invasion ≤1 mm[a]
IB	$T_{1b}N_0M_0$	As above with stromal invasion >1 mm
Stage II	$T_2N_0M_0$	Tumor confined to the vulva and/or perineum, >2 cm in greatest dimension, nodes are negative
Stage III	$T_3N_0M_0$ $T_3N_1M_0$ $T_1N_1M_0$ $T_2N_1M_0$	Tumor of any size with: 1. Adjacent spread to the lower urethra and/or the vagina and/or the anus 2. Unilateral regional lymph node metastasis
Stage IVA	$T_1N_2M_0$ $T_2N_2M_0$ $T_3N_2M_0$ $T_4,$ any N, M_0	Tumor invades any of the following: Upper urethra, bladder mucosa, rectal mucosa, pelvic bone, or bilateral regional node metastasis
Stage IVB	Any T, any N, M_1	Any distant metastasis including pelvic lymph nodes

TNM Classification

T:	Primary Tumor	N:	Regional Lymph Nodes
T_x	Primary tumor cannot be assessed		Regional lymph nodes are the femoral and inguinal nodes
T_0	No evidence of primary tumor	N_x	Regional lymph nodes cannot be assessed
T_{is}	Carcinoma *in situ* (preinvasive carcinoma)	N_0	No lymph node metastasis
T_1	Tumor confined to the vulva and/or perineum 2 cm or less in greatest dimension	N_1	Unilateral regional lymph node metastasis
T_2	Tumor confined to the vulva and/or perineum more than 2 cm in greatest dimension	N_2	Bilateral regional lymph node metastasis
T_3	Tumor involves any of the following: Lower urethra, vagina, anus	**M:**	**Distant Metastasis**
T_4	Tumor involves any of the following: Bladder mucosa, rectal mucosa, upper urethra, pelvic bone	M_x	Presence of distant metastasis cannot be assessed
		M_0	No distant metastasis
		M_1	Distant metastasis (pelvic lymph node metastasis is M1)

[a]The depth of invasion is defined as the measurement of the tumor from the epithelial–stromal junction of the adjacent most superficial dermal papilla to the deepest point of invasion.

FIGO, International Federation of Gynecology and Obstetrics.

morphology of the positive nodes were not taken into account (21,22,87,91,92), and **the final problem was that most reports indicate that bilaterality of positive nodes is not an independent prognostic factor** (21,22,87,91,92).

A new FIGO Staging System for Vulvar Cancer was introduced in 2009 (Table 13.8), to address the above issues. Stage IA remains unchanged, but Stages I and II have been combined. The 2009 staging system also shifted patients who have distal vaginal, distal urethral or anal involvement from the T3 to the T2 category and (if N_0) from FIGO stage III to FIGO stage II. This shift classifies patients more accurately according to prognosis (which is dominated by the nodal status) but the new T2 category now includes patients who are treated with surgery alone, together with lesions that may be treated with initial radiation to preserve urethral or anal function.

Table 13.8 FIGO Surgical Staging for Vulvar Cancer (2009)

FIGO Stage	TNM	Clinical/Pathologic Findings
Stage I		Tumor confined to the vulva
IA	T_{1a}, N_0, M_0	Lesions ≤2 cm in size, confined to the vulva or perineum and with stromal invasion ≤1.0 mm[a], no nodal metastasis.
IB	T_{1b}, N_0, M_0	Lesions >2 cm in size or with stromal invasion >1.0 mm[a], confined to the vulva or perineum, with negative nodes.
Stage II	T_2, N_0, M_0	Tumor of any size with extension to adjacent perineal structures (1/3 lower urethra, 1/3 lower vagina, anus) with negative nodes.
Stage III		Tumor of any size with or without extension to adjacent perineal structures (1/3 lower urethra, 1/3 lower vagina, anus) with positive inguino-femoral lymph nodes.
IIIA	T_1,T_2, N_{1a}, M_0 T_1, T_2, N_{1b}, M_0	(i) 1–2 lymph node metastasis (<5 mm), or (ii) 1 lymph node metastasis(es) (≥5 mm).
IIIB	T_1, T_2, N_{2a}, M_0 T_1, T_2, N_{2b}, M_0	(i) ≥3 lymph node metastasis (<5 mm), or (ii) ≥2 lymph node metastasis(es) (≥5 mm).
IIIC	T_1, T_2, N_{2c}, M_0	With positive nodes with extracapsular spread.
Stage IV		Tumor invades other regional (2/3 upper urethra, 2/3 upper vagina), or distant structures.
IVA	T_1, T_2, T_3, N_3, M_0	Tumor invades any of the following: (i) upper urethral and/or vaginal mucosa, bladder mucosa, rectal mucosa, or fixed to pelvic bone, or (ii) fixed or ulcerated inguino-femoral lymph nodes.
IVB	Any T, any N, M_1	Any distant metastasis including pelvic lymph nodes.

TNM Classification

T:	Primary Tumor	N:	Regional Lymph Nodes
Tis	Carcinoma *in situ* (not in FIGO system)	N_0	No spread to lymph nodes
T_1	Tumor confined to vulva or perineum	N_1	Spread to 1 or 2 lymph nodes
T_{1a}	Tumor invasive ≤1 mm and ≤2 cm	N_{1a}	Spread to 1 or 2 lymph nodes and tumor <5 mm
T_{1b}	Tumor >2 cm or invasive >1 mm	N_{1b}	Spread to 1 or 2 lymph nodes and tumor ≥5 mm
T_2	Tumor any size and growing into anus or lower third of the vagina or urethra	N_2	Spread to groin lymph nodes with the following features:
T_3	Tumor any size, growing into the upper urethra, bladder or rectum or into pubic bone	N_{2a}	Spread to ≥3 lymph nodes and each area of spread <5 mm
M:	**Distant Metastasis**	N_{2b}	Spread to ≥2 lymph nodes and each area of spread ≥5 mm
M_0	No distant spread	N_{2c}	Spread to lymph nodes and has started growing through the outer covering of at least one lymph node (extracapsular spread)
M_1	Spread to distant sites, including spread to pelvic lymph nodes	N_3	Spread to lymph nodes causing open sores (ulceration) or causing the lymph node to be stuck (fixed) to tissue beneath

FIGO no longer includes stage 0.

[a]The depth of invasion is defined as the measurement of the tumor from the epithelial-stromal junction of the adjacent most superficial dermal papilla to the deepest point of invasion.

FIGO Committee on Gynecologic Oncology. Revised FIGO staging for carcinoma of the vulva, cervix, and endometrium. *Int J Gynecol Obstet.* 2009;105:103–104.

Edge SB, Byrd DR, Compton CC, et al., eds. Vulva. In: *AJCC Cancer Staging Manual.* 7th ed. New York, NY: Springer, 2010, pp 379–381.

The number and morphology of positive nodes have been taken into account in Stage III, and the bilaterality of positive nodes has been discounted. Dutch workers reported that the new FIGO staging system led to a 42% downstaging, and did provide a better reflection of prognosis (93).

Treatment

After the pioneering work of Taussig (12) in the United States and Way (10,13) in Great Britain, **en bloc radical vulvectomy and bilateral dissection of the groin and pelvic nodes became the standard treatment for most patients with operable vulvar cancer**. If the disease involved the anus, rectovaginal septum, or proximal urethra, some type of pelvic exenteration was combined with this dissection.

Although the survival rate improved markedly with this aggressive surgical approach, **several factors have led to modifications of this "standard" treatment plan during the past 25 years**. These factors include earlier presentation of women in Western countries, and increasing concern among both patients and doctors about the physical and psychosexual morbidity associated with radical vulvectomy.

Modern management of vulvar cancer requires an experienced, multidisciplinary team approach, which is available only in tertiary referral centers. **Successful centralization of the management of patients with vulvar occurred in the eastern part of the Netherlands following the release of national guidelines by the Dutch Society of Obstetrics and Gynecology in 2000.** In the decade prior to the release of the guidelines, 62% of patients (123 of 198) were treated in an oncology center, but this increased to 93% (172 of 184) from 2000 to 2008. The 5-year relative survival improved from 69% to 75% with the centralization of care, and after adjustment for age and stage, being treated in a specialized oncology center was found to be an independent prognostic factor (94).

The shortcomings of treatment in nonreferral units were highlighted in a British study. Investigators retrospectively reviewed the records of 411 patients with squamous cell carcinoma who had been notified to the Central Intelligence Unit of the West Midlands during two 3-year periods: 1980 to 1982 and 1986 to 1988 (95). **The women were treated at 35 different hospitals, 16 of which averaged 1 case or less per year. Fifteen different operations were used,** the most common of which were simple vulvectomy (35%) and radical vulvectomy with bilateral inguinal lymphadenectomy (34%). Hemivulvectomy was performed in only five patients (1.2%). Only 190 of the 411 patients (46%) had a lymphadenectomy performed, and a unilateral dissection was performed in only 9 patients (2.1%). Survival data for all FIGO stages compared unfavorably with the GOG data from tertiary units in the United States (87): 78% versus 98% for stage I disease; 53% versus 85% for stage II; 27% versus 74% for stage III; and 13% versus 31% for stage IV. **Omission of lymphadenectomy was the single most important prognostic factor, but treatment in a hospital with less than 20 cases in total was a poor prognostic factor in univariate analysis** (95).

Management of Early Vulvar Cancers

The modern approach to the management of patients with carcinoma confined to the vulva should be individualized (15,17,89,96). There is no "standard" treatment applicable to every patient, and emphasis is on performing the most conservative operation consistent with cure of the disease.

In considering the appropriate operation, it is necessary to determine independently the appropriate management of the following:

1. **The primary lesion**
2. **The groin lymph nodes**

Before any surgery, all patients should have colposcopy of the cervix, vagina, and vulva, because preinvasive (and rarely invasive) lesions may be present at other sites along the lower genital tract.

Management of the Primary Lesion

The two factors to take into account in determining the management of the primary tumor are the following:

1. **The condition of the remainder of the vulva**
2. **The presence or absence of multifocal invasive disease**

Table 13.9 Invasive Vulvar Recurrence versus Histopathologic Resection Margins				
	Histologic Margins		Recurrence	
	≥8	<8	>8	<8
	No.	No.	No.	No.
Heaps et al., 1990 (100)	91	44	0	21
de Hullu et al., 2002 (99)	39	40	0	9
Chan et al., 2007 (101)	30	53	0	12
Tantipalakorn et al., 2009 (89)	92	24	6	7
Total	252	161	2.4%	49 (30.4%)

Although radical vulvectomy has been regarded as the standard treatment for the primary vulvar lesion, this operation is associated with significant disturbances of sexual function and body image. Andersen and Hacker (97) reported that, when compared with healthy adult women, sexual arousal was reduced to the eighth percentile and body image to the fourth percentile in women who had undergone vulvectomy.

Since the early 1980s, several investigators have advocated a radical local excision rather than a radical vulvectomy for the primary lesion in patients with T_1 and T_2 tumors (14–20,89,96,98,99). Regardless of whether a radical vulvectomy or a radical local excision is performed, the surgical margins adjacent to the tumor will be the same, and **an analysis of the available literature indicates that the incidence of local invasive recurrence is low if the histopathologic margin (after fixation) is at least 8 mm** (Table 13.9) (89,99–101). Allowing for 20% tissue shrinkage with formalin fixation, this translates to a surgical margin of at least 1 cm.

When vulvar cancer arises in the presence of VIN or some nonneoplastic epithelial disorder, radical local excision should be performed for the invasive disease, and the associated disease should be treated in the most appropriate manner. For example, **topical steroids may be required for squamous hyperplasia or lichen sclerosus, whereas VIN should be treated by superficial local excision and primary closure or split thickness skin grafting.**

Radical local excision of the invasive lesion is most appropriate for lesions on the lateral or posterior aspects of the vulva (Fig. 13.5), where preservation of the clitoris is feasible. **For patients with anterior lesions, surgical resection that includes clitorectomy can have serious psychosexual consequences,** particularly in younger patients. Chan et al. (102) identified 41 patients with squamous carcinoma of the anterior vulva not involving the clitoris. Thirteen patients (32%) had clitoral sparing modified radical vulvectomy and 28 (68%) had radical vulvectomy. The 13 patients who had clitoral sparing surgery included 8 with stage I, two with stage II, two with stage III, and one with stage IV disease. After a median follow-up of 59 months, none of the 13 patients having conservative surgery had locoregional failure.

In young patients with actual involvement of the clitoris or in whom surgical margins would be <5 mm, consideration should be given to treating the primary lesion with a small field of radiation therapy. Small vulvar lesions can often be controlled with 60 to 64 Gy of external radiation, typically using an appositional electron field; if there is suspicion of persistent disease, biopsy can be performed after therapy to confirm complete response (103).

Local Control Rates after Surgical Management of Early Lesions

Two recent papers have looked at single institutional experiences with T_1 and T_2 squamous cell carcinoma of the vulva (89,96).

In the study from Kentucky, 61 patients with a lateral T_1 lesion and 61 patients with a lateral T_2 lesion were seen from 1963 to 2003 (96). Radical vulvectomy was performed on 60 patients (49%) and radical hemivulvectomy on 62 (51%). Ipsilateral inguinal node metastases were present in 11% of patients (7 of 61) with a T_1 lesion, and 31% (19 of 61) of patients with a T_2 lesion. Disease-free survival of patients with T_1 and T_2 lesions was 98% and 93%, respectively at 5 years. **Local or distant recurrence was not more common in patients treated by radical vulvectomy or radical hemivulvectomy.**

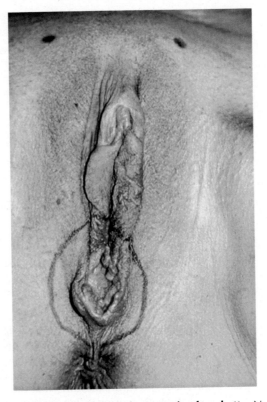

Figure 13.5 **Small (T$_1$) vulvar carcinoma at the posterior fourchette.** Note that the remainder of the vulva is normal.

The 49% incidence of radical vulvectomy in this study is not surprising, because the study dates back to 1963, which is about 20 years before radical local excision was being advocated. More concerning is a 2008 SEER study of 523 patients, which reported that 46–54% of patients with vulvar cancer in the United States still underwent a radical or total vulvectomy (104).

Our experience at the Royal Hospital for Women in Sydney suggests that radical vulvectomy is rarely necessary. Of 121 patients with 1994 FIGO stages I and II vulvar cancer managed from 1987 through 2005, radical local excision was performed in 116 patients (95.9%) (89). Only five patients (4.1%) underwent radical vulvectomy, in all cases for tumor multifocality. **With a median follow-up of 84 months, the overall survival at 5 years was 96.4%.**

Technique for Radical Local Excision

Radical local excision implies a wide and deep excision of the primary tumor. An elliptical incision should be drawn using a marking pen, with the skin in its natural position. Surgical margins around the tumor should be at least 1 cm. The incision should be carried down to the inferior fascia of the urogenital diaphragm, which is coplanar with the fascia lata and the fascia over the pubic symphysis. The surgical defect is closed in two layers. For perineal lesions, proximity to the anus may preclude adequate surgical margins, and consideration should be given to preoperative or postoperative radiation in such cases. For periurethral lesions, the distal half of the urethra may be resected without loss of continence. Figure 13.6 shows the satisfactory cosmetic result achieved in the treatment of the lesion shown in Figure 13.5.

Management of the Groin Lymph Nodes

Appropriate management of the regional lymph nodes is the single most important factor in decreasing the mortality from early vulvar cancer. With respect to lymph node metastases, two facts are apparent:

1. **The only patients without significant risk of lymph node metastases are those with a tumor up to 2 cm in diameter, that invades the stroma to a depth no greater than 1 mm** (Table 13.5).

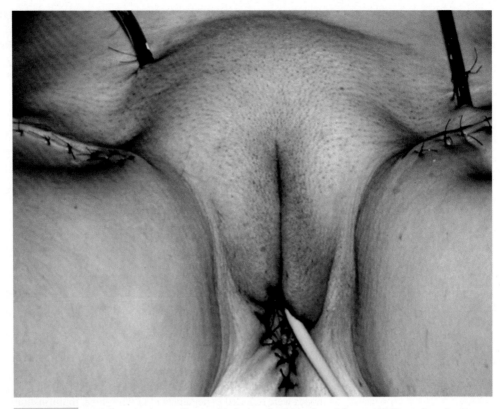

Figure 13.6 **Satisfactory cosmetic result after radical local excision and bilateral groin dissection** (for the small posterior vulvar carcinoma shown in Fig. 13.2).

2. **Patients in whom recurrent disease develops in an undissected groin have a very high mortality rate** (Table 13.10) (17,23,32,78,80,105–107).

The safest treatment for all patients with a 2 cm tumor with more than 1 mm of stromal invasion, and all patients with a tumor greater than 2 cm in diameter, is inguinofemoral lymphadenectomy. A wedge or Keyes biopsy of the primary tumor should be obtained, and the depth of invasion determined. If it is less than 1 mm on the biopsy specimen, and the lesion is 2 cm or less in diameter, the entire lesion should be locally excised and serially sectioned to determine the depth of invasion. If there is still no invasive focus deeper than 1 mm, groin dissection may be omitted. Although there have been case reports positive nodes in a patient with Stage 1A vulvar cancer (108,109), the incidence is extremely low.

Table 13.10 Death from Recurrence in an Undissected Groin		
Author	*Recurrence*	*Dead of Disease*
Rutledge et al., 1970 (105)	4	3
Magrina et al., 1979 (78)	4	3
Hoffman et al., 1983 (80)	4	4
Hacker et al., 1984 (17)	3	3
Monaghan and Hammond, 1984 (23)	4	4
Lingard et al., 1992 (106)	7	7
Burke et al., 1995 (107)	4	3
van der Zee, 2008 (32)	7[a]	6
Total	**37**	**33 (89.2%)**

[a]At least 12 months follow-up.

Table 13.11 Incidence of Positive Contralateral Nodes in Patients with Lateral T$_1$ Squamous Carcinomas

Author	Unilateral Lesions	Contralateral Nodes Positive	Percentage
Wharton et al., 1974 (112)	25	0	0
Parker et al., 1975 (77)	41	0	0
Magrina et al., 1979 (78)	77	2	2.6
Iversen et al., 1981 (16)	112	0	0
Buscema et al., 1981 (113)	38	0	0
Hoffman et al., 1983 (80)[a]	70	0	0
Hacker et al., 1984 (17)	60	0	0
Struyk et al., 1989 (84)	53	0	0
De Simone et al., 2007 (96)	61	0	0
Total	**537**	**2**	**0.37**

[a]Information not contained in reference but obtained from personal communication.

If groin dissection is indicated in patients with early vulvar cancer, it should be a thorough inguinofemoral lymphadenectomy (110). The GOG reported six groin recurrences among 121 patients with T$_1$N$_0$ or N$_1$ tumors after a superficial (inguinal) dissection, even though the inguinal nodes were reported as negative (111). This large, multi-institutional study indicates that modification of the groin dissection increases groin recurrences and, therefore, mortality.

It is not necessary to perform a bilateral groin dissection if the primary lesion is unilateral (defined as 2 cm or more from the midline) and the ipsilateral nodes are negative (Table 13.11) (16,17,77,78,80,84,96,112,113).

Retrospective analysis of a GOG study investigating sentinel lymph node localization before definitive groin dissection was undertaken to determine the safety of unilateral dissection in patients with near midline lesions (114). Sixty-five patients had lesions within 2 cm of the midline, and all underwent bilateral groin dissection. Bilateral drainage was identified in 58% of cases (38 of 65). No nodal metastases were found in the contralateral groin in the 27 patients with ipsilateral drainage identified at lymphatic mapping.

Lesions involving the anterior labia minora should have bilateral dissection because of the more frequent contralateral lymph flow from this region (115).

Measurement of Depth of Invasion

The Nomenclature Committee of the International Society of Gynecologic Pathologists has recommended that depth of invasion be measured from the most superficial dermal papilla adjacent to the tumor to the deepest focus of invasion. This method was originally proposed by Wilkinson et al. (79). Tumor thickness is also commonly measured (77,116), and Fu (117) estimated that the average difference between tumor thickness and depth of invasion as determined by the Wilkinson method was 0.3 mm.

Technique for Groin Dissection

A linear incision is made 1 cm above and parallel to the groin crease along the medial three quarters of a line drawn between the anterior superior iliac spine and labiocrural fold (Fig. 13.7). This incision will be directly over the fossa ovalis (Fig. 13.8). Studies of bipedal lymphangiograms have demonstrated that **there are no lymph nodes adjacent to the anterior superior iliac spine** (118). On the basis of embryologic and anatomical studies, Micheletti et al. (119) have proposed that the superficial circumflex iliac vessels could represent the lateral surgical landmark. The incision is carried through the subcutaneous tissues to the superficial (Camper's) fascia. This layer can be definitively identified, because the superficial circumflex iliac and superficial external pudendal

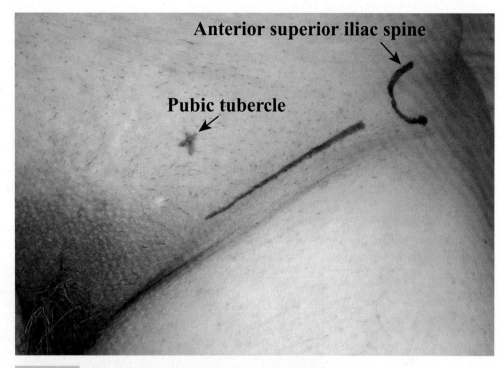

Figure 13.7   Skin incision for groin dissection through a separate incision. The incision is made 1 cm above the groin crease along the medial three quarters of a line drawn between the anterior superior iliac spine and the labiocrural fold.

veins run immediately below it. The superficial fascia is incised and grasped with artery forceps to place it on traction, and the fatty tissue between it and the fascia lata is removed over the femoral triangle (Fig. 13.9). **To avoid skin necrosis, all subcutaneous tissue above Camper fascia must be preserved.** The dissection is carried 1 cm above the inguinal ligament to include all the inguinal nodes.

The saphenous vein is usually tied off at the apex of the femoral triangle and at its point of entry into the femoral vein. Some authors have suggested that saphenous vein sparing may decrease postoperative morbidity (120,121), although in a study of 64 patients, 31 of whom underwent saphenous sparing, Zhang et al. (121) reported no difference in the incidence of postoperative fever, acute cellulitis, seroma, or lymphocyst formation.

The fatty tissue containing the femoral lymph nodes is removed from within the fossa ovalis. **There are only one to three femoral lymph nodes, and they are always situated medial to the femoral vein in the opening of the fossa ovalis** (122). Hence, there is no need to remove the fascia lata lateral to the femoral vessels. Cloquet's node is not consistently present but should be checked for by retraction of the inguinal ligament cephalad over the femoral canal. The wound is closed in two layers, tacking the superficial fascia to the deep fascia. The author no longer places a drain in the groin.

Postoperative Management

In spite of the age and general medical condition of most patients with vulvar cancer, the surgery is usually remarkably well tolerated. However, a postoperative mortality rate of about 1% can be expected, usually as a result of pulmonary embolism or myocardial infarction. A low-residue diet may be commenced on the first postoperative day, and **bed rest is advisable for 2 to 3 days to allow immobilization of the wounds to foster healing**. Pneumatic calf compression and subcutaneous *heparin* or *clexane* should be used to help prevent deep venous thrombosis, and active, nonweight-bearing leg movements should be encouraged. Perineal swabs should be given until the patient is fully mobilized, at which stage sitz baths or whirlpool therapy is helpful. A Foley catheter is usually left in the bladder until the patient is ambulatory.

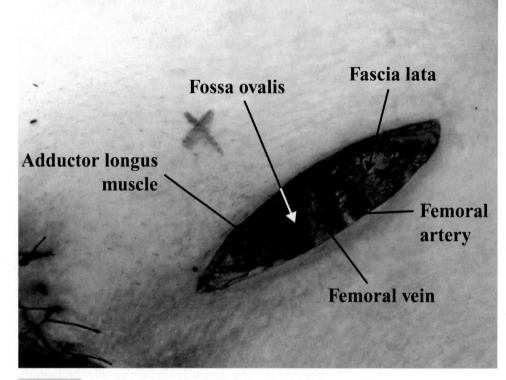

Figure 13.8 Groin incision is directly over the fossa ovalis.

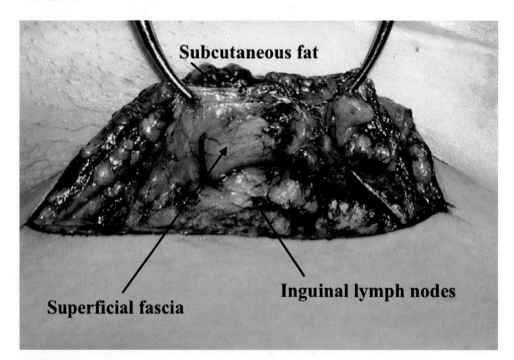

Figure 13.9 **Camper fascia kept on traction with forceps while the underlying node-bearing fatty tissue is dissected out of the femoral triangle.** Note the preservation of the subcutaneous tissue above the superficial fascia. This ensures that skin necrosis will not occur.

Early Postoperative Complications

The major immediate morbidity is related to the groin dissection. With the separate incision approach, and sparing of all subcutaneous fat above the superficial fascia, the incidence of wound breakdown is very low, patients mainly at risk being heavy smokers and diabetics. **The most common problem is lymphocyst formation,** which occurs in about 40% of cases (123). These seem to have become more common since introducing the practice of leaving the fascia lata over the muscles in the floor of the femoral triangle. If large, lymphocysts are best managed by making a linear incision 1 to 2 cm long, and inserting a corrugated drain until the skin flaps have adhered to the underlying tissues. Early mobilization and long walks before the groin is completely healed seem to increase the incidence of lymphocysts.

Other early postoperative complications include cellulitis, urinary tract infection, deep venous thrombosis, pulmonary embolism, myocardial infarction, hemorrhage, and, rarely, osteitis pubis.

Late Complications

The major late complication is chronic leg edema, which has been reported in up to 69% of patients (91). At the Royal Hospital for Women in Sydney, the self-reported incidence of lymphedema after groin dissection was 62% (124). In about 50% of patients, the onset of lymphedema occurred within 3 months, while about 85% experienced the onset within 12 months. Lymphedema was significantly related to the occurrence of early complications, particularly cellulitis (124).

Recurrent lymphangitis or cellulitis of the leg occurs in about 10% of patients. It can develop very quickly, and may need hospitalization and intravenous antibiotics. **Urinary stress incontinence,** with or without **genital prolapse,** occurs in about 10% of patients and may require corrective surgery. **Introital stenosis** can lead to dyspareunia and may require a vertical relaxing incision, which is sutured transversely. An uncommon late complication is **femoral hernia,** which can usually be prevented during surgery by closure of the femoral canal with a suture from the inguinal ligament to Cooper ligament. **Pubic osteomyelitis** and **rectovaginal or rectoperineal fistulae** are rare late complications.

Lymphatic Mapping

The major morbidity associated with the modern management of vulvar cancer is chronic lower limb lymphedema, which occurs in about 60% of patients following groin dissection, and is a lifelong affliction. Hence, for the last 30 years, there has been much interest in eliminating or modifying the groin dissection for patients with negative nodes.

Several noninvasive methods for detecting lymph node metastases have been disappointing, including positron emission tomography (125), computerized tomographic scanning (126), and magnetic resonance imaging (127). Ultrasonic scanning, particularly when combined with fine needle aspiration cytology, shows more promise, but false negatives and false positives still occur (126,128).

For the past decade or more, researchers have been investigating the feasibility of using sentinel node identification to avoid complete inguinofemoral lymphadenectomy in selected patients with vulvar cancer. This concept was initially introduced by Cabanas (129) for the management of men with penile cancer in 1977, and subsequently pioneered for the management of melanomas by Morton et al. (130) in 1992. The hypothesis is that if the sentinel node is negative, all other nodes will be negative, so the patient can be spared the morbidity of full groin dissection.

The sentinel node (or nodes) is identified by the **injection of intradermal isosulfan blue dye** around the primary vulvar lesion, in combination with **intradermal radioactive ^{99m}Tc-labeled sulfur colloid** (32,131,132). After the injections, the node(s) is isolated in the groin by dissection (to identify the blue node or nodes) (Fig. 13.10) and gamma counting. **Ultrastaging, using serial sectioning and immunoperoxidase staining for cytokeratin, is undertaken if the sentinel node is negative on routine hematoxalin and eosin staining.**

In the past 5 years, three large national groups have reported their results on the use of sentinel node identification to obviate the need for groin dissection in patients with early vulvar cancer (32, 131,132).

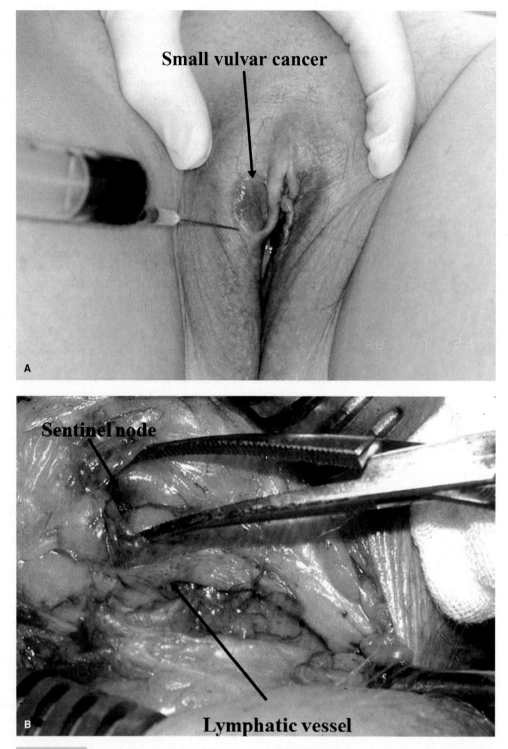

Figure 13.10 Lymphaticmapping utilizing an intradermal injection of blue dye immediately preoperatively **(A).** Note the *blue* lymphatic vessel and blue sentinel node at groin dissection **(B).**

The Groningen multicenter observational study, which was published in 2008, used both radiotracer and blue dye (32). Eligible patients were those with squamous cell carcinomas <4 cm diameter. If the sentinel node was negative on ultrastaging, groin dissection was omitted and the patient was observed clinically every 2 months for 2 years. From March 2000 to June 2006, 403 assessable patients were recruited to the study, and they underwent 623 groin dissections. Metastatic sentinel nodes were found in 163 groins (26.2%). Routine pathologic examination detected 95 (58.3%)

cases and ultrastaging detected a further 68 (41.7%). **In eight of 276 patients in the observational study, groin recurrence was observed after a negative sentinel node procedure. The actuarial groin recurrence rate after 2 years was 3%** (95%, CI 1–6%). All patients with a groin recurrence underwent bilateral inguinofemoral lymphadenectomy and adjuvant (chemo)radiation. **Six of the eight patients died of disease,** while two remained disease-free at 6 and 50 months after recurrence. The median time to recurrence was 12 months (range 5 to 16 months). As expected, both short-term and long-term morbidity were significantly decreased in patients undergoing sentinel node biopsy only.

The results of the multicenter German study were also published in 2008 (131). Between 2003 and 2006, 127 women with T1–T3 vulvar cancer were entered onto the study. Radiotracer and blue dye were used in 72 patients (56.6%), radiotracer alone in 47 (37%), and blue dye alone in 8 (6.3%). In two cases (1.6%), no sentinel nodes were detected. **All patients underwent complete inguinofemoral lymphadenectomy. Positive nodes were identified in 39 cases (30.7%) at groin dissection, but three patients had a negative sentinel node, giving a false-negative rate of 7.7%.** In one additional midline tumor, the sentinel node was positive on one side, but falsely negative on the other, so **the actual false-negative rate for this study should be 10.3%**.

The GOG study was published in 2012 (132). Between 1999 and 2009, 452 eligible patients with squamous carcinomas 2 to 6 cm diameter were recruited. None had clinically suspicious groin nodes, and all underwent complete inguinofemoral lymphadenectomy. Blue dye was used for all patients, and radiotracer was mandated 2 years after study activation. The incidence of positive groin nodes among women with at least one sentinel node identified was 31.6% (132 of 418) and **the false-negative rate was 8.3% (11 of 132)**.

A single institution study from Poland highlights the need to continue to utilize sentinel node biopsy within a research protocol (133). Fifty-six patients with squamous cell carcinomas of the vulva 4 cm or less in diameter underwent sentinel node detection with radiotracer and blue dye, and 109 inguinofemoral lymphadenectomies were performed. Sentinel nodes were identified in 76% of patients with blue dye (82 of 108), and 99% with the radiotracer (106 of 107) ($p < 0.0001$). Positive sentinel nodes were found in 17% of groins (19 of 109), and there were 7 false-negative sentinel nodes, giving a **false-negative rate of 27%**. The authors concluded that in their setting, they could not recommend sentinel node biopsy as a reliable alternative to complete groin dissection. They felt that it was likely that "the main factor responsible for the high false-negative rate was the surgeon's experience. Although all the operations were performed by surgeons with at least 15 years' experience, the procedure was performed only a few times by each surgeon." This highlights the problem of introducing a technically challenging procedure for an uncommon disease.

If a sentinel node is positive, additional groin treatment is mandatory. In a review of the Groningen study, investigators reported that **there was no cutoff in the size of the metastatic focus in the sentinel node below which the chances of nonsentinel node metastases were close to zero** (134).

Sentinel node biopsy is considered to be standard practice in patients with early breast cancer, and in spite of false-negative rates of around 10%, isolated axillary failures are rare. This is because the majority of node-negative patients with breast cancer receive some type of adjuvant therapy that can effectively treat any micrometastases (135). This is not true for patients with vulvar cancer, where adjuvant radiation is not given to patients with negative nodes.

Recurrence in a groin following inguinofemoral lymphadenectomy and negative nodes is rare (Table 13.12) (22,71,89,99,110,136,137) but all attempts at modified groin dissection, including superficial inguinal dissection, have resulted in a groin recurrence rate of about 5% (Table 13.13) (68,96,107,110,111,138–140). The false-negative rate for vulvar sentinel node biopsy ranges from 3–27% (131–133), and in the hands of the average operator, is likely to be at least 7–10% (131,132). **About 80–90% of patients who develop a recurrence in an undissected groin will die from their disease, so while sentinel node biopsy will decrease the incidence of lymphedema, it is also important for the patient to be aware of the rate and consequences of a false-negative result.** Hence, **properly informed consent is crucial.**

Three studies have evaluated patient preferences in this regard. Firstly, de Hullu et al. (141) sent structured questionnaires both to patients who had been treated for vulvar cancer and to gynecologists. The response rate among patients was 91% (107 of 118). **Sixty percent of the patients preferred complete lymphadenectomy in preference to a 5% false-negative rate of the sentinel**

Table 13.12 Groin Recurrence Rate in Patients with Negative Nodes at Inguinofemoral Lymphadenectomy

Author	Number	Groin Recurrence (%)
Hacker et al., 1983 (22)	75	0 (0)
Burger et al., 1995 (136)	119	0 (0)
Bell et al., 2000 (137)	39	0 (0)
Rouzier et al., 2002 (71)	126	3[a] (2.4)
De Hulla et al., 2002 (99)	171	2[a] (1.2)
Bosquet et al., 2005 (110)	200	0 (0)
Tantipalakorn et al., 2009 (89)	102	0 (0)
Total	832	5 (0.6)

[a]Skin bridge recurrence.

node procedure. Their preference was not related to age or the side effects they had experienced. The response among gynecologists was 80% (80 of 100), of whom 60% were willing to accept a 5–20% false-negative rate for the sentinel node procedure. The authors concluded that **although gynecologists may consider this a promising approach, the majority of vulvar cancer patients would not advise its introduction, because they were not prepared to take any risk of missing a lymph node metastasis.**

Secondly, **a recent study of 60 patients with vulvar cancer from the Royal Hospital for Women in Sydney revealed similar findings. Although 73% of these women reported lymphedema, 80% indicated they would choose complete lymphadenectomy rather than take a 5% risk of a false-negative sentinel node procedure** (142). In fact, 53% (32 of 60) of the women said they would take no risk at all, and 10% said they would take a 1 in 1,000,000 chance.

Thirdly, **a Dutch group examined quality of life in patients from the Groningen study** (143). They compared 35 patients who underwent sentinel node biopsy only with 27 patients who underwent inguinofemoral lymphadenectomy because of a positive sentinel node. **In spite of increased lymphedema in the latter group, they found no difference in quality of life between the two groups.** They compared their results to those of two studies of a healthy population of women 60 years or older, and again found no difference. They admitted that their study did not support their original hypothesis that decreased long-term morbidity would translate into an improved quality of life, and **suggested that surviving cancer may change a patient's conceptualization of quality of life**.

If the sentinel lymph node procedure is performed after proper informed consent, it is important to undertake complete inguinofemoral lymphadenectomy if a sentinel node is not detected. This is

Table 13.13 Groin Recurrence Rate in Patients Having Negative Nodes at Modified Groin Dissection

Author	Number	Groin Recurrence (%)
Berman et al., 1989 (138)	49	0 (0)
Stehman et al., 1992 (111)	121	7 (5.8)
Gordinier et al., 2003 (68)	104	9 (8.7)
Kirby et al., 2005 (139)	65	3 (4.6)
Bosquet et al.,[a] 2005 (110)	17	1 (5.8)
Woolderink et al., 2006 (140)	91	6 (6.6)
DiSimone et al., 2007 (96)	96	1 (1.6)
Total	543	27 (5)

[a]Personal communication from Dr Karl Podratz.

particularly likely to occur for lesions close to the midline, when bilateral groin dissection would normally be required (28,144).

An Italian group recently reported the successful use of microsurgical lymphatic venous anastomosis to prevent lower limb lymphedema in patients undergoing inguinofemoral lymphadenectomy for vulvar cancer (145). There were only eight patients and seven historical controls in the study, and larger series of patients will be needed to clarify the utility of this technique.

In the author's opinion, an undissected groin should be followed with ultrasonography every 3 months for the first 12 months to allow early detection of any enlarging lymph nodes.

Management of a Patient with Positive Groin Nodes

Traditionally, patients with positive groin nodes had a pelvic lymphadenectomy, but in 1977, the GOG initiated a prospective trial in which patients with positive groin nodes were randomized to either ipsilateral pelvic node dissection or postoperative radiation to the bilateral pelvic and inguinal nodes (25). Radiation therapy consisted of 45 to 50 Gy to the midplane of the pelvis at a rate of 180 to 200 cGy/d. The survival rate for the radiation group (68% at 2 years) was significantly better than that for the pelvic lymphadenectomy group (54% at 2 years; $p = 0.03$). **A significant survival advantage was only seen in patients with clinically evident groin nodes or more than one positive groin node.** Groin recurrence occurred in 3 of 59 patients (5.1%) treated with radiation, compared with 13 of 55 (23.6%) treated with pelvic lymphadenectomy ($p = 0.02$). Four patients who received radiation had a pelvic recurrence compared with one who had lymphadenectomy, suggesting that there may be an advantage to resecting bulky pelvic lymph nodes before radiation.

Homesley's data highlight the value of prophylactic groin irradiation in preventing groin recurrence in patients with grossly involved or multiple positive groin nodes.

In the 1990s, several investigators demonstrated that there was a correlation between the morphology of positive groin nodes and outcome after lymphadenectomy and postoperative radiation. Origoni et al. (92) demonstrated that for patients with positive lymph nodes, there was a significant difference in survival, depending on the size of the involved nodes and the presence or absence of extracapsular spread. **Patients whose involved nodes were less than 5 mm in diameter had a 5-year survival rate of 90.9%, compared with 41.6% for nodes 5 to 15 mm in diameter and 20.6% for nodes larger than 15 mm diameter** ($p = 0.001$). Similarly, if nodal involvement remained intracapsular, the 5-year survival rate was 85.7%, compared with 25% if there was extracapsular spread ($p = 0.001$).

Similar results were obtained by the group at Gateshead, who reported that in a multivariate analysis, the only significant variables were FIGO stage (III, IVA, or IVB) and the presence or absence of extracapsular spread (146). Van der Velden et al. (147) demonstrated that **even for patients with one positive node, the presence of extracapsular spread decreased the survival rate from 88% (14 of 16 patients) to 44% (7 of 16 patients).** In 2006, Raspagliesi et al. reported a 10-year survival of 55% in lymph node positive patients with <50% of nodal replacement, compared to 34.3% in lymph node positive patients with >50% nodal replacement ($p < 0.01$) (72). They had a 10-year survival of 71% for patients with intracapsular metastases, and 29.8% for those with extracapsular spread ($p < 0.0004$).

These authors did not describe details of radiation therapy dose and technique and did not report on the relationship between regional morphology and the incidence of regional recurrence. In other settings (e.g., head and neck cancers), extracapsular extension is recognized as an indication for increased radiation dose (148).

From the foregoing observations, our **recommendations for the management of patients with positive groin nodes are as follows:**

1. **Patients with one micrometastasis (metastatic deposit ≤5 mm diameter) should be observed after radical lymphadenectomy.** The prognosis for this group of patients is excellent (18). Even if a unilateral groin dissection has been performed for a lateral lesion, there seems to be no indication for dissection of the other groin, because contralateral lymph node involvement is likely only if there are multiple ipsilateral inguinal node metastases (25,73). Dutch workers have also reported no benefit for adjuvant radiation for patients with one positive node without extracapsular spread (149).

2. **Patients with three or more micrometastases, one macrometastasis (>5 mm diameter), or any evidence of extracapsular spread should receive bilateral groin and pelvic radiation.**

3. **There are insufficient data on patients with two micrometastases to draw definitive conclusions.** If these patients are observed, it may be prudent to observe the contralateral groin with ultrasound for the first 6 to 12 months if it has not been dissected.

Advanced Disease

Vulvar cancer may be considered to be advanced on the basis of a T$_3$ or a T$_4$ primary tumor or the presence of bulky, positive groin nodes. Patients with T2 lesions that extensively involve the distal vagina, distal urethra or anus are also considered with this group, because the desire to preserve anal or urethral function may justify multidisciplinary treatment with radiation, with or without concurrent chemotherapy or surgery. Advanced vulvar cancer is uncommon in developed countries, and most data derive from single institutional experience or single-arm multi-institutional reports.

Management should be individualized, and a multidisciplinary team approach is desirable. As with early stage disease, it is advantageous to independently determine the most appropriate treatment for (i) the primary tumor and (ii) groin and pelvic lymph nodes.

Management of the Groin and Pelvic Lymph Nodes

All patients with advanced vulvar cancer should have detailed clinical examination and tomographic imaging of the groin, pelvis, and abdomen before surgery. Patients can then be triaged into three groups, as follows:

1. **Patients with no clinically or radiologically suspicious nodes.** There are **two possible approaches** to these patients. **They may be treated with bilateral inguinofemoral lymphadenectomy, performed through separate groin incisions.** If there are negative nodes or up to two micrometastases (<5-mm tumor deposits) without extracapsular spread, the groins may be eliminated from any subsequent radiation fields. As with early stage disease, if there is one macrometastasis (>5-mm tumor deposit), three or more micrometastases, or extracapsular spread, pelvic and groin radiation is indicated. **An alternative approach that may be preferred in selected patients is to treat the groins with primary radiation, along with the vulvar lesion.** This approach requires thorough review of tomographic imaging to verify that there are no suspicious nodes and careful treatment planning to assure adequate coverage of the inguinofemoral and distal pelvic lymph nodes. Several authors have demonstrated that recurrence in the groin is very rare under these circumstances (150,151).

2. **Patients with clinically or radiologically suspicious resectable nodes.**
   i. **All enlarged groin nodes should be removed** through a separate incision approach and sent for frozen-section diagnosis. If metastatic disease is confirmed, full lymphadenectomy should not be carried out.
   ii. **Any enlarged pelvic nodes seen on CT scan should be removed** by an extraperitoneal approach.
   iii. **Full pelvic and groin irradiation should be given** as soon as the groin incisions are healed, usually within 3 weeks.
   iv. **If the frozen section reveals no metastatic disease** in the removed nodes, **full groin dissection should be performed.** We have reported our experience with resection of bulky positive nodes rather than full groin dissection for patients with advanced vulvar cancer (31). Seventeen patients treated by nodal debulking in Australia were compared with 23 similar patients treated by full groin dissection at the Academic Medical Hospital in Amsterdam. Both groups of patients received groin and pelvic radiation postoperatively. **Both disease-specific survival and groin recurrence-free intervals were superior in the group having nodal debulking** although with the small numbers in both series, the differences were not statistically significant.

3. **Patients with fixed, unresectable groin nodes** (Fig. 13.11). These patients should be treated with primary groin and pelvic radiation, probably combined with chemotherapy. It may be appropriate to resect a residual groin mass following radiation if

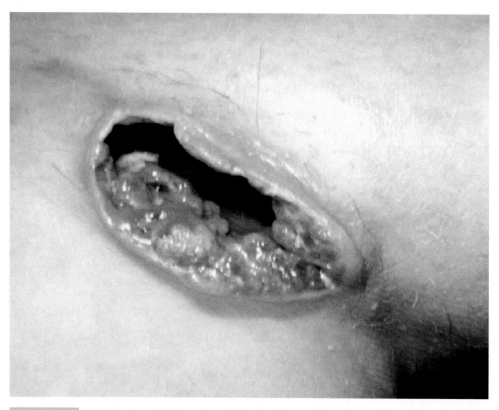

Figure 13.11 A fixed ulcerated lymph node in the right groin.

there is an incomplete response to radiation and no other evidence of metastatic disease (152).

An algorithm for the management of patients with advanced vulvar cancer is shown in Figure 13.12.

Management of the Primary Tumor

Surgery

If the tumor involves the distal vagina and/or urethral orifice and can be resected with clear surgical margins without need for a stoma, primary surgical resection is the best option. Radical vulvectomy often will be required, although a modified radical vulvectomy to allow adequate clearance around the lesion while preserving some normal vulva may also be appropriate.

Traditionally, the *en bloc* **approach** through a trapezoid or butterfly incision has been used (153) (Fig. 13.13), and this may still be useful if there is extensive disease anteriorly. More commonly **the separate incision approach is used,** which involves using three separate incisions, one for the radical vulvectomy and one for each groin dissection (26).

Technique for *En Bloc* Radical Vulvectomy and Groin Dissection

The operation is usually performed with the patient in the low lithotomy position, and groin and vulvar dissections can proceed simultaneously with two teams of surgeons if appropriate. The skin incision has been significantly modified from the original Stanley Way technique to allow primary skin closure. The groin dissection is accomplished initially, with the abdominal incision carried down to the aponeurosis of the external oblique muscle, approximately 2 cm above the inguinal ligament. A skin flap is raised over the femoral triangle, with preservation of the subcutaneous fat above the superficial (Camper) fascia. The technique for groin dissection has been described earlier.

The vulvar incision is carried posteriorly along each labiocrural fold, or within a 1-cm margin of the primary lesion. The technique for vulvectomy is described in the next section.

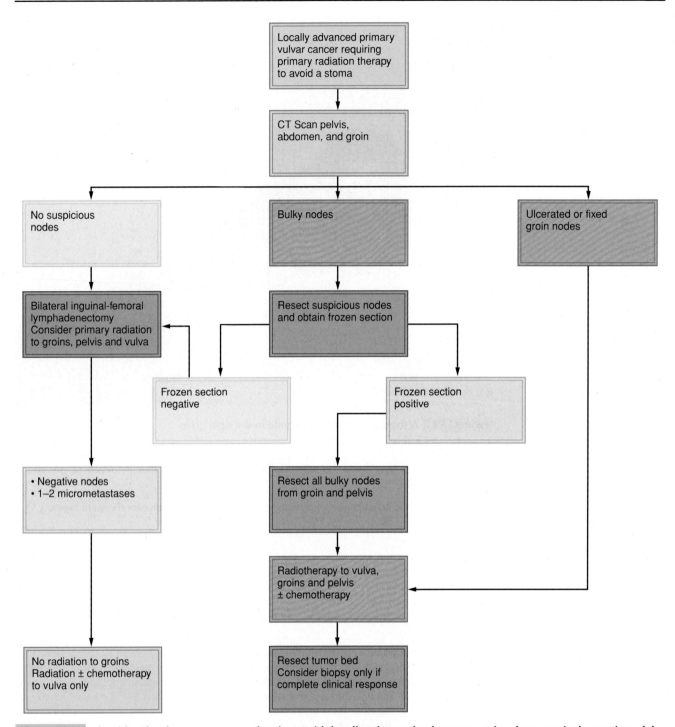

Figure 13.12 Algorithm for the management of patients with locally advanced vulvar cancer, in whom surgical resection of the primary tumor would necessitate a stoma.

Technique for Radical Vulvectomy

If the radical vulvectomy is performed through a separate incision, the lateral incision is basically elliptical. Each lateral incision should commence on the mons pubis anteriorly and extend through the fat and superficial fascia to the fascia over the pubic symphysis. It is then easy to develop bluntly the plane immediately above the pubic symphysis and fascia lata. The skin incision is extended posteriorly along the labiocrural folds to the perianal area and carried down to the fascia lata. The medial incision is placed to clear the tumor with margins of at least 1 cm. If necessary,

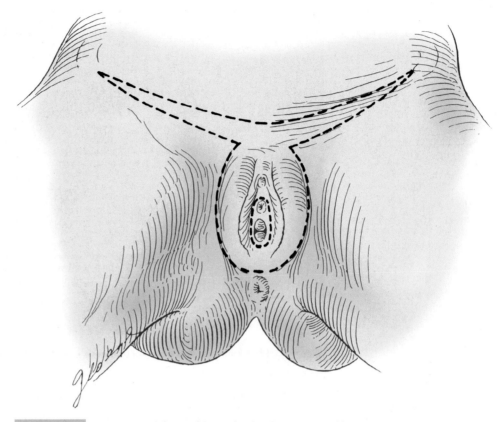

Figure 13.13 Incision used for *en bloc* radical vulvectomy and bilateral groin dissection.

the distal half of the urethra may be resected without compromising continence. If the tumor is involving the urethra or the vagina, dissection around the tumor is facilitated by transection of the vulva, thereby improving exposure of the involved area.

The specimen includes the bulbocavernosus muscles and the vestibular bulb. Because of the vascularity, it is desirable to perform most of the dissection by diathermy after the initial skin incision. In addition, the vessels supplying the clitoris should be clamped and tied, as should the internal pudendal vessels posterolaterally.

Closure of Large Defects

It is usually possible to close the vulvar defect without tension. If a more extensive dissection has been required because of a large primary lesion, a number of options are available to repair the defect. These include the following:

1. **An area may be left open to granulate,** which it usually does over a period of 6 to 8 weeks (154). This is particularly useful around the urethra, where sutures can cause urethral deviation and misdirection of the urinary stream.

2. **Full-thickness skin flaps may be devised** (155). An example is the rhomboid flap, which is best suited for covering large defects of the posterior vulva (156).

3. **Unilateral or bilateral gracilis myocutaneous grafts** may be developed (Fig. 13.14). These are most useful when an extensive area from the mons pubis to the perianal area has been resected. Because the graft brings a new blood supply to the area, it is particularly applicable if the vulva is poorly vascularized from prior surgical resection or radiation (157).

4. **If extensive defects exist in the groin and vulva, the tensor fascia lata myocutaneous graft may be applicable** (158).

Management of patients for whom primary tumor involves the anus or proximal urethra.

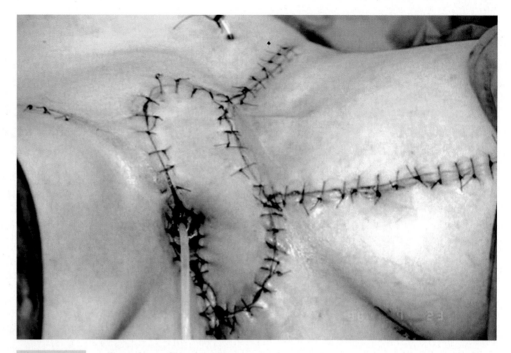

Figure 13.14   Unilateral gracilis myocutaneous graft used to cover a large lateral vulvar defect.

Pelvic Exenteration

When the primary disease involves the anus, rectum, rectovaginal septum, or proximal urethra, **adequate surgical clearance of the primary tumor is possible only by some type of infralevator exenteration, (anterior, posterior, or total), combined with radical vulvectomy and bilateral groin dissection**. Such radical surgery is usually inappropriate for these patients; even in medically fit, suitable surgical candidates, psychological (97,159) and postoperative morbidity are high. Nevertheless, a 5-year survival rate of approximately 50% can be expected with this approach (160–162). Spread to regional lymph nodes and complete resection are the most important prognostic factors following pelvic exenteration (162).

Preoperative Radiation Therapy

Boronow (27) was the first to suggest a combined radiosurgical approach as an alternative to pelvic exenteration for patients with advanced vulvar cancer. A second report of this experience, published in 1987, had three major refinements: (i) The use of external-beam therapy for all cases, with more selective use of brachytherapy; (ii) more conservative vulvar surgery; and (iii) resection of bulky N_2 and N_3 nodes without full groin dissection to minimize lymphedema. The 5-year survival rate for 37 primary cases was 75.6%, and for 11 recurrent cases 62.6%. Seventeen of 40 vulvectomy specimens (42.5%) contained no residual disease. There were a number of major complications in this early series, particularly in patients who received brachytherapy using techniques that are rarely used today.

In 1984, Hacker et al. (28) reported the use of preoperative teletherapy in eight patients with advanced vulvar cancer; brachytherapy was reserved for patients with persistent disease that would otherwise necessitate exenteration (Figs. 13.15 and 13.16). Rather than performing radical vulvectomy for all patients, only the tumor bed was resected, on the assumption that any microscopic foci originally present in the vulva would have been sterilized by the radiation. In specimens from one-half of the patients, there was no residual disease. Long-term morbidity was low with the predominant use of teletherapy, and no patient developed a fistula. Four patients, including two whose primary tumor was fixed to bone, were long-term survivors (28).

In 1989, Thomas et al. (163) was the first to report on the use of chemoradiation for patients with advanced vulvar cancer. Several subsequent studies have reported that complete pathologic response rates of between 31% and 55% can be achieved in these patients even with modest doses of radiation (164–170). However the pathologic response rates seen with chemoradiation were not obviously superior to those achieved with radiation alone.

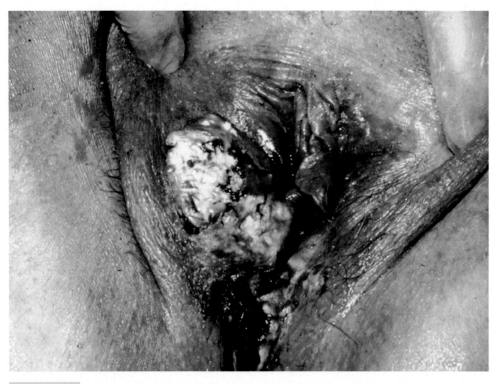

Figure 13.15 **Advanced squamous cell carcinoma of the vulva involving the anal canal.** A primary surgical approach would have necessitated radical vulvectomy, anoproctectomy, and permanent colostomy.

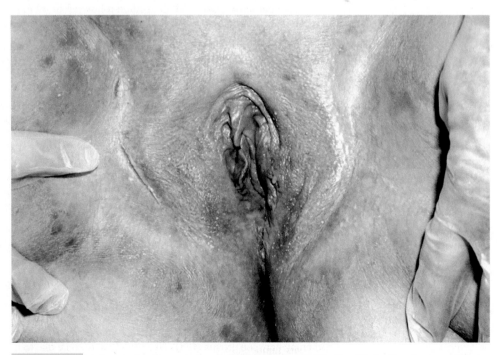

Figure 13.16 **Advanced vulvar cancer shown in Figure 13.15 after 50.4 cGy of external-beam radiation therapy.** Resection of the tumor bed showed microscopic residual disease. The radiation therapy prevented the need for a permanent stoma.

In 2008, Beriwal et al. (171) reported 18 patients having preoperative intensity-modulated radiotherapy and chemotherapy for locally advanced vulvar cancer. The median dose of radiation was 46 Gy and patients had a scheduled treatment break of 11 to 18 days. Fourteen patients had surgery performed, with a pathologic complete response in 9 patients (64%) and a partial response in 5 (36%).

In 2012, the GOG reported a phase II trial of radiation and concurrent weekly *cisplatin* (40 mg/m^2) for patients with locally advanced vulvar cancer (168). Of the 58 eligible patients entered in the trial, 79% completed the planned total dose of 57.6 Gy in 32 fractions; 69% completed radiation therapy and had at least five cycles of chemotherapy. Following completion of radiation, patients had a surgical resection of residual tumor or biopsy to confirm a complete clinical response. **A complete clinical response was achieved in 37 of the 58 patients (64%); of these 37 patients, 29 (78%) also had a complete pathologic response confirmed by biopsy.** However, 5 of these 29 had failed locoregionally by the time of the data analysis. **With a median follow-up of 24.8 months, 31 women (53.4%) were alive without evidence of recurrence.**

A number of other small studies have evaluated the role of preoperative chemoradiation in patients with locally advanced vulvar cancer (169,170,172). These confirm that **patients who have had an apparent complete clinical response to 40 to 45 Gy have a better outcome than those who do not completely respond.** Some studies suggest that the severity of acute cutaneous reactions are greater with chemoradiation, and may be related to the type of chemotherapy delivered (163,169,170,172). A number of different chemotherapeutic regimens have been used including different schedules and combinations of *cisplatin* alone, *cisplatin* plus *5-fluorouracil,* and *cisplatin* plus *mitomycin-C.* However, these single institution studies are all relatively small and heterogeneous, limiting the ability to draw generalizable conclusions.

Neoadjuvant Chemotherapy

In 2006, a study from Indianapolis reported the use of neoadjuvant chemotherapy for patients whose vulvar cancer involved the anus and or urethra (173). Ten patients received *cisplatin* and *5-fluorouracil (5-FU)*, and three received *cisplatin* alone. Patients receiving *cisplatin* alone showed no measurable response, while all patients receiving *cisplatin* and *5-FU* achieved at least a partial response. With a median follow-up of 49 months (3 to 90 months) **nine patients receiving *cisplatin* and *5-FU* followed by surgery remained disease-free, and a stoma was averted in all cases**.

A prospective, multicenter study of neoadjuvant chemotherapy for locally advanced vulvar cancer was reported from Buenos Aires in 2012 (174). Thirty-five patients were recruited to the study, and a variety of different chemotherapeutic regimens were used. Twenty-seven patients (77%) underwent radical surgery, including two who required posterior exenteration for persistent rectal involvement. **Twenty-four patients (68.6%) were without evidence of disease, with a median follow-up of 49 months (range 4 to 155 months).**

Summary

With the experience currently accrued, **preoperative radiation, with or without concurrent chemotherapy, should be regarded as the treatment of choice for patients with advanced vulvar cancer who would otherwise require some type of pelvic exenteration.**

There is a need to accrue more experience with neoadjuvant chemotherapy in this setting. If it could be shown to be at least comparable to radiation, it would become the treatment of choice, because of the significant morbidity associated with the latter.

Role of Radiation Therapy in Vulvar Cancer

Radiation therapy is playing an increasingly important role in the management of patients with vulvar cancer, but a "Patterns of Care" study among members of the Gynecologic Cancer Intergroup revealed differences in the indications for treatment, treatment fields, and use of chemotherapy between groups (175). This was thought to be due to the rarity of the disease, and the lack of randomized trials.

The indications for radiation therapy in patients with this disease are still evolving. At present, radiation seems to be clearly indicated in the following situations:

1. **For patients with advanced disease** who would otherwise require pelvic exenteration. Data indicate that high complete response rates can be achieved with radiation therapy,

with or without chemotherapy. High local control rates have been achieved in selected patients with 40 to 50 Gy followed by organ sparing surgery. In cases where surgery would still risk organ dysfunction, radiation alone (using a higher dose of 60 Gy or more for gross disease) may be the initial treatment of choice, reserving radical surgery for local recurrence.

2. **After surgery, to treat the pelvic lymph nodes and groins** in patients with more than two micrometastases, one macrometastasis, or extracapsular spread.

3. **After surgery, to help prevent local recurrence** and improve survival **in patients with involved surgical margins** (<5 mm) (176,177). Faul et al. (177) from Pittsburgh retrospectively reviewed 62 patients with invasive vulvar carcinoma who had either positive or close (≤8 mm) margins of excision. Half the patients ($n = 31$) were treated with adjuvant radiation to the vulva, and half were observed after surgery. Local recurrence occurred in 58% of the observed patients and 16% following adjuvant radiation. **Twelve patients who had postoperative radiation therapy for positive vulvar margins had a significantly lower 5-year local recurrence rate than 16 patients who had no postoperative radiation (80% vs. 37%, respectively).** Postoperative radiation was also associated with a significantly better overall survival ($p = 0.001$). Patients who had close margins had a significantly better local control but no significant improvement in survival if they had postoperative radiation.

Possible roles for radiation therapy include the following:

1. **As primary therapy for patients with small primary tumors, particularly clitoral or periclitoral lesions** in young and middle-aged women, in whom surgical resection would have significant psychological consequences (103).

2. **As an alternative to groin dissection in patients with N_0 lymph nodes.** In 1992, the GOG reported the results of a phase III trial in which patients with T_1, T_2, or T_3 tumors and N_0 or N_1 groin nodes were randomized between surgical resection (and postoperative irradiation for patients with positive groin nodes) and primary groin irradiation (178). The study was closed prematurely after 5 of 26 patients in the groin irradiation arm had recurrences in the groin. Of 23 patients randomized to surgical resection, five had groin node metastases and received postoperative radiation to the ipsilateral groin and hemipelvis; at a median follow-up of approximately 3 years, none of the patients treated with initial lymphadenectomy had a groin recurrence. These results probably do not generalize to current practice. In the GOG study, pretreatment imaging to detect enlarged groin nodes was not performed, and the radiation technique did not take adequate account of the depth of the nodes (179). The dose of radiation was 5,000 cGy given in daily 200-cGy fractions to a depth of 3 cm below the anterior skin surface. Subsequent **retrospective clinical reviews have suggested that radiation alone can control microscopic nodal disease if adequate coverage of the inguinal and femoral nodes is confirmed** (150,151).

Recurrent Vulvar Cancer

Most treatment failures are diagnosed within 2 years (110), and in patients with early disease, most recurrences are on the vulva. Distant metastases do occur, particularly in the presence of multiple lymph node metastases (22,180).

Rouzier et al. (71) from France identified three patterns of local recurrence with very different prognoses: (i) primary tumor site recurrence (up to and including 2 cm from the vulvectomy scar); (ii) **remote vulvar recurrence (>2 cm from the primary tumor site)**; and (iii) **skin bridge recurrence**. Their study included 215 patients, and the local relapse-free survival was 78.6% at 5 years. Patients with positive margins who did not receive radiotherapy and patients with greater than 1-mm stromal invasion who did not have a groin dissection were excluded from analysis.

Local recurrence at a site distant from the primary tumor (which could be considered a new primary lesion), had a good prognosis, 66.7% of patients surviving 3 years. **By contrast, survival after recurrence at the primary tumor site was poor,** only 15.4% of patients surviving 3 years. None of seven patients with a skin bridge recurrence was alive at 1 year.

Review of our own data from the Royal Hospital for Women in Sydney has confirmed that these patterns of local recurrence are distinct entities, although we saw no skin bridge recurrences (89). In our experience, **primary site recurrences** occurred at a median interval of 21 months, and were more commonly associated with surgical margins <8 mm. By contrast,

remote site vulvar recurrences occurred at a median interval of 69 months, and were commonly associated with lichen sclerosus or VIN. In contrast to Rouzier, **our patients with both primary and remote site recurrence had an excellent prognosis**.

Local vulvar recurrences are usually amenable to further surgical resection (26,71,181). A variety of plastic surgical techniques may facilitate adequate surgical resection, particularly for larger recurrences. Myocutaneous grafts which may be used include the gluteal thigh flap, the rectus abdominous flap, the gracilis flap, and the tensor fascia lata flap (182).

Radiation therapy also has been used to treat vulvar recurrences. Hoffman et al. (183) reported 10 patients treated in this manner, and 9 were still alive with a mean follow-up of 28 months. However, 6 of the 10 had severe radionecrosis at a median of 8.5 months after radiation, and the authors concluded that although this treatment was highly effective, it was also highly morbid. Many of the cases in this series were treated with brachytherapy. **When brachytherapy is used in this region, great care must be taken not to have radiation sources close to vulvar skin or mucous membranes,** because the dose of radiation close to interstitial needles can be 5 to 10 times greater than the prescribed dose. For this reason, and because reports of patients treated with brachytherapy for vulvar cancer tend to have high rates of necrosis, many gynecologic radiation oncologists avoid its use in this region. **Modern conformal external beam radiation techniques such as intensity-modulated radiotherapy (IMRT) deliver a more homogeneous dose to vulvovaginal target tissues,** and would be expected to have a much lower risk of necrosis; however, few data specific to locally recurrent disease treated are available.

Regional and distant recurrences are difficult to manage (176). Although survival rates are low, some patients are cured with surgery and regional radiation therapy (184). Chemotherapeutic agents that have activity against squamous carcinomas may be offered for distant metastases. The most active agents are *cisplatin, methotrexate, cyclophosphamide, bleomycin,* and *mitomycin C,* but response rates are low and the duration of response is usually disappointing (185).

Recently, a targeted therapy was used for the first time in patients with vulvar cancer. The epidermal growth factor receptor (EGFR) inhibitor, *erlotinib,* was trialed in 41 patients, 11 (27.5%) of whom had a partial response and 16 (40%) had stable disease. Responses were of short duration, but toxicities were acceptable (186).

Prognosis

With appropriate management, the prognosis for vulvar cancer is generally good, the overall 5-year survival rate in operable cases being approximately 70%. Survival correlates with the 1988 FIGO clinical stage of disease (Table 13.14) (22,105,152,187–190) and also with lymph node status. In the 26th FIGO annual report, patients with negative lymph nodes had a 5-year survival rate of 80.7%; the survival rate fell to 13.3% for patients with four or more positive nodes (Table 13.15) (191). The GOG staged 588 patients with vulvar cancer by the 1988 FIGO surgical staging criteria, and reported 5-year survival rates of 98%, 85%, 74%, and 31% for stages I, II, III, and IV, respectively (87). There are insufficient data currently available to give figures for the 2009 FIGO staging system.

The number of positive groin nodes is the single most important prognostic variable (22,24,25,91,93,191), and **the survival rate for patients with positive pelvic nodes is only about**

Table 13.14 Five-Year Survival versus FIGO Clinical Stage for Patients Treated with Curative Intent			
FIGO Clinical Stage	*No.*	*Dead of Disease*	*Corrected 5-Year Survival (%)*
I	376	36	90.4
II	310	71	77.1
III	238	116	51.3
IV	111	91	18
Total	**1,035**	**314**	**69.7**

FIGO, International Federation of Gynecology and Obstetrics.

Data compiled from **Rutledge et al., 1970** (105); **Boutselis, 1972** (187); **Morley, 1976** (153); **Japeze et al., 1977** (188); **Benedet et al., 1979** (189); **Hacker et al., 1983** (22); **Cavanagh et al., 1986** (190).

Table 13.15 Five-Year Survival versus Lymph Node Status for Squamous Cell Carcinoma of the Vulva

Lymph Node Status	Patients	5-Year Survival (%)	Hazard Ratio (95% CI)
Negative	302	80.7	Reference
1 positive	66	62.9	2.1 (1.2–3.4)
2 positive	43	30.4	6 (3.7–9.8)
3 positive	24	19.2	5.3 (3–9.5)
4+ positive	62	13.3	2.6 (1.9–3.7)

Modified from the 26th FIGO Annual Report on the Results of Treatment in Gynecological Cancer (190).

11% (85). Patients with one microscopically positive node have a good prognosis (22,24), but patients with three or more positive nodes have a poor prognosis (22,101). Extracapsular spread is a poor prognostic factor (92,146,147).

Before the report of GOG-37 (25), patients who had pelvic node metastases were usually treated with surgery alone. The poor outcome of such patients in the control arm of GOG-37 and other early experience led clinicians to place these patients in the stage IVB category; however, there is evidence that many patients with pelvic node metastases can be cured if they receive postoperative or definitive radiation therapy. Microscopic pelvic node metastases are rarely detected today because elective node dissections are not performed; however, **a recent review of patients treated with definitive radiation therapy for grossly involved pelvic lymph nodes demonstrated an overall survival rate of 43% at 5 years despite extensive locoregional disease** (192). These data suggest that patients with regional disease confined to the groin and distal pelvis should be treated with curative intent whenever possible.

Workers at the Norwegian Radium Hospital evaluated the prognostic significance of DNA ploidy in 118 patients (193), and aberrant expression of the cell cycle kinase inhibitors p16, p21, and p27 among 224 patients with squamous cell carcinomas of the vulva (194). **A low level of p16 protein, a high level of p21 protein, and aneuploidy were associated with a shorter disease-specific survival.** Dutch workers have shown that overexpression of cyclooxygenase 2 (COX-2) is also associated with a poor disease-specific survival (195).

There is often a tendency to undertreat patients over the age of 80, on the false assumption that they will die of other causes before the cancer recurs. **It is a fundamental error to treat any patient on the basis of chronologic rather than biologic age,** and British workers reported a 25% recurrence rate for patients with vulvar cancer over 80 years treated according to their standard protocol, compared to a 53% recurrence rate when there was a protocol violation (196).

A study from Amsterdam reported 75 patients aged 80 years or older, 57 (76%) of whom had standard treatment for vulvar cancer (197). When preoperatively available parameters of all patients were assessed in relation to survival in the total group, Eastern Cooperative Oncology Group (ECOG) performance status was the only independent prognostic variable. When all clinical and histopathologic variables were assessed in the subgroup that had standard treatment, both **ECOG performance status and extracapsular lymph node involvement were independent prognostic variables for overall survival. Age was not a significant prognostic variable.**

Table 13.16 Microstaging of Vulvar Melanomas

Clark's Levels, 1969 (204)		Chung et al., 1975 (201)	Breslow, 1970 (205)
I	Intraepithelial	Intraepithelial	<0.76 mm
II	Into papillary dermis	≤1 mm from granular layer	0.76–1.50 mm
III	Filling dermal papillae	1.1–2 mm from granular layer	1.51–2.25 mm
IV	Into reticular dermis	>2 mm from granular layer	2.26–3 mm
V	Into subcutaneous fat	Into subcutaneous fat	>3 mm

Stage	Primary Tumor (T)	Lymph Node (N)	Metastases (M)
Table 13.17 Revised 2002 American Joint Committee on Cancer (AJCC) Staging for Cutaneous Melanoma			
0	*In situ* (Tis)	No nodes	None
IA	<1 mm no ulceration/Clark's II and III (T1a)	No nodes	None
IB	<1 mm + ulceration/Clark's IV and V (T1b) 1.01–2 mm no ulceration (T2a)	No nodes	None
IIA	1.01–2 mm + ulceration (T2b) 2.01–4 mm no ulceration (T3a)	No nodes	None
IIB	2.01–4 mm+ ulceration (T3b) >4 mm no ulceration	No nodes	None
IIC	>4 mm + ulceration (T4b)	No nodes	None
IIIA	Any thickness, no ulceration	1 node micrometastasis (n1a)	None
IIIB	Any thickness, with ulceration Any thickness, no ulceration Any thickness, ± ulceration	1 node micrometastasis (n1a) Up to 3 nodes micrometastases (n2a) In-transit met/satellites + positive nodes (n2c)	None None
IIIC	Any thickness, with ulceration Any thickness, ± ulceration	Up to 3 nodes macrometastases (n2b) ≥4 metastatic nodes/matted nodes/in-transit with positive nodes (n3)	None None
IV	Any thickness	Any nodes	Present

Follow-up

Patients with vulvar cancer should be seen every 3 months for 2 years, every 6 months for 5 years, and at least annually for life. Data from the Mayo Clinic have shown that **in 35% of cases, vulvar cancer recurs 5 years or more after diagnosis** (110). Virtually all these late recurrences are on the vulva, and many start as *in situ* disease, which can often be resected in the office under local anesthesia if diagnosed early enough. **Patients should be taught self-examination,** and told to seek attention if they develop any vulvar irritation or visual change.

Melanoma

Vulvar melanomas are rare. Most arise *de novo* (198), but they may arise from a pre-existing junctional nevus. **They occur predominantly in postmenopausal white women, most commonly on the labia minora or the clitoris** (Fig. 13.17).

A recent study compared 762 patients with a vulvar/vaginal melanoma with 55,485 patients with a cutaneous melanoma (199). The data were obtained from the SEER database from 1973 to 2008. **Compared to cutaneous melanomas, patients with vulvar/vaginal melanomas were more likely to be older (68 vs. 52 years; $p < 0.0001$), and to present with advanced disease (8.4% vs. 2.7%; $p < 0.008$).**

Most vulvar melanomas are asymptomatic. Some patients have itching or bleeding, and a few present with a groin mass. Amelanotic varieties occasionally occur. **Any pigmented lesion on the vulva should be excised or biopsied, unless it has been present and unchanged for some years.**

There are three basic histologic types: (i) The **superficial spreading melanoma,** which tends to remain relatively superficial early in its development; (ii) the **mucosal lentiginous melanoma,** a flat freckle, which may become quite extensive but also tends to remain superficial; and (iii) the **nodular melanoma,** which is a raised lesion that penetrates deeply and may metastasize widely. A Swedish study of 219 cases reported that the mucosal lentiginous melanoma was the most frequent type (57%) (200).

Staging

The FIGO staging used for squamous lesions is not applicable for melanomas, because these lesions are usually much smaller and the prognosis is related to the depth of penetration rather than to the diameter of the lesion (201–203). The leveling system established by Clark et al. (204) for cutaneous melanomas is less readily applicable to vulvar lesions because of the different skin morphology. Chung et al. (201) proposed a modified system that retained Clark's

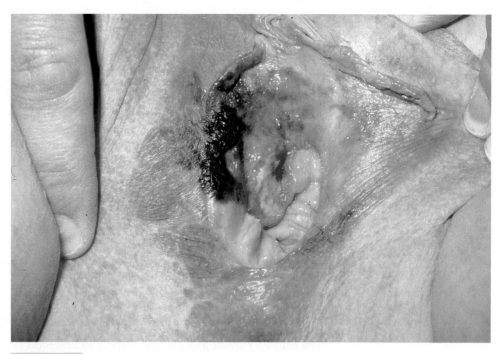

Figure 13.17 Melanoma of the vulva involving the right labium minus.

definitions for levels I and V but arbitrarily defined levels II, III, and IV, using measurements in millimeters. Breslow (205) measured the thickest portion of the melanoma from the surface of intact epithelium to the deepest point of invasion. A comparison of these systems is shown in Table 13.14.

A revised American Joint Committee on Cancer (AJCC) Staging System for cutaneous melanomas came into effect in 2002 (206) (Table 13.15). Prognostic factors taken into account include primary tumor thickness (replacing level of invasion), ulceration, number of metastatic lymph nodes, micrometastatic disease based on sentinel lymph node biopsy or elective node dissection, the site(s) of distant disease, and serum lactate dehydrogenase (LDH) levels. This system appears to be most applicable for vulvar melanomas (207).

Treatment

Management of the Primary Lesion

Although vulvar melanomas are rare, it has become apparent from several small series that **the same surgical principles that apply to cutaneous melanomas should also be used for vulvar melanomas** (207). More conservative surgery for cutaneous melanomas commenced in the 1980s (208,209), and although vulvar melanomas carry a much worse prognosis, this trend has been followed (210–215).

In 1992, Trimble et al. (212) reported on 59 patients who underwent radical vulvectomy and 19 who underwent more conservative resections. Survival was not improved by the more radical approach. In 1994, the GOG conducted a prospective clinicopathologic study of 71 evaluable patients with melanoma of the vulva diagnosed between 1983 and 1990 (214). All patients were required to have had at least a radical hemivulvectomy. **Seven of 37 patients (19%) having radical vulvectomy developed a local recurrence, compared with 3 of 34 (9%) having a hemivulvectomy.** Subsequently, a multicenter US study of 77 patients in 2011 (207), and a Mayo Clinic report of 36 patients in 2013 (215) confirmed the validity of conservative vulvar resection, as for squamous lesions.

As melanomas commonly involve the clitoris and labia minora, the vaginourethral margin of resection is a common site of failure. If necessary, the distal urethra may have to be resected to obtain an inner margin of at least 1 cm. Podratz et al. (203) demonstrated a 10-year survival rate of 61% for lateral lesions, compared with 37% for medial lesions (p < 0.027).

Management of the Groin Lymph Nodes

The advisability of groin node dissection is controversial. **The Intergroup Surgical Melanoma Program conducted a prospective, multi-institutional, randomized trial of elective lymph node dissection versus observation for intermediate thickness cutaneous melanomas** (1 to 4 mm) (216). There were 740 patients entered into the trial, and **elective lymph node dissection resulted in a significantly better 5-year survival rate for the 522 patients 60 years of age or younger** (88% vs. 81%; $p < 0.04$), the 335 **patients with tumors 1 to 2 mm thick** (96% vs. 86%; $p < 0.02$), the 403 **patients without tumor ulceration** (95% vs. 84%; $p < 0.01$), and the 284 **patients with tumors 1 to 2 mm thick and no ulceration** (97% vs. 87%; $p < 0.005$).

Current practice patterns in cutaneous melanomas utilize sentinel node biopsy, with ultrastaging, to assess lymph node status (217,218), and this approach has also been explored in vulvar melanomas (219,220). De Hullu et al. reported 9 patients with vulvar melanoma who underwent a **sentinel node procedure** (219). **Two of nine patients (22%) developed a groin recurrence after having negative sentinel nodes,** compared to 0 of 24 patients who were treated conventionally ($p = 0.06$). The authors postulated that the recurrences were due to in-transit metastases.

As with sentinel nodes in squamous carcinoma of the vulva, sentinel node biopsy in patients with vulvar melanoma is a compromise operation, but in a well-informed patient, in the hands of an experienced team, and with ultrastaging of the negative nodes, lymphatic mapping would seem to be significantly superior to no node dissection for patients with more than 1 mm of stromal invasion. **Lesions with less than 1 mm of invasion may be treated with radical local excision alone** (207,212).

The author's current policy is to perform a radical local excision with 1-cm margins for the primary lesion. In patients with more than 1 mm of stromal invasion, at least an ipsilateral inguinofemoral lymphadenectomy is performed. Sentinel node biopsy is reserved for the few patients who do not want to take the 50–60% risk of developing lymphedema.

Adjuvant Therapy

Interferon alpha-2b (IFN-α-2b) **was the first agent to show significant value as an adjuvant for melanoma in a randomized controlled trial** (221). The ECOG entered 287 patients onto an adjuvant trial of high-dose *IFN-α-2b* after surgery for deep primary (>4 mm) or regionally metastatic melanoma. With a median follow-up of 6.9 years, there was a significant prolongation of relapse-free and overall survival for the group receiving interferon, and the proportion of patients who remained disease free improved from 26% to 37%.

The results were confirmed in a larger intergroup trial that compared the efficacy of high-dose *IFN-α-2b* for 1 year with vaccination using GM2 conjugated to keyhole limpet hemocyanin (222). Eight hundred and eighty patients were randomized, and the trial was closed after interim analysis indicated inferiority of the vaccination compared with high-dose *interferon-α-2b*.

High-dose interferon regimens cause significant morbidity (223), and a 2012 systematic review of adjuvant interferon therapy in patients with high-risk, resected primary melanomas showed no overall survival benefit (223). However, a significant improvement in disease-free survival for high-dose interferon or pegylated interferon treatment was shown.

A 2013 study from the Mayo Clinic reported promising preliminary results in one patient with a 5-cm anterior vulvar melanoma using two cycles of *carboplatin* and *paclitaxel* (CP) plus *bevacizumab* preoperatively. After resection, the patient received two further cycles of CP, and remained disease free at 2 years (215).

Because of the rarity of vulvar melanomas, **consideration should be given to entering these patients onto clinical trials for cutaneous melanomas.**

Prognosis

The behavior of vulvar melanomas can be quite unpredictable, but the overall prognosis is poor. **The mean 5-year survival rate for reported cases of vulvar melanoma ranges from 21.7%** (198) **to 54%** (200). Patients with lesions invading to 1 mm or less have an excellent prognosis, but as depth of invasion increases, prognosis worsens. Chung et al. (201) reported a corrected 5-year survival rate of 100% for patients with level II lesions, 40% for level III or IV lesions, and 20% for level V lesions. Tumor volume has been reported to correlate with prognosis, with patients whose lesion has a volume less than 100 mm^3 having an excellent prognosis (224). DNA ploidy and angio-invasion have been shown to be independent prognostic factors for disease-free survival (225).

Bartholin Gland Carcinoma

Primary carcinoma of Bartholin gland accounts for approximately 5% of vulvar malignancies. Because of its rarity, individual experience with the tumor is limited, and recommendations for management must be based on literature reviews (69,226).

The bilateral Bartholin glands are greater vestibular glands situated posterolaterally in the vulva. Their main duct is lined with stratified squamous epithelium, which changes to transitional epithelium as the terminal ducts are reached. Because tumors may arise from the gland or the duct, **a variety of histologic types may occur, including adenocarcinomas, squamous carcinomas, and, rarely, transitional cell, adenosquamous, and adenoid cystic carcinomas**. One case of small cell neuroendocrine cancer of the Bartholin gland has been reported (227).

Classification of a vulvar tumor as a Bartholin gland carcinoma has typically required that it fulfills criteria proposed by **Honan in 1897. These criteria are as follows:**

1. **The tumor is in the correct anatomic position.**
2. **The tumor is located deep in the labium majus.**
3. **The overlying skin is intact.**
4. **There is some recognizable normal gland present.**

Strict adherence to these criteria may result in under diagnosis. Large tumors may ulcerate through the overlying skin and obliterate the residual normal gland. Although transition between normal and malignant tissue is the best criterion, some cases are diagnosed on the basis of their histologic characteristics and anatomic location.

Bartholin gland carcinomas are often misdiagnosed initially as a Bartholin cyst or abscess. A study from Tampa reported that 8 of 11 cases had initially been treated for an infectious process before referral (228). Other differential diagnoses of any pararectovaginal neoplasm should include cloacogenic carcinoma and secondary neoplasm (226).

The **adenoid cystic variety** accounts for approximately 10% of Bartholin gland carcinomas (229–231). It is **a slow-growing tumor with a marked propensity for perineural and local invasion**. The perineural infiltration is quite characteristic and may account for the pruritus and burning sensation that many patients experience long before a palpable mass is evident (231).

Treatment

If the tumor does not involve adjacent structures, Bartholin gland carcinomas should be treated by radical resection of the primary lesion and ipsilateral inguinofemoral lymphadenectomy (226). Extensive dissection is sometimes required in the ischiorectal fossa, and this may be facilitated by performing an *en bloc* resection of the primary lesion and the groin (Fig. 13.18). In the M. D. Anderson Hospital experience, postoperative radiation to the vulva decreased the likelihood of local recurrence from 27% (6 of 22) to 7% (1 of 14) (226). If the ipsilateral groin nodes are positive, bilateral groin and pelvic radiation may be indicated, based on the same criteria as apply for squamous cell carcinomas.

Radical local excision, with or without ipsilateral inguinal-femoral lymphadenectomy, is also the treatment of choice for adenoid cystic carcinomas, and adjuvant radiation is recommended for positive margins or perineural invasion.

In 2007, **a study from the Massachusetts General Hospital reported 10 women with Bartholin gland carcinoma who were treated with chemoradiation to the primary tumor and regional lymph nodes** (232). There were four patients with stage I disease, one with stage II, three with stage III, and two with stage IV. The 5-year survival was 66%, and the authors concluded that chemoradiation offered an effective alternative to surgery.

Primary chemoradiation or neoadjuvant chemotherapy should certainly be used if the tumor is fixed to the inferior pubic ramus or involves adjacent structures, such as the anal sphincter or rectum, in order to avoid exenterative surgery (233,234).

Prognosis

Because of the deep location of the gland, cases tend to be more advanced than squamous carcinomas at the time of diagnosis, but stage for stage, the prognosis is similar.

Adenoid cystic tumors are less likely to metastasize to lymph nodes and carry a somewhat better prognosis. However, late recurrences may occur in the lungs, liver, or bone, so 10- and 15-year survival rates are more appropriate when evaluating these tumors (235,236).

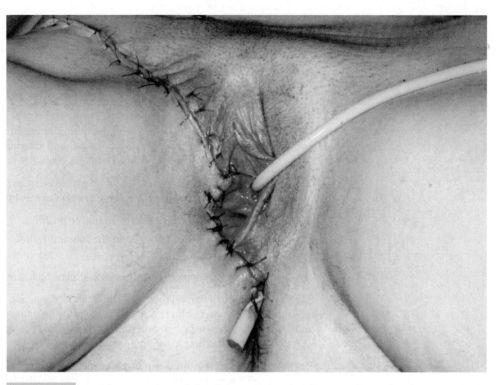

Figure 13.18 *En bloc* **resection of the right groin and right-posterior vulva for a Bartholin gland carcinoma.** Note the preservation of the clitoris and right anterior labium minus.

Other Vulvar Adenocarcinomas

Adenocarcinomas of the vulva usually arise in a Bartholin gland or occur in association with Paget's disease. They may rarely arise from the skin appendages, paraurethral glands, minor vestibular glands, aberrant breast tissue, endometriosis, or a misplaced cloacal remnant (117).

A particularly aggressive type is the **adenosquamous carcinoma**. This tumor has a number of synonyms, including cylindroma, pseudoglandular squamous cell carcinoma, and adenoacanthoma of the sweat gland of Lever. **The tumor has a propensity for perineural invasion, early lymph node metastasis, and local recurrence.** Underwood et al. (237) reported a crude 5-year survival of 5.6% (1 of 18) for adenosquamous carcinoma of the vulva, compared with 62.3% (48 of 77) for patients with squamous cell carcinoma. Treatment should include radical local excision and at least unilateral groin dissection. Postoperative radiation may be appropriate.

A Chinese study recently reported 12 patients with a vulvar sweat gland carcinoma seen between 1958 and 2009 (238). In three cases (27%), the sweat gland carcinoma was underlying Paget's disease, and one case (9%) was an adenoid cystic carcinoma in a sweat gland. A variety of treatments were used over this period, and 5 of the 12 (45%) had unilateral or bilateral lymphadenectomy. Eleven patients were available for follow-up, seven (64%) of whom survived at least 5 years.

Basal Cell Carcinoma

Basal cell carcinoma is the most common human malignant neoplasm. As with melanomas, its incidence is strongly correlated with sun exposure, and nearly 85% of cases occur in the head and neck region. Of 3,604 cases of basal cell carcinoma seen at the University of Florence, Italy, between 1995 and 2003, 63 cases (1.7%) arose on the vulva (239). They represented 20.5% of vulvar cancers (63 of 307) seen at the University during that period, and were **the second most common vulvar cancer after squamous cell carcinomas**.

As with other basal cell carcinomas, vulvar lesions may appear as a "rodent ulcer" with rolled edges, but **the presentation is variable. The lesions may simulate an inflammatory dermatosis, such as eczema or psoriasis, or an infectious process such as chronic candidiasis** (239,240). **Basal cell carcinoma should be suspected whenever lesions thought to be inflammatory do not respond to the usual treatment** (239). Most lesions are smaller than 2 cm in diameter, but giant lesions occasionally occur (241).

Basal cell carcinoma usually affects postmenopausal white women, a Vancouver study reporting a mean age of 74 years (242). **They are slow-growing, locally invasive tumors, and radical local excision usually is adequate treatment**. They are moderately radiosensitive, so radiation may be useful in selected cases. **Metastasis to regional lymph nodes has been reported but is rare** (243,244), and there has been one reported case with hematogenous spread (241). The local recurrence rate is 10–20% (240,244).

Basosquamous Carcinoma

Approximately 3–5% of basal cell carcinomas contain a malignant squamous component, the so-called **basosquamous carcinoma. These lesions are more aggressive and should be treated as squamous carcinomas** (243). **Another subtype of basal cell carcinoma is the** *adenoid basal cell carcinoma,* which must be differentiated from the more aggressive adenoid cystic carcinoma arising in a Bartholin gland or the skin (244).

Verrucous Carcinoma

Verrucous carcinomas are most commonly found in the oral cavity, but may be found on any moist membrane composed of squamous epithelium (245). They are a distinct entity, with no association with HPV infection, and a peculiar distribution pattern of cytokeratins AE1 and AE3 on immunohistochemical staining (246).

Grossly, the tumors have a cauliflower-like appearance (Fig. 13.19), and the diameter of reported lesions ranges from 1 to 15 cm (247). **Microscopically, they contain multiple papillary fronds that lack the central connective tissue core that characterizes condylomata acuminata.** The gross and microscopic features of a verrucous carcinoma are very similar to those of the **giant condyloma of Buschke–Loewenstein,** and they probably represent the same disease entity (117). Adequate biopsy from the base of the lesion is required to differentiate a verrucous carcinoma

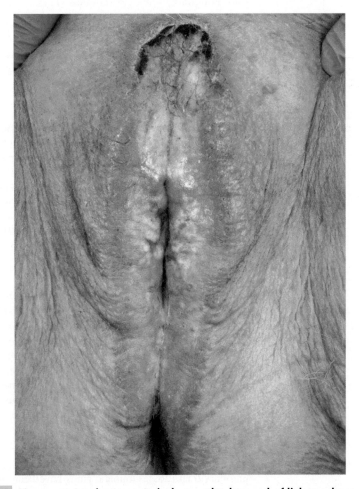

Figure 13.19   Verrucous carcinoma anteriorly, on a background of lichen sclerosus.

from a benign condyloma acuminatum or a squamous cell carcinoma with a verrucous growth pattern.

Clinically, verrucous carcinomas usually occur in postmenopausal women, and they are slowly growing but locally destructive lesions. Even bone may be invaded. Metastasis to regional lymph nodes is rare but has been reported (248). VIN or invasive squamous cell carcinoma may be seen in association with a verrucous carcinoma. A Greek study of 17 cases diagnosed over a 12-year period reported coexistence of verrucous and squamous carcinoma of the vulva in six cases (35%) (249).

Radical local excision is the standard treatment. Usually, any enlarged nodes are due to inflammatory hypertrophy (250), but this should be evaluated with fine-needle aspiration cytology and/or excisional biopsy.

Radiation therapy is contraindicated because it may induce anaplastic transformation with subsequent regional and distant metastasis (251). Japaze et al. reported a corrected 5-year survival of 94% for 17 patients treated with surgery alone, compared with 42% for seven patients treated with surgery and radiation (250). If there is a recurrence, further surgical excision is indicated, and this may occasionally necessitate some type of exenteration.

Vulvar Sarcoma

Sarcomas represent 1–2% of vulvar malignancies and comprise a heterogenous group of tumors. A paper from Johns Hopkins reported seven cases of vulvar sarcoma among 453 patients with vulvar malignancies seen from 1977 to 1997, an incidence of 1.5% (252). **Leiomyosarcomas** are the most common, representing three of nine cases (33%) recently reported from the Queensland Centre for Gynaecological Cancer (253). Other histologic types include **fibrosarcomas, neurofibrosarcomas, liposarcomas, rhabdomyosarcomas, angiosarcomas, epithelioid sarcomas, and malignant schwannomas** (117).

The primary treatment is wide surgical excision (252–255), with or without groin dissection. Adjuvant radiation may be helpful for high-grade tumors and locally recurrent low-grade lesions (252). **The overall survival rate is approximately 70%.** There were no recurrences in the series from Johns Hopkins (252), with follow-up ranging from 60 to 172 months. Only one of their patients had a groin dissection.

Leiomyosarcoma

These usually appear as enlarging, often painful masses in the labium majus. In a 1979 review of 32 smooth muscle tumors of the vulva, Tavassoli and Norris reported that recurrence was associated with three main determinants: diameter greater than 5 cm, infiltrating margins, and five or more mitotic figures per 10 high-power fields (HPF). The absence of one, or even all, of these features did not guarantee that recurrence would not occur (256). A study from the Massachusetts General Hospital suggested that a vulvar smooth muscle tumor should be considered a sarcoma when three or all of the following four features were present: **(i) over 5 cm in greatest dimension; (ii) infiltrative margins; (iii) at least 5 mitoses/10 HPF; and (iv) moderate to severe cytologic atypia** (257). **Lymphatic metastases are uncommon, and radical local excision is the usual treatment.**

Proximal-type Epithelioid Sarcoma of the Vulva

These lesions are much less common than distal epithelioid sarcomas, which characteristically develop in the soft tissues of the extremities of young adults. The vulvar lesions exhibit an aggressive pattern of local recurrence in spite of negative margins, and also have a propensity for early metastasis to lymph nodes and distant sites (258–261). Ulbright et al. described two cases and reviewed three other reports. They concluded that these tumors may mimic a Bartholin cyst, thus leading to delayed diagnosis (259). **Treatment consists of radical excision of the tumor, and at least ipsilateral groin dissection. Systemic therapy is ineffective.** Four of the five patients described by Ulbright died of metastatic disease.

Rhabdomyosarcoma

They are the most common soft tissue sarcomas in childhood, and 20% involve the pelvis or genitourinary tract (262). Dramatic gains have been made in the treatment of these tumors since the late 1970s. Previously, **radical pelvic surgery was the standard approach, but results were** poor. A multimodality approach has evolved, principally as a result of four successful protocols organized by the Intergroup Rhabdomyosarcoma Study Group (IRSG). Survival rates have improved significantly, with a corresponding decrease in morbidity (263).

Arndt et al. summarized the results of these four protocols in 2001. There were 151 patients entered on the studies, and the vulva was the least common primary site, there being only 20 (13%) vulvar rhabdomyosarcomas. Only five (25%) of the patients were 15 years or older, and the histologic subtypes were embryonal, eight (40%); botryoid, three (15%); and alveolar/undifferentiated nine, (45%). **All were managed with chemotherapy (*vincristine, dactinomycin* ± *cyclophosphamide* ± *doxorubicin*), with or without radiation therapy.** Wide local excision of the tumor, with or without inguinofemoral lymphadenectomy, was carried out before or after the chemotherapy.

Patients with local and/or regional rhabdomyosarcoma of the female genital tract have an excellent prognosis, with an estimated 5-year overall survival of 87% (263).

Malignant Schwannoma

Five cases of malignant schwannoma in the vulvar region have been reported. The patients ranged in age from 25 to 45 years. Four of the five were free of tumor from 1 to 9 years after radical surgery, and the fifth patient died of multiple pulmonary metastases (117).

Dermatofibrosarcoma Protuberans

This is a rare, **low-grade cutaneous malignancy** of the dermal connective tissue that occasionally involves the vulva (264–266). A clinicopathologic review of 13 cases seen at the M. D. Anderson Cancer Center from 1978 to 2007 revealed an age range of 23 to 76 years (mean 46 years), and a size range of 1.2 to 15 cm (median 4 cm) (264). Following surgical resection, local recurrence occurred in seven patients (53.8%), and one (7.7%) developed distant metastases. With a follow-up of 2 to 444 months, nine patients (69%) were alive and free of disease, and one (7.7%) had died without disease. They suggested the use of *imatinib* (**Gleevac**) **for patients with recurrent disease not amenable to surgery. Mohs micrographic surgery,** to ensure precise margin control, **is commonly used for these lesions on the trunk and extremities, and has also been described for a vulvar lesion** (267).

Synovial Cell Sarcoma

This is another rare tumor. A case was reported from Boston which started as a "pea-sized" mass, but grew rapidly to 8 cm diameter at presentation. The patient was treated with preoperative radiation, conservative resection with gracilis myocutaneous graft reconstruction, interstitial brachytherapy boost, and postoperative chemotherapy with six cycles of *doxorubicin, ifosfamide,* and *mesna*. She remained free of disease at 14 months (268).

Lymphoma

The genital tract may be involved primarily by malignant lymphomas, but involvement more commonly is a manifestation of systemic disease. **In the lower genital tract, the cervix is most commonly involved, followed by the vulva and the vagina** (117). Most patients are in their third to sixth decade of life, and approximately three-fourths of the cases involve diffuse large cell or histiocytic non-Hodgkin lymphomas. The remainder are nodular or Burkitt lymphomas (269). **Treatment is by surgical excision followed by chemotherapy and/or radiation,** and the overall 5-year survival is approximately 70% (269).

Endodermal Sinus Tumor

Malignant germ cell tumors at an extragonadal site presumably arise from arrested or aberrant migration of primordial germ cells from the embryonic yolk sac endoderm to the genital ridges (117). **Most vulvar germ cell tumors are endodermal sinus tumors,** and there have been 11 cases reported (270). Most patients were young adults with a median age of 24 years, unlike vaginal yolk sac tumors, which usually occur in infants. Unlike their ovarian counterpart, **they are not always associated with elevated serum alpha fetoprotein levels** (270,271). **Using *cisplatin*-based chemotherapy protocols during the past two decades, all reported patients have been cured, regardless of the type of surgery performed,** which ranged from radical local excision to radical vulvectomy and lymph node dissection (270).

Merkel Cell Carcinoma

Merkel cell carcinomas are **primary small cell carcinomas of the skin** that resemble oat cell carcinomas of the lung. They metastasize widely and have a very poor prognosis (272,273). They should be **locally excised and treated with *cisplatin*-based chemotherapy**.

Secondary Vulvar Tumors

Eight percent of vulvar tumors are metastatic (117). **The most common primary site is the cervix, followed by the endometrium, kidney, and urethra.** Most patients in whom vulvar metastases develop have advanced primary tumors at presentation, and in approximately one-fourth of the patients, the primary lesion and the vulvar metastasis are diagnosed simultaneously (274).

References

1. **Siegel R, Ma J, Zou Z, et al.** Cancer statistics 2014. *CA Cancer J Clin.* 2014;64:9–29.
2. **Judson PL, Habermann EB, Baxter NN, et al.** Trends in the incidence of invasive and in situ vulvar carcinoma. *Obstet Gynecol.* 2006;107:1018–1022.
3. **Hampl M, Deckers-Figiel S, Hampl JA, et al.** New aspects of vulvar cancer: Changes in localization and age of onset. *Gynecol Oncol.* 2008;109:340–345.
4. **Jones RW, Baranyai J, Stables S.** Trends in squamous cell carcinoma of the vulva: The influence of vulvar intraepithelial neoplasia. *Obstet Gynecol.* 1997;90:448–452.
5. **Baandrup L, Varbo A, Munk C, et al.** In situ and invasive squamous cell carcinoma of the vulva in Denmark 1978–2007-a nationwide population-based study. *Gynecol Oncol.* 2011;122:45–49.
6. **Madeleine MM, Daling JR, Carter JJ, et al.** Cofactors with human papillomavirus in a population-based study of vulvar cancer. *J Natl Cancer Inst.* 1997;89:1516–1523.
7. **Kumar S, Shah JP, Malone JM, Jr.** Vulvar cancer in women less than fifty in United States, 1980–2005. *Gynecol Oncol.* 2009;112: 283–284; author reply 234.
8. **Smith JS, Backes D, Hoots BE, et al.** Human papillomavirus type-distribution in vulvar and vaginal cancers and their associated precursors. *Obstet Gynecol.* 2009;113:917–924.
9. **Blair-Bell W, Datnow MM.** Primary malignant diseases of the vulva, with special reference to treatment by operation. *J Obstet Gynaecol Brit Empire.* 1936;43:755–763.
10. **Way S.** The anatomy of the lymphatic drainage of the vulva and its influence on the radical operation for carcinoma. *Ann R Coll Surg Eng.* 1948;3:187–209.
11. **Bassett A.** Traitement chirurgical operatoire de l'epithelioma primitif du clitoris: Indications-technique-results. *Revue de Chirurgie.* 1912; 46:546–552.
12. **Taussig F.** Cancer of the vulva: An analysis of 155 cases. *Am J Obstet Gynecol.* 1940;40:764–770.
13. **Way S.** Carcinoma of the vulva. *Am J Obstet Gynecol.* 1960;79: 692–697.
14. **Hacker NF.** Radical resection of vulvar malignancies: A paradigm shift in surgical approaches. *Curr Opin Obstet Gynecol.* 1999;11:61–64.
15. **de Hulla JA, Oonk MH, van der Zee AG.** Modern management of vulvar cancer. *Curr Opin Obstet Gynecol.* 2004;16:65–72.
16. **Iversen T, Abeler V, Aalders J.** Individualized treatment of stage I carcinoma of the vulva. *Obstet Gynecol.* 1981;57:85–89.
17. **Hacker NF, Berek JS, Lagasse LD, et al.** Individualization of treatment for stage I squamous cell vulvar carcinoma. *Obstet Gynecol.* 1984;63:155–162.
18. **DiSaia PJ, Creasman WT, Rich WM.** An alternate approach to early cancer of the vulva. *Am J Obstet Gynecol.* 1979;133:825–832.
19. **Burke TW, Stringer CA, Gershenson DM, et al.** Radical wide excision and selective inguinal node dissection for squamous cell carcinoma of the vulva. *Gynecol Oncol.* 1990;38:328–332.
20. **Burrell MO, Franklin EW, 3rd, Campion MJ, et al.** The modified radical vulvectomy with groin dissection: An eight-year experience. *Am J Obstet Gynecol.* 1988;159:715–722.
21. **Curry SL, Wharton JT, Rutledge F.** Positive lymph nodes in vulvar squamous carcinoma. *Gynecol Oncol.* 1980;9:63–67.
22. **Hacker NF, Berek JS, Lagasse LD, et al.** Management of regional lymph nodes and their prognostic influence in vulvar cancer. *Obstet Gynecol.* 1983;61:408–412.
23. **Monaghan JM, Hammond IG.** Pelvic node dissection in the treatment of vulval carcinoma-is it necessary? *Br J Obstet Gynaecol.* 1984; 91:270–274.
24. **Hoffman JS, Kumar NB, Morley GW.** Prognostic significance of groin lymph node metastases in squamous carcinoma of the vulva. *Obstet Gynecol.* 1985;66:402–405.
25. **Homesley HD, Bundy BN, Sedlis A, et al.** Radiation therapy versus pelvic node resection for carcinoma of the vulva with positive groin nodes. *Obstet Gynecol.* 1986;68:733–740.
26. **Hacker NF, Leuchter RS, Berek JS, et al.** Radical vulvectomy and bilateral inguinal lymphadenectomy through separate groin incisions. *Obstet Gynecol.* 1981;58:574–579.
27. **Boronow RC.** Therapeutic alternative to primary exenteration for advanced vulvovaginal cancer. *Gynecol Oncol.* 1973;1:233–255.
28. **Hacker NF, Berek JS, Juillard GJ, et al.** Preoperative radiation therapy for locally advanced vulvar cancer. *Cancer.* 1984; 54:2056–2061.
29. **Koay EJ, Jhingran A, Klopp AH, et al.** Factors associated with long-term survival in locally-advanced squamous cell carcinoma of the vulva treated with definitive radiation therapy. *Int J Radiat Oncol Biol Phys.* 2013;87:S129.
30. **Koh WJ, Wallace HJ, 3rd, Greer BE, et al.** Combined radiotherapy and chemotherapy in the management of local-regionally advanced vulvar cancer. *Int J Radiat Oncol Biol Phys.* 1993;26:809–816.
31. **Hyde SE, Valmadre S, Hacker NF, et al.** Squamous cell carcinoma of the vulva with bulky positive groin nodes-nodal debulking versus full groin dissection prior to radiation therapy. *Int J Gynecol Cancer.* 2007;17:154–158.
32. **Van der Zee AG, Oonk MH, De Hullu JA, et al.** Sentinel node dissection is safe in the treatment of early-stage vulvar cancer. *J Clin Oncol.* 2008;26:884–889.
33. **Rodriguez M, Sevin BU, Averette HE, et al.** Conservative trends in the surgical management of vulvar cancer: A University of Miami patient care evaluation study. *Int J Gynecol Cancer.* 1997;7:151–157.
34. **Magrina JF, Gonzalez-Bosquet J, Weaver AL, et al.** Primary squamous cell cancer of the vulva: Radical versus modified radical vulvar surgery. *Gynecol Oncol.* 1998;71:116–121.
35. **Sideri M, Jones RW, Wilkinson EJ, et al.** Squamous vulvar intraepithelial neoplasia: 2004 modified terminology, ISSVD Vulvar Oncology Subcommittee. *J Reprod Med.* 2005;50:807–810.
36. **Bloss JD, Liao SY, Wilczynski SP, et al.** Clinical and histologic features of vulvar carcinomas analyzed for human papillomavirus status: Evidence that squamous cell carcinoma of the vulva has more than one etiology. *Hum Pathol.* 1991;22:711–718.
37. **Hording U, Junge J, Daugaard S, et al.** Vulvar squamous cell carcinoma and papillomaviruses: Indications for two different etiologies. *Gynecol Oncol.* 1994;52:241–246.
38. **Lanneau GS, Argenta PA, Lanneau MS, et al.** Vulvar cancer in young women: Demographic features and outcome evaluation. *Am J Obstet Gynecol.* 2009;200:645 e1–e5.

39. **Toki T, Kurman RJ, Park JS, et al.** Probable nonpapillomavirus etiology of squamous cell carcinoma of the vulva in older women: A clinicopathologic study using in situ hybridization and polymerase chain reaction. *Int J Gynecol Pathol.* 1991;10:107–125.

40. **Scurry J.** Does lichen sclerosus play a central role in the pathogenesis of human papillomavirus negative vulvar squamous cell carcinoma? The itch-scratch-lichen sclerosus hypothesis. *Int J Gynecol Cancer.* 1999;9:89–97.

41. **van de Nieuwenhof HP, van der Avoort IA, de Hullu JA.** Review of squamous premalignant vulvar lesions. *Crit Rev Oncol Hematol.* 2008;68:131–156.

42. **Scurry J, Campion M, Scurry B, et al.** Pathologic audit of 164 consecutive cases of vulvar intraepithelial neoplasia. *Int J Gynecol Pathol.* 2006;25:176–181.

43. **van de Nieuwenhof HP, Massuger LF, van der Avoort IA, et al.** Vulvar squamous cell carcinoma development after diagnosis of VIN increases with age. *Eur J Cancer.* 2009;45:851–856.

44. **Eva LJ, Ganesan R, Chan KK, et al.** Differentiated-type vulval intraepithelial neoplasia has a high-risk association with vulval squamous cell carcinoma. *Int J Gynecol Cancer.* 2009;19:741–744.

45. **Sturgeon SR, Curtis RE, Johnson K, et al.** Second primary cancers after vulvar and vaginal cancers. *Am J Obstet Gynecol.* 1996;174:929–933.

46. **Jones RW, Rowan DM, Stewart AW.** Vulvar intraepithelial neoplasia: Aspects of the natural history and outcome in 405 women. *Obstet Gynecol.* 2005;106:1319–1326.

47. **Rodke G, Friedrich EG, Jr., Wilkinson EJ.** Malignant potential of mixed vulvar dystrophy (lichen sclerosus associated with squamous cell hyperplasia). *J Reprod Med.* 1988;33:545–550.

48. **Carli P, De Magnis A, Mannone F, et al.** Vulvar carcinoma associated with lichen sclerosus. Experience at the Florence, Italy, Vulvar Clinic. *J Reprod Med.* 2003;48:313–318.

49. **Fanning J, Lambert HC, Hale TM, et al.** Paget's disease of the vulva: Prevalence of associated vulvar adenocarcinoma, invasive Paget's disease, and recurrence after surgical excision. *Am J Obstet Gynecol.* 1999;180:24–27.

50. **Lam C, Funaro D.** Extramammary Paget's disease: Summary of current knowledge. *Dermatol Clin.* 2010;28:807–826.

51. **Wilkinson EJ, Brown HM.** Vulvar Paget disease of urothelial origin: A report of three cases and a proposed classification of vulvar Paget disease. *Hum Pathol.* 2002;33:549–554.

52. **Syed AH, Rana SH.** *Blaustein's Pathology of the Female Genital Tract.* 5th ed. Springer; 2002.

53. **Niikura H, Yoshida H, Ito K, et al.** Paget's disease of the vulva: Clinicopathologic study of type 1 cases treated at a single institution. *Int J Gynecol Cancer.* 2006;16:1212–1215.

54. **MacLean AB, Makwana M, Ellis PE, et al.** The management of Paget's disease of the vulva. *J Obstet Gynaecol.* 2004;24:124–128.

55. **Lee RA, Dahlin DC.** Paget's disease of the vulva with extension into the urethra, bladder, and ureters: A case report. *Am J Obstet Gynecol.* 1981;140:834–836.

56. **Black D, Tornos C, Soslow RA, et al.** The outcomes of patients with positive margins after excision for intraepithelial Paget's disease of the vulva. *Gynecol Oncol.* 2007;104:547–550.

57. **Cai Y, Sheng W, Xiang L, et al.** Primary extramammary Paget's disease of the vulva: The clinicopathological features and treatment outcomes in a series of 43 patients. *Gynecol Oncol.* 2013;129:412–416.

58. **Fishman DA, Chambers SK, Schwartz PE, et al.** Extramammary Paget's disease of the vulva. *Gynecol Oncol.* 1995;56:266–270.

59. **Brown RS, Lankester KJ, McCormack M, et al.** Radiotherapy for perianal Paget's disease. *Clin Oncol (R Coll Radiol).* 2002;14:272–284.

60. **Fontanelli R, Papadia A, Martinelli F, et al.** Photodynamic therapy with M-ALA as non surgical treatment option in patients with primary extramammary Paget's disease. *Gynecol Oncol.* 2013;130:90–94.

61. **Tonguc E, Gungor T, Var T, et al.** Treatment of recurrent vulvar Paget disease with imiquimod cream: A case report and review of the literature. *Arch Gynecol Obstet.* 2011;283:97–101.

62. **Ewing T, Sawicki J, Ciaravino G, et al.** Microinvasive Paget's disease. *Gynecol Oncol.* 2004;95:755–758.

63. **Karam A, Dorigo O.** Treatment outcomes in a large cohort of patients with invasive Extramammary Paget's disease. *Gynecol Oncol.* 2012;125:346–351.

64. **Scheistroen M, Trope C, Kaern J, et al.** DNA ploidy and expression of p53 and C-erbB-2 in extramammary paget's disease of the vulva. *Gynecol Oncol.* 1997;64:88–92.

65. **Hacker NF, Nieberg RK, Berek JS, et al.** Superficially invasive vulvar cancer with nodal metastases. *Gynecol Oncol.* 1983;15:65–77.

66. **Chu J, Tamimi HK, Figge DC.** Femoral node metastases with negative superficial inguinal nodes in early vulvar cancer. *Am J Obstet Gynecol.* 1981;140:337–339.

67. **Podczaski E, Sexton M, Kaminski P, et al.** Recurrent carcinoma of the vulva after conservative treatment for "microinvasive" disease. *Gynecol Oncol.* 1990;39:65–68.

68. **Gordinier ME, Malpica A, Burke TW, et al.** Groin recurrence in patients with vulvar cancer with negative nodes on superficial inguinal lymphadenectomy. *Gynecol Oncol.* 2003;90:625–628.

69. **Leuchter RS, Hacker NF, Voet RL, et al.** Primary carcinoma of the Bartholin gland: A report of 14 cases and review of the literature. *Obstet Gynecol.* 1982;60:361–368.

70. **Iversen T, Aalders JG, Christensen A, et al.** Squamous cell carcinoma of the vulva: A review of 424 patients, 1956–1974. *Gynecol Oncol.* 1980;9:271–279.

71. **Rouzier R, Haddad B, Plantier F, et al.** Local relapse in patients treated for squamous cell vulvar carcinoma: Incidence and prognostic value. *Obstet Gynecol.* 2002;100:1159–1167.

72. **Raspagliesi F, Hanozet F, Ditto A, et al.** Clinical and pathological prognostic factors in squamous cell carcinoma of the vulva. *Gynecol Oncol.* 2006;102:333–337.

73. **Gonzalez Bosquet J, Magrina JF, Magtibay PM, et al.** Patterns of inguinal groin metastases in squamous cell carcinoma of the vulva. *Gynecol Oncol.* 2007;105:742–746.

74. **Ghebre RG, Posthuma R, Vogel RI, et al.** Effect of age and comorbidity on the treatment and survival of older patients with vulvar cancer. *Gynecol Oncol.* 2011;121:595–599.

75. **Tabbaa ZM, Gonzalez J, Sznurkowski JJ, et al.** Impact of the new FIGO 2009 staging classification for vulvar cancer on prognosis and stage distribution. *Gynecol Oncol.* 2012;127:147–152.

76. **Green TH, Jr.** Carcinoma of the vulva. A reassessment. *Obstet Gynecol.* 1978;52:462–469.

77. **Parker RT, Duncan I, Rampone J, et al.** Operative management of early invasive epidermoid carcinoma of the vulva. *Am J Obstet Gynecol.* 1975;123:349–355.

78. **Magrina JF, Webb MJ, Gaffey TA, et al.** Stage I squamous cell cancer of the vulva. *Am J Obstet Gynecol.* 1979;134:453–459.

79. **Wilkinson EJ, Rico MJ, Pierson KK.** Microinvasive carcinoma of the vulva. *Int J Gynecol Pathol.* 1982;1:29–39.

80. **Hoffman JS, Kumar NB, Morley GW.** Microinvasive squamous carcinoma of the vulva: Search for a definition. *Obstet Gynecol.* 1983;61:615–618.

81. **Boice CR, Seraj IM, Thrasher T, et al.** Microinvasive squamous carcinoma of the vulva: Present status and reassessment. *Gynecol Oncol.* 1984;18:71–76.

82. **Ross MJ, Ehrmann RL.** Histologic prognosticators in stage I squamous cell carcinoma of the vulva. *Obstet Gynecol.* 1987;70:774–784.

83. **Rowley KC, Gallion HH, Donaldson ES, et al.** Prognostic factors in early vulvar cancer. *Gynecol Oncol.* 1988;31:43–49.

84. **Struyk APHB, Bouma JJ, van Lindert ACM.** Early stage cancer of the vulva: A pilot investigation on cancer of the vulva in gynecologic oncology centers in the Netherlands. *Proceedings of the International Gynecological Cancer Society.* 1989;2:303.

85. **van der Velden J HN.** Update on vulvar carcinoma. In: **ML Rothenberg, editor.** *Gynecologic Oncology: Controversies and New Developments.* Boston: Kluwer, 1994:101–119.

86. **Classification and staging of malignant tumors in the female pelvis.** *Int J Gynecol Obstet.* 1971;9:172–176.

87. **Homesley HD, Bundy BN, Sedlis A, et al.** Assessment of current International Federation of Gynecology and Obstetrics staging of vulvar carcinoma relative to prognostic factors for survival (a Gynecologic Oncology Group study). *Am J Obstet Gynecol.* 1991;164:997–1003; discussion 1003–1004.

88. **Hacker NF.** Revised FIGO staging for carcinoma of the vulva. *Int J Gynaecol Obstet.* 2009;105:105–106.

89. **Tantipalakorn C, Robertson G, Marsden DE, et al.** Outcome and patterns of recurrence for International Federation of Gynecology and Obstetrics (FIGO) stages I and II squamous cell vulvar cancer. *Obstet Gynecol.* 2009;113:895–901.

90. **Rouzier R, Preti M, Sideri M, et al.** A suggested modification to FIGO stage III vulvar cancer. *Gynecol Oncol.* 2008;110: 83–86.

91. **Podratz KC, Symmonds RE, Taylor WF, et al.** Carcinoma of the vulva: Analysis of treatment and survival. *Obstet Gynecol.* 1983;61:63–74.

92. **Origoni M, Sideri M, Garsia S, et al.** Prognostic value of pathological patterns of lymph node positivity in squamous cell carcinoma of the vulva stage III and IVA FIGO. *Gynecol Oncol.* 1992;45:313–316.

93. **van der Steen S, de Nieuwenhof HP, Massuger L, et al.** New FIGO staging system of vulvar cancer indeed provides a better reflection of prognosis. *Gynecol Oncol.* 2010;119:520–525.

94. **van den Einden LC, Aben KK, Massuger LF, et al.** Successful centralisation of patients with vulvar carcinoma: A population-based study in The Netherlands. *Eur J Cancer.* 2012;48:1997–2003.

95. **Rhodes CA, Cummins C, Shafi MI.** The management of squamous cell vulval cancer: A population based retrospective study of 411 cases. *Br J Obstet Gynaecol.* 1998;105:200–205.

96. **DeSimone CP, Van Ness JS, Cooper AL, et al.** The treatment of lateral T1 and T2 squamous cell carcinomas of the vulva confined to the labium majus or minus. *Gynecol Oncol.* 2007;104:390–395.

97. **Andersen BL, Hacker NF.** Psychosexual adjustment after vulvar surgery. *Obstet Gynecol.* 1983;62:457–462.

98. **Farias-Eisner R, Cirisano FD, Grouse D, et al.** Conservative and individualized surgery for early squamous carcinoma of the vulva: The treatment of choice for stage I and II (T1–2N0–1M0) disease. *Gynecol Oncol.* 1994;53:55–58.

99. **De Hullu JA, Hollema H, Lolkema S, et al.** Vulvar carcinoma. The price of less radical surgery. *Cancer.* 2002;95:2331–2338.

100. **Heaps JM, Fu YS, Montz FJ, et al.** Surgical-pathologic variables predictive of local recurrence in squamous cell carcinoma of the vulva. *Gynecol Oncol.* 1990;38:309–314.

101. **Chan JK, Sugiyama V, Pham H, et al.** Margin distance and other clinico-pathologic prognostic factors in vulvar carcinoma: A multivariate analysis. *Gynecol Oncol.* 2007;104:636–641.

102. **Chan JK, Sugiyama V, Tajalli TR, et al.** Conservative clitoral preservation surgery in the treatment of vulvar squamous cell carcinoma. *Gynecol Oncol.* 2004;95:152–156.

103. **Jones RW, Matthews JH.** Early clitoral carcinoma successfully treated by radiotherapy and bilateral inguinal lymphadenectomy. *Int J Gynecol Cancer.* 1999;9:348–350.

104. **Stroup AM, Harlan LC, Trimble EL.** Demographic, clinical, and treatment trends among women diagnosed with vulvar cancer in the United States. *Gynecol Oncol.* 2008;108:577–583.

105. **Rutledge F, Smith JP, Franklin EW.** Carcinoma of the vulva. *Am J Obstet Gynecol.* 1970;106:1117–1130.

106. **Lingard D, Free K, Wright RG, et al.** Invasive squamous cell carcinoma of the vulva: Behaviour and results in the light of changing management regimens. A review of clinicohistological features predictive of regional lymph node involvement and local recurrence. *Aust N Z J Obstet Gynaecol.* 1992;32:137–145.

107. **Burke TW, Levenback C, Coleman RL, et al.** Surgical therapy of T1 and T2 vulvar carcinoma: Further experience with radical wide excision and selective inguinal lymphadenectomy. *Gynecol Oncol.* 1995;57:215–220.

108. **Van Der Velden J, Kooyman CD, Van Lindert AC, et al.** A stage Ia vulvar carcinoma with an inguinal lymph node recurrence after local excision. A case report and literature review. *Int J Gynecol Cancer.* 1992;2:157–159.

109. **Vernooij F, Sie-Go DM, Heintz AP.** Lymph node recurrence following stage IA vulvar carcinoma: Two cases and a short overview of literature. *Int J Gynecol Cancer.* 2007;17:517–520.

110. **Gonzalez Bosquet J, Magrina JF, Gaffey TA, et al.** Long-term survival and disease recurrence in patients with primary squa-

mous cell carcinoma of the vulva. *Gynecol Oncol.* 2005;97:828–833.

111. **Stehman FB, Bundy BN, Dvoretsky PM, et al.** Early stage I carcinoma of the vulva treated with ipsilateral superficial inguinal lymphadenectomy and modified radical hemivulvectomy: A prospective study of the Gynecologic Oncology Group. *Obstet Gynecol.* 1992;79:490–497.

112. **Wharton JT, Gallager S, Rutledge FN.** Microinvasive carcinoma of the vulva. *Am J Obstet Gynecol.* 1974;118:159–162.

113. **Buscema J, Stern JL, Woodruff JD.** Early invasive carcinoma of the vulva. *Am J Obstet Gynecol.* 1981;140:563–569.

114. **Coleman RL, Ali S, Levenback CF, et al.** Is bilateral lymphadenectomy for midline squamous carcinoma of the vulva always necessary? An analysis from Gynecologic Oncology Group (GOG) 173. *Gynecol Oncol.* 2013;128:155–159.

115. **Iversen T, Aas M.** Lymph drainage from the vulva. *Gynecol Oncol.* 1983;16:179–189.

116. **Sedlis A, Homesley H, Bundy BN, et al.** Positive groin lymph nodes in superficial squamous cell vulvar cancer. A Gynecologic Oncology Group Study. *Am J Obstet Gynecol.* 1987;156:1159–1164.

117. **Fu YS.** Nonepithelial and metastatic tumors of the lower genital tract. In: *YS Fu, editor. Pathology of the Uterine Cervix, Vagina, and Vulva.* Philadelphia, PA: Saunders, 2002:471–539.

118. **Nicklin JL, Hacker NF, Heintze SW, et al.** An anatomical study of inguinal lymph node topography and clinical implications for the surgical management of vulval cancer. *Int J Gynecol Cancer.* 1995;5:128–133.

119. **Micheletti L, Levi AC, Bogliatto F, et al.** Rationale and definition of the lateral extension of the inguinal lymphadenectomy for vulvar cancer derived from an embryological and anatomical study. *J Surg Oncol.* 2002;81:19–24.

120. **Dardarian TS, Gray HJ, Morgan MA, et al.** Saphenous vein sparing during inguinal lymphadenectomy to reduce morbidity in patients with vulvar carcinoma. *Gynecol Oncol.* 2006;101: 140–142.

121. **Zhang X, Sheng X, Niu J, et al.** Sparing of saphenous vein during inguinal lymphadenectomy for vulval malignancies. *Gynecol Oncol.* 2007;105:722–726.

122. **Micheletti L, Borgno G, Barbero M, et al.** Deep femoral lymphadenectomy with preservation of the fascia lata. Preliminary report on 42 invasive vulvar carcinomas. *J Reprod Med.* 1990;35:1130–1133.

123. **Gaarenstroom KN, Kenter GG, Trimbos JB, et al.** Postoperative complications after vulvectomy and inguinofemoral lymphadenectomy using separate groin incisions. *Int J Gynecol Cancer.* 2003;13: 522–527.

124. **Ryan M, Stainton MC, Slaytor EK, et al.** Aetiology and prevalence of lower limb lymphoedema following treatment for gynaecological cancer. *Aust N Z J Obstet Gynaecol.* 2003;43:148–151.

125. **De Hullu JA, Pruim J, Que TH, et al.** Noninvasive detection of inguinofemoral lymph node metastases in squamous cell cancer of the vulva by L. *Int J Gynecol Cancer.* 1999;9:141–146.

126. **Land R, Herod J, Moskovic E, et al.** Routine computerized tomography scanning, groin ultrasound with or without fine needle aspiration cytology in the surgical management of primary squamous cell carcinoma of the vulva. *Int J Gynecol Cancer.* 2006; 16:312–317.

127. **Kataoka MY, Sala E, Baldwin P, et al.** The accuracy of magnetic resonance imaging in staging of vulvar cancer: A retrospective multicentre study. *Gynecol Oncol.* 2010;117:82–87.

128. **Abang Mohammed DK, Uberoi R, de B Lopes A, et al.** Inguinal node status by ultrasound in vulva cancer. *Gynecol Oncol.* 2000;77:93–96.

129. **Cabanas RM.** An approach for the treatment of penile carcinoma. *Cancer.* 1977;39:456–466.

130. **Morton DL, Wen DR, Wong JH, et al.** Technical details of intraoperative lymphatic mapping for early stage melanoma. *Arch Surg.* 1992; 127:392–399.

131. **Hampl M, Hantschmann P, Michels W, et al.** Validation of the accuracy of the sentinel lymph node procedure in patients with vulvar cancer: Results of a multicenter study in Germany. *Gynecol Oncol.* 2008;111:282–288.

132. **Levenback CF, Ali S, Coleman RL, et al.** Lymphatic mapping and sentinel lymph node biopsy in women with squamous cell carcinoma

of the vulva: A gynecologic oncology group study. *J Clin Oncol.* 2012;30:3786–3791.

133. **Radziszewski J, Kowalewska M, Jedrzejczak T, et al.** The accuracy of the sentinel lymph node concept in early stage squamous cell vulvar carcinoma. *Gynecol Oncol.* 2010;116:473–477.

134. **Oonk MH, van Hemel BM, Hollema H, et al.** Size of sentinel-node metastasis and chances of non-sentinel-node involvement and survival in early stage vulvar cancer: Results from GROINSS-V, a multicentre observational study. *Lancet Oncol.* 2010;11:646–652.

135. **Levenback CF.** How safe is sentinel lymph node biopsy in patients with vulvar cancer? *J Clin Oncol.* 2008;26:828–829.

136. **Burger MP, Hollema H, Emanuels AG, et al.** The importance of the groin node status for the survival of T1 and T2 vulval carcinoma patients. *Gynecol Oncol.* 1995;57:327–334.

137. **Bell JG, Lea JS, Reid GC.** Complete groin lymphadenectomy with preservation of the fascia lata in the treatment of vulvar carcinoma. *Gynecol Oncol.* 2000;77:314–318.

138. **Berman ML, Soper JT, Creasman WT, et al.** Conservative surgical management of superficially invasive stage I vulvar carcinoma. *Gynecol Oncol.* 1989;35:352–357.

139. **Kirby TO, Rocconi RP, Numnum TM, et al.** Outcomes of Stage I/II vulvar cancer patients after negative superficial inguinal lymphadenectomy. *Gynecol Oncol.* 2005;98:309–312.

140. **Woolderink JM, de Bock GH, de Hullu JA, et al.** Patterns and frequency of recurrences of squamous cell carcinoma of the vulva. *Gynecol Oncol.* 2006;103:293–299.

141. **de Hullu JA, Ansink AC, Tymstra T, et al.** What doctors and patients think about false-negative sentinel lymph nodes in vulvar cancer. *J Psychosom Obstet Gynaecol.* 2001;22:199–203.

142. **Farrell R, Gebski V, Hacker NF.** Quality of life after complete lymphadenectomy for vulvar cancer: do women prefer sentinel node biopsy. *Int J Gynecol Cancer.* 2014;24:813–819.

143. **Oonk MH, van Os MA, de Bock GH, et al.** A comparison of quality of life between vulvar cancer patients after sentinel lymph node procedure only and inguinofemoral lymphadenectomy. *Gynecol Oncol.* 2009;113:301–305.

144. **Louis-Sylvestre C, Evangelista E, Leonard F, et al.** Sentinel node localization should be interpreted with caution in midline vulvar cancer. *Gynecol Oncol.* 2005;97:151–154.

145. **Morotti M, Menada MV, Boccardo F, et al.** Lymphedema microsurgical preventive healing approach for primary prevention of lower limb lymphedema after inguinofemoral lymphadenectomy for vulvar cancer. *Int J Gynecol Cancer.* 2013;23:769–774.

146. **Paladini D, Cross P, Lopes A, et al.** Prognostic significance of lymph node variables in squamous cell carcinoma of the vulva. *Cancer.* 1994;74:2491–2496.

147. **van der Velden J, van Lindert AC, Lammes FB, et al.** Extracapsular growth of lymph node metastases in squamous cell carcinoma of the vulva. The impact on recurrence and survival. *Cancer.* 1995;75: 2885–2890.

148. **Peters LJ, Goepfert H, Ang KK, et al.** Evaluation of the dose for postoperative radiation therapy of head and neck cancer: First report of a prospective randomized trial. *Int J Radiat Oncol Biol Phys.* 1993;26:3–11.

149. **Fons G, Groenen SM, Oonk MH, et al.** Adjuvant radiotherapy in patients with vulvar cancer and one intra capsular lymph node metastasis is not beneficial. *Gynecol Oncol.* 2009;114:343–345.

150. **Katz A, Eifel PJ, Jhingran A, et al.** The role of radiation therapy in preventing regional recurrences of invasive squamous cell carcinoma of the vulva. *Int J Radiat Oncol Biol Phys.* 2003;57:409–418.

151. **Petereit DG, Mehta MP, Buchler DA, et al.** A retrospective review of nodal treatment for vulvar cancer. *Am J Clin Oncol.* 1993;16:38–42.

152. **Montana GS, Thomas GM, Moore DH, et al.** Preoperative chemoradiation for carcinoma of the vulva with N2/N3 nodes: A gynecologic oncology group study. *Int J Radiat Oncol Biol Phys.* 2000;48:1007–1013.

153. **Morley GW.** Infiltrative carcinoma of the vulva: Results of surgical treatment. *Am J Obstet Gynecol.* 1976;124:874–888.

154. **Simonsen E, Johnsson JE, Trope C.** Radical vulvectomy with warm-knife and open-wound techniques in vulvar malignancies. *Gynecol Oncol.* 1984;17:22–31.

155. **Low JJ, Hacker NF.** Vulvar reconstruction in gynecologic oncology. *Hung J Gynecol Oncol.* 1999;3:105–112.

156. **Barnhill DR, Hoskins WJ, Metz P.** Use of the rhomboid flap after partial vulvectomy. *Obstet Gynecol.* 1983;62:444–447.

157. **Ballon SC, Donaldson RC, Roberts JA, et al.** Reconstruction of the vulva using a myocutaneous graft. *Gynecol Oncol.* 1979; 7:123–127.

158. **Chafe W, Fowler WC, Walton LA, et al.** Radical vulvectomy with use of tensor fascia lata myocutaneous flap. *Am J Obstet Gynecol.* 1983;145:207–213.

159. **Andersen BL, Hacker NF.** Psychosexual adjustment following pelvic exenteration. *Obstet Gynecol.* 1983;61:331–338.

160. **Cavanagh D, Shepherd JH.** The place of pelvic exenteration in the primary management of advanced carcinoma of the vulva. *Gynecol Oncol.* 1982;13:318–322.

161. **Grimshaw RN, Aswad SG, Monaghan JM.** The role of anovulvectomy in locally advanced carcinoma of the vulva. *Int J Gynecol Cancer.* 1991;1:15–18.

162. **Forner DM, Lampe B.** Exenteration in the treatment of Stage III/IV vulvar cancer. *Gynecol Oncol.* 2012;124:87–91.

163. **Thomas G, Dembo A, DePetrillo A, et al.** Concurrent radiation and chemotherapy in vulvar carcinoma. *Gynecol Oncol.* 1989;34:263–267.

164. **Moore DH, Thomas GM, Montana GS, et al.** Preoperative chemoradiation for advanced vulvar cancer: A phase II study of the Gynecologic Oncology Group. *Int J Radiat Oncol Biol Phys.* 1998; 42:79–85.

165. **Landoni F, Maneo A, Zanetta G, et al.** Concurrent preoperative chemotherapy with 5-fluorouracil and mitomycin C and radiotherapy (FUMIR) followed by limited surgery in locally advanced and recurrent vulvar carcinoma. *Gynecol Oncol.* 1996;61:321–327.

166. **Landrum LM, Skaggs V, Gould N, et al.** Comparison of outcome measures in patients with advanced squamous cell carcinoma of the vulva treated with surgery or primary chemoradiation. *Gynecol Oncol.* 2008;108:584–590.

167. **Cunningham MJ, Goyer RP, Gibbons SK, et al.** Primary radiation, cisplatin, and 5-fluorouracil for advanced squamous carcinoma of the vulva. *Gynecol Oncol.* 1997;66:258–261.

168. **Moore DH, Ali S, Koh WJ, et al.** A phase II trial of radiation therapy and weekly cisplatin chemotherapy for the treatment of locally-advanced squamous cell carcinoma of the vulva: A gynecologic oncology group study. *Gynecol Oncol.* 2012;124:529–533.

169. **Rogers LJ, Howard B, Van Wijk L, et al.** Chemoradiation in advanced vulval carcinoma. *Int J Gynecol Cancer.* 2009;19:745–751.

170. **Mak RH, Halasz LM, Tanaka CK, et al.** Outcomes after radiation therapy with concurrent weekly platinum-based chemotherapy or every-3–4-week 5-fluorouracil-containing regimens for squamous cell carcinoma of the vulva. *Gynecol Oncol.* 2011;120:101–107.

171. **Beriwal S, Coon D, Heron DE, et al.** Preoperative intensity-modulated radiotherapy and chemotherapy for locally advanced vulvar carcinoma. *Gynecol Oncol.* 2008;109:291–295.

172. **Eifel PJ, Morris M, Burke TW, et al.** Preoperative continuous infusion cisplatinum and 5-fluorouracil with radiation for locally advanced or recurrent carcinoma of the vulva. *Gynecol Oncol.* 1995;59:51–56.

173. **Geisler JP, Manahan KJ, Buller RE.** Neoadjuvant chemotherapy in vulvar cancer: Avoiding primary exenteration. *Gynecol Oncol.* 2006;100:53–57.

174. **Aragona AM, Cuneo N, Soderini AH, et al.** Tailoring the treatment of locally advanced squamous cell carcinoma of the vulva: Neoadjuvant chemotherapy followed by radical surgery: Results from a multicenter study. *Int J Gynecol Cancer.* 2012;22:1258–1263.

175. **Gaffney DK, Du Bois A, Narayan K, et al.** Patterns of care for radiotherapy in vulvar cancer: A Gynecologic Cancer Intergroup study. *Int J Gynecol Cancer.* 2009;19:163–167.

176. **Podratz KC, Symmonds RE, Taylor WF.** Carcinoma of the vulva: Analysis of treatment failures. *Am J Obstet Gynecol.* 1982;143:340–351.

177. **Faul CM, Mirmow D, Huang Q, et al.** Adjuvant radiation for vulvar carcinoma: Improved local control. *Int J Radiat Oncol Biol Phys.* 1997;38:381–389.

178. **Stehman FB, Bundy BN, Thomas G, et al.** Groin dissection versus groin radiation in carcinoma of the vulva: A Gynecologic Oncology Group study. *Int J Radiat Oncol Biol Phys.* 1992;24:389–396.

179. **Koh WJ, Chiu M, Stelzer KJ, et al.** Femoral vessel depth and the implications for groin node radiation. *Int J Radiat Oncol Biol Phys.* 1993;27:969–974.

180. **Lataifeh I, Nascimento MC, Nicklin JL, et al.** Patterns of recurrence and disease-free survival in advanced squamous cell carcinoma of the vulva. *Gynecol Oncol.* 2004;95:701–705.

181. **Hopkins MP, Reid GC, Morley GW.** The surgical management of recurrent squamous cell carcinoma of the vulva. *Obstet Gynecol.* 1990;75:1001–1005.

182. **Weikel W, Schmidt M, Steiner E, et al.** Surgical therapy of recurrent vulvar cancer. *Am J Obstet Gynecol.* 2006;195:1293–1302.

183. **Hoffman M, Greenberg S, Greenberg H, et al.** Interstitial radiotherapy for the treatment of advanced or recurrent vulvar and distal vaginal malignancy. *Am J Obstet Gynecol.* 1990;162:1278–1282.

184. **Tilmans AS, Sutton GP, Look KY, et al.** Recurrent squamous carcinoma of the vulva. *Am J Obstet Gynecol.* 1992;167:1383–1389.

185. **Marx GM, Friedlander ML, Hacker NF.** Cytotoxic drug treatment of vulval and vaginal cancer. *CME J Gynecol Oncol.* 2001;6:67–72.

186. **Horowitz NS, Olawaiye AB, Borger DR, et al.** Phase II trial of erlotinib in women with squamous cell carcinoma of the vulva. *Gynecol Oncol.* 2012;127:141–146.

187. **Boutselis JG.** Radical vulvectomy for invasive squamous cell carcinoma of the vulva. *Obstet Gynecol.* 1972;39:827–836.

188. **Japaze H, Garcia-Bunuel R, Woodruff JD.** Primary vulvar neoplasia: A review of in situ and invasive carcinoma, 1935–1972. *Obstet Gynecol.* 1977;49:404–411.

189. **Benedet JL, Turko M, Fairey RN, et al.** Squamous carcinoma of the vulva: Results of treatment, 1938 to 1976. *Am J Obstet Gynecol.* 1979;134:201–207.

190. **Cavanagh D, Roberts WS, Bryson SC, et al.** Changing trends in the surgical treatment of invasive carcinoma of the vulva. *Surg Gynecol Obstet.* 1986;162:164–168.

191. **Beller U, Quinn MA, Benedet JL, et al.** Carcinoma of the vulva. FIGO 26th Annual Report on the Results of Treatment in Gynecological Cancer. *Int J Gynaecol Obstet.* 2006;95(1):S7–S27.

192. **Thaker N, Klopp AH, Jhingran A, et al.** Survival outcomes for patients with pelvic lymph node-positive Stage IVB vulvar cancer: Time to reconsider the FIGO staging system? *Int J Radiat Oncol Biol Phys.* 2013;87:S129.

193. **Kaern J, Iversen T, Trope C, et al.** Flow cytometric DNA measurements in squamous cell carcinoma of the vulva: An important prognostic method. *Int J Gynecol Cancer.* 1992;2:169–174.

194. **Knopp S, Bjorge T, Nesland JM, et al.** p16INK4 a and p21Waf1/Cip1 expression correlates with clinical outcome in vulvar carcinomas. *Gynecol Oncol.* 2004;95:37–45.

195. **Fons G, Burger MP, ten Kate FJ, et al.** Assessment of promising protein markers for vulva cancer. *Int J Gynecol Cancer.* 2009;19:756–760.

196. **Talaat A, Brinkmann D, Nagar Y, et al.** Experience in the management of patients older than 80 years with vulval cancer. *Int J Gynecol Cancer.* 2009;19:752–755.

197. **Hyde SE, Ansink AC, Burger MP, et al.** The impact of performance status on survival in patients of 80 years and older with vulvar cancer. *Gynecol Oncol.* 2002;84:388–393.

198. **Blessing K, Kernohan NM, Miller ID, et al.** Malignant melanoma of the vulva: Clinicopathological features. *Int J Gynecol Cancer.* 1991;1:81–87.

199. **Mert I, Semaan A, Winer I, et al.** Vulvar/vaginal melanoma: An updated surveillance epidemiology and end results database review, comparison with cutaneous melanoma and significance of racial disparities. *Int J Gynecol Cancer.* 2013;23:1118–1125.

200. **Ragnarsson-Olding BK, Nilsson BR, Kanter-Lewensohn LR, et al.** Malignant melanoma of the vulva in a nationwide, 25-year study of 219 Swedish females: Predictors of survival. *Cancer.* 1999;86:1285–1293.

201. **Chung AF, Woodruff JM, Lewis JL, Jr.** Malignant melanoma of the vulva: A report of 44 cases. *Obstet Gynecol.* 1975;45:638–646.

202. **Phillips GL, Twiggs LB, Okagaki T.** Vulvar melanoma: A microstaging study. *Gynecol Oncol.* 1982;14:80–88.

203. **Podratz KC, Gaffey TA, Symmonds RE, et al.** Melanoma of the vulva: An update. *Gynecol Oncol.* 1983;16:153–168.

204. **Clark WH, Jr., From L, Bernardino EA, et al.** The histogenesis and biologic behavior of primary human malignant melanomas of the skin. *Cancer Res.* 1969;29:705–727.

205. **Breslow A.** Thickness, cross-sectional areas and depth of invasion in the prognosis of cutaneous melanoma. *Ann Surg.* 1970;172:902–908.

206. **Kim CJ, Reintgen DS, Balch CM, AJCC Melanoma Staging Committee.** The new melanoma staging system. *Cancer Control.* 2002;9:9–15.

207. **Moxley KM, Fader AN, Rose PG, et al.** Malignant melanoma of the vulva: An extension of cutaneous melanoma? *Gynecol Oncol.* 2011;122:612–617.

208. **Aitken DR, Clausen K, Klein JP, James AG.** The extent of primary melanoma excision. A re-evaluation–how wide is wide? *Ann Surg.* 1983;198:634–641.

209. **Day CL, Jr., Mihm MC, Jr., Sober AJ, et al.** Narrower margins for clinical stage I malignant melanoma. *N Engl J Med.* 1982;306:479–482.

210. **Rose PG, Piver MS, Tsukada Y, et al.** Conservative therapy for melanoma of the vulva. *Am J Obstet Gynecol.* 1988;159:52–55.

211. **Davidson T, Kissin M, Westbury G.** Vulvo-vaginal melanoma–should radical surgery be abandoned? *Br J Obstet Gynaecol.* 1987;94:473–476.

212. **Trimble EL, Lewis JL, Jr., Williams LL, et al.** Management of vulvar melanoma. *Gynecol Oncol.* 1992;45:254–258.

213. **Verschraegen CF, Benjapibal M, Supakarapongkul W, et al.** Vulvar melanoma at the M. D. Anderson Cancer Center: 25 years later. *Int J Gynecol Cancer.* 2001;11:359–364.

214. **Phillips GL, Bundy BN, Okagaki T, et al.** Malignant melanoma of the vulva treated by radical hemivulvectomy. A prospective study of the Gynecologic Oncology Group. *Cancer.* 1994;73:2626–2632.

215. **Janco JM, Markovic SN, Weaver AL, et al.** Vulvar and vaginal melanoma: Case series and review of current management options including neoadjuvant chemotherapy. *Gynecol Oncol.* 2013;129:533–537.

216. **Balch CM, Soong SJ, Bartolucci AA, et al.** Efficacy of an elective regional lymph node dissection of 1 to 4 mm thick melanomas for patients 60 years of age and younger. *Ann Surg.* 1996;224:255–263; discussion 263–256.

217. **Gershenwald JE, Colome MI, Lee JE, et al.** Patterns of recurrence following a negative sentinel lymph node biopsy in 243 patients with stage I or II melanoma. *J Clin Oncol.* 1998;16:2253–2260.

218. **Messina JL, Sondak VK.** Refining the criteria for sentinel lymph node biopsy in patients with thinner melanoma: A roadmap for the future. *Cancer.* 2010;116:1403–1405.

219. **de Hullu JA, Hollema H, Hoekstra HJ, et al.** Vulvar melanoma: Is there a role for sentinel lymph node biopsy? *Cancer.* 2002;94:486–491.

220. **Dhar KK, Das N, Brinkman DA, et al.** Utility of sentinel node biopsy in vulvar and vaginal melanoma: Report of two cases and review of the literature. *Int J Gynecol Cancer.* 2007;17:720–723.

221. **Kirkwood JM, Strawderman MH, Ernstoff MS, et al.** Interferon alfa-2b adjuvant therapy of high-risk resected cutaneous melanoma: The Eastern Cooperative Oncology Group Trial EST 1684. *J Clin Oncol.* 1996;14:7–17.

222. **Kirkwood JM, Ibrahim JG, Sosman JA, et al.** High-dose interferon alfa-2b significantly prolongs relapse-free and overall survival compared with the GM2-KLH/QS-21 vaccine in patients with resected stage IIB-III melanoma: Results of intergroup trial E1694/S9512/C509801. *J Clin Oncol.* 2001;19:2370–2380.

223. **Gray RJ, Pockaj BA, Kirkwood JM.** An update on adjuvant interferon for melanoma. *Cancer Control.* 2002;9:16–21.

224. **Beller U, Demopoulos R, Beckman EM.** Vulvovaginal melanoma. A clinicopathologic study. *J Reprod Med.* 1986;31:315–319.

225. **Scheistroen M, Trope C, Koern J, et al.** Malignant melanoma of the vulva. Evaluation of prognostic factors with emphasis on DNA ploidy in 75 patients. *Cancer.* 1995;75:72–80.

226. **Copeland LJ, Sneige N, Gershenson DM, et al.** Bartholin gland carcinoma. *Obstet Gynecol.* 1986;67:794–801.

227. **Obermair A, Koller S, Crandon AJ, et al.** Primary Bartholin gland carcinoma: A report of seven cases. *Aust N Z J Obstet Gynaecol.* 2001;41:78–81.

228. **Cardosi RJ, Speights A, Fiorica JV, et al.** Bartholin's gland carcinoma: A 15-year experience. *Gynecol Oncol.* 2001;82:247–251.

229. **Lelle RJ, Davis KP, Roberts JA.** Adenoid cystic carcinoma of the Bartholin's gland: The University of Michigan experience. *Int J Gynecol Cancer.* 1994;4:145–149.

230. **Yang SY, Lee JW, Kim WS, et al.** Adenoid cystic carcinoma of the Bartholin's gland: Report of two cases and review of the literature. *Gynecol Oncol.* 2006;100:422–425.

231. **DePasquale SE, McGuinness TB, Mangan CE, et al.** Adenoid cystic carcinoma of Bartholin's gland: A review of the literature and report of a patient. *Gynecol Oncol.* 1996;61:122–125.

232. **Lopez-Varela E, Oliva E, McIntyre JF, et al.** Primary treatment of Bartholin's gland carcinoma with radiation and chemoradiation: A report on ten consecutive cases. *Int J Gynecol Cancer.* 2007;17:661–667.

233. **Massad LS, De Geest K.** Multimodality therapy for carcinoma of the Bartholin gland. *Gynecol Oncol.* 1999;75:305–307.

234. **Downs LS, Ghosh K, Dusenbery KE, et al.** Stage IV carcinoma of the Bartholin gland managed with primary chemoradiation. *Gynecol Oncol.* 2002;87:210–212.

235. **Rosenberg P, Simonsen E, Risberg B.** Adenoid cystic carcinoma of Bartholin's gland: A report of five new cases treated with surgery and radiotherapy. *Gynecol Oncol.* 1989;34:145–147.

236. **Copeland LJ, Sneige N, Gershenson DM, et al.** Adenoid cystic carcinoma of Bartholin gland. *Obstet Gynecol.* 1986;67:115–120.

237. **Underwood JW, Adcock LL, Okagaki T.** Adenosquamous carcinoma of skin appendages (adenoid squamous cell carcinoma, pseudoglandular squamous cell carcinoma, adenocanthoma of sweat gland of Lever) of the vulva: A clinical and ultrastructural study. *Cancer.* 1978;42:1851–1858.

238. **Hou JL, Wu LY, Zhang HT, et al.** Clinicopathologic characteristics of 12 patients with vulvar sweat gland carcinoma. *Int J Gynecol Cancer.* 2010;20:874–878.

239. **de Giorgi V, Salvini C, Massi D, et al.** Vulvar basal cell carcinoma: Retrospective study and review of literature. *Gynecol Oncol.* 2005;97:192–194.

240. **Fleury AC, Junkins-Hopkins JM, Diaz-Montes T.** Vulvar basal cell carcinoma in a 20-year-old: Case report and review of the literature. *Gynecol Oncol Case Rep.* 2012;2:26–27.

241. **Dudzinski MR, Askin FB, Fowler WC, Jr.** Giant basal cell carcinoma of the vulva. *Obstet Gynecol.* 1984;63:57S–60S.

242. **Benedet JL, Miller DM, Ehlen TG, et al.** Basal cell carcinoma of the vulva: Clinical features and treatment results in 28 patients. *Obstet Gynecol.* 1997;90:765–768.

243. **Hoffman MS, Roberts WS, Ruffolo EH.** Basal cell carcinoma of the vulva with inguinal lymph node metastases. *Gynecol Oncol.* 1988;29:113–119.

244. **Mulayim N, Foster Silver D, Tolgay Ocal I, et al.** Vulvar basal cell carcinoma: Two unusual presentations and review of the literature. *Gynecol Oncol.* 2002;85:532–537.

245. **Partridge EE, Murad T, Shingleton HM, et al.** Verrucous lesions of the female genitalia. II. Verrucous carcinoma. *Am J Obstet Gynecol.* 1980;137:419–424.

246. **Gualco M, Bonin S, Foglia G, et al.** Morphologic and biologic studies on ten cases of verrucous carcinoma of the vulva supporting the theory of a discrete clinico-pathologic entity. *Int J Gynecol Cancer.* 2003;13:317–324.

247. **Crowther ME, Lowe DG, Shepherd JH.** Verrucous carcinoma of the female genital tract: A review. *Obstet Gynecol Surv.* 1988;43:263–280.

248. **Gallousis S.** Verrucous carcinoma. Report of three vulvar cases and review of the literature. *Obstet Gynecol.* 1972;40:502–507.

249. **Haidopoulos D, Diakomanolis E, Rodolakis A, et al.** Coexistence of verrucous and squamous carcinoma of the vulva. *Aust N Z J Obstet Gynaecol.* 2005;45:60–63.

250. **Japaze H, Van Dinh T, Woodruff JD.** Verrucous carcinoma of the vulva: Study of 24 cases. *Obstet Gynecol.* 1982;60:462–466.

251. **Demian SD, Bushkin FL, Echevarria RA.** Perineural invasion and anaplastic transformation of verrucous carcinoma. *Cancer.* 1973;32:395–401.

252. **Ulutin HC, Zellars RC, Frassica D.** Soft tissue sarcoma of the vulva: A clinical study. *Int J Gynecol Cancer.* 2003;13:528–531.

253. **Jones IS C, Crandon A, Sanday K.** Vulvar sarcomas: A 25 plus-year experience from Queensland. *Open J Obstet Gynecol.* 2013;3:37–40.

254. **Curtin JP, Saigo P, Slucher B, et al.** Soft-tissue sarcoma of the vagina and vulva: A clinicopathologic study. *Obstet Gynecol.* 1995;86:269–272.

255. **Aartsen EJ, Albus-Lutter CE.** Vulvar sarcoma: Clinical implications. *Eur J Obstet Gynecol Reprod Biol.* 1994;56:181–189.

256. **Tavassoli FA, Norris HJ.** Smooth muscle tumors of the vulva. *Obstet Gynecol.* 1979;53:213–217.

257. **Nielsen GP, Rosenberg AE, Koerner FC, et al.** Smooth-muscle tumors of the vulva. A clinicopathological study of 25 cases and review of the literature. *Am J Surg Pathol.* 1996;20:779–793.

258. **Argenta PA, Thomas S, Chura JC.** Proximal-type epithelioid sarcoma vs. malignant rhabdoid tumor of the vulva: A case report, review of the literature, and an argument for consolidation. *Gynecol Oncol.* 2007;107:130–135.

259. **Ulbright TM, Brokaw SA, Stehman FB, et al.** Epithelioid sarcoma of the vulva. Evidence suggesting a more aggressive behavior than extra-genital epithelioid sarcoma. *Cancer.* 1983;52:1462–1469.

260. **de Visscher SA, van Ginkel RJ, Wobbes T, et al.** Epithelioid sarcoma: Still an only surgically curable disease. *Cancer.* 2006;107:606–612.

261. **Spillane AJ, Thomas JM, Fisher C.** Epithelioid sarcoma: The clinicopathological complexities of this rare soft tissue sarcoma. *Ann Surg Oncol.* 2000;7:218–225.

262. **Bell J, Averette H, Davis J, et al.** Genital rhabdomyosarcoma: Current management and review of the literature. *Obstet Gynecol Surv.* 1986;41:257–263.

263. **Arndt CA, Donaldson SS, Anderson JR, et al.** What constitutes optimal therapy for patients with rhabdomyosarcoma of the female genital tract? *Cancer.* 2001;91:2454–2468.

264. **Behranwala KA, Latifaj B, Blake P, et al.** Vulvar soft tissue tumors. *Int J Gynecol Cancer.* 2004;14:94–99.

265. **Edelweiss M, Malpica A.** Dermatofibrosarcoma protuberans of the vulva: A clinicopathologic and immunohistochemical study of 13 cases. *Am J Surg Pathol.* 2010;34:393–400.

266. **Soergel TM, Doering DL, O'Connor D.** Metastatic dermatofibrosarcoma protuberans of the vulva. *Gynecol Oncol.* 1998;71:320–324.

267. **Doufekas K, Duncan TJ, Williamson KM, et al.** Mohs micrographic surgery for dermatofibrosarcoma protuberans of the vulva. *Obstet Gynecol Int.* 2009;2009:547672.

268. **Holloway CL, Russell AH, Muto M, et al.** Synovial cell sarcoma of the vulva: Multimodality treatment incorporating preoperative external-beam radiation, hemivulvectomy, flap reconstruction, interstitial brachytherapy, and chemotherapy. *Gynecol Oncol.* 2007;104:253–256.

269. **Harris NL, Scully RE.** Malignant lymphoma and granulocytic sarcoma of the uterus and vagina. A clinicopathologic analysis of 27 cases. *Cancer.* 1984;53:2530–2545.

270. **Kurucu N, Kosucu P, Imamoglu M, et al.** Primary vulvar endodermal sinus tumor: A case report and review of the literature. *Pediatr Int.* 2011;53:396–399.

271. **Khunamornpong S, Siriaunkgul S, Suprasert P, et al.** Yolk sac tumor of the vulva: A case report with long-term disease-free survival. *Gynecol Oncol.* 2005;97:238–242.

272. **Bottles K, Lacey CG, Goldberg J, et al.** Merkel cell carcinoma of the vulva. *Obstet Gynecol.* 1984;63:61S–65S.

273. **Husseinzadeh N, Wesseler T, Newman N, et al.** Neuroendocrine (Merkel cell) carcinoma of the vulva. *Gynecol Oncol.* 1988;29:105–112.

274. **Dehner LP.** Metastatic and secondary tumors of the vulva. *Obstet Gynecol.* 1973;42:47–57.

Vaginal Cancer

Neville F. Hacker
Patricia J. Eifel

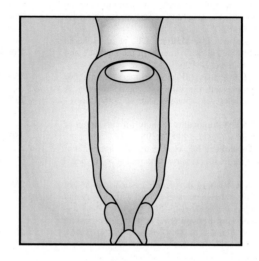

Primary carcinomas of the vagina represent 1–2% of malignant neoplasms of the female genital tract. In the United States, it is estimated that there will be 3,170 new cases diagnosed in 2014, and 880 deaths from the disease (1). Incidence rates in the United States from 1998 through 2003 were 0.18 per 100,000 female population for *in situ* cases, and 0.69 per 100,000 females for invasive cases; median ages were 58 and 68 years, respectively (2). Unlike cervical cancer, more than 50% of patients are diagnosed in the seventh, eighth, and ninth decades of life. Like cervical cancer, squamous cell histology accounts for 70–80% of cases (2,3).

Until the late 1930s, vaginal cancer was in general considered to be incurable. Most patients presented with disease that had spread beyond the vagina, and radiation therapy techniques were poorly developed. **With modern radiation therapy techniques, cure rates of even advanced cases should now be comparable with those for cervical cancer** (4–6). According to the 26th International Federation of Gynecology and Obstetrics (FIGO) Annual Report, the overall 5-year survival rate has increased from 34.1% between 1959 and 1963 to 53.6% between 1999 and 2001 (3).

Fu (7) **reported that 84% of carcinomas involving the vagina were secondary, usually from the cervix (32%);** endometrium (18%); colon and rectum (9%); ovary (6%); or vulva (6%). Of 164 squamous cell carcinomas, 44 (27%) were primary and 120 (73%) were secondary. Among the latter, 95 (79%) originated from the cervix; 17 (14%) from the vulva; and 8 (7%) from the cervix and the vulva. This apparent discrepancy is partly related to the FIGO classification and staging of malignant tumors of the female pelvis. The staging requires that a tumor that has extended to the portio and reached the area of the external os should be regarded as a carcinoma of the cervix, whereas a tumor that involves the vulva and vagina should be classified as a carcinoma of the vulva. **Endometrial carcinomas and choriocarcinomas commonly metastasize to the vagina, whereas tumors from the bladder or rectum may invade the vagina directly.**

Primary Vaginal Tumors

The histologic types of primary vaginal tumors are shown in Table 14.1 (8–20). Squamous cell carcinomas are the most common, although adenocarcinomas, melanomas, and sarcomas are also seen.

Table 14.1 Primary Vaginal Cancer: Reported Incidence of Histologic Types

Histologic Types	Number	Percentage
Squamous cell	1,054	82.6
Adenocarcinoma (including clear cell)	123	9.6
Melanoma	42	3.3
Sarcoma	40	3.1
Undifferentiated	8	0.6
Small cell	5	0.4
Lymphoma	4	0.3
Carcinoid	1	0.1
Total	**1,277**	**100**

Data compiled from **Perez et al., 1974** (8); **Pride and Buchler, 1977** (9); **Ball and Berman, 1982** (10); **Houghton and Iversen, 1982** (11); **Benedet et al., 1983** (12); **Peters et al., 1985** (13); **Rubin et al., 1985** (14); **Sulak et al., 1988** (15); **Eddy et al., 1991** (16); **Ali et al., 1996** (17); **Tjalma et al., 2001** (18); **Tewari et al., 2001** (19), **Hellman et al., 2006** (20).

Squamous Cell Carcinoma

Squamous cell carcinoma is the most common vaginal cancer. The mean age of the patients is approximately 67 years, although the disease occasionally is seen in the third and fourth decades of life (6,8,11,14). About 80% of patients are older than 50 years (3).

Etiology

Women who have been treated for a prior anogenital cancer, particularly of the cervix, have a high relative risk of developing vaginal cancer, although the absolute risk is low (21).

In a population-based study of 156 women with in situ or invasive vaginal cancer, Daling et al. determined that they had many of the same risk factors as patients with cervical cancer, including a strong relationship with human papillomavirus (HPV) infection (21). The presence of antibodies to HPV 16 was strongly related to this risk. **A study of 341 cases from the Radiumhemmet reported that the disease seemed to be etiologically related to cervical cancer, and thus HPV infection, in young patients, but in older patients, there was no such association** (22). The rate of vaginal HPV infection in women posthysterectomy is similar to the rate of cervical HPV infection in women who have a uterus. **The relative rarity of invasive vaginal cancer suggests that the cervical transformation zone is an important, but not necessary, factor in malignant transformation** (23).

As many as 30% of patients with primary vaginal carcinoma have a history of in situ or invasive cervical cancer treated at least 5 years earlier (10,15,17). In a report from the University of South Carolina (11), a past history of invasive cervical cancer was present in 20% of the cases and of cervical intraepithelial neoplasia (CIN) in 7%. The median interval between the diagnosis of cervical cancer and the diagnosis of vaginal cancer was 14 years, with a range of 5 years, 8 months to 28 years. Sixteen percent of the patients had a history of prior pelvic irradiation.

There are three possible mechanisms for the occurrence of vaginal cancer after cervical neoplasia:

1. **Occult residual disease**
2. **New primary disease arising in an "at-risk" lower genital tract**
3. **Radiation carcinogenicity**

Colposcopy of the vagina should always be performed before surgical treatment for cervical cancer, and this should detect any extension of intraepithelial neoplasia from the cervix to the upper vagina. Adequate vaginal margins should be taken, and occult residual disease prevented.

There is controversy regarding the distinction between a new primary vaginal cancer and a recurrent cervical cancer. Some authorities use a 5-year cutoff because 95% of cervical cancer recurrences will occur within this period (24–26) but others prefer a 10-year interval (12).

Prior pelvic radiation therapy has been considered a possible cause of some vaginal carcinomas (22,27). In a series of 314 patients with squamous cell carcinoma of the vagina reported from

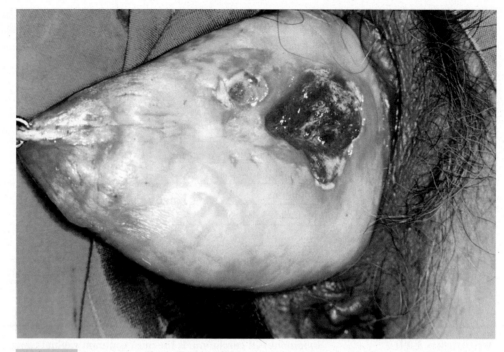

Figure 14.1 **Squamous cell carcinoma of the vagina in a patient with a procidentia.** The cancer was apparently related to long-term pessary use.

Sweden, 44 (14%) had received previous pelvic or vaginal radiation 5 to 55 years earlier. Although in many cases the radiation had been given for another HPV-related cancer, in 22 cases, the previous radiation had been for uterine or ovarian cancers (22). Judicious use of pelvic radiation may be particularly important in young patients, who may live long enough to develop a second neoplasm in the irradiated vagina (27).

The true malignant potential of vaginal intraepithelial neoplasia (VAIN) is unclear because after diagnosis, the condition is usually treated. Benedet and Saunders (28) reviewed 136 cases of carcinoma in situ of the vagina seen over a 30-year period. Four cases (3%) progressed to invasive vaginal cancer in spite of various methods of treatment. Rome and England reported 9 cases (6.8%) of early invasive vaginal cancer detected during the initial management of 132 cases of VAIN (29).

Chronic local irritation from long-term use of a pessary may be associated with vaginal cancer (Fig. 14.1) (7), although pessaries are used less commonly in modern gynecology.

Screening

For screening to be cost effective, the incidence of the disease must be sufficient to justify the cost of screening. In the United States, the age-adjusted incidence of vaginal cancer is 0.6 per 100,000 women, making routine screening of all patients inappropriate (30). **Women with a history of cervical intraepithelial or invasive neoplasia are at increased risk, and should be monitored with Pap smears and careful examination of the entire vagina.**

As many as 59% of patients with a vaginal cancer have had a prior hysterectomy (5,10), **but when age and prior cervical disease are controlled for, there is no increased risk of vaginal cancer in women who have had a hysterectomy for benign disease** (31).

Symptoms and Signs

Most patients with vaginal cancer present with painless vaginal bleeding and discharge. The bleeding is usually postmenopausal but may be postcoital. In the large series reported from the Radiumhemmet, 14% of patients were asymptomatic, and the diagnosis was made either by routine examination (7%) or by abnormal cytology (7%) (20).

Because the bladder neck is close to the vagina, bladder pain and frequency of micturition occur earlier than with cervical cancer. Posterior tumors may produce tenesmus. Approximately 5% of patients present with pelvic pain because of extension of disease beyond the vagina.

Most lesions are situated in the upper one-third of the vagina, usually at the apex or on the posterior wall (21,22,25–27,32). Macroscopically, the lesions are usually exophytic (fungating or polypoid), but they may be endophytic. Surface ulceration usually occurs late in the course of the disease.

Diagnosis

The diagnosis of carcinoma of the vagina is easily missed on first examination, particularly if the lesion is small and situated in the lower two-thirds of the vagina, where it may be covered by the blades of the speculum. Definitive diagnosis is usually made by biopsy of a gross lesion, which can often be performed in the office without anesthesia. In elderly patients or in those with some degree of vaginal stenosis, examination under anesthesia may be necessary to allow adequate biopsy and clinical staging. The latter may require cystoscopy or proctoscopy, depending on the location of the tumor.

In patients with an abnormal Pap smear and no gross abnormality, careful vaginal colposcopy and the liberal use of Lugol iodine to stain the vagina are necessary. This is initially performed in the office, but may need to be repeated with the patient under regional or general anesthesia to allow excision of colposcopically abnormal areas.

For definitive diagnosis of early vaginal carcinoma, it may be necessary to resect the entire vaginal vault and submit it for careful histologic evaluation, because the lesion may be partially buried by closure of the vault at the time of hysterectomy. This is usually done with a cold knife, but Fanning et al. have reported the successful use of the loop electrosurgical procedure for partial upper vaginectomy in 15 patients (33). Inadvertent cystotomy may occur, and this requires immediate repair.

Hoffman et al. at the University of South Florida reported on 32 patients who underwent upper vaginectomy for VAIN 3 (34). Occult invasive carcinoma was found in nine patients (28%). In five cases, the depth of invasion was less than 2 mm, but in four cases, invasion ranged from 3.5 mm to full-thickness involvement.

Staging

The FIGO staging for vaginal carcinoma is shown in Table 14.2. **The staging is clinical** and is based on the findings at general physical and pelvic examination, cystoscopy, proctoscopy, chest x-ray, and possible skeletal radiographs if the latter are indicated because of bone pain.

Because it is difficult to determine accurately any spread into subvaginal tissues, particularly from anterior or posterior lesions, **observer differences are common**. This is reflected in the wide range of stage distributions reported and the wide range of survival rates within a given stage. The distribution by FIGO stage from 16 series is shown in Table 14.3. Less than one-third of patients present with disease confined to the vagina, although Hellman et al. reported that significantly more patients were diagnosed at an early stage in the last 20 years of their study, compared to the first 20 years (20).

Because there have been no clinical series correlating the risk of lymph node involvement with the depth of invasion, there is no official definition of microinvasive disease. Peters et al. (35) suggested the following criteria for microinvasive carcinoma of the vagina: focal invasion

Table 14.2 Carcinoma of the Vagina: FIGO Nomenclature	
Stage I	The carcinoma is limited to the vaginal wall
Stage II	The carcinoma has involved the subvaginal tissue but has not extended to the pelvic wall
Stage III	The carcinoma has extended to the pelvic wall
Stage IV	The carcinoma has extended beyond the true pelvis or has involved the mucosa of the bladder or rectum; bullous edema as such does not permit a case to be allotted to stage IV
IVA	Tumor invades bladder and/or rectal mucosa and/or direct extension beyond the true pelvis
IVB	Spread to distant organs

FIGO Annual Report. *Int J Gynecol Obstet.* 2006;95:S29; *Int J Gynecol Obstet.* 2009;105:3–4.

Table 14.3 Primary Vaginal Carcinoma: Distribution by Stage of Disease		
Stage	*Number*	*Percentage*
I	611	29
II	769	36.5
III	451	21.4
IV	275	13.1
Total	**2,106**	**100**

Data compiled from **Ball and Berman, 1982** (10); **Houghton and Iversen, 1982** (11); **Benedet et al., 1983** (12); **Peters et al., 1985** (13); **Rubin et al., 1985** (14); **Kucera et al., 1991** (36); **Eddy et al., 1991** (16); **Kirkbride et al., 1995** (6); **Stock et al., 1995** (37); **Chyle et al., 1996** (4); **Ali et al., 1996** (17); **Perez et al., 1999** (26); **Tjalma et al., 2001** (18); and **Tewari et al., 2001** (19); **Hellman et al., 2006** (20); **Sinha et al., 2009** (32); **Hiniker et al., 2013** (38).

associated with VAIN 3, no lymph-vascular invasion, free margins on partial or total vaginectomy, and a maximum depth of invasion of less than 2.5 mm, measured from the overlying surface. Eddy et al. (39) reported six patients who met these criteria and were treated by either partial or total vaginectomy. In one of the six, a bladder recurrence developed at 35 months.

Patterns of Spread

Vaginal cancer spreads by the following routes:

1. **Direct extension** to the pelvic soft tissues, adjacent organs (bladder and rectum), and pelvic bones.
2. **Lymphatic dissemination** to the pelvic, and later the para-aortic lymph nodes. Lesions in the distal one-third of the vagina may metastasize directly to the inguinofemoral lymph nodes, with the pelvic nodes involved secondarily, or they may spread directly to pelvic nodes. Posterior vaginal lesions may involve perirectal nodes.

   Using lymphoscintigraphy, pretreatment lymphatic mapping and sentinel node identification were performed in 11 patients at the M. D. Anderson Cancer Center. Five patients (45%) had sentinel nodes identified in the groin only, four (36%) in the pelvis only, and two (18%) had sentinel nodes identified in both the groin and the pelvis (40). No relationship was observed between sentinel node location and primary tumor location.

3. **Hematogenous dissemination** to distant organs, including lungs, liver, and bone. Hematogenous dissemination is usually a late phenomenon in vaginal cancer, and the disease usually remains confined to the pelvis for most of its course.

There is little information available on the incidence of lymph node metastases in vaginal cancer, because most patients are treated with radiation therapy. Rubin et al. (14) reported that 16 of 38 patients (42.1%) with all stages of disease had lymphangiographic abnormalities, but many of these abnormalities were not confirmed histologically. **Al-Kurdi and Monaghan** (41) **performed lymph node dissections on 35 patients and reported positive pelvic nodes in 10 patients (28.6%). Positive inguinal nodes were present in 6 of 19 patients (31.6%), with disease involving the lower vagina.** Stock et al. reported positive pelvic nodes in 10 of 29 patients (34.5%) with all stages of disease who underwent bilateral pelvic lymphadenectomy as part of their therapy or staging. Positive para-aortic nodes were present in one of eight patients (12.5%) undergoing para-aortic dissection (37).

Preoperative Evaluation

Apart from the standard staging investigations, a computed tomographic (CT) or magnetic resonance imaging (MRI) scan of the pelvis and abdomen is useful for evaluation of the status of the primary tumor, liver, pelvic and para-aortic lymph nodes, and ureters. **A high-quality pelvic MRI usually gives better definition of the extent of the primary tumor than CT, and is particularly helpful in detecting bladder or rectal infiltration.** However, MRI can underestimate the extent of rectal mucosal infiltration, and must always be supplemented with a careful pelvic examination prior to treatment planning.

The group in St. Louis compared CT and F-18 fluorodeoxy glucose positron emission tomography (FDG-PET) for the detection of the primary tumor and lymph node metastases in patients with carcinoma of the vagina (42). In a series of 21 patients with an intact primary tumor, **CT demonstrated abnormally enlarged lymph nodes in 17%, while 35% had abnormal uptake with FDG-PET**. In the same series, CT visualized the primary tumor in only nine cases (43%), while FDG-PET demonstrated abnormal uptake at the primary site in all 21 (100%). Uptake in the bladder can obscure the extent of disease, particularly in the region of the anterior vaginal wall.

Treatment

Experience with the management of primary vaginal cancer is limited by the rarity of the disease. Most gynecologic oncology centers in the United States see only two to five new cases per year, and even in some European centers, where referral of oncology cases tends to be more centralized, only one new case per month can be expected (43). **Therapy must be individualized, and varies depending on the stage of disease and the site of vaginal involvement, further limiting physician experience.**

Anatomic factors and psychological considerations place significant constraints on treatment planning. The proximity of the vagina to the rectum, bladder, and urethra limits the dose of radiation that can be safely delivered, and restricts the surgical margins that can be attained, unless an exenterative procedure is performed. **For most patients, maintenance of a functional vagina is an important factor in the planning of therapy.**

Primary Surgery

Primary surgery has a limited role in the management of patients with vaginal cancer because of the radicality required to achieve clear surgical margins, but in selected cases, satisfactory results can be achieved (20,32,37,40,44–46). Surgery may be useful in the following circumstances:

1. **In patients with stage I disease involving the upper posterior vagina.** If the uterus is still in situ, these patients require radical hysterectomy, partial vaginectomy, and bilateral pelvic lymphadenectomy. If the patient has had a hysterectomy, radical upper vaginectomy and pelvic lymphadenectomy can be performed after development of the paravesicular and pararectal spaces and dissection of each ureter out to its point of entry into the bladder.

   A Chinese report described four patients who had laparoscopic radical hysterectomy, pelvic lymphadenectomy, and total vaginectomy for stage I vaginal carcinoma (45). Vaginal reconstruction was performed using the sigmoid colon. All patients were clinically free of disease with a mean follow-up of 46 months (range 40 to 54 months).

   A surgical approach to conserve reproductive and sexual function was described from Italy (46). Three nulliparous women under 40 years of age with stage I squamous cell carcinoma confined to the upper third of the vagina underwent radical tumorectomy and pelvic lymphadenectomy. A fourth patient underwent partial hemivaginectomy plus ipsilateral paracolpectomy and pelvic lymphadenectomy. One patient with microscopic involvement of the paracolpium received adjuvant radiation after laparoscopic ovarian transposition. With a follow-up of 9 to 51 months, all patients were regularly menstruating, sexually active, and clinically free of disease.

   Although this approach has obvious appeal, the number of cases is very limited, and such an approach should be limited to small lesions, particularly if located in the upper vagina. The authors recommended more intensive follow-up, particularly aimed at early detection of any locoregional relapse or a second tumor of the lower genital tract (46).

2. **In young patients who require radiation therapy.** Pretreatment laparotomy or laparoscopy in such patients may allow ovarian transposition, surgical staging, and resection of any lymph nodes larger than 2 cm diameter.

3. **In patients with stage IVA disease, particularly if a rectovaginal or vesicovaginal fistula is present.** Primary pelvic exenteration is a suitable treatment option for such patients, provided they are medically fit, and the tumor is not fixed to the pelvic sidewall. Eddy et al. (16) reported a 5-year disease-free survival in three of six patients with stage IVA disease treated with preoperative radiation followed by anterior or total pelvic exenteration. In sexually active patients, vaginal reconstruction should be performed simultaneously.

4. **In patients with a central recurrence after radiation therapy.** Surgical resection, which usually necessitates pelvic exenteration, is the only option for this group of patients.

Neoadjuvant Chemotherapy followed by Radical Surgery

Benedetti Panici et al. from Italy reported 11 patients with FIGO stage II vaginal cancer who were treated with *paclitaxel* 175 mg/m^2 and *cisplatin* 75 mg/m^2 every 21 days for three courses, followed by radical hysterectomy, radical vaginectomy, and pelvic lymphadenectomy. If the distal third of the vagina was involved, an inguinal-femoral lymphadenectomy was also performed (44). One patient had a positive pelvic node and received external pelvic radiation. Three patients (27%) achieved a complete clinical response and seven (64%) a partial clinical response to the chemotherapy. With a median follow-up of 75 months, nine patients (82%) remained free of disease.

Radiation Therapy

Radiation therapy is the treatment of choice for all patients except those previously listed. In most cases, a combination of teletherapy and intracavitary or interstitial brachytherapy is used to achieve optimal control rates (4–6,8,19,20,26,37). Although several reports suggest that local control can sometimes be achieved with brachytherapy alone for highly selected stage I and II lesions, local recurrence rates of 20–30% are higher than expected for these early lesions and suggest that some treatment with external beam is usually indicated (5,6,26,47). For larger lesions, treatment is usually started with approximately 4,000 to 5,000 cGy of external beam irradiation to treat the pelvic lymph nodes and to obtain initial shrinkage of primary tumor. Radiation fields should be carefully tailored to the primary site and must take into account movement of the vagina with variations in bladder and rectal filling. Radiopaque fiducial markers inserted in the vagina assist in external beam treatment planning and document the original extent of disease for brachytherapy planning. **If the distal one-third of the vagina is involved, the groin nodes should be treated. As with cervical cancer, patients who have involved common iliac or para-aortic nodes should be treated with extended fields.**

The most challenging part of treatment is the final boost treatment that must be given to achieve control of initial sites of gross disease. A wide variety of highly specialized techniques can be used to deliver additional radiation to the primary site, while minimizing the dose to adjacent critical structures. In most cases, this additional dose is achieved using intracavitary or interstitial brachytherapy.

If the uterus is intact and the lesion involves the upper vagina, an intrauterine tandem and appropriate vaginal applicator can be used. In patients who have had a hysterectomy, superficial apical lesions may be treated using a vaginal domed cylinder. A cylinder with peripheral channels may be used for superficial lesions in the midvagina. **Because of its steep fall-off in radiation dose deep to a cylinder, intracavitary treatment should rarely be used for lesions that are thicker than 3 to 5 mm at the time of brachytherapy. Interstitial brachytherapy techniques permit coverage of more deeply invasive lesions;** however, when interstitial therapy is used for apical lesions, laparoscopy or open guidance may be needed (5,19,26).

In general, brachytherapy is preferred over an external beam boost if the tumor target volume can be adequately covered without overdosing critical structures. When the location of the target makes it impossible to treat the entire tumor to high dose without placing needles in or very close to critical structures, it may be better to complete the treatment using highly conformal techniques, such as intensity modulated radiation therapy (IMRT). In particular, **massive, fixed tumors and tumors that involve the rectovaginal septum or bladder may be treated more effectively with additional external beam irradiation using IMRT.**

There is limited reported experience with chemoradiation for vaginal cancer (6,48), although many centers routinely use this combined therapy, as is being done for cervical carcinoma. In our centers, *cisplatin* 35 to 40 mg/m^2 given on the first day of each week of external beam therapy is used. The small number of cases makes it virtually impossible to conduct a randomized, prospective study to compare standard radiation with chemoradiation for patients with vaginal cancer.

Complications of Therapy

Major complications of therapy are usually reported in 10–15% of patients treated for primary vaginal cancer, whether the treatment is by surgery or radiation. Extensive tumor involvement can cause tissue injury and scarring, but the close proximity of the rectum, bladder, and urethra predispose these structures to treatment-related injuries in the form of radiation cystitis, radiation proctitis, recto or vesicovaginal fistulas, and rectal strictures or ulceration. Frank et al. (5) reported overall actuarial rates of major complications of 10% and 17% at 5 and 10 years, respectively. Eight of 11 major rectal complications occurred in patients whose tumors involved the posterior wall and all of the major bladder complications occurred in patients whose tumors involved the anterior wall. The risk of major complications was also strongly correlated with tumor stage and with a history of smoking. **The risk of functional damage to the vagina after treatment of vaginal cancer is high,** particularly for patients with large, destructive cancers. Localized radiation necrosis is occasionally seen during the first 3 to 6 months after treatment but fibrosis and vaginal stenosis are more common causes of sexual dysfunction.

Stryker (49) reported vaginal morbidity in 9 of 15 patients (60%) undergoing external beam therapy plus intracavitary brachytherapy, and 3 of 10 patients (30%) undergoing external beam therapy plus interstitial brachytherapy. He suggested that when combining external beam therapy with brachytherapy, interstitial techniques were preferable, although **the probability of late vaginal morbidity may be related to radiation dose rate and radiation fractionation, as well as technique.** These factors vary widely between practitioners, and detailed quality-of-life studies comparing outcome with tumor characteristics and treatment techniques are needed.

Patients who are sexually active should be encouraged to continue regular intercourse, but those who are not sexually active, or for whom intercourse is temporarily too painful, should be encouraged to use topical estrogen and a vaginal dilator, at least every second night.

Prognosis

A compilation of large published series reveals a mean overall 5-year survival rate for vaginal cancer of about 52%, which reflects the challenges involved in treating this disease, and the late stage at presentation (Table 14.4). For patients with stage I disease, the 5-year survival rate in combined series is approximately 74%. In the 26th volume of the FIGO *Annual Report on the Results of Treatment in Gynecological Cancer,* the 5-year survival for 224 patients with vaginal cancer was as follows: Stage I, 77.6%; stage II, 52.2%; stage III, 42.5%; stage IVA, 20.5%; stage IVB, 12.9% (3).

Better results have been reported from individual centers. In a report of 193 cases of primary vaginal squamous cell carcinoma from the M. D. Anderson Cancer Center in Houston, Frank et al. reported 5-year disease-specific survival rates of 85% for 50 patients with FIGO stage I disease, 78% for 97 patients with stage II, and 58% for 46 patients with stages III to IV (5). Five-year disease-specific survival rates were 82% and 60% for patients with tumors ≥4 cm and >4 cm, respectively ($p = 0.0001$). Kirkbride et al. (6) from the **Princess Margaret Hospital in Toronto reported on 138 patients** with invasive vaginal carcinoma. **The 5-year cause-specific survival rates by stage were 77% for stages I/II and 56% for stages III/IV.** In a multivariate analysis, only tumor size and stage of disease were significant variables.

Most recurrences of vaginal cancer are in the pelvis (50), so high-quality radiation therapy including brachytherapy performed by an experienced brachytherapist and possibly concurrent chemotherapy may improve the results. Chyle et al. (4) reported that **cure after first relapse was uncommon, with a 5-year survival rate of only 12%.**

Because of the rarity of the disease, patients with vaginal cancer should be referred centrally to a limited number of tertiary referral units so that increasing experience can be gained in their management.

Table 14.4 Primary Vaginal Carcinoma: 5-Year Survival Rates

Stage	No.	5-Year Survival	Percentage
I	509	378	74.3
II	622	333	53.5
III	377	128	34
IV	163	24	15.3
Total	1,671	864	51.7

Data compiled from **Pride et al., 1979** (9); **Houghton and Iversen, 1982** (11); **Benedet et al., 1983** (12); **Rubin et al., 1985** (14); **Kucera et al., 1991** (36); **Eddy et al., 1991** (16); **Kirkbride et al., 1995** (6); and **Tewari et al., 2001** (19); **Perez et al., 1999** (26); **Otton et al., 2004** (51); **Frank et al., 2005** (5); **Hellman et al., 2006** (20); **Tran et al., 2007** (52).

Adenocarcinoma

Approximately 10% of primary vaginal carcinomas are adenocarcinomas. They tend to affect a younger population of women than squamous cancers, regardless of whether or not exposure to *diethylstilbestrol (DES) in utero* has occurred (53). Adenocarcinomas may arise in areas of vaginal adenosis, particularly in patients exposed to *DES in utero* (54), but they probably also arise in Wolffian rest elements, periurethral glands, and foci of endometriosis. Vaginal adenosis is the sequestration of müllerian glandular epithelium into the vaginal mucosa during embryogenesis. It is thought to arise as a consequence of disrupted development and has been reported in non–*DES*-exposed women from infancy to old age (54). Intestinal metaplasia occasionally occurs in tissues of müllerian origin, and primary vaginal adenocarcinoma of intestinal type has been described (55). **Secondary tumors from such sites as the colon, endometrium, or ovary should be considered when vaginal adenocarcinoma is diagnosed.**

Diethylstilbestrol Exposure *In Utero*

In 1970, Herbst and Scully (56) reported on seven women with clear cell adenocarcinoma of the vagina, seen in Boston over a 4-year period. Their ages ranged from 15 to 22 years. One year later, Herbst et al. reported an association with maternal *DES* ingestion during pregnancy in six of the seven cases (57). *DES* was used to maintain high-risk pregnancies, such as diabetic or twin pregnancies, in women with a history of spontaneous abortion.

A Registry for Research on Hormonal Transplacental Carcinogenesis was established in 1971 to investigate all aspects of clear cell adenocarcinoma of the vagina and cervix. More than 500 cases were reported to the Registry, although **only about two-thirds of cases had a history of prenatal exposure to *DES***. In all instances, the mother had been treated in the first half of the pregnancy (58). An additional 10% of the mothers had received some unknown medication, but in 25% of cases, there was no indication of any maternal hormone ingestion. The oldest reported *DES*-exposed patient with vaginal clear cell carcinoma was 52 years. The use of *DES* for pregnant patients was discontinued in the United States in 1971, and since the 1990s, the incidence of clear cell adenocarcinoma of the vagina has substantially declined.

The estimated risk of clear cell adenocarcinoma in an exposed offspring was 1:1,000 or less, and 70% of cases were stage I at diagnosis. Although *DES* exposure *in utero* rarely led to vaginal adenocarcinoma, vaginal adenosis occurred in about 45% of patients, and 25% of exposed women had structural changes to the cervix and vagina, such as a transverse vaginal septum, a cervical collar, a cockscomb (a raised ridge, usually on the anterior cervix), or cervical hypoplasia.

Two types of cells have been described in vaginal adenosis and cervical ectropion: The mucinous cell, which resembles the endocervical epithelium, and the tuboendometrial cell (59). **Areas of vaginal adenosis and cervical ectropion are progressively covered with metaplastic squamous epithelium as the individual matures, and areas of adenosis may disappear completely and be replaced by normally glycogenated squamous epithelium.**

Treatment of Adenocarcinoma

Adenocarcinomas may be treated in a similar way to squamous carcinomas. **The cohort of DES-related cancers is now over 55 years, and rarely seen in clinical practice.** In the past, radical hysterectomy, pelvic lymphadenectomy, vaginectomy, and replacement of the vagina with a split-thickness skin graft were used very successfully for early-stage DES-related cancers, and a combination of wide local excision, retroperitoneal lymphadenectomy, and local irradiation was also effective (60). Local surgical excision alone for small primary tumors was associated with a higher incidence of local and regional recurrence, as about 16% of patients with DES-related stage I disease had positive pelvic nodes (61).

If radiation alone is used, a pretreatment staging laparotomy or laparoscopy to allow resection of any bulky nodes and ovarian transposition may facilitate an optimal functional outcome. Freezing of embryos with a view to a subsequent surrogate pregnancy may be considered if ovarian function is in jeopardy and the patient has a suitable partner.

Prognosis

Herbst et al. (61) reported a 5-year survival rate for DES-related patients with clear cell carcinoma of the vagina, regardless of the mode of therapy of 78%. **The survival rate correlated well with stage of disease: 87% for patients with stage I, 76% for patients with stage II, and 30% for those with stage III disease.**

In contrast, the prognosis of patients with primary non–DES-related adenocarcinomas appears to be relatively poor. Twenty-six patients, with a median age of 54 years, were reported from the M. D. Anderson Cancer Center in 2007 (62). The 5-year overall survival for these patients was 34%, compared to 58% for squamous cell carcinomas treated over the same period (p < 0.01), and pelvic disease control was 31%, compared to 81% for squamous carcinomas (p < 0.01). At 5 years, 39% of adenocarcinomas had developed distant metastases, compared to 15% of squamous carcinomas (p < 0.01).

Small Cell Carcinoma

Primary small cell carcinoma of the vagina is extremely rare, but as many as 5% of such tumors arise in extrapulmonary sites. In the female genital tract, such tumors arise most commonly in the cervix, followed by the ovary, endometrium, vagina, and vulva (63). As with other primary sites, small cell carcinoma of the vagina has a proclivity for distant failure and a poor prognosis. Management should be with concurrent chemoradiation, and probably systemic chemotherapy.

Verrucous Carcinoma

Verrucous carcinomas of the vagina are rare, but their clinical and pathologic features are similar to those of their vulvar counterparts (64). They are large, warty tumors that are locally aggressive but have a minimal tendency to metastasize. Wide surgical excision of the tumor is the treatment of choice. Crowther et al. (64), in a literature review, reported a successful outcome in four of five patients with small lesions treated by wide excision. For larger lesions, exenteration or vaginectomy was successful in seven of seven patients, but there were three postoperative deaths. Regional lymphadenectomy is not required, provided there is no suspicious lymphadenopathy. Radiation therapy has been implicated in the rapid transformation of such lesions to a more malignant tumor, and Crowther et al. (64) reported recurrence in all four patients treated with primary radiation therapy.

Vaginal Melanoma

Malignant melanomas of the vagina are rare, with fewer than 250 reported cases to 2002 (65). The 26th FIGO Annual Report documents 13 cases (4%) among 324 cases of vaginal cancer (3). They presumably arise from melanocytes that are present in the vagina in 3% of normal women (66).

A recent report of 201 patients diagnosed from 1998 to 2008 from the Surveillance, Epidemiology, and End Results (SEER) registry, revealed a median age of 68 years (range 28 to 100 years). The population was 73% white, 11% African-American, and 16% Asian/American Indian (67).

Clinically, most patients present with vaginal bleeding, a vaginal mass, or vaginal discharge (68, 69). The lesions most commonly arise in the distal part of the vagina, particularly on the anterior wall (69,70). They may be nonpigmented and are frequently ulcerated, making them easily confused with squamous carcinomas.

Most are deeply invasive. Expressing the lesion in terms of Chung's level of invasion (as defined for vulvar melanomas) (71), Chung et al. (70) reported that 13 of 15 (87%) vaginal melanomas were at level IV. A more recent study from Houston reported that 20 of 26 cases (77%) were level IV lesions (72). Approximately 60% of Chung's cases exhibited spread of melanocytic cells into the adjacent epithelium, and in approximately 30% of the cases, the lateral spread was extensive (70).

Radical surgery has traditionally been the mainstay of treatment, and has often involved anterior, posterior, or total pelvic exenteration, depending on the location of the lesion. Small upper vaginal lesions have been treated with radical hysterectomy, subtotal vaginectomy, and pelvic lymphadenectomy, whereas small distal lesions have been treated by partial vaginectomy, total or partial vulvectomy, with or without bilateral inguinofemoral lymphadenectomy.

More recently, conservative operations (e.g., wide local excision) have been used, followed frequently by pelvic radiotherapy (65,69,73–75), and there appears to be no significant benefit in terms of survival or disease-free interval for radical versus conservative surgery. The most important issue is to remove all gross disease whenever possible (75). Postoperative radiation therapy is effective for prevention of local recurrence; hypofractioned schedules of more than 400 cGy per radiation fraction may be more effective than conventional schedules of 180 to 200 cGy per fraction (76). The results of treatment with cytotoxic chemotherapy have been disappointing, and most patients die with distant metastases (72).

The overall prognosis for patients with vaginal melanoma is poor because most patients have deeply penetrating lesions with a high probability of distant metastasis. The recent SEER study reported an overall survival at 2 and 5 years of 24% and 15%, respectively (67). The presence of lymph node metastases at diagnosis was associated with a worse prognosis ($p = 0.02$), and adjuvant radiation did not offer any survival advantage over surgery alone. Reid et al. (69) and Buchanan et al. (74) noted that the size of the lesion was the best prognostic indicator. **Among 13 5-year survivors who had their tumor size noted, 11 (84.6%) had lesions less than 3 cm in maximal diameter.** Among 10 5-year survivors who had depth of invasion noted, only 2 (20%) had invasion of greater than 2 mm (69).

Adjuvant therapy with *interferon alfa-2b* has been shown to improve relapse-free and overall survival in patients with high-risk cutaneous melanomas (77), but there are as yet no data on this treatment for vaginal melanomas.

After a recurrence is noted, prognosis is extremely poor.

Vaginal Sarcoma

Leiomyosarcoma

Vaginal sarcomas, such as **fibrosarcomas** and **leiomyosarcomas,** are rare tumors. They are usually bulky lesions and occur most commonly in the upper vagina. Tavassoli and Norris (78) reported 60 smooth muscle tumors of the vagina, only 5 of which recurred. All recurrences were seen in tumors more than 3 cm in diameter with moderate to marked cytologic atypia and more than five mitoses per 10 high-power fields. **A review of vaginal leiomyosarcomas in 2000 revealed fewer than 70 cases reported in the English literature (79). The average age at presentation was 47 years, and the overall 5-year survival was 43%.**

Surgical excision is the mainstay of treatment. If the lesion is well differentiated and the surgical margins are not involved, as is likely with tumors of low malignant potential, the likelihood of cure is good. For frankly malignant lesions, lymphatic and hematogenous dissemination are common. Adjuvant pelvic radiation may be indicated in selected cases (80).

Rhabdomyosarcoma

Rhabdomyosarcoma, a malignant tumor of the rhabdomyoblasts, is the most common soft tissue tumor in children. Rhabdomyosarcoma of the female genital tract is one of the most curable forms of the disease, but accounts for less than 4% of all pediatric rhabdomyosarcomas (81).

Sarcoma botryoides (embryonal rhabdomyosarcoma) is a highly malignant, grapelike tumor. The term *botryoides* comes from the Greek word *botrys,* which means "grapes," and, grossly, the tumor usually appears as a polypoid mass extruding from the vagina. Microscopically, the characteristic feature is the presence of cross-striated rhabdomyoblasts (strap cells). **More than 75% of vulvovaginal rhabdomyosarcomas are of the botryoid histologic type (81,82). In the female genital tract, sarcoma botryoides is usually found in the vagina during infancy and early childhood, in the cervix during the reproductive years, and in the corpus uteri during the postmenopausal period.**

Approaches to management have varied over the years, but **radical surgery, including pelvic exenteration for primary management, has progressively been replaced by chemotherapy and more conservative surgery and radiation. The most influential group in this regard has been the Intergroup Rhabdomyosarcoma Study Group (IRSG),** which conducted four consecutive trials commencing in 1972 (82). The initial study (1972 to 1978) involved radical surgical resection followed by chemotherapy, with or without radiotherapy. In the second study (1978 to 1984), multiagent chemotherapy was given first to reduce tumor size, with the objective of allowing more conservative surgery and organ preservation. Radiotherapy was reserved for those patients with residual disease after surgery. In both the third (1984 to 1991) and fourth (1991 to 1997) studies, chemotherapy was intensified, with the aim of further reducing the extent of necessary surgery. After induction chemotherapy, clinical and radiologic responses were closely monitored and local treatment given only if residual tumor persisted (82).

The IRSG grouping classification is shown in Table 14.5. Chemotherapy was given according to the tumor group. **Patients with group I, II, or III tumors received 12 months of treatment with either VAC** (*vincristine, actinomycin D,* and *cyclophosphamide*), **VAI** (*vincristine, actinomycin D, and ifosfamide*) **plus VAC, or VIE** (*vincristine, ifosfamide and etoposide*) **plus VAC. Patients with group IV tumors were randomized to receive VM** (*vincristine* and *melphelan*) **or ID** (*ifosfamide* and *doxyrubicin*) as initial therapy, followed by **VAC** plus RT.

Table 14.5 IRSG Grouping Classification	
Group I	Localized disease, completely excised, no microscopic residual tumor
	A. Confined to site of origin, completely resected
	B. Infiltrating beyond site of origin, completely resected
Group II	Total gross resection
	A. Gross resection with evidence of microscopic local residual disease
	B. Regional disease with involved lymph nodes, completely resected with no macroscopic residual tumor
	C. Microscopic local and/or lymph node residual disease
Group III	Incomplete resection or biopsy with gross residual disease
Group IV	Distant metastases

IRSG, Intergroup Rhabdomyosarcoma Study Group.

As with surgery, radiotherapy has been more limited in recent years with a view to decreasing morbidity and preserving reproductive capability. Since 1990, only residual disease has been included in the brachytherapy-treated volume at the Gustave Roussy Institute in Paris (81). **Ovarian transposition should be undertaken surgically prior to radiation therapy.** Tumors larger than 40 mm after chemotherapy are not candidates for exclusive brachytherapy (81).

In a review of the records of 82 cases of vaginal rhabdomyosarcoma treated on IRSG protocols I to IV, **the estimated 5-year survival was over 85% for patients with locoregional tumors** (82).

Other Vaginal Sarcomas

A variety of other malignant mesodermal tumors have been reported to arise in the vagina, including **malignant fibrous histiocytoma** (83); **angiosarcoma** (84); and **hemangiopericytoma** (85). Petur and Young suggested that the latter tumors probably represent extrauterine endometrial stromal sarcomas (86).

Endodermal Sinus Tumor (Yolk Sac Tumor)

These rare germ cell tumors are occasionally found in extragonadal sites such as the vagina. Leverger et al. (87) reported 11 such cases from the Institut Gustave Roussy. **The average age of the patients was 10 months,** and the presenting symptom was vaginal bleeding. Diagnosis was made by examination and biopsy with the patient under anesthesia. All children had high serum alpha-fetoprotein levels. From 1977 to 1983, **six of eight children were cured,** with an average follow-up of 3 years. Treatment consisted of primary chemotherapy to reduce the tumor volume, followed by partial colpectomy, radiation therapy, or both.

Carcinoma of the Female Urethra

Primary carcinoma of the female urethra is a rare malignancy, accounting for less than 0.1% of all female genital malignancies (88). The disease has been reported from the third to the ninth decades of life, with a **median age of approximately 65 years**. The most common presenting symptoms are urethral bleeding, hematuria, dysuria, urinary obstruction, and a mass at the introitus (89). Uncommon presenting symptoms include urinary incontinence, perineal pain, and dyspareunia.

Most tumors involve the anterior or distal urethra and may be confused with a urethral caruncle or mucosal prolapse. Histologically, these distal lesions are usually squamous cell carcinomas. Tumors involving the posterior or proximal urethra are usually adenocarcinomas or transitional cell carcinomas. The relative frequency of the various histologic variants is shown in Table 14.6. Urethral carcinomas, often of clear cell type, occasionally arise in a urethral diverticulum (90).

There is no FIGO staging for the disease, and several staging classifications have been suggested (91–94). The TNM staging system is shown in Table 14.7. **Distal tumors spread to the lymph nodes of the groin, whereas proximal tumors tend to spread to pelvic nodes; treatment planning**

Table 14.6 Histology of Urethral Carcinomas		
Type	*No.*	*Percentage*
Squamous cell	133	53
Adenocarcinoma	54	21.5
Transitional cell	48	19.1
Undifferentiated	8	3.2
Melanoma	5	2
Sarcoma	1	0.4
Non-Hodgkin lymphoma	1	0.4
Unknown	1	0.4
Total	**251**	**100**

Data compiled from **Bracken et al., 1976** (93); **Benson et al., 1982** (90); **Weghaupt et al., 1984** (88); **Prempree et al., 1984** (91); **Grigsby, 1998** (95); **Eng et al., 2003** (96) and **Thyarihally et al., 2005** (89).

should take this into consideration. Bladder neck involvement is a common cause of local recurrence, and examination under anesthesia, endoscopic evaluation, and biopsy of the bladder neck should be undertaken as part of the pretreatment workup.

The treatment of urethral cancer must be individualized (88) and requires close multidisciplinary collaboration (89,96,97). For small distal lesions, the distal half of the urethra can be excised without loss of urinary continence. **Bilateral inguinofemoral lymphadenectomy or inguinal radiation therapy should be performed for all but the most superficial distal lesions.** Early lesions arising in the proximal urethra can be effectively treated with definitive radiation therapy to the primary site and regional lymph nodes.

Most patients present with advanced disease. In these cases, even pelvic exenteration yields survival rates of only 10–20% (98). Some investigators have recommended multimodality treatment involving radiation or chemotherapy combined with surgical resection. Many combinations have been suggested but the small size of most experiences makes it difficult to compare the effectiveness of different treatment approaches. **Postoperative radiation therapy with or without chemotherapy may yield higher local control rates than radical surgery alone** (97). Klein et al. (99) from Memorial Sloan-Kettering reported on the use of preoperative radiation followed by anterior exenteration combined with resection of the inferior pubic rami in five women with urethral cancer. Two died with distant metastases, and one died of surgical complications at 1 month. **Neoadjuvant chemotherapy followed by anterior exenteration has been used with some success** (100).

Definitive radiation therapy, with or without concurrent chemotherapy, has been used with some success and may be the treatment of choice, particularly for patients with advanced disease (95,101,102). Milosevic et al. (102) reported a 7-year overall survival rate of 41% for 34 women treated with radiation therapy alone. Patients whose treatment included brachytherapy tended to have better outcomes but also tended to have less advanced tumors. In another series of 44 women, Grigsby (95) reported a 5-year survival rate of 42%. Most of the patients reported in these series had stage III or IV disease and many had gross nodal involvement. In addition, they were treated 20 to 50 years ago, often using techniques that would be considered primitive by current standards. Modern image-guidance, 3D planning and high-energy photon beams would be expected to hold major advantages over earlier techniques, but have only been anecdotally described in the clinical literature.

Experience with chemoradiation is limited to case reports, but the results appear to be favorable (103–105). Chemotherapeutic agents used have included *cisplatin, 5-fluorouracil,* and *mitomycin-C*. In view of the experience with other primary sites, this would seem to be an acceptable initial approach for locally advanced cases.

A Japanese case report described bladder-sparing urethrectomy with resection of the anterior vaginal wall and continent urinary diversion using the appendix (Mitrofanoff procedure) for a 2 cm × 2 cm distal urethral cancer invading the anterior vaginal wall. The patient was 77 years old and 4 years after surgery, she remained disease free (106).

Table 14.7 TNM Staging for Urethral Cancer

Stage		TNM	
Stage 0_a	T_a	N_0	M_0
Stage 0_{is}	T_{is}	N_0	M_0
Stage I	T_1	N_0	M_0
Stage II	T_2	N_0	M_0
Stage III	T_1	N_1	M_0
	T_2	N_1	M_0
	T_3	N_0	M_0
	T_3	N_1	M_0
Stage IV	T_4	N_0	M_0
	T_4	N_1	M_0
	Any T	N_2	M_0
	Any T	N_3	M_0
	Any T	Any N	M_1

TNM Classification

T:	Primary Tumor	M:	Distant Metastases
T_a	Noninvasive papillary, polypoid, or verrucous carcinoma		
T_{is}	Carcinoma in situ	M_x	Presence of distant metastasis cannot be assessed
T_1	Tumor invades subepithelial connective tissue	M_0	No distant metastasis
T_2	Tumor invades the periurethral muscle	M_1	Distant metastasis
T_3	Tumor invades the anterior vagina or bladder neck	**Histopathologic Type**	
T_4	Tumor invades other adjacent organs	Cell types can be divided into transitional, squamous, and glandular	

N:	Regional Lymph Nodes	G:	Histopathologic Grade
N_x	Regional lymph nodes cannot be assessed	G_x	Grade cannot be assessed
N_0	No regional lymph node metastasis	G_1	Well differentiated
N_1	Metastasis in a single lymph node, 2 cm or less in greatest dimension	G_2	Moderately differentiated
N_2	Metastasis in a single lymph node, more than 2 cm but not more than 5 cm in greatest dimension; or multiple lymph nodes, none more than 5 cm in greatest dimension	G_{3-4}	Poorly differentiated or undifferentiated
N_3	Metastasis in a lymph node more than 5 cm in greatest dimension		

Prognosis

Bracken et al. (93) from the M. D. Anderson Hospital reported an overall 5-year survival rate of only 32% for 81 cases of carcinoma of the female urethra. Grigsby (95), from the Mallinckrodt Institute of Radiology in St. Louis, reported a 5-year survival rate of 42% for 44 cases. Treatment was with surgery in seven cases, radiation therapy in 25 cases, and combined surgery and radiation therapy in 12. The severe complication rate was 29% for treatment with surgery, 24% for radiation therapy, and 8% for combined therapy. **The most important clinical factors affecting prognosis were tumor size and histologic type—none of 13 women with adenocarcinomas was alive at 5 years, and only 1 of 10 women with a tumor greater than 4 cm diameter was a 5-year survivor. The main cause of treatment failure was local recurrence.**

Malignant Melanoma of the Urethra

This rare primary urethral tumor accounts for 0.2% of all melanomas. Di Marco et al. (107) reported the Mayo Clinic experience of 11 cases (mean age 68 years) treated from 1950 to 1999. Most patients presented with hematuria or a urethral mass. Four patients were treated by radical surgery, including anterior exenteration in two patients. Two (50%) of the four patients undergoing radical surgery recurred at 4 and 34 months, respectively. The remaining seven patients underwent local excision with partial urethrectomy. This group experienced urethral recurrence in five of the seven patients (71%). No patient received any adjuvant therapy. The authors suggested that radical urethrectomy with bladder preservation and a continent catheterizable stoma may be a more appropriate option. They suggested that the catheterizable stoma could be constructed using an appendicovesicostomy or an ileovesicostomy for urinary diversion.

References

1. **Siegel R, Ma J, Zou Z, et al.** Cancer statistics, 2014. *CA Cancer J Clin.* 2014;64:9–29.
2. **Wu X, Matanoski G, Chen VW, et al.** Descriptive epidemiology of vaginal cancer incidence and survival by race, ethnicity, and age in the United States. *Cancer.* 2008;113:2873–2882.
3. **Beller U, Benedet J, Creasman W, et al.** Carcinoma of the vagina: 26th annual report on the results of treatment in gynecological cancer. *Int J Gynaecol Obstet.* 2006;95(suppl 1):S29–S42.
4. **Chyle V, Zagars GK, Wheeler JA, et al.** Definitive radiotherapy for carcinoma of the vagina: Outcome and prognostic factors. *Int J Radiat Oncol Biol Phys.* 1996;35:891–905.
5. **Frank SJ, Jhingran A, Levenback C, et al.** Definitive radiation therapy for squamous cell carcinoma of the vagina. *Int J Radiat Oncol Biol Phys.* 2005;62:138–147.
6. **Kirkbride P, Fyles A, Rawlings GA, et al.** Carcinoma of the vagina–experience at the Princess Margaret Hospital (1974–1989). *Gynecol Oncol.* 1995;56:435–443.
7. **Fu YS, Reagan J.** *Pathology of the Uterine Cervix, Vagina, and Vulva.* Philadelphia, PA: W B Saunders; 1989.
8. **Perez CA, Arneson AN, Dehner LP, et al.** Radiation therapy in carcinoma of the vagina. *Obstet Gynecol.* 1974;44:862–872.
9. **Pride GL, Schultz AE, Chuprevich TW, et al.** Primary invasive squamous carcinoma of the vagina. *Obstet Gynecol.* 1979;53:218–225.
10. **Ball HG, Berman ML.** Management of primary vaginal carcinoma. *Gynecol Oncol.* 1982;14:154–163.
11. **Houghton CR, Iversen T.** Squamous cell carcinoma of the vagina: A clinical study of the location of the tumor. *Gynecol Oncol.* 1982;13:365–372.
12. **Benedet JL, Murphy KJ, Fairey RN, et al.** Primary invasive carcinoma of the vagina. *Obstet Gynecol.* 1983;62:715–719.
13. **Peters W, Kumar N, Morley G.** Carcinoma of the vagina. Factors influencing outcome. *Cancer.* 1985;55:892–897.
14. **Rubin SC, Young J, Mikuta JJ.** Squamous carcinoma of the vagina: Treatment, complications, and long-term follow-up. *Gynecol Oncol.* 1985;20:346–354.
15. **Sulak P, Barnhill D, Heller P, et al.** Nonsquamous cancer of the vagina. *Gynecol Oncol.* 1988;29:309–320.
16. **Eddy GL, Marks RD, Miller MC, et al.** Primary invasive vaginal carcinoma. *Am J Obstet Gynecol.* 1991;165:292–298.
17. **Ali MM, Huang DT, Goplerud DR, et al.** Radiation alone for carcinoma of the vagina: Variation in response related to the location of the primary tumor. *Cancer.* 1996;77:1934–1939.
18. **Tjalma WA, Monaghan JM, de Barros Lopes A, et al.** The role of surgery in invasive squamous carcinoma of the vagina. *Gynecol Oncol.* 2001;81:360–365.
19. **Tewari KS, Cappuccini F, Puthawala AA, et al.** Primary invasive carcinoma of the vagina: Treatment with interstitial brachytherapy. *Cancer.* 2001;91:758–770.
20. **Hellman K, Lundell M, Silfversward C, et al.** Clinical and histopathologic factors related to prognosis in primary squamous cell carcinoma of the vagina. *Int J Gynecol Cancer.* 2006;16:1201–1211.
21. **Daling JR, Madeleine MM, Schwartz SM, et al.** A population-based study of squamous cell vaginal cancer: HPV and cofactors. *Gynecol Oncol.* 2002;84:263–270.
22. **Hellman K, Silfversward C, Nilsson B, et al.** Primary carcinoma of the vagina: Factors influencing the age at diagnosis. The Radiumhemmet series 1956–1996. *Int J Gynecol Cancer.* 2004;14:491–501.
23. **Castle PE, Schiffman M, Bratti MC, et al.** A population-based study of vaginal human papillomavirus infection in hysterectomized women. *J Infect Dis.* 2004;190:458–467.
24. **Eifel PJ, Jhingran A, Brown J, et al.** Time course and outcome of central recurrence after radiation therapy for carcinoma of the cervix. *Int J Gynecol Cancer.* 2006;16:1106–1111.
25. **Murad TM, Durant JR, Maddox WA, et al.** The pathologic behavior of primary vaginal carcinoma and its relationship to cervical cancer. *Cancer.* 1975;35:787–794.
26. **Perez CA, Grigsby PW, Garipagaoglu M, et al.** Factors affecting long-term outcome of irradiation in carcinoma of the vagina. *Int J Radiat Oncol Biol Phys.* 1999;44:37–45.
27. **Choo YC, Anderson DG.** Neoplasms of the vagina following cervical carcinoma. *Gynecol Oncol.* 1982;23:125–132.
28. **Benedet JL, Saunders BH.** Carcinoma in situ of the vagina. *Am J Obstet Gynecol.* 1984;148:695–700.
29. **Rome RM, England PG.** Management of vaginal intraepithelial neoplasia: A series of 132 cases with long-term follow-up. *Int J Gynecol Cancer.* 2000;10:382–390.
30. **Cramer DW, Cutler SJ.** Incidence and histopathology of malignancies of the female genital organs in the United States. *Am J Obstet Gynecol.* 1974;118:443–460.

31. **Herman JM, Homesley HD, Dignan MB.** Is hysterectomy a risk factor for vaginal cancer? *JAMA.* 1986;256:601–603.

32. **Sinha B, Stehman F, Schilder J, et al.** Indiana University experience in the management of vaginal cancer. *Int J Gynecol Cancer.* 2009;19:686–693.

33. **Fanning J, Manahan KJ, McLean SA.** Loop electrosurgical excision procedure for partial upper vaginectomy. *Am J Obstet Gynecol.* 1999;181:1382–1385.

34. **Hoffman MS, De Cesare LS, Roberts WS, et al.** Upper vaginectomy for in situ and occult, superficially invasive carcinoma of the vagina. *Am J Obstet Gynecol.* 1992;166:30–33.

35. **Peters WA, 3rd, Kumar NB, Morley GW.** Microinvasive carcinoma of the vagina: A distinct clinical entity? *Am J Obstet Gynecol.* 1985;153:505–507.

36. **Kucera H, Vavra N.** Radiation management of primary carcinoma of the vagina: Clinical and histopathological variables associated with survival. *Gynecol Oncol.* 1991;40:12–16.

37. **Stock RG, Chen AS, Seski J.** A 30-year experience in the management of primary carcinoma of the vagina: Analysis of prognostic factors and treatment modalities. *Gynecol Oncol.* 1995;56: 45–52.

38. **Hiniker SM, Roux A, Murphy JD, et al.** Primary squamous cell carcinoma of the vagina: Prognostic factors, treatment patterns, and outcomes. *Gynecol Oncol.* 2013;131:380–385.

39. **Eddy GL, Singh KP, Gansler TS.** Superficially invasive carcinoma of the vagina following treatment for cervical cancer: A report of six cases. *Gynecol Oncol.* 1990;36:376–379.

40. **Frumovitz M, Gayed IW, Jhingran A, et al.** Lymphatic mapping and sentinel lymph node detection in women with vaginal cancer. *Gynecol Oncol.* 2008;108:478–481.

41. **Al-Kurdi M, Monagnan JM.** Thirty-two years experience in management of primary tumors of the vagina. *Br J Obstet Gynecol.* 1981; 88:1145–1150.

42. **Lamoreaux WT, Grigsby PW, Dehdashti F, et al.** FDG-PET evaluation of vaginal carcinoma. *Int J Radiat Oncol Biol Phys.* 2005; 62:733–737.

43. **Kucera H, Mock U, Knocke TH, et al.** Radiotherapy alone for invasive vaginal cancer: Outcome with intracavitary high dose rate brachytherapy versus conventional low dose rate brachytherapy. *Acta Obstet Gynecol Scand.* 2001;80:355–360.

44. **Benedetti Panici P, Bellati F, Plotti F, et al.** Neoadjuvant chemotherapy followed by radical surgery in patients affected by vaginal carcinoma. *Gynecol Oncol.* 2008;111:307–311.

45. **Ling B, Gao Z, Sun M, et al.** Laparoscopic radical hysterectomy with vaginectomy and reconstruction of vagina in patients with stage I of primary vaginal carcinoma. *Gynecol Oncol.* 2008;109: 92–96.

46. **Cutillo G, Cignini P, Pizzi G, et al.** Conservative treatment of reproductive and sexual function in young woman with squamous carcinoma of the vagina. *Gynecol Oncol.* 2006;103:234–237.

47. **Pride GL, Buchler DA.** Carcinoma of vagina 10 or more years following pelvic irradiation therapy. *Am J Obstet Gynecol.* 1977;127: 513–517.

48. **Dalrymple JL, Russell AH, Lee SW, et al.** Chemoradiation for primary invasive squamous carcinoma of the vagina. *Int J Gynecol Cancer.* 2004;14:110–117.

49. **Stryker JA.** Radiotherapy for vaginal carcinoma: A 23-year review. *Br J Radiol.* 2000;73:1200–1205.

50. **Tabata T, Takeshima N, Nishida H, et al.** Treatment failure in vaginal cancer. *Gynecol Oncol.* 2002;84:309–314.

51. **Otton GR, Nicklin JL, Dickie GJ, et al.** Early-stage vaginal carcinoma—an analysis of 70 patients. *Int J Gynecol Cancer.* 2004; 14:304–310.

52. **Tran PT, Su Z, Lee P, et al.** Prognostic factors for outcomes and complications for primary squamous cell carcinoma of the vagina treated with radiation. *Gynecol Oncol.* 2007;105:641–649.

53. **Ballon SC, Lagasse LD, Chang NH, et al.** Primary adenocarcinoma of the vagina. *Surg Gynecol Obstet.* 1979;149:233–237.

54. **Robboy SJ, Hill EC, Sandberg EC, et al.** Vaginal adenosis in women born prior to the diethylstilbestrol era. *Hum Pathol.* 1986; 17:488–492.

55. **Mudhar HS, Smith JH, Tidy J.** Primary vaginal adenocarcinoma of intestinal type arising from an adenoma: Case report and review of the literature. *Int J Gynecol Pathol.* 2001;20:204–209.

56. **Herbst AL, Scully RE.** Adenocarcinoma of the vagina in adolescence. A report of 7 cases including 6 clear-cell carcinomas (so-called mesonephromas). *Cancer.* 1970;25:745–757.

57. **Herbst AL, Ulfelder H, Poskanzer DC.** Adenocarcinoma of the vagina: An association of maternal stilboestrol therapy with tumour appearing in young women. *N Engl J Med.* 1971;284:878–881.

58. **Herbst AL, Cole P, Norusis MJ.** Epidemiologic aspects and factors related to survival in 384 registry cases of clear cell adenocarcinoma of the vagina and cervix. *Am J Obstet Gynecol.* 1979;135:876–886.

59. **Robboy SJ, Young RH, Welch WR, et al.** Atypical vaginal adenosis and cervical ectropion. Association with clear cell adenocarcinoma in diethylstilbestrol-exposed offspring. *Cancer.* 1984;54:869–875.

60. **Senekjian E, Frey K, Anderson D, et al.** Local therapy in stage I clear cell adenocarcinoma of the vagina. *Cancer.* 1987;60:1319–1324.

61. **Herbst AL, Robboy SJ, Scully RE, et al.** Clear-cell adenocarcinoma of the vagina and cervix in girls: Analysis of 170 registry cases. *Am J Obstet Gynecol.* 1974;119:713–724.

62. **Frank SJ, Deavers MT, Jhingran A, et al.** Primary adenocarcinoma of the vagina not associated with diethylstilbestrol (DES) exposure. *Gynecol Oncol.* 2007;105:470–474.

63. **Kaminski JM, Anderson PR, Han AC, et al.** Primary small cell carcinoma of the vagina. *Gynecol Oncol.* 2003;88:451–455.

64. **Crowther ME, Lowe DG, Shepherd JH.** Verrucous carcinoma of the female genital tract: A review. *Obstet Gynecol Surv.* 1998;43: 263–280.

65. **Piura B, Rabinovich A, Yanai-Inbar I.** Primary malignant melanoma of the vagina: Case report and review of literature. *Eur J Gynaecol Oncol.* 2002;23:195–198.

66. **Nigogosyan G, Delapava S, Pickren JW.** Melanoblasts in Vaginal Mucosa. Origin for Primary Malignant Melanoma. *Cancer.* 1964;17: 912–913.

67. **Kirschner AN, Kidd EA, DeWees T, et al.** Treatment approach and outcomes of vaginal melanoma. *Int J Gynecol Cancer.* 2013;23: 1484–1489.

68. **Morrow CP, DiSaia PJ.** Malignant melanoma of the female genitalia: A clinical analysis. *Obstet Gynecol Surv.* 1976;31:233–271.

69. **Reid GC, Schmidt RW, Roberts JA, et al.** Primary melanoma of the vagina: A clinicopathologic analysis. *Obstet Gynecol.* 1989;74: 190–199.

70. **Chung AF, Casey MJ, Flannery JT, et al.** Malignant melanoma of the vagina-report of 19 cases. *Obstet Gynecol.* 1980;55:720–727.

71. **Chung AF, Woodruff JM, Lewis JL, Jr.** Malignant melanoma of the vulva: A report of 44 cases. *Obstet Gynecol.* 1975;45:638–646.

72. **Gupta D, Malpica A, Deavers MT, et al.** Vaginal melanoma: A clinicopathologic and immunohistochemical study of 26 cases. *Am J Surg Pathol.* 2002;26:1450–1457.

73. **Tjalma WA, Monaghan JM, de Barros Lopes A, et al.** Primary vaginal melanoma and long-term survivors. *Eur J Gynaecol Oncol.* 2001;22:20–22.

74. **Buchanan DJ, Schlaerth J, Kurosaki T.** Primary vaginal melanoma: Thirteen-year disease-free survival after wide local excision and review of recent literature. *Am J Obstet Gynecol.* 1998;178:1177–1184.

75. **Miner TJ, Delgado R, Zeisler J, et al.** Primary vaginal melanoma: A critical analysis of therapy. *Ann Surg Oncol.* 2004;11:34–39.

76. **Harwood AR, Cummings BJ.** Radiotherapy for mucosal melanomas. *Int J Radiat Oncol Biol Phys.* 1982;8:1121–1126.

77. **Gray RJ, Pockaj BA, Kirkwood JM.** An update on adjuvant interferon for melanoma. *Cancer Control.* 2002;9:16–21.

78. **Tavassoli FA, Norris HJ.** Smooth muscle tumors of the vagina. *Obstet Gynecol.* 1979;53:689–693.

79. **Ciaravino G, Kapp DS, Vela AM, et al.** Primary leiomyosarcoma of the vagina. A case report and literature review. *Int J Gynecol Cancer.* 2000;10:340–347.

80. **Curtin JP, Saigo P, Slucher B, et al.** Soft-tissue sarcoma of the vagina and vulva: A clinicopathologic study. *Obstet Gynecol.* 1995; 86:269–272.

81. **Magne N, Oberlin O, Martelli H, et al.** Vulval and vaginal rhabdomyosarcoma in children: Update and reappraisal of Institut Gustave Roussy brachytherapy experience. *Int J Radiat Oncol Biol Phys.* 2008;72:878–883.

82. **Arndt CA, Donaldson SS, Anderson JR, et al.** What constitutes optimal therapy for patients with rhabdomyosarcoma of the female genital tract? *Cancer.* 2001;91:2454–2468.

83. **Webb MJ, Symmonds RE, Weiland LH.** Malignant fibrous histio-cytoma of the vagina. *Am J Obstet Gynecol.* 1974;119:190–192.
84. **McAdam JA, Stewart F, Reid R.** Vaginal epithelioid angiosarcoma. *J Clin Pathol.* 1998;51:928–930.
85. **Buscema J, Rosenshein NB, Taqi F, et al.** Vaginal hemangiopericy-toma: A histopathologic and ultrastructural evaluation. *Obstet Gyne-col.* 1985;66:82S–85S.
86. **Petur NG, Young RH.** Mesenchymal tumors and tumor-like lesions of the female genital tract: A selective review with emphasis on recently described entities. *Int J Gynecol Pathol.* 2001;20:105–127.
87. **Leverger G, Flamant F, Gerbaulet A, et al.** [Tumors of the vitel-line sac located in the vagina in children. Apropos of 11 cases]. *Arch Fr Pediatr.* 1983;40:85–89.
88. **Weghaupt K, Gerstner GJ, Kucera H.** Radiation therapy for pri-mary carcinoma of the female urethra: A survey over 25 years. *Gynecol Oncol.* 1984;17:58–63.
89. **Thyavihally YB, Wuntkal R, Bakshi G, et al.** Primary carcinoma of the female urethra: Single center experience of 18 cases. *Jpn J Clin Oncol.* 2005;35:84–87.
90. **Benson RC, Jr., Tunca JC, Buchler DA, et al.** Primary carcinoma of the female urethra. *Gynecol Oncol.* 1982;14:313–318.
91. **Prempree T, Amornmarn R, Patanaphan V.** Radiation therapy in primary carcinoma of the female urethra. II. An update on results. *Cancer.* 1984;54:729–733.
92. **Grabstald H, Hilaris B, Henschke U, et al.** Cancer of the female urethra. *JAMA.* 1966;197:835–842.
93. **Bracken RB, Johnson DE, Miller LS, et al.** Primary carcinoma of the female urethra. *J Urol.* 1976;116:188–192.
94. **Ampil FL.** Primary malignant neoplasm of the female urethra. *Obstet Gynecol.* 1985;66:799–804.
95. **Grigsby PW.** Carcinoma of the urethra in women. *Int J Radiat Oncol Biol Phys.* 1998;41:535–541.
96. **Eng TY, Naguib M, Galang T, et al.** Retrospective study of the treatment of urethral cancer. *Am J Clin Oncol.* 2003;26:558–562.
97. **Dalbagni G, Donat SM, Eschwege P, et al.** Results of high dose rate brachytherapy, anterior pelvic exenteration and external beam radiotherapy for carcinoma of the female urethra. *J Urol.* 2001;166:1759–1761.
98. **Srinivas V, Khan SA.** Female urethral cancer–an overview. *Int Urol Nephrol.* 1987;19:423–427.
99. **Klein FA, Ali MM, Kersh R.** Carcinoma of the female urethra: Combined iridium Ir 192 interstitial and external beam radiotherapy. *South Med J.* 1987;80:1129–1132.
100. **Dayyani F, Pettaway CA, Kamat AM, et al.** Retrospective analysis of survival outcomes and the role of cisplatin-based chemotherapy in patients with urethral carcinomas referred to medical oncologists. *Urol Oncol.* 2012;31(7):1171–1177.
101. **Hahn P, Krepart G, Malaker K.** Carcinoma of female urethra. Manitoba experience: 1958–1987. *Urology.* 1991;37:106–109.
102. **Milosevic MF, Warde PR, Banerjee D, et al.** Urethral carcinoma in women: Results of treatment with primary radiotherapy. *Radiother Oncol.* 2000;56:29–35.
103. **Hara I, Hikosaka S, Eto H, et al.** Successful treatment for squa-mous cell carcinoma of the female urethra with combined radio- and chemotherapy. *Int J Urol.* 2004;11:678–682.
104. **Licht MR, Klein EA, Bukowski R, et al.** Combination radiation and chemotherapy for the treatment of squamous cell carcinoma of the male and female urethra. *J Urol.* 1995;153:1918–1920.
105. **Shah AB, Kalra JK, Silber L, et al.** Squamous cell cancer of female urethra. Successful treatment with chemoradiotherapy. *Urol-ogy.* 1985;25:284–286.
106. **Kobayashi M, Nomura M, Yamada Y, et al.** Bladder-sparing surgery and continent urinary diversion using the appendix (Mitrofanoff procedure) for urethral cancer. *Int J Urol.* 2005;12:581–584.
107. **DiMarco DS, DiMarco CS, Zincke H, et al.** Outcome of surgical treatment for primary malignant melanoma of the female urethra. *J Urol.* 2004;171:765–767.

15 Gestational Trophoblastic Disease

Ross S. Berkowitz
Donald P. Goldstein

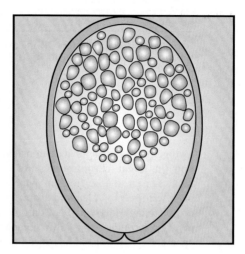

Gestational trophoblastic disease (GTD) includes a spectrum of interrelated tumors, including complete and partial hydatidiform mole, invasive mole, choriocarcinoma, placental site trophoblastic tumor (PSTT) and epithelioid trophoblastic tumor (ETT) that have varying propensities for local invasion and metastasis (1–3). Persistent GTD, also called gestational trophoblastic neoplasia (GTN), is among the rare human malignancies that can be cured in the presence of widespread metastases (1–3). With the exception of PSTT and ETT, all GTN arises from the cytotrophoblast and syncytial cells of the villous trophoblast, and produces abundant amounts of human chorionic gonadotropin (hCG). Measurement of hCG levels serves as a reliable tumor marker for diagnosis, monitoring of treatment response, and follow-up to detect recurrence.

Placental site and epithelioid trophoblastic tumors originate from the intermediate cells of extravillous trophoblast and produce hCG sparsely, making its use as a tumor marker less reliable. Although GTN most commonly ensues after a molar pregnancy, it may follow any gestational event, including therapeutic or spontaneous abortion and ectopic or term pregnancy.

Prior to the development of effective chemotherapy in 1956, the majority of patients with disease localized to the uterus were cured with hysterectomy, and metastatic disease was almost always fatal. Most women can now be cured and their reproductive function preserved if they are managed according to the well-established guidelines summarized in this chapter.

Hydatidiform Mole

Complete Versus Partial Hydatidiform Mole

Hydatidiform moles may be categorized as either complete or partial moles on the basis of gross morphology, histopathology, and karyotype (Table 15.1).

Complete Hydatidiform Mole

Pathology

Complete hydatidiform moles lack identifiable embryonic or fetal tissues, and the chorionic villi exhibit generalized hydatidiform swelling and diffuse trophoblastic hyperplasia.

625

Table 15.1 Features of Complete and Partial Hydatidiform Moles		
	Complete Mole	*Partial Mole*
Fetal or embryonic tissue	Absent	Present
Hydatidiform swelling of chorionic villi	Diffuse	Focal
Trophoblastic hyperplasia	Diffuse	Focal
Scalloping of chorionic villi	Absent	Present
Trophoblastic stromal inclusions	Absent	Present
Karyotype	46XX; 46XY	69XXY; 69XYY

From **Berkowitz RS, Goldstein DP.** The management of molar pregnancy and gestational trophoblastic tumors. In: **Knapp RC, Berkowitz RS, eds.** *Gynecologic oncology.* New York, NY: MacMillan; 1993:425, with permission.

Chromosomes

Cytogenetic studies have demonstrated that complete moles usually have a 46XX karyotype and the molar chromosomes are entirely of paternal origin (androgenetic) (4). Complete moles appear to arise from an ovum in which the nucleus is either absent or inactivated that has been fertilized by a haploid sperm, which duplicates its own chromosomes (5). Although most complete moles have a 46XX chromosomal pattern, approximately 10% have a 46XY karyotype (6). Chromosomes in a 46XY complete mole appear to be entirely of paternal origin, when an apparently empty egg is fertilized by two sperm (dispermy).

Partial Hydatidiform Mole

Pathology

Partial hydatidiform moles are characterized by the following pathologic features (7):

1. Chorionic villi of varying size with focal hydatidiform swelling and cavitation
2. Marked villous scalloping
3. Focal trophoblastic hyperplasia with or without atypia
4. Prominent stromal trophoblastic inclusions
5. Identifiable embryonic or fetal tissues

Chromosomes

Partial moles usually have a triploid karyotype (69 chromosomes), with the extra haploid set of chromosomes derived from the father (8). When a fetus is present in conjunction with a partial mole, it usually exhibits the stigmata of triploidy, including growth retardation and multiple congenital malformations. In a careful review of our pathologic material, Genest et al. (9) concluded that nontriploid partial moles probably do not exist.

Clinical Features

The classical presenting symptoms and signs of patients with complete and partial molar pregnancy are presented in Table 15.2 (10–12). These symptoms have been modified significantly by earlier diagnosis over the past 25 years, with more widespread use of routine ultrasound early in the pregnancy.

Complete Hydatidiform Mole

Vaginal Bleeding

Vaginal bleeding is the most common presenting symptom and occurs in almost all cases. Molar tissues may separate from the decidua and disrupt maternal vessels, and large volumes of retained blood may distend the endometrial cavity. As intrauterine clots undergo oxidation and liquefaction, "prune juice"–like fluid may leak into the vagina. Because vaginal bleeding may be considerable and prolonged, half of these patients present with anemia (hemoglobin <10 g/100 mL).

	Table 15.2 Presenting Symptoms and Signs in Patients with Complete and Partial Molar Pregnancy	
Sign	**Complete Mole**[a] N = 306 (%)	**Partial Moles**[b] N = 81 (%)
Vaginal bleeding	97	73
Excessive uterine size	51	4
Prominent ovarian theca lutein cysts	50	0
Toxemia	27	3
Hyperemesis	26	0
Hyperthyroidism	7	0
Trophoblastic emboli	2	0

Adapted from [a]**Berkowitz RS, Goldstein DP**. Pathogenesis of gestational trophoblastic neoplasms. *Pathobiol Annu* 1981;11:391, and [b]**Berkowitz RS, Goldstein DP, Bernstein MR**. Natural history of partial molar pregnancy. *Obstet Gynecol* 1985;66:677–681.

Excessive Uterine Size

Excessive uterine enlargement relative to gestational age is one of the classic signs of a complete mole, although it was present in only approximately half of our patients. **The endometrial cavity may be expanded by both chorionic tissue and retained blood.** Excessive uterine size is usually associated with markedly elevated levels of hCG, because uterine enlargement results in part from exuberant trophoblastic growth.

Toxemia

Preeclampsia was observed in approximately 27% of our patients. Although preeclampsia is often associated with hypertension, proteinuria, and hyperreflexia, eclamptic convulsions rarely occur. Toxemia develops almost exclusively in patients with excessive uterine size and markedly elevated hCG levels. **The diagnosis of hydatidiform mole should be considered whenever preeclampsia develops early in pregnancy.**

Hyperemesis Gravidarum

Hyperemesis requiring antiemetic and/or intravenous replacement therapy occurred in one-fourth of our patients, particularly those with excessive uterine size and markedly elevated hCG levels. Severe disturbances of electrolytes may develop and require treatment with parenteral fluids.

Hyperthyroidism

Clinically evident hyperthyroidism was observed in approximately 7% of our patients. These patients may present with tachycardia, warm skin, and tremor. The diagnosis can be confirmed by detection of elevated serum levels of free thyroxine (T_4) and triiodothyronine (T_3).

Laboratory evidence of hyperthyroidism is commonly detected in asymptomatic patients with hydatidiform moles. Galton et al. (13) reported 11 patients in whom thyroid function tests were elevated before molar evacuation, but returned rapidly to normal after evacuation.

When hyperthyroidism is suspected, it is important to administer β-adrenergic blocking agents before the induction of anesthesia for molar evacuation, because anesthesia or surgery may precipitate a thyroid storm. The latter may be manifested by hyperthermia, delirium, convulsions, atrial fibrillation, high-output heart failure, or cardiovascular collapse. Administration of β-adrenergic blocking agents prevents or rapidly reverses many of the metabolic and cardiovascular complications of a thyroid storm.

The identity of a thyrotropic factor in hydatidiform moles has not been delineated. Amir et al. measured thyroid function in 47 patients with a complete mole, and reported no correlation between serum hCG levels and the serum free T_4 index or free T_3 index (14). Thus, although some investigators have speculated about a separate chorionic thyrotropin, this substance has not been isolated.

Trophoblastic Embolization

Respiratory distress developed in approximately 2% of our patients with a complete mole. These patients may experience chest pain, dyspnea, tachypnea, tachycardia, and severe respiratory distress after molar evacuation. Auscultation of the chest usually reveals diffuse rales, and the chest radiograph may demonstrate bilateral pulmonary infiltrates. The signs and symptoms of respiratory distress usually resolve within 72 hours of evacuation with cardiopulmonary support. Respiratory insufficiency may result from trophoblastic embolization, as well as from the cardiopulmonary complications of thyroid storm, toxemia, and massive fluid replacement.

Theca Lutein Ovarian Cysts

Prominent theca lutein ovarian cysts (>6 cm in diameter) developed in approximately half of our patients. These cysts contain amber-colored or serosanguineous fluid, and are usually bilateral and multilocular. Their formation may be related to increased serum levels of hCG and prolactin (15). **Ovarian enlargement occurred almost exclusively in patients with markedly elevated hCG values.** Because the uterus also may be excessively enlarged, theca lutein cysts may be difficult to palpate, but ultrasonography can accurately document their presence and size. After molar evacuation, theca lutein cysts normally regress spontaneously within 2 to 4 months.

Prominent theca lutein cysts frequently cause symptoms of marked pelvic pressure, which can be relieved by **laparoscopic decompression** or transabdominal aspiration. If acute pelvic pain develops, laparoscopy should be performed to assess and manage possible cystic torsion or rupture (16).

Prior to the early 1980s, complete moles were usually diagnosed in the second trimester, but the widespread use of ultrasound has shifted the diagnosis to the first trimester (17). With earlier diagnosis, excessive uterine size, hyperemesis, anemia, and preeclampsia were observed at presentation in only 28%, 8%, 5%, and 1% of our patients, respectively. In the 1990s, none of our 74 patients with a complete mole had respiratory distress or hyperthyroidism. However, patients continued to present with vaginal bleeding and markedly elevated hCG levels.

The histopathologic characteristics of complete mole are different in the first trimester (18). First trimester complete moles have less circumferential trophoblastic hyperplasia and smaller villi. These more subtle morphologic alterations may lead to misclassification as partial moles or nonmolar spontaneous abortions. **Immunohistochemistry for p57** (paternally imprinted, maternally expressed gene products) **may be used to confirm the diagnosis of a complete mole** (19). Nuclei of decidual cells (maternally derived tissue) and extravillous trophoblast of all types of gestations stain positively for p57. **Almost all complete moles have absent** (or near absent) **villous stromal and cytotrophoblastic nuclear activity for p57,** while all other types of gestations (including partial moles) show nuclear reactivity in more than 25% of villous stromal and cytotrophoblastic nuclei. Fisher et al reported that maternal chromosome 11 was retained in the rare case of complete mole exhibiting p57 staining (20). This also helps to explain the rare occurrence of familial recurrent complete hydatidiform moles of biparental, rather than the usual androgenetic, origin. **Familial recurrent molar pregnancy is reported to be strongly associated with a mutation in the *NLRP7* gene (21).**

Partial Hydatidiform Mole

Patients with a partial hydatidiform mole usually do not have the clinical features characteristic of complete molar pregnancy. **In general, these patients present with the signs and symptoms of incomplete or missed abortion, and the diagnosis of partial mole may be made only after histologic review of the curettings** (22).

The main presenting sign among 81 patients with a partial mole seen at the New England Trophoblastic Disease Center (NETDC) was vaginal bleeding, which occurred in 59 patients (72.8%) (10). There was absence of a fetal heart beat in 12 patients (14.8%), excessive uterine enlargement in three (3.7%), and preeclampsia in two (2.5%). No patient presented with theca lutein cysts, hyperemesis, or hyperthyroidism. **The presenting clinical diagnosis was incomplete or missed abortion in 74 patients (91.4%) and hydatidiform mole in five patients (6.2%).** Pre-evacuation hCG levels were measured in 30 patients and were greater than 100,000 milli-International Unit/mL in only two patients (6.7%) (10).

Table 15.3 Sequelae of Low- and High-risk Complete Hydatidiform Moles

	No. of Patients (%)	
Outcome	Low-risk	High-risk
Normal involution	486/506 (96)	212/352 (60.2)
Persistent GTN		
Nonmetastatic	17/506 (3.4)	109/352 (31)
Metastatic	3/506 (0.6)	31/352 (8.8)
Totals	**506/858 (59)**	**352/858 (41)**

All patients managed by evacuation without prophylactic chemotherapy.

GTN, gestational trophoblastic neoplasia.

Reproduced from **Goldstein DP, Berkowitz RS, Bernstein MR**. Management of molar pregnancy. *J Reprod Med.* 1981;26:208, with permission.

Natural History

Complete Hydatidiform Mole

Complete moles have a potential for local invasion and distant spread. **After molar evacuation, local uterine invasion occurs in 15% of patients and metastasis in 4%** (11,12).

A review of 858 patients with complete hydatidiform mole revealed that **two-fifths of the patients had** the following signs of marked trophoblastic proliferation at the time of presentation:

1. **hCG level greater than 100,000 milli-International Unit/mL**
2. **Excessive uterine enlargement**
3. **Theca lutein cysts larger than 6 cm in diameter**

Patients with any of these signs are at high risk for postmolar persistent tumor. The sequelae of 858 patients with low- and high-risk complete hydatidiform moles are shown in Table 15.3. After molar evacuation, local uterine invasion occurred in 31%, and metastases in 8.8% of the 352 high-risk patients. For the 506 low-risk patients, local invasion occurred in only 3.4%, and metastases in only 0.6%.

Patients older than 40 years of age are also at increased risk of postmolar GTN. Elias et al. reported that persistent GTN developed in 53% of such women (23).

Partial Hydatidiform Mole

Approximately 2–4% of patients with a partial mole develop persistent postmolar tumor and require chemotherapy to achieve remission (24). Patients who develop persistent disease have no distinguishing clinical or pathologic characteristics.

Diagnosis

Ultrasonography is a reliable and sensitive technique for the diagnosis of complete molar pregnancy. Because the chorionic villi exhibit diffuse hydatidiform swelling, complete moles produce a characteristic vesicular sonographic pattern, usually referred to as a **"swiss cheese" pattern**. Ultrasonography continues to be useful in the detection of first trimester complete moles (25) (Fig. 15.1).

Ultrasonography may contribute to the diagnosis of partial molar pregnancy by demonstrating focal cystic spaces in the placental tissues and an increase in the transverse diameter of the gestational sac (26).

Treatment

After molar pregnancy is diagnosed, the patient should be evaluated carefully for the presence of associated medical complications, including preeclampsia, hyperthyroidism, electrolyte imbalance, and anemia. After the patient is stabilized, a decision must be made concerning the most appropriate method of evacuation.

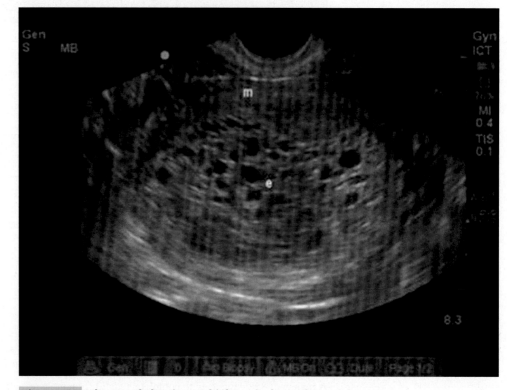

Figure 15.1 Ultrasound showing multiple vesicular endometrial structures consistent with a complete molar pregnancy. A 26-year-old presented at 10 weeks' gestation with irregular vaginal bleeding. Serum hCG was 120,000 milli-International Unit/mL.

Hysterectomy	**If the patient desires surgical sterilization, a hysterectomy may be performed with the mole in situ.** The ovaries may be preserved at the time of surgery, even though theca lutein cysts are present. Prominent ovarian cysts may be decompressed by aspiration. Although hysterectomy eliminates the risks associated with local invasion, it does not prevent distant spread.
Suction Curettage	**Suction curettage is the preferred method of evacuation in patients who desire to preserve fertility, regardless of uterine size.** The procedure involves the following steps:

1. **Oxytocin infusion**—This is begun in the operating room before the induction of anesthesia.
2. **Cervical dilatation**—Laminaria or medical effacement agents are utilized by some clinicians to facilitate dilation. While the cervix is being dilated, the surgeon frequently encounters increased uterine bleeding. Retained blood in the endometrial cavity may be expelled during cervical dilatation. Active uterine bleeding should not deter the prompt completion of cervical dilatation.
3. **Suction curettage**—Evacuation can be facilitated with the use of a large bore cannula. Within a few minutes of commencing suction curettage, the uterus will decrease dramatically in size, and bleeding usually slows. If the uterus is more than 14 weeks in size, one hand may be placed on top of the fundus and the uterus massaged to stimulate uterine contraction and reduce the risk of perforation.
4. **Sharp curettage**—When suction is thought to be complete, a gentle sharp curettage may be performed to remove any residual molar tissue. Aggressive curettage may result in uterine synechiae, but ultrasonography may help to detect any residual tissue.

The specimens obtained on suction and sharp curettage should be submitted separately for pathologic review.

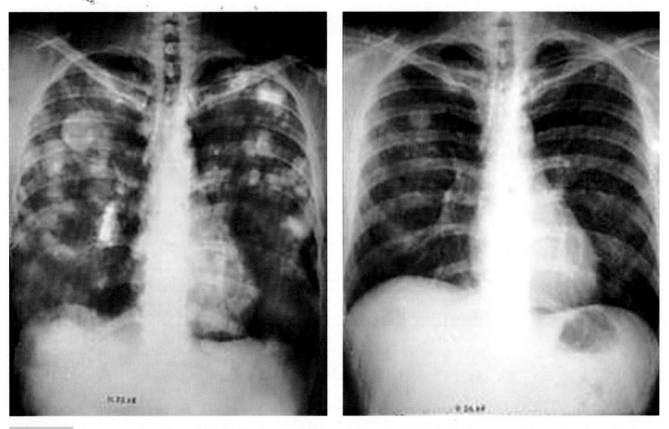

Figure 15.4 Chest x-ray showing multiple pulmonary metastases. A 27-year-old G3 P2 Tab1 presented 8 months after a therapeutic abortion with irregular vaginal bleeding and hemoptysis. Serum hCG was 710,000 milli-International Unit/mL. Following five courses of EMA-CO, the hCG declined to nondetectable levels and the chest x-ray was normal.

stretch the Glisson capsule. Hepatic lesions are hemorrhagic and friable and may rupture, causing exsanguinating intraperitoneal bleeding. Bakri et al. noted that only 5 of 19 patients (26%) with hepatic metastases presented with liver-related complaints such as jaundice, intra-abdominal bleeding, or epigastric pain (41).

Central Nervous System

Ten percent of metastatic trophoblastic disease involves the brain and spinal cord. **Cerebral involvement is usually seen in patients with very advanced disease. Virtually all patients with brain metastases have concurrent pulmonary and vaginal involvement.** Women with brain involvement usually have neurologic symptoms including nausea and vomiting, headache, seizures, slurred speech, visual disturbances, or hemiparesis. Neurologic symptoms in patients with brain metastases range from 87–100% (42–44).

Staging

The current staging system for GTN combines both anatomic staging and a prognostic scoring system (Tables 15.6 and 15.7). It is hoped that this staging system will encourage the objective comparison of data among various centers.

Table 15.6 Staging of Gestational Trophoblastic Neoplasia	
Stage I	Disease confined to uterine corpus
Stage II	GTN extends outside of uterus, but is limited to the genital structures (adnexa, vagina, broad ligament)
Stage III	GTN extends to the lungs, with or without known genital tract involvement
Stage IV	All other metastatic sites

FIGO, International Federation of Obstetrics and Gynecology; GTN, gestational trophoblastic neoplasia.
FIGO Annual Report. *Int J Gynecol Obstet.* 2006;95:S29; *Int J Gynecol Obstet.* 2009;105:3–4.

Table 15.7 Scoring System Based on Prognostic Factors				
	Scores			
	0	**1**	**2**	**4**
Age (yr)	<40	≥40	—	
Antecedent pregnancy	Mole	Abortion	Term	
Interval months from index pregnancy	<4	4–<7	7–<13	≥13
Pretreatment serum hCG (International Unit/L)	$<10^3$	10^3–$<10^4$	10^4–$<10^5$	$>10^5$
Largest tumor size (including uterus)	3–<5 cm	≥5 cm		
Site of metastases	Lung	Kidney/spleen	Gastrointestinal/ liver	Brain
Number of metastases	—	1–4	5–8	>8
Previous failed chemotherapy	—	—	Single drug	2 or more drugs

Format for reporting to FIGO Annual Report: In order to stage and allot a risk factor score, a patient's diagnosis is allocated to a stage as represented by a Roman numeral I, II, III, and IV. This is then separated by a colon from the sum of all the actual risk factor scores expressed in Arabic numerals for example, stage II:4, stage IV:9. This stage and score will be allotted for each patient.

Stage I includes all patients with persistently elevated hCG levels and tumor confined to the uterine corpus.

Stage II comprises all patients with metastases to the vagina and/or pelvis.

Stage III includes all patients with pulmonary metastases with or without uterine, vaginal, or pelvic involvement. The diagnosis is based on a rising hCG level in the presence of pulmonary lesions on a chest film, rather than a computed tomography (CT) scan.

Stage IV patients have far advanced disease with involvement of the brain, liver, kidneys, or gastrointestinal tract. These patients are in the highest-risk category, because they are most likely to be resistant to chemotherapy. In most cases, their disease follows a nonmolar pregnancy and has the histologic pattern of choriocarcinoma. An isolated cerebral metastases noted in a magnetic resonance imaging (MRI) of the head is shown (Fig. 15.5).

Prognostic Scoring System

In addition to anatomic staging, it is important to consider other variables to predict the likelihood of drug resistance, and to assist in the selection of appropriate chemotherapy. A prognostic scoring system, based on one developed by Bagshawe, reliably predicts the potential for resistance to chemotherapy (3).

When the prognostic score is 7 or more, the patient is categorized as high risk and requires intensive combination chemotherapy to achieve remission. Patients with stage I disease usually have a low-risk score, and those with stage IV disease have a high-risk score, so that the distinction between low and high risk applies mainly to patients with stages II or III disease.

Diagnostic Evaluation

Optimal management of GTN requires a thorough assessment of the extent of the disease before the initiation of treatment. Most patients who develop GTN after a molar pregnancy are detected early by hCG monitoring, so detailed investigation is rarely needed. **The diagnosis of postmolar GTN is based on** the following International Federation of Gynecologists and Obstetricians (FIGO) guidelines (45):

1. **A plateau in β-hCG levels** over at least 3 weeks
2. **A 10% or greater rise in β-hCG levels for three or more values over at least 2 weeks**
3. **Persistence of β-hCG levels 6 months after molar evacuation**

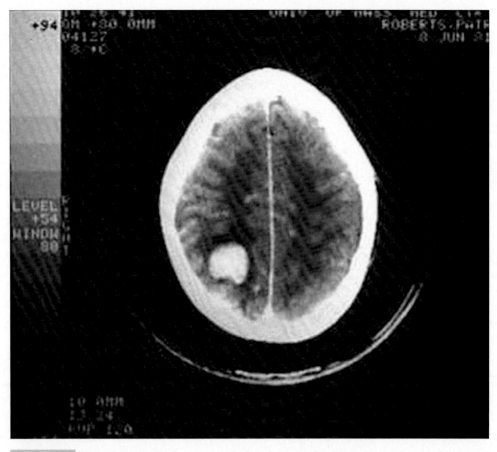

Figure 15.5 **MRI of the brain showing an isolated cerebral metastasis.** A 36-year-old, G2 P2 presented 2 years after a normal-term vaginal birth with several months of irregular vaginal bleeding and acute onset of a severe headache. Serum hCG was 1.2 million milli-International Unit/mL, and the chest x-ray showed multiple pulmonary lesions.

4. **Histologic evidence of choriocarcinoma**

5. **The presence of metastatic disease**

Patients who present with an elevated β-hCG following a nonmolar pregnancy should be considered to have choriocarcinoma until proven otherwise. **Any woman in the reproductive age group who presents with abnormal bleeding or evidence of metastatic disease should undergo hCG testing to rule out GTN.**

All patients with GTN should undergo a careful pretreatment evaluation, including the following:

1. **A complete history and physical examination** including a speculum examination

2. Measurement of the **serum hCG level**

3. **Hepatic, thyroid, and renal function tests**

4. Baseline peripheral **white blood cell and platelet counts**

5. **Stool guaiac testing**

6. **Chest x-ray**

7. **A pelvic ultrasound** to confirm the absence of pregnancy and to detect pelvic disease, myometrial invasion, or retained tissue

The metastatic workup should include the following:

1. **Chest CT, if chest x-ray is positive.** This is not needed if the plain film is negative, because micrometastases do not affect outcome and are not considered a risk factor (46).

2. **Ultrasound or CT scan of the abdomen and pelvis.**

3. **MRI or CT scan of the head.**

4. **Measurement of cerebrospinal fluid (csf) hCG level,** if any metastatic disease is present, or if the patient exhibits neurologic signs and the head MRI or CT scan is negative.

5. **Selective angiography** of abdominal and pelvic organs, if indicated.

6. **Whole body 18 FDG-PET scan** to identify occult disease, if indicated (47).

7. **Review of all available pathology.** Histologic confirmation of the diagnosis of GTN is not required for treatment. Biopsy of a metastatic site may be indicated if the diagnosis is in doubt.

Liver ultrasonography and CT scanning document most hepatic metastases in patients with abnormal liver function tests. CT or MRI of the head facilitate the early diagnosis of asymptomatic cerebral lesions (43). In the absence of lung or vaginal metastasis, the risk of cerebral and hepatic spread is exceedingly low.

In patients with choriocarcinoma and metastatic disease, hCG levels should be measured in the CSF to exclude cerebral involvement if the CT scan of the brain is negative. The plasma/csf hCG ratio tends to be less than 60 in the presence of cerebral metastases (48). A single plasma/csf hCG ratio may be misleading, because rapid changes in plasma hCG levels may not be reflected promptly in the cerebrospinal fluid (49).

Stool guaiac tests should be routinely performed in patients with persistent GTN. If the guaiac test is positive or if the patient reports gastrointestinal symptoms, a complete radiographic evaluation of the gastrointestinal tract should be undertaken.

Pelvic ultrasonography is useful in detecting extensive trophoblastic uterine involvement and may aid in identifying sites of resistant uterine tumor (50). **Because ultrasonography can accurately and noninvasively detect extensive uterine tumor, it may help select patients who will benefit from hysterectomy.** When the uterus contains large amounts of tumor, hysterectomy may substantially reduce the tumor burden, limit the number of cycles of chemotherapy necessary to induce remission, and eliminate the potential for hemorrhage or infection (51).

Management of Gestational Trophoblastic Neoplasia

Stage I

The NETDC protocol for the management of stage I disease is presented in Table 15.8. The selection of treatment is based primarily on the patient's wish regarding fertility.

Patients with stage I (nonmetastatic) GTN who desire sterilization can opt for hysterectomy, although chemotherapy may be necessary to prevent persistent active disease resulting from occult metastases. **Hysterectomy is indicated as primary treatment in all patients with a placental-site or epithelioid trophoblastic tumor, because both are relatively chemoresistant.**

Between July 1965 and December 2012, 566 patients with stage I GTN were treated at the NETDC, of whom 33 patients (5.8%) underwent primary hysterectomy and a course of adjunctive single-agent chemotherapy. All have achieved remission with no further therapy.

Table 15.8 Protocol for Treatment of Stage I Gestational Trophoblastic Neoplasia	
Initial	MTX-FA; if resistant, switch to Act-D or hysterectomy with adjuvant chemotherapy
Resistant	Combination chemotherapy or hysterectomy with adjuvant chemotherapy; local uterine resection; pelvic intra-arterial infusion
Follow-up hCG	Weekly until normal for 3 wks, then monthly until normal for 12 mos
Contraception	12 consecutive mos of normal hCG values

MTX, *methotrexate;* FA, folinic acid; Act-D, *actinomycin D;* hCG, human chorionic gonadotropin.

Modified from **Goldstein DP, Berkowitz RS, eds**. *Gestational Trophoblastic Neoplasms: Clinical Principles of Diagnosis and Management*. Philadelphia, PA: WB Saunders; 1982:1–301, with permission.

Chemotherapy Alone

Single-agent chemotherapy is the preferred treatment in patients with stage I disease who desire to retain fertility. At the NETDC between 1965 and 2012, 532 patients (94%) with stage I disease were treated initially with sequential *Methotrexate and Actinomycin-D*, and 435 (81.8%) achieved a complete remission. One additional patient was treated with combination chemotherapy consisting of *Methotrexate, Act-D*, and *cyclophosphamide (MAC)* because of high prognostic scores. The 97 patients (18.2%) resistant to monotherapy subsequently attained remission after treatment with combination chemotherapy, with or without surgical intervention.

Patients resistant to single-agent chemotherapy who wish to preserve fertility should be transitioned to combination chemotherapy. **If the patient is resistant to both single-agent and combination chemotherapy and wants to retain fertility, local uterine resection may be considered if the lesion is focal and well demarcated.** When local resection is being considered, preoperative imaging with an ultrasonogram, MRI scan, arteriogram, and/or PET scan may help to define the site of the resistant tumor.

Follow-up

All patients with stage I lesions should be followed with:

1. **Weekly measurement of hCG levels** until they are normal for 3 consecutive weeks
2. **Monthly hCG levels** until levels are normal for 12 consecutive months
3. **Effective contraception** during the entire period of hormonal follow-up.

Stages II and III

Low-risk patients are treated initially with primary single-agent chemotherapy, and high-risk patients are managed initially with primary dose-intense combination chemotherapy. A protocol for the management of patients with stage II and III disease is presented in Table 15.9.

Thirty patients with **stage II GTN** were treated at the NETDC between July 1965 and December 2012 and all achieved complete remission. **Initial single-agent chemotherapy induced complete remission in 18 of 22 patients (81.2%) with low-risk disease.** Complete remission was achieved with combination chemotherapy in the four patients resistant to single agents. In eight patients with high-risk stage II GTN, six patients (75%) achieved remission following initial therapy. The remaining two were cured with secondary combination regimens and surgery.

Vaginal Metastases

Vaginal metastases may bleed profusely because they are highly vascular and friable. Yingna et al. (52) reported that 18 of 51 patients (35.3%) with vaginal metastases presented with a vaginal

Table 15.9 Protocol for Treatment of Stages II and III Gestational Trophoblastic	
Neoplasia	
Low-risk[a]	
Initial	MTX-FA; if resistant, switch to *Act-D*
Resistant to both single agents	Combination chemotherapy
High-risk[a]	
Initial	Combination chemotherapy
Resistant	Second-line combination chemotherapy
Follow-up hCG	Weekly until normal for 3 wks, then monthly until normal for 12 mos
Contraception	Until there have been 12 consecutive months of normal hCG levels

[a]Local resection optional.

MTX, *methotrexate;* FA, folinic acid; Act-D, *actinomycin D;* hCG, human chorionic gonadotropin.

Modified from **Goldstein DP, Berkowitz RS, eds**. *Gestational Trophoblastic Neoplasms: Clinical Principles of Diagnosis and Management.* Philadelphia, PA: WB Saunders; 1982:1–301, with permission.

hemorrhage. When bleeding is substantial, it may be controlled by the use of a vaginal pack or by arteriographic embolization.

Pulmonary Metastases

Two hundred and six patients with **stage III GTN** were treated at the NETDC between July 1965 and December 2012. **Of the 138 patients with low-risk stage III GTN, 110 (79.7%) achieved complete remission with initial single-agent chemotherapy.** All 28 patients resistant to initial single-agent chemotherapy achieved remission with combination chemotherapy. Of the 68 patients with high-risk stage III GTN, 59 (86.8%) were cured with initial therapy, and eight of the nine drug-resistant patients were cured with secondary combination chemotherapy.

Thoracotomy

Thoracotomy has a limited role in the management of stage III disease. **If a patient has a persistent viable pulmonary metastasis despite intensive chemotherapy, thoracotomy may be used to excise the resistant focus (53).** A thorough metastatic workup should be performed before surgery to exclude other sites of persistent disease. A PET–CT may be useful to distinguish between viable tumor and fibrotic pulmonary nodules. The latter can persist indefinitely on a chest x-ray after complete gonadotropin remission. **In patients undergoing thoracotomy for a resistant lesion, chemotherapy should be administered postoperatively to treat potential sites of occult micrometastases.**

Hysterectomy

Hysterectomy may be required in patients with metastatic GTN to control uterine hemorrhage or sepsis (51). **In patients with extensive uterine tumor, hysterectomy may substantially reduce the trophoblastic tumor burden and limit the need for multiple courses of chemotherapy.**

Follow-up monitoring for patients with stages II and III disease is the same as for patients with stage I disease.

Stage IV

A protocol for the management of stage IV disease is presented in Table 15.10. These patients are at greatest risk for the development of rapidly progressive and unresponsive tumors despite intensive multimodal therapy. They should all be referred to centers with special expertise in the management of trophoblastic disease.

All patients with stage IV disease should be treated with primary dose-intense combination chemotherapy and the selective use of radiation therapy and surgery. Before 1975, only 6 of 20 patients (30%) with stage IV disease treated at the NETDC attained complete remission. Since 1975, 18 of 23 patients (78.2%) with stage IV tumors have achieved gonadotropin remission. This gratifying improvement in survival has resulted from the use of primary combination chemotherapy in conjunction with radiation and surgical treatment.

Table 15.10 Protocol for Treatment of Stage IV Gestational Trophoblastic Neoplasia

Initial	Combination Chemotherapy
Brain	Whole-head irradiation (3,000 cGy)
	Craniotomy to manage complications
Liver	Resection to manage complications
Resistant[a]	Second-line combination chemotherapy
	Hepatic arterial infusion
Follow-up hCG	Weekly until normal for 3 wks, then monthly until normal for 24 mos
Contraception	Until there have been 24 consecutive months of normal hCG levels

[a]Local resection optional.

hCG, human chorionic gonadotropin.

Modified from **Goldstein DP, Berkowitz RS, eds**. *Gestational Trophoblastic Neoplasms: Clinical Principles of Diagnosis and Management*. Philadelphia, PA: WB Saunders; 1982:1–301, with permission.

Hepatic Metastases

The management of hepatic metastases is particularly challenging and problematic. If a patient is resistant to systemic chemotherapy, hepatic embolization or arterial infusion of chemotherapy may induce complete remission in selected cases. Hepatic resection may be required to control acute bleeding or to excise a focus of resistant tumor.

Cerebral Metastases

If cerebral metastases are diagnosed, whole-brain irradiation (3,000 cGy in ten fractions) should be instituted promptly. As an alternative, high beam localized radiation has proven effective. Yordan et al. (54) reported that deaths as a result of cerebral involvement occurred in 11 of 25 patients (44%) treated with chemotherapy alone, but **there were no deaths in the 18 patients treated with brain irradiation and chemotherapy.** The risk of spontaneous cerebral hemorrhage may be lessened by the concurrent use of combination chemotherapy and brain irradiation, because irradiation may be both hemostatic and tumoricidal.

Craniotomy

Craniotomy may be required to provide acute decompression or to control bleeding, and should be performed to manage life-threatening complications in the hope that the patient ultimately will be cured with chemotherapy. **Cerebral metastases resistant to chemotherapy may be amenable to local resection, particularly if located peripherally.** Most patients with cerebral metastases who achieve sustained remission have no residual neurologic deficits (55).

Salvage Therapy for Drug Resistance

Despite the effectiveness of current regimens, there is a need to identify new agents with the potential to treat resistant GTN. **Although *ifosfamide* and *paclitaxel* have been used successfully, further studies are needed to define their potential role as either first- or second-line therapy** (56,57). Osborne and associates reported that a novel three-drug doublet regimen consisting of *paclitaxel, etoposide,* and *cisplatin* (TE/TP) induced complete remission in two patients with relapsed high risk GTN (58). Wan et al. (59) demonstrated the efficacy of *floxuridine* (FUDR)-containing regimens by inducing remission in all 21 drug-resistant patients. Matsui et al. (60) found that *5-FU in combination with Act-D* could be used effectively as second-line therapy and induced remission in 8 of 10 drug-resistant patients.

The potential role of high dose chemotherapy and autologous bone marrow transplantation or stem cell rescue for patients with drug-resistant disease has yet to be defined, although successful individual cases have been reported (61,62).

Follow-up

Patients with stage IV disease should be followed with:

1. **Weekly hCG levels** until they have been normal for 3 consecutive weeks
2. **Monthly hCG levels** until they have been normal for 24 consecutive months
3. **Effective contraception** during the interval of hormonal follow-up

These patients require prolonged gonadotropin follow-up because they are at increased risk of late recurrence.

An algorithm for the management of GTN is presented in Figure 15.6.

Many hCG assays have some cross-reactivity with LH. Following multiple courses of combination chemotherapy, ovarian steroidal function may be damaged, leading to rising LH levels. Patients who receive combination chemotherapy should be placed on oral contraceptives to suppress LH levels and prevent problems with cross-reactivity.

Phantom hCG

False positive elevations in serum hCG levels caused by circulating heterophilic antibodies can present a diagnostic challenge and lead to unnecessary treatment (63). **Patients with** so-called "phantom choriocarcinoma" or **"phantom hCG" usually exhibit no progressive rise in their hCG levels** and have no clear history of an antecedent pregnancy. The possibility of false-positive hCG levels should be evaluated by sending both urine and serum samples to a reference hCG laboratory. **Because heterophile antibodies are too large to cross the renal tubule, the test for hCG in urine will be negative.**

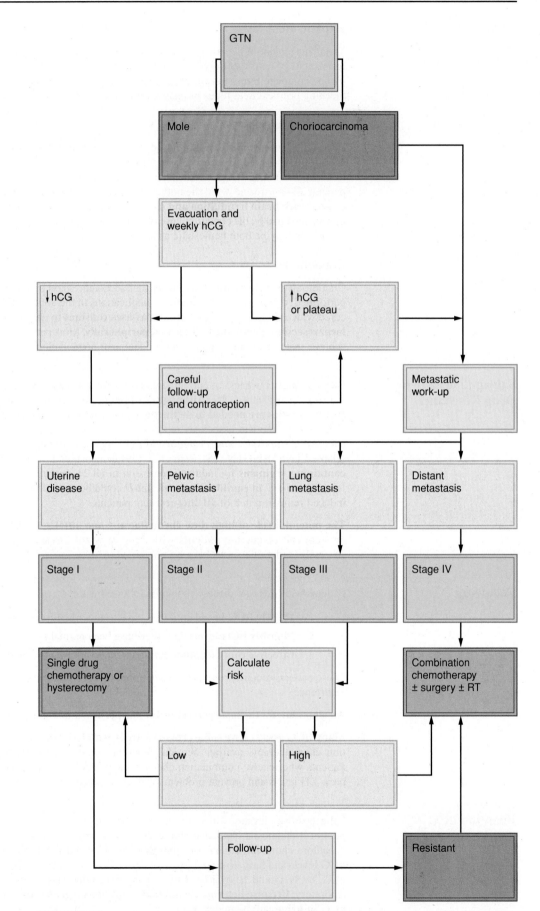

Figure 15.6 **Management of gestational trophoblastic neoplasia.** GTN, gestational trophoblastic neoplasia; hCG, human chorionic gonadotropin; RT, radiation therapy.

Peri- or postmenopausal patients can present with a false-positive hCG elevation presumably resulting from the elaboration of an hCG-like polypeptide by the pituitary gland, particularly when the LH level is markedly elevated. The hCG levels in this situation tend to cluster in the single or low double digit range, and can be readily suppressed with the use of oral contraceptives (64).

Chemotherapy

Single-Agent Chemotherapy

Single-agent chemotherapy with either *Actinomycin-D or Methotrexate* achieve comparable and excellent remission rates in both nonmetastatic and low-risk metastatic GTN (65,66), and there are several protocols available (Table 15.11).

Act-D can be given every other week in a 5-day regimen or in a pulsed fashion. MTX can be given similarly in a 5-day regimen, weekly in a pulsed fashion, or over 8 days alternating with folinic acid (a.k.a. calcium leucovorin). No study has compared all of these protocols with regard to success and morbidity. The GOG performed a prospective randomized study of pulsed *Act-D* versus weekly pulsed *MTX* and reported that pulsed *Act-D* had a significantly higher remission rate in patients with low-risk GTN (67). Shah et al. (68) found that the 8-day *MTX-folinic acid* (*MTX-FA*) regimen was more cost-effective than the biweekly pulsed administration of *Act-D*. The selection of chemotherapy should be influenced by the associated systemic toxicity. **An optimal regimen should maximize response rate while minimizing morbidity and cost.**

In 1964, Bagshawe and Wilde (69) reported that the administration of *MTX-FA* in patients with GTN limited systemic toxicity and was effective and safe (Table 15.12). *MTX-FA* has been the preferred single-agent regimen in the treatment of GTN at the NETDC since 1974 (70). An evaluation of 185 patients treated with this regimen revealed that complete remission was achieved in 162 patients (87.6%), and 132 of the 162 patients (81.5%) required only one course of *MTX-FA* to attain remission. *MTX-FA* induced remission in 147 of 163 patients (90.2%) with stage I GTN and in 15 of 22 patients (68.2%) with low-risk stages II and III GTN. **Resistance to therapy was more common in patients with choriocarcinoma, metastatic disease, and when pretreatment serum hCG levels exceeded 50,000 milli-International Unit/mL.** After treatment with *MTX-FA*, thrombocytopenia, granulocytopenia, and hepatotoxicity developed in only 3 (1.6%), 11 (5.9%), and 26 (14.1%) patients, respectively. *MTX-FA* achieved an excellent therapeutic outcome with minimal toxicity and attained this goal with limited exposure to chemotherapy.

Table 15.11 Single-Drug Treatment

I. Actinomycin D treatment

  A. 5-d *actinomycin D*

  Actinomycin D 12 μg/kg IV daily for 5 d

  CBC, platelet count, aspartate aminotransferase daily

  With response, retreat at the same dose

  Without response, add 2 μg/kg to the initial dose or switch to *methotrexate* protocol

  B. Pulse *actinomycin D*

  Actinomycin D 1.25 mg/m² every 2 wk

II. Methotrexate treatment

  A. 5-d *methotrexate*

  Methotrexate 0.4 mg/kg IV or IM daily for 5 d

  CBC, platelet count daily

  With response, retreat at the same dose

  Without response, increase dose to 0.6 mg/kg or switch to *actinomycin D* protocol

  B. Pulse *methotrexate*

  Methotrexate 40 mg/m² IM weekly

IV, intravenous; CBC, complete blood count; IM, intramuscular.

Table 15.12 Protocol for Therapy with *Methotrexate* and Folinic Acid "Rescue"

Day	Time	Follow-up Tests and Therapy
1	8 AM	CBC, platelet count, AST
	4 PM	*Methotrexate*, 1 mg/kg
2	4 PM	*Folinic acid*, 0.1 mg/kg
3	8 AM	CBC, platelet count, AST
	4 PM	*Methotrexate*, 1 mg/kg
4	4 PM	*Folinic acid*, 0.1 mg/kg
5	8 AM	CBC, platelet count, AST
	4 PM	*Methotrexate*, 1 mg/kg
6	4 PM	*Folinic acid*, 0.1 mg/kg
7	8 AM	CBC, platelet count, AST
	4 PM	*Methotrexate*, 1 mg/kg
8	4 PM	*Folinic acid*, 0.1 mg/kg

CBC, complete blood count; AST, aspartate aminotransferase.

Reproduced from **Berkowitz RS, Goldstein DP, Bernstein MR**. Ten years' experience with *methotrexate* and folinic acid as primary therapy for gestational trophoblastic disease. *Gynecol Oncol.* 1986;23:111, with permission.

Administration of Single-Agent Treatment

The serum hCG level is measured weekly after each course of chemotherapy, and the hCG regression curve serves as the primary basis for determining the need for additional treatment. Courses of single agent chemotherapy are administered at 2-week intervals until the serum β-hCG level becomes undetectable. In patients with low-risk disease, one to three additional courses of consolidation therapy using the last effective agent is recommended (71).

The dosage of *MTX* should be unaltered if the patient's response to the first treatment was adequate. **An adequate response is defined as a fall in the hCG level by 1 log after a single course of chemotherapy.** If the response to the first course was inadequate, the dosage of *MTX* should be increased from 1 to 1.5 mg/kg/d for each of the 4 treatment days. **If the response to two consecutive courses of *MTX-FA* is inadequate, the patient is considered to be resistant to *MTX*,** and *Act-D* should be promptly substituted in patients with nonmetastatic and low-risk metastatic GTN. If the hCG levels do not decline by 1 log after a course of *Act-D*, the patient should be considered resistant to *Act-D* as a single agent, and dose-intensive therapy with combination chemotherapy should be started.

Combination Chemotherapy

MAC

In the past, the preferred combination drug regimen at the NETDC was triple therapy with *MAC*, which included *MTX-FA, Act-D,* and *cyclophosphamide* (72). Triple therapy proved to be inadequate as an initial treatment in patients with metastases and a high-risk prognostic score. Data from the GOG, M. D. Anderson Hospital, and the NETDC, indicated that triple therapy–induced remission in only 21 of 43 patients (49%) with metastases and a high-risk score (7 or more) (73–75). *MAC* **may be useful to treat low-risk patients with prognostic scores in the 5 to 6 range, because only 30% of these women are cured with initial monotherapy.** Characteristically, these patients have hCG levels of >100,000 milli-International Unit/mL, and Doppler ultrasound evidence of large tumor burden (76).

EMA-CO

Etoposide was reported to induce complete remission in 56 of 60 patients (93%) with nonmetastatic and low-risk metastatic GTN (77). **In 1984, Bagshawe first described a new combination regimen that included *etoposide, MTX, Act-D, cyclophosphamide*, and *vincristine* (EMA-CO);** (Table 15.13), and reported an 83% remission in patients with metastases and a high-risk score (78). Bolis et al. (79) confirmed that primary EMA-CO–induced complete remission in 76% of patients with metastatic GTN and a high-risk score. Bower et al. (80) updated the data from

Table 15.13 EMA-CO Regimen for Patients with Gestational Trophoblastic Neoplasia

Regimen

Course 1 (EMA)

Day 1   *VP-16 (etoposide),* 100 mg/m^2, IV infusion in 200 mL of saline over 30-min *Actinomycin D,* 0.5 mg, IV push
Methotrexate, 100 mg/m^2, IV push, followed by a 200 mg/m^2 IV infusion over 12 hr

Day 2   *VP-16 (etoposide),* 100 mg/m^2, IV infusion in 200 mL of saline over 30-min *Actinomycin D,* 0.5 mg, IV push
Folinic acid, 15 mg, IM or orally every 12 hr for 4 doses beginning 24 hr after start of methotrexate

Course 2 (CO)

Day 8   *Vincristine,* 1 mg/m^2, IV push
Cyclophosphamide, 600 mg/m^2, IV in saline

This regimen consists of two courses: (a) course 1 is given on days 1 and 2; (b) course 2 is given on day 8. Course 1 might require overnight hospital stay; course 2 does not. These courses can usually be given on days 1 and 2, 8, 15, and 16, 22, etc., and the intervals should not be extended without cause.

IV, intravenous; IM, intramuscular.

Reproduced from **Bagshawe KD**. Treatment of high-risk choriocarcinoma. *J Reprod Med.* 1984;29:813, with permission.

Charing Cross Hospital and reported in 1997 that EMA-CO–induced complete remission in 130 of 151 patients (86.1%) with high-risk metastatic GTN. Newlands et al. (81) reported **remission using EMA-CO with intrathecal *MTX* in 30 of 35 patients (86%) with brain metastases.** The EMA-CO regimen is usually well tolerated, and treatment seldom has to be suspended because of toxicity, particularly with the judicious use of marrow stimulants.

The EMA-CO regimen is the preferred primary treatment in patients with metastases and a high-risk prognostic score. If patients become resistant to EMA-CO, remission may still be achieved by substituting *etoposide* and *cisplatin* for *cyclophosphamide* and *vincristine* on day 8 (EMA-EP) (82). **EMA-EP–induced complete remission in 12 of 18 patients (66.7%) with EMA-CO-resistance or relapse.** The optimal combination drug protocol will most likely include *etoposide, MTX,* and *Act-D* and perhaps other agents, administered in the most dose-intensive manner. *Vinblastine, bleomycin,* and *cisplatin* effectively induced remission in four of seven patients who were resistant to triple therapy (83).

Duration of Therapy

Patients who require combination chemotherapy must be treated intensively to attain remission. Combination chemotherapy should be given every 2 weeks or as often as toxicity permits until the patient achieves three consecutive normal hCG levels. **After normal hCG levels have been attained, an additional two to four courses should be administered as consolidation therapy to reduce the risk of relapse.**

Secondary Tumors

Investigators have reported an increased risk of secondary tumors, including leukemia, colon cancer, melanoma, and breast cancer, in patients treated with chemotherapy for gestational trophoblastic tumors (84). **The increased risk of secondary tumors has been attributed to the inclusion of *etoposide* in the combination chemotherapy.** The increased incidence of colon cancer, melanoma, and breast cancer was not apparent until at least 5, 10, and 25 years, respectively, and appears to be limited to those patients who received a total dose of 2 g/m^2 of *etoposide.*

Subsequent Pregnancies

Pregnancies after Hydatidiform Mole

Patients with hydatidiform moles can anticipate normal reproduction in the future (85). From July 1, 1965 to May 1, 2013, patients who were treated at the NETDC for complete molar gestation had 1,392 subsequent pregnancies that resulted in 944 full-term live births (67.8%), 103 premature deliveries (7.4%), 11 ectopic pregnancies (0.8%), 7 stillbirths (0.5%), and 20 repeat molar pregnancies

(1.4%). First- and second-trimester spontaneous abortions occurred in 256 pregnancies (18.4%). There were 42 therapeutic abortions (3%). Major and minor congenital malformations were detected in 40 infants (3.8%). **Patients with a complete molar pregnancy should be reassured that they are at no increased risk of obstetric complications, either prenatally or intrapartum in later pregnancies.** Although data concerning subsequent pregnancies after a partial mole are available for only 359 pregnancies, the data are similarly reassuring.

After a patient has a hydatidiform mole, she is at increased risk of molar pregnancy in subsequent conceptions. Approximately 1 in 100 patients have at least two molar gestations. Some patients with repetitive molar pregnancies have a molar pregnancy with different male partners (86). Later molar pregnancies are characterized by worsening histologic type and increased risk of postmolar GTN. Nonetheless, **after two episodes of molar pregnancy, approximately 60% of patients still achieve a normal full-term gestation** (85).

Recommendations for any Subsequent Pregnancy

1. **A pelvic ultrasonogram during the first trimester,** ideally at 10 weeks gestational age, to confirm normal gestational development.

2. **An hCG measurement 6 weeks after completion of the pregnancy** to exclude occult trophoblastic neoplasia.

Pregnancies after Gestational Trophoblastic Neoplasia

Patients with GTN who are treated successfully with chemotherapy can expect normal reproduction in the future (85). Patients who were treated with chemotherapy at the NETDC from July 1, 1965 to May 1, 2013 reported 668 subsequent pregnancies that resulted in 446 term live births (66.8%), 4 premature deliveries (6.6%), 7 ectopic pregnancies (1%), 10 stillbirths (1.5%), and 10 repeat molar pregnancies (1.5%). First- and second-trimester spontaneous abortions occurred in 123 pregnancies (18.4%). There were 28 therapeutic abortions (4.2%). **Major and minor congenital anomalies were detected in only 12 of 5,008 infants (2.4%).** It is particularly reassuring that the frequency of congenital malformations was not increased, although chemotherapeutic agents are known to have teratogenic and mutagenic potential.

References

1. **Berkowitz RS, Goldstein DP.** Chorionic tumors. *N Engl J Med.* 1996;335:1740–1748.
2. **Goldstein DP, Berkowitz RS.** *Gestational Trophoblastic Neoplasms: Clinical Principles of Diagnosis and Management.* Philadelphia, PA: WB Saunders; 1982:1–301.
3. **Bagshawe KD.** Risk and prognostic factors in trophoblastic neoplasia. *Cancer.* 1976;38:1373–1385.
4. **Kajii T, Ohama K.** Androgenetic origin of hydatidiform mole. *Nature.* 1977;268:633–634.
5. **Yamashita K, Wake N, Araki T, et al.** Human lymphocyte antigen expression in hydatidiform mole: Androgenesis following fertilization by a haploid sperm. *Am J Obstet Gynecol.* 1979;135:597–600.
6. **Pattillo RA, Sasaki S, Katayama KP, et al.** Genesis of 46,XY hydatidiform mole. *Am J Obstet Gynecol.* 1981;141:104–105.
7. **Szulman AE, Surti U.** The syndromes of hydatidiform mole: I. cytogenetic and morphologic correlations. *Am J Obstet Gynecol.* 1978;131:665–671.
8. **Lawler SD, Fisher RA, Dent J.** A prospective genetic study of complete and partial hydatidiform moles. *Am J Obstet Gynecol.* 1991;164:1270–1277.
9. **Genest DR, Ruiz RE, Weremowicz S, et al.** Do nontriploid partial hydatidiform moles exist? *J Reprod Med.* 2002;47:363–368.
10. **Berkowitz RS, Goldstein DP, Bernstein MR.** Natural history of partial molar pregnancy. *Obstet Gynecol.* 1985;66:677–681.
11. **Berkowitz RS, Goldstein DP.** Presentation and management of molar pregnancy. In: **Hancock BW, Newlands ES, Berkowitz RS, eds.** *Gestational Trophoblastic Disease.* London: Chapman and Hall; 1997:127–142.
12. **Berkowitz RS, Goldstein DP.** Molar pregnancy. *N Engl J Med.* 2009;360:1639–1645.
13. **Galton VA, Ingbar SH, Jimenez-Fonseca J, et al.** Alterations in thyroid hormone economy in patients with hydatidiform mole. *J Clin Invest.* 1971;50:1345–1354.

14. **Amir SM, Osathanondh R, Berkowitz RS, et al.** Human chorionic gonadotropin and thyroid function in patients with hydatidiform mole. *Am J Obstet Gynecol.* 1984;150:723–728.
15. **Osathanondh R, Berkowitz RS, de Cholnoky C, et al.** Hormonal measurements in patients with theca lutein cysts and gestational trophoblastic disease. *J Reprod Med.* 1986;31:179–183.
16. **Berkowitz RS, Goldstein DP, Bernstein MR.** Laparoscopy in the management of gestational trophoblastic neoplasms. *J Reprod Med.* 1980;24:261–264.
17. **Soto-Wright V, Bernstein M, Goldstein D, et al.** The changing clinical presentation of complete molar pregnancy. *Obstet Gynecol.* 1995;86:775–779.
18. **Mosher R, Goldstein DP, Berkowitz RS, et al.** Complete hydatidiform mole—comparison of clinicopathologic features, current and past. *J Reprod Med.* 1998;43:21–27.
19. **Thaker HM, Berlin A, Tycko B, et al.** Immunochemistry for the imprinted gene product IPL/PHLDA2 for facilitating the differential diagnosis of complete hydatidiform mole. *J Reprod Med.* 2004;49: 630–636.
20. **Fisher R, Nucci MR, Thaker HM, et al.** Complete hydatidiform mole retaining a chromosome 11 of maternal origin: Analysis of a case. *Mod Pathol.* 2004;17:1155–1160.
21. **Dixon P, Trongwongsa P, Abu-Hayyah S, et al.** Mutation in *NLRP7* are associated with diploid biparental hydatidiform moles, but not androgenetic complete moles. *J Med Genet.* 2012;49: 206–211.
22. **Szulman AE, Surti U.** The clinicopathologic profile of the partial hydatidiform mole. *Obstet Gynecol.* 1982;59:597–602.
23. **Elias K, Shoni M, Bernstein MR, et al.** Complete hydatidiform mole in women aged 40–49 years. *J Reprod Med.* 2012;57:254–258.
24. **Feltmate CM, Growdon WB, Wolfberg AJ, et al.** Clinical characteristics of persistent gestational trophoblastic neoplasia after partial hydatidiform molar pregnancy. *J Reprod Med.* 2006;51:902–906.

25. **Benson CB, Genest DR, Bernstein MR, et al.** Sonographic appearance of first trimester complete hydatidiform moles. *Ultrasound Obstet Gynecol.* 2000;16:188–191.

26. **Fine C, Bundy AL, Berkowitz RS, et al.** Sonographic diagnosis of partial hydatidiform mole. *Obstet Gynecol.* 1989;73:414–418.

27. **Goldstein DP, Berkowitz RS.** Prophylactic chemotherapy of complete molar pregnancy. *Semin Oncol.* 1995;22:157–160.

28. **Kim DS, Moon H, Kim KT, et al.** Effects of prophylactic chemotherapy for persistent trophoblastic disease in patients with complete hydatidiform mole. *Obstet Gynecol.* 1986;67:690–694.

29. **Limpongsanurak S.** Prophylactic actinomycin D for high-risk complete hydatidiform mole. *J Reprod Med.* 2001;46:110–116.

30. **Feltmate CM, Batorfi J, Fulop V, et al.** Human chorionic gonadotropin follow-up in patients with molar pregnancy: A time for reevaluation. *Obstet Gynecol.* 2003;101:732–736.

31. **Wolfberg AJ, Feltmate C, Goldstein DP, et al.** Low risk of relapse after achieving undetectable hCG levels in women with complete molar pregnancy. *Obstet Gynecol.* 2004;104:551–554.

32. **Growdon WB, Wolfberg AJ, Feltmate CM, et al.** Postevacuation hCG levels and risk of gestational trophoblastic neoplasia among women with partial molar pregnancies. *J Reprod Med.* 2006;51:871–874.

33. **Schmitt C, Doret M, Massardier J, et al.** Risk of gestational trophoblastic neoplasia after hCG normalization according to hydatidiform type. *Gynecol Oncol.* 2013;130:86–89.

34. **Stone M, Dent J, Kardana A, et al.** Relationship of oral contraception to development of trophoblastic tumor after evacuation of a hydatidiform mole. *Br J Obstet Gynaecol.* 1976;83:913–916.

35. **Berkowitz RS, Goldstein DP, Marean AR, et al.** Oral contraceptives and postmolar trophoblastic disease. *Obstet Gynecol.* 1981;58:474–477.

36. **Curry SL, Schlaerth JB, Kohorn EI, et al.** Hormonal contraception and trophoblastic sequelae after hydatidiform mole (a Gynecologic Oncology Group study). *Am J Obstet Gynecol.* 1989;160:805–811.

37. **Feltmate CM, Genest DR, Wise L, et al.** Placental site trophoblastic tumor: A 17 year experience at the New England Trophoblastic Disease Center. *Gynecol Oncol.* 2001;82:415–419.

38. **Palmer JE, MacDonald M, Wells M, et al.** Epithelioid trophoblastic tumor: A review of the literature. *J Reprod Med.* 2008;53:465–475.

39. **Papadopoulos AJ, Foskett M, Seckl MJ, et al.** Twenty-five years' clinical experience with placental site trophoblastic tumors. *J Reprod Med.* 2002;47:460–464.

40. **Newlands ES, Mulholland PJ, Holden L, et al.** Etoposide and cisplatin/etoposide, methotrexate and actinomycin D (EMA) chemotherapy for patients with high-risk gestational trophoblastic tumors refractory to EMA/cyclophosphamide and vincrisitine chemotherapy and patients presenting with metastatic placental site trophoblastic tumors. *J Clin Oncol.* 2000;18:854–859.

41. **Bakri YN, Subhi J, Amer M, et al.** Liver metastases of gestational trophoblastic tumors. *Gynecol Oncol.* 1993;40:110–113.

42. **Bakri Y, Berkowitz RS, Goldstein DP, et al.** Brain metastases of gestational trophoblastic tumors. *J Reprod Med.* 1994;39:179–184.

43. **Athanassiou A, Begent RH, Newlands ES, et al.** Central nervous system metastases of choriocarcinoma: 23 years' experience at Charing Cross Hospital. *Cancer.* 1983;52:1728–1735.

44. **Liu TL, Deppe G, Chang QT, et al.** Cerebral metastatic choriocarcinoma in the People's Republic of China. *Gynecol Oncol.* 1983;15:166–170.

45. **Kohorn EI.** Negotiating a staging and risk factor scoring system for gestational trophoblastic neoplasia: A progress report. *J Reprod Med.* 2002;47:445–450.

46. **Garner EIO, Garrett A, Goldstein DP, et al.** Significance of chest computed tomography findings in the evaluation and treatment of persistent gestational trophoblastic neoplasms. *J Reprod Med.* 2004;49:422–427

47. **Dhillon T, Palmieri C, Sebire NJ, et al.** Value of whole body 18 FDG_PET to identify the active site of gestational trophoblastic neoplasia. *J Reprod Med.* 2006;51:879–883.

48. **Bagshawe KD, Harland S.** Immunodiagnosis and monitoring of gonadotropin-producing metastases in the central nervous system. *Cancer.* 1976;38:112–118.

49. **Bakri YN, Al-Hawashim N, Berkowitz RS.** Cerebrospinal fluid/serum beta-subunit human chorionic gonadotropin ratio in patients with brain metastases of gestational trophoblastic tumor. *J Reprod Med.* 2000;45:94–96.

50. **Berkowitz RS, Birnholz J, Goldstein DP, et al.** Pelvic ultrasonography and the management of gestational trophoblastic disease. *Gynecol Oncol.* 1983;15:403–412.

51. **Clark RM, Nevadunsky N, Ghosh S, et al.** The evolving role of hysterectomy in gestational trophoblastic neoplasia at the New England Trophoblastic Disease Center. *J Reprod Med.* 2010;55:194–198.

52. **Yingna S, Yang X, Xiuyu Y, et al.** Clinical characteristics and treatment of gestational trophoblastic tumor with vaginal metastasis. *Gynecol Oncol.* 2002;84:416–419.

53. **Fleming EI, Garrett LA, Growdon WB, et al.** The changing role of thoracotomy in gestational trophoblastic neoplasia at the New England Trophoblastic Disease Center. *J Reprod Med.* 2008;53:493–498.

54. **Yordan EL Jr, Schlaerth J, Gaddis O, et al.** Radiation therapy in the management of gestational choriocarcinoma metastatic to the central nervous system. *Obstet Gynecol.* 1987;69:627–630.

55. **Newlands ES, Holden L, Seckl MJ, et al.** Management of brain metastases in patients with high-risk gestational trophoblastic tumors. *J Reprod Med.* 2002;47:465–471.

56. **Jones WB, Schneider JT, Blessing JA, et al.** Treatment of resistant gestational choriocarcinoma with Taxol; report of two cases. *Gynecol Oncol.* 1996;61:126–129.

57. **Sutton GP, Soper JT, Blessing JA, et al.** Ifosfamide alone and in combination in the treatment of refractory malignant gestational trophoblastic disease. *Am J Obstet Gynecol.* 1992;167:489–493.

58. **Osborne R, Covens AS, Mechdani DE, et al.** Successful salvage of relapsed high-risk gestational trophoblastic neoplasia patients using a novel paclitaxel-containing doublet. *J Reprod Med.* 2004;49:655–659.

59. **Wan X, Yang X, Xiang Y, et al.** Floxuridine-containing regimens in the treatment of gestational trophoblastic tumor. *J Reprod Med.* 2004;49:453–457.

60. **Matsui H, Itsuka Y, Suzuka K, et al.** Salvage chemotherapy for high-risk gestational trophoblastic tumor. *J Reprod Med.* 2004;49:438–441.

61. **Giacalone PL, Benos P, Donnadio DF, et al.** High-dose chemotherapy with autologous bone marrow transplantation for refractory metastatic gestational trophoblastic disease. *Gynecol Oncol.* 1995;58:383–387.

62. **Van Besien K, Vershcragen C, Mehra R, et al.** Complete remission of refractory gestational trophoblastic disease with brain metastases treated with multicycle ifosfamide, carboplatin and etoposide (ICE) and stem cell rescue. *Gynecol Oncol.* 1997;65:366–369.

63. **Cole LA, Butler S.** Detection of hCG in trophoblastic disease: The USA hCG Reference Service Experience. *J Reprod Med.* 2002;47:433–444.

64. **Cole LA, Khanlian A, Muller CY.** Normal production of human chorionic gonadotropin in menopause. *N Engl J Med.* 2007;356:1184–1186.

65. **Garrett AP, Garner EO, Goldstein DP, et al.** Methotrexate infusion and folinic acid as primary therapy for nonmetastatic and low-risk metastatic gestational trophoblastic tumors: 15 years of experience. *J Reprod Med.* 2002;47:355–362.

66. **Lurain JR.** Gestational trophoblastic disease. II. Classification and management of gestational trophoblastic neoplasia. *Am J Obstet Gynecol.* 2011;204:11–18.

67. **Osborne R, Fillaci V, Schink J, et al.** Phase III trial of weekly methotrexate versus pulsed Dactinomycin for low-risk gestational trophoblastic neoplasia: A Gynecologic Oncology Group Study. *J Clin Oncol.* 2011;29:825–831.

68. **Shah NT, Barroilhet L, Berkowitz RS, et al.** A cost analysis of first-line chemotherapy for low-risk gestational trophoblastic neoplasia. *J Reprod Med.* 2012;57:211–218.

69. **Bagshawe KD, Wilde C.** Infusion therapy for pelvic trophoblastic tumors. *J Obstet Gynaecol Br Commonw.* 1964;71:565–570.

70. **Berkowitz RS, Goldstein DP, Bernstein MR.** Ten years' experience with methotrexate and folinic acid as primary therapy for gestational trophoblastic disease. *Gynecol Oncol.* 1986;23:111–118.

71. **Lybol C, Sweep FC, Harvey R, et al.** Relapse rates after two versus three consolidation courses of methotrexate in the treatment of low-risk gestational trophoblastic neoplasia. *Gynecol Oncol.* 2012;125:576–579.

647

72. **Berkowitz RS, Goldstein DP, Bernstein MR.** Modified triple chemotherapy in the management of high-risk metastatic gestational trophoblastic tumors. *Gynecol Oncol.* 1984;19:173–181.

73. **Curry SL, Blessing JA, DiSaia PJ, et al.** A prospective randomized comparison of methotrexate, dactinomycin and chlorambucil versus methotrexate, dactinomycin, cyclophosphamide, doxorubicin, melphalan, hydroxyurea and vincristine in "poor prognosis" metastatic gestational trophoblastic disease: A Gynecologic Group study. *Obstet Gynecol.* 1989;73:357–362.

74. **Gordon AN, Gershenson DM, Copeland LJ, et al.** High-risk metastatic gestational trophoblastic disease: Further stratification into two clinical entities. *Gynecol Oncol.* 1989;34:54–56.

75. **DuBeshter B, Berkowitz RS, Goldstein DP, et al.** Metastatic gestational trophoblastic disease: Experience at the New England Trophoblastic Disease Center, 1965 to 1985. *Obstet Gynecol.* 1987;69:390–395.

76. **McGrath S, Short D, Harvey R, et al.** The management and outcome of women with posthydatidiform mole 'low-risk' gestational trophoblastic neoplasia, but hCG levels in excess of 100,000 IU/L. *Br J Cancer.* 2010;102:810–814.

77. **Wong LC, Choo YC, Ma HK.** Primary oral etoposide therapy in gestational trophoblastic disease: An update. *Cancer.* 1986;58:14–17.

78. **Bagshawe KD.** Treatment of high-risk choriocarcinoma. *J Reprod Med.* 1984;29:813–820.

79. **Bolis G, Bonazzi C, Landoni F, et al.** EMA/CO regimen in high-risk gestational trophoblastic tumor (GTT). *Gynecol Oncol.* 1988;31:439–444.

80. **Bower M, Newlands ES, Holden L, et al.** EMA/CO for high-risk gestational trophoblastic tumors: Results from a cohort of 272 patients. *J Clin Oncol.* 1997;15:2636–2643.

81. **Newlands ES, Bagshawe KD, Begent RH, et al.** Results with the EMA/CO (etoposide, methotrexate, actinomycin D, cyclophosphamide, vincristine) regimen in high risk gestational trophoblastic tumors, 1979 to 1989. *Br J Obstet Gynecol.* 1991;98:550–557.

82. **Mao Y, Wan X, Lu W, et al.** Relapsed or refractory gestational trophoblastic neoplasia treated with etoposide and cisplatin/etoposide, methotrexate, and actinomycin D(EP-EMA) regimen. *Int J Gynecol Oncol.* 2007;98:44–47.

83. **DuBeshter B, Berkowitz RS, Goldstein DP, et al.** Vinblastine, cisplatin and bleomycin as salvage therapy for refractory high-risk metastatic gestational trophoblastic disease. *J Reprod Med.* 1989;34:189–192.

84. **Rustin GJ, Newlands ES, Lutz JM, et al.** Combination but not single-agent methotrexate chemotherapy for gestational trophoblastic tumors increases the incidence of second tumors. *J Clin Oncol.* 1996;14:2769–2773.

85. **Garrett LA, Garner EIO, Feltmate CM, et al.** Subsequent pregnancy outcomes in patients with molar pregnancy and persistent gestational trophoblastic neoplasia. *J Reprod Med.* 2008;53:481–486.

86. **Tuncer ZS, Bernstein MR, Wang J, et al.** Repetitive hydatidiform mole with different male partners. *Gynecol Oncol.* 1999;75:224–226.

16 Breast Disease

Armando E. Giuliano
Catherine M. Dang

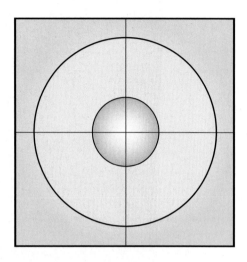

Essential tools for the practicing gynecologist are an understanding of benign and malignant breast diseases, the ability to detect and diagnose breast cancer, and an appreciation of the various treatment options for the breast cancer patient. In this chapter, benign conditions that can masquerade as malignant, are discussed, as well as the diagnosis and management of in situ and invasive breast cancers.

Detection

Physical Examination

Breast malignancies are usually asymptomatic and are discovered only by physical examination or screening mammography. Any physical findings on a routine breast examination must be recorded in the medical record for future reference.

For the breast and nodal examination, the patient should be examined in both the upright and supine positions. Examination should begin with inspection of the breasts with the patient seated comfortably, arms relaxed at her sides. Differences in symmetry or contour of the breasts should be noted, as well as any skin changes such as edema or erythema. Skin dimpling or nipple retraction may become apparent by having the patient raise her arms above her head then press her hands on her hips (Fig. 16.1). The cervical, supraclavicular, and axillary areas should be palpated for enlarged nodes. With the patient still seated, each breast should be examined by using the nondominant hand to support the breast, while palpating with the dominant hand using the flat portion of the fingers rather than the tips. The upper outer quadrant of the breast up to the clavicle, the axillary tail of Spence, and the axilla should be palpated for possible masses. The nipples should be assessed for nipple discharge.

The patient should then be asked to lie down and raise one arm over her head, while keeping the other arm at her side. The breast examination should commence on the side with the raised arm, and proceed systematically from the clavicle to the costal margin. The manner in which the breast is examined is not as important as consistency and diligence; it is important to choose one method that allows for examination of the entire breast that can be repeated methodically. One technique that many clinicians use is to palpate the breast in enlarging concentric circles. Placement of a pillow or towel beneath the scapula to elevate the side examined is important for women with large, pendulous breasts, which tend to fall laterally, making palpation of the lateral breast challenging.

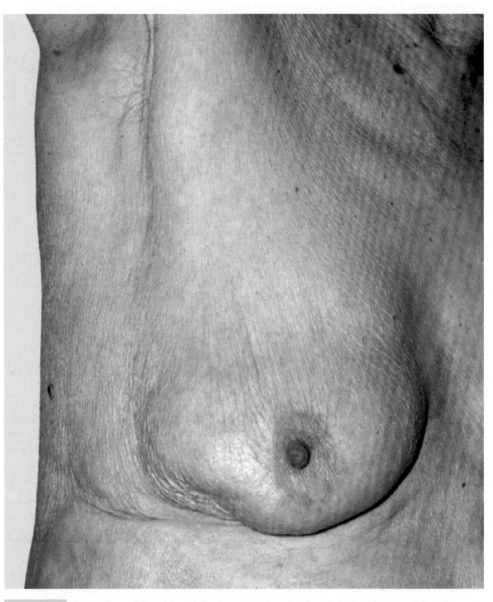

Figure 16.1 Retraction of the skin of the lower, outer quadrant seen only on raising the arm. A small carcinoma was palpable.

The major features in a breast examination to be identified are nodularity, nipple inversion or discharge, skin retraction, tenderness, and dominant masses. Any abnormalities should be documented by identifying the area of concern as the position on the face of a clock, and its distance from the nipple, for example, a right breast lesion at 10 o'clock, 5 cm from the nipple is located in the upper outer quadrant. Many patients, particularly young, premenopausal women, have nodular breast parenchyma. Nodularity is frequently diffuse although it tends to be more prevalent in the upper outer quadrants where there is more breast tissue. Nodules are small, indistinct, and similar in size. **Conversely, breast cancers tend to present as nontender, firm masses with unclear margins, often feeling distinct from the surrounding nodularity. Malignant masses may also be fixed to the chest wall (underlying fascia) or to the skin.** Not all breast cancers possess these characteristics, so **any dominant mass in the breast requires further evaluation**.

Around the time of menses, many women have increased nodularity and engorgement of the breast, which occasionally obscures an underlying lesion. If a patient presents to the physician with concern about a mass that she has palpated and the physician cannot confirm the patient's finding because of breast engorgement, the examination should be repeated after the patient's menses. Mammography or ultrasonography is a useful adjunct in cases where the patient has palpated a mass, yet the clinician is unable to confirm the finding.

Breast Self-examination

Although there is no evidence to date that breast self-examination (BSE) leads to a decreased mortality rate by diagnosing breast cancers at an early stage, its utilization is still advocated by many organizations (1,2). It is viewed as a surveillance tool for women to heighten awareness of the normal composition of the breast, and to detect changes that may occur. BSE can be useful in detecting interval cancers between screenings. BSE should not be used in isolation; it supplements screening by clinical breast examination (CBE) and mammography.

It is advocated by the American Cancer Society (ACS) and the National Comprehensive Cancer Network (NCCN) that BSE begin early, at age 20 years. Starting BSE at an early age allows women to familiarize themselves with the composition of their breasts, increases awareness of breast cancer surveillance, and establishes a good habit. **Women should report any changes to their physicians.** As part of the ACS guidelines for the Early Detection of Breast Cancer, CBE **should be performed every 3 years starting at age 20,** with the option of monthly BSE also starting at age 20. **Premenopausal women may find that monthly examinations are most informative during the week after their menses.** There are complex reasons why many women do not perform BSE, but reassurance and patient education may encourage women to overcome psychological barriers. In women who have been treated for breast cancer, BSE can be used as a supplemental method to aid in detecting recurrence.

Like CBE, the BSE should begin with visual inspection. A woman should inspect her breasts while standing or sitting before a mirror, looking for asymmetry, nipple retraction, or skin dimpling. Skin dimpling is highlighted by elevation of the arms over the head or by pressing the hands against the hips to contract the chest muscles. While standing or sitting, the woman should carefully palpate her breasts using the finger pads of the opposite hand, initially with light pressure then with increasing firmness. This may be performed while showering with soapy hands to increase the sensitivity of palpation. Finally, she should lie down and again palpate each quadrant of the breast extending into the axilla. A good resource for instructions on BSE can be found on website below: **http://www.breastcancer.org/symptoms/testing/types/self_exam/bse_steps.**

Breast Imaging

The two most important imaging techniques are **mammography** and **ultrasonography**. **Magnetic resonance imaging** (MRI) may be used as a screening tool in subsets of women at higher risk of breast cancer, and as a diagnostic tool in certain clinical situations.

Screening Mammography

Screening of asymptomatic women for breast cancer has been shown to reduce the death rate by 20–30%, most likely as a result of earlier detection. Half of the reduction seen in breast cancer deaths in the United States has been attributed to screening mammography (3).

Several randomized controlled trials (RCTs) support the use of mammography for breast cancer screening in women older than 50 years of age. Controversy regarding the benefit of screening women aged 40 to 49 years is primarily related to by the lack of relevant RCTs. Accordingly, in 2009, the US Preventive Services Task Forces recommended that "the decision to start regular biennial screening mammography before the age of 50 years should be an individual one and take patient context into account, including the patient's values regarding specific benefits and harms (4)." **When data regarding screening in women aged 40 to 49 years were combined from the various RCTs and analyzed in a meta-analysis, there was a significant reduction of 18% in the breast cancer mortality rate for this group of women** (5). The Swedish Two-Country Trial demonstrated a 23% reduction in mortality rate for this group of women with screening mammography and 18 years of follow-up (6). A UK study has shown a survival benefit in younger women equivalent to that seen in women over 50 years (7).

The ACS, American Society of Clinical Oncologists (ASCO), and the American College of Radiology recommend that annual mammographic screening should begin at age 40 for women at normal risk (8), **and the National Cancer Institute recommends screening mammography every other year for women 40 and older** (9). Additional screening recommendations exist for women at increased risk of breast cancer; these recommendations include more frequent CBE, initiation of screening at ages younger than 40, and using other modalities as adjuncts to mammography, including ultrasound and MRI. **There is no established upper age limit for breast cancer screening.**

Mammography is the best method of detection for a nonpalpable breast cancer but occasionally misses some palpable and nonpalpable or ultrasonographically detected malignancies. Mammography should not be used in isolation. Neither the technology of mammography nor its interpretation by radiologists is infallible. **The basis of any screening program or workup of breast abnormalities is the physical examination.** Mammography and CBE complement one another; it is recommended that women undergo CBEs around the time of their regularly scheduled annual mammograms (8). Patients should be cautioned that breast compression can be uncomfortable and that steady compression of the breast is necessary to obtain good images.

In addition to mammography used as a screening tool, there are circumstances in which bilateral mammography is mandatory:

1. **In any patient with a dominant mass,** even if biopsy is planned, to assess the ipsilateral lesion and to exclude disease in the contralateral breast.

2. **In any patient with enlarged axillary or supraclavicular nodes,** in order to search for an occult primary breast carcinoma.

3. **Before any cosmetic breast operation** (augmentation, implant exchange, breast reduction) to rule out occult disease.

Mammographic Abnormalities

Mammography can detect microcalcifications, breast densities, and architectural distortions (Fig. 16.2). To standardize the reporting of mammographic findings, **the American College of Radiology developed the Breast-Imaging Reporting and Data System (BI-RADS) classification** (10). There are six categories (1–6) for classifying findings, with category 0 representing an incomplete assessment with the need for additional studies (Table 16.1). Additional imaging recommendations may include magnification, spot compression, and ultrasonography. A patient may

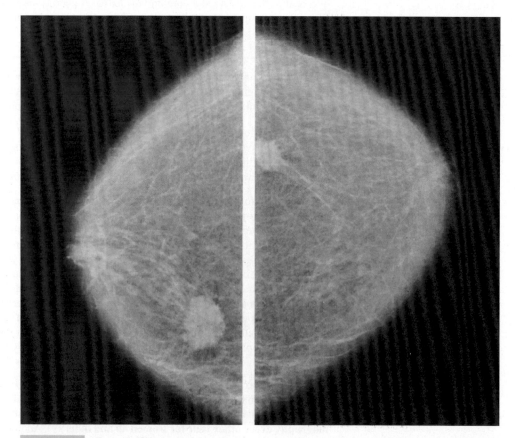

Figure 16.2 Bilateral film screen mammograms showing a typical carcinoma in each breast, illustrating the importance of bilateral mammography in the workup of a clinically apparent mass.

Table 16.1 Mammographic Interpretations and the Breast Imaging Reporting and Data System Classification with Recommendations	
Category 0	Needs additional studies
Category 1	Negative; routine screening mammogram
Category 2	Benign finding; routine screening mammogram
Category 3	Probably a benign finding; repeat mammogram in 6 mos
Category 4	Suspicious abnormality; biopsy
Category 5	Highly suggestive of malignancy; biopsy if palpable or needle localization biopsy if nonpalpable
Category 6	Known biopsy-proven malignancy

have a screening mammogram that shows a questionable abnormality, while spot compression views may indicate the finding is completely normal; this would fall into category 1 "negative."

Mammographic Findings

Microcalcifications are the most frequent mammographic abnormalities necessitating biopsy. The evaluation of microcalcifications includes review of their size, number, location, distribution, and morphology. Microcalcifications that tend to be benign are smooth, round, solid, or lucent-centered spheres. Tubular or rod-shaped calcifications are often associated with ectatic ducts. If further analysis is required, magnification and spot compression views are the primary techniques used. Calcifications that are classified as benign do not require histologic confirmation. **Of concern are calcifications that vary in size and shape (pleomorphic).** Most calcifications in breast cancers form in the intraductal portion of the breast and are small and irregular, with varying levels of maturation or density.

The most common signs of breast cancer seen on mammography are the following:

1. **A cluster of microcalcifications**
2. **A mass seen as an area of increased radiodensity**
3. **An area of architectural distortion in the breast parenchyma**
4. **Skin thickening or edema**
5. **Rarely, asymmetry alone**

These "common signs" can also be seen with benign lesions, leading to a false-positive mammographic rate of 15–20% (11). For example, clusters of microcalcifications are also seen with benign processes such as hyperplasia, adenosis, fibroadenomas, and ductal papillomas. However, for accurate diagnosis, a stereotactic core or excisional biopsy may be required.

Mammography misses approximately 10–15% of cancers. It has a low sensitivity for the detection of infiltrating lobular cancers, and cancers in young women with dense breast parenchyma and little fat (12). If there are suspicious findings on clinical examination, biopsy of the breast must be performed regardless of the mammographic findings (13).

Digital Mammography

Digital mammography (DM) was developed to address some of the limitations of film mammography (FM) (14). **Its advantages include speed and higher contrast resolution,** which in theory is better for detecting densities and masses in dense tissue. The image contrast can be manipulated to aid in the evaluation of dense breasts, which have low contrast. The advantage of FM is spatial resolution, which is better for detecting calcifications. DM also delivers a smaller dose of radiation than FM, but the differences are of minor significance.

Earlier trials did not demonstrate a significant difference in accuracy between digital and conventional mammography, but were limited by sample size. The **Digital Mammographic Imaging Screening Trial** (DMIST) involved 49,500 female volunteers who underwent both conventional and digital mammography. Subset analyses indicated that in women under age 50 and in women with dense breasts, DM may be more accurate in detecting breast cancer (15). **Because digital images can be stored electronically, most facilities have transitioned to DM.** Even though DM may be of benefit in certain subgroups of women, women should not forego annual screening mammograms if DM is not available to them.

Digital Breast Tomosynthesis

Digital breast tomosynthesis (DBT) is a relatively new technology derived from DM. In DBT, a series of cross-sectional images (much like a CT scan) is obtained of the compressed breast, then mathematical algorithms are used to render a 3D mammogram of the breast. This may reduce the effect of tissue overlap and breast density (16). In the United States, approximately 50% of women who undergo screening mammography are categorized as having either "extremely dense" or "heterogeneously dense" breast tissue. **Nine states, including California, have enacted legislation requiring written notification of breast density be given to women with mammographically dense breasts,** so that they may discuss supplemental screening techniques with their physicians (17).

Early studies suggest that the addition of DBT to screening DM may improve breast cancer detection. The Screening with Tomosynthesis OR standard Mammography (STORM) trial prospectively compared conventional DM and DM with the addition of DBT performed in 7,292 asymptomatic women aged 48 and older at a single institution. Each participant's DM and DM plus DBT were read independently by a panel of radiologists. A total of 59 cancers were identified in this cohort: 39 were detected on DM and DM plus DBT; an additional 20 cancers were detected only by DM plus DBT. The incremental increase in cancer detection with the addition of DBT to DM was 2.7 cancers per 1,000 screens and the false-positive recall rate was 141 with DM only versus 73 with DM plus DBT (18). **RCTs are still needed to prove the benefit and cost-effectiveness of the addition of DBT to screening DM.**

Ultrasonography

Breast ultrasonography (US) is a popular imaging technique that is **primarily used as an adjunctive tool. The American College of Radiology Imaging Network Trial found that the addition of physician-performed screening breast ultrasonography to annual screening mammography in 2,809 women with mammographically dense breast tissue would detect an additional 1.1 to 7.2 cancers per 1,000 high-risk women, but would substantially increase the number of false-positive biopsies** (19).

Current breast cancer screening guidelines state that there is no role for surveying the entire breast using ultrasound; the main use of ultrasound should be to focus on an area identified as abnormal by mammography or clinical examination. Ultrasonography can determine whether a lesion is present, or whether a clinical finding is within the spectrum of normal parenchyma, such as a prominent fat lobule. If a lesion does exist, US can be used to further characterize the finding.

There are clinical indications for the use of ultrasound as the primary imaging modality. These include evaluating palpable findings in young patients (teens and early 20s); pregnant women; and women presenting with erythematous, tender breasts (19), where the diagnostic dilemma is between infection and inflammatory breast cancer. Other uses include the evaluation of axillary lymph nodes, the postoperative examination of fluid collections (seroma, hematoma), as an aid in interventional procedures such as needle aspiration or biopsy, and for the preoperative localization of nonpalpable lesions.

Ultrasonography is 95–100% accurate in differentiating solid masses from cysts. It can aid in the evaluation of a benign-appearing, nonpalpable density identified by mammography. If such a lesion proves to be a simple cyst, no further workup is necessary if the patient is asymptomatic. There are certain criteria that must be met for a cyst to be classified as "simple," thus falling into the category of BI-RADS 2: Benign finding. These criteria are (i) anechoic; (ii) well-circumscribed round or oval mass with posterior enhancement; and (iii) thin bilateral edge shadows (20).

Magnetic Resonance Imaging

Magnetic resonance imaging (MRI) produces detailed cross-sectional images of tissues and structures utilizing magnetic fields. The use of screening and diagnostic MRI is gaining more recognition as an adjunct to mammography in specific clinical scenarios. MRI has associated false-negative rates depending on the specific clinical application, and its **specificity is significantly lower than that of mammography.** This is caused by the enhancement of benign lesions such as fat necrosis, fibroadenomas, and fibrocystic changes (21), and **results in an increased recall and biopsy rate.**

Table 16.2 Recommendations for Breast MRI Screening as Adjunct to Mammography
Recommend Annual MRI Screening (based on nonrandomized screening trials and observational studies)
• *BRCA* mutation
• Lifetime risk 20–25% or greater, as defined by risk assessment models largely dependent on family history
• First-degree relative of *BRCA* carrier, but untested
Recommend Annual MRI Screening (based on expert consensus opinion and evidence of lifetime risk of breast cancer)
• Li–Fraumeni syndrome and first-degree relatives
• Radiation to chest between ages 10 and 30 years
• Cowden and Bannayan–Riley–Ruvalcaba syndromes and first-degree relatives

Saslow D, Boetes, Burke W, et al. American Cancer Society (ACS) Guidelines for breast screening with MRI as an adjunct to mammography. *CA Cancer J Clin.* 2007;57;75–89.

As the technology of MRI has become more sophisticated with dedicated breast MRI coils, contrast agents, and protocols (21), breast MRI is increasingly being used in the clinical setting. **MRI is a useful tool** in the setting of equivocal mammographic or ultrasonic findings, **particularly in patients with dense breasts, postlumpectomy scarring, a strong suspicion of infiltrating lobular carcinoma (ILC), scattered calcifications suggestive of extensive ductal carcinoma in situ (DCIS) or extensive intraductal cancer, bloody nipple discharge, or silicone implants** (12).

In women who have an occult primary breast cancer presenting as axillary adenopathy, mammography is limited in its ability to identify the primary breast cancer. There is evidence that **MRI can identify occult breast lesions,** allowing for more accurate staging and the possibility of breast-conserving surgery (22,23). Clinical studies have shown that **MRI can be beneficial in monitoring the response to neoadjuvant chemotherapy** (24), in determining the extent of disease, and for contralateral breast cancer screening (25). **MRI is also used as an adjunct to mammography in screening high-risk women, including those with *BRCA* gene mutations and those with an estimated lifetime risk of breast cancer greater than 20%.** See Table 16.2 for American Cancer Society MRI screening guidelines (26).

Benign Breast Conditions

Fibrocystic Change

Fibrocystic disease is one of the most common breast problems seen in clinical practice. **The term "disease" is misleading and "change" or "condition" is a preferable,** more accurate description. **Fibrocystic change/condition constitutes a spectrum of clinical signs, symptoms, and histologic features.** In a woman with fibrocystic change symptoms, an important part of the evaluation is to exclude malignancy, because the diagnosis of fibrocystic change is otherwise of little clinical significance (27).

Clinical Presentation

Symptoms and Signs

Fibrocystic change is thought to be hormonally related because it appears primarily in women between the ages of 30 and 50 years, subsides after menopause, and can fluctuate with menstrual cycles. Women may present with multiple, tender, palpable masses; usually the breasts are most tender and the masses largest just before the menses, with signs and symptoms abating after menstruation. **It is estimated that 60% of women have clinical findings compatible with the diagnosis of fibrocystic change** (27). Fibrocystic change involves changes in both the stromal and glandular tissues.

Evaluation

Malignancy must be excluded, but often on physical examination, the breasts are diffusely nodular, with areas of increased density, mainly in the upper, outer quadrants, with no dominant masses.

A mammogram should be performed, with possible ultrasound if there is concern about the presence of a mass clinically. **A repeat physical examination after the next menstrual cycle is often valuable** to document resolution of questionable areas. In the case of a dominant mass, a breast biopsy, preferably needle biopsy or aspiration cytology, is recommended to rule out malignancy. Large cysts may be aspirated if symptomatic.

Any clear, watery, straw-colored, or greenish nipple discharge should be tested for blood by means of a standard guaiac or Hemoccult test. If the discharge is from multiple ducts, bilateral and nonbloody, it is most likely benign. Copious discharge may be a sign of malignancy.

Pathology

The histologic features of fibrocystic change are variable (27). Changes such as fibrosis, cyst formation, hyperplasia (overgrowth of the cells that line the ducts), adenosis (enlargement of breast lobules), and sclerosing adenosis can be seen microscopically. One or more of these histologic features can be found in 50–60% of asymptomatic women (27). **In the case of epithelial hyperplasia, it is important to distinguish between usual and atypical hyperplasia. Atypical hyperplasia is associated with an increased risk of future breast cancer.**

Cancer and Fibrocystic Change

The conclusion that there is an association between fibrocystic change and cancer was originally drawn because fibrocystic change and malignancy were commonly found together in the same breast (28). However, because 50–60% of women have fibrocystic change and one in every eight women has breast cancer during her lifetime, it is not surprising that these two entities frequently coexist.

Not all women with fibrocystic change are at an increased risk for cancer. Those with histologic features such as fibrosis, cysts, apocrine metaplasia, and mild hyperplasia are at no increased risk (29,30). Histologic features such as sclerosing adenosis and solid or papillary hyperplasia increase the risk slightly (1.5 to 2 times). **Women who have atypical hyperplasia, either lobular or ductal, have at least five times the average risk.**

Benign Tumors

Intraductal Papilloma

An intraductal papilloma is a benign lesion that can cause serous, serosanguinous, or bloody nipple discharge (31). It is **the most common etiology of bloody nipple discharge without an associated mass.** True polyps of epithelial-lined breast ducts, intraductal papillomas are often solitary and found in the subareolar location, arising in a major duct close to the nipple. Intraductal papillomas are most frequently observed in women aged 30 to 50 years and typically are not palpable because they are rarely larger than 5 mm. Compression of the breast close to the nipple in the affected quadrant often produces the discharge.

Because malignancies may present with bloody nipple discharge, mammography should be performed to rule out other abnormalities, and biopsy is usually necessary. **Fiberoptic ductoscopy is an endoscopic technique that has been developed over the past 15 years for evaluating bloody nipple discharge; it allows direct visualization of the ductal system through a nipple orifice.** For diagnosis of nipple discharge, fiberoptic ductoscopy has demonstrated an 88% sensitivity, 77% specificity, 83% positive predictive value, and 82% negative predictive value (32). **The technique is not widely used in clinical practice** because of limited expertise, high cost, and poor reproducibility.

In addition to ductoscopy, ductal lavage is another screening procedure for women with nipple discharge. Ductal lavage involves irrigation of the duct with saline and cytologic evaluation of the irrigant. Cytologic analysis of ductal lavage alone has a positive predictive value of 72% and a negative predictive value of 50%, but when combined with fiberoptic ductoscopy, the positive predictive value increases to 86% and the negative predictive value increases to 87% (32). There are limitations to the utilization of this technique including patient discomfort, low cytologic yield, and limited accuracy.

Treatment

Local excision of the draining duct is the treatment of choice. This can be performed using local anesthesia through a circumareolar incision by reflecting the nipple away from the breast tissue. A lacrimal probe can be used to assist in locating the offending duct. If it is not possible to identify the duct, total ductal excision of the subareolar duct can be performed through the same incision. The subsequent risk of invasive breast cancer is increased with the presence of atypical hyperplasia in a papilloma, with the risk similar to that of proliferative disease with atypia (33). **Papillomas may have malignant epithelium either *in situ* or invasive (34).**

Papillomatosis, defined as a minimum of five papillomas within an excised segment of breast tissue, is benign. Papillomatosis may present as nipple discharge, imaging abnormality, or even a palpable mass. Surgical excision alone is sufficient (32). There is an increased risk of cancer in patients with papillomatosis.

Fibroadenoma

Fibroadenomas are the most common benign breast mass in women (27). They are noncancerous growths composed of epithelial and stromal elements. They rarely occur after menopause, but occasionally calcified fibroadenomas are found in postmenopausal women. It is believed that they are influenced by estrogenic stimulation (27).

Symptoms and Signs

Clinically, a young patient usually notices a mass while showering or dressing. Most masses are 1 to 3 cm in diameter, but they can grow to an extremely large size (i.e., the giant fibroadenoma). On physical examination, they are firm, rubbery, smooth, and freely mobile. Fibroadenomas may be multiple. On mammography, they may appear as circumscribed, oval, or round masses. Occasionally, coarse calcifications can be seen within a fibroadenoma. On ultrasonography, they characteristically appear as circumscribed, homogeneous, hypoechoic oval masses with occasional lobulations, and are wider rather than tall. On MRI, they typically appear as smooth masses with high signal intensity on T2-weighted images.

Although the risk of cancer in a fibroadenoma is extremely low, some clinicians choose to biopsy (with fine-needle aspiration [FNA], core needle, or excisional biopsy) any solid mass in patients older than 30 years for definitive diagnosis. A lesion that is benign on ultrasonography and mammography is benign more than 99% of the time. **Some clinicians will omit biopsies in younger women with lesions characteristic of fibroadenomas** and will follow these patients with serial ultrasonography (27).

Complex fibroadenomas are fibroadenomas that contain cysts, sclerosing adenosis, papillary apocrine changes, or epithelial calcifications. In a clinical follow-up study by Dupont et al. (35), complex fibroadenomas were shown to be associated with a slightly increased risk of breast cancer. **Patients who have simple fibroadenomas without complex histologic features are at no increased risk for development of invasive cancer.**

Treatment

Although complete excision under local anesthesia can treat the lesion and confirm the absence of malignancy, excision is not often necessary. A fibroadenoma diagnosed by clinical examination, imaging and needle biopsy may be followed if the lesion remains stable. If a fibroadenoma increases in size, it should be excised. Excision is recommended for fibroadenomas that are greater than 2 or 3 cm to rule out phyllodes tumor. **Fibroadenomas may diminish in size or even totally resolve, particularly in younger women;** therefore excision can be avoided (36).

Benign Phyllodes Tumor

Phyllodes tumors are fibroepithelial breast tumors characterized by stromal overgrowth and hypercellularity combined with an epithelial component, grossly forming a leaf-like structure. Clinically, phyllodes tumors tend to occur in women aged 35 to 55 years, and comprise less than 1% of breast tumors (37). These lesions usually appear as isolated masses that are difficult to distinguish from fibroadenomas (38). Size is not a diagnostic criterion, although **phyllodes tumors tend to be larger than fibroadenomas, often with a history of rapid growth.** Both appear as well circumscribed, oval or lobulated masses, with round borders on mammography and ultrasonography. **There are no good clinical or radiographic criteria by which to distinguish a phyllodes tumor from a fibroadenoma (37,38).**

Pathology

Phyllodes tumors are classified as benign, borderline, or malignant based on the histologic criteria first described in 1978 (39). These histologic criteria are based on features **such as the number of mitoses, pushing or infiltrative tumor margins, degree of stromal overgrowth, and**

degree of stromal cellular atypia. These are all used in combination to distinguish between the benign and malignant spectrum (40). Even with histologic criteria, definitive distinction between fibroadenoma, benign phyllodes tumor, and malignant phyllodes tumor can be very difficult, and the correlation of histologic grade to clinical behavior and outcome has been challenging. **Even "benign" phyllodes tumors tend to recur locally, particularly if the tumor is simply enucleated.** Malignant phyllodes tumors have a higher local recurrence rate and can metastasize, usually to the lungs (40,41); for this reason, these tumors were originally called cystosarcoma phyllodes. Axillary lymph node metastases are extremely unusual despite the large size of some phyllodes tumors that are classified as "malignant."

Treatment

Because of the high propensity for local recurrence, the treatment of phyllodes tumors should consist of a wide, local excision (40–42). Large tumors not amenable to breast conservation and malignant tumors with particularly infiltrative margins may require total mastectomy without axillary node dissection; however, mastectomy should be avoided whenever possible. These malignant tumors are rarely multicentric and rarely metastasize to lymph nodes. **Typically, a phyllodes tumor is discovered by histologic examination after a patient has undergone an excisional biopsy of a mass believed to be a fibroadenoma.** When the pathologic diagnosis is phyllodes tumor, a complete re-excision of the area should be undertaken so that the prior biopsy site and any residual tumor are excised. There is no role for adjuvant therapy, either radiation therapy or chemotherapy.

Breast Cancer

Breast cancer is the most common cancer in women under the age of 60, and is second only to lung cancer as the leading cause of cancer deaths in women. It accounts for 29% of all new cancers in women. In 2013 in the United States, an estimated 232,340 new cases of invasive breast cancer will be diagnosed in women, with approximately 39,620 deaths (43). **The overall lifetime risk for development of breast cancer in women in the United States is one in eight or 12.38%** (43).

During the past 50 years, there has been a significant increase in the incidence of breast cancer in the United States. This correlates with the increased use of screening mammography (44). Breast cancer incidence rates increased after 1980, but decreased by 3.5% per year from 2001 to 2004 probably as a result of declining use of hormonal replacement therapy (HRT) by postmenopausal women, and delays in diagnosis caused by a decrease in mammographic utilization (45).

The mortality rate has dropped slightly, thought to result in part from mammographic screening and improvements in systemic therapy (3). Screening mammography has also resulted in a decrease in the size of breast cancer at diagnosis, with close to one-third of cancers being 1 cm or less in diameter (46). Not surprisingly, nodal involvement has decreased and the proportion of DCIS cases has increased. It is predicted that in the next decade, these trends will continue.

Predisposing Factors

One of the fundamental steps in determining a patient's risk for breast cancer is to obtain a detailed history. This allows the physician to plan preventive and diagnostic strategies, as well as to educate the patient about breast cancer. Intrinsic and extrinsic factors contribute to increasing a woman's risk. Intrinsic characteristics include genetic and familial elements, age, endogenous hormonal exposures, and benign breast lesions with high-risk histologies. Extrinsic characteristics include environmental exposures, diet, and exogenous hormonal exposures.

Age

Breast cancer is rare before the age of 25 years, accounting for less than 1% of all cases. After the age of 30 years, there is a sharp increase in the incidence, with a small plateau between the ages of 45 and 50 years, consistent with the involvement of hormonal factors (47). The risk of breast cancer in the next decade of life is 0.44% for a 30-year-old woman, 1.45% for a 40-year old, 2.31% for a 50-year old, 3.49% for a 60-year old, and 3.84% for a 70-year old (48).

Prior History of Breast Cancer

One of the strongest single risk factors for the development of breast cancer is the previous diagnosis of a contralateral breast cancer. The risk of subsequent contralateral breast cancer in a patient with unilateral breast cancer has been reported to range from 0.5–1% per year (49–52). **Young age (49,50,52) and lobular histology (50–52) have been associated with a greater likelihood of**

contralateral breast cancer and adjuvant chemotherapy with a decreased likelihood (51,52). In patients diagnosed with unilateral breast cancer, breast MRI has been shown to detect clinically and mammographically occult contralateral cancers in 3.1% of cases at the time of diagnosis (25).

Family History

A family history of breast cancer increases a patient's overall relative risk (53). However, the risk is not significantly increased for women with first-degree relatives (mother, sister) with postmenopausal breast cancers, whereas **women whose mothers or sisters had bilateral premenopausal breast cancer have a high likelihood of acquiring the disease**. If the patient's mother or sister had unilateral premenopausal breast cancer, the likelihood of the patient developing breast cancer is approximately 30%. If a woman has several first-degree relatives with breast cancer, the risk increases.

Inherited Syndromes of Breast Cancer

The majority of breast cancers occur sporadically, with only approximately 5–10% attributable to a breast cancer susceptibility gene (54). Two breast cancer susceptibility genes, *BRCA1* mapped to chromosome 17q21, and *BRCA2* on chromosome 13q12 to 13, are high penetrance tumor suppressor genes inherited in an autosomal-dominant fashion (55,56). Mutations in these genes account for only about 15% of all familial breast cancers, suggesting that other breast cancer susceptibility genes exist (57).

The estimated lifetime risk of breast cancer for women who have *BRCA1* mutations ranges from 36% to as high as 87%, with a pooled estimate of 70% (56–59). **The cumulative risk of ovarian cancer in *BRCA1* carriers has been reported to be between 27% and 45%** (58–60). **For *BRCA2* mutation carriers, lifetime estimated breast cancer risk is 60% (range 45–84%) and lifetime estimated ovarian cancer risk is 20%** (59). ***BRCA2* mutations are also associated with a 6% lifetime risk of male breast cancer. Furthermore, 10–20% of *BRCA1–2* mutation carriers treated with breast conservation at initial diagnosis will develop contralateral breast cancer within 10 years.** The likelihood of contralateral breast cancer increases with young age at diagnosis and number of first-degree relatives with breast cancer (59,61). **Breast cancers that occur in women with *BRCA1* mutations are mostly estrogen-receptor (ER) negative (up to 90%) and of high nuclear grade** (59). *BRCA* mutations are also associated with increased risk for the development of additional cancers such as colon, pancreatic, uterine, and cervical (59,62).

The prevalence of *BRCA1* and *BRCA2* in the general population is unknown but is estimated to be less than 0.12% and 0.044%, respectively (59). **In Ashkenazi Jewish women without breast cancer, the prevalence of these mutations is as high as 2%** (63). In women diagnosed with breast cancer before the age of 32, the incidence of *BRCA1* or *BRCA2* mutations is approximately 12% and in Ashkenazi women diagnosed with breast cancer before age 40, the incidence is 20% (64,65). There are a large number of potential mutations and other genetic modifiers, and the penetrance of the various mutations is highly variable. It is being studied by the Consortium of Investigators of Modifiers of BRCA1/2 (CIMBA) (66).

There are other hereditary syndromes associated with breast cancer with mostly autosomal dominant transmission, such as Li–Fraumeni, Cowden disease, Muir–Torre, a variant of hereditary nonpolyposis colon cancer (HNPCC), ataxia–telangiectasia (autosomal recessive), and Peutz–Jeghers syndromes. Each syndrome is associated with an abnormal gene responsible for producing a recognizable phenotype. In clinical practice, these syndromes contribute to only a small fraction of hereditary breast cancers. **The American Society of Clinical Oncology has specific guidelines for genetic testing for cancer susceptibility that are summarized in** Table 16.3 (67).

The American Society of Breast Surgeons (ASBS) issued a statement in 2006 defining patients at high risk for breast cancer. Persons in this high-risk population were those with early onset breast cancer (before age 50), two primary breast cancers, a family history of early onset breast cancer, a previously identified *BRCA1/BRCA2* mutation in the family, a personal or family history of ovarian cancer, or Ashkenazi Jewish heritage (https://www.breastsurgeons. org/statements/PDF_Statements/BRCA_Testing.pdf). Patients included in this group have a 10% or greater risk of harboring a *BRCA1* or *BRCA2* mutation, which is the traditional cutoff for testing.

Reproductive and Hormonal Factors

It is thought that lifetime exposure to endogenous estrogen plays a promotional role in the development of breast cancer (68–70). Women with breast cancer begin menses at a younger median age (70), and the **longer a woman's reproductive phase, the higher the risk of breast cancer** (68).

Table 16.3 American Society of Clinical Oncology: Genetic Testing for Cancer Susceptibility Guidelines

ASCO recommends that genetic testing only be offered when:

- The patient has very early onset of cancer or a strong family history
- The test can be adequately interpreted
- Medical management of the patient (or family member) will be influenced by the result

Patients must be given appropriate informed consent including information about the test performed and the implications of a negative and positive result.

There should be pre- and posttest counseling that includes a discussion about the options available to genetic carriers. Such options include surveillance and early detection with radiographic or physical examination, which have inherent limitations, and risk reduction strategies such as chemoprevention or prophylactic surgery, which have presumed but unproven efficacy.

Criteria defining patients at high risk of hereditary breast-ovarian cancer syndrome:

- Family with >2 breast cancers and one or more cases of ovarian cancer diagnosed at any age
- Family with >3 breast cancers diagnosed before age 50
- Sister pairs with 2 or more of the following cancers diagnosed before age 50:
  - 2 breast cancers, 2 ovarian cancers, 1 breast, and 1 ovarian cancer

Adapted from a **Statement of the American Society of Clinical Oncology: Genetic testing for cancer susceptibility.** *J Clin Oncol.* 1996;14:1730–1736; **American Society of Clinical Oncology policy statement update: Genetic testing for cancer susceptibility.** *J Clin Oncol.* 2003;12:2397–2406.

There is no clear association between the risk of breast cancer and duration of menses or menstrual irregularity. Studies of the effect of lactation have been inconclusive, but childbearing definitely has an effect on breast cancer risk (69). **Women who have never been pregnant have an increased risk compared to women who are parous, and late age at first birth also increases the risk of breast cancer** (69).

Meta-analyses of prospective cohort studies have demonstrated a small, increased risk of breast cancer for women who have ever taken oral contraceptives (odds ratio 1.08; 95% confidence interval: 0.99 to 1.17). Furthermore, every 10 years of oral contraceptive use is associated with a 14% increase in breast cancer risk (71). Other analyses suggest that **the risk declines with cessation of oral contraceptive use and, after 10 or more years from cessation, there appears to be no excess risk.** Breast cancers in women who had used oral contraceptives tended to be less advanced clinically and localized to the breast (72).

The association between breast cancer and HRT in postmenopausal women has been investigated in two large randomized trials. In the Women's Health Initiative (WHI) study, investigators demonstrated that **women randomized to combination estrogen plus progesterone HRT, had a significantly increased incidence of breast cancer, stroke, and pulmonary embolus compared with those randomized to a placebo** (73). HRT however, significantly decreased the incidence of colorectal cancer and femoral neck fractures. The WHI trial was stopped prematurely after it became apparent that the risks outweighed the benefits. **The risk of breast cancer has been shown to be greater for combination versus estrogen-only HRT.** However, women receiving estrogen-only HRT after hysterectomy in this study were at an increased risk for stroke (74). The Million Women Study in the United Kingdom recruited 1,084,110 women and also demonstrated that current use of HRT was associated with an increased risk of breast cancer (75).

Soon after the report of the WHI, the use of HRT in the United States decreased by 38%, with approximately 20 million fewer prescriptions written in 2003 than 2002 (76). Analysis of data from the National Cancer Institute's Surveillance, Epidemiology and End Results (SEER) registries indicates that the age-adjusted incidence rate of breast cancer in women fell by 6.7% in 2003. **This decrease in breast cancer incidence seems to be temporally related to the drop in the use of HRT by postmenopausal women. This decrease occurred primarily in non-Hispanic white women who were the primary users of HRT** (77). Follow-up data from the WHI study has demonstrated that the risk of breast cancer associated with combination HRT began to decrease toward baseline risk levels at 2 years from HRT cessation (78).

In counseling women with complaints of postmenopausal symptoms, the decision to initiate combination HRT must be individualized. For some patients, the improved quality of life and protection against fractures outweigh the potential risks. The individual risk of breast cancer in a particular postmenopausal patient should be considered before initiating HRT. If HRT is to be prescribed, low dosage formulations should be used with the understanding that the risk for harm will likely increase with prolonged use, and the survival benefit will diminish over time. For women at high risk for fractures, bisphosphonates are a suitable alternative. **Any postmenopausal woman on HRT should be aware of the increased risks of breast cancer, and should be counseled to be particularly diligent regarding breast cancer awareness and screening.**

Diet, Obesity, and Exercise

Regarding diet and breast cancer, **the majority of epidemiologic studies are case-control studies and cohort studies. Few RCTs have been conducted and are problematic because the randomized dietary plan has to be adhered to for a many years.** The association between breast cancer risk and dietary fat intake, for example, has been inconsistent. One large meta-analysis of 11 prospective cohort studies found no evidence of a positive association between fat intake and risk of breast cancer when those in the highest quintile of total fat intake were compared with those in the lowest quintile (79). Similarly, a large RCT involving 40 US centers from the WHI study followed 48,835 postmenopausal women for 8 years who were randomly assigned to a dietary modification group or a control group (80). The dietary modifications included five servings of fruits and vegetables, six servings of grains, and total fat to 20% of energy requirements daily. In the group of women who had a low-fat diet, there was no statistically significant reduction in invasive breast cancer risk. The results were confounded by relatively few women meeting the low-fat dietary target (only 14.4% at year 6). **Future studies were encouraged because it may take years for the benefits of a low-fat diet to be manifested.**

One large prospective study in the United States of 90,655 premenopausal women found no association between **fiber intake** and the risk of breast cancer, whereas a study in the United Kingdom of 35,792 women demonstrated a reduced risk of breast cancer for premenopausal women who consumed more than 30 g of fiber per day as compared to those who consumed less than 20 g/d (81,82). Studies on soy intake have also yielded mixed results. **Historically, breast cancer incidence has been lower in Asia where dietary soy intake is significantly higher than in a typical American diet.** This may be counterintuitive because soy protein is broken down into estrogenic compounds. A recent meta-analysis of four studies of breast cancer recurrence and 14 studies of breast cancer incidence demonstrated that soy consumption was inversely associated with breast cancer incidence (RR = 0.89, 95% CI: 0.79 to 0.99). However, the protective effect of soy was only observed among studies conducted in Asian populations (RR = 0.76, 95% CI: 0.65 to 0.86), not in Western populations (RR = 0.97, 95% CI: 0.87 to 1.06). Soy intake was also inversely associated with risk of breast cancer recurrence (RR = 0.84, 95% CI: 0.70 to 0.99) (83). **Studies of natural antioxidants, the dietary carotenoids, and vitamins A, C, E, and D have also been conflicting.** While early observational studies suggested an association between low levels of 25-hydroxy vitamin D and breast cancer, pooled analyses of subsequent observational studies have not demonstrated a reduction in breast cancer risk associated with vitamin D supplementation (84).

The evidence for obesity as a risk factor for breast cancer development is much greater. Obesity, as defined by a body mass index (BMI) greater than or equal to 30 kg/m^2, is a rapidly growing problem that has been associated with increased risk of cancer development. Increased adiposity has been associated with increased levels of proinflammatory cytokines and adipose tissue-derived cytokines leptin and adiponectin, which can initiate a number of molecular pathways associated with cancer development (85). **The Million Women Study in the United Kingdom,** for example, **demonstrated a linear correlation between increasing BMI and increasing risk of postmenopausal breast cancer incidence and mortality** (86). This increased risk has not been demonstrated for premenopausal breast cancer (86,87).

Exercise has been shown to reduce the risk of postmenopausal breast cancer (88). A recent study of 64,777 women from the Nurses' Health Study Cohort II evaluated premenopausal exercise habits and showed that the most active women (running 3.25 hours or walking 13 hours per week) had a 23% reduction in the risk for premenopausal breast cancer (89). A large systematic review supports the decreased risk of breast cancer with exercise: 62 studies were evaluated with the conclusion that **increased physical activity led to an overall risk reduction for breast cancer**

of 25%, with a dose-dependent effect noted in 28 of the studies (90). This reduction in risk was seen in both premenopausal and postmenopausal women.

The metabolic effect of exercise and its impact on breast cancer risk biomarkers are being investigated in a randomized, multicenter SHAPE-2 trial of 243 sedentary, postmenopausal women with BMI 25 to 35 kg/m^2 (overweight or obese). Participants have been randomized to one of three groups: Diet alone, exercise alone, or diet plus exercise. The results of the SHAPE-2 trial may lead to more specific lifestyle guidelines for breast cancer prevention (91).

Observational studies have shown that moderate exercise may reduce the risk of breast cancer recurrence and mortality and may be protective against second breast cancers (92). The Health, Eating, Activity, and Lifestyle (HEAL) study of 688 women with early stage breast cancer found that women who expended the equivalent of brisk walking 2 to 3 hours per week had a hazard ratio for death of 0.33 compared with sedentary women (93). Likewise, the WHI study demonstrated lower breast cancer-specific mortality for women who engaged in 3 hours per week of fast walking after their cancer diagnosis, even if they were sedentary previously (HR 0.61, 95% CI 0.44 to 0.87, $p = 0.01$) (94).

Alcohol

Regular alcohol consumption of as little as half a drink (1 drink = 10 g) per day has been linked to an increased risk of breast cancer. This increase is seen irrespective of the type of alcoholic beverage consumed. The Million Women Study in the United Kingdom found that consumption of an average of 1 drink per day in middle-aged women was associated with a 12% increase in breast cancer risk (95). The Nurses Health Study in the United States found that after 2.4 million person-years of follow-up, 7,690 cases of invasive breast cancer were diagnosed among the 105,986 original participants, and that consumption of as little as 0.5 to 1 drink per week was associated with an increased breast cancer risk (RR 1.15, CI, 1.06 to 1.24). Furthermore, alcohol intake early or late in adult life is an independent risk factor for breast cancer (96).

Radiation Exposure

Prior radiation exposure to the thoracic area, especially during adolescence or early adulthood (when breasts are developing), has been shown to increase the risk of breast cancer. In Japan, female atomic bomb survivors have been noted to have an increased risk of breast cancer, and the risk was greatest for women who were exposed as children (97). Multiple studies, including the Childhood Cancer Survivor Study, have demonstrated **an increased risk for women who have undergone treatment for Hodgkin disease.** In this study, the 30-year incidence of invasive breast cancer among 878 female survivors of Hodgkin disease was 18% (98). **The increased risk is primarily age related, with the highest risk associated with treatment at ages 10 to 20 years.** This increased risk warrants high-risk surveillance with annual screening breast MRI, in addition to annual mammography (26). Lower doses of therapeutic radiation, such as with fluoroscopy previously used to treat tuberculosis, have also been associated with an increased risk (99).

Diagnosis

The majority of breast tumors are found in the upper, outer quadrant, where there is more breast tissue. Breast cancer is often discovered by the patient. The findings on mammography may suggest that a palpable lesion is malignant. On the other hand, screening mammography may detect an abnormality without a palpable tumor. Rarely, the patient may present with an axillary mass and no obvious carcinoma in the breast.

A breast mass in a woman of any age must be approached as a possible carcinoma. At times, the only clue to an underlying malignancy may be a subtle finding of an area of thickening amid normal nodularity. Obvious clues to malignancy include nipple retraction, skin dimpling, involved nodes, or ulceration, but these are late signs and are not common at presentation.

After obtaining the history and physical examination, **the "triple test" should be utilized to evaluate a palpable mass. Triple test refers to the combination of physical examination, breast imaging** (usually mammogram ± ultrasound) **and pathologic diagnosis** employing cytology by means of FNA, or histology by means of a core-needle biopsy (CNB) or excisional biopsy. **The diagnostic accuracy is approximately 100% when all three are concordant** (100,101). Indications for an excisional biopsy include cytologic or histologic atypia on needle biopsy, any discordance between any of the three modalities, or the patient's desire to eliminate a source for concern. Algorithms for the evaluation of breast masses in premenopausal and postmenopausal women are presented in Figs. 16.3 and 16.4. The **ACS** reports that 80% of breast biopsies are benign (http://www.cancer.org).

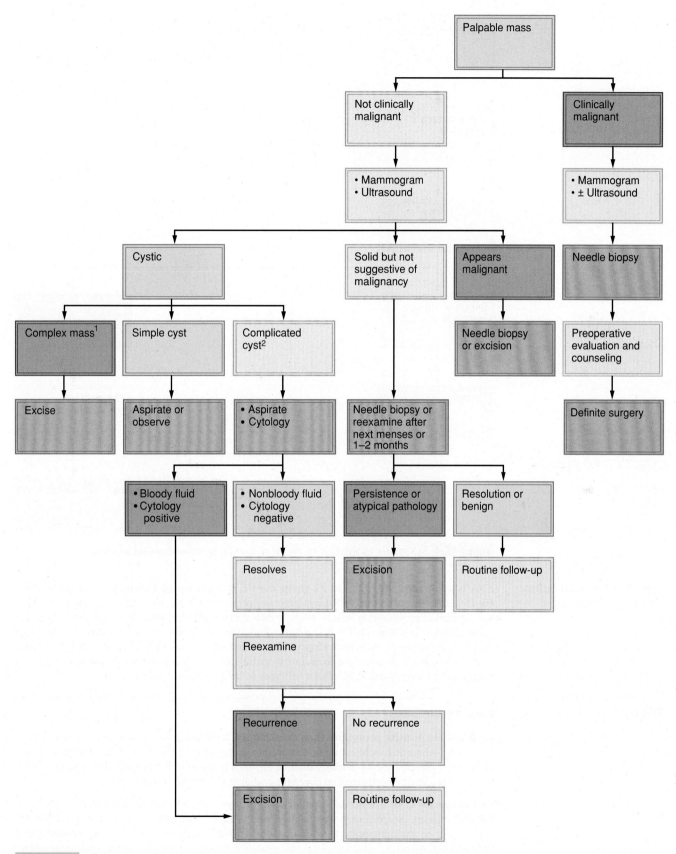

Figure 16.3 Schematic evaluation of breast masses in premenopausal women. [1]Complex mass—a cystic mass with a solid component that may be malignant. [2]Complicated cyst—usually multiple simple cysts or cysts with septations.

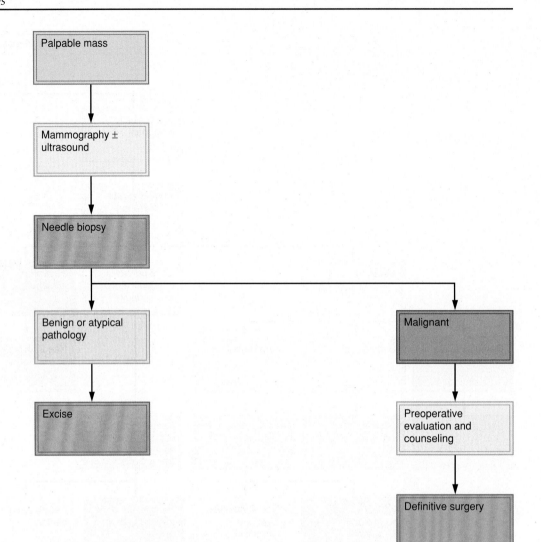

Figure 16.4 Schematic evaluation of breast masses in postmenopausal women.

Fine-Needle Aspiration Cytologic Testing	**FNA is performed with a 20- or 22-gauge needle, and has a high diagnostic accuracy, with a 10–15% false-negative rate.** FNA has a rare but persistent false-positive rate, often in association with epithelial proliferative lesions such as ductal or lobular hyperplasia (102,103). A negative FNA cytologic diagnosis that is discordant with CBE and imaging must be followed with either core needle biopsy or excisional biopsy. FNA is limited by the availability of a skilled cytopathologist and the inability of the technique to distinguish between noninvasive and invasive breast cancer and between ductal and lobular subtypes of invasive breast cancer (104).
Biopsy	**Core-Needle Biopsy**
	CNB is a less invasive procedure than open biopsy. It utilizes an 8- to 14-gauge needle to obtain specimens. Abnormal architecture and invasion can be identified in these tissue samples, unlike FNA (105). Specific tumor markers such as estrogen receptor (ER), progesterone receptor (PR), or HER2/*neu* can be performed on core biopsy-diagnosed breast cancers (106).
	Indications for CNB are the same as for open biopsy and CNB may be performed handheld for palpable masses. Suspicious nonpalpable lesions can be biopsied using stereotactic CNB for lesions seen on mammography, or with ultrasonic or MRI guidance for lesions seen on ultrasound or MRI, respectively. CNB using ultrasonic guidance is simpler and less expensive than stereotactic CNB, and does not require special equipment (105).
	A number of studies have shown sensitivity and specificity ranging from of 85–100% for image-guided CNB. The sensitivity and negative predictive values of CNB are less for

mammographic calcifications (0.84 and 0.94, respectively) than for the diagnosis of masses (0.96 and 0.99, respectively) (104,105). When CNB is used to sample microcalcifications, radiography of the specimen must be performed to ensure the calcifications are present in the tissue removed. A microclip is usually placed after CNB to indicate the biopsied area and a postbiopsy mammogram is obtained. CNB usually does not result in architectural distortion, which may alter the interpretation of future mammograms.

Certain technical issues may not allow CNB to be employed, such as very superficial or posterior lesions. **Mammographic lesions in a very small breast are usually not amenable to stereotactic core biopsy, and breast implants can make CNB more challenging.** Depending on the location of the lesion in relation to the implant, open biopsy is sometimes recommended to avoid implant rupture. Vacuum-assisted devices with CNB allow for multiple samples to be obtained without withdrawing and reinserting the needle.

Open Biopsy

A minority of patients requires surgical biopsy if the lesion is not amenable to CNB, the sample is inadequate, or the pathologic results are equivocal. Likewise, follow-up open biopsy is indicated if benign diagnoses of atypical ductal hyperplasia (ADH), flat epithelial atypia, atypical lobular hyperplasia (ALH), lobular carcinoma in situ (LCIS), intraductal papilloma, or radial scar are made after CNB, because of the coexistence of malignancy in up to 20–30% of such cases (107).

Image-Guided Open-Biopsy

Nonpalpable lesions detected by a mammogram, ultrasound, or MRI that are not amenable to CNB require open biopsy after preoperative localization by imaging. This requires the collaborative effort of the surgeon and the radiologist and entails the placement of a needle or specialized wire into the suspicious area. To further assist in localization, many radiologists also inject a biologic dye. The surgeon reviews the films and localizes the abnormality with respect to the tip of the wire or needle and plans the operation accordingly.

Open biopsy can usually be performed in the outpatient setting with the aid of intravenous (IV) sedation and local anesthesia. The following steps are undertaken:

1. **IV sedation** is used to ease anxiety. **Local anesthesia** is used to infiltrate the skin and subcutaneous tissue surrounding the mass or wire-localized abnormality.

2. **An incision is often made directly over the mass or localized area, at the site of the wire insertion, or periareolar.** The incision should be placed cosmetically so that a partial mastectomy can be performed through the same incision. If the tumor is far from the areola, circumareolar incisions are best avoided.

3. After the skin and underlying tissues have been incised, **the mass or localized area can be gently grasped** with a stay suture or **with Allis forceps** and delivered into the operative field.

4. **Whenever possible, the lesion should be totally excised.** An incisional biopsy may be performed for large masses, but a frozen section should be done to confirm that malignant tissue has been obtained. It is important not to remove too much additional breast tissue, because the main purpose of the procedure is to achieve a tissue diagnosis.

5. **In the case of abnormalities localized by mammography, a postexcisional mammogram of the surgical specimen** should be performed to be certain that the lesion in question has been excised.

6. **After adequate hemostasis has been achieved, the wound should be irrigated, the specimen confirmed to contain the lesion by mammography, and the incision closed.** The most superficial subcutaneous fat is reapproximated with fine, absorbable sutures, usually a 3–0 or 4–0 vicryl. The skin is best closed with an absorbable subcuticular suture, with either Steri-Strips or Dermabond applied to the incision to achieve the most cosmetically pleasing result.

Two-Step Approach

The two-step approach involves the initial biopsy, either by needle or open procedures, followed by subsequent definitive treatment. Women who are diagnosed with breast cancer on biopsy can discuss the various treatment options and seek out additional consultations, if desirable, before undergoing definitive treatment. For most patients, being engaged in the planning of therapy is an important psychological aspect in the healing process.

Pathology and Natural History

Breast cancer constitutes a heterogeneous group of histopathologic lesions. Regardless of the histologic type, most breast cancers arise in the terminal duct lobular unit. **The classification of the World Health Organization (WHO) is most widely used for invasive breast cancers, and it recognizes invasive carcinoma as "ductal" and "lobular."** The WHO classification scheme is based on cytologic features and growth patterns of the invasive tumor cells, with the distinction between lobular and intraductal carcinoma based on the histologic appearance rather than the site of origin (108). Breast cancer may be either **invasive (infiltrating lobular carcinoma, ILC),** which indicates invasion into the breast stroma with the potential for lymph node and distant metastases, or *in situ* **(DCIS or LCIS),** which indicates the inability to spread to other sites.

The most common histologic diagnosis of invasive breast carcinoma is infiltrating ductal carcinoma (IDC). This histologic type accounts for 60–75% of breast cancers in the United States (109). This diagnosis is actually a diagnosis by default, because this tumor type is defined as a type of cancer that does not fall into any of the other categories of invasive mammary carcinoma (108), as recognized by defined histologic features (mucinous, tubular, medullary). **Mammographically, it is often characterized by a stellate appearance with microcalcifications.** The classic macroscopic appearance of infiltrating ductal carcinoma is a firm, often rock-hard mass that has gritty, chalky streaks within the substance of the tumor. This consistency is caused by the fibrotic response of the surrounding stroma. Microscopically, the appearance is highly heterogeneous with regard to growth pattern, cytologic features, mitotic activity, and extent of in situ component.

The second most common histologic diagnosis is infiltrating lobular carcinoma (ILC), which comprises 5–15% of cases (109). It may present as a mammographic abnormality or palpable mass, as with invasive ductal carcinoma, but the extent of disease may be underestimated by the physical or radiographic findings. Invasive lobular carcinoma often presents as multifocal disease in the ipsilateral breast, with **coexistent LCIS in approximately 5–15% of cases** (110). **The incidence of contralateral breast cancer in ILC patients ranges from 6–47%** (109). Macroscopically, some invasive lobular carcinomas may appear as firm, gray-white masses similar to invasive ductal cancers, while others may have only a rubbery consistency of the breast tissue. **Microscopically, invasive lobular cancer is characterized by small, uniform neoplastic cells infiltrating the stroma in a single-file pattern, with little or no desmoplastic stromal reaction** (108). Other types of invasive breast carcinoma are far less common, and are subtypes of infiltrating ductal carcinoma.

Medullary carcinoma accounts for approximately 2–5% of cases, and is often well circumscribed grossly, with a dense lymphocytic infiltrate microscopically (109). They are usually slow growing, less aggressive cancers. The distant recurrence-free survival was 89% at 14 years in one series, compared with 64% for usual infiltrating ductal carcinomas (111). **Tubular carcinoma** is a well-differentiated breast cancer with limited metastatic potential and an excellent prognosis, occurring in about 1% of breast cancers (109). **Mucinous (colloid) carcinoma accounts for fewer than 5% of all breast cancers, and is also associated with a favorable prognosis** (109). Grossly, the tumors are well circumscribed and may have areas that appear mucinous or gelatinous. Microscopically, small clusters or sheets of tumor cells are dispersed in pools of extracellular mucin (108,109).

Papillary carcinoma is used to describe a predominantly noninvasive ductal carcinoma; **invasive papillary carcinomas are rare, accounting for approximately 1% of breast cancers** (108,109). An extremely rare form of breast cancer is adenoid cystic carcinoma, which is similar histologically to the salivary gland tumor. They often present as a palpable mass with no clinicoradiologic features. **These cancers metastasize late and tend to be well differentiated** (109,112).

Growth Patterns

The tumor growth rate of a breast cancer varies widely among patients and at different stages of the disease. Many mathematical models have been devised based on the natural history of breast cancer, assumptions of tumor growth rate, the probability of detecting a tumor of a given size, and the rate of clinical surfacing (113). Doubling time of breast cancer has been estimated to range from several weeks for rapidly growing tumors to months for slowly growing ones. **Based on seminal studies, the mean doubling time for mammary carcinomas has been estimated to be 5.4 months, with a standard deviation of 4 months** (114). To give an example for clinical application, if it is assumed that the doubling time is 100 days, the doubling time is constant (which is

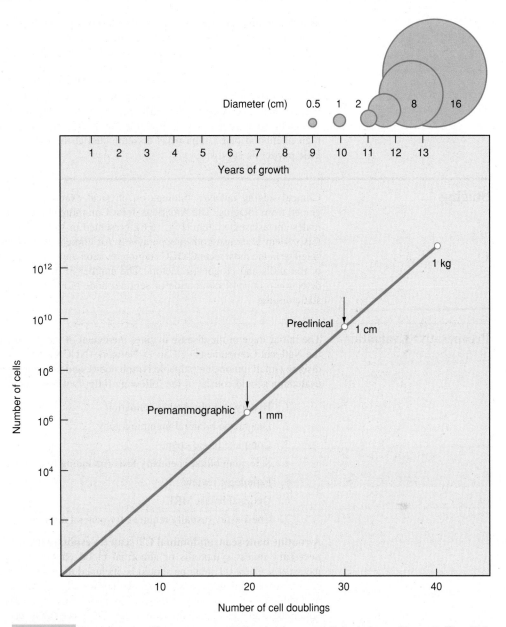

Figure 16.5 **Growth rate of breast cancer, indicating long preclinical phase.** (From **Gullino PM**. Natural history of breast cancer: Progression from hyperplasia to neoplasia as predicted by angiogenesis. *Cancer.* 1977;39:2699. Copyright 1977 American Cancer Society. Reprinted by permission of Wiley-Liss, Inc., a subsidiary of John Wiley & Sons, Inc.)

not often the case), and the tumor originated from one cell, it would take 8 years to result in a 1-cm tumor (Fig. 16.5) (115). Before the tumor is clinically apparent, tumor cells may be circulating through the body.

Many clinicians view breast cancer as a systemic disease at the time of diagnosis, but **this pessimistic view is not justified.** A more realistic approach is to view breast cancer as a two-compartment disease: One consists of the primary breast tumor with its possible local and regional extension, and the other consists of the systemic metastases, with their life-threatening consequences.

Biology of Breast Cancer

The biology of breast cancer is highly variable. **Some view breast cancer as a local disease** that progresses in a predictable manner to develop distant metastases over time, known as the **"Halstedian" theory,** named after the prominent surgeon who popularized the radical mastectomy. **With this view, aggressive local control is necessary for survival. Others view breast cancer** as a "systemic" disease, with distant metastases present before a patient is diagnosed. With the systemic view, it is thought that some tumors have the ability to metastasize and others do not; the emphasis is on systemic therapy with the belief that local recurrences are treated as they develop and have no bearing on the development of future distant disease or on survival. **Another theory, known as the "spectrum theory," is a synthesis of the two views: Breast cancer is a heterogeneous disease, with some cancers remaining localized throughout their course, while others are systemic from the outset** (116). With this view, unless initial local control is sufficient, some tumors will gain the ability to disseminate. It is acknowledged that if there is a high likelihood that a tumor has disseminated at the time of diagnosis, local control will have little impact on survival.

Staging

Clinical staging involves findings on physical examination, with incorporation of information gained from imaging. The American Joint Committee on Cancer (AJCC) uses the TNM (tumor–nodes–metastases) system (Fig. 16.6), presented in Tables 16.4 and 16.5 (117). The advantage of this system is its use both preoperatively for clinical staging and postoperatively for pathologic staging. In the most recent AJCC staging revision, new areas are incorporated regarding evaluation of the axilla and prognostic factors: The number of positive axillary nodes; the method used for detection (clinical examination or sentinel node biopsy [SNB]); and the presence of micrometastatic disease.

Preoperative Evaluation

The initial stage of the disease dictates the extent of the preoperative workup (118). According to the National Comprehensive Cancer Network (NCCN), for most patients with TNM stage I or II disease (small tumors, no palpable lymph nodes, and no symptoms of metastases), the preoperative evaluation should consist of the following (http://www.nccn.org):

1. History and physical examination
2. Diagnostic bilateral mammography
3. Complete blood count
4. Screening blood chemistry tests (including liver function tests)
5. Pathologic review
6. Optional breast MRI
7. Chest x-ray (usually required for general anesthesia)

A routine bone scan, abdominal CT scan (to evaluate the liver) and chest CT imaging are not necessary unless symptoms or abnormal blood chemistry suggests bone, liver, or pulmonary metastases. Chest CT imaging should be included for any patient presenting with clinical stage III or IV disease. Although the NCCN guidelines for clinical stage III workup recommend a bone scan or abdominal CT scan only if dictated by symptoms or laboratory values, most physicians will obtain these studies in patients with locally advanced breast cancer.

Patients with clinical stage IV disease should have both a bone scan and abdominal CT scan; if metastases are evident on imaging or there is obvious bone marrow dysfunction, most physicians will recommend a bone marrow biopsy. **Routine bone marrow biopsy is viewed by some to be an important prognostic test that may supplant axillary dissection for staging breast cancer patients** (119). Brain MRI or CT scan of the head should be performed in patients with ER-negative or human epidermal growth factor receptor 2 (HER2)-positive breast cancer subtypes, as they are more likely to metastasize to the brain (120) than other subtypes.

Positron emission tomography (PET) uses a glucose analog tracer, fluorodeoxyglucose (FDG), which is taken up by cells in proportion to their rate of glucose metabolism (121); malignant cells have increased glucose uptake in comparison to normal tissues. As of November 2004, the Centers for Medicare and Medicaid Services had approved FDG-PET scanning for the following indications: (i) Staging patients with distant metastasis; (ii) restaging patients with locoregional recurrence; or (iii) monitoring response to therapy in women with either metastasis or locally advanced breast cancer when a change in treatment has been planned.

FDG-PET is not recommended for axillary staging in patients with an initial diagnosis of breast cancer because FDG-PET cannot detect small metastases (i.e., <1 cm) (121,122). In a meta-analysis of 26 studies, PET had a lower mean sensitivity and specificity than SNB for the detection of axillary lymph node metastasis (122).

American Joint Committee on Cancer

Breast Cancer Staging

7th EDITION

T1

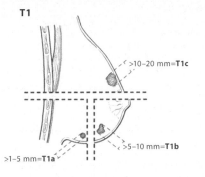

>10–20 mm=**T1c**

>5–10 mm=**T1b**

>1–5 mm=**T1a**

T2

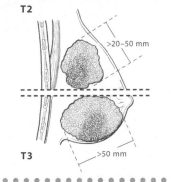

>20–50 mm

T3

>50 mm

T4a

Direct extension to chest wall not including pectoralis muscle.

Primary Tumor (T)

TX	Primary tumor cannot be assessed
T0	No evidence of primary tumor
Tis	Carcinoma in situ
Tis (DCIS)	Ductal carcinoma in situ
Tis (LCIS)	Lobular carcinoma in situ
Tis (Paget's)	Paget's disease of the nipple NOT associated with invasive carcinoma and/or carcinoma in situ (DCIS and/or LCIS) in the underlying breast parenchyma. Carcinomas in the breast parenchyma associated with Paget's disease are categorized based on the size and characteristics of the parenchymal disease, although the presence of Paget's disease should still be noted

T1	Tumor ≤ 20 mm in greatest dimension
T1mi	Tumor ≤ 1 mm in greatest dimension
T1a	Tumor > 1 mm but ≤ 5 mm in greatest dimension
T1b	Tumor > 5 mm but ≤ 10 mm in greatest dimension
T1c	Tumor > 10 mm but ≤ 20 mm in greatest dimension
T2	Tumor > 20 mm but ≤ 50 mm in greatest dimension
T3	Tumor > 50 mm in greatest dimension

T4	Tumor of any size with direct extension to the chest wall and/or to the skin (ulceration or skin nodules) Note: Invasion of the dermis alone does not qualify as T4
T4a	Extension to the chest wall, not including only pectoralis muscle adherence/invasion
T4b	Ulceration and/or ipsilateral satellite nodules and/or edema (including peau d'orange) of the skin, which do not meet the criteria for inflammatory carcinoma
T4c	Both T4a and T4b
T4d	Inflammatory carcinoma (see "Rules for Classification")

Distant Metastases (M)

M0	No clinical or radiographic evidence of distant metastases
cM0(i+)	No clinical or radiographic evidence of distant metastases, but deposits of molecularly or microscopically detected tumor cells in circulating blood, bone marrow, or other nonregional nodal tissue that are no larger than 0.2 mm in a patient without symptoms or signs of metastases
M1	Distant detectable metastases as determined by classic clinical and radiographic means and/or histologically proven larger than 0.2 mm

ANATOMIC STAGE/PROGNOSTIC GROUPS

Stage 0	Tis	N0	M0
Stage IA	T1*	N0	M0
Stage IB	T0	N1mi	M0
	T1*	N1mi	M0
Stage IIA	T0	N1**	M0
	T1*	N1**	M0
	T2	N0	M0
Stage IIB	T2	N1	M0
	T3	N0	M0
Stage IIIA	T0	N2	M0
	T1*	N2	M0
	T2	N2	M0
	T3	N1	M0
	T3	N2	M0
Stage IIIB	T4	N0	M0
	T4	N1	M0
	T4	N2	M0
Stage IIIC	Any T	N3	M0
Stage IV	Any T	Any N	M1

Notes

* T1 includes T1mi.
** T0 and T1 tumors with nodal micrometastases only are excluded from Stage IIA and are classified Stage IB.
* M0 includes M0(i+).
* The designation pM0 is not valid; any M0 should be clinical.
* If a patient presents with M1 prior to neoadjuvant systemic therapy, the stage is considered Stage IV and remains Stage IV regardless of response to neoadjuvant therapy.
* Stage designation may be changed if postsurgical imaging studies reveal the presence of distant metastases, provided that the studies are carried out within 4 months of diagnosis in the absence of disease progression and provided that the patient has not received neoadjuvant therapy.
* Postneoadjuvant therapy is designated with "yc" or "yp" prefix. Of note, no stage group is assigned if there is a complete pathologic response (CR) to neoadjuvant therapy, for example, ypT0ypN0cM0.

Financial support for AJCC 7th Edition Staging Posters provided by the American Cancer Society

American Cancer Society®

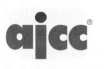

Copyright 2009 American Joint Committee on Cancer • Printed with permission from the AJCC.

1 of 2

Figure 16.6 Breast Cancer is staged using the TNM (Tumor-Nodes-Metastasis) system as presented in the American Joint Commission on Cancer (AJCC) Staging Manual, 2010, 7th ed. (117). (*continued*)

669

American Joint Committee on Cancer

Breast Cancer Staging

7th EDITION

Regional Lymph Nodes (N)

CLINICAL

NX   Regional lymph nodes cannot be assessed (for example, previously removed)

N0   No regional lymph node metastases

N1   Metastases to movable ipsilateral level I, II axillary lymph node(s)

N2   Metastases in ipsilateral level I, II axillary lymph nodes that are clinically fixed or matted; or in clinically detected* ipsilateral internal mammary nodes in the absence of clinically evident axillary lymph node metastases

N2a   Metastases in ipsilateral level I, II axillary lymph nodes fixed to one another (matted) or to other structures

N2b   Metastases only in clinically detected* ipsilateral internal mammary nodes and in the absence of clinically evident level I, II axillary lymph node metastases

N3   Metastases in ipsilateral infraclavicular (level III axillary) lymph node(s) with or without level I, II axillary lymph node involvement; or in clinically detected* ipsilateral internal mammary lymph node(s) with clinically evident level I, II axillary lymph node metastases; or metastases in ipsilateral supraclavicular lymph node(s) with or without axillary or internal mammary lymph node involvement

N3a   Metastases in ipsilateral infraclavicular lymph node(s)

N3b   Metastases in ipsilateral internal mammary lymph node(s) and axillary lymph node(s)

N3c   Metastases in ipsilateral supraclavicular lymph node(s)

Notes

*   "Clinically detected" is defined as detected by imaging studies (excluding lymphoscintigraphy) or by clinical examination and having characteristics highly suspicious for malignancy or a presumed pathologic macrometastasis based on fine needle aspiration biopsy with cytologic examination. Confirmation of clinically detected metastatic disease by fine needle aspiration without excision biopsy is designated with an (f) suffix, for example, cN3a(f). Excisional biopsy of a lymph node or biopsy of a sentinel node, in the absence of assignment of a pT, is classified as a clinical N, for example, cN1. Information regarding the confirmation of the nodal status will be designated in site-specific factors as clinical, fine needle aspiration, core biopsy, or sentinel lymph node biopsy. Pathologic classification (pN) is used for excision or sentinel lymph node biopsy only in conjunction with a pathologic T assignment.

PATHOLOGIC (PN)*

pNX   Regional lymph nodes cannot be assessed (for example, previously removed, or not removed for pathologic study)

pN0   No regional lymph node metastasis identified histologically

Note: Isolated tumor cell clusters (ITC) are defined as small clusters of cells not greater than 0.2 mm, or single tumor cells, or a cluster of fewer than 200 cells in a single histologic cross-section. ITCs may be detected by routine histology or by immunohistochemical (IHC) methods. Nodes containing only ITCs are excluded from the total positive node count for purposes of N classification but should be included in the total number of nodes evaluated.

pN0(i–)   No regional lymph node metastases histologically, negative IHC

pN0(i+)   Malignant cells in regional lymph node(s) no greater than 0.2 mm (detected by H&E or IHC including ITC)

pN0(mol–)   No regional lymph node metastases histologically, negative molecular findings (RT-PCR)

pN0(mol+)   Positive molecular findings (RT-PCR)**, but no regional lymph node metastases detected by histology or IHC

pN1   Micrometastases; or metastases in 1–3 axillary lymph nodes; and/or in internal mammary nodes with metastases detected by sentinel lymph node biopsy but not clinically detected***

pN1mi   Micrometastases (greater than 0.2 mm and/or more than 200 cells, but none greater than 2.0 mm)

pN1a   Metastases in 1–3 axillary lymph nodes, at least one metastasis greater than 2.0 mm

pN1b   Metastases in internal mammary nodes with micrometastases or macrometastases detected by sentinel lymph node biopsy but not clinically detected***

pN1c   Metastases in 1–3 axillary lymph nodes and in internal mammary lymph nodes with micrometastases or macrometastases detected by sentinel lymph node biopsy but not clinically detected

pN2   Metastases in 4–9 axillary lymph nodes; or in clinically detected**** internal mammary lymph nodes in the absence of axillary lymph node metastases

pN2a   Metastases in 4–9 axillary lymph nodes (at least one tumor deposit greater than 2.0 mm)

pN2b   Metastases in clinically detected**** internal mammary lymph nodes in the absence of axillary lymph node metastases

pN3   Metastases in 10 or more axillary lymph nodes; or in infraclavicular (level III axillary) lymph nodes; or in clinically detected**** ipsilateral internal mammary lymph nodes in the presence of one or more positive level I, II axillary lymph nodes; or in more than three axillary lymph nodes and in internal mammary lymph nodes with micrometastases or macrometastases detected by sentinel lymph node biopsy but not clinically detected***; or in ipsilateral supraclavicular lymph nodes

pN3a   Metastases in 10 or more axillary lymph nodes (at least one tumor deposit greater than 2.0 mm); or metastases to the infraclavicular (level III axillary lymph) nodes

pN3b   Metastases in clinically detected**** ipsilateral internal mammary lymph nodes in the presence of one or more positive axillary lymph nodes; or in more than three axillary lymph nodes and in internal mammary lymph nodes with micrometastases or macrometastases detected by sentinel lymph node biopsy but not clinically detected***

pN3c   Metastases in ipsilateral supraclavicular lymph nodes

Notes

*   Classification is based on axillary lymph node dissection with or without sentinel lymph node biopsy. Classification based solely on sentinel lymph node biopsy without subsequent axillary lymph node dissection is designated (sn) for "sentinel node," for example, pN0(sn).

**   RT-PCR: reverse transcriptase/polymerase chain reaction.

***   "Not clinically detected" is defined as not detected by imaging studies (excluding lymphoscintigraphy) or not detected by clinical examination.

****   "Clinically detected" is defined as detected by imaging studies (excluding lymphoscintigraphy) or by clinical examination and having characteristics highly suspicious for malignancy or a presumed pathologic macrometastasis based on fine needle aspiration biopsy with cytologic examination.

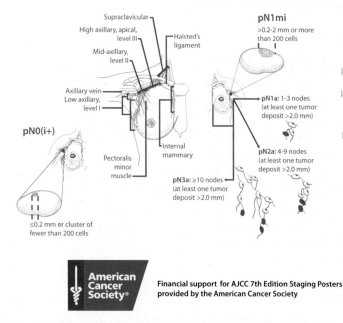

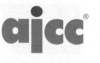

American Cancer Society®

Financial support for AJCC 7th Edition Staging Posters provided by the American Cancer Society

Copyright 2009 American Joint Committee on Cancer • Printed with permission from the AJCC.

2 of 2

Figure 16.6 *Continued.* **Breast Cancer is staged using the TNM (Tumor-Nodes-Metastasis) system as presented in the American Joint Commission on Cancer (AJCC) Staging Manual, 2010, 7th ed.** (117).

Table 16.4 TNM (Tumor–Nodes–Metastases) System for Staging of Breast Cancer

Primary Tumor (T)

TX	Primary tumor cannot be assessed
T_0	No evidence of primary tumor
T_{is}	Carcinoma *in situ* T_{is} (DCIS) Ductal carcinoma *in situ* T_{is} (LCIS) Lobular carcinoma *in situ* T_{is} (Paget) Paget's disease of the nipple with no tumor
T_1	Tumor 2 cm or less in greatest dimension T_{1mic} Microinvasion 0.1 cm or less in greatest dimension T_{1a} Tumor more than 0.1 cm but not more than 0.5 cm in greatest dimension T_{1b} Tumor more than 0.5 cm but not more than 1 cm in greatest dimension T_{1c} Tumor more than 1 cm but not more than 2 cm in greatest dimension
T_2	Tumor more than 2 cm but not more than 5 cm in greatest dimension
T_3	Tumor more than 5 cm in greatest dimension
T_4	Tumor of any size with direct extension to (a) chest wall or (b) skin, only as described below T_{4a} Extension to chest wall, not including pectoralis muscle T_{4b} Edema (including peau d'orange) or ulceration of the skin of the breast, or satellite skin nodules confined to the same breast T_{4c} Both (T_{4a} and T_{4b}) T_{4d} Inflammatory carcinoma (see section on Inflammatory Carcinoma)

Regional Lymph Nodes (N)

NX	Regional lymph nodes cannot be assessed (e.g., previously removed)
N_0	No regional lymph node metastasis
N_1	Metastasis in movable ipsilateral axillary lymph node(s)
N_2	Metastasis in ipsilateral axillary lymph node(s) fixed or matted, or in clinically apparent[a] ipsilateral internal mammary nodes in the absence of clinically evident axillary lymph node metastasis N_{2a} Metastasis in ipsilateral axillary lymph nodes fixed to one another (matted) or to other structures N_{2b} Metastasis only in clinically apparent[a] ipsilateral internal mammary nodes and in the absence of clinically evident axillary lymph node metastasis
N_3	Metastasis in ipsilateral infraclavicular lymph node(s), or in clinically apparent[a] ipsilateral internal mammary lymph node(s) and in the presence of clinically evident axillary lymph node metastasis; or metastasis in ipsilateral supraclavicular lymph node(s) with or without axillary or internal mammary lymph node involvement N_{3a} Metastasis in ipsilateral infraclavicular lymph node(s) and axillary lymph node(s) N_{3b} Metastasis in ipsilateral internal mammary lymph node(s) and axillary lymph node(s) N_{3c} Metastasis in ipsilateral supraclavicular lymph node(s)

Pathologic Classification (pN)

pNX	Regional lymph nodes cannot be assessed (e.g., previously removed, or not removed for pathologic study)
pN_0	No regional lymph node metastasis histologically, no additional examination for isolated tumor cells $pN_{0(I-)}$ No regional lymph node metastasis histologically, negative IHC $pN_{0(I+)}$ No regional lymph node metastasis histologically, positive IHC, no IHC cluster greater than 0.2 mm $pN_{0(mol-)}$ No regional lymph node metastasis histologically, negative molecular findings (RT-PCR) $pN_{0(mol+)}$ No regional lymph node metastasis histologically, positive molecular findings (RT-PCR) pN^{1mi} Micrometastasis (>0.2 mm, none >2 mm)
pN_1	Metastasis in one to three axillary lymph nodes and/or in internal mammary nodes with microscopic disease detected by sentinel lymph node dissection but not clinically apparent pN_{1a} Metastasis in one to three axillary lymph nodes pN_{1b} Metastasis in internal mammary nodes with microscopic disease detected by sentinel lymph node dissection but not clinically apparent pN_{1c} Metastasis in one to three axillary lymph nodes and in internal mammary lymph nodes with microscopic disease detected by sentinel lymph node dissection but not clinically apparent

(Continued)

Table 16.4 TNM (Tumor–Nodes–Metastases) System for Staging of Breast Cancer (*Continued*)

Pathologic Classification (pN) *(Continued)*

pN$_2$	Metastasis in four to nine axillary lymph nodes, or in clinically apparent internal mammary lymph nodes in the absence of axillary lymph node metastasis
	pN$_{2a}$ Metastasis in four to nine axillary lymph nodes (at least one tumor deposit >2 mm)
	pN$_{2b}$ Metastasis in clinically apparent internal mammary lymph nodes in the absence of axillary lymph node metastasis
pN$_3$	Metastasis in 10 or more axillary lymph nodes, or in infraclavicular lymph nodes, or in clinically apparent ipsilateral internal mammary lymph nodes in the presence of one or more positive axillary lymph nodes; or in more than three axillary lymph nodes with clinically negative microscopic metastasis in internal mammary lymph nodes; or in ipsilateral supraclavicular lymph nodes
	pN$_{3a}$ Metastasis in 10 or more axillary lymph nodes (at least one tumor deposit >2 mm), or metastasis to the infraclavicular lymph nodes
	pN$_{3b}$ Metastasis in clinically apparent ipsilateral internal mammary lymph nodes in the presence of one or more positive axillary lymph nodes; or in more than three axillary lymph nodes and in internal mammary lymph nodes with microscopic disease detected by sentinel lymph node dissection but not clinically apparent
	pN$_{3c}$ Metastasis in ipsilateral supraclavicular lymph nodes

Distant Metastasis (M)

MX	Distant metastasis cannot be assessed
M$_0$	No distant metastasis
M$_1$	Distant metastasis

Note: Paget's disease associated with a tumor is classified according to the size of the tumor.

[a]"Clinically apparent" is defined as detected by imaging studies (excluding lymphoscintigraphy) or by clinical examination.

IHC, immunohistochemistry; RT-PCR, reverse transcription—polymerase chain reaction.

Used with the permission of the American Joint Committee on Cancer (AJCC), Chicago, IL. *AJCC Cancer Staging Manual.* 7th ed. New York, NY: Springer-Verlag; 2010 (117).

Table 16.5 TNM (Tumor–Nodes–Metastases) Stage Grouping of Breast Cancer

Stage 0	T$_{is}$	N$_0$	M$_0$
Stage I	T$_1$[a]	N$_0$	M$_0$
Stage IIA	T$_0$	N$_1$	M$_0$
	T$_1$[a]	N$_1$	M$_0$
	T$_2$	N$_0$	M$_0$
Stage IIB	T$_2$	N$_1$	M$_0$
	T$_3$	N$_0$	M$_0$
Stage IIIA	T$_0$	N$_2$	M$_0$
	T$_1$[a]	N$_2$	M$_0$
	T$_2$	N$_2$	M$_0$
	T$_3$	N$_1$	M$_0$
	T$_3$	N$_2$	M$_0$
Stage IIIB	T$_4$	N$_0$	M$_0$
	T$_4$	N$_1$	M$_0$
	T$_4$	N$_2$	M$_0$
Stage IIIC	Any T	N$_3$	M$_0$
Stage IV	Any T	Any N	M$_1$

[a]T$_1$ includes T$_{1mic}$.

Used with the permission of the American Joint Committee on Cancer (AJCC), Chicago, IL. *AJCC Cancer Staging Manual.* 7th ed. New York, NY: Springer-Verlag; 2010 (117).

Treatment of Breast Cancer

Surgery

The traditional treatment of breast cancer has been primarily surgical, but has evolved to a multidisciplinary approach, requiring the collaborative effort of surgeons, pathologists, radiologists, oncologists, and others.

The modern era of breast surgery began with Halsted and the development of the radical mastectomy, based on his understanding of breast cancer as a locally infiltrative process that spread primarily via the lymphatics (123). The radical mastectomy involved resection of the entire breast with overlying skin, the underlying pectoral muscles, and the axillary lymph nodes in continuity (Fig. 16.7) (124). This operation was designed initially to treat patients with palpable axillary lymph nodes and locally advanced disease. **Although effective in local control of the tumor, this surgery failed to cure many patients,** most likely because of their advanced stage at presentation.

During the 20th century, more extensive variations of the radical mastectomy were adopted in order to remove more regional tissue. Some of the variations included supraclavicular dissection (125) and supraclavicular, internal mammary, and mediastinal lymph node dissections, with resulting higher morbidity and mortality rates (126). The extended radical mastectomy, first described by Urban (127) added an *en bloc* internal mammary node dissection to the standard operation. **This surgery did not improve survival rates but increased morbidity.**

The modified radical mastectomy (MRM) was progressively adopted when it was recognized that the mortality was caused by the systemic dissemination of neoplastic cells preoperatively. It completely removed the breast and axillary nodes, the pectoralis muscles were preserved, and there was no need for skin grafting (Fig. 16.7B). The modified operation was functionally and cosmetically superior.

Total or simple mastectomy is the removal of the entire breast, nipple, and areolar complex, with preservation of the pectoralis muscles and axillary lymph nodes. Usually included in the specimen are the lymph nodes in the upper, outer portion of the breast and lower axilla.

To refute the Halstedian concept, a randomized trial comparing the Halsted mastectomy to less extensive surgery, with or without radiation therapy, was conducted. The National Surgical Adjuvant Breast and Bowel Project (NSABP) B-04 study randomly assigned patients with clinically negative axillary nodes to radical mastectomy, total mastectomy with postoperative irradiation, or total mastectomy with delayed dissection if positive nodes developed. Patients with clinically positive axillary nodes were randomly assigned to radical mastectomy or total mastectomy with postoperative irradiation. After 25 years of follow-up, there was no significant difference among the three groups of women with negative nodes or between the two groups of women with positive nodes with respect to disease-free survival, distant disease-free survival, or overall survival (128). Therefore, **the radical mastectomy was shown to have no advantage over total mastectomy in terms of local control or overall survival; in addition, the removal of lymph nodes was shown to have no effect on survival.**

Breast-Conserving Surgery

Breast-conserving surgery developed from the same desire as did the MRM: defining the extent of surgery required to treat invasive breast cancer without compromising outcome. One of its major goals is to preserve the cosmetic appearance of the breast. **Radiation therapy without surgical treatment has been shown to result in high local failure rates** (129).

Two pivotal prospective randomized trials have compared standard surgery to a combination of less extensive operations, with or without radiation. In the **Milan study,** patients were randomly assigned to either (i) the standard Halsted radical mastectomy or (ii) quadrantectomy, axillary lymph node dissection (ALND), and postoperative radiation (130,131). **Patients with tumors less than or equal to 2 cm with clinically negative axillary nodes ($T_1N_0M_0$) were eligible for this trial.** The two groups, totaling 701 women, were comparable with respect to age, tumor size, menopausal status, and nodal involvement (132). **After 20 years of follow-up, there was no statistically significant difference between the two groups regarding contralateral breast cancer, second primary cancer in the ipsilateral breast, distant metastases, or overall survival** (Table 16.6) (131); **however chest wall recurrences were significantly more common in the breast conserving group (8.8% vs. 2.3%).**

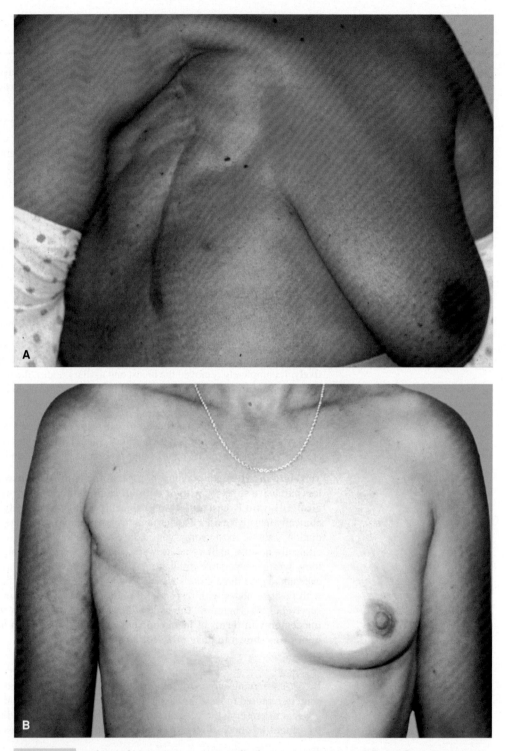

Figure 16.7 Defects after mastectomy (A) radical mastectomy (B) modified radical mastectomy.

The NSABP conducted a similar trial, B-06, for patients with tumors less than or equal to 4 cm, either without palpable nodes, or with palpable nonfixed axillary lymph nodes (i.e., stage I or II: T_1 or T_2, and N_0 or N_1) (132). Patients were assigned randomly to (i) the MRM; (ii) lumpectomy (segmental mastectomy) and ALND; or (iii) lumpectomy, ALND, and postoperative radiation therapy (Fig. 16.8). Tumor-free specimen margins were required to maintain eligibility. A total of 1,851 women were randomized among the three treatment arms and the groups were comparable. **After 20 years of follow-up, the NSABP B-06 trial provided clear evidence that the combined lumpectomy, ALND, and postoperative radiation therapy was as effective as**

Table 16.6 Halsted Radical Mastectomy versus Breast-Conserving Surgery: Results of 20-Year Follow-up

	Halsted (%)	Quadrantectomy + RT (%)
No. of patients	349	352
Contralateral-breast carcinoma	9.7	8.2
Distant metastases	23.8	23.3
Other primary cancers	8.6	8.8
Overall survival	43.6	44.3

RT, radiation therapy.

From **Veronesi U, Cascinelli N, Mariani L, et al.** Twenty-year follow-up of a randomized study comparing breast-conserving surgery with radical mastectomy for early breast cancer. *N Engl J Med.* 2002;347: 1227–1232.

the MRM **for the management of patients with early stage breast cancer** (133). Although there was no significant difference in overall survival among the three treatment arms, there were significant differences in local control. The in-breast recurrence rate for patients randomized to lumpectomy and radiation therapy was 14.3% versus 39.2% for patients randomized to lumpectomy alone. This trial established the safety of breast-conserving surgery for early-stage breast cancer, and showed the importance of postoperative radiation for reducing the risk of in-breast recurrences. **A National Institute of Health (NIH) Consensus Conference in 1991 endorsed breast-conserving surgery as the preferred treatment for early-stage breast cancer** (134).

Axillary Lymph Node Staging

Axillary nodal involvement remains the most significant prognostic factor for recurrence and survival for patients with early-stage breast cancer. The management of the axilla continues to evolve. In patients with palpable axillary lymph node, level I and II ALND should be performed. **As part of breast-conserving surgery, the axillary dissection preferably should be performed through a separate incision.** The three levels of nodes in the axilla are based on their relationship to the pectoralis minor muscle. Level I and II axillary dissection involves removal of all the fatty and lymph node-bearing tissue lateral and posterior to the medial border of the pectoralis minor

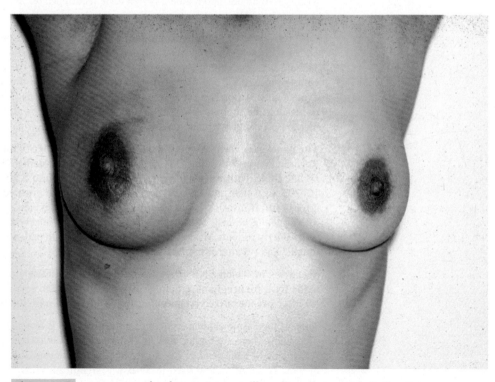

Figure 16.8 Appearance after lumpectomy, axillary dissection, and radiation therapy.

muscle. It is very rare for so-called "skip metastases" to be present in the higher levels of the axilla without involvement of the lower levels (135). If palpable nodes are encountered medial to the pectoralis minor (level III), a complete dissection should be performed, usually necessitating transection of the pectoralis minor muscle. Alternatively, axillary ultrasound and ultrasonically directed needle biopsy can be used to confirm axillary lymph node involvement if neoadjuvant chemotherapy is being considered (136).

Although axillary nodal dissection is accurate for staging, there are known morbidities associated with the procedure such as paresthesias, wound complications, and lymphedema. The latter occurs in approximately 10–20% of patients. **Since the advent of mammography, tumor size, and positive nodal involvement at diagnosis have been diminishing. Only 30% of breast cancer patients have involved axillary nodes detected by standard pathologic techniques** (44). This has led some authorities to question the value of routine ALND in patients with early stage breast cancer.

The technique of sentinel node biopsy (SNB), a minimally invasive procedure, is based on the observation that specific areas drain via lymphatic channels to one or two primary nodes before involving other lymph nodes within a nodal basin. By injecting radioisotope or blue dye into the region of the tumor or under the areola and performing a limited axillary dissection, these primary or sentinel nodes can be identified, either by visual inspection or by the use of a handheld gamma counter. When the H&E-stained sentinel nodes are negative, most institutions perform immunohistochemistry (IHC). **The hypothesis is that if the sentinel node is free of tumor histopathologically, the rest of the axillary nodes will also be free, thereby avoiding the need for a complete ALND** (137–139).

In experienced hands, the false-negative rate is low, and can be nearly 0% with proper patient selection and adherence to technical detail (138). **The safety and efficacy of SNB has been confirmed in several RCTs.** Veronesi's group in Milan randomized 516 patients with pathologically negative sentinel nodes to SNB alone or SNB followed by completion ALND and found no significant difference in 10-year disease-free survival (89.9% SNB alone vs. 88.8% SNB + ALND) (140). The NSABP-B-32 trial randomized 5,611 women at 80 institutions across the United States and Canada with clinically negative axillae to one of two groups: SNB + routine completion of ALND or SNB alone (followed by ALND only if the sentinel node harbored metastases on H&E staining). At a mean follow-up of 95.6 months, there were equivalent rates of overall survival (96.4% SNB + ALND vs. 95% SNB alone) 8-year disease-free survival (82.4% SNB + ALND vs. 81.5% SNB alone), and regional lymph node recurrence (8 SNB +ALND vs. 14 SNB alone) in the two groups (141).

In 2005, the ASCO published guideline recommendations for SNB in early-stage breast cancer (142). These guidelines were based on 69 studies in which SNB was compared to ALND. There was sufficient evidence for the panel to **recommend the use of SNB in early-stage breast cancer patients with clinically negative nodes, provided the procedure was performed by an experienced team.** The panel recommended that suspicious palpable nodes found during dissection should be submitted as SLNs. A completion ALND was advised for any patient with SLN metastases, including micrometastasis (>0.2 to <2 mm).

The panel gave recommendations regarding the use of SNB in certain clinical circumstances. Regarding cases involving DCIS, the panel **recommended SNB for mastectomy patients with DCIS, DCIS with microinvasion, or DCIS larger than 5 cm.** Although DCIS is noninvasive, 10–20% of patients will be subsequently found to have invasive disease as a result of a sampling error (140). If invasion is discovered after a mastectomy, the opportunity to stage the axilla with SLND would be lost. Other special clinical circumstances in which SNB is recommended are (i) in elderly patients; (ii) in obese patients; (iii) in male patients; (iv) in patients with multicentric tumors; and (v) after prior excisional biopsy.

Scenarios in which SNB is *not* recommended include (i) patients with a clinically positive axilla (N_1); (ii) pregnant patients; (iii) prior axillary surgery; (iv) inflammatory breast cancer; (v) after preoperative systemic therapy; and (vi) in patients with tumors larger than 5 cm.

There is increasing evidence supporting the use of SNB in some of these circumstances, including pregnancy. There are limited reports of the safety of radioisotopes in pregnant patients (144–146). A study of 14 breast cancer patients found that the uterine dose of radiation from an average dose of 99m-Tc sulfur colloid used in SNB was significantly less than the average daily background dose of radiation (147). A study of the pharmacokinetics of methylene blue dye found that the estimated maximal dose to the fetus was only about 5% of the administered dose (148). Further research is needed to confirm the safety of SNB in pregnancy.

Regarding the technical aspects of the procedure, the panel supported the **Guidelines for Performance of Sentinel Lymphadenectomy for Breast Cancer** developed by the ASBS (**https://www. breastsurgeons.org/statements/slnd.php**). The ASBS maintains that a SLN identification rate of 85% and a false-negative rate of 5% or less are necessary in order to abandon axillary dissection. The American Society of Breast Surgeons (ASBS) recommends that surgeons perform a minimum of 20 SNB cases followed by completion ALND, or have proper mentoring, before relying on the procedure to avoid ALND. The ASCO panel has pointed out that the lowest false-negative rates were obtained with the combined methods of isotope and blue dye, but do not believe that ASCO should present separate guidelines for the technical performance of the procedure.

Historically, level I and II ALND has been performed for patients found to have sentinel lymph node metastases. The benefit of ALND has been questioned because of the morbidity of ALND, and the NSABP B-04 trial, which demonstrated no benefit in overall or disease-free survival up to 25 years in node-positive women with breast cancer randomized to one of three treatment arms: Radical mastectomy, simple mastectomy with axillary and chest wall irradiation, and simple mastectomy alone (149).

The multicenter American College of Surgeons Oncology Group (ACOSOG) Z0011 trial randomized patients with T1 or T2, clinically node negative breast cancer with axillary metastases identified in 1 to 2 sentinel lymph nodes to completion ALND followed by tangential whole breast radiation therapy (445 patients) or whole breast radiation therapy without further axillary surgery (446 patients). All patients underwent lumpectomy with negative margins and most received adjuvant systemic therapy, 97% in SNB (no further surgery) group versus 96% in ALND group. Of those in the ALND group, 27% had additional nonsentinel lymph node metastases. **At a median follow-up of more than 6 years, there was no statistically significant difference in 5-year overall survival (91.8% ALND vs. 92.5% SNB) or axillary recurrence between the two groups** (150). Therefore, in select patients who are undergoing lumpectomy and whole breast irradiation for early-stage breast cancer and who are found to have 1 to 2 positive sentinel lymph nodes, completion of ALND may be omitted.

Adjuvant Radiation Therapy	**Adjuvant radiation after breast-conserving procedures is essential for the achievement of recurrence rates equivalent to those obtained with mastectomy.** Radiation therapy, when combined with radical surgery, improves local control, but overall survival rates are not affected (132,133,151). In NSABP B-06, the in-breast recurrence rate for patients randomized to lumpectomy and radiation therapy was 14.3% versus 39.2% for patients randomized to lumpectomy alone.

In 2005, the Early Breast Cancer Trialists' Collaborative Group (EBCTCG) presented the findings from 78 randomized clinical trials evaluating the extent of surgery and the use of radiation (152). This large meta-analysis analyzed data on 42,000 women, and **was able to show that improved local control with radiotherapy at 5 years resulted in a significant improvement in breast cancer survival at 15 years.** For every four local recurrences that could be avoided over 15 years, one fewer breast cancer death would occur. Local treatments had the greatest effects in the patients who were at greatest risk for local recurrence.

Postoperative radiation therapy is recommended as part of breast cancer treatment to reduce local recurrence rates; there are also indications for its use in postmastectomy patients who are at higher risk for locoregional failure (151–156). ASCO issued guidelines in 2001 recommending postmastectomy radiation for women with four or more positive lymph nodes, tumors greater than 5 cm in diameter, or operable stage III disease. ASCO guidelines state that there is insufficient evidence at this time for postmastectomy radiation for patients with high-risk, node-negative disease, including premenopausal women with tumors greater than 2 cm in diameter, 1 to 3 positive lymph nodes, evidence of vascular invasion, invasion of the skin or pectoral fascia, or close/positive margins (156).

Clinical trials evaluating breast-conserving surgery and intraoperative radiation therapy (IORT) for localized breast cancer have been completed. The rationale for IORT is based on the desire to minimize length of treatment and the finding that 85% of recurrent breast cancer is confined to the same quadrant as the primary tumor (157). Because it requires wide mobilization of the breast tissue after lumpectomy and immediate delivery of radiation therapy to the operative bed, IORT can prolong operative times. Three main methods of IORT delivery are available: **Electron**

beam intraoperative radiotherapy via linear accelerators (ELIOT), brachytherapy, and photon radiosurgical systems.

The potential advantages of IORT are that it ensures 100% compliance with radiation therapy, facilitates breast conservation in areas where access to radiation centers is limited, sterilizes the lumpectomy cavity immediately and minimizes radiation dose to the skin, lungs, and heart. The primary concern regarding IORT is that the final pathologic status of the surgical margins and axillary lymph nodes is unknown at the time of radiation delivery, since IORT does not treat the lymphatics or regional lymph nodes, and re-excision or mastectomy may be necessary for positive margins (158).

In the **European Institute of Oncology trial,** 1,822 patients with tumors <2.5 cm underwent quadrantectomy and IORT with electrons. At a mean follow-up of 36 months, the rate of local recurrence was 2.3% and the incidence of new ipsilateral breast cancer was 1.3%. **Five- and 10-year survival rates were comparable to those for conventional whole breast radiation therapy** (159). The prospective, multicenter targeted intraoperative radiotherapy versus whole breast radiotherapy for breast cancer **(TARGIT-A) trial** randomized patients aged 45 and older undergoing lumpectomy to either IORT or whole breast, external beam radiation. Of the 996 patients who received IORT, 14% subsequently received whole breast radiation at the discretion of the treating physicians, and 1,025 received whole breast radiation alone. **At 4 years of follow-up, there was no statistical difference in local recurrence in the two treatment arms** (160). **Whether or not the therapeutic effect of IORT will remain equivalent to traditional whole breast radiation therapy with longer follow-up remains to be determined.**

Accelerated Partial Breast Irradiation (APBI) has evolved as a result of the observation that most recurrences after breast-conserving surgery occur in close proximity to the surgical site and the demand for shorter and more limited treatment (161). Results from studies using interstitial catheter brachytherapy to deliver APBI have shown good local tumor control rates, but the technique can be cumbersome and difficult to learn. **The MammoSite balloon catheter was developed as a single catheter delivery device** that allows a shorter period of radiation treatment, usually 5 days instead of 5 to 6 weeks, as an alternative to external beam radiation or seed brachytherapy. **The balloon catheter is placed in the lumpectomy cavity** and filled with saline/contrast. Before treatment is initiated, the position of the balloon is checked to ensure adequate conformity to the lumpectomy cavity. The radiation source is advanced into the catheter and radiation therapy is delivered twice a day for 5 days. The radiation source is removed between treatments. After completion of therapy, the balloon catheter is removed. **With the success of the MammoSite catheter, additional brachytherapy catheters have become available for use.**

The ASBS recommendations for eligibility criteria are age greater than 45, invasive ductal carcinoma or DCIS, tumor size of 3 cm or less, negative microscopic surgical margins, and negative nodal status **(http://www.breastsurgeons.org/statements/PDF_Statements/APBI.pdf)**. Additional factors to be considered for MammoSite use are adequate skin spacing (usually 7 mm) and catheter conformity to surgical cavity. **Early results have been promising with 5-year local recurrence rates comparable to those achieved with conventional whole-breast radiation,** with decreased toxicity and good to excellent cosmetic results in the majority of patients (162,163). Randomized studies in progress will determine the role of APBI.

Adjuvant Systemic Therapy

Patients may have clinically undetectable systemic micrometastases at the time of primary surgery that are responsible for later recurrences, as evidenced by the lower survival rates for women with metastatic nodal disease. **Approximately 20% of patients with node negative, early breast cancer may recur.**

Early randomized clinical trials conducted by the NSABP and by Bonadonna et al. in Milan have demonstrated that **polychemotherapy increased both recurrence-free survival and overall survival in women with node positive breast cancer** (164,165). These and subsequent trials established the efficacy of *cyclophosphamide, methotrexate,* and *5-fluorouracil* (CMF) as the standard adjuvant regimen in the 1970s. In the 1980s, the *anthracyclines, adriamycin* and *epirubicin* began to be used. *Tamoxifen* was used for ovarian suppression in ER-positive breast cancer. **The Early Breast Cancer Trialists' Collaborative Group (EBCTCG) conducted a meta-analysis of 123 trials of adjuvant therapy that involved 100,000 women and found a 20–25% relative reduction and 6% absolute reduction in breast cancer mortality at 10 years for both CMF and *anthracycline*-based chemotherapy regimens (FAC or FEC)** (166). The benefits were independent of *tamoxifen* use, nodal status, ER status, and other tumor characteristics and were greater in younger women, with reductions in annual breast cancer death rates of 38% for women diagnosed under the age of 50, and 20% for women aged 50 to 69 years.

The *anthracycline* regimens were more effective than the CMF regimens, with moderate, but highly significant reductions in the annual recurrence rate of 11% ($p = 0.001$), and annual breast cancer death rate of 16% ($p < 0.00001$) (166). **Four cycles of *doxorubicin* and *cyclophosphamide (AC)* have been shown to offer an equivalent disease-free survival and overall survival to 6 months of traditional CMF in two NSABP trials (B-15 and B-23)** (167,168). None of the trials involved the newer agents such as *taxanes, raloxifene, trastuzumab,* or *aromatase* inhibitors (AIs).

Newer chemotherapeutic agents have emerged in the 1990s, most notably, members of the *taxane* family, including *paclitaxel (Taxol) and docetaxel (Taxotere)*. The *taxanes* have been shown to have good activity in patients with metastatic breast cancer and are not cross-resistant to *anthracyclines.* For these reasons, the NSABP B-28 trial and the Cancer and Leukemia Group B (CALGB) 9344 trial were conducted to evaluate the efficacy of the *taxanes.* Results from NSABP B-28 demonstrated that **the addition of *paclitaxel* after *AC* resulted in a 17% reduction in the risk of recurrence, but had no statistically significant impact on overall survival** (169). By contrast, both disease-free and overall survival rates were improved in node-positive patients who were randomized to receive *AC* in combination with sequential *paclitaxel* compared with *AC* alone in a large, cooperative, randomized study (170). **Results of the US Oncology (USO) 9735 trial suggest that the combination of *docetaxel* and *cyclophosphamide (TC)* is associated with a superior disease-free survival than *AC* for patients with stages I to III breast cancer** (171). **The CALGB 9741 trial demonstrated that dose-dense regimens,** in which chemotherapeutic agents were given every 2 weeks with granulocyte colony-stimulating factor (GCSF) **improved disease-free survival (HR = 0.74, $p = 0.0072$) and overall survival (RR = 0.69, $p = 0.014$)** compared with conventional three-weekly regimens (172).

A recent meta-analysis of 19 randomized clinical trials found that *taxane*-based **regimens yielded a 17% relative reduction in disease recurrence and mortality compared with *anthracycline*-based regimens in patients with early stage and operable breast cancers** (173). Investigation is ongoing to optimize *taxane*-based regimens, and to better identify subgroups of patients that may particularly benefit.

Amplification of the *HER2/neu* gene, a member of the tyrosine-kinase pathway family, or overexpression of the HER2/*neu* protein occurs in approximately 15–25% of breast cancers and is associated with aggressive tumor behavior (173). *Trastuzumab* (Herceptin) is a humanized monoclonal antibody against the HER2/*neu* growth factor receptor that has been shown to have clinical activity in women with metastatic HER2/*neu* positive breast cancer. It is administered intravenously every 3 weeks (174,175). In the **international, multicenter Herceptin Adjuvant (HERA) trial,** 5,102 patients who had completed locoregional therapy and at least four cycles of chemotherapy for early-stage invasive breast cancer with HER2/*neu* overexpression were randomized to one of three groups: Observation only ($n = 1,698$), 1 year of *trastuzumab* ($n = 1,703$), or 2 years of *trastuzumab* ($n = 1,553$). **Interim analysis at 1 year demonstrated benefit in disease-free survival for patients receiving *trastuzumab*,** and patients in the observation group were invited to cross over to treatment with *trastuzumab* for 1 or 2 years. Intention-to-treat analysis of the HERA trial has demonstrated a 4-year disease free survival of 78.6% in the 1 year of *trastuzumab* group versus 72.2% in the observation group, 52% of whom crossed over to receive *trastuzumab* after 1 year. There was no significant difference in overall survival between the 1-year *trastuzumab* and observation groups, 89.3% and 87.7%, respectively (176). The HERA study found that **2 years of *trastuzumab* was associated with more severe adverse events (including decreased left ventricular ejection fraction) and is not more effective than 1 year of therapy** (177).

Newer agents that inhibit activation of the HER2/*neu* pathway have been developed. *Pertuzumab,* a monoclonal antibody that inhibits dimerization, and therefore, activation of the HER2/*neu* receptor signaling pathway, has been used successfully in conjunction with *trastuzumab* and *docetaxel* to improve progression-free survival by 6.1 months in patients with metastatic HER2-positive metastatic breast cancer in the randomized, double-blind, placebo-controlled CLEOPATRA study (178). *Pertuzamab* is approved for use in metastatic or *trastuzumab*-resistant HER2/*neu* positive breast cancer but may have efficacy in the adjuvant setting as well.

Lapatinib is an oral drug that inhibits the intracellular portion of the HER2/*neu* receptor and is Food and Drug Administration (FDA) approved for the treatment of *trastuzumab*-resistant metastatic

HER2/*neu* positive breast cancer when used in conjunction with *capecitabine*. It is being investigated as a component of neoadjuvant chemotherapy for HER2 positive operable breast cancer in the phase 3 NSABP B-41 trial (179).

Predicting Chemotherapy Benefit

A number of prognostic factors may be used to predict the risk of future recurrence or death from breast cancer, including age, tumor size, number of involved axillary nodes, and HER2-*neu* status. One validated computer-based model (**Adjuvant! Online; http://www.adjuvantonline. com**) is available to the clinician to estimate 10-year disease-free and overall survival. In this model, HER2/*neu* status is not included. The estimates for recurrence and death vary based on various treatment options from no additional therapy to the most aggressive form of polychemotherapy.

Although chemotherapy has been shown to benefit women with node negative, ER-positive disease in large clinical trials such as NSABP B-14 and B-20 (163,164,168,169), **there are many patients who would not derive much additional benefit and would in fact be over treated.**

Two gene-based approaches have become available to aid in the determination of those most likely to benefit from additional chemotherapy. One such tool is a 21-gene assay using reverse transcription polymerase chain reaction (RT-PCR) on RNA isolated from paraffin-embedded breast cancer tissue (**Oncotype DX**) (180). **This tool is able to quantify the 10-year risk of recurrence in** *tamoxifen***-treated patients with node-negative, ER-positive disease.** The 21-gene assay yields a numeric recurrence score (RS), which can be stratified according to risk for recurrence: low (RS $\leq$ 18), intermediate (RS 19 to 30), or high (RS $\geq$ 31). The prognostic value of Oncotype DX in ER-positive, node negative breast cancer was validated with specimens from the NSABP B-14 study, in which 51% of women were found to have a Low RS and a 10-year risk of recurrence of only 6.8%, with minimal benefit from the addition of chemotherapy to endocrine therapy. High RS (27%) was associated with a 30.5% risk of relapse at 10 years, and the greatest benefit from adjuvant chemotherapy. **In the high RS group, the addition of chemotherapy conferred a 28% improvement in recurrence-free survival.** The benefit of adjuvant chemotherapy in the intermediate RS group (22%) was less clear, and the intermediate RS group had a 14% recurrence rate at 10 years (181).

Subsequent analyses have suggested that **the value of the 21-gene assay is the potential to reclassify patients to the low-risk category who would otherwise have been considered high risk by NCCN guidelines or Adjuvant! Online.** The 21-gene assay has also been used in patients with one to three lymph node metastases (N1), and ER-positive cancers (182). While the 21-gene assay is the most commonly used of the new genomic predictors, prospective validation of the assay is ongoing, specifically to address the problematic intermediate RS group (TAILORx trial), and its validity in node-positive, ER-positive breast cancer, (RxPONDER) (183).

A microarray-based genomic assay has been developed that analyzes a 70-gene expression profile (Mammaprint) from frozen or paraffin-embedded breast tissue to predict those early-stage breast cancer patients who are more likely to develop distant metastases. Unlike the 21-gene assay, the 70-gene expression profile was developed using tumor samples from women with stage I and II breast cancer, regardless of nodal or ER status, who did *not* receive adjuvant systemic therapy. The 70-gene profile yields either a High-Risk or Low-Risk result. The Low-Risk category is associated with 95% and 85% recurrence-free survivals at 5 and 10 years, respectively, and a 95% overall 10-year survival without any adjuvant therapy. **High risk predicts 5- and 10-year recurrence free survival rates of 61% and 51%, respectively, and a 10-year overall survival rate of 55%** (184). A retrospective multivariate analysis has demonstrated that women with a High-Risk 70-gene expression profile should derive substantial benefit from adjuvant chemotherapy, unlike women with a Low-Risk profile (185). The prognostic and predictive validity of Mammaprint is under investigation in the prospective, randomized MINDACT trial, involving multiple sites in Europe (186).

Adjuvant Hormone Therapy

In the EBCTCG overview, the effects of hormonal therapy for early breast cancer on recurrence and 15-year survival were investigated (164). **For women with ER-positive disease, adjuvant** *tamoxifen* **given for 5 years reduced the annual breast cancer recurrence rate by 31%, independent of patient age, use of chemotherapy, or other tumor characteristics.** *Tamoxifen* therapy for 5 years was significantly more effective than 1 or 2 years of therapy. **Among women with ER-positive disease who were allocated to 5 years of** *tamoxifen,* **there was a 41% reduction**

in the annual recurrence rate. Most of the effect on recurrence was seen during the first 5 years; most of the effect on breast cancer mortality was seen after this time period.

For years, *tamoxifen* was the gold standard of hormonal therapy for patients with breast cancer. Aromatase inhibitors (AIs) were first studied in the metastatic setting for postmenopausal women with hormone-receptor positive disease (187). These agents act to markedly reduce the circulating estrogen levels in postmenopausal women. In 1996, a randomized double-blind multi-center trial was initiated to investigate the efficacy of the AI, *anastrozole* (*Arimidex*) in the adjuvant setting. **The trial known as *Arimidex*, *Tamoxifen*, Alone or in Combination (ATAC)** compared *tamoxifen* with *Arimidex* alone and in combination with *tamoxifen* as adjuvant endocrine therapy for postmenopausal patients with operable, invasive, early-stage (stage I and II) breast cancer. **Results of the ATAC trial demonstrated *Arimidex* to be better tolerated and more effective in improving disease-free survival and time to recurrence than *tamoxifen* after a median follow-up of 100 months** (188). There was a yearly increased fracture episode rate with *anastrozole* over *tamoxifen* (2.93% vs. 1.90%, respectively), but this effect did not continue after therapy was completed. **None of the known associated risks of *tamoxifen*, thromboembolism, endometrial cancer, or vaginal bleeding, were seen with *anastrozole*.**

Other AIs, such as *letrozole* (*Femara*) and *exemestane* (*Aromasin*), are alternatives for postmenopausal patients with hormone-sensitive breast cancer. Most recent ASCO practice guidelines recommend incorporating AIs into adjuvant regimens. Specifically, AIs are recommended as primary, sequential (*tamoxifen* for 2 to 3 years followed by AI), or extended (*tamoxifen* for 5 years followed by AI) therapy. AIs are recommended as initial therapy for postmenopausal women, and as initial treatment for women intolerant of *tamoxifen*. Conversely, women intolerant of AIs should receive *tamoxifen*. **Women with hormone receptor-negative tumors should not receive adjuvant hormonal therapy** (189).

Endocrine therapy in combination with chemotherapy synergistically lowers the risk of breast cancer recurrence. ***Anthracycline*-based chemotherapy reduces 15-year mortality rates for women with ER-positive disease.** A meta-analysis has demonstrated that **5 years of *tamoxifen* after *anthracycline*-based chemotherapy further reduced the 15-year mortality rates:** For patients under 50 with ER-positive disease, the final mortality reduction was almost 60%, and for patients aged 50 to 69, the reduction was almost 50% (164).

In practice, oncologists are using systemic adjuvant therapy for most patients with early-stage breast cancer larger than **1 cm and patients with node-positive disease.** Factors that determine the patient's risk of recurrence are tumor size, ER and PR status, HER2/*neu* status, nuclear grade, histologic type, and proliferative rate (190–192). Other biochemical and biologic factors such as ploidy, S-phase fraction, and cathepsin D levels appear to have some prognostic significance (Table 16.7), especially in node-negative patients (180). **The NCCN guidelines recommend considering the 21-gene assay (Oncotype DX) in cases of tumors 0.6 to 1 cm with unfavorable features, and in certain cases of tumors >1 cm.** The 21-gene assay is best used in patients who would receive questionable benefit from the addition of chemotherapy.

Table 16.7 Prognostic Factors in Node-negative Breast Cancers

Factor	Increased Risk of Recurrence
Size	Larger tumors
Histologic grade	High-grade tumors
DNA ploidy	Aneuploid tumors
Labeling index	High index (>3%)
S-phase fraction	High fraction (>5%)
Lymphatic/vascular invasion	Present
p53 tumor suppressor gene	High expression
HER2/*neu* oncogene expression	High expression
Epidermal growth factor	High levels
Angiogenesis	High microvessel density

In patients with large tumors or tumors with aggressive features, such as HER2/*neu* overexpression, the decision to offer adjuvant chemotherapy is obvious. Patients with nodal disease should be considered for adjuvant chemotherapy. Most patients with tumors larger than 0.5 cm (or larger than 1 cm in the cases of tubular or mucinous tumors) and positive ER status should be offered hormonal therapy. Table 16.7 summarizes these prognostic factors and their effect on recurrence (190–192).

To aid in the discussion with patients regarding the use of adjuvant therapy, risk reductions in breast cancer mortality should be translated into absolute benefits by calculating the number of deaths avoided per 100 women. For instance, if the 10-year risk of death from breast cancer is 10%, and if adjuvant chemotherapy reduces the mortality rate by 30%, the absolute increase in the number of patients alive will be 3/100 treated. On the other hand, if the 10-year risk of death is 50%, the same proportional reduction in mortality would mean 15 extra lives saved.

The current recommendations for adjuvant chemotherapy and hormonal therapy in breast cancer can be summarized as follows (Table 16.8):

1. **Premenopausal women who have ER-negative tumors should be treated with adjuvant chemotherapy.**

2. **Premenopausal women with ER-positive tumors should be treated with hormonal therapy (*tamoxifen*) in addition to chemotherapy.**

3. **Postmenopausal patients who have negative lymph nodes and positive hormone receptor levels should be treated with adjuvant endocrine therapy (preferably AIs) or both chemotherapy and endocrine therapy. Those with positive lymph nodes should receive both endocrine therapy and chemotherapy.**

4. **Postmenopausal women who have negative hormone receptor levels may be treated with adjuvant chemotherapy.**

5. **All women with invasive breast cancer and HER2/*neu* over-expression should undergo chemotherapy treatment with *trastuzumab*.**

6. **The 21-gene RT-PCR assay (Oncotype Dx) should be considered in patients with ER-positive/HER2/*neu* negative breast cancers >0.5 cm in size with sentinel node negative or micrometastatic disease; therapy should be guided by the Recurrence Score.**

The decision for adjuvant therapy ultimately rests with a well-educated and well-informed patient.

Table 16.8 Summary of Adjuvant Systemic Therapy for Women with Breast Cancer

Patient Age	Estrogen-Receptor Status	Level of Risk	Adjuvant Systemic Therapy
<50 yrs	Negative	Any	Chemotherapy
	Positive	Low	Hormonal therapy or chemotherapy or chemotherapy and hormonal therapy
	Positive	Moderate or high	Chemotherapy and hormonal therapy or investigational therapies
	Unknown	Any	Chemotherapy and hormonal therapy
≥50 yrs	Negative	Any	Chemotherapy
	Positive	Low	*Tamoxifen* or chemotherapy and hormonal therapy
	Positive	Moderate or high	Chemotherapy and hormonal therapy or investigational therapies
	Unknown	Any	Chemotherapy and hormonal therapy

Chemotherapy consists of *fluorouracil, doxorubicin,* and *cyclophosphamide* (FAC); *doxorubicin* and *cyclophosphamide* (AC); or *cyclophosphamide, methotrexate,* and *fluorouracil* (CMF). Hormonal therapy consists of *tamoxifen* or ovarian ablation (either surgical or chemical).

From **Hortobagyi GN**. Drug therapy: Treatment of breast cancer. *N Engl J Med.* 1998;339:974–984. Copyright ©1998 Massachusetts Medical Society. All rights reserved.

Metastatic Disease

Although the natural history of breast cancer can involve metastases to any organ, 85% of metastases involve the bone, lungs, or liver (193), with bone the most common site. Bone metastases can give rise to pathologic fractures and hypercalcemia.

Treatment for metastatic disease may include surgery (if locally recurrent disease), chemotherapy, hormonal therapy, or radiation treatment. Workup for metastatic disease should be tailored to specific complaints. Once one site is involved, metastases in other organs are highly likely. The initial workup for patients presenting with recurrent or stage IV disease should include liver function tests, chest imaging, bone scan, x-rays of symptomatic bones, biopsy documentation of first recurrence if feasible, and possible CT scan/PET imaging or MRI. Whether a patient has received prior chemotherapy or endocrine therapy will determine future treatment options. **For patients with a systemic recurrence of breast cancer, cure is no longer possible, and the goal of treatment is to prolong survival without jeopardizing quality of life.**

The treatment algorithm and various therapeutic options in metastatic breast disease are complex; to discuss them in detail is beyond the scope of this chapter, but a few notable therapies will be addressed.

Bisphosphonates

According to the NCCN guidelines for recurrent or metastatic breast cancer, patients should be initially stratified according to the presence or absence of bony metastases. The two subsets of patients should then be further stratified by HER2/*neu* and hormone receptor status. **Women with bony metastasis, especially with lytic lesions, should be offered a bisphosphonate with calcium and vitamin D.** The use of bisphosphonates in this setting has no impact on overall survival, but it provides supportive care (194).

Hormonal Therapies

Metastatic disease may respond to hormonal manipulation (195). The usual course of disease is progression after an initial response to hormonal therapy. Sequential therapy using other drugs should be instituted in a stepwise fashion, with responses typically diminishing with each new line of therapy. Even patients with ER-negative/PR-negative disease who have metastasis limited to bone or soft tissue may be considered for a trial of endocrine therapy, but the response rate is extremely low. Women with bulky, progressive visceral metastases should initially receive cytotoxic chemotherapy rather than hormonal therapy, even if ER-positive.

In premenopausal patients, who progress on *tamoxifen*, the preferred second-line therapy is ovarian ablation with oophorectomy, radiation, or hormonal therapy using a luteinizing hormone-releasing hormone (LHRH) agonist, such as *goserelin (Zoladex)*. The combination of *tamoxifen* and *goserelin* has been shown in a meta-analysis of four randomized trials to provide a significant survival and progression-free benefit, with a 30% reduction in the risk of an event with the combined therapy (196). Premenopausal women with ER-positive disease who have undergone ovarian ablation/suppression should be treated following postmenopausal guidelines.

Many postmenopausal women with hormone receptor-positive breast cancer benefit from sequential endocrine therapies. There are several AIs that are effective and well tolerated in metastatic disease, such as **anastrozole (Arimidex), letrozole (Femara), or exemestane (Aromasin)**. *Fulvestrant (Faslodex)* is a new ER antagonist that downregulates the ER, and has none of the estrogen agonist effects of *tamoxifen* (i.e., endometrial proliferation). **It is indicated for postmenopausal patients with metastatic breast cancer previously treated with an antiestrogen, who progress on therapy.** *Fulvestrant* appears to be at least as effective as *anastrozole* for the second-line treatment of patients with metastatic breast cancer (197). mTOR inhibitors, which inhibit the phosphatidylinositol 3-kinase/mammalian target of the *rapamycin* (PI3 K/mTOR) pathway that is thought to be a mechanism for resistance to endocrine therapy, have been used in endocrine-resistant, metastatic breast cancer. Specifically, **trials of the combination of the mTOR inhibitor *everolimus* (Afinitor) and *tamoxifen* or *everolimus* and *exemestane* have been shown to be more effective than *tamoxifen* or *exemestane* alone in preventing disease progression in patients with ER-positive metastatic breast cancer** (198).

Targeted Therapies

Patients who have **HER2/*neu*** positive metastatic disease may benefit from treatment with ***trastuzumab*** as a single agent or ***lapatinib (Tykerb)*** in combination with ***capecitabine (Xeloda)***, an oral form of *5-FU* (199). ***Lapatinib,*** also an oral agent, is a tyrosine kinase inhibitor of HER2/*neu* and epidermal growth factor receptor. In a phase III open-label trial, **the combination of *lapatinib* plus *capecitabine* proved to be superior to *capecitabine* alone in women with HER2-positive metastatic breast cancer that had progressed after therapies including *trastuzumab, anthracycline,* and a *taxane*** (199). Time to progression was increased by 50% in patients receiving combination therapy, with a median time to progression of 8.4 months, compared to 4.4 months with *capecitabine* alone.

Other Breast Diseases

Preinvasive (*In Situ*) Breast Carcinoma

Both lobular and ductal carcinomas may be confined by the basement membrane of the ducts or lobules. The goal of treatment for pure *in situ* disease is preventing invasive disease from occurring or diagnosing developing invasive disease that is localized to the breast. If microinvasion or invasion is found on pathologic review of the specimen, the patient should be treated appropriately for invasive disease.

Lobular Carcinoma *In Situ*

LCIS is typically an incidental finding at biopsy for a mass, or mammographic abnormality unrelated to the LCIS. **The true incidence of LCIS is unknown as a result of the lack of clinical and mammographic signs.** Most cases occur in premenopausal women. **It is viewed as a marker of increased risk for breast cancer, not limited to the involved side.** Most subsequent cancers that develop are invasive ductal carcinomas, with **ILCs** representing the minority. The risk of developing invasive cancer is approximately 1% annually, a risk that indefinitely persists (200).

Biopsy-proven LCIS is usually managed with surveillance by CBE bi-annually, yearly mammography, and possibly breast MRI. **Patients should be informed of their increased risk, and bilateral prophylactic mastectomy should be considered in women with a strong family history or a proven *BRCA 1/2* mutation** (200).

***Tamoxifen* is approved by the FDA as a chemopreventive agent in women with LCIS.** In the NSABP P-1 Study, women at an increased risk for breast cancer were given *tamoxifen* as a chemopreventive agent for 5 years. Women with LCIS who took *tamoxifen* had over a 50% reduction in the occurrence of invasive cancer compared to women in the placebo group. Women who are found to have LCIS on biopsy should be counseled regarding chemoprevention (201).

Ductal Carcinoma *In Situ*

Ductal carcinoma *in situ* typically occurs in postmenopausal women. Since the implementation of mammography as a screening tool (202), the incidence has increased from approximately 5,000 cases annually in the 1980s to approximately 60,000 cases in 2012 (45,202). Mammographically, DCIS typically appears as a cluster of branched or Y-shaped microcalcifications, although it sometimes presents as a palpable mass. DCIS is characterized by a clonal proliferation of malignant epithelial cells that do not invade beyond the basement membrane.

Unlike patients with LCIS, **30–60% of patients will develop invasive cancer in the same breast when treated with excisional biopsy alone** (203). Axillary metastases occur in fewer than 5% of patients. The occurrence of metastases indicates that an invasive component has been missed on biopsy. **Approximately 15–20% of patients with DCIS diagnosed on core-needle biopsy will be upstaged to infiltrating ductal carcinoma following excision** (143).

For years, the standard treatment for DCIS was total mastectomy, but most women in the United States are now treated with breast-conserving surgery following the shift toward this approach for invasive cancer (202). There have been no randomized trials comparing mastectomy with breast-conserving surgery for DCIS.

The NSABP B-17 randomized trial compared lumpectomy with or without postoperative radiation for DCIS. After 8 years of follow-up, the overall recurrence rate for either DCIS or invasive carcinoma in the ipsilateral breast was reduced by more than half, from 26.8% to 12.1% in the patients who received radiation (204). The benefit of radiation was greatest for recurrent invasive carcinoma, with an 8-year reduction from 13.4% to 3.9%. The benefit of radiation was seen with all patient subgroups, including those with small nonpalpable tumors detected by mammography.

The NSABP-24 randomized clinical trial evaluated adjuvant *tamoxifen* therapy in addition to lumpectomy and radiation. The trial involved 1,800 women with DCIS who were randomly assigned to lumpectomy and radiation therapy, followed by 5 years of *tamoxifen* or placebo. After 7 years of follow-up, the addition of *tamoxifen* significantly reduced the rate of all breast cancer events (ipsilateral and contralateral, *in situ* and invasive) by 39%, from 16% in the placebo group to 10% in the *tamoxifen* group ($p = 0.0003$) (205).

As a result of the variability in behavior of DCIS, concerns regarding overtreatment of DCIS exist. In response, a multigene expression assay (Oncotype DX) has been developed to predict the risk of recurrence without radiation therapy. Like the Oncotype DX for invasive, ER-positive breast cancer, the Oncotype DX assay for DCIS generates a numeric DCIS Score that can be stratified into low, intermediate, and high-risk categories. The DCIS Score has been found to be statistically significantly associated with the risk of developing an in-breast recurrence of either DCIS or invasive breast cancer, (HR = 2.31, 95% CI: 1.15 to 4.49, $p = 0.02$) and specifically in-breast, invasive breast cancer recurrence (HR = 3.68, 95% CI: 1.34 to 9.62, $p = 0.01$). Ten-year risks of in-breast recurrence for each of the risk categories were 10.6% for low risk, 26.7% for intermediate risk, and 25.9% for high risk (206).

Paget's Disease

Paget's disease of the breast, first described in 1874, is a rare manifestation of breast cancer with associated nipple changes similar to eczema, with itching and ulceration (207). Characteristic large cells with irregular nuclei, called Paget cells, invade the nipple and surrounding areola. There is debate as to the origin of Paget cells: either the cells originate from underlying carcinoma in the breast and then migrate into the major ducts of the nipple–areolar complex, or the cells originate in the epidermis. Initially there may be no visible changes, but patients often notice a discharge of serum and blood from the involved ducts. Paget's disease is often mistaken for a dermatitis, which can lead to a delay in diagnosis.

The underlying malignancy determines the overall prognosis for patients with Paget's disease. Paget's disease associated with DCIS alone has a very favorable prognosis, whereas those cases with infiltrating ductal carcinoma and involved lymph nodes have less favorable outcomes depending on the pathological stage of the invasive cancer.

Traditional treatment has been total mastectomy and lymph node dissection, although breast-conserving surgery is being performed at some institutions. Results of studies of breast-conserving surgery have generally been translated to the treatment of Paget's disease with underlying DCIS only. One small study treated patients with Paget's disease presenting without a palpable mass or radiographic abnormality with segmentectomy of the nipple–areolar complex followed by radiotherapy. The local control rate at 10 and 15 years was 87%, with a cause-specific survival of 97% (208). Another single institutional study showed breast-conserving surgery in Paget's disease cases to be equivalent to mastectomy regarding recurrence-specific, disease-specific, and overall survival with proper patient selection (209).

Inflammatory Carcinoma

Inflammatory breast carcinoma (IBC) is a rare but aggressive form of breast cancer, characterized by the rapid onset of inflammation of the breast with accompanying redness, warmth, and edema. The differential diagnosis includes mastitis and cellulitis of the breast. The distinguishing pathologic finding associated with IBC is metastatic invasion of the dermal and subdermal lymphatics. However, the diagnosis of IBC is primarily clinical and absence of lymphatic invasion does not exclude the diagnosis.

Mammographically, the breast shows skin thickening with an infiltrative process. Often there is no detectable palpable mass because the tumor, which is often very poorly differentiated, infiltrates through the breast with ill-defined margins. According to the AJCC staging guidelines (Tables 16.4 and 16.5), even if no mass is apparent, IBC by definition is classified as T4d lesion (the primary tumor size) (117). Then, depending on the degree of nodal involvement and presence of distant metastasis, patients with IBC are staged as IIIb, IIIc, or IV.

The initial step in management is a skin biopsy with excision of a small portion of underlying tissue, followed by complete staging with bilateral mammograms (± ultrasound), bone scan, CT imaging, and optional breast MRI. Primary surgical treatment in the face of inflammatory carcinoma is associated with high local failure rates, and survival is not improved. The treatment of IBC involves a combined-modality approach using chemotherapy, radiation therapy and, at times, surgery. If a good response is achieved with induction chemotherapy, one of the combined-modality options includes a modified radical mastectomy with postoperative radiation therapy to the chest wall, internal mammary nodes and supraclavicular nodes, followed by additional chemotherapy (210). If there is no response to induction chemotherapy, mastectomy is not recommended. Despite the improvements in IBC treatment, **the prognosis remains poor**.

Future Fertility

Approximately 25% of breast cancer cases occur in premenopausal women (211) and for these patients, counseling regarding future childbearing is important. Infertility can be a significant problem for those treated with adjuvant chemo and endocrine therapy, and the rates of amenorrhea may be as high as 40–70% (212). Even if amenorrhea resolves, **many cancer survivors have limited ovarian reserve** (213).

In the recommendations set forth by ASCO, **the only option not considered experimental is to undergo a cycle of ovarian stimulation, oocyte retrieval and embryo creation for cryopreservation before starting chemotherapy** (214). Another option, not as successful as in vitro fertilization, is **cryopreservation of oocytes, which may be used if the woman does not have a partner**. Epidemiologic data have not found a detrimental effect of subsequent pregnancy, even if conception takes place 6 months after therapy (215).

Prognosis

The most reliable predictor of survival for patients with breast cancer is the stage of disease at the time of diagnosis. Based on recent data collected on women diagnosed from 1995 to 1998 from the American College of Surgeons National Cancer Data Base, **the 5-year survival rate for stage I disease is almost 100%**. For patients with stage IIA disease, the 5-year survival rate is 92%, and for stage IIB, it is 82%. As the level of nodal involvement increases or tumor size increases, the survival rates decrease. Patients with stage IIIA breast cancer have a 5-year survival of 67%, stage IIIB 54%, and stage IV 20%.

Two significant prognostic indicators are the status of the axillary lymph nodes and the tumor size (190,191). **Histologic subtype is of prognostic significance;** tubular or mucinous carcinomas have a more favorable prognosis (108,109). Nuclear grade, lymphovascular invasion, younger age at diagnosis, and proliferation indices such as mitotic index, S-phase fraction, Ki-67 have all been shown to be of prognostic significance (190,191,216–219).

The presence of estrogen and progesterone receptors (ER-/PR-positive) may indicate less aggressive disease, although these factors are more predictive than prognostic. The main utility of these factors is in determining which patients should receive hormonal therapy. **Her2/*neu* oncogene amplification is associated with more aggressive disease,** and its presence in an invasive breast cancer indicates that *trastuzumab* therapy would be of benefit.

Chemoprevention

In an NSABP trial of adjuvant *tamoxifen* for breast cancer, *tamoxifen* was found to decrease the incidence of contralateral breast cancers as a secondary end point (220). As a consequence, the NSABP conducted a randomized, controlled trial, the Breast Cancer Prevention Trial (BCPT), which investigated the efficacy of *tamoxifen* as a chemopreventive agent in women who were at high risk for breast cancer based on their risk profile. **With over 13,000 women enrolled, the group of women who received *tamoxifen* for 5 years experienced a 50% reduction in both noninvasive and invasive breast cancers, compared with those taking a placebo** (221). Offsetting these benefits were a two- to threefold increase in the risk of endometrial cancer and increased risk of deep venous thrombosis, particularly in postmenopausal women.

Raloxifene, a second-generation selective ER modulator, has been used for the prevention of osteoporosis in postmenopausal women. It exhibits antiestrogenic properties in the breast and possibly in the endometrium, as well as protective, estrogenic properties in the bone. Secondary end points from studies of *raloxifene* have demonstrated its ability to reduce the risk of invasive breast cancer. This has led to the development of the multicenter, randomized, double-blind trial named **Study of *Tamoxifen* and *Raloxifene* (STAR)** NSABP P-2 to directly compare the effectiveness of *raloxifene* with that of *tamoxifen* in postmenopausal women who are at increased risk for developing breast cancer (222,223). **The study showed that *raloxifene* was as effective as *tamoxifen,* and had a lower risk of thromboembolic events and cataracts** (224).

References

1. **Semiglazov VF, Moiseyenko VM, Bavli JL, et al.** The role of breast self-examination in early breast cancer detection (results of the 5-years USSR/WHO randomized study in Leningrad). *Eur J Epidemiol.* 1992;8:498–502.

2. **Thomas DB, Gao DL, Ray RM, et al.** Randomized trial of breast self-examination in Shanghai: Final results. *J Natl Cancer Inst.* 2002; 94:1445–1457.

3. **Berry DA, Cronin KA, Plevritis SK, et al.** Effect of screening and adjuvant therapy on mortality from breast cancer. *N Engl J Med.* 2005;353:1784–1792.

4. **U.S. Preventative Services Task Force.** Screening for breast cancer: U.S. Preventative Services Task Force recommendation statement. *Ann Intern Med.* 2009;151:716–726.

5. **Hendrick RE, Smith RA, Rutledge JH, et al.** Benefit of screening mammography in women aged 40–49: A new meta-analysis of randomized controlled trials. *J Natl Cancer Inst Monogr.* 1997;22: 87–92.

6. **Larsson LG, Andersson I, Bjurstam N, et al.** Updated overview of the Swedish randomized trials on breast cancer screening with mammography: Age group 40–49 at randomization. *J Natl Cancer Inst Monogr.* 1997;22:57–61.

7. **UK trial of early detection of Breast Cancer Group.** 16-year mortality from breast cancer in the UK Trial of Early Detection of Breast Cancer. *Lancet.* 1999;353:1909–1914.

8. **Smith RA, Brooks D, Cokkinides V, et al.** Cancer screening in the United States, 2013: A review of current American Cancer Society guidelines, current issues in cancer screening, and new guidance on cervical cancer screening and lung cancer screening. *CA Cancer J Clin.* 2013;63:88–105.

9. **National Cancer Institute at the National Institute of Health.** Breast Cancer Screening. http://www.cancer.gov/cancertopics/pdq/ screening/breast/HealthProfessional. Updated 06/21/2013.

10. **American College of Radiology.** *Breast-imaging reporting and data system (BI-RADS) mammography.* 4th ed. Reston, Virginia: American College of Radiology. 2003.

11. **Christiansen CL, Wang F, Barton MB, et al.** Predicting the cumulative risk of false-positive mammograms. *J Natl Cancer Inst.* 2000; 92:1657–1666.

12. **Bleicher RJ, Morrow M.** MRI and breast cancer: Role in detection, diagnosis and staging. *Oncology.* 2007;21:1521–1530.

13. **Mann BD, Giuliano AE, Bassett LW, et al.** Delayed diagnosis of breast cancer as a result of normal mammograms. *Arch Surg.* 1983;118:23–24.

14. **Shtern F.** Digital mammography and related technologies: A perspective from the National Cancer Institute. *Radiology.* 1992;183:629–630.

15. **Pisano ED, Gatsonis C, Hendrick E, et al.** Diagnostic performance of digital versus film mammography for breast cancer screening. *N Engl J Med.* 2005;353:1773–1783.

16. **Houssami N, Skaane P.** Overview of the evidence on digital breast tomosynthesis in breast cancer detection. *Breast.* 2013;22:101–108.

17. **Price ER, Hargreaves J, Lipson JA, et al.** The California breast density information group: A collaborative response to the issues of breast density, breast cancer risk, and breast density notification legislation. *Radiology.* 2013;269(3):887–892. (Epub ahead of print) doi:10.1148/radiol.13131217.

18. **Berg WA, Blume JD, Cormack JB, et al.** Combined screening with ultrasound and mammography vs mammography alone in women at elevated risk of breast cancer. *JAMA.* 2008;299:2151–2163.

19. **Yang W, Dempsey PJ.** Diagnostic breast ultrasound: Current status and future directions. *Radiol Clin N Am.* 2007;46:845–861.

20. **Levy L, Suissa M, Chiche JF, et al.** BIRADS ultrasonography. *Eur J Radiol.* 2007;61:202–211.

21. **Orel SG, Schnall MD.** MR imaging of the breast for the detection, diagnosis, and staging of breast cancer. *Radiology.* 2001;200:13–30.

22. **Esserman L, Wolverton D, Hylton N.** MR imaging and breast cancer. *Endocr Relat Cancer.* 2002;9:141–153.

23. **Orel S.** Who should have breast magnetic resonance imaging evaluation? *J Clin Oncol.* 2008;26:703–711.

24. **Segara D, Krop IE, Garber JE, et al.** Does MRI predict pathologic tumor response in women with breast cancer undergoing preoperative chemotherapy? *J Surg Oncol.* 2007;96:474–480.

25. **Lehman CD, Gatsonis C, Kuhl CK, et al.** MRI Evaluation of the contralateral breast in women with recently diagnosed breast cancer. *N Engl J Med.* 2007;356:1295–1303.

26. **American Cancer Society (ACS).** Guidelines for breast screening with MRI as an adjunct to mammography. *CA Cancer J Clin.* 2007; 57:75–89.

27. **Santen RJ, Mansel R.** Benign breast disorders. *N Engl J Med.* 2005; 353:275–285.

28. **Page DL, Dupont WD.** Anatomic markers of human premalignancy and risk of breast cancer. *Cancer.* 1990;66:1326–1335.

29. **Morrow M, Jordan VC, eds.** *Managing Breast Cancer Risk.* Ontario, CA: BC Decker; 2000.

30. **Hartman LC, Sellers TA, Frost MH, et al.** Benign breast disease and the risk of breast cancer. *N Engl J Med.* 2005;353:329–337.

31. **Schnitt SJ, Connolly JL.** Pathology of benign breast disorders. In: **Harris JR, Lippman ME, Morrow M, et al., eds.** *Diseases of the Breast.* Philadelphia, PA: Lippincott Williams & Wilkins; 2004:77–99.

32. **Shen KW, Wu J, Lu JS, et al.** Fiberoptic ductoscopy for patients with nipple discharge. *Cancer.* 2000;89:1512–1519.

33. **Page DL, Salhany KE, Jensen RA, et al.** Subsequent breast carcinoma risk after biopsy with atypia in a breast papilloma. *Cancer.* 1996;78:258–266.

34. **Mulligan AM, O'Malley FP.** Papillary lesions of the breast. *Adv Anat Pathol.* 2007;14:108–119.

35. **Dupont WD, Page DL, Parl FF, et al.** Long-term risk of breast cancer in women with fibroadenoma. *N Engl J Med.* 1994;331: 10–15.

36. **Dixon JM, Dobie V, Lamb J, et al.** Assessment of the acceptability of conservative management of fibroadenoma of the breast. *Br J Surg.* 1996;83:264–265.

37. **Jacklin RK, Ridgway PF, Ziprin P, et al.** Optimizing preoperative diagnosis in phyllodes tumour of the breast. *J Clin Pathol.* 2006; 59:454–459.

38. **Krishnamurthy S, Ashfaq R, Shin HJ, et al.** Distinction of phyllodes tumor from fibroadenoma. *Cancer.* 2000;90:342–449.

39. **Pietruszka M, Barnes L.** Cystosarcoma phyllodes: A clinicopathologic analysis of 42 cases. *Cancer.* 1978;41:1974–1983.

40. **Zissis C, Apostolikas N, Konstantinidou A, et al.** The extent of surgery and prognosis of patients with phyllodes tumor of the breast. *Breast Cancer Res Treat.* 1998;48:205–210.

41. **Chen WH, Cheng SP, Tzen CY, et al.** Surgical treatment of phyllodes tumors of the breast: Retrospective review of 172 cases. *J Surg Oncol.* 2005;91:185–194.

42. **Taira N, Takabatake D, Aogi K, et al.** Phyllodes tumor of the breast: Stromal overgrowth and histological classification are useful prognosis-predictive factors for local recurrence in patients with a positive surgical margin. *Jpn J Clin Oncol.* 2007;37:730–736.

43. **Siegel R, Naishadham D, Jemal A.** Cancer statistics, 2013. *CA Cancer J Clin.* 2013;63:11–30. doi:10.3322/caac.21166.

44. **Hoeksema MJ, Law C.** Cancer mortality rates fall: A turning point for the nation. *J Natl Cancer Inst.* 1996;88:1706–1707.

45. **Jemal A, Ward E, Thun MJ.** Recent trends in breast cancer incidence rates by age and tumor characteristics among U.S. women. *Breast Cancer Res.* 2007;9:R28.

46. **Cady B, Stone MD, Schuler JG, et al.** The new era in breast cancer: Invasion, size, and nodal involvement dramatically decreasing as a result of mammographic screening. *Arch Surg.* 1996;131: 301–308.

47. **Pike MC, Spicer DV, Dahmoush L, et al.** Estrogens, progestogens, normal breast cell proliferation, and breast cancer risk. *Epidemiol Rev.* 1993;15:48–65.

48. **Howlader N, Noone AM, Krapcho M, et al., eds.** *SEER Cancer Statistics Review, 1975–2010,* National Cancer Institute. Bethesda, MD, http://seer.cancer.gov/csr/1975_2010/.

49. **Healey EA, Cook EF, Orav EJ, et al.** Contralateral breast cancer: Clinical characteristics and impact on prognosis. *J Clin Oncol.* 1993;11:1545–1552.

50. **Mariani L, Coradini D, Biganzoli E, et al.** Prognostic factors for metachronous contralateral breast cancer: A comparison of the linear Cox regression model and its artificial neural network extension. *Breast Cancer Res.* 1997;44:167–178.

51. Bernstein JL, Thompson WD, Risch N, et al. Risk factors predicting the incidence of second primary breast cancer among women diagnosed with first primary breast cancer. *Am J Epidemiol.* 1992;136:925–936.

52. Broët P, de la Rochefordière A, Scholl SM, et al. Contralateral breast cancer: Annual incidence and risk parameters. *J Clin Oncol.* 1995;13:1578–1583.

53. Tchou J, Morrow M. Overview of clinical risk assessment. In: *Managing Breast Cancer Risk.* Ontario, CA: BC Decker; 2000:3–25.

54. Claus EB, Schildkraut JM, Thompson WD, et al. The genetic attributable risk of breast and ovarian cancer. *Cancer.* 1996; 77:2318–2324.

55. Miki Y, Swensen J, Shattuck-Eidens D, et al. A strong candidate for the breast and ovarian susceptibility gene BRCA1. *Science.* 1994; 266:66–71.

56. Wooster R, Bignell G, Lancaster J, et al. Identification of the breast cancer susceptibility gene BRCA2. *Nature.* 1995;378:789–792.

57. Antoniou AC, Pharoah PD, McMullan G, et al. A comprehensive model for familial breast cancer incorporating BRCA1, BRCA2, and other genes. *Br J Cancer.* 2002;86:76–83.

58. Fodor FH, Weston A, Bleiweiss IJ, et al. Frequency and carrier risk associated with common BRCA1 and BRCA2 mutations in Ashkenazi Jewish breast cancer patients. *Am J Hum Genet.* 1998;63:45–51.

59. Narod SA. BRCA mutations in the management of breast cancer: The state of the art. *Nat Rev Clin Oncol.* 2010;7(12):702–707.

60. Antoniou A, Pharoah PD, Narod S, et al. Average risks of breast and ovarian cancer associated with BRCA1 and BRCA2 mutations detected in case series unselected for family history: A combined analysis of 22 studies. *Am J Hum Genet.* 2003;72:1117–1130.

61. Metcalfe K, Gershman S, Lynch HT, et al. Predictors of contralateral breast cancer in BRCA1 and BRCA2 mutation carriers. *Br J Cancer.* 2011;104(9):1384–1392.

62. Iqbal J, Ragone A, Lubinski J, et al. The incidence of pancreatic cancer in BRCA1 and BRCA2 mutation carriers. *Br J Cancer.* 2012; 107(12):2005–2009.

63. Struewing JP, Hartge P, Wacholder S, et al. The risk of cancer associated with specific mutations of BRCA1 and BRCA2 among Ashkenazi Jews. *N Engl J Med.* 1997;336:1401–1408.

64. Krainer M, Silva-Arrieta S, FitzGerald MG, et al. Differential contributions of BRCA1 and BRCA2 to early-onset breast cancer. *N Engl J Med.* 1997;336:1416–1421.

65. FitzGerald MG, Macdonald DJ, Krainer M, et al. Germ-line mutations in Jewish and non-Jewish women with early-onset breast cancer. *N Engl J Med.* 1996;334:143–149.

66. Antoniou AC, Beesley J, McGuffog L, et al. Common breast cancer susceptibility alleles and the risk of breast cancer for BRCA1 and BRCA2 mutation carriers: Implications for risk prediction. *Cancer Res.* 2010;70(23):9742–9754.

67. American Society of Clinical Oncology. Policy statement update: Genetic testing for cancer susceptibility. *J Clin Oncol.* 2003;12: 2397–2406.

68. Pike MC, Krailo MD, Henderson BD, et al. Hormonal risk factors, "breast tissue age" and the age incidence of breast cancer. *Nature.* 1983;303:767–770.

69. Trapido EJ. Age at first birth, parity, and breast cancer risks. *Cancer.* 1983;51:946–948.

70. Collaborative Group on Hormonal Factors in Breast Cancer. Menarche, menopause, and breast cancer risk: Individual participant meta-analysis, including 118 964 women with breast cancer from 117 epidemiological studies. *Lancet Oncol.* 2012;13(11):1141–1151.

71. Zhu H, Lei X, Feng J, et al. Oral contraceptive use and risk of breast cancer: A meta-analysis of prospective cohort studies. *Eur J Contracept Reprod Health Care.* 2012;17(6):402–414.

72. Collaborative Group on Hormonal Factors in Breast Cancer. Breast cancer and hormonal contraceptives: Collaborative reanalysis of individual data on 53,297 women with breast cancer and 100,239 women without breast cancer from 54 epidemiological studies. *Lancet.* 1996;347:1713–1727.

73. Writing Group for the Women's Health Initiative Investigators. Risks and benefits of estrogen plus progestin in healthy postmenopausal women: Principal results from the Women's Health Initiative randomized controlled trial. *JAMA.* 2002;288:321–333.

74. Women's Health Initiative Steering Committee. Effects of conjugated equine estrogen in postmenopausal women with hysterectomy:

The Women's Health Initiative Randomized controlled trail. *JAMA.* 2004;291:1701–1712.

75. Beral V; Million Women Study Collaborators. Breast cancer and hormone-replacement therapy in the Million Women Study. *Lancet.* 2003;362:419–427.

76. Hersh AL, Stefanick ML, Stafford RS. National use of postmenopausal hormone therapy: Annual trends and response to recent evidence. *JAMA.* 2004;291:47–53.

77. Krieger N, Chen JT, Waterman PD. Decline in US breast cancer rates after the Women's Health Initiative: Socioeconomic and racial/ethnic differentials. *Am J Public Health.* 2010;100(suppl 1):S132–S139.

78. Heiss G, Wallace R, Anderson GL, et al.; WHI Investigators. Health risks and benefits 3 years after stopping randomized treatment with estrogen and progestin. *JAMA.* 2008;299(9):1036–1045.

79. Alexander DD, Morimoto LM, Mink PJ, et al. Summary and meta-analysis of prospective studies of animal fat intake and breast cancer. *Nutr Res Rev.* 2010;23(1):169–179.

80. Prentice RL, Thomson CA, Caan B, et al. Low-fat dietary pattern and risk of invasive breast cancer. *JAMA.* 2006;295:629–642.

81. Cho E, Spiegelman D, Hunter DJ, et al. Premenopausal dietary carbohydrate. Glycemic index, glycemic loan, and fiber in relation to risk of breast cancer. *Cancer Epidemiol Biomarkers Prev.* 2003;12: 1153–1158.

82. Cade JE, Burley VJ, Greenwood DC; UK Women's Cohort Study Steering Group. Dietary fibre and risk of breast cancer in the UK Women's Cohort Study Steering Group. *Int J Epidemiol.* 2007; 36:431–438.

83. Dong JY, Qin LQ. Soy isoflavones consumption and risk of breast cancer incidence or recurrence: A meta-analysis of prospective studies. *Breast Cancer Res Treat.* 2011;125(2):315–323.

84. Chlebowski RT. Nutrition and physical activity influence on breast cancer incidence and outcome. *Breast.* 2013;22(suppl2):S30–S37.

85. Vucinick I, Stains JP. Obesity and cancer risk: Evidence, mechanisms, and recommendations. *Ann N Y Acad Sci.* 2012;1271(1): 37–43.

86. Reeves GK, Pirie K, Beral V, et al. Cancer incidence and mortality in relation to body mass index in the Million Women Study: Cohort study. *BMJ.* 2007;335:1134.

87. Lahmann PH, Hoffmann K, Allen N, et al. Body size and breast cancer risk: Findings from the European Prospective Investigation into Cancer and Nutrition (EPIC). *Int J Cancer.* 2004;111: 762–771.

88. Monninkhof EM, Elias SG, Vlems FA, et al. Physical activity and breast cancer: A systematic review. *Epidemiology.* 2007;18: 137–157.

89. Maruti SS, Willett WC, Feskanich D, et al. A prospective study of age-specific physical activity and premenopausal breast cancer. *J Natl Cancer Inst.* 2008;100:728–737.

90. Friedenreich CM, Cust AE. Physical activity and breast cancer risk: Impact of timing, type and dose of activity and population subgroup effects. *Br J Sports Med.* 2008;42:636–647.

91. Van Gemert WA, Lestra JI, Schuit AJ, et al. Design of the SHAPE-2 study: The effect of physical activity, in addition to weight loss, on biomarkers of postmenopausal breast cancer risk. *BMC Cancer.* 2013;13:395.

92. McTiernan A, Irwin M, VonGruenigen V. Weight, physical activity, diet, and prognosis in breast and gynecologic cancers. *J Clin Oncol.* 2010;28:4074–4080.

93. Irwin ML SA, McTiernan A, Ballard-Barbash R. Influence of pre- and postdiagnosis physical activity on mortality in breast cancer survivors: The health, eating, activity, and lifestyle study. *J Clin Oncol.* 2008;26:3958–3964.

94. Irwin ML, McTiernan A, Manson JE, et al. Physical activity and survival in postmenopausal women with breast cancer: Results of the women's health initiative. *Cancer Prev Res.* 2011;4:522–529.

95. Allen NE, Beral V, Casabonne D, et al.; Million Women Study Collaborators. Moderate alcohol intake and cancer incidence in women. *J Natl Cancer Inst.* 2009;101:296–305.

96. Chen WY, Rosner B, Hankinson SE, et al. Moderate alcohol consumption during adult life, drinking patterns, and breast cancer risk. *JAMA.* 2011;306:1884–1890.

97. Land CE, Tokunaga M, Koyama K, et al. Incidence of female breast cancer among atomic bomb survivors, 1950–1985. *Radiat Res.* 1994;138:209–223.

98. **Castellino SM, Geiger AM, Mertens AC, et al.** Morbidity and mortality in long-term survivors of Hodgkin lymphoma: A report from the Childhood Cancer Survivor Study. *Blood.* 2011;117:1806–1816.

99. **Miller AB, Howe GR, Sherman GJ, et al.** Mortality from breast cancer after irradiation during fluoroscopic examinations in patients being treated for tuberculosis. *N Engl J Med.* 1989;321:1285–1289.

100. **Morris AA, Pommier RF, Schmidt WA, et al.** Accurate evaluation of palpable masses by the triple test score. *Arch Surg.* 1998;133: 930–934.

101. **Kaufman Z, Shpitz B, Shapiro M, et al.** Triple approach in the diagnosis of dominant breast masses: Combined physical examination, mammography, and fine-needle aspiration. *J Surg Oncol.* 1994; 56:254–257.

102. **Ariga R, Bloom K, Reddy VB, et al.** Fine-needle aspiration of clinically suspicious palpable breast masses with histopathologic correlation. *Am J Surg.* 2002;184:410–413.

103. **Ishikawa T, Hamaguchi Y, Tanabe M, et al.** False-positive and false-negative cases of fine-needle aspiration cytology for palpable breast lesions. *Breast Cancer.* 2007;14:388–392.

104. **Tse GM, Tan PH.** Diagnosing breast lesions by fine needle aspiration cytology or core biopsy: Which is better? *Breast Cancer Res Treat.* 2010;123:1–8.

105. **OFlynn EA, Wilson AR, Michell MJ.** Image-guided breast biopsy: State-of-the-art. *Clinical Radiology.* 2010;65:259–270.

106. **Li S, Yang X, Zhang Y, et al.** Assessment accuracy of core needle biopsy for hormone receptors in breast cancer: A meta-analysis. *Breast Cancer Res Treat.* 2012;135:325–334.

107. **Degnim AC, King TA.** Surgical Management of high-risk breast lesions. *Surg Clinic North Am.* 2013;93:329–340.

108. **International Agency for Research on Cancer.** *WHO Classification of Tumours of the Breast (IARC WHO Classification of Tumors).* 4th ed. World Health Organization: 2012.

109. **Corben AD.** Pathology of invasive breast disease. *Surg Clin North Am.* 2013;93:363–392.

110. **Jolly S, Kestin LL, Goldstein NS, et al.** The impact of lobular carcinoma *in situ* in association with invasive breast cancer on the rate of local recurrence in patients with early-stage breast cancer treated with breast-conserving therapy. *Int J Radiat Oncol.* 2006;66: 365–371.

111. **Huober J, Gelber S, Goldhirsch A, et al.** Prognosis of medullary breast cancer: Analysis of 13 International Breast Cancer Study Group (IBCSG) trials. *Ann Oncol.* 2012;23:2843–2851.

112. **Soon SR, Yong WS, Ho GH, et al.** Adenoid cystic breast carcinoma: A salivary gland-type tumour with excellent prognosis and implications for management. *Pathology.* 2008;40:413–415.

113. **Plevritis SK.** A mathematical algorithm that computes breast cancer sizes and doubling times detected by screening. *Math Biosci.* 2001; 171:155–178.

114. **Kusama S, Spratt JS, Donegan WL, et al.** The gross rates of growth of human mammary carcinoma. *Cancer.* 1972;30:594–599.

115. **Tubiana M, Pejovic JM, Renaud A, et al.** Kinetic parameters and the course of the disease in breast cancer. *Cancer.* 1981;47:937–943.

116. **Punglia RS, Morrow M, Winer EP, et al.** Local therapy and survival in breast cancer. *N Engl J Med.* 2007;356:2399–2405.

117. **Greene FL, Page DL, Fleming ID, eds.** *AJCC Cancer Staging Manual.* 7th ed. New York, NY: Springer-Verlag; 2010.

118. **National Comprehensive Cancer Network.** Breast cancer: In NCCN clinical practice guidelines in oncology. V.2. 2013; http://www.nccn.org.

119. **Diel IJ, Kaufmann M, Costa SD, et al.** Micrometastatic breast cancer cells in bone marrow at primary surgery: Prognostic value in comparison with nodal status. *J Natl Cancer Inst.* 1996;88: 1652–1664.

120. **Lim E, Lin NU.** New insights and emerging therapies for breast cancer brain metastases. *Oncology.* 2012;26:652–659.

121. **Groheux D, Espe M, Giacchtti S, et al.** Performance of FDG PET/CT in the clinical management of breast cancer. *Radiology.* 2013; 266:388–405.

122. **Cooper KL, Harnan S, Meng Y, et al.** Positron emission tomography (PET) for assessment of axillary lymph node status in early breast cancer: A systematic review and meta-analysis. *Eur J Surg Oncol.* 2011;37:187–198.

123. **Halsted WS.** The results of radical operation for cure of cancer of the breast. *Ann Surg.* 1907;46:1–19.

124. **Meyer W.** Carcinoma of the breast: Ten years experience with my method of radical operation. *JAMA.* 1905;45:219–313.

125. **Dahl-Iversen E, Tobiassen T.** Radical mastectomy with parasternal and supraclavicular dissection for mammary carcinoma. *Ann Surg.* 1969;170:889–891.

126. **Lewis FJ.** Extended or super radical mastectomy for cancer of the breast. *Minn Med.* 1953;36:763–766.

127. **Urban JA.** Extended radical mastectomy for breast cancer. *Am J Surg.* 1963;106:399–404.

128. **Fisher B, Jeong JH, Anderson S, et al.** Twenty-five-year follow-up of a randomized trial comparing radical mastectomy, total mastectomy, and total mastectomy followed by irradiation. *N Engl J Med.* 2002;347:567–575.

129. **Prosnitz LR, Goldenberg IS, Packard RA, et al.** Radiation therapy as initial treatment for early stage cancer of the breast without mastectomy. *Cancer.* 1977;39:917–923.

130. **Veronesi U, Saccozzi R, Del Veccio M, et al.** Comparing radical mastectomy with quadrantectomy, axillary dissection and radiotherapy in patients with small cancers of the breast. *N Engl J Med.* 1981; 305:6–11.

131. **Veronesi U, Cascinelli N, Mariani L, et al.** Twenty-year follow-up of a randomized study comparing breast-conserving surgery with radical mastectomy for early breast cancer. *N Engl J Med.* 2002;347: 1227–1232.

132. **Fisher B, Bauer M, Margolese R, et al.** Five-year results of a randomized clinical trial comparing total mastectomy and segmental mastectomy with or without radiation in the treatment of cancer. *N Engl J Med.* 1985;312:665–673.

133. **Fisher B, Anderson S, Bryant J, et al.** Twenty-year follow-up of a randomized trial comparing total mastectomy, lumpectomy, and lumpectomy plus irradiation for the treatment of invasive breast cancer. *N Engl J Med.* 2002;347:1233–1241.

134. **NIH Consensus Conference.** Treatment of early-stage breast cancer. *JAMA.* 1991;265:391–395.

135. **Veronesi U, Rilke F, Luini A, et al.** Distribution of axillary node metastases by level of invasion: An analysis of 539 cases. *Cancer.* 1987;59:682–687.

136. **Sauer T, Suciu V.** The role of preoperative axillary lymph node fine needle aspiration in locoregional staging of breast cancer. *Ann Pathol.* 2012;32:e24–28, 410–414.

137. **Giuliano AE, Kirgan DM, Guenther JM, et al.** Lymphatic mapping and sentinel lymphadenectomy for breast cancer. *Ann Surg.* 1994;220:391–401.

138. **Giuliano AE, Jones RC, Brennan M, et al.** Sentinel lymphadenectomy in breast cancer. *J Clin Oncol.* 1997;15:2345–2350.

139. **Giuliano AE, Haigh PI, Brennan MB, et al.** Prospective observational study of sentinel lymphadenectomy without further axillary dissection in patients with sentinel node-negative breast cancer. *J Clin Oncol.* 2000;18:2553–2559.

140. **Veronesi U, Viale G, Paganelli G, et al.** Sentinel lymph node biopsy in breast cancer: Ten-year results of a randomized controlled study. *Ann Surg.* 2010;251:595–600.

141. **Krag DN, Anderson SJ, Julian TB, et al.** Sentinel-lymph-node resection compared with conventional axillary-lymph-node dissection in clinically node-negative patients with breast cancer: Overall survival findings from the NSABP B-32 randomised phase 3 trial. *Lancet Oncol.* 2010;11:927–933.

142. **Lyman GH, Giuliano AE, Somerfield MR, et al.** ASCO guideline recommendations for sentinel lymph node biopsy in early-stage breast cancer. *J Clin Oncol.* 2005;23:7703–7720.

143. **Yen TW, Hunt KK, Ross MI, et al.** Predictors of invasive breast cancer in patients with an initial diagnosis of ductal carcinoma *in situ*: A guide to selective use of sentinel lymph node biopsy in management of ductal carcinoma *in situ. J Am Coll Surg.* 2005;200: 516–526.

144. **Keleher A, Wendt R 3rd, Delpassand E, et al.** The safety of lymphatic mapping in pregnant cancer patients using Tc-99m sulfur colloid. *Breast J.* 2004;10:492–495.

145. **Gentilini O, Cremonesi M, Trifirò G, et al.** Safety of sentinel node biopsy in pregnant patients with breast cancer. *Ann Oncol.* 2004;15: 1348–1351.

146. **Gentilini O, Cremonesi M, Toesca A, et al.** Sentinel lymph node biopsy in pregnant patients with breast cancer. *Eur J Nucl Med Mol Imaging.* 2010;37:78–83.

147. **Spanheimer PM, Graham MM, Sug SL, et al.** Measurement of uterine radiation exposure from lymphoscintigraphy indicates safety of sentinel lymph node biopsy during pregnancy. *Ann Surg Oncol.* 2009;16:1143–1147.

148. **Pruthi S, Haakenson C, Brost BC, et al.** Pharmacokinetics of methylene blue dye for lymphatic mapping in breast cancer–implications for use in pregnancy. *Am J Surg.* 2011;201:70–75.

149. **Fisher B, Montague E, Redmond C, et al.** Comparison of radical mastectomy with alternative treatments for primary breast cancer. A first report of results from a prospective randomized clinical trial. *Cancer.* 1977;39:2827–2839.

150. **Giuliano AE, Hunt KK, Ballman KV, et al.** Axillary dissection vs no axillary dissection in women with invasive breast cancer and sentinel node metastasis: A randomized clinical trial. *JAMA.* 2011; 305:569–575

151. **Arrigada R, Le MG, Rochard F, et al.** Conservative treatment versus mastectomy in early breast cancer: Patterns of failure with 15 years of follow-up data. Institut Gustave-Roussy Breast Cancer Group. *J Clin Oncol.* 1996;14:1558–1564.

152. **Clarke M, Collins R, Darby S, et al.** Effects of radiotherapy and of differences in the extent of surgery for early breast cancer on local recurrence and 15-year survival: An overview of the randomized trials. *Lancet.* 2005;366:2087–2106.

153. **Overgaard M, Hansen PS, Overgaard J, et al.** Postoperative radiotherapy in high-risk premenopausal women with breast cancer who receive adjuvant chemotherapy. *N Engl J Med.* 1997;337:949–955.

154. **Overgaard M, Jensen MB, Overgaard J, et al.** Postoperative radiotherapy in high-risk postmenopausal breast-cancer patients given adjuvant tamoxifen: Danish Breast Cancer Cooperative Group DBCG 82c randomized trial. *Lancet.* 1999;353:1641–1648.

155. **Ragaz J, Olivotto IA, Spinelli JJ, et al.** Locoregional radiation therapy in patients with high-risk breast cancer receiving adjuvant chemotherapy: 20-year results of the British Columbia randomized trial. *J Natl Cancer Inst.* 2005;97:116–126.

156. **Lee CM, Jagsi R.** Postmastectomy radiation therapy: Indications and controversies. *Surg Clin North Am.* 2011;87:511–526.

157. **Fisher ER, Anderson S, Redmon C, et al.** Ipsilateral breast tumor recurrence and survival following lumpectomy and irradiation: Pathological findings from NSABP protocol B-06. *Semin Surg Oncol.* 1992;8:161–166.

158. **Barry M, Sacchini V.** Evaluating the role of intra-operative radiation therapy in the modern management of breast cancer. *Surg Oncol.* 2012;21:159–163.

159. **Veronesi U, Orecchia R, Luini A, et al.** Intraoperative radiotherapy during breast conserving surgery: A study on 1822 cases treated with electrons. *Breast Cancer Res Treat.* 2010;124:141–151.

160. **Vaidya JS, Joseph DJ, Tobias JS, et al.** Targeted intraoperative radiotherapy versus whole breast radiotherapy for breast cancer (TARGIT-A trial): An international, prospective, randomized, non-inferiority phase 3 trial. *Lancet.* 2010;376:91–102.

161. **Pawlik TM, Bucholz TA, Kuerer HM.** The biologic rationale for and emerging role of accelerated partial breast irradiation for breast cancer. *J Am Coll Surg.* 2004;199:479–492.

162. **Benitez PR, Keisch ME, Vicini F, et al.** Five-year results: The initial clinical trial of Mammosite balloon brachytherapy for partial breast irradiation in early-stage breast cancer. *Am J Surg.* 2007;194: 456–462.

163. **Chao KK, Vicini FA, Wallace M, et al.** Analysis of treatment efficacy, cosmesis, and toxicity using the Mammosite breast brachytherapy catheter to deliver accelerated partial-breast irradiation: The william beaumont hospital experience. *Int J Radiat Oncol Biol Phys.* 2007;69:32–40.

164. **Fisher B, Redmond C, Elias EG, et al.** Adjuvant chemotherapy for breast cancer: An overview of NSABP findings. *Int Adv Surg Oncol.* 1982;5:65–90.

165. **Bonadonna G, Valagussa P, Moliterni A, et al.** Adjuvant cyclophosphamide, methotrexate, and fluorouracil in node-positive breast cancer: The results of 20 years of follow up. *N Engl J Med.* 1995; 332:901–906.

166. **Early Breast Cancer Trialists' Collaborative Group (EBCTCG), Peto R, Davies C, et al.** Comparisons between different polychemotherapy regimens for early breast cancer: Meta-analyses of long-term outcome among 100,000 women in 123 randomised trials. *Lancet.* 2012;379:432–444.

167. **Fisher B, Brown AM, Dimitrov NV, et al.** Two months of doxorubicin-cyclophosphamide with and without interval reinduction therapy compared with 6 months of cyclophosphamide, methotrexate, and fluorouracil in tamoxifen-nonresponsive tumors: Results from the National Surgical Adjuvant Breast and Bowel Project B-15. *J Clin Oncol.* 1990;8:1483–1496.

168. **Fisher B, Anderson S, Tan-Chiu E, et al.** Tamoxifen and chemotherapy for axillary node-negative, estrogen-receptor negative breast cancer: Findings from National Surgical Adjuvant Breast and Bowel Project B-23. *J Clin Oncol.* 2001;19:931–942.

169. **Mamounas EP, Bryant J, Lembersky B, et al.** Paclitaxel after doxorubicin plus cyclophosphamide as adjuvant chemotherapy for node-positive breast cancer: Results from NSABP B-28. *J Clin Oncol.* 2005;23:3686–3696.

170. **Henderson IC, Berry DA, Demetri GD, et al.** Improved outcomes from adding sequential paclitaxel but not from escalating doxorubicin dose in an adjuvant chemotherapy regimen for patients with node-positive primary breast cancer. *J Clin Oncol.* 2003;21:976–983.

171. **Jones SE, Savin MA, Holmes FA, et al.** Phase III trial comparing doxorubicin plus cyclophosphamide with docetaxel plus cyclophosphamide as adjuvant therapy for operable breast cancer. *J Clin Oncol.* 2006;24:5381–5387.

172. **Citron ML, Berry DA, Cirrincione C, et al.** Randomized trial of dose-dense versus conventionally scheduled and sequential versus concurrent combination chemotherapy as postoperative adjuvant treatment of node-positive primary breast cancer: First report of Intergroup trial C9741/Cancer and Leukemia Group B Trial 9741. *J Clin Oncol.* 2003;21:1431–1439.

173. **Qin YY, Li H, Guo XJ, et al.** Adjuvant chemotherapy, with or without taxanes, in early or operable breast cancer: A meta-analysis of 19 randomized trials with 30698 patients. *PLoS One.* 2011;6:e26946. doi:1-.1371/journal.pone.0026946.

174. **Slamon DJ, Godolphin W, Jones LA, et al.** Studies of the HER-2/*neu* proto-oncogene in human breast and ovarian cancer. *Science.* 1989;244:707–712.

175. **Slamon DJ, Leyland-Jones B, Shak S, et al.** Use of chemotherapy plus a monoclonal antibody against HER2 for metastatic breast cancer that overexpresses HER2. *N Engl J Med.* 2001;344:783–792.

176. **Gianni L, Dafni U, Gelber RD, et al.** Treatment with trastuzumab for 1 year alter adjuvant chemotherapy in patients with HER2-positive early breast cancer: A 4-year follow-up of a randomised controlled trial. *Lancet Oncol.* 2011;12:236–244.

177. **Goldhirsch A, Gelber RD, Piccart-Gebhart MJ, et al.** 2 years versus 1 year of adjuvant trastuzumab for HER2-positive breast cancer (HERA): An open-label, randomised controlled trial. *Lancet.* 2013;382:1021–1028.

178. **Swain SM, Kim SB, Cortes J, et al.** Pertuzumab, trastuzumab, and docetaxel for HER2-positive metastatic breast cancer (CLEOPATRA study): Overall survival results from a randomised, double-blind, placebo-controlled, phase 3 study. *Lancet Oncol.* 2013;14:461–471.

179. **Robidoux A, Tang G, Rastogi P, et al.** Lapatinib as a component of neoadjuvant therapy for HER2-positive operable breast cancer (NSABP protocol B-41): An open-label, randomised phase 3 trial. *Lancet Oncol.* 2013;14:1183–1192. doi:10.1016/S1470–2045(13)70411-X. [Epub ahead of print].

180. **Paik S, Shak S, Tang G, et al.** A multigene assay to predict recurrence of tamoxifen-treated, node-negative breast cancer. *N Engl J Med.* 2004;351:2817–2826.

181. **Paik S, Tang G, Shak S, et al.** Gene expression and benefit of chemotherapy in women with node disease, estrogen receptor-positive breast cancer. *J Clin Oncology.* 2006;24:3726–3734.

182. **Stemmer SM, Klang SH, Ben-Baruch N, et al.** The impact of the 21-gene Recurrence Score assay on clinical decision-making in node-positive (up to 3 positive nodes) estrogen receptor-positive breast cancer patients. *Breast Cancer Res Treat.* 2013;140:83–92.

183. **Goncalves R, Bose R.** Using multigene tests to select treatment for early-stage breast cancer. *J Natl Compr Canc Netw.* 2013;11: 174–182.

184. **van de Vijver MJ, He YD, van't Veer LJ, et al.** A gene-expression signature as a predictor of survival in breast cancer. *N Engl J Med.* 2002;347:1999–2009.

185. **Knauer M, Mook S, Rutgers EJ, et al.** The predictive value of the 70-gene signature for adjuvant chemotherapy in early breast cancer. *Breast Cancer Res Treat.* 2010;120:655–661.

186. Rutgers E, Piccart-Gebhart MJ, Bogaerts J, et al. The EORTC 10041/BIG 03-04 MINDACT trial is feasible: Results of the pilot phase. *Eur J Cancer.* 2011;47:2742–2749.

187. Buzdar AU, Jonat W, Howell A, et al. Anastrozole versus megestrol acetate in the treatment of postmenopausal women with advanced breast carcinoma: Results of a survival update based on a combined analysis of data from two mature phase III trials. Arimidex Study Group. *Cancer.* 1998;83:1142–1152.

188. Forbes JF, Cuzick J, Buzdar A, et al. Effect of anastrozole and tamoxifen as adjuvant treatment for early-stage breast cancer: 100-month analysis of the ATAC trial. *Lancet.* 2008;9:45–53.

189. Burstein HJ, Prestrud AA, Seidenfeld J, et al.; American Society of Clinical Oncology. American Society of Clinical Oncology clinical practice guideline: Update on adjuvant endocrine therapy for women with hormone receptor-positive breast cancer. *J Clin Oncol.* 2010;28:3784–3796.

190. Cianfrocca M, Goldstein LJ. Prognostic and predictive factors in early-stage breast cancer. *Oncologist.* 2004;9:606–616.

191. Fisher ER, Anderson S, Tan-Chiu E, et al. Fifteen-year prognostic discriminants for invasive breast carcinoma: National Surgical Adjuvant Breast and Bowel Project Protocol-06. *Cancer.* 2001;91:1679–1687.

192. Fisher ER, Redmond C, Fisher B, et al. Pathologic findings from the National Surgical Adjuvant Breast and Bowel Projects (NSABP): Prognostic discriminants for eight-year survival for node-negative invasive breast cancer patients. *Cancer.* 1990;65:2121–2128.

193. Lee YT. Breast carcinoma: Pattern of metastasis at autopsy. *Surg Oncol.* 1983;23:175–180.

194. Hillner BE, Ingle JN, Chlebowski RT, et al. American Society of Clinical Oncology 2003 update on the role of bisphosphonates and bone health issues in women with breast cancer. *J Clin Oncol.* 2003;21:4042–4057.

195. Taylor CW, Green S, Dalton WS, et al. Multicenter randomized clinical trial of goserelin versus surgical ovariectomy in premenopausal patients with receptor-positive metastatic breast cancer: An Intergroup study. *J Clin Oncol.* 1998;16:994–999.

196. Klijn JG, Blamey RW, Boccardo F, et al. Combined tamoxifen and luteinizing hormone-releasing hormone (LHRH) agonist versus LHRH agonist alone in premenopausal advanced breast cancer: A meta-analysis of four randomized trials. *J Clin Oncol.* 2001;19:343–353.

197. Robertson JF, Osborne CK, Howell A, et al. Fulvestrant versus anastrozole for the treatment of advanced breast carcinoma in postmenopausal women. *Cancer.* 2003;98:229–238.

198. Vinayak S, Carlson RW. mTOR inhibitors in the treatment of breast cancer. *Oncology.* 2013;27:38–44.

199. Geyer CE, Forster J, Lindquist D, et al. Lapatinib plus capecitabine for HER2-positive advanced breast cancer. *N Engl J Med.* 2006;355:2733–2743.

200. Oppong BA, King TA. Recommendations for women with lobular carcinoma in situ (LCIS). *Oncology.* 2011;25:1051–1056.

201. Fisher B, Costantino JP, Wickerham DL, et al. Tamoxifen for prevention of breast cancer: Report of the National Surgical Adjuvant Breast and Bowel Project P-1 Study. *J Natl Cancer Inst.* 1998;90:1371–1388.

202. Burstein HJ, Polyak K, Wong JS, et al. Ductal carcinoma *in situ* of the breast. *N Engl J Med.* 2004;350:1430–1441.

203. Page DL, Dupont WD, Rogers LW, et al. Intraductal carcinoma of the breast: Follow-up after biopsy only. *Cancer.* 1982;49:751–758.

204. Fisher B, Dignam J, Wolmark N, et al. Lumpectomy and radiation therapy for the treatment of intraductal breast cancer: Findings from the NSABP B-17. *J Clin Oncol.* 1998;16:441–452.

205. Fisher B, Land S, Mamounas E, et al. Prevention of invasive breast cancer in women with ductal carcinoma *in situ:* An update of the national surgical adjuvant breast and bowel project experience. *Semin Oncol.* 2001;28:400–418.

206. Solin LJ, Gray R, Baehner FL, et al. A multigene expression assay to predict local recurrence risk for ductal carcinoma in situ of the breast. *J Natl Cancer Inst.* 2013;105:701–710.

207. Paget J. Disease of the mammary areola preceding cancer of the mammary gland. *St. Bartholomew Hospital Report.* 1874;10:87–89.

208. Marshall JK, Griffith KA, Haffty BG, et al. Conservative management of Paget disease of the breast with radiotherapy. *Cancer.* 2003;97:2142–2149.

209. Kawase K, Dimaio DJ, Tucker SL, et al. Paget's disease of the breast: There is a role for breast-conserving therapy. *Ann Surg Oncol.* 2005;12:1–7.

210. Yamauchi H, Woodward WA, Valero V, et al. Inflammatory breast cancer: What we know and what we need to learn. *Oncologist.* 2012;17:891–899.

211. Schover LR. Premature ovarian failure and its consequences: Vasomotor symptoms, sexuality, and fertility. *J Clin Oncol.* 2008;26:753–758.

212. Bines J, Oleske DM, Cobleigh MA. Ovarian function in premenopausal women treated with adjuvant chemotherapy for breast cancer. *J Clin Oncol.* 1996;14:1718–1729.

213. Lutchman Singh K, Muttukrishna S, Stein RC, et al. Predictors of ovarian reserve in young women with breast cancer. *Br J Cancer.* 2007;96:1806–1816.

214. Lee SJ, Schover LR, Partridge AH, et al. American Society of Clinical Oncology recommendations on fertility preservation in cancer patients. *J Clin Oncol.* 2006;24:2917–2931.

215. Ives A, Saunders C, Bulsara M, et al. Pregnancy after breast cancer: Population-based study. *BMJ.* 2007;334:194.

216. Brown RW, Allred CD, Clark GM, et al. Prognostic value of Ki-67 compared to S-phase fraction in axillary node-negative breast cancer. *Clin Cancer Res.* 1996;2:585–592.

217. Neville AM, Bettelheim R, Gelber RD, et al. Factors predicting treatment responsiveness and prognosis in node-negative breast cancer. The International (Ludwig) Breast Cancer Study Group. *J Clin Oncol.* 1992;10:696–705.

218. Wegner CR, Clark GM. S-phase fraction and breast cancer–a decade of experience. *Breast Cancer Res Treat.* 1998;51:255–265.

219. Nixon AJ, Neuberg D, Hayes DF, et al. Relationship of patient age to pathologic features of the tumor and prognosis for patients with stage I or II breast cancer. *J Clin Oncol.* 1994;12:888–894.

220. Fisher B, Costantino J, Redmond C, et al. A randomized clinical trial evaluating tamoxifen in the treatment of patients with node-negative breast cancer who have estrogen-receptor-positive tumors. *N Engl J Med.* 1989;320:479–484.

221. Fisher B, Constantino JP, Wickerham DL, et al. Tamoxifen for prevention of breast cancer: Report of the National Surgical Adjuvant Breast and Bowel Project P-1 study. *J Natl Cancer Inst.* 1998;90:1371–1388.

222. Dunn BK, Ford LG. From adjuvant therapy to breast cancer prevention: BCPT and STAR. *Breast J.* 2001;7:144–157.

223. Rhodes DJ, Hartmann LC, Perez EA. Breast Cancer Prevention Trials. *Curr Oncol Rep.* 2000;2:558–565.

224. Vogel VG, Costantino JP, Wickerham DL, et al. Effects of tamoxifen vs raloxifene on the risk of developing invasive breast cancer and other disease outcomes. *JAMA.* 2006;295:2727–2741.

17 Cancer in Pregnancy

Frédéric Amant
Laszlo Ungar

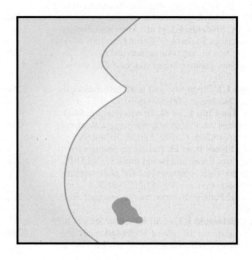

Cancer is diagnosed in 1 per 1,000 to 2,000 pregnancies, and is likely to increase with childbearing being delayed until higher maternal age in developed countries (1,2). **Pregnancy does not predispose to cancer and cancers occurring during pregnancy are those typical of women of reproductive age.** The most frequently encountered cancers during pregnancy include breast, cervical, hematologic malignancies, and melanoma (2,3). Lung and gastric cancers are less frequent, but are associated with a worse prognosis (4,5). Cancer diagnosis and treatment during pregnancy is a challenge for the obstetrician, the oncologist, and the perinatologist. **Treatment decisions must take into account maternal and fetal concerns.** Whether or not to terminate the pregnancy is an individual decision and depends on the parental opinion, the oncologic prognosis, and the urgency of cancer treatment initiation.

Diagnosis

Time between symptoms and cancer diagnosis may be delayed by physiologic gestational symptoms (6,7). Pregnant patients with fatigue, anemia, vaginal bleeding, vaginal discharge, or breast lumps deserve a careful clinical examination. **Complaints of pregnant patients are not necessarily physiologic, and careful examination and further investigation are mandatory.** In the absence of symptoms, palpation of regional lymph nodes or breasts, and visualization and Pap smear of the cervix may help in early detection.

The maternal prognosis per stage does not seem to be worse during pregnancy. Historical data are underpowered to provide valid data for most tumor types. In contrast, studies comparing breast cancer in the pregnant and nonpregnant states, stratified for the most important prognostic factors, have shown no significant differences in survival rates (8,9).

Staging

Staging examinations are performed as in nonpregnant women and are important for their impact on therapeutic decisions. **Nonionizing examinations, including ultrasound and magnetic resonance imaging (MRI), should be preferred during pregnancy** (10). If needed, diagnostic ionizing imaging modalities can be performed with appropriate fetal shielding. Ionizing examinations of distant parts of the maternal body expose the fetus to low dosages, and the accumulated radiation dose may harm the fetus. **The general rule when performing radiologic and nuclear medical examinations during pregnancy is that the radiation doses should be kept as low as reasonably achievable (ALARA-principle), and where possible should be avoided.**

In the absence of safety data, contrast agents should not be used, which is unlikely to alter the diagnostic accuracy. For the evaluation of adnexal masses, contrast administration is mainly used to assess the presence of solid components in a cystic mass, and to a lesser extent, to evaluate nonenhancement in a torted mass. **The presence of solid components in a cystic mass can generally be derived from gray-scale and Doppler sonography.** It is unlikely that intravenous *gadolinium* would be considered critical for MRI of an adnexal mass in pregnancy (11). For cervical cancer, MRI is the reference diagnostic examination to determine tumor size in three dimensions. **Stromal invasion, vaginal, and parametrial extension can be visualized without the use of** *gadolinium* (12).

During normal pregnancy, tumor markers including CA15-3, squamous cell carcinoma (SCC) antigen, and CA125 can be elevated (13). A recent review reported that elevated titers were found in 3–20% of patients for CA15–3 (maximum 56 unit/mL in the third trimester), 3–10.5% for SCC (maximum 4.3 µg/L in the third trimester), and up to 35% for CA125 (maximum 550 unit/mL in the first trimester). **Inhibin B, anti-müllerian hormone (AMH), and lactate dehydrogenase (LDH) levels are not elevated in maternal serum during normal pregnancy** (13).

Interdisciplinary Review

The treatment of pregnant cancer patients is not a typical daily practice, and the experience is diluted among specialists and centers. Apart from this limited experience per clinician, the complexity of conflicting maternal and fetal interests deserves an interdisciplinary discussion, to include radiologists and obstetricians/perinatologists (Fig. 17.1). **An initial interdisciplinary discussion on the choice of imaging modality is a good strategy to avoid overlapping examinations and accumulation of radiation exposure** (14).

A second interdisciplinary discussion should individualize the treatment, which should adhere as much as possible to standard care (14). Fetal concerns are assessed by the obstetricians and perinatologists, who address the long-term morbidity of prematurity. **Where possible, the standard maternal treatment and the prevention of prematurity should be the goal. An interdisciplinary setting is the best guarantee to maximize fetal and maternal outcomes.**

Surgery during Pregnancy

A stable maternal condition is the best guarantee for fetal well-being. Abdominal surgery is preferably planned for the second trimester, because the risk of miscarriage is decreased and the size of the uterus still allows a certain degree of access. Monitoring of hemodynamic parameters is crucial to prevent hypoxia, hypotension, and hypoglycemia. **From 20 weeks gestational age onward, the pregnant patient is positioned in the "left lateral tilt" position.**

Pregnant patients may undergo laparoscopic surgery for pelvic conditions safely up to about 28 weeks (15,16). Specific risks in pregnancy include hypercapnia related to the use of carbon dioxide, perforation of an enlarged uterus, and reduced blood flow caused by the increased intraabdominal pressure. **A maximum laparoscopic procedure time of 90 minutes, a pneumoperitoneum with a maximum intra-abdominal pressure of 10 to 13 mm Hg, an open introduction, and an experienced surgeon are prerequisites.** Apart from adequate analgesia, tocolytic agents are indicated postoperatively when manipulation of the pregnant uterus has been unavoidable. **After surgery on upper parts of the body, tocolytics should not be routinely prescribed.**

Radiation during Pregnancy

Fetal exposure to radiation is associated with deterministic and stochastic effects. Radiotherapy exposes the fetus to higher radiation doses than diagnostic procedures. Deterministic

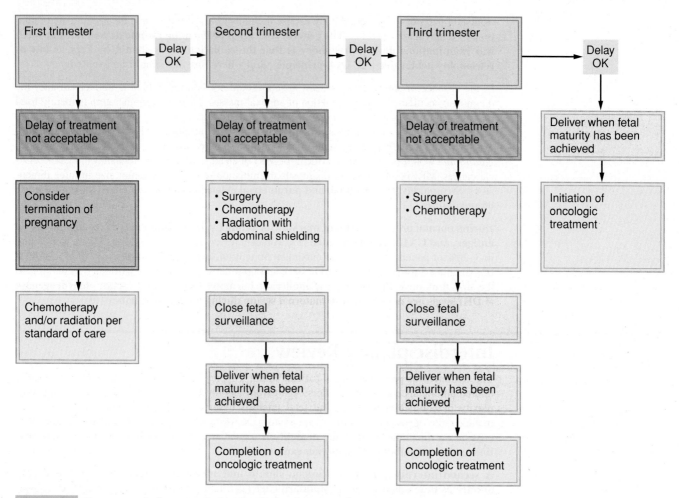

Figure 17.1 Management of cancer during the three trimesters of pregnancy.

effects occur when a certain threshold has been exceeded, shortly after the radiation has been given. **Possible deterministic effects during pregnancy include fetal malformations, growth restriction, microcephaly, mental retardation, and fetal demise.** Stochastic risk of radiotherapy cannot be exactly predicted, and there is no threshold for toxic effects. These manifest years later, and cannot definitively be associated with the radiation exposure. **Radiation exposure during fetal life results in a slightly greater risk of childhood cancer and leukemia.** A fetal dose of 0.01 Gy will increase their incidence from 2 to 3 per 1,000 to 3 to 4 per 1,000 (17).

When applied during the first trimester, pelvic radiotherapy causes spontaneous abortion. When applied during the second trimester, pelvic radiotherapy evokes death of the fetus within the first month after external beam therapy (18). The advantages and disadvantages of hysterotomy before radiotherapy should be assessed on an individual basis. When hysterotomy is performed before initiating radiotherapy, there is no need to alter the radiation fields, there is less psychological distress, and fewer obstetrical complications (bleeding, diffuse intravascular coagulation) (19). Abdominal surgery may potentially delay treatment should a wound infection occur, and there is a small risk of wound metastasis. Postoperative adhesions may enhance radiation toxicity (18).

Chemotherapy during Pregnancy

Pharmacokinetics

During pregnancy multiple changes in physiology occur that affect the major pharmacokinetic processes, including absorption, distribution, metabolism, and excretion. Changes in drug metabolism begin at 4 weeks of gestation and progressively increase, mainly under the influence of progesterone and estrogen. These alterations are more pronounced in the third trimester of pregnancy and may alter the efficacy and toxicity of antineoplastic drugs administered during pregnancy (20,21).

The maternal gastrointestinal absorption of drugs may be altered because of changes in gastric secretion and motility. Changes in gastric pH influence the degree of ionization and solubility of many drugs, modifying their absorption rate and altering drug bioavailability. During normal pregnancy, maternal drug metabolism may be altered by elevation of endogenous hormones such as progesterone and estrogen. Their increased secretion can induce or inhibit the hepatic microsomal oxidase system and elevated or reduced rates of hepatic metabolism may result in altered transformation of drugs. The cholestatic effect of estrogen may interfere with biliary drug clearance (20–22).

Therapeutic concentrations of the active drug may be affected by hemodynamic changes that take place throughout pregnancy. Cardiac output and blood volume increase by 50%, primarily as a result of an increase in plasma volume of 45%, leading to an increase in hepatic and renal perfusion, and an increased glomerular filtration rate, which may cause increased renal elimination. Total body water increases by 5–8%, resulting from the expansion of the extracellular fluid space and the growth of new tissue. Body water accumulates in the fetus, placenta, and amniotic fluid, which collectively contribute to an increase in the distribution volume and this may lower the concentration of drugs and increase their elimination half-life (20–22).

As pregnancy advances, the plasma volume expands at a greater rate than the increase in albumin production, creating a dilutional hypoalbuminemia, which may increase the fraction of unbound drugs (20).

Physiologic pharmacokinetic changes in humans result in a decrease in plasma drug exposure, as measured by area under the curve (AUC) and peak plasma concentrations, because of the increased plasma volume and renal clearance (20).

Theoretically, a reduced plasma drug concentration could lead to suboptimal treatment. The largest follow-up study in breast cancer showed no significant difference in survival between women with cancer during pregnancy and stage-matched nonpregnant women (8,9). Therefore, **despite the dilution of chemotherapy during pregnancy, data have not shown a worse outcome in pregnant women who receive chemotherapy, so doses should be based on actual weight and height during pregnancy.**

Transplacental Passage of Chemotherapeutic Drugs

The placenta is an active organ providing nutrition and protection for the fetus. Transplacental transfer of substances is mediated by passive diffusion, active transport, facilitated diffusion, and phagocytosis and pinocytosis (23,24).

The placenta, and more specifically, the syncytiotrophoblast and fetal capillary endothelium, express ATP-binding cassette (ABC) efflux transporters, including P-glycoprotein (P-gp: MDR 1/ABCB1), breast cancer resistance protein (BCRP/ABCG2), and multidrug resistance protein 1 to 3 and 5 (MRP 1 to 3 and 5/ABCC 1 to 3 and 5), which actively extrude substrates into the maternal circulation. **One of the major roles of these efflux transporters in the placenta is to limit fetal overexposure to toxins, drugs, or xenobiotics, thus protecting the fetus pharmacokinetically and pharmacodynamically.** Most of the chemotherapeutic drugs (e.g., anthracyclines, taxanes) are substrates of these ABC drug transporters.

The data on transplacental passage are in agreement with the expectations based on physicochemical drug characteristics. Because all drugs that are substrates of ABC transporters have a limited transplacental transfer, a major role for the active transporters in the protection of the fetus from toxic agents is suggested (25).

The placenta reduces transplacental passage of all studied drugs, albeit at variable rates. Transplacental transfer of *doxorubicin* and *epirubicin* averages less than 10% (26). Taxanes display a favorable toxicity profile during the second and third trimesters, because less than 2% of maternal plasma concentrations are measured in fetal plasma (27,28). Approximately 20% of the vinca alkaloids and the active metabolite of *cyclophosphamide* cross the placenta (26). In contrast, fetal plasma concentrations of *carboplatin* reach up to 60% of maternal plasma levels (27).

Obstetric Management

A pregnancy complicated by cancer is a high-risk pregnancy and should be managed as such. A checklist for obstetricians is available (14). A 3-week interval between the last cycle of chemotherapy and the delivery will avoid problems associated with hematopoietic suppression in the mother and child, and the accumulation of cytotoxic drugs in the neonate. For all patients, a term delivery (37 weeks' gestation or longer) should be the aim whenever possible. **Chemotherapy during pregnancy followed by term delivery is preferable to late preterm delivery without chemotherapy.** A vaginal birth should also be the objective whenever possible. **It is acceptable in cases of cervical intraepithelial neoplasia (CIN) (29), but in the presence of invasive cervical cancer, an operative delivery is preferable.** The literature has documented seven fatal recurrences in the episiotomy site after vaginal delivery (18).

A classical (corporeal) uterine incision, avoiding the lower uterine segment in order to prevent wound metastasis, is preferable. Cesarean section enables additional surgical treatment of the cancer, when indicated. After surgery for vulvar cancer, vulvar scarring and the risk of vulvar laceration may be an indication for cesarean section. In the presence of vulvar cancer, tumor location and diameter will determine the safest route for delivery.

Fetal Outcome after Antenatal Exposure to Chemotherapy

Timing of oncologic treatment is a crucial factor in determining the fetal outcome. During the period of organogenesis, the fetus is especially vulnerable to cytotoxic agents. After the period of organogenesis, different developmental steps still take place, for example, the development of the central nervous system. Therefore, the fetal outcome in the short and long term is of particular interest.

Short-term Outcome

Spontaneous abortion, fetal death, and major malformations (toes, eyes, ears, and palate) are associated with the administration of chemotherapy during the first trimester. **If chemotherapy is administered after the first trimester, there is no increased risk of congenital malformations compared to the background population** (2,30,31). *In utero* exposure to chemotherapy during the second and the third trimester of pregnancy is related to low birth weight and intrauterine growth restriction (2,3,8). In a series of 413 women exposed to chemotherapy for breast cancer during pregnancy, 50% had a spontaneous or induced premature delivery (8).

Long-term Outcome

There are few published studies concerning the long-term outcome of *in utero* exposure to chemotherapy or radiotherapy. In a series of 40 children for whom parents completed a questionnaire, health and cognitive outcomes were reassuring after antenatal exposure to chemotherapy (32). In a prospective study of 70 children with *in utero* exposure to chemotherapy, **general health, cognitive development, and cardiac outcome showed levels comparable to the general population,** with a median follow-up of 22 months (31). A bias related to prematurity was suggested, because the IQ-scores increased with gestational age. **Prematurity is associated with impaired cognitive functioning, and should be avoided whenever possible** (33,34).

A longer follow-up and more children are needed, but **the available data suggest that fear of the long-term effects in children should not be a reason to withhold chemotherapy during pregnancy** (31).

Management of Cervical Intraepithelial Neoplasia in Pregnancy

The American Society for Colposcopy and Cervical Pathology (ASCCP) has provided consensus guidelines for the management of abnormal cervical cytology and biopsies during pregnancy, which we have summarized below (35,36). **The main treatment strategy for CIN during pregnancy is observation.** Pregnancy does not influence cervical lesions, and progression to invasive disease during pregnancy is very rare (0–0.4%) (37). **When progression does occur, a higher stage than microinvasion has not been documented.** Colposcopy and directed biopsies can be safely performed during pregnancy, but endocervical curettage is contraindicated (36). Physiologic cervical changes during pregnancy, such as increased vascularity, hypertrophy, and hyperplasia of the endocervical glands, may mimic CIN, so colposcopy should be performed by an experienced colposcopist. Several physiologic cellular changes, such as degenerated decidual cells (Arias-Stella phenomena) and trophoblastic cells with variably staining cytoplasm and an enlarged nucleus may mimic high-grade squamous intraepithelial lesions (HSIL), and lead to false-positive Pap smears if the pathologist is unaware of the pregnant state.

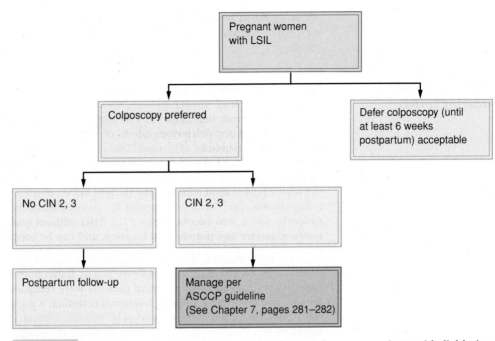

Figure 17.2 Management of pregnant women with low-grade squamous intraepithelial lesion (LSIL) according to the 2013 American Society for Colposcopy and Cervical Pathology (ASCCP) guideline. CIN, cervical intraepithelial neoplasia.

In the case of atypical squamous cells of undetermined significance (ASC-US) or low-grade squamous intraepithelial lesion (LSIL) on a Pap smear during pregnancy, the likelihood of finding CIN 2 to 3 on postpartum follow-up is only 3.7% (38). **Colposcopic examination for such patients can therefore be safely postponed until at least 6 weeks postpartum.**

In cases of HSIL on cervical cytology, prenatal colposcopy (with directed biopsy) is recommended. When CIN 2 to 3 is biopsy proven, or when the colposcopist is certain of the absence of invasion based on colposcopy alone, repeat cytology and colposcopy may be performed every 12 weeks to exclude disease progression. **Treatment of CIN 2 or 3 during pregnancy, such as by ablation or excision, is contraindicated. The authors recommend conization only if the suspicion for microinvasion is high, or the colposcopic examination has been unsatisfactory** (Fig. 17.2). The risks of obstetric complications such as hemorrhage, cervical incompetence, and fetal loss from conization depend on the gestational age, and should be discussed with the patient. A superficial, flat cone is desirable to reduce these risks.

Management of Cancer in Pregnancy

Invasive Cervical Cancer	Invasive cervical cancer belongs among the common cancers diagnosed during pregnancy. The estimated incidence is about 3.3 to 11.1 per 100,000 deliveries (18). Of all the cancer types, cervical cancer treatment during pregnancy is the most challenging, because the uterus itself is involved.
Symptoms	**Pregnancy is an opportunity to screen for cervical cancer.** Similar to the nonpregnant patient, some early cancers will be asymptomatic, but the most common symptom is (postcoital) vaginal bleeding, although an abnormal vaginal discharge (bloody, watery, malodorous, or purulent) can be present (39). Symptoms may be misinterpreted as pregnancy related, and the diagnosis delayed if the level of suspicion is low.
Staging	Pregnant women are more likely to present with early disease because of regular, pregnancy-related obstetric examinations (40). Stensheim et al. reported no differences in the extent of cervical cancer when comparing 80 pregnant patients with 111 lactating and 5,865 nonpregnant patients (1). **The International Federation of Obstetrics and Gynecology (FIGO) staging of cervical cancer is**

primarily based on clinical examination, including examination under anesthesia if necessary. More accurate information on the extent of disease is usually required for treatment planning.

Magnetic Resonance Imaging (MRI)

MRI is the reference diagnostic examination which can help determine tumor size in three dimensions, extent of stromal invasion, amount of healthy stroma, vaginal and parametrial invasion, and lymph node infiltration (12). As stated by the American College of Radiology, data have not documented any deleterious effects of MRI exposure on the developing fetus in any trimester of the pregnancy (41). *Gadolinium* (a category C drug according to the U.S. Food and Drug Administration) should be used only if absolutely essential, although no adverse effects to the neonate have been reported after *gadolinium* exposure in any trimester (42). *Gadolinium* crosses the placenta and is excreted by the fetal kidney into amniotic fluid. It is unknown how long it stays in this space, with the potential for dissociation of the *gadolinium* ion from its chelated molecule, which then becomes toxic (41). MRI without *gadolinium* allows an assessment of tumor diameter and parametrial invasion, and can be used safely during pregnancy.

MRI for determination of locoregional spread of cervical cancer during pregnancy has been described by Zanetta et al. in six patients, and by Balleyguier et al. in 12 (43,44). The MRI features of cervical cancer in pregnant patients were comparable to those in the nonpregnant patient, and allowed for tailored treatment planning. A good correlation between MRI findings and pathology specimens was found (43). Possible difficulties reported for MRI interpretation during pregnancy were physiologic hyperintensity of the cervix, making the tumor either iso- or hypointense; fetal movement impairing image quality (especially for small lesions); and scanning without gadolinium (44). A possible pitfall may be mistaking dilated pelvic veins for pelvic adenopathy when evaluating the axial plane, which can be prevented by examining the other planes. As with the nonpregnant patient, estimation of tumor size may be difficult if the patient has previously undergone diagnostic conization.

Pelvic Lymph Node Assessment

Lymph node status is one of the most significant prognostic factors for patients with cervical cancer (45,46). Information on lymph node involvement can be obtained by MRI or surgical staging. Histopathologic assessment remains the most accurate method for assessment of nodal status, and laparoscopic lymphadenectomy for pregnant women with stage I disease is feasible in experienced hands. In 31 reported cases, maternal and neonatal morbidity has been low (47). As the uterine volume increases, a complete lymphadenectomy becomes more difficult, especially after 22 to 25 weeks of gestational age.

Treatment

Given the limited experience, cervical cancer treatment during pregnancy remains experimental, and should only be offered to motivated patients after sufficient information has been given (Fig. 17.3). An unwanted pregnancy, poor prognosis, and the patient's preference are possible indications to sacrifice the pregnancy and undertake immediate standard treatment.

Stage IA

Cervical conization is indicated only when invasive disease cannot be ruled out. The optimal time to perform a conization during pregnancy is between 14 and 20 weeks. A conization may be both diagnostic and therapeutic for stage IA1 cervical cancer. Surgical expertise is needed, because positive margins are frequently reported (48,49). Delivery should be vaginal after cervical conization with negative margins, unless there are obstetric indications for cesarean section.

Stage IA2 to IB1, Tumor 2 cm or Smaller

A pelvic lymphadenectomy may be performed for tumors smaller than 2 cm, diagnosed before a gestational age of 22 to 25 weeks. If there are positive nodes, termination of the pregnancy and standard treatment should be recommended. When pelvic lymph nodes are negative, a large cone or simple trachelectomy has been recommended. Both procedures appear to give good obstetric and oncologic outcomes, with low complication rates (50).

The rationale for removal of the parametrium is to obtain clear margins around the tumor, and to prevent local recurrence due to any residual cancer in parametrial lymph nodes. Billingsley et al. reported a patient with a stage IA2 cervical cancer who had negative margins on cone biopsy, no

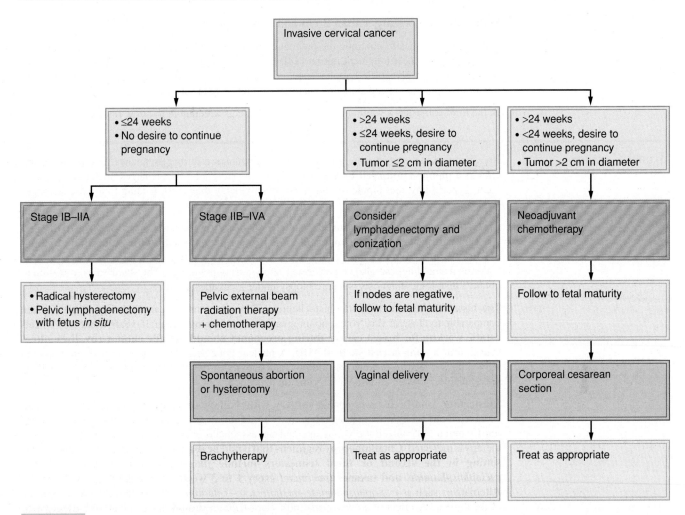

Figure 17.3 **Management of cervical cancer in pregnancy.**

vascular space invasion, but was found to have a single positive parametrial lymph node at radical hysterectomy (51).

Several studies have shown a parametrial invasion rate of less than 1% if the primary tumor is ≤2 cm, the lymph nodes are negative, and stromal invasion is ≤10 mm, supporting the option of less radical surgery in such patients (50,52). **Although radical trachelectomy during pregnancy is technically feasible and oncologically safe, the fetal loss is 33% (5/15) within 16 days,** and it is associated with significant blood loss (47,53,54).

A possible alternative, especially late in the second trimester, is to adopt a waiting policy if the lymph nodes are negative. An average treatment delay of 16 weeks has been reported to not jeopardize maternal outcome (47), but this defies biologic credibility, and most would find this delay unacceptable, even in the nonpregnant state.

Neoadjuvant chemotherapy **is an option for achieving disease control until fetal maturation has occurred, followed by radical hysterectomy postpartum** (55). A prospective evaluation of the efficacy of neoadjuvant chemotherapy during pregnancy is difficult, because the number of cases is small. A retrospective review of 50 cases has shown that neoadjuvant chemotherapy allowed the pregnancy to continue to an average of 33.2 weeks (18). Response was complete in 6.25%, partial in 62.5%, stable in 28.1%, and the disease progressed in 3.1% of cases.

Combination therapy achieved better response rates. The recommended regimen is platinum-based chemotherapy (*cisplatin* 75 mg/m^2), preferably with *paclitaxel* (175 mg/m^2) at three-weekly intervals (56). *Carboplatin* (AUC 5 to 6) has a more favorable toxicity profile with less nephrotoxicity and ototoxicity, and similar efficacy (57). There are few reports of *paclitaxel* during pregnancy, but preclinical studies have shown minimal transplacental passage of the drug (20).

Stages IB1 Tumor Larger than 2 cm and Higher Stages

If the patient wishes to continue the pregnancy in the first or second trimester, neoadjuvant chemotherapy is the best treatment option (18). Before 22 to 25 weeks, a pelvic lymphadenectomy, with or without a paraaortic lymphadenectomy, may be performed. If the nodes are positive, termination of pregnancy and standard treatment should be recommended.

In the third trimester, a waiting policy of a few weeks is acceptable to allow fetal maturity.

Breast Cancer

Breast cancer is the most common cancer type encountered during pregnancy. **It typically presents as a painless lump felt by the woman,** but physiologic breast changes, including engorgement, hypertrophy, and nipple discharge commonly delay diagnosis, leading to a more advanced stage at presentation.

Breast ultrasonography is safe and differentiates solid from cystic masses. **Its high sensitivity and specificity make breast ultrasonography the preferred examination for evaluation of palpable breast masses and lymph node regions during pregnancy.** Mammography, with proper abdominal shielding, can also be performed safely during pregnancy. The standard examination to obtain a histologic diagnosis is a core biopsy under local anesthesia.

The histopathologic and immunohistochemical findings of breast cancer during pregnancy are comparable to those in very young nonpregnant women (younger than 35 years) (32,58,59). **Metastatic workup for breast cancer during pregnancy should include chest x-ray, liver ultrasound, and a noncontrast skeletal MRI.** A nuclear bone scan with adequate hydration, and an indwelling catheter to prevent retention of radioactivity in the bladder, can be used when MRI is not available, or when additional information is needed.

Mastectomy and breast-conserving surgery with axillary or sentinel lymphadenectomy can be carried out safely during pregnancy and should follow the same guidelines as for nonpregnant women (14). Given the young age and the associated poor prognostic risk factors, chemotherapy is indicated. **Chemotherapy regimens that could be used in the adjuvant or neoadjuvant setting in the second or third trimesters include** *fluorouracil–epirubicin/doxorubicin–cyclophosphamide,* **and taxanes (***paclitaxel* **every 1 to 3 weeks or** *docetaxel* **every 3 weeks).** Alternatives such as *cyclophosphamide–methotrexate–5-fluorouracil* should not be used because of the third space effect of *methotrexate* (60). *Trastuzumab* **should not be given to patients with HER2-positive tumors because it blocks HER2 receptors in the fetal kidney, causing oligo- and anhydramnios** (14).

Ovarian Cancer

Atypical proliferative mucinous tumors of the ovary, also called "borderline" mucinous ovarian tumors, have a benign behavior if confined to the ovary (61). These tumors should be discriminated from metastatic pancreatobiliary adenocarcinomas (displaying a paradoxically benign or borderline appearance in the ovary), and ovarian deposits of low-grade appendiceal mucinous neoplasms in the setting of pseudomyxoma peritonei (61). **Treatment of these tumors during pregnancy is by unilateral salpingo-oophorectomy.** Depending on the tumor diameter, gestational age, and expertise of the surgeon, a laparoscopic or open approach may be used.

Serous tumors of low malignant potential may shed cells, resulting in noninvasive or invasive peritoneal implants. **As in nonpregnant patients, surgical staging consists of unilateral salpingo-oophorectomy, omentectomy, and peritoneal biopsies.** During pregnancy, thorough exploration of pelvic peritoneum may be difficult, so primary salpingo-oophorectomy and planned restaging laparoscopy may be appropriate (62).

Most cases of invasive epithelial ovarian cancer during pregnancy are diagnosed at an early stage because of the routine ultrasonic scanning. If the patient wishes to preserve the pregnancy, unilateral salpingo-oophorectomy and surgical staging, including pelvic and para-aortic lymphadenectomy if feasible, should be undertaken early in the second trimester. Adjuvant platinum-based chemotherapy may be required, as in the nonpregnant state.

For mucinous tumors, grading is not reliable, and the treatment is based on the microscopic growth pattern. While an expansile growth pattern relates to an excellent outcome after extirpation of the cyst only, tumors with infiltrative growth are malignant. Staging for the latter includes a lymphadenectomy with possible adjuvant chemotherapy (63,64).

For patients diagnosed with advanced ovarian cancer, the poor maternal prognosis makes termination of pregnancy a viable option. Standard treatment is impossible if preservation of the pregnancy is the intent. **Any cytoreductive surgery will unnecessarily jeopardize fetal health and is not recommended. Neoadjuvant chemotherapy until fetal maturity and complete cytoreduction after delivery are the only viable options.** A combination of *paclitaxel* and *carboplatin* should be the treatment of choice (18). The teratogenic effects of *thalidomide* are explained by the inhibition of angiogenesis; consequently, *bevacizumab* is not recommended during pregnancy.

Germ cell and sex-cord stromal tumors are usually stage I when diagnosed during pregnancy. Unilateral salpingo-oophorectomy and surgical staging (without lymphadenectomy) will usually be appropriate. Indications for adjuvant chemotherapy should be the same as for nonpregnant patients. The fetal safety of etoposide is doubtful, and alternatives during pregnancy for the *bleomycin–etoposide–cisplatin* combination include *paclitaxel–carboplatin* or *cisplatin–vinblastine–bleomycin* (18).

Vulvar Cancer

Carcinoma of the vulva diagnosed and treated during pregnancy is a rare event. **In most cases, standard treatment is possible, including the sentinel node procedure and chemotherapy** (18). Vulvar or inguinal radiotherapy during pregnancy is not possible because of the close fetal proximity.

Two cases have been reported from the Royal Hospital for Women in Sydney (65). The first patient had a 5- × 2-cm ulcerated lesion under the clitoris, and was treated by radical anterior vulvectomy and bilateral groin dissection at 22 weeks. The nodes were negative, and she was delivered by cesarean section at term because of some anterior scarring. She remained free of disease at 39 months. The second patient had multifocal disease and underwent modified radical vulvectomy and bilateral groin dissection at 17 weeks. She had one 25-mm lymph node replaced with tumor. After fetal viability was assured by amniocentesis in the 35th week, she underwent cesarean section and ovarian transposition. Radiation therapy to the groins and pelvis was given 6 weeks postoperatively, and she remained alive and free of disease at 28 months.

The surgical techniques and indications for lymphadenectomy should follow the same guidelines as in nonpregnant women. Special attention should be paid to hemostasis because of the increased vascularity during pregnancy. Surgical margins should be 8 mm microscopically in order to avoid postoperative recurrence (66).

When vulvar cancer is diagnosed after 30 weeks, an observational policy, with close monitoring until fetal maturity, may be reasonable.

Malignant Melanoma

About one-third of all melanomas in women occur during childbearing age. Malignant melanoma is the most common type of malignancy during pregnancy in Australia (67). **The skin changes that occur in pregnancy can make diagnosis more difficult, but any suspicious lesion should be fully evaluated.**

The effects of pregnancy hormones on malignant melanoma remain controversial, although studies that have corrected for thickness of the primary tumor have shown no significant difference in survival between pregnant and nonpregnant women (68,69). **O'Meara et al. reported no difference in stage, tumor thickness, lymph node involvement, or survival** (68). With early diagnosis and treatment, excellent outcomes should be expected.

Treatment of early stage melanoma is surgical excision. Resection of regional lymph nodes or sentinel lymph node biopsy is possible during pregnancy, but should be performed only when necessary (70). Given the limited efficacy of adjuvant immunotherapy with *interferon alpha*, its use is not recommended during pregnancy.

For metastatic disease, treatment with B-*raf*-inhibitors is an established treatment for malignant melanomas that carry an activating mutation of the protooncogene B-*raf*. One case of a patient who received *vemurafenib* for metastatic disease during pregnancy has been reported (71). A 34% intrauterine growth restriction was observed, and *vemurafenib* treatment could not be ruled out as a contributing factor. A cesarean section was performed at 30 weeks, and postpartum blood samples showed that the neonatal serum concentration of the drug was approximately 50% of the maternal concentration. This was considerably higher than expected from animal experiments.

The potential for metastasis to the placenta warrants careful histologic evaluation of the placenta by pathologists. With placental involvement, the fetal risk of metastatic melanoma is approximately 22%. Neonates delivered with concomitant placental involvement should be considered at high risk, and followed with vigilance (72).

Hematologic Malignancy

Hematologic malignancies during pregnancy are rare. Hodgkin disease is the most common type (incidence 1:6,000 pregnancies), followed by non-Hodgkin lymphoma and leukemia (incidence 1:75,000 to 100,000 pregnancies) (73). Diagnosis by lymph node biopsy can be performed safely in the pregnant patient, and any suspicious adenopathy should be assessed regardless of the gestational age. **Hodgkin lymphoma and non-Hodgkin lymphoma should be treated as in nonpregnant patients.**

If chemotherapy is indicated during the first trimester, termination of pregnancy is typically recommended. In cases of low-grade or indolent lymphoma, or if a patient desires to maintain the pregnancy, treatment should be delayed until the second trimester (74). **Women treated for lymphoma during pregnancy have the same survival as their nonpregnant counterparts** (74). An overview of chemotherapeutic regimens and targeted therapies for hematologic malignancies during pregnancy can be found in the Lancet Series (73).

Leukemia in pregnancy is rare and presents a very difficult challenge. **Treatment for leukemia should be started as soon as possible regardless of the gestational age, because delay or modification of therapy worsens maternal prognosis** (75). In early pregnancy, termination is considered the best course of action, given the teratogenicity of antineoplastic agents, and the potential for maternal complications during periods of extreme pancytopenia and immunosuppression (76). Leukapheresis can be performed without causing major maternal or fetal morbidity, and is indicated in the presence of significant leukocytosis and leukostasis-related complications, such as impending vascular occlusion (77). The hypercoagulable state of pregnancy can be aggravated by myeloproliferative neoplasms, and thromboprophylaxis should be considered.

References

1. **Stensheim H, Moller B, van Dijk T, et al.** Cause-specific survival for women diagnosed with cancer during pregnancy or lactation: A registry-based cohort study. *J Clin Oncol.* 2009;27:45–51.
2. **Van Calsteren K, Heyns L, De Smet F, et al.** Cancer during pregnancy: An analysis of 215 patients emphasizing the obstetrical and the neonatal outcomes. *J Clin Oncol.* 2010;28:683–689.
3. **Cardonick E, Iacobucci A.** Use of chemotherapy during human pregnancy. *Lancet Oncol.* 2004;5:283–291.
4. **Azim HA, Jr., Peccatori FA, Pavlidis N.** Lung cancer in the pregnant woman: To treat or not to treat, that is the question. *Lung Cancer.* 2010;67:251–256.
5. **Lee HJ, Lee IK, Kim JW, et al.** Clinical characteristics of gastric cancer associated with pregnancy. *Dig Surg.* 2009;26:31–36.
6. **Voulgaris E, Pentheroudakis G, Pavlidis N.** Cancer and pregnancy: A comprehensive review. *Surg Oncol.* 2011;20:e175–e185.
7. **Han SN, Van Calsteren K, Heyns L, et al.** Breast cancer during pregnancy: A literature review. *Minerva Ginecol.* 2010;62:585–597.
8. **Loibl S, Han SN, von Minckwitz G, et al.** Treatment of breast cancer during pregnancy: An observational study. *Lancet Oncol.* 2012;13:887–896.
9. **Amant F, von Minckwitz MG, Han SN, et al.** Prognosis of women with primary breast cancer diagnosed during pregnancy: Results from an international collaborative study. *J Clin Oncol.* 2013;31: 2532–2539.
10. **Patel SJ, Reede DL, Katz DS, et al.** Imaging the pregnant patient for nonobstetric conditions: Algorithms and radiation dose considerations. *Radiographics.* 2007;27:1705–1722.
11. **Telischak NA, Yeh BM, Joe BN, et al.** MRI of adnexal masses in pregnancy. *AJR Am J Roentgenol.* 2008;191:364–370.

12. **Nicolet V, Carignan L, Bourdon F, et al.** MR imaging of cervical carcinoma: A practical staging approach. *Radiographics.* 2000; 20:1539–1549.
13. **Han SN, Lotgerink A, Gziri MM, et al.** Physiologic variations of serum tumor markers in gynecological malignancies during pregnancy: A systematic review. *BMC Med.* 2012;10:86.
14. **Amant F, Loibl S, Neven P, et al.** Breast cancer in pregnancy. *Lancet.* 2012;379:570–579.
15. **Pearl J, Price R, Richardson W, et al.; Society of American Gastrointestinal Endoscopic Surgeons.** Guidelines for diagnosis, treatment, and use of laparoscopy for surgical problems during pregnancy. *Surg Endosc.* 2011;25:3479–3492.
16. **Balthazar U, Steiner AZ, Boggess JF, et al.** Management of a persistent adnexal mass in pregnancy: What is the ideal surgical approach? *J Minim Invasive Gynecol.* 2011;18:720–725.
17. **Doll R, Wakeford R.** Risk of childhood cancer from fetal irradiation. *Br J Radiol.* 1997;70:130–139.
18. **Amant F, Halaska MJ, Fumagalli M, et al.** Gynecologic cancers in pregnancy: Guidelines of a second international consensus meeting. *Int J Gynecol Cancer.* 2014;24(3):394–403.
19. **Sood AK, Sorosky JI, Mayr N, et al.** Radiotherapeutic management of cervical carcinoma that complicates pregnancy. *Cancer.* 1997;80:1073–1038.
20. **Van Calsteren K, Verbesselt R, Ottevanger N, et al.** Pharmacokinetics of chemotherapeutic agents in pregnancy: A preclinical and clinical study. *Acta Obstet Gynecol Scand.* 2010;89:1338–1345.
21. **Amant F, Han SN, Gziri MM, et al.** Chemotherapy during pregnancy. *Curr Opin Oncol.* 2012;24:580–586.

22. **Gedeon C, Koren G.** Designing pregnancy centered medications: Drugs which do not cross the human placenta. *Placenta.* 2006;27: 861–868.

23. **Ceckova-Novotna M, Pavek P, Staud F.** P-glycoprotein in the placenta: Expression, localization, regulation and function. *Reprod Toxicol.* 2006;22:400–410.

24. **Ni Z, Mao Q.** ATP-binding cassette efflux transporters in human placenta. *Curr Pharm Biotechnol.* 2011;12:674–685.

25. **Van Calsteren K, Verbesselt R, Van Bree R, et al.** Substantial variation in transplacental transfer of chemotherapeutic agents in a mouse model. *Reprod Sci.* 2011;18:57–63.

26. **Van Calsteren K, Verbesselt R, Beijnen J, et al.** Transplacental transfer of anthracyclines, vinblastine, and 4-hydroxy-cyclophosphamide in a baboon model. *Gynecol Oncol.* 2010;119:594–600.

27. **Van Calsteren K, Verbesselt R, Devlieger R, et al.** Transplacental Transfer of Paclitaxel, Docetaxel, Carboplatin, and Trastuzumab in a Baboon Model. *Int J Gynecol Cancer.* 2010;20:1456–1464.

28. **Berveiller P, Vinot C, Mir O, et al.** Comparative transplacental transfer of taxanes using the human perfused cotyledon placental model. *Am J Obstet Gynecol.* 2012;207:514–517.

29. **Morice P, Narducci F, Mathevet P, et al.** French recommendations on the management of invasive cervical cancer during pregnancy. *Int J Gynecol Cancer.* 2009;19:1638–1641.

30. **Ring AE, Smith IE, Jones A, et al.** Chemotherapy for breast cancer during pregnancy: An 18-year experience from five London teaching hospitals. *J Clin Oncol.* 2005;23:4192–4197.

31. **Amant F, Van Calsteren K, Halaska MJ, et al.** Long-term cognitive and cardiac outcomes after prenatal exposure to chemotherapy in children aged 18 months or older: An observational study. *Lancet Oncol.* 2012;13:256–264.

32. **Hahn KM, Johnson PH, Gordon N, et al.** Treatment of pregnant breast cancer patients and outcomes of children exposed to chemotherapy in utero. *Cancer.* 2006;107:1219–1226.

33. **Voigt B, Pietz J, Pauen S, et al.** Cognitive development in very vs. moderately to late preterm and full-term children: Can effortful control account for group differences in toddlerhood? *Early Hum Dev.* 2012;88:307–313.

34. **van Baar AL, Vermaas J, Knots E, et al.** Functioning at school age of moderately preterm children born at 32 to 36 weeks' gestational age. *Pediatrics.* 2009;124:251–257.

35. **Wright TC, Jr., Massad LS, Dunton CJ, et al.** 2006 consensus guidelines for the management of women with cervical intraepithelial neoplasia or adenocarcinoma in situ. *Am J Obstet Gynecol.* 2007; 197:340–345.

36. **Massad LS, Einstein MH, Huh WK, et al.** 2012 updated consensus guidelines for the management of abnormal cervical cancer screening tests and cancer precursors. *Obstet Gynecol.* 2013;121:829–846.

37. **Paraskevaidis E, Koliopoulos G, Kalantaridou S, et al.** Management and evolution of cervical intraepithelial neoplasia during pregnancy and postpartum. *Eur J Obstet Gynecol Reprod Biol.* 2002;104: 67–69.

38. **Dunn TS, Bajaj JE, Stamm CA, et al.** Management of the minimally abnormal papanicolaou smear in pregnancy. *J Low Genit Tract Dis.* 2001;5:133–137.

39. **Nguyen C, Montz FJ, Bristow RE.** Management of stage I cervical cancer in pregnancy. *Obstet Gynecol Surv.* 2000;55:633–643.

40. **Zemlickis D, Lishner M, Degendorfer P, et al.** Maternal and fetal outcome after invasive cervical cancer in pregnancy. *J Clin Oncol.* 1991;9:1956–1961.

41. **Kanal E, Barkovich AJ, Bell C, et al.** ACR guidance document for safe MR practices: 2007. *AJR Am J Roentgenol.* 2007;188: 1447–1474.

42. **Sundgren PC, Leander P.** Is administration of gadolinium-based contrast media to pregnant women and small children justified? *J Magn Reson Imaging.* 2011;34:750–757.

43. **Zanetta G, Pellegrino A, Vanzulli A, et al.** Magnetic resonance imaging of cervical cancer in pregnancy. *Int J Gynecol Cancer.* 1998;8:265–269.

44. **Balleyguier C, Fournet C, Ben HW, et al.** Management of cervical cancer detected during pregnancy: Role of magnetic resonance imaging. *Clin Imaging.* 2013;37:70–76.

45. **Delgado G, Bundy B, Zaino R, et al.** Prospective surgical-pathological study of disease-free interval in patients with stage IB squamous cell carcinoma of the cervix: A Gynecologic Oncology Group study. *Gynecol Oncol.* 1990;38:352–357.

46. **Benedetti-Panici P, Maneschi F, Scambia G, et al.** Lymphatic spread of cervical cancer: An anatomical and pathological study based on 225 radical hysterectomies with systematic pelvic and aortic lymphadenectomy. *Gynecol Oncol.* 1996;62:19–24.

47. **Morice P, Uzan C, Gouy S, et al.** Gynaecological cancers in pregnancy. *Lancet.* 2012;379:558–569.

48. **Dunn TS, Ginsburg V, Wolf D.** Loop-cone cerclage in pregnancy: A 5-year review. *Gynecol Oncol.* 2003;90:577–580.

49. **Yahata T, Numata M, Kashima K, et al.** Conservative treatment of stage IA1 adenocarcinoma of the cervix during pregnancy. *Gynecol Oncol.* 2008;109:49–52.

50. **Rob L, Skapa P, Robova H.** Fertility-sparing surgery in patients with cervical cancer. *Lancet Oncol.* 2011;12:192–200.

51. **Billingsley CC, Kohler MF, Creasman WT, et al.** A case of parametrial lymph node involvement in stage 1A2 squamous cell carcinoma of the cervix treated with radical hysterectomy and a review of the literature. *J Low Genit Tract Dis.* 2012;16:145–148.

52. **Schmeler KM, Frumovitz M, Ramirez PT.** Conservative management of early stage cervical cancer: Is there a role for less radical surgery? *Gynecol Oncol.* 2011;120:321–325.

53. **Karateke A, Cam C, Celik C, et al.** Radical trachelectomy in late pregnancy: Is it an option? *Eur J Obstet Gynecol Reprod Biol.* 2010; 152:112–113.

54. **Ungar L, Smith JR, Palfalvi L, et al.** Abdominal radical trachelectomy during pregnancy to preserve pregnancy and fertility. *Obstet Gynecol.* 2006;108:811–814.

55. **Karam A, Feldman N, Holschneider CH.** Neoadjuvant cisplatin and radical cesarean hysterectomy for cervical cancer in pregnancy. *Nat Clin Pract Oncol.* 2007;4:375–380.

56. **Zagouri F, Sergentanis TN, Chrysikos D, et al.** Platinum derivatives during pregnancy in cervical cancer: A systematic review and meta-analysis. *Obstet Gynecol.* 2013;121:337–343.

57. **Moore KN, Herzog TJ, Lewin S, et al.** A comparison of cisplatin/paclitaxel and carboplatin/paclitaxel in stage IVB, recurrent or persistent cervical cancer. *Gynecol Oncol.* 2007;105:299–303.

58. **Halaska MJ, Pentheroudakis G, Strnad P, et al.** Presentation, management and outcome of 32 patients with pregnancy-associated breast cancer: A matched controlled study. *Breast J.* 2009;15:461–467.

59. **Middleton LP, Amin M, Gwyn K, et al.** Breast carcinoma in pregnant women: Assessment of clinicopathologic and immunohistochemical features. *Cancer.* 2003;98:1055–1060.

60. **Amant F, Deckers S, Van Calsteren K, et al.** Breast cancer in pregnancy: Recommendations of an international consensus meeting. *Eur J Cancer.* 2010;46:3158–3168.

61. **Han G, Soslow RA.** Nonserous ovarian epithelial tumors. *Surgical Pathology Clinics.* 2011;4:397–459.

62. **Fauvet R, Brzakowski M, Morice P, et al.** Borderline ovarian tumors diagnosed during pregnancy exhibit a high incidence of aggressive features: Results of a French multicenter study. *Ann Oncol.* 2012;23:1481–1487.

63. **Muyldermans K, Moerman P, Amant F, et al.** Primary invasive mucinous ovarian carcinoma of the intestinal type: Importance of the expansile versus infiltrative type in predicting recurrence and lymph node metastases. *Eur J Cancer.* 2013;49:1600–1608.

64. **He SY, Shen HW, Xu L, et al.** Successful management of mucinous ovarian cancer by conservative surgery in week 6 of pregnancy: Case report and literature review. *Arch Gynecol Obstet.* 2012;286:989–993.

65. **Gitsch G, van Eijkeran MJ, Hacker NF.** Surgical therapy of vulvar cancer in pregnancy. *Gynecol Oncol.* 1995;56:312–316.

66. **Heaps JM, Fu YS, Montz FJ, et al.** Surgical-pathologic variables predictive of local recurrence in squamous cell carcinoma of the vulva. *Gynecol Oncol.* 1990;38:309–314.

67. **Lee Y, Roberts C, Dobbins T, et al.** Incidence and outcomes of pregnancy-associated cancer in Australia, 1994–2008: A population-based linkage study. *BJOG.* 2012;119(13):1572–1582.

68. **O'Meara AT, Cress R, Xing G, et al.** Malignant melanoma in pregnancy. A population-based evaluation. *Cancer.* 2005;103: 1217–1226.

69. **Lens M, Bataille V.** Melanoma in relation to reproductive and hormonal factors in women: Current review on controversial issues. *Cancer Causes Control.* 2008;19:437–442.

70. **Andtbacka RH, Donaldson MR, Bowles TL, et al.** Sentinel lymph node biopsy for melanoma in pregnant women. *Ann Surg Oncol.* 2013;20:689–696.

71. **Maleka A, Enblad G, Sjors G, et al.** Treatment of metastatic malignant melanoma with vemurafenib during pregnancy. *J Clin Oncol.* 2013;31:e192–e193.

72. **Alexander A, Samlowski WE, Grossman D, et al.** Metastatic melanoma in pregnancy: Risk of transplacental metastases in the infant. *J Clin Oncol.* 2003;21:2179–2186.

73. **Brenner B, Avivi I, Lishner M.** Haematological cancers in pregnancy. *Lancet.* 2012;379:580–587.

74. **Pereg D, Koren G, Lishner M.** The treatment of Hodgkin's and non-Hodgkin's lymphoma in pregnancy. *Haematologica.* 2007;92:1230–1237.

75. **Chelghoum Y, Vey N, Raffoux E, et al.** Acute leukemia during pregnancy: A report on 37 patients and a review of the literature. *Cancer.* 2005;104:110–117.

76. **Shapira T, Pereg D, Lishner M.** How I treat acute and chronic leukemia in pregnancy. *Blood Rev.* 2008;22:247–259.

77. **Ali R, Ozkalemkas F, Ozkocaman V, et al.** Successful pregnancy and delivery in a patient with chronic myelogenous leukemia (CML), and management of CML with leukapheresis during pregnancy: A case report and review of the literature. *Jpn J Clin Oncol.* 2004;34:215–217.

MEDICAL AND SURGICAL TOPICS

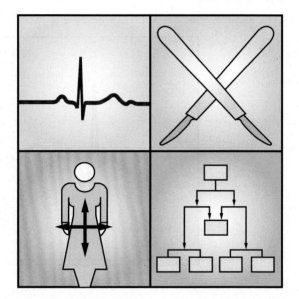

18 Preoperative Evaluation, Medical Management, and Critical Care

Spencer R. Adams
M. Iain Smith
Roger M. Lee
Reza Khorsan
Patricia Eshaghian
Samuel A. Skootsky

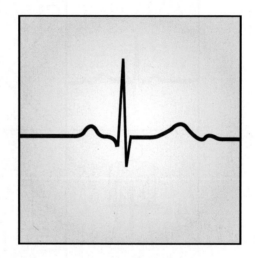

Most patients with gynecologic cancer are middle-aged to elderly and have a high incidence of coexisting medical problems at the time of presentation. The medical status of all patients requiring aggressive surgery needs to be optimized preoperatively, to ensure the optimal postoperative outcome. The early identification, evaluation, and management of emerging medical problems are essential. This chapter discusses the preoperative evaluation of the surgical patient, and the postoperative management of some of the most common medical problems encountered by patients with gynecologic cancers.

Preoperative Evaluation

The cornerstone of all perioperative medical management is the anticipation of specific problems. Careful and accurate assessment of preoperative risk is the first step in developing a perioperative plan that maximizes successful outcomes.

Cardiovascular

Surgery can represent a major cardiovascular stress because of depression in myocardial contractility, changes in sympathetic tone induced by general anesthetic agents, and rapid changes in intravascular volume that occur as a result of blood loss and "third spacing" of fluids. The magnitude of cardiovascular stress depends on patient characteristics, the nature and site of the operation, the duration of the operation, and whether it is elective or emergent. Perioperative myocardial ischemia and infarction are the most significant predictors of adverse cardiovascular outcomes in the years following surgery.

Cardiovascular Risk Factors

Multiple studies have been published over the last 30 years assessing clinical risks for cardiac events during surgery (1–5). The risk of perioperative cardiovascular complications depends on the

Table 18.1 Revised Cardiac Risk Index

1. Ischemic heart disease (history of myocardial infarction, history of positive cardiac stress test, use of nitroglycerin, current chest pain thought secondary to coronary ischemia, or ECG with abnormal Q waves).

2. Congestive heart failure (history of heart failure, pulmonary edema, paroxysmal nocturnal dyspnea, peripheral edema, bilateral rales, S_3, or x-ray with pulmonary vascular redistribution).

3. Cerebral vascular disease (history of transient ischemic attack [TIA] or stroke).

4. Diabetes mellitus treated preoperatively with insulin.

5. Chronic kidney disease with a preoperative creatinine greater than 2 mg/dL.

6. High-risk surgery (abdominal aortic aneurysm or other vascular surgery, thoracic, abdominal, or orthopedic surgery).

Adapted from **Lee TH, Marcantonio ER, Mangione CM, et al**. Derivation and prospective validation of a simple index for prediction of cardiac risk of major noncardiac surgery. *Circulation*. 1999;100:1043–1049.

patient's underlying health and the nature of the planned surgery. A commonly used "simple index" called the **Revised Cardiac Risk Index identifies five clinical variables as independent predictors of cardiac complications** (Table 18.1). This simple index is among the best validated ways to estimate cardiovascular risk and forms the foundation of the 2007 revision of the American College of Cardiology (ACC) and the American Heart Association (AHA) guidelines on perioperative cardiovascular evaluation and care for noncardiac surgery (5,6).

The 2007 ACC/AHA guidelines (in addition to the 2009 ACCF/AHA focused update on perioperative β-blockade) offer a simplified yet comprehensive approach to the assessment of cardiac risks for patients undergoing noncardiac surgery (6,7). An algorithm based on this approach is shown in Figure 18.1. This approach represents a consensus view derived from a review of the literature to date and is periodically updated on the ACC website (http://www.acc.org). **An important overriding theme of these guidelines is that cardiac stress testing and interventions (such as coronary stenting or coronary bypass graft surgery) are rarely necessary simply to lower the risk of surgery. Such interventions are likely unnecessary unless they would have been performed if the patient were not undergoing surgery.** No test should be performed unless it is likely to influence patient treatment.

If the patient has an active cardiac condition that indicates major clinical risk (Table 18.2), **the surgery should be delayed or cancelled until the condition is stabilized unless the surgery is emergent** (6,8). For stable patients, the algorithm can be used as follows: obtain information from the patient and use the **Revised Cardiac Risk Index** to determine how many of the clinical risk factors (from Table 18.1) the patient has. **One point is assigned for each of the six possible clinical risk factors. Based on how many points are assigned, patients can be characterized as high risk (3 or more points), intermediate risk (1 to 2 points), or low risk (0 points).**

The first step is to determine the urgency of surgery. If emergent surgery is needed, there is no time for any cardiac assessment beyond what history is available and the patient should proceed immediately to the operating room. For urgent or elective surgery, there is more time to accurately assess a patient's cardiac risks. **If the patient has an active cardiac condition** (Table 18.2), **all but emergency surgeries should be delayed until the cardiac condition is properly evaluated and treated.**

Table 18.2 Major Active Cardiac Conditions

1. Unstable coronary syndromes (unstable or severe angina [Canadian class III or IV], acute [<7 d] or recent [7–30 d] myocardial infarction with evidence of important ischemic risk by clinical symptoms or noninvasive study)

2. Decompensated heart failure

3. Significant, uncontrolled arrhythmias (high-grade atrioventricular block, symptomatic ventricular arrhythmias in the presence of underlying heart disease)

4. Severe valvular heart disease (especially severe aortic stenosis)

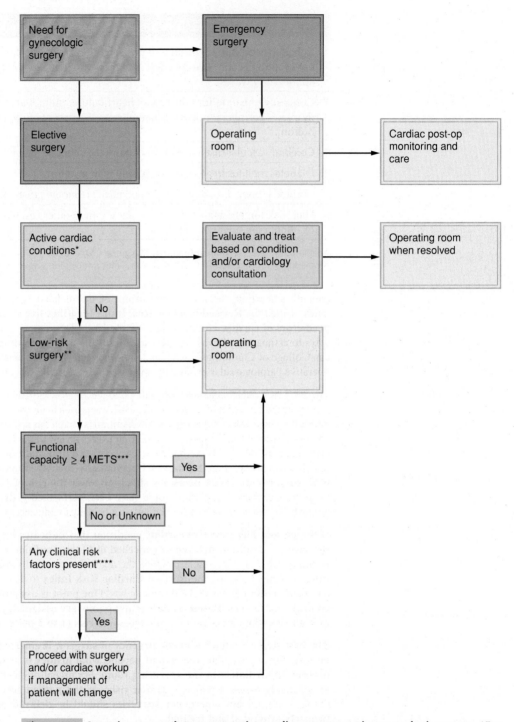

Figure 18.1 **Stepwise approach to preoperative cardiac assessment in gynecologic surgery.** *For active cardiac conditions, refer Table 18.2; **risk of surgery is shown in Table 18.3 ***MET, metabolic equivalent (see Table 18.4) ****Clinical Risk Factors refers to Table 18.1. (From **Fliesher LA, Beckman JA, Brown KA, et al**. ACC/AHA 2007 guidelines on perioperative cardiovascular evaluation and care for noncardiac surgery: A report of the American College of Cardiology/ American Heart Association Task Force on Practice Guidelines (Writing Committee to Revise the 2002 Guidelines on Perioperative Cardiovascular Evaluation for Noncardiac Surgery). *Circulation*. 2007;116:e418–e499.)

Table 18.3 Cardiac Risk Stratification for Noncardiac Surgical Procedures

High (reported cardiac risk often greater than 5%)

Emergent major operations, particularly in the elderly

Aortic and other major vascular surgery

Peripheral vascular surgery

Anticipated prolonged surgical procedures associated with large fluid shifts and/or blood loss

Intermediate (reported cardiac risk generally less than 5%)

Carotid endarterectomy

Head and neck surgery

Intraperitoneal and intrathoracic surgery

Orthopedic surgery

Prostate surgery

Low (reported cardiac risk generally less than 1%)

Endoscopic procedures

Superficial procedure

Cataract surgery

Breast surgery

Often patients need very little evaluation and no additional cardiac testing. Patients who are undergoing low-risk surgery (Table 18.3) do not need further evaluation. Patients with good functional capacity (metabolic equivalents [METs] levels ≥4) (Table 18.4) without symptoms and active conditions can proceed with gynecologic surgery without further evaluation (Fig. 18.1) (9).

If the patient has poor or unknown functional capacity, the presence of clinical risk factors from the Revised Cardiac Risk Index will help to determine the need for further evaluation.

Table 18.4 Estimated Energy Requirements for Various Activities

1–4 Metabolic Equivalents (METs)

Can you take care of yourself?

Eat, dress, or use the toilet?

Walk indoors around the house?

Walk a block or two on level ground at 2–3 mph (3.2–4.8 km/hr)?

Do light work around the house like dusting or washing dishes?

5–10 Metabolic Equivalents (METs)

Climb a flight of stairs or walk up a hill?

Walk on level ground at 4 mph (6.4 km/hr)?

Run a short distance?

Do heavy work around the house like scrubbing floors or lifting or moving heavy furniture?

Participate in moderate recreational activities like golf, bowling, dancing, doubles tennis, or throwing a baseball or football?

>10 Metabolic Equivalents (METs)

Participate in strenuous sports like swimming, singles tennis, football, basketball, or skiing?

MET, Metabolic Equivalent, which can be used as a measure of energy requirements and may be used in treadmill reports.

Adapted from the Duke Activities Status Index. **Hlatky MA, Doineau RE, Higginbotham MB, et al**. *Am J Cardiol*. 1989;64:651–654.

The most challenging patients to evaluate preoperatively are those with at least one cardiac risk factor and with poor or uncertain functional capacity undergoing intermediate risk surgeries (most gynecologic surgeries). **Evidence from a randomized trial suggests that preoperative cardiac stress testing is of no value in patients with only one or two cardiac risk factors** (10). Preoperative stress testing is best reserved for patients with three or more cardiac risk factors in whom preoperative revascularization is feasible, and would have been considered regardless of whether or not the patient was having surgery. The guidelines emphasize that stress testing should be performed only if it will change management (6,11). Perioperative β-blockade will be discussed in more detail below, but based on the evidence, **β-blockade cannot be recommended for patients with intermediate risk and extreme caution should be used if these drugs are newly prescribed preoperatively.** *Dipyridamole-thallium* imaging or *dobutamine* stress echocardiography can be considered for noninvasive testing in these patients (12,13). If noninvasive testing shows only minor abnormalities (minimal areas of myocardial ischemia), the patient can proceed with surgery with medical management including β-blockade, if appropriate. With optimal medical therapy, these patients have no greater incidence of perioperative cardiac events than those with no evidence of ischemia (14). If stress testing reveals moderate or severe abnormalities, subsequent care should include cardiology consultation. Considerations would include cancellation or delay of surgery, coronary revascularization followed by noncardiac surgery, or intensified care in such patients (6).

Myocardial Infarction	**Even with careful and accurate preoperative assessment and preparation, postoperative myocardial infarction (MI) can still occur after surgery under general anesthesia.** The risk factors for perioperative MI are related to the underlying risk of ischemic heart disease. Before the advent of more modern management of ischemic heart disease, the risk of a second MI after anesthesia and general surgery was considered too high during the first few months post-MI (15). Current cardiologic practice, including revascularization, angioplasty, or very aggressive medical therapy with lipid-lowering agents and use of β-blockers, makes this rule less useful. **It is now commonly believed that with proper management, patients can undergo surgery 6 weeks after MI if necessary.**

Traditionally, it has been felt that coronary revascularization with coronary artery bypass surgery lowered the risk in patients with coronary artery disease (CAD) (16,17). Recent evidence, however, suggests that **only certain patients with severe CAD benefit from coronary revascularization** (significant left main stenosis, three-vessel CAD with a decreased left ventricular ejection fraction [EF < 50%], two-vessel CAD with proximal left anterior descending artery stenosis and either EF < 50% or ischemia on stress-testing, or active acute coronary syndromes such as acute MI) (6). **If none of the factors listed above are present, aggressive medical therapy, including β-blockade if appropriate, is as effective as revascularization at reducing surgical risk, including postoperative MI and long-term mortality, even in high-risk ischemic patients** (e.g., patients with significantly abnormal preoperative *dobutamine* stress echocardiograms) (18,19). Studies show that prophylactic percutaneous coronary intervention (PCI) confers no additional benefit when added to rigorous medical therapy in patients with stable CAD (stable angina) (20).

With the increasing use of PCI, elective or nonurgent surgery should be delayed for at least 14 days after balloon angioplasty. When a stent is placed, dual oral antiplatelet therapy with *aspirin* and *clopidogrel* is needed to reduce the risk of stent restenosis and stent thrombosis. Therefore, *clopidogrel* and *aspirin* therapy should be instituted following placement of a coronary stent and elective or nonurgent surgery should be delayed at least 30 days after the placement of a baremetal coronary stent, and 365 days after the placement of a drug-eluting stent. **When surgery is undertaken, perioperative *aspirin* should be continued in each of these situations** (6,21). In fact, perioperative *aspirin* therapy should be continued in all patients with previous cardiac stent placement if possible (discussed in detail below).

A postoperative MI can be painless. The risk of MI is throughout the first week, but the incidence is thought to peak on the third postoperative day. Perioperative MI is associated with significant perioperative mortality (30–50%) and reduced long-term survival (22,23), so appropriate surveillance is prudent in high-risk patients.

Electrocardiography (ECG), beginning in the immediate postoperative period and continuing at least through postoperative day 3, is prudent (24,25). Cardiac *troponin* assays are now part of the universal definition for MI. They should be monitored in high-risk patients and often can detect postoperative MI earlier than other tests (6,26–30). Because the risk of perioperative MI is increased in patients who are subjected to intraoperative hypotension, measures must be taken to maintain high-risk patients in a normotensive state during surgery. **If intraoperative hypotension occurs, the patient should be considered at high risk of postoperative MI and monitored appropriately.**

Theoretically, β-blockers would be expected to facilitate the development of intraoperative hypotension because of the additive myocardial depressive effect of these medications with general anesthesia. However, **abrupt discontinuation of β-blocker medication can be associated with a dangerous rebound syndrome (i.e., acute hypertension and coronary ischemia), with the incidence of the syndrome peaking at 4 to 7 days after discontinuation of the drug** (31,32). Patients tolerate general anesthesia in the presence of continued β-blocker treatment. All patients on chronic β-blocker therapy should continue β-blockers in the perioperative period (7). While several studies in the 1990s suggested that perioperative β-blocker use reduced postoperative nonfatal MI and mortality in many patients including those with intermediate risk, subsequent research has cast great doubt on this claim (33–35). **The largest placebo-controlled trial of perioperative β-blocker use to date (the POISE trial) showed an increase in mortality and stroke in those receiving β-blockers compared with placebo** (35). This study caused the ACC and AHA to publish a focused update in which the only definite recommendation for perioperative β-blockade was that β-blockers be continued in patients who were already receiving chronic β-blocker therapy, because ischemia can be precipitated by abrupt discontinuation (31,32). Although β-blockers may still be considered in high-risk patients with inducible ischemia, CAD, or multiple coronary risk factors (at least 3 points on the Revised Cardiac Risk Index), the ACC/AHA update emphasizes the mixed evidence and potential dangers of aggressive treatment (7).

If β-blockers are prescribed for high-risk patients, the recommended target heart rate for effective β-blockade is below 65, but not lower than 50 beats per minute. The appropriate duration of β-blockade is debated, but should certainly begin before surgery and continue throughout the hospitalization. If possible, there may be additional benefit if β-blockers can be started 1 month before surgery to titrate the heart rate, and be continued after hospitalization for at least 30 days if adequate postoperative medical follow-up can be arranged (34,36).

There is substantial evidence that perioperative statin therapy reduces cardiovascular risk in patients undergoing vascular surgery (37–39). **Statins should not be stopped abruptly in patients on chronic therapy, as there appears to be a rebound effect during which the risk of cardiovascular events increases after abrupt cessation (40). Aspirin therapy should be continued in the perioperative period in most cases where there is a risk of cardiovascular complications.** *Aspirin* discontinuation has been shown to result in an increase in adverse cardiac events occurring an average of 10 days after *aspirin* cessation (41,42). There is a theoretical increase in bleeding risk in patients taking *aspirin,* but a meta-analysis of studies comparing surgical bleeding in patients taking low-dose *aspirin* found no difference in the severity of bleeding events (with the exception of intracranial surgery and possibly transurethral prostatectomy) or mortality (42). **For most surgeries *aspirin* can be safely continued in the perioperative period.**

Congestive Heart Failure

Heart failure is associated with a poorer outcome after noncardiac surgery (1,2,5). The cause of heart failure should be identified if possible, as this may have implications concerning perioperative risk (6). It may be reasonable to perform an echocardiogram in symptomatic patients, but the utility of this is still questionable (43). Patients with moderate or severe congestive heart failure should be treated before surgery with appropriate medications to optimize their cardiovascular status. **Perioperative use of a pulmonary artery (Swan–Ganz) catheter is no longer recommended,** as studies have not shown clear benefit to these devices in managing high-risk surgical patients (44).

Arrhythmias

Cardiac arrhythmias that are hemodynamically significant or symptomatic should be treated and stabilized prior to elective or nonurgent surgery. Atrial fibrillation is the most frequently seen arrhythmia, and may require electrical or pharmacologic cardioversion. Alternatively, a rate-control strategy can be attempted with β-blockers, calcium channel blockers, or *digoxin.* Ventricular arrhythmias, such as simple premature ventricular contractions, complex ventricular ectopy, or nonsustained tachycardia usually require no therapy unless they are associated with hemodynamic compromise or occur in the presence of left ventricular dysfunction or ongoing cardiac ischemia (45,46). **Careful evaluation for underlying cardiopulmonary disease, drug toxicity, metabolic disturbances, and infection should be undertaken in patients who have any arrhythmia in the perioperative period (47).**

Conduction Disturbances

High-grade Conduction Abnormalities

Patients who do not have permanent pacemakers and who have third-degree heart block at the time of presentation are at substantial risk of cardiopulmonary arrest during surgery. Typically, they are unable to mount an appropriate pulse response to the vasodilatation and decreased myocardial contractility induced by general anesthesia, or to the volume depletion induced by surgical blood loss. Patients with high-grade conduction abnormalities, including complete heart block, may require temporary or permanent transvenous pacing.

Bifascicular Block

In patients with lower degrees of heart block, specifically bifascicular block (right heart block with left axis deviation), the risk of development of a higher degree of ventricular block during surgery is not significantly increased, provided there is no history of previous third-degree heart block or syncope. Such patients rarely require insertion of a temporary pacemaker (48). Patients with bifascicular block who have a history of third-degree heart block should be managed for complete heart block with preoperative cardiologic evaluation and likely pacemaker insertion.

A new bifascicular block developing in the setting of acute MI carries a high risk of progression to complete heart block. Therefore, if this problem occurs after surgery, the patient should be considered at significant risk for the development of complete atrioventricular block. Such patients require a cardiology consultation and insertion of a temporary pacemaker.

Pacemakers

Patients with permanently implanted pacemakers should have a preoperative pacemaker evaluation to allow examination of all pacemaker functions. This precaution ensures that backup demand pacemaker failure will not be uncovered unexpectedly with the vagotonic stimuli associated with general anesthesia in abdominal surgery. Patients with implanted defibrillators typically have their devices turned off shortly before surgery and then turned back on shortly afterward.

Even newer pacemakers and defibrillators can sense the electromagnetic impulses created by electrocautery, especially when the electrocautery plate is close to the pacemaker unit. It is prudent to place the indifferent electrocautery electrode as far as possible from the chest and to use electrocautery sparingly. An added precaution consists of keeping a magnet available in the operating room to convert a pacemaker rapidly from the demand to a fixed pacing mode. Inappropriate discharges from the implanted defibrillator are avoided by having the device turned off during the time of surgery (49). Those with permanent pacemakers should have their device assessed for proper function after surgery (6).

Endocarditis Prophylaxis

Guidelines for the prevention of infective endocarditis (IE) do not recommend administration of antibiotics solely to prevent endocarditis for patients who undergo a genitourinary (GU) or gastrointestinal (GI) tract procedure. As a result of a lack of published data demonstrating a benefit from prophylaxis, current guidelines differ substantially from previous guidelines, and far fewer patients should be recommended for IE prophylaxis than previously thought (50). Very few data exist on the risk or prevention of IE with a GI or GU tract procedure. Enterococci are part of the normal flora of the GI tract and are the primary bacteria from this area likely to cause IE. In patients with the highest risk cardiac conditions (prosthetic cardiac valve, previous IE, or congenital heart disease) who are to receive antibiotic therapy to prevent wound infection, it may be reasonable to include an antibiotic that is active against enterococci, such as penicillin, ampicillin, or vancomycin. However, no published studies demonstrate that such therapy will prevent enterococcal IE (50).

Hypertension

The significance of mild to moderate hypertension (stage 1 or 2 with systolic blood pressure below 180 mm Hg and diastolic blood pressure below 110 mm Hg) in patients undergoing surgery remains controversial. This controversy stems from the difficulty in sorting out the risk of hypertension *per se* from the risk of hypertension in the setting of hypertensive or atherosclerotic heart disease.

Numerous studies have shown that uncomplicated mild to moderate hypertension (stage 1 or 2), regardless of treatment status, is not an independent risk factor for perioperative

Table 18.5 Causes of Perioperative Hypertension

Cause	Recognition
Chronic hypertension	History, medication review
Laryngoscopy and intubation	Situation
Inadequate anesthesia	Situation
Inadequate ventilation	Arterial blood gas
Pain or anxiety	Patient examination and interview
Bladder distension	Bladder palpation
Emergence from anesthesia	Situation
Excessive fluid administration	Operating room records, patient examination
Postoperative fluid mobilization	Situation, patient examination
Acute cardiac events (e.g., congestive heart failure)	Patient examination, electrocardiogram, chest radiograph
Pheochromocytoma (rare—can be occult)	Unusual clinical responses
Malignant hyperthermia	Unusual clinical responses, fever

complications (1,2,51,52). The presence of hypertension may be of consequence, because it has been reported that patients with preoperative hypertension may demonstrate marked intraoperative blood pressure lability and postoperative hypertensive episodes (53). Certain medications used for the treatment of chronic hypertension, including angiotensin-converting enzyme (ACE) inhibitors and angiotensin II receptor antagonists (ARBs), seem to make intraoperative hypertension more likely (54,55).

It is generally agreed that **severe hypertension** (stage 3 with systolic pressure greater than 180 mm Hg, diastolic greater than 110 mm Hg) **should be controlled with effective oral medications in the days to weeks prior to undertaking an elective operation.** Another option for **severe hypertension** is the use of rapidly acting intravenous agents, which usually can bring blood pressure under control in a few hours. **One randomized trial was unable to demonstrate a benefit to delaying surgery in a select patient group with severe hypertension** (56).

The causes of perioperative hypertension are presented in Table 18.5. Patients with both hypertensive and atherosclerotic heart disease may be at greater risk than those with uncomplicated hypertension alone. As is the case for cardiac complications, the type of surgery is important in understanding the risk of hypertension. Hypotension as a result of any cause remains a concern in patients with CAD.

Hypertensive management begins with identification, followed by development of a plan for control (57). Most antihypertensive medications should be given on the morning of surgery. If tolerated by blood pressure, it is important to continue β-blockers and *clonidine* to avoid withdrawal and potential heart rate or blood pressure rebound. Because of the possible problem of intraoperative hypotension, several authors have suggested holding ACE inhibitors and ARBs on the morning of surgery (58,59). Most clinicians hold diuretics to avoid volume depletion. Although diuretic use is associated with volume depletion and hypokalemia, the importance of correcting mild degrees of diuretic-induced hypokalemia in the absence of significant heart disease is controversial (60). Potassium repletion should never be rapid, and is safest by the oral route or by adjustment of medication.

In the postoperative period, many patients, especially the elderly, need less antihypertensive medication because of the salutary effects of bed rest and relative sodium restriction. If blood pressure is not elevated, it is wise to plan on reinstating drugs stepwise, beginning with the most active agent at approximately half the usual dose and finally adding the diuretic, if used, sometime later. An exception to this would be the use of β-blockers, which, because of the concern about rebound hypertensive effects and cardiac ischemia if they are stopped abruptly, should be continued in the postoperative setting. Likewise, *clonidine* should be continued in the perioperative period to avoid rebound hypertension. Patients whose only antihypertensive drugs are *thiazide* diuretics are best observed in the immediate postoperative period. **Patients who need additional antihypertensive therapy in the immediate preoperative period should not be treated with diuretics because of the risk of associated hypovolemia and hypokalemia.**

Pulmonary

It is estimated that pulmonary complications are at least as common as cardiac complications after noncardiac surgery (61,62). Atelectasis, postoperative pneumonia, respiratory failure, and exacerbation of an underlying pulmonary condition can all develop after abdominal and pelvic surgery. Pulmonary complications are often associated with the highest costs and the longest hospital stays after surgeries (A). Clinicians should attempt to identify patients at increased risk for pulmonary complications, and reduce these risks whenever possible (Fig. 18.2).

Pulmonary Risk Factors

Pulmonary risk factors are typically grouped as "procedure related" or "patient related." For "procedure-related" risks, it has been shown that **the closer a procedure is to the diaphragm, the greater the perioperative pulmonary risks** (63). This is presumably caused by the higher likelihood of diaphragmatic dysfunction, or related postoperative pain and shallow inspiration. For this reason **upper abdominal surgeries create more postoperative risk than lower abdominal procedures**.

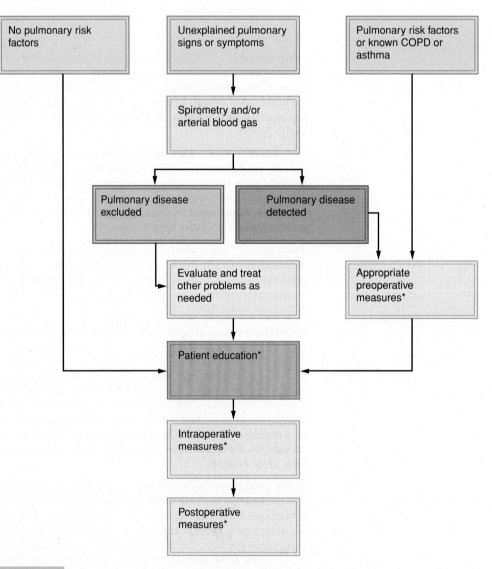

Figure 18.2 Pulmonary evaluation and postoperative care. *Measures to reduce pulmonary complications (see Table 18.6). COPD, chronic obstructive pulmonary disease.

General anesthesia, emergency surgery, and prolonged surgeries (greater than 3 hours in duration) increase the risk of postoperative pulmonary complications (63). There is some evidence that minimizing and changing to shorter-acting neuromuscular blockers during an operation can reduce postoperative pulmonary complications (64,65). Although comparative data are limited, most clinicians believe that epidural anesthesia and analgesia and the use of laparoscopic rather than open surgery should reduce postoperative pulmonary risks.

A review of multiple studies has confirmed several patient-related risk factors for postoperative pulmonary complications: advanced age; ASA (American Society of Anesthesiologists) class ≥2; heart failure; functional dependence; and chronic obstructive pulmonary disease (COPD). A serum albumin level <3.5 mg/dL and overt malnutrition were also associated with increased pulmonary complications, and current smoking seems to increase postoperative pulmonary risks (66).

Although COPD is a known risk factor for postoperative pulmonary complications, there is considerable debate about the routine use of spirometry to screen for this condition before nonthoracic surgery. The American College of Physicians (ACP) recommends spirometry only if the history and physical examination suggest an undefined lung condition (67). A history of prolonged cigarette smoking, dyspnea, chronic cough, sputum production, wheezing, or prolonged expiration and hyperinflation noted on examination would all be suggestive findings for COPD. Patients with these findings should typically receive pulmonary function testing with spirometry (and possibly a blood gas), whether an operation was intended or not.

Although COPD increases the risk of postoperative complications, it does not typically make these risks prohibitive. Even patients with severe COPD can tolerate abdominal surgery when properly prepared (68). When patients with COPD are identified before elective operations, every effort should be made to optimize their lung function and minimize any other perioperative risks.

Studies have not shown asthmatic patients to have significant risks of serious postoperative complications when managed appropriately (69). Obesity considered in isolation is not associated with increased pulmonary risks. However, many of the comorbidities often seen with obesity, such as obstructive sleep apnea, are known to increase perioperative risk (70). Sleep apnea patients are often prescribed positive pressure airway masks to assist their breathing at home during sleep. This equipment should be available in the postoperative period to assist with any apneic breathing episodes. Obese patients (and other patients with unusual upper airway anatomy) may present difficulties for intubation, and fiber optic instruments may be needed in the operating room. Pulmonary hypertension, whether associated with sleep apnea or not, is associated in some studies with increased postoperative risks in noncardiac surgery (71).

Pulmonary Risk Reduction

Physicians should attempt to reduce perioperative risks whenever possible (Table 18.6). Some identified risks (such as location of surgery, type of anesthesia, age, poor general health status, and fixed airways obstruction) cannot be improved. Smoking cessation should be encouraged. Several studies have shown increased reduction in postoperative complications (both pulmonary and nonpulmonary) with each week of smoking cessation prior to surgery (72). Patients with asthma should be optimized to their baseline pulmonary status before surgery. National guidelines recommend bringing asthmatics under "good control" prior to any elective surgery (73). This may involve bronchodilator use, inhaled steroids, and/or oral steroids.

COPD management typically involves inhaled β-agonists and anticholinergics. Noninvasive ventilation has been used successfully in postoperative patients with COPD (74). Both COPD and asthmatic patients should continue their home medications during their postoperative course. Exacerbations of either during the postoperative period can be treated with additional doses of inhaled or nebulized bronchodilators and systemic corticosteroids (oral or intravenous) if needed. For acute COPD exacerbations, antibiotics are usually indicated and have been shown to improve outcomes in patients with a change in sputum volume or purulence, and in patients who require mechanical ventilation. There is strong evidence that noninvasive ventilation helps avoid mechanical ventilation and improves outcomes and mortality in patients with severe dyspnea and clinical signs of respiratory muscle fatigue or respiratory acidosis (75).

Because low lung volumes produced by anesthesia, operative site pain, and bowel distension all contribute to respiratory dysfunction in the postoperative period, clinicians have prescribed deep-breathing exercises, intermittent positive pressure breathing (IPPB), and simple incentive

Table 18.6 Measures to Reduce Pulmonary Complications
Preoperative
Identification of patients at risk
Patient education to ensure optimal preoperative and postoperative compliance and performance
Cessation of smoking for at least 6 weeks
Instruction in incentive spirometry
Bronchodilation (e.g., β-adrenergic agonist by inhaler)
Inhaled or possibly oral steroids for asthmatics
Antibiotics for bronchitis
Control of secretions
Intraoperative
Avoidance of prolonged anesthesia (>3 hr) if possible
Possible use of regional anesthesia
Use of shorter-acting neuromuscular blockers
Maintenance of bronchodilation
Possible use of laparoscopic procedures
Postoperative
Lung expansion maneuvers: incentive spirometry. Possible use of intermittent or continuous positive pressure breathing techniques
Early ambulation
Pain control, possible use of regional analgesia
Attention to the effects of analgesia on respiration

spirometry to attempt lung expansion in the postoperative period. Although the actual value of these techniques was never carefully studied, most clinicians believe that their benefits exceed any small risks (76). Adequate pain control is important to improve deep breathing and lung expansion after abdominal surgery. **Systematic reviews emphasized more judicious use of nasogastric tubes in the postoperative period to reduce postoperative pneumonia and atelectasis** (77). Guidelines suggest that these tubes be used selectively for nausea and vomiting, inability to tolerate oral intake, or for symptomatic abdominal distension.

Diabetes Mellitus

According the Centers for Disease Control and Prevention, in 2010 diabetes mellitus affected approximately 25.6 million or 11.3% of all people 20 years of age and older. Type I diabetes is an autoimmune disease that attacks pancreatic beta cells. People with type I diabetes have a near-total lack of *insulin* as a result of pancreatic beta cell destruction and become ketoacidotic if *insulin* is withheld. Although common in juveniles, type I diabetes can occur in adults. **People with type II diabetes are not insulin deficient in an absolute sense** and are not generally prone to ketoacidosis. The problem in type II diabetes is usually one of relative *insulin* resistance. *Insulin* treatment is not limited to type I disease because **many patients with type II do require some insulin therapy**. Patients with type II diabetes are usually older and overweight. Both groups may experience the complications listed in Table 18.7. Many elderly patients have mild type II diabetes of recent onset related to obesity, are well controlled with diet or oral hypoglycemic drugs, and have few overt complications, but may have occult atherosclerotic vascular disease.

The management of diabetes begins with some understanding of the factors that influence perioperative glucose metabolism. *Insulin* **is the principal glucose-lowering hormone; cortisol, glucagon, growth hormone, and catecholamines are the principal glucose-raising hormones.** In the preoperative period, stress and the "dawn" phenomenon may elevate blood glucose. The dawn phenomenon is early morning hyperglycemia resulting from nocturnal surges of growth hormone. **During**

Table 18.7 Complications of Diabetes Mellitus

Complication	Importance
Cataracts	Decreased vision
Retinopathy	Decreased vision
Nephropathy	Nephrotic syndrome, hyperkalemia, metabolic acidosis, reduced glomerular filtration rate
Peripheral neuropathy	Decreased peripheral nociception, susceptibility to foot ulceration and subsequent infection
Autonomic neuropathy	Orthostatic hypotension, gastropathy (delayed gastric emptying, diarrhea), uropathy (urinary retention, overflow incontinence, infection), cardiorespiratory arrest
Coronary artery disease	Silent ischemia, myocardial infarction
Vascular disease	Peripheral arterial insufficiency, coronary artery disease, stroke

surgery, cortisol, epinephrine, and growth hormone levels rise. In this period, there is hyperglycemia in diabetic and nondiabetic patients alike. This is caused by glycogenolysis, inhibition of glucose uptake, and decreased insulin release. After surgery, in nondiabetic patients, the hyperglycemia is brought under control by increased endogenous insulin release over a period of 4 to 6 hours. Patients with diabetes may need additional exogenous *insulin.*

In addition to these hormonal factors, several other factors are important in modulating the blood glucose level in the perioperative period. **Inactivity, stress, and intravenous glucose infusions tend to raise blood glucose. Decreased caloric intake and semistarvation tend to lower blood glucose.** Because the net effect of these factors is sometimes difficult to anticipate, it is important to monitor blood glucose levels frequently.

Oral Hypoglycemics

There are many more oral agents being used to treat diabetes than in the past (Table 18.8). **Sulfonylureas such as *glyburide (Diabeta)* remain the most popular.** Most sulfonylureas are excreted primarily by the kidney. These drugs are typically withheld 24 to 48 hours before surgery, depending on their half-life. They can be restarted when the patient starts eating.

The biguanide *metformin (Glucophage)* is used frequently. *Metformin* should be used with extreme caution (and is frequently held) in the perioperative period and probably should be avoided altogether in systemically ill gynecologic oncology patients. There is a serious risk of lactic acidosis if renal function declines as a result of chemotherapy, dehydration, congestive heart failure, sepsis, radiologic contrast agents, or third spacing. It should not be used in patients with liver disease.

Acarbose (Precose) is a complex oligosaccharide glucosidase inhibitor that delays the digestion of ingested carbohydrates. There is little use for this drug in the perioperative period. *Repaglinide (Prandin)* is a meglitinide that stimulates release of insulin from the pancreas. It is used to cover mealtime blood sugar and may have a limited role in blood sugar management during the perioperative period. Its safe use depends on stable renal and hepatic function.

The thiazolidinedione *rosiglitazone (Avandia)* improves peripheral use of glucose by improving *insulin* sensitivity. This class of medication has a risk of fluid retention. It is not recommended for patients with NYHA class III or IV status. The use of thiazolidinediones around the perioperative period should be exercised with caution, especially in patients with cardiac disease or in those who have received more intravenous fluids during the perioperative period.

Exenatide (Byetta) is a glucagon-like peptide-1 receptor agonist that acts like an incretin mimetic agent. It enhances insulin secretion from pancreatic beta cells, suppresses glucagon secretion, and slows gastric emptying. This medication can be continued perioperatively when a patient is starting to take oral nutrition. *Liraglutide (Victoza)* is formulated as weekly injectable medication, which may not be ideal for inpatient blood sugar management.

The latest oral diabetic medication is dipeptidyl peptidase-4 (DPP-4) enzyme inhibitor, *Sitagliptin (Januvia).* DDP-4 breaks down incretin hormones. *Sitagliptin,* therefore, increases the level of incretin hormones (glucose-dependent insulinotropic polypeptide [GIP] and glucagon-like

Table 18.8 Characteristics of Oral Hypoglycemics

Agent	Brand	Dose Range (mg)	Half-life (hr)	Metabolism
Sulfonylureas				
Tolbutamide	Orinase	500–3,000	4.5–6.5	Renal
Chlorpropamide	Diabinese	100–500	36	Renal
Tolazamide	Tolinase	100–1,000	7	Renal
Glyburide	DiaBeta	2.5–30	10	Liver/renal
Glipizide	Glucotrol	5–4	2–10.3	Renal
Glimepiride	Amaryl	1–8	5–9.2	Renal/fecal
Biguanide				
Metformin	Glucophage	500–2,500	6.2	Renal
Glucosidase inhibitors				
Acarbose	Precose	75–300	2	Fecal/renal
Miglitol	Glyset	75–300	2	Renal
Meglitinides				
Repaglinide	Prandin	0.5–16	1	Fecal/renal
Nateglinide	Starlix	180–360	1.5	Renal/fecal
Thiazolidinediones				
Rosiglitazone	Avandia	4–8	3–4	Renal/fecal
Pioglitazone	Actos	15–45	16–24	Fecal/renal
Glucagon-like peptide-1				
Exenatide	Byetta	0.010–0.020	2.4	Renal
Liraglutide	Victoza	0.6–1.8	13	Fecal/renal
DDP-4 inhibitor				
Sitagliptin	Januvia	50–100	12.4	Renal
Saxagliptin	Onglyza	2.5–5	2.5	Renal/fecal
Linagliptin	Tradjenta	5	>100	Liver

DDP-4, dipeptidyl peptidase-4.

peptide-1 [GLP-1]) by inhibiting their breakdown. Incretins enhance glucose-dependent insulin secretion, glucose-dependent suppression of inappropriately high glucagon secretion, slowing of gastric emptying, reduction of food intake, and promotion of beta-cell activity. This medication is not useful during the perioperative period if patients are nil per os (NPO). Dose adjustment is needed for renal insufficiency patients.

Insulin

Insulin **is the mainstay of in-hospital management of diabetes because it is easily titrated during management.** In spite of many oral and other subcutaneous diabetic therapies, *insulin* remains an important tool in the inpatient management of diabetes. There are various types of *insulin* available for treatment of diabetes (Table 18.9). The use of different *insulin* types depends on the goals of treatment. **Long-acting** *insulins* **like** *glargine* **and** *detemir* are used to cover basal blood sugar needs. **Short-acting** *insulins* **like ultrashort-acting** *insulin* **or regular** *insulin* are used to cover mealtime blood sugar or any elevated blood sugar not covered by the basal *insulin*.

Management

Hyperglycemia is known to impair neutrophil function, wound healing, and to increase the risk of wound infection (78–83). In addition, it impairs cardiac ischemic preconditioning (a protective mechanism for ischemic insult), enhances neuronal damage following ischemia,

Table 18.9 Characteristics of Insulin				
Type of Insulin	Brand	Onset of Action	Time of Peak Effect	Duration of Action
Ultra Short Acting				
Lispro	Humulog	5–15 min	30–90 min	4–6 hrs
Aspart	Novolog	5–15 min	30–90 min	4–6 hrs
Glulisine	Apidra	5–15 min	30–90 min	4–6 hrs
Short Acting				
Regular	Humulin R Novolin R	30–60 min	2–3 hrs	8–10 hrs
Intermediate Acting				
NPH	Humulin Novolin	2–4 hrs	4–10 hrs	12–18 hrs
Long Acting				
Glargine	Lantus	2–4 hrs	No peak	20–24 hrs
Detemir	Levemir	2–4 hrs	No Peak	6–24 hrs

NPH, neutral protamine Hagedorn.

decreases nitric oxide, increases platelet activation, increases inflammatory markers, and increases reactive oxygen species, all of which have a significant impact on a patient's morbidity and mortality (84). Several studies have shown that hyperglycemic patients have a higher mortality, increased risk of infection, poorer functional recovery, more postoperative complications, and longer length of stay (85–92). **Previous studies have shown that tight glycemic control improved mortality, decreased risk of infection, and decreased length of ICU stay** (93–101). One study of critically ill surgical ICU patients showed that **tight glycemic control with blood glucose at or around 110 mg/dL reduced blood stream infections, acute renal failure (ARF) requiring dialysis, blood transfusion, length of mechanical ventilation and critical care, and in-hospital mortality** (94). Mortality at 12 months was reduced in the intensive *insulin* therapy patient (94). Subsequent studies of tight glycemic control in critically ill patients have failed to show improved mortality. Some of the studies showed increased mortality in the tighter glycemic control group and increased risk of severe hypoglycemia (95,96). In a meta-analysis of 26 trials, the pooled relative risk of death was 0.93 (95% CI 0.83 to 1.04) comparing intensive therapy to conventional therapy, and half reported hypoglycemia with a relative risk of 6 (95% CI 4.5 to 8). Surgical ICU patients appear to benefit from intensive insulin therapy with relative risk of 0.63 (9% CI 0.44 to 0.91) (97).

In light of these recent studies, **the American Association of Clinical Endocrinologists and American Diabetic Association recommend controlling preprandial blood sugar to <140 mg/dL and random blood sugar <180 mg/dL in critical care patients.** Some surgical ICU patients can have tighter blood sugar control, with preprandial blood sugar between 80 and 110 mg/dL. For noncritical care patients, the goal of preprandial blood sugar should be <140 mg/dL and random blood sugar should be <180 mg/dL (Table 18.10).

Details of the management of the diabetic patient who is taking an oral hypoglycemic agent are presented in Table 18.11. A patient with well-controlled diabetes who takes sulfonylureas is at risk of hypoglycemia if sulfonylureas are given while the caloric intake is reduced. Sulfonylureas should be held on the morning of surgery or longer if the medication has a long duration of action. **Dextrose infusion should be given to prevent any hypoglycemia.** Glucose monitoring should be performed at regular intervals to ensure that the blood sugar falls within an acceptable range. **Any hyperglycemia can be treated with supplemental *insulin*.** When oral nutrition is reinstated, sulfonylureas can be resumed. Thiazolidinediones can be continued during the perioperative period, but should not be used if the patient received excessive amounts of fluids or developed NYHA Class III or IV heart failure. Glucosidase inhibitors, meglitinides, glucagon-like peptide-1, and DDP-4 inhibitors can be resumed only when the patient is on oral nutrition. *Metformin* should not be used during the perioperative period for the reasons mentioned above.

Table 18.10 Target Goals of Inpatient Blood Glucose Control

American Association of Clinical Endocrinologists and American Diabetes Association

Critical Care Patients	
Preprandial	<140 mg/dL 80–110 mg/dL in selected surgical patients
Random	<180 mg/dL
Noncritical Care Patients	
Preprandial	<140 mg/dL
Random	<180 mg/dL

Alternatively, patients can be started on a basal-bolus *insulin* regimen perioperatively instead of resuming oral hypoglycemic medications. A patient's oral nutritional intake is often unpredictable because of postoperative nausea and vomiting. Postoperative hyperglycemia is common due to stress hormone release. Total *insulin* need is between 0.3 and 0.6 unit/kg/d depending on the patient's insulin-resistance status (102,103). Half of that *insulin* dose should be given as basal *insulin* with *glargine* or *detemir*. The other half should be divided into four doses given every 6 hours or before each meal and at bedtime, using ultra short-acting or short-acting *insulin*. Any additional hyperglycemia should be covered with supplemental *insulin* with a corrective scale. Basal *insulin* dosage can be increased daily by 10–20% if blood sugar is not controlled, or it can be decreased daily by 10–20% if the patient has episodes of hypoglycemia.

Patients on *insulin* treatment should not be on sliding scale insulin only, as that strategy produces fluctuating high and low blood sugar levels, and the blood sugar may be still inadequately controlled (102,104–106). In a randomized controlled trial comparing sliding-scale *insulin* to a basal-bolus *insulin* regimen, the latter resulted in significantly improved glycemic control, without significant risk of hypoglycemia (102).

The management of the diabetic patient who routinely takes *insulin* at home is presented in Table 18.12. **Because caloric intake is reduced on the day of surgery, total daily *insulin* dose should be reduced. Usually, half the dose of basal *insulin* is given the night before or the morning of surgery to cover endogenous glucose production.** Patients should be started on a dextrose infusion to prevent hypoglycemia. Glucose monitoring should be performed to make sure that the patient's blood sugar is within an acceptable range. Postoperatively, patients are likely to

Table 18.11 Details of Perioperative Diabetes Management for Well-Controlled Patients Taking Oral Hypoglycemics

Preoperative

1. Plan for surgery early in the day
2. Hold oral hypoglycemic on day of surgery; long-acting drugs (e.g., chlorpropamide) should be held for 48 hrs
3. Measure early AM glucose (use corrective dose insulin for glucose >140 mg/dL)

Intraoperative

4. Measure intraoperative glucose frequently (e.g., every 1 hr) and start insulin drip to keep blood glucose <140 mg/dL

Postoperative

5. Measure recovery room glucose (use corrective dose insulin for glucose <140 mg/dL)
6. Measure postoperative glucose every 6 hrs (use corrective dose insulin to keep blood glucose <140 mg/dL)
7. Return to home regimen in AM if eating adequately
8. Alternatively, consider starting basal-bolus insulin regimen if concerns about resuming oral agents

Table 18.12 Details of Perioperative Insulin Management for Well-Controlled Patients Taking Insulin

Preoperative

1. Plan for surgery early in the day
2. Measure early AM glucose (use corrective dose insulin to keep glucose <140 mg/dL)
3. Use one-half of long-acting basal insulin
4. Start D5W at 50–100 mL/hr

Intraoperative

5. Measure intraoperative glucose frequently (e.g., every 2 hrs) and make adjustments

Postoperative

6. Measure recovery room glucose (use corrective dose insulin to keep glucose <140 mg/dL)
7. Measure postoperative glucose every 6 hrs (use corrective dose insulin to keep glucose <140 mg/dL)
8. Use rapid short-acting insulin according to corrective dose scale as needed
9. Use one-half of long-acting basal insulin when NPO
10. Continue above regimen until patient begins to eat (usually next morning)
11. Return to home regimen incrementally beginning in AM if eating

D5W, dextrose in 5% water; NPO, nil per os (nothing by mouth).

have increased stress hormone levels and are on a dextrose infusion; thus, hyperglycemia is often seen despite the patient being on nil orally. Frequent blood sugar monitoring is needed for management of these hyperglycemic episodes with corrective dose *insulin*. After patients recover from the surgery and start to take oral nutrition, they can be resumed on their home *insulin* regimen. Caution should be exercised with any changes in the patient's nutritional status.

In critically ill patients or those with uncontrolled diabetes, continuous *insulin* infusion is a better strategy for glycemic control (93–101). Continuous *insulin* infusion with glucose infusion maintains normal insulin sensitivity during the perioperative period and decreases blood cortisol, glucagons, fat oxidation, and free fatty acids when compared with controls (107). An *insulin* infusion can be started at 1 unit/hr and the rate titrated by 0.5 unit/hr increments to keep blood glucose levels below 140 mg/dL. Five percent dextrose infusion with or without potassium at a rate of 50 to 100 mL/hr should be given to avoid any hypoglycemia.

Despite studies that have not shown improved mortality with tighter blood sugar control in critically ill patients, keeping the blood glucose levels below 180 mg/dL is believed to decrease infection risk and improve morbidity. Postoperative diabetic management can be difficult and many hospitals have endocrinology consultants available to assist surgical teams in managing postoperative diabetic patients with hyperglycemia.

Thyroid Disorders

Hypothyroidism

Hypothyroidism is common and may go undetected in patients being prepared for surgery (108). Symptoms include cold intolerance, recent or progressive constipation, hoarseness, fatigability, and changes in cognition. Signs include associated goiter, skin dryness, and a delayed relaxation phase of peripheral reflexes (best demonstrated in the Achilles tendon). Studies have suggested that unrecognized mild to moderate hypothyroidism is clinically important, but fears of hyponatremia, prolonged respirator dependency, hypothermia, delayed recovery from anesthesia, or death are probably unwarranted (109,110). One retrospective study suggested that such patients have more intraoperative hypotension, postoperative ileus and confusion, and that infection is less often accompanied by fever (109).

For patients who are suspected before surgery of being hypothyroid, thyroid hormone levels should be measured. **Hypothyroid patients should be treated with replacement hormone and rendered euthyroid before surgery.** In urgent situations, patients who are not myxedematous should be given 1 or 2 days of oral replacement before surgery, with careful postoperative follow-up (111–113).

Hyperthyroidism

Hyperthyroidism can be a dramatic illness, with tachycardia, fever, and exophthalmos associated with goiter. Other common symptoms and signs include weight loss, fatigue, diarrhea, heat intolerance, tremor, hyperreflexia, and muscle weakness. **Hyperthyroidism may be occult in older patients.** Unexplained tachycardia, weight loss, arrhythmias, or fever may be the only clinical indicators and should always raise suspicions of unrecognized hyperthyroidism in surgical patients. With proper preparation, hyperthyroid patients undergoing thyroid surgery do well (114). There are scant data concerning the problems of the hyperthyroid patient undergoing nonthyroidal surgery, such as radical hysterectomy. Exacerbation of the illness into a "thyroid storm" is the usual concern. Because of this, **when any patient is suspected before surgery of being hyperthyroid, thyroid hormone levels should be measured. If the diagnosis is confirmed, elective surgery should be delayed until treatment has produced a euthyroid state** (113,115). In the postoperative period, thyroid hormone levels should be measured when any patient has persistent unexplained tachycardia, fever, or tachyarrhythmias.

Corticosteroids

Patients taking corticosteroids or those who took them in the recent past should be evaluated for the need of supplemental corticosteroid coverage. Patients taking less than the equivalent of 5-mg *prednisone* **daily should not have adrenal suppression** (116–118). There is variability between patients in their response to suppression of the hypothalamic–pituitary–adrenal (HPA) axis by exogenous steroid. In a prospective cohort study, 75 patients were given short-term, high-dose glucocorticoid treatment of at least 25 mg *prednisone* daily for 5 to 30 days (119). Forty-five percent of the patients experienced HPA suppression. Of those patients, the majority recovered within 14 days. However, a couple of patients remained suppressed at 3 and 6 months.

In a retrospective study, 279 patients were taking *prednisone* or its equivalent steroid at doses of 5 to 30 mg/d for between 1 week and 15 years (120). Human corticotropin-releasing hormone (CRH) was used to assess HPA suppression. **There was a trend toward an inverse correlation between dosage and duration of therapy and the plasma cortisol response to CRH.** There were numerous patients taking high-dose steroids for more than 100 weeks who still had an intact HPA axis. Despite this variability, **suppression of the HPA axis should be anticipated in patients taking more than 25 mg of** *hydrocortisone,* **5 mg of** *prednisone,* **or 0.75 mg** *dexamethasone* **per day for more than 3 weeks** (121).

To further clarify whether patients on chronic steroids have suppressed HPA axis, a **cortrosyn (ACTH) stimulation test** can be performed. Baseline cortisol and ACTH levels should be obtained, then 250 µg of ACTH is given intramuscularly or intravenously. A cortisol level is obtained 30 minutes after ACTH is given. If the stimulated cortisol level does not rise above 18 µg/mL, the patient is suspected of having a suppressed HPA axis and stress dose steroid should be given perioperatively (119,122–124). In addition to an abnormal ACTH stimulation test, patients who have findings of Cushing syndrome or findings of adrenocortical insufficiency such as hypotension, hyponatremia, or hyperkalemia should be considered for stress dose steroids perioperatively.

Corticosteroid supplementation for patients suspected of adrenal suppression will depend on the type of surgery performed. Patients having minor surgeries like hernia repair or colonoscopy should be able to take their usual dose of oral steroid on the day of surgery without additional supplementation. Patients undergoing moderate surgical stress, such as hysterectomy, should take their usual steroid dose on the morning of the surgery and be supplemented with 50 mg intravenous *hydrocortisone* on call to surgery, followed by 25 mg intravenously every 8 hours for three doses. They should resume their usual oral steroids the following morning. Patients undergoing major surgery, such as primary cytoreduction for advanced ovarian cancer, should take their usual steroid dose on the morning of surgery and be supplemented with 100 mg intravenous *hydrocortisone* on call to surgery, followed by 50 mg intravenously every 8 hours, tapering the dose by half each day over the next 24 to 48 hours. The patient can resume oral steroids in the morning after tapered off intravenous stress dose hydrocortisone (125,126). For those patients who continue to not be able to take oral medications, equivalent dose of intravenous hydrocortisone should be given in the mornings.

Thromboembolic Disease Prevention

Almost all hospitalized patients are at risk for venous thromboembolism (VTE) and should receive some type of prophylaxis to reduce these adverse events. Surgical patients, in particular, are at increased risk for deep venous thrombosis (DVT) and associated pulmonary embolism (PE) related to immobility and the operative stimulation of the coagulation cascade. One older analysis of historical data suggested that nearly a third of hospitalized surgical patients might develop VTE, and perhaps 1% may develop fatal PE if no prophylaxis was given (127). More recent data collected by the American Heart Association suggest that up to two million Americans will develop a DVT each year, with almost one-third of them also developing a PE, resulting in 60,000 deaths annually (128).

Although young, ambulatory patients without additional risks who undergo short (<30 minutes) surgeries may not need specific interventions other than early mobilization, almost all other postoperative patients should receive some type of thromboprophylaxis. Gynecologic surgical patients known to be at particularly high risk include those with malignant disease; those undergoing open abdominal (vs. vaginal or laparoscopic) surgery; elderly patients; and those who have had previous venous thrombotic events. A more complete list of risk factors for venous thromboembolic disease in hospitalized patients is shown in Table 18.13.

Preventive therapy for venous thrombosis in the setting of gynecologic surgery **includes graded compression stockings and mechanical compression devices** placed on the lower extremities, and various subcutaneous anticoagulation regimens with **unfractionated *heparin*, low molecular weight *heparins*, and newer agents such as *fondaparinux*.** Higher doses of the latter agents may have associated risks for postoperative bleeding.

There are conflicting reports on the relative protective benefits of each of these treatments. **At least one randomized trial showed that proper use of compression stockings may be as effective as subcutaneous *heparin* in major surgeries for gynecologic malignancies** (129). Other trials have suggested that higher doses of subcutaneous unfractionated *heparin* (three times a day) or low molecular weight heparin may be more protective than lower doses of unfractionated heparin, especially in cases of malignancy (130). Some surgeons have advocated the use of pneumatic compression devices and subcutaneous anticoagulants in their highest risk patients, although there are no clear data that these treatments are additive in effectiveness in gynecology patients.

Thromboprophylaxis in hospitalized patients is typically continued at least until hospital discharge. **One study of patients with gynecologic malignancies undergoing open abdominal surgery**

Table 18.13 Factors Related to Increased Risk of Thromboembolic Disease
Inherited disorders (e.g., deficiency of antithrombin III, Factor C or S, or the Factor V Leiden Mutation)
Acquired or inherited thrombophillia
Nephrotic syndrome
Paroxysmal nocturnal hemoglobinuria
Cancer
Stasis (e.g., congestive heart failure)
Age > 40 yrs
Estrogen therapy
Sepsis
Bed rest
Trauma
Stroke and/or lower extremity paralysis
Myeloproliferative disorder
Inflammatory bowel disease
Obesity
Prior thromboembolism
Central venous catheter
Erythropoiesis stimulating agents
Pregnancy and the postpartum period

Table 18.14 Recommendations for Venous Thromboembolic Prophylaxis in Gynecologic Surgery: Ninth (2012) American College of Chest Physicians Guidelines for Antithrombotic Therapy for Prevention and Treatment of Thrombosis

1. For general and abdominal–pelvic surgery patients at very low risk for VTE, we recommend that no specific pharmacologic (Grade 1B) or mechanical (Grade 2C) prophylaxis be used other than early ambulation.

2. For general and abdominal–pelvic surgery patients at low risk for VTE, we suggest mechanical prophylaxis, preferably with IPC, over no prophylaxis (Grade 2C).

3. For general and abdominal–pelvic surgery patients at moderate risk for VTE who are not at high risk for major bleeding complications, we suggest LMWH (Grade 2B), LDUH (Grade 2B), or mechanical prophylaxis, preferably with IPC (Grade 2 C), over no prophylaxis.

4. For general and abdominal–pelvic surgery patients at moderate risk for VTE who are at high risk for major bleeding complications or those in whom the consequences of bleeding are thought to be particularly severe, we suggest mechanical prophylaxis, preferably with IPC, over no prophylaxis (Grade 2C).

5. For general and abdominal–pelvic surgery patients at high risk for VTE who are not at high risk for major bleeding complications, we recommend pharmacologic prophylaxis with LMWH (Grade1B) or LDUH (Grade 1B) over no prophylaxis. We suggest that mechanical prophylaxis with ES or IPC should be added to pharmacologic prophylaxis (Grade 2C) .

6. For high-VTE-risk patients undergoing abdominal or pelvic surgery for cancer who are not otherwise at high risk for major bleeding complications, we recommend extended-duration pharmacologic prophylaxis (4 wks) with LMWH over limited-duration prophylaxis (Grade 1B).

7. For high-VTE-risk general and abdominal pelvic surgery patients who are at high risk for major bleeding complications or those in whom the consequences of bleeding are thought to be particularly severe, we suggest use of mechanical prophylaxis, preferably with IPC, over no prophylaxis until the risk of bleeding diminishes and pharmacologic prophylaxis may be initiated (Grade 2C).

8. For general and abdominal–pelvic surgery patients at high risk for VTE in whom both LMWH and unfractionated heparin are contraindicated or unavailable and who are not at high risk for major bleeding complications, we suggest low-dose aspirin (Grade 2C), fondaparinux (Grade 2C), or mechanical prophylaxis, preferably with IPC (Grade 2C), over no prophylaxis.

9. For general and abdominal–pelvic surgery patients, we suggest that an IVC filter should not be used for primary VTE prevention (Grade 2C).

10. For general and abdominal–pelvic surgery patients, we suggest that periodic surveillance with VCU should not be performed (Grade 2C).

VTE, venous thromboembolism; IPC, intermittent pneumatic compression; LMWH, low molecular weight heparin; LDUH, low-dose unfractionated heparin; VCU, venous compression ultrasonography.

Evidence Grades: 1A, Strong Recommendation, High Quality Evidence; 1B, Strong Recommendation, Moderate Quality Evidence; 1C, Strong Recommendation, Low Quality Evidence; 2C, Weak Recommendation, Low Quality Evidence.

Sources: **Gould MK, Garcia DA, Wren SM, et al.; American College of Chest Physicians.** Prevention of VTE in Nonorthopedic Surgical Patients Antithrombotic Therapy and Prevention of Thrombosis. 9th ed. American College of Chest Physicians. Evidence-Based Clinical Practice Guidelines. *Chest.* 2012;141:e227S–e277S; **Guyatt GH, Norris SL, Schulman S, et al.** Methodology for the Development of Antithrombotic Therapy and Prevention of Thrombosis Guidelines Methodology for the Guidelines: Antithrombotic Therapy and Prevention of Thrombosis. 9th ed. American College of Chest Physicians Evidence-Based Clinical Practice Guidelines *Chest.* 2012;141:53S–70S.

has suggested that 4 weeks of postoperative prophylaxis is cost-effective, and improves patient outcomes (131). Additional studies are needed to determine optimal length of VTE prophylaxis in high-risk populations.

A recent consensus statement summarizes recommendations for prevention of VTE in postoperative gynecologic patients (Table 18.14).

Preoperative Testing

The question of how much preoperative laboratory testing is warranted is the subject of considerable interest and debate (132,133). Two randomized trials on patients undergoing cataract surgery, and one randomized trial on ambulatory surgical patients that included orthopedic, general, plastic, ophthalmologic, urologic, spinal, and neurosurgical patients showed no difference in adverse events between patients with and without preoperative laboratory testing (134–136). A recent review of the effectiveness of preoperative testing in noncardiac elective surgical patients has revealed a scarcity of evidence supporting preoperative testing, but has suggested that testing based on pathologic findings in a patient's medical history and physical examination would be prudent (137). Many previous studies have demonstrated that unless clinical indicators are

Table 18.15 Surgical Grade	
	Example
Grade 1 (minor)	Excision of skin, drainage of breast abscess
Grade 2 (intermediate)	Primary repair of inguinal hernia, knee arthroscopy, tonsillectomy/ adenoidectomy, varicose vein stripping
Grade 3 (major)	Total abdominal hysterectomy, thyroidectomy, lumbar surgery, endoscopic resection of prostate
Grade 4 (major+)	Joint replacement, lung resection, radical neck surgery, colonic resection
Neurosurgery	—
Cardiovascular surgery	—

Adapted from http://www.nice.org.uk/Guidance/CG3/Guidance/pdf/English.

present, preoperative test results will usually be normal, falsely positive, or truly positive with no significant clinical outcome on perioperative complications (136,138–142).

The National Institute for Clinical Excellence of the United Kingdom developed guidelines in 2003 in an attempt to give some directions for clinicians on preoperative testing for elective surgery. The guidelines incorporated as much evidence as possible, but the evidence base is often lacking, so recommendations are frequently based on experts' opinions and consensus (143). These guidelines categorize patients by age; surgical grade (minor, intermediate, major, major+); anesthetic grade as per American Society of Anesthesiologists (ASA); and comorbidity (cardiac, respiratory, and renal) (Tables 18.15 and 18.16). Preoperative test recommendations cover chest x-ray, complete blood count, electrocardiogram (ECG), coagulation studies, blood chemistry, renal function tests, blood glucose, urine analysis, blood gases, and lung function tests. The complete guidelines are available online (143).

Patients who are under 40 years, healthy, and undergoing minor surgery generally do not need any preoperative testing. Gynecologic oncology patients are at least Surgical Grade 3— major surgery. Such patients often have clinical indicators that support additional testing, particularly when they are 60 years or older, have higher ASA Class, and/or multiple comorbidities. A preoperative ECG should be obtained on all women over 60 years, or younger if the patient has cardiac disease. A complete blood count and chemistries are recommended. Glucose level is not recommended by the guidelines in many patients, but is usually warranted to exclude diabetes because of the increased morbidity and mortality associated with inpatient hyperglycemia. Chest x-ray is generally not recommended, but can be considered if the patient has respiratory symptoms or an abnormal chest examination. Urinalysis should be considered in all gynecologic patients. Coagulation studies are not recommended in the majority of the patients, except for those patients with hepatic comorbidity or cardiac comorbidity in ASA Class 3 status. For those patients with metastatic liver cancer or who are significantly malnourished, coagulation studies prior to surgery are reasonable. Blood gases can be considered in patients with multiple comorbidities. Pulmonary function tests are not recommended for gynecologic patients even if they have respiratory comorbidity (Tables 18.17–18.19).

The guidelines on preoperative testing are a general roadmap for the clinician. Combining the patient's medical conditions and symptoms with the guidelines will provide a more focused approach to preoperative testing.

Table 18.16 American Society of Anesthesiologists (ASA) Class	
ASA Class 1	Healthy patient without clinical comorbidity or medical conditions
ASA Class 2	Patients with mild systemic disease
ASA Class 3	Patients with severe systemic disease
ASA Class 4	Patients with severe systemic disease that is constant threat to life

Adapted from http://www.nice.org.uk/Guidance/CG3/Guidance/pdf/English.

	Age (yrs)			
	≥16 to <40	≥40 to <60	≥60 to <80	≥80
Test	**ASA Class 2 with cardiovascular disease**			
Chest x-ray	C	C	C	C
ECG	Y	Y	Y	Y
CBC	Y	Y	Y	Y
Coagulation	N	N	N	N
Renal function	Y	Y	Y	Y
Glucose	N	N	N	N
Urine analysis	C	C	C	C
Blood gas	C	C	C	C
PFT	N	N	N	N
	ASA Class 3 with cardiovascular disease			
Chest x-ray	C	C	C	C
ECG	Y	Y	Y	Y
CBC	Y	Y	Y	Y
Coagulation	C	C	C	C
Renal function	Y	Y	Y	Y
Glucose	N	N	N	N
Urine analysis	C	C	C	C
Blood gas	C	C	C	C
PFT	N	N	N	N

Table 18.17 Grade 3 Surgery (Major) with Cardiovascular Disease

ASA, American Society of Anesthesiologists; C, Considered; ECG, electrocardiogram; Y, Yes; CBC, complete blood count; N, No; PFT, pulmonary function test.

Adapted from http://www.nice.org.uk/Guidance/CG3/Guidance/pdf/English.

Screening for Hemostatic Defects

A good history and physical examination are most helpful in screening patients for hemostatic defects before operations. Some of the most important information involves the outcome of prior hemostatic stress and the family history. Minor surgical procedures should not have required transfusion, and a history of postoperative bleeding 2 or 3 days after surgery is also suspicious. Many patients have had tooth extractions. Bleeding should not last more than 24 hours and should not start again after stopping. **A familial history of bleeding or suspected bleeding should be investigated.** Patients should be questioned about nosebleeds, intestinal bleeding, and heavy menstrual bleeding. Large ecchymosis and mucosal bleeding on examination can be a cause for concern.

Studies suggest that screening for hemostatic defects has no benefit in patients without a history of oral anticoagulation use or significant liver disease that impairs the liver's ability to synthesize coagulation factors, even in neurological patients (144–146). Despite the lack of evidence, coagulation screening tests are still frequently ordered preoperatively. **A platelet count, INR (international normalized ratio), and PTT (partial thromboplastin time) are the most commonly ordered tests for this purpose.** A low platelet count can be caused by decreased production, sequestration into the spleen, or increased destruction. For platelet counts less than 100,000/cc, platelet transfusions may be necessary before the operation, depending on additional risks. Certain commonly prescribed drugs (such as *aspirin* and nonsteroidal anti-inflammatory drugs [NSAIDs]) can inhibit platelet function and should be held for a week before the operation if possible. As stated previously, low-dose *aspirin* therapy should be continued in many patients with cardiovascular disease, and communication between the primary care physician and surgeon is essential in weighing the risks of adverse cardiac events and bleeding. Renal dysfunction is another common cause of acquired platelet dysfunction.

Table 18.18 Grade 3 Surgery (Major) with Respiratory Disease			
	Age (yrs)		
	≥16 to <40	≥40 to <60	≥60 to <80	≥80

Test	ASA Class 2 with respiratory disease			
Chest x-ray	C	C	C	C
ECG	C	C	C	Y
CBC	Y	Y	Y	Y
Coagulation	N	N	N	N
Renal function	C	C	Y	Y
Glucose	N	N	N	N
Urine analysis	C	C	C	C
Blood gas	C	C	C	C
PFT	N	C	C	C
Test	**ASA Class 3 with respiratory disease**			
Chest x-ray	C	C	C	C
ECG	C	C	Y	Y
CBC	Y	Y	Y	Y
Coagulation	C	C	C	C
Renal function	Y	Y	Y	Y
Glucose	C	C	C	C
Urine analysis	C	C	C	C
Blood gas	C	C	C	C
PFT	C	C	C	C

ASA, American Society of Anesthesiologists; C, Considered; ECG, electrocardiogram; Y, Yes; CBC, complete blood count; N, No; PFT, pulmonary function test.

Adapted from http://www.nice.org.uk/Guidance/CG3/Guidance/pdf/English.

Elevated INR and PTT values reflect blood coagulation protein deficiencies or inhibitors. Patients with elevated values may require plasma factor replacement before surgery to minimize their bleeding risks, and further hematologic testing is warranted to identify the specific deficiency or inhibitor.

There are some patients with normal screening laboratory tests who have suggestive histories or examinations for hemostatic defects. One possible culprit might be **Von Willebrand disease—an inheritable coagulation defect in platelet function and the most common hereditary bleeding disorder.** Identification and perioperative management of this and other more uncommon bleeding disorders may require further laboratory testing and the expertise of a hematologist (147).

Perioperative Antibiotics for Wound Infection Prophylaxis

A dose of intravenous antibiotics such as *vancomycin, cefazolin,* or *cefotetan* should be given within 1 hour of incision to decrease the risk of surgical site infections (148). Additional doses can be given at intervals of one or two times the half-life of the drug if there is extended surgery. If bowel resection is anticipated, mechanical bowel preparation on the day before surgery has been the traditional practice. More recent studies have shown no difference in infection or postoperative complication rates among patients with or without a mechanical bowel preparation (149,150), and a recent clinical practice guideline has recommended omission of mechanical bowel preparation for patients undergoing elective colorectal surgery (151).

Table 18.19 Grade 3 Surgery (Major) with Renal Disease				
	Age (yrs)			
	≥16 to <40	≥40 to <60	≥60 to <80	≥80
Test	**ASA Class 2 with renal disease**			
Chest x-ray	C	C	C	C
ECG	C	C	Y	Y
CBC	Y	Y	Y	Y
Coagulation	C	C	C	C
Renal function	Y	Y	Y	Y
Glucose	C	C	C	C
Urine analysis	C	C	C	C
Blood gas	C	C	C	C
PFT	N	N	N	N
	ASA Class 3 with renal disease			
Chest X-ray	C	C	C	C
ECG	C	C	Y	Y
CBC	Y	Y	Y	Y
Coagulation	C	C	C	C
Renal function	Y	Y	Y	Y
Glucose	C	C	C	C
Urine analysis	C	C	C	C
Blood gas	C	C	C	C
PFT	N	N	N	N

ASA, American Society of Anesthesiologists; C, Considered; ECG, electrocardiogram; Y, Yes; CBC, complete blood count; PFT, pulmonary function test; N, No.

Adapted from http://www.nice.org.uk/Guidance/CG3/Guidance/pdf/English.

Postoperative Management

Cardiovascular

Hypertension

High blood pressure, both labile and persistent, is a common problem for acutely ill patients. Perioperative hypertensive episodes occur commonly in hypertensive patients and occasionally in normotensive patients because of pain, anxiety, stress, medications, and other factors (Table 18.5). **Perioperative hypertension is most common during laryngoscopy and induction (primarily because of sympathetic stimulation) and immediately after surgery,** often in the recovery room.

Patients with pre-existing hypertension usually require some continuation of their daily antihypertensive medication when they are brought into the hospital or are critically ill, but the dosages may need titration and diuretic use for blood pressure control is infrequent. Many agents can be converted to an intravenous form or administered with minimal fluid down a gastric tube if the patient is not eating or drinking. The use of β-blockers as antihypertensives in the acute care setting may have additional benefits by decreasing the risks of atrial fibrillation and myocardial ischemia in vulnerable patients, and these agents are often selected as first-line agents for this reason. Some studies suggested that routine use of these agents might decrease cardiovascular mortality after noncardiac surgery in patients at risk (152). At the minimum, care should be taken that β-blockers are not discontinued suddenly, as this can cause rebound hypertension and associated problems. Sublingual, short-acting calcium channel blockers (e.g., *nifedipine*) should be avoided because their use can lead to reflex tachycardia and myocardial ischemia.

Corticosteroid medications can cause hypertension in susceptible patients. Mild antihypertensive medication may be necessary until the steroid dose is lowered or discontinued.

Many hypertensive episodes resolve spontaneously. **Patients with pain and anxiety are best treated with appropriate analgesics and anxiolytics.** When evaluating the hypertensive postoperative patient, adequacy of ventilation and stable cardiac status should be verified by examination, arterial blood gases, and ECG. **Bladder distension may cause elevated blood pressure and should be relieved. A patient may require a continuous intravenous infusion to control severe hypertension. Intravenous drugs with short half-lives should be chosen to allow safe titration** (the vasodilator *nitroprusside* or short-acting β-blockers are two popular choices) and the patient should be changed to longer-acting agents as their condition stabilizes (153).

Myocardial Injury and Ischemia

Patients undergoing oncologic treatment may have underlying coronary artery disease (CAD). The variable stresses in the postoperative period, such as inflammation, increased hypercoagulable state, and hypoxemia, can lead to myocardial injury or ischemia. One study of unselected patients aged over 50 years undergoing noncardiac surgery showed that the risk of postoperative cardiac events was nearly 1.5% (5). **Most postoperative MIs occur during the first 3 days, at a time when patients may be receiving narcotics that may mask the symptoms of ischemia.**

Patients experiencing postoperative MI have an increased risk of hospital mortality. These patients need to be managed promptly by a surgeon and a consulting cardiologist, and observed closely in a monitored bed for any complicating features such as arrhythmia, pulmonary edema, and shock. **In addition to correcting anemia, hypoxia, and starting β-blockers in those that can tolerate them, the treatment of such acute coronary syndromes involves the use of anticoagulants such as *aspirin* and *heparin*.** The use of these agents must be balanced against the risk of postoperative bleeding. MIs are typically divided into ST segment or non-ST segment elevation injuries, depending on the ECG appearance. MI patients with ST elevation or with hemodynamic instability have improved outcomes if they can receive rapid angiography and angioplasty, while those in a stable condition with non-ST segment elevations can often be managed medically (at least initially). Unless contraindicated, **all patients with postoperative MI should be on *aspirin*, β-blockers, HMG co A reductase inhibitors, and ACE inhibitors by the time of discharge** (154).

Arrhythmia

Every physician working in an acute care hospital should be familiar with the use of a defibrillator and the algorithms developed by the American Heart Association for Advanced Life Support (155). Fluid shifts, electrolyte changes, and myocardial ischemia can put the patient receiving treatment for gynecologic malignancy at increased risk for heart rhythm abnormalities.

The tachyarrhythmias, both ventricular and supraventricular, can be quite dangerous and should be electrically cardioverted immediately if the blood pressure is low, or the patient is unstable. In less urgent situations, a variety of antiarrhythmic medications are available for chemical conversion and stabilization. Many of these medications are proarrhythmic as well, and a search for an underlying cause of the rhythm disturbance is indicated to reduce the propensity for recurrence. **Often, when the electrolyte imbalance or other precipitant has been corrected, the heart rhythm normalizes, and these agents can be discontinued. Persistent or unstable ventricular arrhythmias are often managed in the acute setting with intravenous *amiodarone*. Supraventricular tachycardias** may respond to vagal maneuvers or a rapid bolus of *adenosine*.

Atrial fibrillation is the most common postoperative tachyarrhythmia and deserves special mention. After the blood pressure is stabilized in a patient with atrial fibrillation, attempts should be made to control the heart rate. **Popular drugs for rate control include β-blockers** (if left ventricular function is preserved), *diltiazem,* or *digoxin*. If the rhythm persists after other precipitants are corrected (e.g., hypokalemia, hypoxemia, fluid overload), many clinicians would attempt chemical or electrical conversion if the atrial fibrillation has not been present more than 48 hours. Restoration of normal sinus rhythm often improves cardiac output (CO), and mitigates the risk of stroke from left atrial thrombus formation in the fibrillating chamber. **Patients with atrial fibrillation lasting longer than a few days and who have no contraindication should be considered for anticoagulation, to decrease their risk of a stroke** (156).

Bradyarrhythmias often arise from excessive vagal stimulation. Nausea, bladder distension, pain, and endotracheal tube manipulation can all stimulate excessive vagal tone. As with tachyarrhythmias, attention to blood pressure is paramount. **Those patients who develop hypotension should receive *atropine* and catecholamines. Patients not responding to these agents may need urgent transvenous pacemaker placement.** Transcutaneous pacing can be attempted if available at the bedside.

Shock

Shock is defined as a clinical syndrome in which the patient shows signs of decreased perfusion of vital organs. Typical findings include alterations in mental status, cold and clammy skin, oliguria, and metabolic acidosis. Patients with shock have a substantial decrease in blood pressure, but no absolute value is used to define shock.

The therapeutic approach to these patients is facilitated by a functional classification of shock states. Each class of shock has its own pathophysiologic process, and requires a different management strategy. **Traditionally, four varieties of shock have been described:**

1. **Hypovolemic shock**—secondary to fluid losses and decreased cardiac filling pressures (e.g., postoperative bleeding or intravascular fluid redistribution).
2. **Distributive shock**—secondary to inappropriate "vasodilation" and venous pooling (e.g., sepsis syndrome, anaphylaxis, decreased vasomotor tone from spinal anesthesia, and adrenal insufficiency from steroid withdrawal).
3. **Cardiogenic shock**—secondary to decreased myocardial contractility and function (e.g., acute MI or ischemia, or congestive cardiac failure).
4. **Obstructive shock**—secondary to mechanical obstructions in the cardiovascular circuit (e.g., PE, cardiac tamponade).

Common causes of shock in the perioperative management of gynecologic malignancy include the following:

1. **Hemorrhage (hypovolemic)**
2. **Sepsis (distributive)**
3. **Postoperative MI (cardiogenic)**
4. **Pulmonary embolus (obstructive)**

A careful physical examination, review of laboratory and test results, and consideration of the clinical situation often suggests the etiology of a particular shock syndrome. Therapy should begin promptly, as information is being gathered. In the past, invasive hemodynamic monitoring with pulmonary artery catheters was often used to diagnose and manage these conditions. This has declined significantly as studies have shown no clear benefit to their use (157).

Regardless of whether measured directly with a pulmonary catheter, or deduced from less invasive data, each of the shock states has an expected hemodynamic profile. Therapy is targeted to the underlying defect in cardiovascular performance:

1. **Hypovolemic shock** is treated with crystalloid or colloid infusion to increase cardiac filling and CO and perfusion to vital organs. There is no clear evidence that colloids have any benefits over crystalloids for this purpose (158). Hypovolemic shock is the most common form of shock in the surgical patient, and treatment of the hypotensive, oliguric patient typically begins with a "fluid trial."
2. **Distributive shock** often requires vasopressor management with catecholamines active at the alpha receptors on the vasculature. This helps restore adequate resistance to create a perfusing blood pressure. Equally important is to commence treatment of the presumed cause of the vasodilation: Prompt antibiotics and source control for cases of suspected sepsis, steroids if secondary adrenal insufficiency is a possibility, or withdrawal of the offending agent and anti-inflammatory treatment if an allergic reaction is suspected. There are published guidelines for the treatment of septic shock (159).
3. **Cardiogenic shock** is characterized by inadequate CO, such that inotropic management with catecholamine and dopaminergic compounds is often necessary to maintain adequate contractility. Vasodilator therapy can be helpful in cardiogenic shock because it unburdens the failing heart's afterload. This allows contractility to improve without excessive cardiac work, which might exacerbate myocardial ischemia.

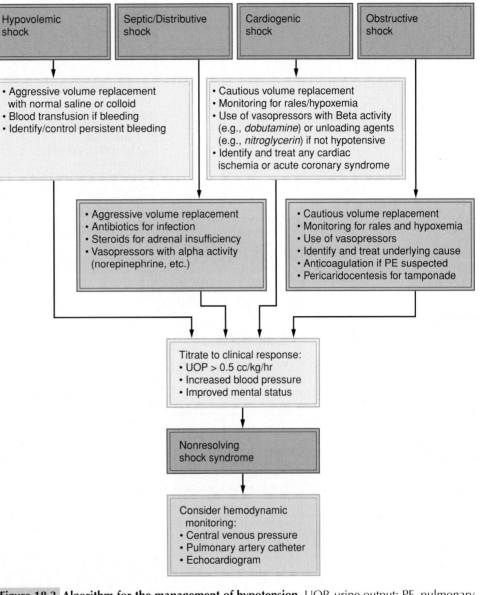

Figure 18.3 **Algorithm for the management of hypotension.** UOP, urine output; PE, pulmonary embolism.

4. **Obstructive shock** can be difficult to manage and might require a combination of measures to maintain adequate filling pressures and contractility. Like distributive shock, it is important to attempt reversal of the precipitant quickly (e.g., anticoagulation for PE, pericardiocentesis for tamponade) because the patient's ultimate outcome depends on this.

An algorithm for the management of shock syndromes is shown in Figure 18.3, and critically ill patients may often develop mixed shock states.

Respiratory Failure

Respiratory failure can be defined as a failure of gas exchange, that is, failure of the respiratory system to accomplish the exchange of oxygen and carbon dioxide between ambient air and red blood cells in amounts required to meet the body's metabolic needs. **Respiratory syndromes characterized by difficulty in oxygenation of the blood are grouped under the umbrella term, hypoxic respiratory failure and those with difficulty removing carbon dioxide from the blood are described as ventilatory failure.** It is often helpful for assessment and therapy to consider these as separate entities, although in reality they are closely connected. The arterial blood gas is used to determine the degree and type of gas exchange failure, and should be performed as part of the initial evaluation. Patients with respiratory failure commonly have abnormal mental status

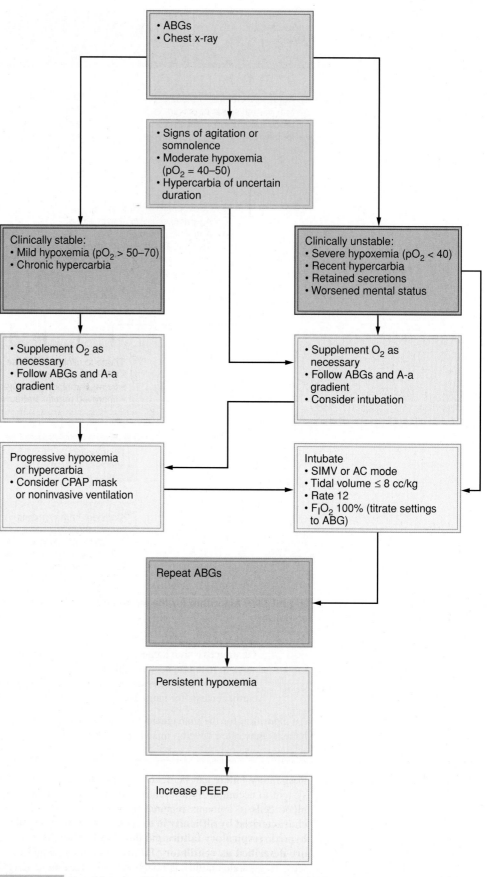

Figure 18.4 Algorithm for the management of respiratory failure. ABG, arterial blood gases; CPAP, continuous positive airway pressure; PEEP, positive end-expiratory pressure; SIMV, synchronized intermittent mandatory ventilation; AC, assist control; F₁O₂, fraction of inspired oxygen; A-a gradient, alveolar-arterial gradient.

(agitation, somnolence, and disorientation) and physical findings may include tachycardia, hypertension, and occasionally cyanosis and sweating (Fig. 18.4).

Common causes of respiratory failure in the perioperative management of gynecologic cancer patients include the following:

1. **Nervous system depression secondary to sedative or analgesic medications**
2. **Bronchospasm**
3. **Pneumonia**
4. **Pulmonary edema**
5. **Lymphangitic spread of cancer**
6. **Respiratory muscle weakness**

Hypoxic Respiratory Failure

Hypoxic respiratory failure is usually caused by a mismatch between inhaled gas and blood circulation in the lung parenchyma. Blood circulating in areas of mismatch is relatively deoxygenated. **The degree of hypoxic respiratory failure can be characterized by the alveolar-arterial oxygen gradient. This "gradient" is the difference between the alveolar and arterial concentrations of oxygen.**

The arterial blood oxygen concentration is directly measured on blood gas. The alveolar oxygen concentration is calculated by a formula accounting for the fraction of oxygen in inspired air (adjusted for any oxygen supplementation, barometric pressure and water vapor pressure) and the amount of carbon dioxide expected in the alveolar gas (adjusted for the carbon dioxide concentration in the blood measured on blood gas and the expected exchange into the alveolus to maintain metabolic processes).

This formula is called the **"alveolar gas equation"**:

$$\text{Alveolar } PO_2 = [FiO_2 \times (\text{barometric pressure} - \text{water pressure*})] - [(PaCO_2 \text{ arterial}) \times 1.25]$$

*713 mm Hg at sea level.

This calculation will vary depending on altitude, oxygen supplementation, and the CO_2 concentration in the blood. As an example: at sea level and on no oxygen supplementation, and with a normal CO_2 concentration on blood gas ($pCO_2 = 40$ mm Hg) this calculation gives an alveolar oxygen concentration of 100 mm Hg.

The measured arterial concentration of oxygen on blood gas would then be subtracted from this calculated value of the **alveolar oxygen concentration**:

$$\text{Alveolar} - \text{arterial gradient} = \text{alveolar } PO_2 - \text{arterial } PO_2$$

The alveolar-arterial difference in oxygen concentration increases with age, but typically does not exceed 20 mm Hg. A gradient wider than 20 mm Hg is the hallmark of hypoxic respiratory failure.

Treatment of hypoxic respiratory failure involves improving oxygenation of arterial blood, and attempting correction of the underlying mismatch in lung function. **Interventions to improve oxygenation include supplemental oxygen by nasal cannula or mask, or by positive-pressure breathing for refractory hypoxemia.** Positive airway pressure serves in part to inflate partially or totally collapsed regions of the lung, often with a dramatic improvement in oxygenation. On a mechanical ventilator, different manipulations can be made to increase airway pressures. Most commonly, this is done by increasing positive end-expiratory pressure (PEEP). **Additional measures to help reverse underlying ventilation–perfusion mismatch in hypoxic respiratory failure are as follows:**

1. **Bronchodilators for bronchospasm**
2. **Diuretics for excess lung edema**
3. **Antibiotics for pneumonia**
4. **Chest physiotherapy for atelectasis**
5. **Anticoagulants for PE**

Ventilatory Failure

Ventilatory failure occurs in patients who fail to "excrete" adequate carbon dioxide from their lungs. These problems typically do not arise from mismatch at the alveolar–capillary level, but more likely from failure of the lungs to effectively pump gas out of the respiratory circuit. As PCO_2 builds up in the alveoli, the arterial PCO_2 begins to rise as well. **Hypercarbia on the blood gas measurement is the hallmark of ventilatory failure.** "Pump" dysfunction can occur anywhere from the medulla, to the diaphragm, to the thickened or destroyed airways of the patient with COPD. Typical scenarios for the oncologic patient include the oversedated patient with an inadequate respiratory rate, or the weakened patient unable to pump air adequately through diseased lungs.

Treatment of ventilatory failure consists of reversing any precipitants and if these are not readily correctable, providing an adequate tidal volume and respiratory rate with a mechanical ventilator. This is typically administered through an endotracheal tube with a mechanical ventilator, although this can also be done with the use of noninvasive masks to administer continuous or phasic positive airway pressure in certain situations (74).

Chronic Respiratory Failure

Some patients with gynecologic malignancy may have adapted to chronic respiratory insufficiency. These patients with chronic lung disease may have abnormal alveolar–arterial oxygen gradients or carbon dioxide tensions as their baseline equilibrium. Chronic hypoxemia often leads to elevated hemoglobin and improved oxygen delivery chemistry, and these patients are not in acute distress unless their PO_2 dips into the 50 mm Hg range. **Chronic lung disease can lead to carbon dioxide retention, which is compensated by a metabolic alkalosis to maintain blood pH near normal. Increasing oxygen supplementation beyond that necessary to maintain hemoglobin saturations at the patient's baseline can sometimes lead to worsening (acute on chronic) PCO_2 levels and acidemia in these patients.** Conversely, improving ventilation by mechanical means to a "normal" PCO_2 on blood gas measurement may lead to dangerous alkalemia in a patient with chronic lung disease who was in acid–base balance at a higher PCO_2. **The goal of oxygenation and ventilation in patients with chronic respiratory insufficiency should be to maintain their baseline status.**

Adult Respiratory Distress Syndrome

One pattern of severe respiratory failure that deserves special mention is the adult respiratory distress syndrome (ARDS). **This is a pattern of lung injury that can be precipitated by direct damage (aspiration) or can occur as part of a septic syndrome and resulting lung inflammation. It is characterized by severe hypoxemia and decreased lung compliance, thought to be secondary to diffuse capillary leakage into the lung parenchyma.** The chest radiograph has the appearance of pulmonary edema, although direct measurement with a pulmonary catheter typically shows low or normal left-sided filling pressures. Management typically involves mechanical ventilation with lower tidal volumes to minimize lung distension, and to avoid fluid overload (160,161). **Despite aggressive support, the mortality rate from this syndrome remains high (162).**

Mechanical Ventilation

Physicians working with critically ill patients need to understand the principles of mechanical ventilation. Postoperative patients sometimes remain on mechanical ventilation until they are stabilized. Even apparently stable oncologic patients on the wards are often at risk for hypoxic and ventilatory failure that can progress to the need for mechanical ventilation.

Mechanical ventilation is typically performed by placement of an endotracheal tube, although tight-fitting masks are sometimes used in patients who are awake and alert enough (noninvasive positive-pressure ventilation) (74). There has been a proliferation in the types and terminology for mechanical ventilation over the years, often leading to some confusion. Despite many modalities, little is known about improved benefits of one ventilator setting versus another in terms of long-term patient outcome.

A basic understanding of ventilator management can be divided into two realms (much like the understanding of respiratory failure): Ventilation and oxygenation. **Management of ventilation requires adjusting *when* the machine delivers a breath** (with every patient effort or on a timer), **and *how* it delivers that breath** (either as a preset volume, or applying a preset pressure). These settings are chosen to help the clinician accomplish two goals: full or partial support of the patient's breathing efforts, and adequate ventilation without excessive airway pressures. **Management of oxygenation requires adjustment of the fraction of inspired oxygen delivered into the lungs and the end-expiratory airway pressure settings.** These values are set to achieve adequate blood oxygen saturation without damaging the lungs.

When the machine is set to deliver a full mechanical breath with each patient effort, the patient is receiving fully supported ventilation. Typically, a backup respiratory rate is set, but the patient can breathe as often as she wants and receive a fully supported tidal breath each time. This is typically called **assist control (AC) ventilation.** Alternately, the machine can be set to deliver only a certain number of breaths each minute and the patient needs to breathe without full machine support for any additional respirations above the set rate. This is considered partially supported ventilation and is most typically set as **synchronized intermittent mandatory ventilation (SIMV).**

The mechanical breath itself can be delivered as a preset volume with each breath. This is often called "volume control ventilation." This ensures an adequate tidal volume, but risks increased airway pressures if the lungs become difficult to inflate because of increased airway resistance or lung stiffness. High airway pressures can cause barotrauma, such as pneumothorax, and it is recommended to keep peak airway pressures less than 35 cm H_2O if possible (163). Instead of volume control, the mechanical breath can be administered as a preset pressure; this is usually termed pressure control (or in a slightly different mode, pressure support). This avoids the risks of increased airway pressures, but may provide smaller (or larger) tidal volumes with each breath if lung mechanics (or patient effort) changes. Some of the more sophisticated ventilators can adjust pressures with each breath to meet a targeted volume in a mode called pressure-regulated volume control. Regardless of which mode is chosen, blood gases are typically followed for patients on mechanical ventilation, and adjustments are made in the aforementioned settings to keep the patient's arterial carbon dioxide level near her baseline value.

When adjusting oxygenation settings on the ventilator, most critical care physicians attempt to lower the fraction of inspired oxygen (F_IO_2) to below 65%. Values above this for prolonged periods are believed to be damaging to lung parenchyma (164). The addition of PEEP often increases the functional reserve capacity of the diseased lung and allows F_IO_2 reductions. PEEP should be titrated to maximize oxygenation in respiratory failure, although some caution is needed because higher values can begin to precipitate barotrauma from increased peak pressures. In some forms of acute respiratory failure, such as ARDS, additional measures may be tried for refractory hypoxemia, including neuromuscular paralysis or changing patients to the prone position. These interventions have shown only mixed results in improving long-term outcomes (161,165,166).

After the cause of respiratory failure is improved or improving and the patient is judged hemodynamically stable, attempts to remove the patient from mechanical ventilation should begin. This process is known as weaning, although it does not need to be as slow as this appellation suggests. Clinicians have looked at many screening methods for identifying patients who are ready to come off mechanical ventilation, but none offers perfect sensitivity or specificity. Traditional weaning criteria such as negative inspiratory force less than 25 cm and minute ventilation less than 10 L/min have shown poor predictive value. Many physicians think that the bedside test with best predictive accuracy may be the rapid shallow breathing index (167). This "index" is derived by dividing respiratory rate (breaths per minute) by tidal volume (L) measured with the patient removed briefly from ventilatory support. A rapid shallow breathing index value of less than 100 breaths/min/L would suggest that the patient may be ready for extubation.

In the end, the most useful test to determine a patient's readiness for extubation is probably a trial of spontaneous breathing with little or no support from the ventilator. This is often performed with minimal pressure support (7 cm of H_2O per breath or less) or by having the patient breathe through the endotracheal tube without any ventilator support at all. Patients who can tolerate 30 minutes to 2 hours of such unsupported breathing should be considered for extubation if their airways remain patent, their secretions can be managed, and their oxygenation and ventilation can be maintained (168). Early extubation can help avoid nosocomial pneumonia and other complications associated with the mechanical ventilator and a prolonged ICU stay.

Renal Insufficiency, Fluids, and Electrolytes

Acute Kidney Injury

Acute kidney injury (AKI) or acute renal failure (ARF) remains a serious postoperative complication in surgical patients. Surgical patients are particularly predisposed to AKI because of the physiologic insult induced by the surgical procedure, pre-existing comorbidity, and sepsis. The overall incidence of AKI in surgical patients is estimated at 1–2%, although it is higher in at-risk groups (Table 18.20), and mortality rates remain high despite advances in dialysis and supportive care (169). The most consistent preoperative factor contributing to AKI is pre-existing renal impairment (170). The best form of treatment is prevention.

While a number of definitions of AKI exist and new markers such as serum cystatin C have been developed, the most common sign of new or worsening renal dysfunction in clinical practice is a rising serum creatinine concentration or a low urinary output. Oliguria is defined as a urine output of less than 400 mL/d. Acute renal failure typically reflects an abrupt loss and sustained decline

Table 18.20 Risk Factors for Developing Perioperative Acute Renal Failure

1. Pre-existing renal impairment (chronic kidney disease)

2. Hypertension

3. Cardiac disease

4. Diabetes mellitus

5. Jaundice or liver disease

in the glomerular filtration rate, which manifests as an increasing serum creatinine to twice its baseline value (171). In the hospital setting, acute oliguria or renal failure is usually caused by hypovolemia, decreased CO, postoperative kidney injury, or the use of nephrotoxic drugs (172).

Prerenal causes are responsible for the majority of cases (up to 90%) of ARF in surgical patients (170). Patients are at increased risk for AKI from etiologies arising from cancer treatment such as severe vomiting or diarrhea, nephrotoxic chemotherapy, or tumor lysis syndrome. The cancer itself may cause ureteral obstruction (Table 18.21) (173).

Table 18.21 Common Causes of Acute Renal Failure in Surgical Cancer Patients

I. Prerenal

   a. Hypotension

   b. Hypovolemia (diarrhea, vomiting, anemia)

   c. Heart failure

   d. Sepsis

   e. Drugs: angiotensin converting enzyme (ACE) inhibitors, nonsteroidal anti-inflammatory drugs (NSAIDs)

II. Intrinsic (Renal)

   a. Acute tubular necrosis

      1. ischemia (shock, severe sepsis)

      2. nephrotoxic agents (radiographic contrast, aminoglycosides, *cisplatin,* amphotericin)

      3. pigment nephropathy—rhabdomyolysis (myoglobin)

   b. Acute interstitial nephritis

      1. allergic nephritis (drugs such as antibiotics)

      2. cancer infiltration

   c. Glomerulonephritis

      1. Amyloidosis

      2. IgA nephropathy

      3. membranous glomerulonephritis

   d. Renal tubular obstruction

      1. urate crystals (tumor lysis syndrome)

      2. light chains (multiple myeloma)

      3. drugs—*acyclovir, methotrexate*

III. Postrenal

   a. Bladder dysfunction—drugs, nerve injury

   b. Uretral obstruction—cancer

Adapted from **Carmichael P, Carmichael AR**. Acute renal failure in the surgical setting. *ANZ J Surg.* 2003;73: 144–153; and **Darmon M, Ciroldi M, Thiery G, et al.** Clinical review: Specific aspects of acute renal failure in cancer patients. *Crit Care.* 2006;10:211–217.

The causes of ARF are grouped into three categories: Prerenal, intrinsic, and postrenal (Table 18.21). Initial evaluation should attempt to place the patient into one of these categories. **Prerenal failure and intrinsic renal failure caused by ischemia and nephrotoxins (acute tubular necrosis [ATN]) are responsible for most cases** (170). The physical examination should include measurement of orthostatic blood pressure changes, assessment of jugular venous distention, evaluation for a palpable bladder, and checking a postvoid residual urine volume as determined by bladder catheterization. Laboratory evaluation should include determinations of urinary and serum sodium and creatinine concentrations (to calculate the fractional excretion of sodium [$F_{ex}Na$]; see below), serum metabolic panel and total CK level, urine osmolality, and microscopic urinalysis. The results of urinary electrolytes may be unreliable and should be interpreted with caution in patients with glycosuria, pre-existing renal disease, and in those receiving diuretics.

Postrenal causes of oliguria or ARF arise from obstruction of the urinary tract. If this remains a suspicion even after a urethral catheter has been placed, a renal ultrasound should be ordered, which may show characteristic dilation of the collection system (hydronephrosis) above the obstruction. Although quite specific, this finding may not be present in all cases of ureteral obstruction, and additional radiographic tests may be needed (174). Percutaneous or cystoscopic stenting is often performed for cases of acute ureteral obstruction.

Prerenal azotemia can often be diagnosed with urinary indices. It tends to be associated with high urine osmolality, low urinary sodium, and a high urine-to-plasma creatinine ratio. **The best discriminator between prerenal and other causes of ARF is the $F_{ex}Na$** (175). This can be easily calculated from serum and urine sodium and creatinine concentrations as follows:

$$F_{ex}Na = \frac{Urine \times plasma\ creatinine}{Plasma\ sodium \times urine\ creatinine} \times 100$$

Prerenal azotemia is associated with a $F_{ex}Na$ of less than 1%, whereas obstructive uropathy (postrenal) and most forms of intrinsic renal failure (except pigment- or radiocontrast-induced ATN) are associated with $F_{ex}Na$ levels greater than 2%. Patients with a history or physical examination suggestive of volume depletion, or urinary indices consistent with prerenal azotemia, should be treated with aggressive fluid administration with frequent reexamination for evidence of volume overload. Characteristic urinary indices for prerenal and other causes of ARF are listed in Table 18.22.

If prerenal and postrenal causes of renal dysfunction are excluded, the patient likely has intrinsic disease of the kidney. Most of these cases are caused by ATN, although a small percentage of patients may have interstitial nephritis or a form of glomerulonephritis (171). Urinalysis in conjunction with urine microscopy may suggest the etiology. **Red blood cell casts** in the sediment are diagnostic of **glomerulonephritis, "muddy" and cellular casts are suggestive of ATN,** and **eosinophils** in the urine (stained with Wright stain) **are often indicative of interstitial nephritis** induced by drugs.

Table 18.22 Urinary Diagnostic Indices[a]

	Prerenal Azotemia	Acute Oliguric Renal Failure	Acute Nonoliguric Renal Failure	Acute Obstructive Uropathy	Acute Glomerulonephritis
Urine osmolality, mOsm/kg H_2O	518 ± 35	369 ± 20	343 ± 17	393 ± 39	385 ± 61
Urine sodium, mEq/L	18 ± 3	68 ± 5	50 ± 5	69 ± 10	22 ± 6
Urine/plasma urea nitrogen	18 ± 7	3 ± 0.5	7 ± 1	8 ± 4	11 ± 4
Urine/plasma creatinine	45 ± 6	17 ± 2	17 ± 2	16 ± 4	43 ± 7
Fractional excretion of filtered sodium	0.4 ± 0.1	7 ± 1.4	3 ± 0.5	6 ± 2	0.6 ± 0.2

[a]Values are expressed as mean ± standard error of the mean (SEM).

Adapted from **Miller TR, Anderson RJ, Linas SC, et al**. Urinary diagnostic indices in acute renal failure: A prospective study. *Ann Intern Med.* 1978; 89:47–50, with permission.

Acute tubular necrosis is usually caused by ischemia, nephrotoxic agents, or untreated pre-renal azotemia. Many drugs are known nephrotoxins, including radiocontrast agents and many chemotherapeutic drugs. Clinicians should attempt to avoid nephrotoxicity by careful dosing and avoidance of hypovolemia. Administration of intravenous fluids (isotonic saline or sodium bicarbonate) shortly before administering radiocontrast dye, for instance, decreases the risk of nephropathy from contrast agents. While still controversial, studies suggest a possible reduction in nephrotoxicity of contrast agents with the use of *N*-acetylcysteine (176,177).

One cause of intrinsic renal failure that should be considered in any oncologic patient being treated with chemotherapy is **tumor lysis syndrome. This condition is caused by the rapid destruction of large numbers of tumor cells (often just after the initiation of chemotherapy), and results in the sudden release of intracellular phosphate and other intracellular ions** (173). Metabolic abnormalities including hyperphosphatemia, hypocalcemia, hyperkalemia, hyperuricemia, and increased serum creatinine can be seen. **Acute renal failure develops as a result of the uric acid crystal formation in the renal tubules.** The syndrome is most commonly seen in high-grade hematologic malignancies such as lymphoma, but it can occur in solid malignancies that respond dramatically to chemotherapeutic agents. Prophylactic measures include hydration, drugs that reduce uric acid levels such as *allopurinol,* and urate oxidases such as *rasburicase.* Urgent hemodialysis is often indicated (178).

Management of patients with ARF includes discontinuation of any nephrotoxic agents and appropriate adjustment of continuing medications to the patient's new creatinine clearance. Adequate fluid resuscitation to ensure euvolemia is critical, as is the assessment for volume overload if renal function continues to deteriorate. Careful attention to volume status, serum electrolytes, and acid–base status is warranted. Nephrology consultation is recommended for all patients in whom the diagnosis is uncertain or the ARF persists. Many clinicians use diuretics to maintain urine output (179). This strategy may make volume management easier, but is controversial as several studies suggest that diuretics are potentially detrimental and do not improve mortality or make it less likely that the patient will require renal replacement therapy with dialysis (180).

Sometimes the use of renal replacement therapy (hemodialysis) is needed, as there are no effective pharmacologic agents for the treatment of established ARF. Indications for hemodialysis include hyperkalemia; pulmonary edema and volume overload that cannot be corrected; acidemia; and uremic symptoms (encephalopathy, bleeding from platelet dysfunction, or pericarditis). The selection of modality of renal replacement therapy (intermittent vs. continuous) and the optimal timing of initiation and dose of therapy remain unclear (181). Patients who are hemodynamically unstable might benefit from continuous renal replacement techniques (continuous venovenous hemodialysis or ultrafiltration) rather than intermittent therapy (182). An algorithm for managing oliguria and rising serum creatinine (ARF) is shown in Figure 18.5.

Prevention of ARF in the surgical setting is the key. Several preventative measures are essential for high-risk patients (especially those with pre-existing impairment). These include (i) optimizing volume status; (ii) keeping the mean arterial pressure >80 mm Hg; (iii) reducing the risk of nosocomial infections by rapid removal of intravascular and bladder catheters; (iv) appropriate use of antibiotics; (v) aggressive treatment of any sepsis; and (vi) restricted use or avoidance of potentially nephrotoxic agents (169).

Acid–Base Disorders

Disorders of acid–base homeostasis are common in critical care medicine, and accurate interpretation of these disorders is important for successful management. For an exhaustive review of acid–base disorders, the reader is referred to several excellent summaries (183–185).

The human body requires tight regulation of acid–base balance despite ongoing metabolic processes that produce substantial acid loads. It does this with several buffering systems, all of which are in balance and correct any disturbances. **The most important (and most easily measured) is the bicarbonate–carbonic acid equilibrium. This buffering system is reflected in serum bicarbonate levels and carbon dioxide tension** (which is in equilibrium with serum carbonic acid). Changes in these measurements from baseline reflect changes in acid or base balance.

Changes in serum carbon dioxide tension (PCO_2) reflect either primary lung disorders (hyperventilation or hypoventilation) with resulting respiratory disturbances in acid–base balance, or attempts by the lungs to compensate for metabolic disturbances causing changes in bicarbonate concentration in the blood. Hyperventilation as a primary disturbance results in a low PCO_2 in the blood and resulting **respiratory alkalemia.** Hypoventilation as a primary disturbance

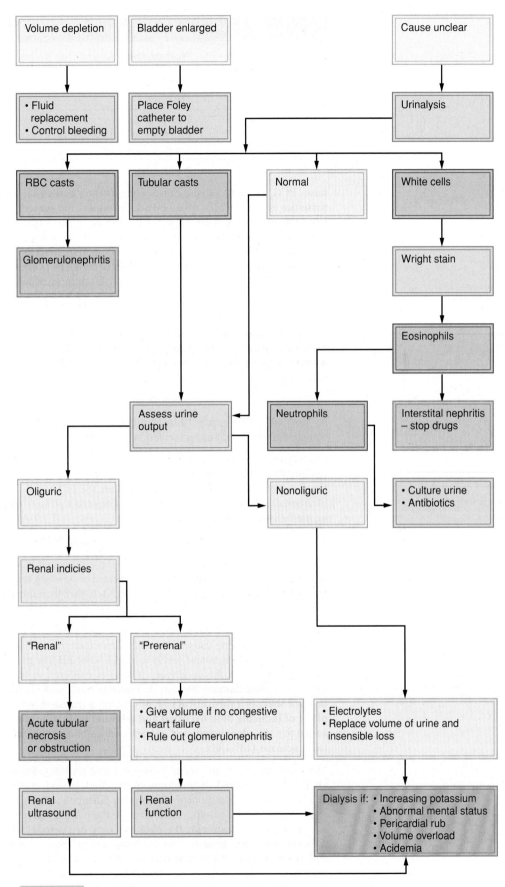

Figure 18.5 Algorithm for the management of a rising serum creatinine.

Table 18.23 Causes of Metabolic Acidosis		
Elevated Anion Gap	*Normal Anion Gap*	*Normal-Hyperkalemic Acidosis*
Renal failure	Renal tubular acidosis	Early renal failure
Ketoacidosis	Diarrhea	Hydronephrosis
Lactic acidosis	Posthypocapnic acidosis Carbonic anhydrase inhibitors Ureteral diversions	Addition of HCl Sulfur toxicity

raises PCO_2 in the blood and causes a **respiratory acidemia. When the primary acid–base disturbance is caused by a metabolic disturbance, the patient's ventilatory system attempts to keep the pH balanced by hyperventilation or hypoventilation,** thereby creating compensatory changes in the PCO_2. By studying the serum pH and comparing changes in the serum PCO_2 to changes in the serum bicarbonate concentration, the clinician is often able to distinguish primary respiratory alkalemia and acidemia (and their duration) from secondary compensation (185,186). Bedside nomograms have been designed for this purpose as well.

Primary changes in the serum bicarbonate concentration often reflect metabolic processes initially less obvious than primary lung disturbances. **Metabolic acidosis is defined as a decrease in serum bicarbonate level, and occurs as a primary disorder or as a compensation for a respiratory disturbance. Typically, the first step in evaluating a patient with a primary metabolic acidosis is to measure serum electrolytes and calculate the anion gap.** A formula for the anion gap using serum electrolyte concentrations is as follows.

$$\text{Anion gap} = (Na^+) - (Cl^- + HCO_3^-)$$

A "normal" anion gap is 10 to 14 mEq/L. Selected causes of metabolic acidosis with elevated and normal anion gaps are presented in Table 18.23.

The second step in evaluating a metabolic acidosis is assessment of the adequacy of the patient's ventilatory response. The normal mechanism of compensation for decreased serum bicarbonate is hyperventilation, which lowers the PCO_2 and offsets the impact of the decreased bicarbonate on serum pH. The expected response to a primary metabolic acidosis can be estimated by the following equation (186):

$$\text{Expected } PCO_2 = 1.5 \text{ (measured } HCO_3^-) + 8 \text{ (range } \pm 2)$$

Patients who have metabolic acidosis and whose measured PCO_2 levels fall below those expected on the basis of this equation should be suspected of having a second disturbance (i.e., an additional respiratory alkalosis). In patients with a PCO_2 higher than this expected level, additional respiratory acidosis should be suspected as complicating their metabolic disturbance (186).

The treatment of metabolic acidosis depends on its severity. In most cases, identification and treatment of the underlying cause is the only direct therapy necessary. In patients who have profound disturbances and bicarbonate levels less than 10 or pH less than 7.2, especially if there is associated hypotension or the underlying disease is expected to worsen, bicarbonate therapy can be considered. **Bicarbonate therapy is controversial, and should be undertaken with caution, because there is a theoretical risk of causing a transient worsening of the cerebrospinal fluid pH or of inducing fluid overload and rebound metabolic alkalosis.** Some researchers have suggested that the administration of exogenous bicarbonate may worsen the outcome in patients with lactic acidosis (187,188).

Metabolic alkalosis can occur in hospitalized patients. Perhaps most commonly, metabolic alkalosis is associated with volume contraction. In such conditions, sodium reabsorption by the kidney is linked to bicarbonate reabsorption. Metabolic alkalosis does not resolve until the patient regains intravascular volume. **To determine the primary precipitant of metabolic alkalosis and the appropriate treatment, the clinician may use urinary chloride measurements to divide patients into two groups** (provided the patient has not received recent diuretic therapy): (i) **Patients with very low urinary chlorides.** These include those who have received nasogastric drainage, diuretic therapy, were vomiting, or have lingering alkalosis after hypercapnic lung failure. These "chloride-responsive" patients should be treated with normal saline solution; (ii) **patients with higher urinary chloride concentrations.** These patients do not respond to

Table 18.24 Differential Diagnosis to Metabolic Alkalosis in Gynecologic Oncology Patients
A. Sodium chloride responsive (urinary chloride <10 mmol/L)
1. GI disorders
Vomiting
Gastric drainage
Diarrhea
2. Diuretic therapy
3. Correction of chronic hypercapnia
B. Sodium chloride resistant (urinary chloride >15 mmol/L)
1. Profound potassium depletion
C. Unclassified
1. Alkali administration
2. Milk–alkali syndrome
3. Massive blood or plasma transfusion
4. Nonparathyroid hypercalcemia
5. Glucose ingestion after starvation
6. Large doses of carbenicillin or penicillin

Adapted from **Schrier RW, ed**. *Renal and Electrolyte Disorders*. 2nd ed. Boston, MA: Little Brown; 1980:146.

sodium chloride, and must be managed by treatment of the underlying disease (184). Table 18.24 lists the causes of metabolic alkalosis.

Maintenance Fluids

Proper management of water and electrolyte therapy is an integral component in the care of surgical and oncologic patients, particularly those who are not taking oral hydration or nourishment. In the average adult who is taking fluids orally, the average daily loss of water is approximately 3 L (2 L as urine and 1 L as insensible losses from perspiration, respiration, and feces). The condition of critically ill patients may be complicated by additional ongoing losses, derangements in renal function, increased insensible losses, and disturbances in free water metabolism induced by the underlying disease. **Successful management of these patients requires frequent monitoring of volume status and serum electrolytes.** Predictable losses of fluids and electrolytes must be replaced, particularly those from nasogastric suctioning, and the increased insensible losses associated with fever and diarrhea (189).

Several simple guidelines can be kept in mind when managing fluid replacement in the hospitalized patient. **In a patient with no pre-existing renal disease and no disorder of water or electrolyte metabolism, a reasonable maintenance fluid regimen is 3 L daily of a half-normal saline solution with 20 mEq of potassium chloride in each liter. In the presence of significant renal impairment (glomerular filtration rate <25 mL/min), potassium therapy should not be given routinely, replacement being based on serial determinations of serum potassium.** In patients suspected of having a defect in free water excretion (see below), it is prudent to decrease the free-water content of the initial maintenance fluids (typically by giving normal saline at half the rate). Gastric fluid is composed of hypotonic saline solution (one-fourth to one-half normal saline) with 5 to 10 mEq/L of potassium. Gastric fluid losses should be replaced with replacement fluids in addition to the maintenance prescription.

Hyponatremia and Hypernatremia

Hyponatremia is a common disorder in gynecologic oncology patients. Serum sodium concentration reflects total body water content. Total body sodium content is reflected in extracellular fluid volume. Hyponatremia represents a relative water excess. Disorders of sodium excess or deficit are expressed as either extracellular volume overload or depletion. **Hyponatremia is common, affecting up to 15% of hospitalized patients.** The most common causes of hyponatremia in hospitalized patients are hypovolemia and the syndrome of inappropriate antidiuresis (SIAD) also known as syndrome of inappropriate antidiuretic hormone (SIADH) (190). **Hyponatremic conditions are best grouped into three different categories:**

1. **Hyponatremia associated with extracellular volume depletion (hypovolemia).** Hypovolemic patients block free-water excretion by increasing antidiuretic hormone secretion. All forms of intravascular volume depletion in patients with normal renal function predispose to this form of hyponatremia, especially when losses are replaced with hypotonic fluids. Typically, the urinary sodium level is low (<20 mEq/L) and signs of volume depletion are present (191).

2. **Hyponatremia with normal volume status (euvolemia).** This is seen in patients with SIAD and patients with hypothyroidism. The cause of SIAD should be determined, and can include certain malignancies, intrathoracic disorders, central nervous system disorders, and a variety of drugs including several chemotherapeutic agents. In SIAD, urinary sodium levels are typically greater than 30 to 35 mEq/L and urine osmolality greater than 100 (191).

3. **Hyponatremia with increased total-body sodium and increased extracellular volume (hypervolemia).** The hallmark of these disorders is edema and urinary sodium levels are often low reflecting the decreased effective arterial volume in these conditions. Patients with this category of hyponatremia usually have congestive heart failure, nephrotic syndrome, or cirrhotic liver disease (191).

The treatment of hyponatremia is tailored to its pathophysiology. Immediate treatment depends on the patient's symptoms, the rate at which the hyponatremia has developed, and the absolute serum sodium concentration. **Patients with diminished extracellular volume should be treated with an infusion of normal saline. Patients with normal or increased extracellular volume can be managed initially with free-water restriction (192). Those with persisting or worsening hyponatremia and adequate extracellular volume should be managed acutely with** *furosemide* **to induce a hypotonic diuresis,** and with replacement of urine output with normal saline infusion.

Therapy with hypertonic saline is rarely necessary and is reserved for patients with profound hyponatremia typically associated with seizures or markedly diminished mental status. An algorithm detailing an approach to the patient with hyponatremia is presented in Figure 18.6.

Hypernatremia, less commonly encountered in hospitalized patients, represents relative total-body water deficit (193). Usually it is the result of inadequate water replacement in a patient unable to take fluids spontaneously. This might be exaggerated or precipitated by failure of the kidneys to adequately reabsorb water (concentrate urine), a condition termed *nephrogenic diabetes insipidus.* **Hypercalcemia affects the kidney's ability to concentrate. Hyperglycemia can worsen water losses** by causing an osmotic diuresis. Treatment of hypernatremia is directed at providing adequate hypotonic fluids (often as "free water" or fluids with very minimal solute), and treating hypercalcemia and hyperglycemia. Rarely, patients may have disorders of antidiuretic hormone manufacture and secretion in the hypothalamus and posterior pituitary **(central diabetes insipidus).** Such patients must receive exogenous hormone to maintain water balance.

Hypokalemia and Hyperkalemia

Disturbances in serum potassium concentration are common and important because of the pivotal role played by this ion in maintaining transmembrane potentials of the heart. **Because 98% of total-body potassium is intracellular, small changes in serum potassium concentration may reflect very large excesses or deficits in total-body potassium content.** For instance, a decrease in the plasma potassium concentration to 3 mEq/L may reflect a 100- to 200-mEq deficit in total-body potassium content; a decrease to 2 mEq/L may reflect a total-body deficit of 300 to 500 mEq of potassium.

Changes in hydrogen ion concentration may have an impact on the distribution of potassium between the intracellular and extracellular spaces. **In acidemic patients, there is a shift in potassium from intracellular to extracellular sites.** In a patient who is acidemic and hypokalemic, the plasma potassium concentration is not appropriately diminished, and the total-body potassium deficit will be underestimated.

Possible causes of hypokalemia include decreased dietary intake or insufficient replacement in maintenance fluids, often worsened by diarrhea, nasogastric suction, or diuretic therapy.

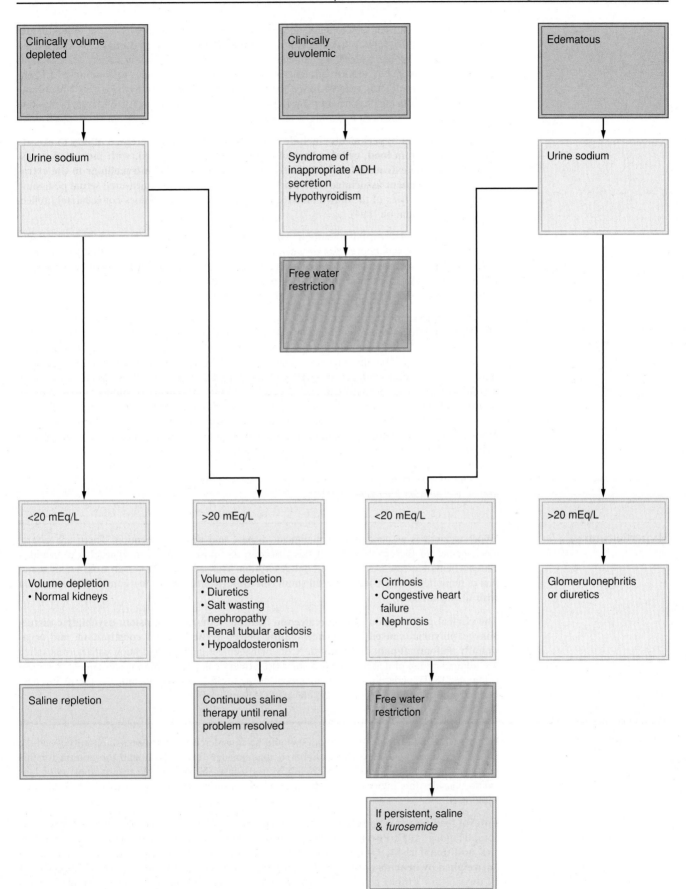

Figure 18.6 Algorithm for the evaluation of hyponatremia. ADH, antidiuretic hormone.

Hypokalemia may present as weakness, ileus, or muscular cramps. Of most concern, **hypokalemia increases myocardial irritability and can precipitate dangerous arrhythmias** (194). Treatment involves reversal of the underlying cause and repletion of the potassium deficit. Potassium is replaced relatively slowly in most circumstances to allow cell membranes to equilibrate. **In general, patients should not receive more than 10 mEq/hr intravenously.** Patients undergoing potassium therapy in the presence of renal failure have a diminished capacity to excrete potassium, and added caution is needed to avoid the dangers of hyperkalemia.

Common causes of hyperkalemia include renal insufficiency and decreased ability to excrete the daily potassium load, cellular breakdown (including hemolysis), with increased potassium release into extracellular fluids, and redistribution from the intracellular to the extracellular compartment associated with acidemia. Occasionally, high measured serum potassium results from hemolysis of the drawn blood sample in the test tube and does not accurately reflect the serum concentration (194).

Patients with elevated serum potassium typically have no symptoms. The condition is usually noted on screening laboratory tests or when changes are noted on an ECG. **Although variable, ECG changes associated with elevated serum potassium include peaked T-waves, a prolonged PR interval, and widening of the QRS complex.** These changes often herald dangerous serum potassium levels that need correction to avert cardiac arrest.

The initial approach to hyperkalemia is to identify and remove the precipitating cause and rapidly assess any ECG changes. In patients with mild hyperkalemia (serum $K^+ < 6$ mEq/L) and minimal ECG changes, treatment of the underlying cause and careful monitoring of the serum potassium levels may be the only therapy necessary. **In patients with potassium levels greater than 6.5 mEq/L and evidence of QRS widening, rapid steps should be taken to decrease serum potassium levels with the use of oral or rectal potassium exchange resins such as *sodium polystyrene sulfonate (Kayexalate)* and a loop diuretic such as *furosemide*. If there is associated renal failure, urgent arrangements for dialysis are indicated.** In patients with prolonged QRS duration approaching sine-wave configuration, or in patients who are hypotensive, **the following treatments can "temporize"** until more definitive treatment can be arranged: *calcium gluconate* to stabilize myocardial cell membranes, **intravenous *glucose* and *insulin*** (one unit of *insulin* for each gram of *glucose* in an ampule of *glucose*), high-dose inhaled *albuterol*, and *sodium bicarbonate* (191).

Hypercalcemia

Hypercalcemia is associated with malignant disease and deserves mention. There are several mechanisms for the development of this disorder, the most common in gynecologic oncology patients being increased osteoclastic bone resorption. This is believed to result from tumor secretion of humoral factors. **Clear cell and small cell tumors of the ovary are commonly associated with this syndrome.**

The clinical presentation of hypercalcemia includes lethargy, confusion, psychiatric disturbances, polyuria (caused by a concentrating defect in the kidney), constipation, and occasionally abdominal pain and nausea. Acute management includes hydration with normal saline and administration of a loop diuretic to increase urinary calcium excretion. Subsequent treatment is targeted to the underlying cause (treatment of the tumor) and may include the use of **intravenous bisphosphonates** to control the elevated calcium level (194).

Nutrition

Patients who cannot eat for several days should be considered for nutritional support (beyond the minimal calories available in glucose-based maintenance fluids). Although the criteria for this intervention are not well defined and clinical trials have shown variable results, most clinicians would consider this intervention after several days without adequate calories and several more anticipated.

Enteral feeding is preferred because it may protect patients from GI bleeding and infectious complications (195). **Parenteral feeding usually requires central line placement and carries additional risks. One large trial in postsurgical patients showed these risks to be outweighed by benefits only when the patients required parenteral feeding for longer than 14 days** (196). Various enteral and parenteral feeding formulas are available, and adjustments in constituents are often needed to avoid many of the fluid and electrolyte problems described previously.

Blood Replacement

Anemia/Red Blood Cells

Anemia can be an additional stress on the cardiovascular system and may worsen myocardial ischemia or heart failure. **Appropriate preoperative or perioperative transfusion may reduce cardiac morbidity in patients with significant CAD or heart failure** (6). Some studies suggest that even mild preoperative anemia is associated with increased risk of postoperative cardiac events and mortality in elderly patients undergoing noncardiac surgery (197). There are many published studies regarding blood transfusions.

Guidelines emphasize that decisions regarding transfusion should be based on symptoms of anemia rather than hemoglobin concentration alone (198,199). However, most physicians still use hemoglobin concentrations to decide when to transfuse. **A growing body of evidence shows that a "restrictive" transfusion strategy is safe and possibly leads to better outcomes** and should be applied to most patients, including postoperative surgical patients and those with pre-existing cardiovascular disease. Specifically, **transfusion should be considered only for stable patients with a hemoglobin level of 8 g/dL or less or symptoms of anemia** (angina, orthostatic hypotension, tachycardia not responsive to fluid resuscitation, or congestive heart failure) (198,200). **Some evidence shows that in patients in the intensive care unit, a transfusion threshold of 7 g/dL is safe and leads to better outcomes** (201).

Studies suggest that a restrictive transfusion strategy may protect patients from a host of adverse outcomes that are associated with perioperative blood transfusion, including increased morbidity and mortality, increased length of stay, increased rates of infection, and transfusion reactions (202,203). Based on this evidence, some hospitals and healthcare systems have developed blood management programs aimed at reducing the incidence of transfusions for greater patient safety and cost savings (202). **The evidence base regarding what transfusion threshold to use in patients with acute coronary syndromes remains poor** and no specific recommendations can be made in this patient population (198).

In summary, **a conservative or "restrictive" approach with respect to transfusion for the vast majority of patients is as effective and possibly safer than a more liberal transfusion policy.** Guidelines for perioperative transfusion practices have been published (198,199).

Packed red blood cells (PRBCs) are almost always used when red cell transfusion is indicated. The possible indications for transfusion of red blood cells include the following:

1. **A decreasing hematocrit value in a patient who, because of bone marrow failure, is unlikely to begin producing red blood cells in the near future.** There is no specific information available in the literature to define exactly when a transfusion should be given in patients with bone marrow failure. There are good data showing that in the absence of symptoms directly referable to anemia, transfusion should be considered only in those with a hemoglobin concentration of 8 g/dL or less (7 g/dL or less in ICU patients) (198,200,201). These recommendations apply to postoperative surgical patients and patients with a history of pre-existing cardiovascular disease (198,200). No recommendations for transfusion triggers can be made yet for patients with acute coronary syndromes.

2. **Anemia in a patient with such symptoms as chest pain, orthostatic hypotension, tachycardia unresponsive to fluid resuscitation, congestive heart failure, or other evidence of inadequate perfusion and oxygenation of major organs.** Monitoring such parameters as blood pressure, heart rate, oxygen saturation, urine output, and ECG is recommended to assess whether vital organs have adequate perfusion (204).

Platelets

Platelet concentrates are prepared by removal of platelets from whole-blood fractions. Platelets may also be obtained by pheresis from a single donor.

Platelet transfusions are indicated in patients with the following:

1. **Platelet counts less than 50,000/mL^3 who show evidence of bleeding** (204).

2. **In certain patients (see below) with platelet counts less than 10,000/mL^3 as prophylaxis against acute bleeding.**

Each whole blood fraction unit of platelets should be expected to raise the recipient's platelet count approximately 5,000 to 10,000/mL^3. Prophylactic platelet transfusions are indicated only in patients whose platelet count is expected to recover in the future, because platelets express human leukocyte antigens and induce antibodies in the recipient. After prolonged platelet therapy, most patients become resistant to platelet transfusions, presumably because of immune destruction of all transfused platelets.

Plasma Fractions

Several plasma fractions are available for transfusion. The two most commonly used fractions are fresh frozen plasma (FFP) and cryoprecipitate.

Fresh Frozen Plasma   **All the blood-clotting proteins present in the original unit of blood are contained in FFP,** and it is an adequate source of all coagulation factors for the treatment of mild coagulation factor deficiencies. **FFP may be used to rapidly reverse *warfarin* toxicity if bleeding is present.** FFP should be given to bleeding patients if the INR or activated partial thromboplastin time (aPTT) is elevated (204). Plasma may be used to reverse the coagulopathy associated with massive blood loss and red cell replacement by restoring the lost coagulation factors. **In patients undergoing transfusion of multiple units of red blood cells, the INR and aPTT should be monitored for evidence of coagulopathy, and FFP given as needed to correct this.** It may require several "units" of FFP to restore clotting factors to adequate levels. The half-life of transfused clotting factors is measured in hours, and bleeding risks can recur when these factors are consumed.

Cryoprecipitate   Cryoprecipitate is produced by the freezing of plasma, followed by thawing, which produces a precipitate **rich in factor VIII and fibrinogen**. This cryoprecipitate fraction contains approximately 250 mg of fibrinogen per unit and 80 clotting units of factor VIII. Cryoprecipitate units are smaller in volume than FFP, and can be useful adjuncts in treating certain bleeding conditions such as disseminated intravascular coagulation (DIC). Cryoprecipitate should be given to patients who are bleeding when fibrinogen concentrations are less than 80 mg/dL (204).

Clotting Disorders

Massive Blood Transfusion

Pelvic surgeons may at times encounter unexpected and dramatic intraoperative bleeding. This may require large amounts of transfused blood, typically given as PRBC units. **"Massive transfusion" is typically defined as replacing the entire blood volume (5 to 6 L in a 70-kg patient) over a 24-hour period, or half the blood volume over a 3-hour period. "Washout" coagulopathy has been shown in some studies to begin when greater than 10 units of packed red cells have been transfused** (205,206). Such rapid blood transfusion can result in a **dilutional coagulopathy,** as these transfused units do not contain adequate amounts of blood proteins or platelets. **This can be worsened by the hypothermia and acidosis** brought on by hypovolemic shock.

The INR, aPTT, fibrinogen concentration, and platelet counts should be followed closely in these cases. Transfusions are indicated to maintain the INR and aPTT levels less than 1.5 times control values, a fibrinogen level greater than 100 mg/dL, and a platelet count greater than 50,000 (206).

Disseminated Intravascular Coagulation

DIC is a syndrome that complicates the course of a variety of disease states and is characterized by the pathologic activation of the coagulation cascade and the fibrinolytic system. **It occurs most commonly in critically ill patients with sepsis or liver disease. In gynecologic oncology patients, it may be associated with certain mucin-producing adenocarcinomas** (207).

In its acute form, DIC appears rapidly, and is manifested by bleeding from multiple sites, including venipunctures, surgical wounds, gingiva, GI tract, and skin. More rarely, DIC can take a chronic course over a period of months, with thrombotic complications more common than bleeding complications. This form is more typical of the syndrome associated with adenocarcinomas.

Direct evidence of DIC requires demonstration of intravascular fibrin deposition. The laboratory diagnosis of DIC depends on indirect evidence of coagulation activity. **The most common laboratory abnormalities in this disorder are decreased platelet count; elevated INR and aPTT; elevated D-dimer (a breakdown product of fibrin); and decreased fibrinogen concentration** (207,208).

The primary treatment of DIC is aimed at controlling the underlying cause. **Typical treatment would include empiric antibiotic therapy when sepsis is suspected, treatment of other** conditions adversely affecting coagulation, and replacement with appropriate clotting factors** in patients with active bleeding. Some of the controversial options, such as anticoagulation, factor replacement, *epsilon aminocaproic acid* with *heparin,* and antiplatelet drugs may be considered, but should be guided by a hematologic specialist (207).

Adverse Effects of Blood Transfusions	In addition to the possible adverse outcomes associated with a "liberal" blood transfusion strategy described previously, several other adverse effects of blood transfusions are possible. **These possible adverse effects include transfusion reactions, bacterial contamination, transmission of infectious diseases, and transfusion-related lung injury (TRALI).**
Acute Hemolytic and Nonhemolytic Reactions	Acute hemolytic and nonhemolytic transfusion reactions are possible. **Nonhemolytic transfusion reactions are often characterized by fever, chills, or urticaria.** Hemolytic transfusion reactions can be life threatening because of associated hypotension, DIC and renal failure. These reactions are often manifested by fever, chest pain, back pain, hypotension, tachycardia, and red urine indicating hemoglobinuria (204). **When a patient undergoing a red cell transfusion has any signs or symptoms suggestive of a hemolytic transfusion reaction, the transfusion should be stopped immediately and the remaining aliquot of blood sent to the blood bank, along with a sample of the patient's blood for culture and repeat cross-matching.** Tests to screen for DIC, a urinalysis for hemoglobin, and a blood sample for bilirubin should be obtained. In patients with symptoms of a hemolytic transfusion reaction who, on analysis, show no evidence of hemolysis, a hypersensitivity reaction to transfused leukocytes or plasma proteins contaminating the red cells should be suspected. The incidence of hemolytic transfusion reactions can be minimized by careful attention to clerical information, ensuring that the patient is receiving blood cross-matched to her blood sample and careful cross-matching in the blood bank.
Transmission of Infection	The safety of the blood supply in terms of transmission of viral diseases has improved markedly with the development of better screening techniques. **While not zero, the risk of tranfusion-transmitted viral infections, hepatitis B and C and human immunodeficiency virus (HIV), is very low** (209). **Bacterial contamination (most commonly from platelets) and subsequent sepsis are the most common infectious complications of blood transfusions, and remain a leading cause of transfusion mortality** (204,210). This diagnosis should be considered in any patient with fever or hemodynamic instability following a transfusion. **Cytomegalovirus can still be a problem,** although seroconverters are typically asymptomatic. The use of pooled products, such as platelets and plasma, increases the risks because multiple donors are required. **Autologous blood donation may be considered for elective surgery in certain patients, but its use is declining.**
Transfusion-related Lung Injury	Transfusion-related Lung Injury (TRALI) is characterized by noncardiogenic pulmonary edema within 6 hours of blood product transfusion. **TRALI is thought to occur as the result of an immune response of the recipient to leukocyte antibodies in the transfused blood, inducing capillary leak syndrome** (211). This syndrome can be fatal, and is thought to be on the rise. The risk is higher in patients who have received plasma from multiparous female donors. Hypoxia, fever, and dyspnea typically appear a few hours after transfusion. No specific therapy is available, and treatment is limited to stopping the transfusion and supportive measures (204,211).
Thromboembolism	
Detection of Deep Venous Thrombosis	**Clinical signs and symptoms of VTE are notoriously unreliable and detection of thromboembolic disease when it occurs is a challenging problem.** DVT of the lower extremity classically presents as a swollen, painful leg, but this may be completely absent in some patients. **Lower extremity venous clot is now typically screened with compression ultrasonography of the femoral, popliteal, and calf vein trifurcation.** This method is more than 90% sensitive for proximal thrombosis, but much less sensitive for calf thrombosis. Clinicians should perform serial testing with this method, or use **contrast venography (gold standard test)** if clinical suspicion remains high (212).

Detection of Pulmonary Embolus

Pulmonary embolism can be a life-threatening emergency. Autopsy studies suggest that PE may account for as many as 5% of unexpected deaths in hospitalized patients (213). **Presenting symptoms and signs of PE may include pleuritic chest pain, shortness of breath, cough with or without hemoptysis, and, in the case of a very large embolus, acute clinical decompensation or syncope and hypotension.** Patients are often tachycardic and hypoxic, the ECG may show evidence of right heart strain, and the chest radiograph may show an infarct with effusion. These same symptoms and signs may be present in other conditions, such as pneumonia and myocardial ischemia. Conversely, **a PE may be completely asymptomatic.** Because of this variable presentation, clinicians must be vigilant, particularly in their relatively immobile postoperative patients (214).

The reference standard for the diagnosis of PE remains direct angiography, although this test is rarely performed today. The two most commonly performed tests for suspected PE are the ventilation-perfusion (VQ) scan of the lung and the CT angiogram of the chest. In the case of VQ scanning, a large study in hospitalized patients showed that VQ test results were often inconclusive when compared to conventional pulmonary angiography (215). An entirely negative test was helpful in excluding a pulmonary embolus (risk <1%), and a classic positive test obviated further testing, but the test results were more typically intermediate or low probability. Combining results of the VQ scan with pretest clinical probability did improve the accuracy if clinical suspicion correlated with the scan results. **One advantage of VQ scanning is the absence of the contrast nephropathy risk which is associated with CT angiography. Hence, VQ scanning is often preferred in patients with marginal renal function.**

CT angiography performed with multidetector CT scanners and delayed venography of the thighs has been shown to be sensitive and specific for VTE detection in recent trials. If the patient's renal function can tolerate angiographic dye, this test has largely supplanted VQ scanning at most centers. The predictive value of this test (like the VQ scan) decreases if the test result conflicts with the pretest suspicion (216).

In the outpatient or emergency room setting, assays for increased blood levels of D-dimer (one of the byproducts of the coagulation cascade) are sensitive tests for VTE and can be used to screen for DVT or PE. **This test is relatively nonspecific in the hospitalized, postoperative, and cancer patients,** who often have many other reasons for elevated D-dimer levels (217).

Treatment

When documented, DVT or PE requires immediate treatment to decrease the risk of complications (PE or recurrent embolism). Patients who do not have an overriding contraindication to anticoagulation should be treated immediately with *heparin* **before the diagnosis is confirmed.** Traditionally this has been treated with intravenous *unfractionated heparin* in a large initial bolus, followed by a continuous *heparin* infusion adjusted to achieve an aPTT approximately two to three times that of the control value. **Several trials have shown that treatment with** *low-molecular-weight heparin* **is equal to, if not better than, treatment with standard** *unfractionated heparin* **for PE** (218). Postsurgical and intensive care unit patients are more often treated with an unfractionated heparin infusion that is more easily reversed because of a shorter drug half-life.

Systemic thrombolytic therapy can be considered in cases of acute PE with hypotension or shock unresponsive to fluid resuscitation, which is most often seen in massive PE. Many postoperative patients are at high risk for bleeding from lytic therapy, and this treatment should be carefully considered as it carries an estimated 20% risk of major hemorrhage and 3–5% risk of hemorrhagic stroke (219). Some centers may have the ability to perform catheter-directed thrombolytic therapy. There is no evidence that intrapulmonary arterial infusion confers greater benefit than peripheral venous infusion, but it is associated with bleeding at the catheter insertion site (220).

If a patient with a pulmonary embolus has active bleeding, or a high risk of bleeding and cannot be anticoagulated, a filter can be inserted into the inferior vena cava (IVC) to prevent recurrent pulmonary emboli. A percutaneously placed filter into the IVC can be used for those patients who develop recurrent pulmonary emboli despite adequate anticoagulation (218). Retrievable IVC filters have been developed that can be removed several months after placement (221).

When a patient with a pulmonary embolus has been stabilized, treatment with intravenous *heparin* is often transitioned to an **oral vitamin K antagonist (such as** *warfarin***),** for continued outpatient treatment. The *warfarin* oral dosage is titrated to an INR of 2 to 3. **A newer oral anticoagulant, rivaroxaban, an oral factor Xa inhibitor, has been approved for the treatment of**

acute PE. It is administered at a fixed dose and does not require laboratory monitoring. Rivaroxaban should not be used in patients with a creatinine clearance of 30 mL/min or less, significant hepatic impairment, or during pregnancy. Presently, there is no specific antidote to rivaroxaban. **Alternatively** a patient may go home on subcutaneous injections **of low-molecular-weight *heparin* or *fondaparinux*.**

The optimal duration of anticoagulation for deep venous thrombosis or PE remains controversial, but these **medications should be continued for at least 3 to 6 months**. Studies suggest that the risk of recurrent thrombosis can persist indefinitely, particularly in patients with an underlying malignancy (222). For select patients, clinicians may consider lengthy or even lifelong treatment with anticoagulation.

Infection

About 8–10% of gynecologic surgical patients will develop a hospital acquired infection. Central line associated blood stream infections, ventilator associated pneumonia, and catheter associated urinary tract infections account for greater than 80% of hospital acquired infections, and are associated with 5–35% mortality rates (223,224). These infections increase patients' morbidity and mortality, risk of long-term disability, length of hospital stay, and financial burden (224). Prevention of these infections is important.

Surgical site infections can be limited by giving gynecologic surgical patients prophylactic antibiotics 15 to 60 minutes prior to skin incision (223). Antibiotics of choice should cover Gram-positive bacteria for skin flora. If surgery involves the bowels, expanding the antibacterial coverage to include Gram-negative bacteria is prudent. Studies and published guidelines have suggested that first- and second-generation cephalosporins are reasonable for gynecologic patients. If patients have a *penicillin* allergy, *clindamycin* with *ciprofloxacin, levofloxacin,* or *aztreonam* are reasonable choices (223–226).

To limit hospital acquired infections, judicious use of central lines and Foley catheters should be implemented. These devices should be removed as soon as they are no longer needed. Maximal sterile barrier technique and use of *chlorhexidine* skin preparation are a must when placing central lines. Preferably, Foley catheters should be placed in the operating room for gynecologic surgical patients. Subsequent care of central lines and Foley catheters should include sterile techniques. For ventilated patients, promoting good hand hygiene prior to manipulating the airways, scheduled oral care with *chlorhexidine,* placing patients in a semirecumbent position, and daily assessment of readiness to extubate will help to limit incidence of ventilator-associated pneumonia (224,227).

When infections do occur, antibiotics should be chosen initially on the basis of probable infecting organisms, and changed if necessary when the results of culture and sensitivity testing are known (228).

Fever in the Neutropenic Patient

Febrile neutropenia is one of the most serious adverse events related to antineoplastic chemotherapy, and causes significant morbidity and mortality. When the absolute granulocyte count falls below 1,000/mm³, the incidence of infection rises and infected patients frequently decompensate rapidly. Many clinicians use prophylactic antibiotics in an attempt to decrease the frequency and mortality of this condition. While the guidelines advise against the use of prophylactic antibiotics, several studies provide evidence for the benefit of prophylactic *levofloxacin* (229–231). In patients with solid tumors receiving moderately myelosuppressive chemotherapy, prophylactic *levaquin* reduces the incidence of febrile neutropenia and all-cause mortality in the first cycle of treatment (232). Controversy about issues such as cost, toxicity, and antibiotic resistance remain (233–235).

Patients with established neutropenia who become febrile can decompensate rapidly and should be treated immediately with empiric broad-spectrum intravenous antibiotics, regardless of whether or not there are focal signs of infection. Frequently encountered pathogens in the neutropenic patient include *Staphylococcus aureus* and gram-negative enteric organisms such as *Escherichia coli, Klebsiella,* and *Pseudomonas.*

There are many combinations of empiric antibiotics that achieve the goal of covering likely pathogens in the febrile neutropenic patient (229,236,237). **For hospitalized, low-risk patients who have fever and neutropenia during cancer chemotherapy, empiric therapy with oral *ciprofloxacin* and *amoxicillin-clavulanate* appears to be safe and effective** (236). This approach is as effective as intravenous therapy and may be the preferred approach (237). If intravenous antibiotics are considered necessary, a broad-spectrum semisynthetic *penicillin,* sometimes combined with an aminoglycoside and *vancomycin,* may be used. **If febrile neutropenia persists despite several days of broad-spectrum antibiotics, guidelines suggest the empiric addition of antifungal agents** (229). Meticulous daily follow-up and adjustment of antibiotic coverage is critical and likely more important than the precise initial combination chosen.

Use of growth factor rescue for febrile neutropenia has been studied, and the use of *granulocyte colony-stimulating factor (G-CSF)* can shorten the duration of neutropenia. G-CSF is sometimes prescribed prophylactically during courses of chemotherapy, although this usage remains controversial in many treatment regimens (238,239).

Fungemia

Fungemia is a life-threatening postoperative complication of surgery and severe medical illness. **Typical patients at risk include those receiving multiple antibiotics and hyperalimentation.** Central venous access lines and Foley catheters can provide entry sites for fungal organisms. Additional important risk factors include cancer, chemotherapy, corticosteroids, and hyperglycemia (240,241). **The clinical presentation of disseminated disease is identical to that of gram-negative sepsis.** These patients may have signs of local fungal disease, such as oral thrush. The principal organisms found are *Candida* species. There are now several antifungal agents available to treat invasive disease (242). Patients with localized fungal infections should be aggressively treated with topical agents.

"Blind Loop Syndrome" and Small Intestinal Bacterial Overgrowth

The "blind loop syndrome" refers to symptoms from small intestinal bacterial overgrowth (SIBO) as a result of impaired motility or stasis in the small intestine. In gynecologic oncology, this condition usually occurs when a blind loop is artificially created by performing a side-to-side anastomosis to relieve a small bowel obstruction. **Excessive colonization of the small intestine by bacteria can interfere with the metabolism and the absorption of carbohydrates, proteins, lipids, and vitamins.** Carbohydrate malabsorption can be due to mucosal injury and the loss of activity of enzymes (disaccharidases) in the brush border, as well as bacterial fermentation of sugars. Intestinal mucosal injury can alter gut permeability, leading to protein-losing enteropathy. **Deconjugation of bile acids can lead to malabsorption of fat and fat-soluble vitamins (A, D, E).** Cobalamin (vitamin B_{12}) deficiency can occur as a result of use of the vitamin by anaerobic bacteria.

While SIBO is generally considered a malabsorption syndrome, clinical manifestations vary in each patient. Common symptoms include bloating, abdominal discomfort, foul-smelling diarrhea, nutritional deficiencies, and progressive weight loss. Diagnosis requires a high degree of suspicion and the most common diagnostic tests include hydrogen breath testing and duodenal aspiration with quantitative bacterial culture (243).

Treatment of SIBO consists of antibiotic therapy, treating the underlying disease surgically if possible, dietary manipulation, and correction of nutritional deficiencies. Empiric antibiotic therapy is the mainstay of treatment. The goal of antibiotic therapy is to reduce the flora, leading to symptomatic improvement. Recommended antibiotic regimens reflect the predominant organisms associated with SIBO, and cover both aerobic and anaerobic enteric bacteria (244). The optimal antibiotic regimen is not known due to a lack of high-quality studies. *Rifaximin, metronidazole,* and *ciprofloxacin* **have all been shown to be effective** (245). A 7- to 10-day course is usually sufficient to improve symptoms, and the effect may last for months. Recurrence is common, and patients often require repeated courses or regular treatment (e.g., the first 5 to 10 days of every month) with rotating antibiotic regimens (243,246).

In the case of a blind loop or fistula, **surgery may be necessary, if feasible, in patients who fail to respond to dietary manipulation and antibiotics, and have ongoing significant weight loss and diarrhea**. The identification and correction of nutritional deficiencies are necessary. A high-fat, low-carbohydrate, low-fiber diet has been advocated (247). As lactase deficiency develops in many adult patients with SIBO, lactose-containing foods should often be avoided. Deficiencies of calcium, magnesium, iron, vitamin B12, and fat-soluble vitamins including vitamin D should be tested for and corrected if necessary (243). The role of probiotics in treating SIBO remains unclear but is not recommended, as studies have shown conflicting evidence (247,248). **A team approach including the surgeon, GI specialist with experience in SIBO, nutritionist, and infectious disease consultant is the key to effective management of this complex condition.**

References

1. **Goldman L, Caldera DL, Nussbaum SR, et al.** Multifactorial index of cardiac risk in noncardiac surgical procedures. *N Engl J Med.* 1977;297:845–850.
2. **Detsky AS, Abrams HB, McLaughlin JR, et al.** Predicting cardiac complications in patients undergoing non-cardiac surgery. *J Gen Intern Med.* 1986;1:211–219.
3. **Hollenberg M, Mangano DT, Browner WS, et al.** Predictors of postoperative myocardial ischemia in patients undergoing noncardiac surgery: The Study of Perioperative Ischemia Research Group. *JAMA.* 1992;268:205–209.
4. **Mangano DT, Browner WS, Hollenberg M, et al.** Association of perioperative myocardial ischemia with cardiac morbidity and mortality in men undergoing noncardiac surgery: The Study of Perioperative Ischemia Research Group. *N Engl J Med.* 1990;323:1781–1788.
5. **Lee TH, Marcantonio ER, Mangione CM, et al.** Derivation and prospective validation of a simple index for prediction of cardiac risk of major noncardiac surgery. *Circulation.* 1999;100:1043–1049.
6. **Fleisher LA, Beckman JA, Brown KA, et al.** ACC/AHA 2007 guidelines on perioperative cardiovascular evaluation and care for noncardiac surgery: A report of the American College of Cardiology/American Heart Association Task Force on Practice Guidelines (Writing Committee to Revise the 2002 Guidelines on Perioperative Cardiovascular Evaluation for Noncardiac Surgery). *Circulation.* 2007;116:e418–e499.
7. **Fleisher LA, Beckman JA, Brown KA, et al.** 2009 ACCF/AHA focused update on perioperative beta blockade incorporated into the ACC/AHA 2007 guidelines on perioperative cardiovascular evaluation and care for noncardiac surgery: A report of the American College of Cardiology Foundation/American Heart Association Task Force on Practice Guidelines. *Circulation.* 2009;120(21):e169–e276.
8. **Mangano DT, Goldman L.** Preoperative assessment of patients with known or suspected coronary disease. *N Engl J Med.* 1995;333:1750–1756.
9. **Romero L, de Virgilio C.** Preoperative cardiac risk assessment. *Arch Surg.* 2001;136:1370–1376.
10. **Poldermans D, Bax JJ, Schouten O, et al.; Dutch Echocardiographic Cardiac Risk Evaluation Applying Stress Echo Study Group.** Should major vascular surgery be delayed because of preoperative cardiac testing in intermediate-risk patients receiving beta-blockade with tight heart rate control? *J Am Coll Cardiol.* 2006;48(5):964–969.
11. **American College of Physicians.** Guidelines for assessing and managing the perioperative risk from coronary artery disease associated with major noncardiac surgery. *Ann Intern Med.* 1997;127:309–312.
12. **Palda VA, Detsky AS.** Perioperative assessment and management of risk from coronary artery disease. *Ann Intern Med.* 1997;127:313–328.
13. **Kertai MD, Boersma E, Bax JJ, et al.** A meta-analysis comparing the prognostic accuracy of six diagnostic tests for predicting perioperative cardiac risk in patients undergoing major vascular surgery. *Heart.* 2003;89:1327–1334.
14. **Boersma E, Poldermans D, Bax JJ, et al.; DECREASE Study Group (Dutch Echocardiographic Cardiac Risk Evaluation Applying Stress Echocardiography).** Predictors of cardiac events after major vascular surgery: Role of clinical characteristics, dobutamine echocardiography, and beta-blocker therapy. *JAMA.* 2001;285(14):1865–1873.
15. **Steen PA, Tinker JH, Tarhan S.** Myocardial infarction after anesthesia and surgery. *JAMA.* 1978;239:2566–2570.
16. **Mahar LJ, Steen PA, Tinker JH, et al.** Preoperative myocardial infarction in patients with coronary artery disease with and without aorta-coronary bypass grafts. *J Thorac Cardiovasc Surg.* 1978;76:533–537.
17. **McCollum CH, Garcia-Rinald R, Graham JM, et al.** Myocardial revascularization prior to subsequent major surgery in patients with coronary artery disease. *Surgery.* 1977;81:302–304.
18. **McFalls EO, Ward HB, Moritz TE, et al.** Coronary-artery revascularization before elective major vascular surgery. *N Engl J Med.* 2004;351:2795–2804.
19. **Poldermans D, Schouten O, Vidakovic R, et al.; DECREASE Study Group.** A clinical randomized trial to evaluate the safety of a noninvasive approach in high-risk patients undergoing major vascular surgery: The DECREASE-V Pilot Study. *J Am Coll Cardiol.* 2007;49(17):1763–1769.
20. **Boden WE, O'Rourke RA, Teo KK, et al.; COURAGE Trial Research Group.** Optimal medical therapy with or without PCI for stable coronary disease. *N Engl J Med.* 2007;356(15):1503–1516.
21. **Douketis JD, Berger PB, Dunn AS, et al.; American College of Chest Physicians.** The perioperative management of antithrombotic therapy. *Chest.* 2008;133(6 suppl):299S–339S.
22. **Mangano DT, Browner WS, Hollenberg M, et al.** Association of perioperative myocardial ischemia with cardiac morbidity and mortality in men undergoing noncardiac surgery. The Study of Perioperative Ischemia Research Group. *N Engl J Med.* 1990;323:1781–1788.
23. **Mangano DT, Browner WS, Hooenberg M, et al.** Long-term cardiac prognosis following noncardiac surgery. The Study of Perioperative Ischemia Research Group. *JAMA.* 1992;268:233–239.
24. **Devereaux PJ, Goldman L, Yusuf S, et al.** Surveillance and prevention of major perioperative ischemic cardiac events in patients undergoing noncardiac surgery: A review. *CMAJ.* 2005;173:779–788.
25. **Charlson ME, MacKenzie CR, Ales K, et al.** Surveillance for postoperative myocardial infarction after noncardiac operations. *Surg Gynecol Obstet.* 1988;167:407–414.
26. **Landesberg G, Beattie WS, Mosseri M, et al.** Postoperative myocardial infarction. *Circulation.* 2009;119:2936–2944.
27. **Jaffe AS.** A small step for man, a leap forward for postoperative management. *J Am Coll Cardiol.* 2003;42:1555–1557.
28. **Thygesen K, Alpert JS, White HD, for the Joint ESC/ACCF/AHA/WHF Task Force for the Redefinition of Myocardial Infarction.** Universal definition of myocardial infarction. *J Am Coll Cardiol.* 2007;50:2173–2195.
29. **Lee TH, Thomas EJ, Ludwig LE, et al.** Troponin T as a marker for myocardial ischemia in patients undergoing major noncardiac surgery. *Am J Cardiol.* 1996;77:1031–1036.
30. **Lopez-Jimenez F, Goldman L, Sacks DB, et al.** Prognostic value of cardiac troponin T after noncardiac surgery: 6 month follow-up data. *J Am Coll Cardiol.* 1997;29:1241–1245.
31. **Psaty BM, Koepsell TD, Wagner EH, et al.** The relative risk of incident coronary artery disease associated with recently stopping the use of beta-blockers. *JAMA.* 1990;263:1653–1657.
32. **Shammash JB, Trost JC, Gold JM, et al.** Perioperative beta-blocker withdrawal and mortality in vascular surgery patients. *Am Heart J.* 2001;141:148–153.
33. **Mangano DT, Layug EL, Wallace A, et al.** Effect of atenolol on mortality and cardiovascular morbidity after non-cardiac surgery. *N Engl J Med.* 1996;335:1713–1720.
34. **Poldermans D, Boersma E, Bax JJ, et al.** The effect of bisoprolol on perioperative mortality and myocardial infarction in high-risk patients undergoing vascular surgery: Dutch Echocardiographic Cardiac Risk Evaluation Applying Stress Echocardiograph Study Group. *N Engl J Med.* 1999;341:1789–1794.
35. **POISE Study Group.** Effect of extended-release metoprolol succinate in patients undergoing non-cardiac surgery (POISE trial): A randomized controlled trial. *Lancet.* 2008;371:1839–1847.
36. **Auerbach AD, Goldman L.** β-blockers and reduction of cardiac events in noncardiac surgery, scientific review. *JAMA.* 2002;287:1435–1444.
37. **Lindenauer PK, Pekow P, Wang K, et al.** Lipid-lowering therapy and in-hospital mortality following major noncardiac surgery. *JAMA.* 2004;291(17):2092–2099.
38. **Schouten O, Boersma E, Hoeks SE, et al.; Dutch Echocardiographic Cardiac Risk Evaluation Applying Stress Echocardiography Study Group.** Fluvastatin and perioperative events in patients undergoing vascular surgery. *N Engl J Med.* 2009;361(10):980–989.
39. **Winchester DE, Wen X, Xie L, et al.** Evidence of preprocedural statin therapy: A meta-analysis of randomized trials. *J Am Coll Cardiol.* 2010;56(14):1099–1109.
40. **Schouten O, Hoeks SE, Welten GM, et al.** Effect of statin withdrawal on frequency of cardiac events after vascular surgery. *Am J Caridiol.* 2007;100(2):316–320.

41. **Eberli D, Chassot PG, Sulser T, et al.** Urological surgery and antiplatelet drugs after cardiac and cerebrovascular accidents. *J Urol.* 2010;183(6):2128–2136.

42. **Burger W, Chemnitius JM, Kneissl GD, et al.** Low-dose aspirin for secondary cardiovascular prevention – cardiovascular risks after its perioperative withdrawal versus bleeding risks with its continuation – review and meta-analysis. *J Intern Med.* 2005;257(5):399–414.

43. **Halm EA, Browner WS, Tubau JF, et al.** Echocardiography for assessing cardiac risk in patients having noncardiac surgery. Study of Perioperative Ischemia Research Group. (published correction appears in *Ann Intern Med* 1997;126:494). *Ann Int Med.* 1996;125:433–441.

44. **Sandham JD, Hull RD, Brant RF, et al.** A randomized, controlled trial of the use of pulmonary-artery catheter in high-risk surgical patients. *N Engl J Med.* 2003;348:5–14.

45. **O'Kelly B, Browner WS, Massie B, et al.** Ventricular arrhythmias in patients undergoing noncardiac surgery. The Study of Preoperative Ischemia Research Group. *JAMA.* 1992;268:217–221.

46. **Mahla E, Rotman B, Rehak P, et al.** Perioperative ventricular dysrhythmias in patients with structural heart disease undergoing noncardiac surgery. *Anesth Analg.* 1998;86:16–21.

47. **Melduni RM, Koshino Y, Shen W.** Management of arrhythmias in the perioperative setting. *Clin Geriatr Med.* 2012;28:729-743.

48. **Pastore JO, Yurchak PM, Janis KM, et al.** The risk of advanced heart block in surgical patients with right bundle branch block and left axis deviation. *Circulation.* 1978;57:677–680.

49. **American Society of Anesthesiologists.** Practice advisory for the perioperative management of patients with cardiac implantable electronic devices: Pacemakers and implantable cardioverter-defibrillators: An updated report. Task Force on Perioperative Management of Patients with Cardiac Implantable Electronic Devices. *Anesthesiology.* 2011;114(2):247–261.

50. **Wilson W, Taubert KA, Gewitz M, et al.** Prevention of infective endocarditis: Guidelines from the American Heart Association: A guideline from the American Heart Association Rheumatic Fever, Endocarditis, and Kawasaki Disease Committee, Council on Cardiovascular Disease in the Young, and the Council on Clinical Cardiology, Council on Cardiovascular Surgery and Anesthesia, and the Quality of Care and Outcomes Research Interdisciplinary Working Group. *Circulation.* 2007;116:1736–1754.

51. **Bedford RF, Feinstein B.** Hospital admission blood pressure: A predictor for hypertension following endotracheal intubation. *Anesth Analg.* 1980;59:367–370.

52. **Ashton CM, Petersen NJ, Wray NP, et al.** The incidence of perioperative myocardial infarction in men undergoing noncardiac surgery. *Ann Intern Med.* 1993;118:504–510.

53. **Charlson ME, MacKenzie CR, Gold JP, et al.** Preoperative characteristics predicting intraoperative hypotension and hypertension among hypertensives and diabetics undergoing noncardiac surgery. *Ann Surg.* 1990;212:66–81.

54. **Brabant SM, Bertrand M, Eyraud D, et al.** The hemodynamic effects of anesthetic induction in vascular surgery patients chronically treated with angiotensin II receptor antagonists. *Anesth Analg.* 1999;89:1388–1392.

55. **Colson P, Saussine M, Seguin JR, et al.** Hemodynamic effects of anesthesia in patients chronically treated with angiotensin-converting enzyme inhibitors. *Anesth Analg.* 1992;74:805–808.

56. **Weksler N, Klein M, Szendro G, et al.** The dilemma of immediate preoperative hypertension: To treat and operate, or to postpone surgery? *J Clin Anesth.* 2003;15:179–183.

57. **Marik PE, Varon J.** Perioperative hypertension: A review of current and emerging therapeutic agents. *J Clin Anesth.* 2009;21:220–229.

58. **Comfere T, Sprung J, Kumar MM, et al.** Angiotensin system inhibitors in a general surgical population. *Anesth Analg.* 2005;100:636–644.

59. **Bertrand M, Godet G, Meersschaert K, et al.** Should the angiotensin II antagonists be discontinued before surgery? *Anesth Analg.* 2001;92:26–30.

60. **Vitez TS, Soper LE, Wong KC, et al.** Chronic hypokalemia and intraoperative dysrhythmias. *Anesthesiology.* 1986;63:130–133.

61. **Fleischmann KE, Goldman L, Young B.** Association between cardiac and noncardiac complications in patients undergoing noncardiac surgery: Outcomes and effects o length of stay. *Am J Med.* 2003;115:515–520.

62. **Dimick JB, Chen SL, Taheri PA, et al.** Hospital costs associated with surgical complications: A report from the private-sector national quality improvement panel. *J Am Coll Surg.* 2004;199:531–537.

63. **Smetana GW, Lawrence VA, Cornell JE, for the American College of Physicians.** Preoperative pulmonary risk stratification for noncardiothoracic surgery: Systemic review for the American College of Physicians. *Ann Intern Med.* 2006;144:581–595.

64. **Berg H, Roed J, Viby-Morgenson J, et al.** Residual neuromuscular block is a risk factor for postoperative pulmonary complications: A prospective, randomized, and blinded study of postoperative pulmonary complications after atracurium, vecuronium and pancuronium. *Acta Anaesthesiol Scand.* 1997;41:1095–1103.

65. **Murphy GS, Szokol JW, Marymont JH, et al.** Residual neuromuscular blockade and respiratory events in the post anesthesia unit. *Anesth Analg.* 2008 107:130–137

66. **Qassem T.** Risk assessment for and strategies to reduce perioperative pulmonary complications. *Ann Intern Med.* 2006;145:553.

67. **American College of Physicians.** Preoperative pulmonary function testing. *Ann Intern Med.* 1990;112:793–794.

68. **Wong DH, Weber EC, Schell MJ.** Factors associated with postoperative pulmonary complications in patients with severe chronic obstructive disease. *Anesth Analg.* 1995;80:276–284.

69. **Warner DO, Warner MA, Barnes RD.** Perioperative respiratory complications in patients with asthma. *Anesthesiology.* 1996;85:460–467.

70. **Gross JB, Bachenberg KL, Nanumof JL, et al.** Practice guidelines for the perioperative management of patients with obstructive sleep apnea: A report of the American Society of Anesthesiologists Task force on Perioperative Management of Patients with Obstructive Sleep Apnea. *Anesthesiology.* 2006;104:1081–1093.

71. **Ramakrishna G, Sprung J, Ravi BS.** Impact of pulmonary hypertension on the outcomes of noncardiac surgery: Predictors of perioperative morbidity and mortality. *J Am Coll Cardiol.* 2005;45:1691–1699.

72. **Mills E, Eyawo O, Lockhart I, et al.** Smoking Cessation reduces postoperative complications: A systematic review and meta analysis. *Am J Med.* 2011;124:144–154.

73. **National Asthma Education and Prevention Program.** Expert Panel Report 3 (EPR-3): Guidelines for the Diagnosis and Management of Asthma-Summary Report 2007. *J Allergy Clin Immunol.* 2007;120(5suppl):S94–S138.

74. **Leisching T, Kwok H, Hill N.** Acute applications of noninvasive positive pressure ventilation. *Chest.* 2003;124:699–713.

75. **Brochard L1, Mancebo J, Wysocki M, et al.** Noninvasive ventilation for acute exacerbations of COPD. *N Engl J Med.* 1995;333:817–822.

76. **Guimaraes MM, El Dib R, Smith AF, et al.** Incentive spirometry for prevention of postoperative pulmonary complications in upper abdominal surgery. *Cochrane Database Syst Rev.* 2009;(3):CD006058.

77. **Nelson R, Tse B, Edwards S.** Systematic review of prophylactic nasogastric decompression after abdominal operations. *Br J Surg.* 2005;92:673–680.

78. **Marhoffer W, Stein M, Maeser E, et al.** Impairment of polymorphonuclear leukocyte function and metabolic control of diabetes. *Diabetes Care.* 1992;15:256–260.

79. **Alexiewicz JM, Kumar D, Smogorzewski M, et al.** Polymorphonuclear leukocytes in non-insulin-dependent diabetes mellitus: Abnormalities in metabolism and function. *Ann Intern Med.* 1995;123:919–924.

80. **Rassias AJ, Marrin CA, Arruda J, et al.** Insulin infusion improves neutrophil function in diabetic cardiac surgery patients. *Anesth Analg.* 1999;88:1011–1016.

81. **Pozzilli P, Leslie R.** Infections and diabetes: Mechanism and prospects for prevention. *Diabet Med.* 1994;11:935–941.

82. **Loots M, Lamme E, Mekkes J, et al.** Cultured fibroblasts from chronic diabetic wounds on the lower extremity (non-insulin-dependent diabetes mellitus) show disturbed proliferation. *Arch Dermatol Res.* 1999;291:93–99.

83. **Turina M, Fry DE, Polk HC.** Acute hyperglycemia and the innate immune system: Clinical, cellular, and molecular aspects. *Crit Care Med.* 2005;33:1624–1633.

84. **Clement S, Braithwaite SS, Magee MF, et al.; for the American Diabetes Association Diabetes in Hospitals Writing Committee.**

Management of diabetes and hyperglycemia in hospitals. *Diabetes Care.* 2004;27:553–591.

85. **Bakkum-Gamez JN, Dowdy SC, Borah BJ, et al.** Predictors and costs of surgical site infections in patients with endometrial cancer. *Gynecol Oncol.* 2013;130:100–106.

86. **Kwon S, Thompson R, Dellinger P, et al.** Importance of perioperative glycemic control in general surgery: A report from the Surgical Care and Outcomes Assessment Program. *Ann Surg.* 2013;257(1): 8–14.

87. **Pomposelli JJ, Baxter JK 3rd, Babineau TJ, et al.** Early postoperative glucose control predicts nosocomial infection rate in diabetic patients. *JPEN J Parenter Enteral Nutr.* 1998;22:77–81.

88. **Umpierrez GE, Isaacs SD, Barzargan N, et al.** Hyperglycemia: An independent marker of in-hospital mortality in patients with undiagnosed diabetes. *J Clin Endocrinol Metab.* 2002;87:978–982.

89. **Suleiman M, Hammerman H, Boulos M, et al.** Fasting glucose is an important independent risk factor for 30-day mortality in patient with acute myocardial infarction: A prospective study. *Circulation.* 2005;111:754–760.

90. **Krinsley JS.** Association between hyperglycemia and increased hospital mortality in a heterogeneous population of critically ill patients. *Mayo Clin Proc.* 2003;78:1471–1478.

91. **Finney SJ, Zekveld C, Elia A, et al.** Glucose control and mortality in critically ill patients. *JAMA.* 2003;290:2041–2047.

92. **Vilar-Compte Diana, Alvarez de Iturbe I, Martín-Onraet A, et al.** Hyperglycemia as a risk factor for surgical site infections in patients undergoing mastectomy. *Am J Infect Control.* 2008;36: 192–198.

93. **Furnary A, Zerr K, Grunkemeier G, et al.** Continuous intravenous insulin infusion reduces the incidence of deep sternal wound infection in diabetic patients after cardiac surgical procedures. *Ann Thorac Surg.* 1999;67:352–362.

94. **van den Berghe G, Wouters P, Weekers F, et al.** Intensive insulin therapy in critically ill patients. *N Engl J Med.* 2001;345:1359–1367.

95. **Wiener RS, Wiener DC, Larson RJ.** Benefits and risks of tighter control in critically ill adults: A meta-analysis. *JAMA.* 2008;300: 933–944.

96. **Finfer S, Chittock DR, Su SY, et al.; NICE-SUGAR Study Investigators.** Intensive versus conventional glucose control in critically ill patients. *N Engl J Med.* 2009;360:1283–1297.

97. **Krinsley JS, Grover A.** Severe hypoglycemia in critically ill patients: Risk factors and outcomes. *Crit Care Med.* 2007;35: 2262–2267.

98. **Griesdale DE, de Souza RJ, van Dam RM, et al.** Intensive insulin therapy and mortality among critically ill patients: A meta-analysis including NICD-SUGAR study data. *CMAJ.* 2009;180:821–827.

99. **van den Berghe G, Wiler A, Hermans G, et al.** Intensive insulin therapy in the medical ICU. *N Engl J Med.* 2006;354:449–461.

100. **Kirnsley JS.** Effect of intensive glucose management protocol on the mortality of critically ill adult patients. *Mayo Clin Proc.* 2004;79: 992–1000.

101. **Lazar HL, Chipkin SR, Fitzgerald CA, et al.** Tight glycemic control in diabetic coronary artery bypass graft patients improves perioperative outcomes and decreases recurrent ischemic events. *Circulation.* 2004;109:1497–1502.

102. **Umpierrez GE, Smiley D, Zisman A, et al.** Randomized study of basal-bolus insulin therapy in the in-patient management of patients with type 2 diabetes (RABBIT 2 trial). *Diabetes Care.* 2007;30: 2181–2186.

103. **Inzucchi S.** Management of hyperglycemia in the hospital setting. *N Engl J Med.* 2006;355:1903–1911.

104. **Queale WS, Seidler AJ, Brancati FL.** Glycemic control and sliding scale insulin use in medical in-patients with diabetes mellitus. *Arch Intern Med.* 1997;157:545–552.

105. **Baldwin D, Villanueva G, McNutt R, et al.** Eliminating inpatient sliding-scale insulin: A reeducation project with medical house staff. *Diabetes Care.* 2005;28:1008–1011.

106. **Golightly LK, Jones MA, Hamamura DH, et al.** Management of diabetes mellitus in hospitalized patients: Efficiency and effectiveness of sliding-scale insulin therapy. *Pharmacotherapy.* 2006;26: 1421–1432.

107. **Nygren J, Thorell A, Soop M, et al.** Perioperative insulin and glucose infusion maintains normal insulin sensitivity after surgery. *Am J Physiol.* 1998;275:E140–E148.

108. **Drucker DJ, Burrow GN.** Cardiovascular surgery in the hypothyroid patient. *Arch Intern Med.* 1985;145:1585–1587.

109. **Ladenson PW, Levin AA, Ridgway ED, et al.** Complications of surgery in hypothyroid patients. *Am J Med.* 1984;77:261–266.

110. **Weinberg AD, Brennan MD, Gorman CA, et al.** Outcome of anesthesia and surgery in hypothyroid patients. *Arch Intern Med.* 1983;143:893–897.

111. **Schiff RL, Welsh GA.** Perioperative evaluation and management of the patient with endocrine dysfunction. *Med Clin N Am.* 2003;87: 175–192.

112. **Stathatos N, Wartofsky L.** Perioperative management of patients with hypothyroidism. *Endocrinol Metab Clin N Am.* 2003;32: 503–518.

113. **Kohl BA, Schwartz Stanley.** How to Manage Perioperative Endocrine Insufficiency. *Anesthesiol Clin.* 2010;28(1):139-155.

114. **Lennquist S, Jörtsö E, Anderberg B, et al.** Beta-blockers compared with antithyroidal drugs as preoperative treatment in hyperthyroidism: Drug tolerance, complications, and postoperative thyroid function. *Surgery.* 1985;98:1141–1147.

115. **Langley RW, Burch HB.** Perioperative management of the thyrotoxic patient. *Endocrinol Metab Clin N Am.* 2003;32:519–534.

116. **Bromberg JS, Alfrey EJ, Barker CF, et al.** Adrenal suppression and steroid supplementation in renal transplant recipients. *Transplantation.* 1991;51:385–390.

117. **LaRochelle GE, LaRochelle AG, Ratner RE, et al.** Recovery of the hypothalamic-pituitary adrenal (HPA) axis in patients with rheumatic diseases receiving low-dose prednisone. *Am J Med.* 1993;95:258–264.

118. **Glowniak JV, Loriaux DL.** A double-blind study of perioperative steroid requirements in secondary adrenal insufficiency. *Surgery.* 1997;121:123–129.

119. **Henzen C, Suter A, Lerch E, et al.** Suppression and recovery of adrenal response after short-term, high-dose glucocorticoid treatment. *Lancet.* 2000;355:542–545.

120. **Schlaghecke R, Kornelly E, Santen R, et al.** The effect of long-term glucocorticoid therapy on pituitary-adrenal responses to exogenous corticotropin-releasing hormone. *N Engl J Med.* 1992;326: 226–230.

121. **Cooper M, Stewart P.** Corticosteroid insufficiency in acutely ill patients. *N Engl J Med.* 2003;348:727–734.

122. **Dickstein G, Shechner C, Nicholson WE, et al.** Adrenocorticotropin stimulation test: Effects of basal cortisol level, time of day, and suggested new sensitive low dose test. *J Clin Endocrinol Metab.* 1991; 72:77–78.

123. **Oelkers W.** Adrenal insufficiency. *N Engl J Med.* 1996;335:1206–1212.

124. **Dorin RI, Qualls CR, Crapo LM.** Diagnosis of adrenal insufficiency. *Ann Intern Med* 2003;139:194–204.

125. **Salem M, Tainsh RE, Bromberg J, et al.** Perioperative glucocorticoid coverage: A reassessment 42 years after emergence of a problem. *Ann Surg.* 1994;219:416–425.

126. **Coursin D, Wood K.** Corticosteroid supplementation for adrenal insufficiency. *JAMA.* 2002;287:236–340.

127. **Clagett GP, Reisch JS.** Prevention of venous thromboembolism in general surgical patients: Results of meta-analysis. *Ann Surg.* 1988; 208:227–240.

128. **Hirsh J, Hoak J.** Management of deep vein thrombosis and pulmonary embolism. A statement for healthcare professionals. Council on Thrombosis (in consultation with the Council on Cardiovascular Radiology), American Heart Association. *Circulation.* 1996;93:2212–2245.

129. **Maxwell GL, Synan I, Dodge R, et al.** Pneumatic compression versus low molecular weight heparin in gynecologic oncology surgery: A randomized trial. *Obstet Gynecol.* 2001;98:989–995.

130. **Heilmann L, von Tempelhoff GF, Schneider D.** Prevention of thrombosis in gynecologic malignancy. *Clin Appl Thromb/Hemost.* 1998;4:153–159.

131. **Uppal S, Hernandez E, Dutta M, et al.** Prolonged postoperative venous thrombo-embolism prophylaxis is cost-effective in advanced ovarian cancer patients. *Gynecol Oncol.* 2012;127(3):631–637.

132. **Smetana GW, Macpherson DS.** The case against routine preoperative laboratory testing. *Med Clin North Am.* 2003;89:7–40.

133. **Pasternack LR.** Preoperative screening for ambulatory patients. *Anesthesiol Clin North Am.* 2003;21:229–242.

134. **Cavallini GM, Saccarola P, D'Amico R, et al.** Impact of preoperative testing on ophthalmologic and systemic outcomes in cataract surgery. *Eur J Ophthalmol.* 2004;14(5):369–374.

135. **Chung F, Yuan H, Yin L, et al.** Elimination of preoperative testing in ambulatory surgery. *Anesth Analg.* 2009;108:467-475.

136. **Schein O, Katz J, Bass E.** The value of routine preoperative testing before cataract surgery. *N Engl J Med.* 2000;342:168–175.

137. **Johansson T, Fritsch G, Flamm M, et al.** Effectiveness of non-cardiac preoperative testing in non-cardiac elective surgery: A systematic review. *Br J Anaesth* 2013;110(6):926–939.

138. **Munro J, Booth A, Nicholl J.** Routine preoperative testing: A systematic review of the evidence. *Health Technol Assess.* 1997;1:i–iv; 1–62.

139. **Ajimura FY, Maia AS, Hachiya A, et al.** Preoperative laboratory evaluation of patients aged over 40 years undergoing elective non-cardiac surgery. *Sao Paulo Med J.* 2005;123:50–53.

140. **Joo HS, Wong J, Naik VN, et al.** The value of screening preoperative chest x-rays: A systematic review. *Can J Anesth.* 2005;52: 568–574.

141. **Reynolds TM.** National Institute for Health and Clinical Excellence guidelines on preoperative tests: The use of routine preoperative tests for elective surgery. *Ann Clin Biochem.* 2006;43:13–16.

142. **Narr BJ, Warner ME, Schroeder DR, et al.** Outcomes of patients with no laboratory assessment before anesthesia and a surgical procedure. *Mayo Clin Proc.* 1997;72:505–509.

143. **CG3 Preoperative Tests.** Available online at: http://www.nice.org.uk/Guidance/CG3/Guidance/pdf/English. Accessed August 30, 2013.

144. **Suchman A, Mushin A.** How well does the activated partial thromboplastin time predict post operative hemorrhage? *JAMA.* 1986;256: 750–753.

145. **Eckman MH, Erban JK, Singh SK, et al.** Screening for the risk of bleeding or thrombosis. *Arch Intern Med.* 2003;138(3):W15–W24.

146. **Seicean A, Schiltz NK, Seicean S, et al.** Use and utility of preoperative hemostatic screening and patient history in adult neurosurgical patients. *J Neurosurg.* 2012;116:1097–1105.

147. **Tuohy E, Litt E, Alikhan R.** Treatment of patients with von Willebrand disease. *J Blood Med* 2011;2:49–57.

148. **ACOG Committee on Practice Bulletins-Gynecology.** ACOG practice bulletin No. 104: Antibiotic prophylaxis for gynecologic procedures. *Obstet Gynecol.* 2009;113(5):1180–1189.

149. **Jung B, Pahlman L, Nystrom PO, et al.** Multicentre randomized clinical trial of mechanical bowel preparation in elective colonic resection. *Br J Surg.* 2007;94:689–695.

150. **Van't Sant HP, Slieker JC, Hop WCJ, et al.** The influence of mechanical bowel preparation in elective colorectal surgery for diverticulitis. *Tech Coloproctol.* 2012;16(4):309–314.

151. **Eskicioglu C, Forbes SS, Fenech DS, et al.; Best Practice in General Surgery Committee.** Preoperative bowel preparation for patients undergoing elective colorectal surgery: A clinical practice guideline endorsed by the Canadian Society of Colon and Rectal Surgeons. *Can J Surg.* 2010;53(6):385–395.

152. **Lindenauer PK.** Perioperative beta-blocker therapy and mortality after major noncardiac surgery. *N Engl J Med.* 2005;353:349–361.

153. **Chobanian AV, Bakris GL, Black HR, et al.** The Seventh Report of the Joint National Committee on Prevention, Detection, Evaluation, and Treatment of High Blood Pressure: The JNC 7 report. *JAMA.* 2003;289:2560–2572.

154. **Adebola OA.** Management of perioperative myocardial infarction in noncardiac surgical patients. *Chest.* 2006;130:584–596.

155. **Advanced life support: Part 4.** *Circulation.* 2005;112(22suppl 22): III–25–III–54.

156. **Anderson JL, Halperin JL, Albert NM, et al.** Management of patients with atrial fibrillation (compilation of 2006 ACF/AHA/ESC and 2011 ACCF/AHA/HRS recommendations): A report of the American College of Cardiology/American Heart Association Task Force on Practice Guidelines. *J Am Coll Cardiol.* 2013;61(18):1935–1944.

157. **Shah MR, Hasselblad V, Stevenson LW, et al.** Impact of the pulmonary artery catheter in critically ill patients: Meta-analysis of randomized clinical trials. *JAMA.* 2005;294:1664–1670.

158. **Finfer S, Bellomo R, Boyce N, et al.** A comparison of albumin and saline for fluid resuscitation in the intensive care unit. *N Engl J Med.* 2004;350:2247–2256.

159. **Dellinger RP, Levy MM, et al.** Surviving Sepsis Campaign: International guidelines for management of severe sepsis and septic shock: 2012. *Crit Care Med.* 2012;41:580–637.

160. **Calfee CS, Matthay MA.** Nonventilatory treatments for acute lung injury and ARDS. *Chest.* 2007;131:913–920.

161. **Girard T, Bernard GR.** Mechanical ventilation in ARDS: A state of the art review. *Chest.* 2007;131:921–929.

162. **Villar J, Blanco J, Añón JM, et al.** The ALIEN study: Incidence and outcome of acute respiratory distress syndrome in the era of lung protective ventilation. *Intensive Care Med.* 2011;37(12):1932–1941.

163. **Slutsky AS.** Mechanical ventilation. American College of Chest Physicians' Consensus Conference. *Chest.* 1993;104:1833–1859.

164. **Bitterman H.** Bench to Bedside Review: Oxygen as a drug. *Crit Care.* 2009 13(1):205.

165. **Guerin C.** Prone positioning in severe acute respiratory distress syndrome. *N Engl J Med.* 2013;268(23):2159-2168.

166. **Papazian C, Forel JM, Gacouin A, et al.** Neuromuscular blockers in early acute respiratory distress syndrome. *N Engl J Med.* 2010; 303:1107–1116.

167. **Tobin MJ, Jubran A.** Variable performance of weaning-predictor tests. Variable performance of weaning-predictor tests: Role of Bayes' theorem and spectrum and test-referral bias. *Intensive Care Med.* 2006;32:2002–2012.

168. **MacIntyre NR, Cook DL, Ely EW Jr, et al.** Evidence-based guidelines for weaning and discontinuing ventilatory support: A collective task force facilitated by the American College of Chest Physicians; the American Association for Respiratory Care; And the American College of Critical Care Medicine. *Chest.* 1993;120:375s–395s.

169. **Carmichael P, Carmichael AR.** Acute renal failure in the surgical setting. *ANZ J Surg.* 2003;73:144–153.

170. **Novis BK, Roizen MF, Aronson S, et al.** Association of preoperative risk factors with postoperative acute renal failure. *Anesth Analg.* 1994;78:143–149.

171. **Thadhani R, Pascual M, Bonvnetre J.** Acute renal failure. *N Engl J Med.* 1996;334:1448–1460.

172. **Hou SH, Bushinsky DA.** Hospital acquired renal insufficiency: A prospective study. *Am J Med.* 1983;74:243–248.

173. **Darmon M, Ciroldi M, Thiery G, et al.** Clinical review: Specific aspects of acute renal failure in cancer patients. *Crit Care.* 2006; 10:211–217.

174. **Millet PJ, Pelle-Francoz D.** Nondilated obstructive acute renal failure: Diagnostic procedures and therapeutic management. *Radiology.* 1986;160:659–662.

175. **Miller TR, Anderson RJ, Linas SL, et al.** Urinary diagnostic indices in acute renal failure: A prospective study. *Ann Intern Med.* 1978;89:47–50.

176. **Barrett JB, Parfrey PS.** Preventing nephropathy induced by contrast medium. *N Engl J Med* 2006;354:379–386.

177. **Tepel M, van der Giet M, Schwarzfeld C.** Prevention of radiographic-contrast agent-induced reductions in renal function by acetylcysteine. *N Engl J Med.* 2000;343:180–184.

178. **Tiu RV, Mountantonakis SE, Dunbar AJ, et al.** Tumor lysis syndrome. *Semin Thromb Hemost.* 2007;33:397–407.

179. **Klahir S, Miller S.** Acute oliguria. *N Engl J Med.* 1998;338:671–675.

180. **Bagshaw SM, Delaney A, Haase M, et al.** Loop diuretics in the management of acute renal failure: A systematic review and meta-analysis. *Crit Care Resusc.* 2007;9:60–68.

181. **Weisbord SD, Palevsky PM.** Acute renal failure in the intensive care unit. *Semin Respir Crit Care Med.* 2006;27:262–273.

182. **Yagi N, Paginini E.** Acute dialysis and continuous renal replacement: The emergence of new technology involving the nephrologist in the intensive care setting. *Semin Nephrol.* 1997;17:306–320.

183. **Adrogué HJ, Madias NE.** Management of life-threatening acid-base disorders. First of two parts. *N Engl J Med.* 1998;338:26–34.

184. **Adrogué HJ, Madias NE.** Medical progress: Management of life-threatening acid-base disorders. Second of two parts. *N Engl J Med.* 1998;338:107–111.

185. **Ayers P, Warrington L.** Diagnosis and treatment of simple acid-base disorders. *Nutr Clin Pract.* 2008;23:122–127.

186. **Narins RG, Emmett M.** Simple and mixed acid base disorders. *Medicine (Baltimore).* 1980;59:161–187.

187. **Cooper DJ, Walley KR, Wiggs BR, et al.** Bicarbonate does not improve the hemodynamics in critically ill patients who have lactic

acidosis. A prospective, controlled study. *Ann Intern Med.* 1990; 112:492–498.

188. **Stacpoole PW.** Lactic acidosis: The case against bicarbonate therapy. *Ann Intern Med.* 1986;105:276–279.

189. **McLaughlin ML, Kassirer JP.** Rational treatment of acid-base disorders. *Drugs.* 1990;39:841–855.

190. **Kumar S, Berl T.** Sodium. *Lancet.* 1998;352:220–228.

191. **Adrogue HJ, Madias NE.** Hyponatremia. *N Engl J Med.* 2000;342: 1581–1589.

192. **Goh KP.** Management of hyponatremia. *Am Fam Physician.* 2004; 69:2387–2394.

193. **Adrogué HJ, Madias NE.** Hypernatremia. *N Engl J Med.* 2000; 342:1493–1499.

194. **Kapoor M, Chan GZ.** Fluid and electrolyte abnormalities. *Crit Care Clin.* 2001;17:503–529.

195. **Souba WW.** Nutritional support. *N Engl J Med.* 1997;336:41–48.

196. **Sanström R, Drott C, Hyltander A, et al.** The effect of postoperative intravenous feeding (TPN) on outcome following major surgery evaluated in a randomized study. *Ann Surg.* 1993;217: 185–195.

197. **Wu WC, Schifftner TL, Henderson WG, et al.** Preoperative hematocrit levels and postoperative outcomes in older patients undergoing noncardiac surgery. *JAMA.* 2007;297:2481–2488.

198. **Carson JL, Grossman BJ, Kleinman S, et al.** Red blood cell transfusion: A clinical practice guideline from the AABB. *Ann Intern Med.* 2012;157:49–58.

199. **Napolitano LM, Kurek S, Luchette FA, et al.; American College of Critical Care Medicine of the Society of Critical Care Medicine.** Clinical practice guideline: Red blood cell transfusion in adult trauma and critical care. *Crit Care Med.* 2009;37:3124–3157.

200. **Carson JL, Terrin ML, Novec H, et al.** Liberal or restrictive transfusion in high-risk patients after hip surgery. *N Engl J Med.* 2011; 365:2453–2462.

201. **Hébert PC, Wells G, Blajchman MA, et al.** A multicenter, randomized, controlled clinical trial of transfusion requirements in critical care. Transfusion Requirements in Critical Care Investigators, Canadian Critical Care Trials Group. *N Engl J Med.* 1999;340: 409–417.

202. **Kumar A.** Perioperative management of anemia: Limits of blood transfusion and alternatives to it. *Cleve Clin J Med.* 2009;76(suppl 4): S112–S118.

203. **Murphy GJ, Barnaby CR, Rogers CA, et al.** Increased mortality, postoperative morbidity, and cost after red blood cell transfusion in patients having cardiac surgery. *Circulation.* 2007;116:2544–2552.

204. **Nuttall GA, Brost BC, Connis RT, et al.** Practice guidelines for perioperative blood transfusion and adjuvant therapies: An Updated Report by the American Society of Anesthesiologists Task Force on Perioperative Blood Transfusion and Adjuvant Therapies. *Anesthesiology.* 2006;105:198–208.

205. **Hellstern P, Haubelt H.** Indications for plasma in massive transfusion. *Thromb Res.* 2002;107:s19–s22.

206. **Stainsby D, Maclennan S, Thomas D, et al.** British Committee for Standards in Haematology. Guidelines on the management of massive blood loss. *Br J Haematol.* 2006;135:634–641.

207. **Levi M.** Disseminated intravascular coagulation. *Crit Care Med.* 2007;35:2191–2195.

208. **Levi M, ten Cate H, van der Poll, et al.** Pathogenesis of disseminated intravascular coagulation in sepsis. *JAMA.* 1993;270: 975–979.

209. **Busch MP, Kleinman SH, Nemo GJ.** Current and emerging infectious risks of blood transfusion. *JAMA.* 2003;289:959–962.

210. **Sandler SG, Yu H, Rassai N.** Risks of blood transfusion and their prevention. *Clin Adv Hematol Oncol.* 2003;1:307–313.

211. **Silliman CC, Ambruso DR, Boshkov LK.** Transfusion-related acute lung injury. *Blood.* 2005;105:2266–2273.

212. **Hirsch J.** How we diagnose and treat deep vein thrombosis. *Blood.* 2002;99:3102–3110.

213. **Alikhan R.** Fatal pulmonary embolism in hospitalized patients; A necroscopy review. *J Clin Pathol.* 2004;57:1254–1257.

214. **Tapson VF.** Acute pulmonary embolism. *N Engl J Med.* 2008;358: 1037–1052.

215. **The PIOPED Investigators.** Value of the ventilation/perfusion scan in acute pulmonary embolism. Results of the prospective investigation of pulmonary embolism diagnosis (PIOPED). *JAMA.* 1990;263: 2753–2759.

216. **Stein PD, Fowler SE, Goodman LR, et al.** Multidetector computed tomography for acute pulmonary embolism. *N Engl J Med.* 2006; 354:2317–2327.

217. **Goodacre S, Sampson FC, Sutton AJ, et al.** Variation in the diagnostic performance of D-Dimer for suspected deep vein thrombosis. *QJM* 2005;98:513–27.

218. **Kearon C, Kahn SR, Agnelli G, et al.; American College of Chest Physicians.** Antithrombotic therapy for venous thromboembolic disease. American College of Chest Physicians Evidence-Based practice guidelines (8th ed). *Chest.* 2008;133:454S–545S.

219. **Goldhaber SZ, Visani L, De M.** Rosa Acute pulmonary embolism: Clinical outcomes in the International Cooperative Pulmonary Embolism Registry (ICOPER). *Lancet.* 353(1999):1386–1389.

220. **Verstraete M, Miller GA, Bounameaux H, et al.** Intravenous and intrapulmonary recombinant tissue-type plasminogen activator in the treatment of acute massive pulmonary embolism. *Circulation.* 1988; 77(2):353–360.

221. **Dentali F, Ageno W, Imberti D.** Retrievable vena caval filters: Clinical experience. *Curr Opin Pulm Med.* 2006;12:304–309.

222. **Baglin T, Luddington R, Brown K, et al.** Incidence of recurrent venous thromboembolism in relation to clinical and thrombophilic risk factors: A prospective cohort study. *Lancet.* 2003;362:523–526.

223. **Clifford V, Daley A.** Antibiotic prophylaxis in obstetric and gynaecologic procedures: A review. *Aust N Z J Obstet Gynaecol.* 2012;52: 412–419.

224. **Flodgren G, Contemo LO, Mayhew A, et al.** Interventions to improve professional adherence to guidelines for prevention of device-related infections. *Cochrane Database Syst Rev.* 2013;3:CD006559.

225. **Kushnir CL, Diaz-Montes TP.** Perioperative care in gynecologic oncology. *Curr Opin Obstet Gynecol.* 2013;25:23–28.

226. **Van Eyk N, van Schalkwyk J.** Antibiotic prophylaxis in Gynaecologic Procedures. *J Obstet Gynaecol Can.* 2012;34(4):382–391.

227. **Krein SL, Kowalski CP, Hofer TP, et al.** Preventing Hospital-Acquired Infections: A National Survey of Practices Reported by U.S. Hospitals in 2005 and 2009. *J Gen Intern Med.* 27(7):773–779.

228. **O'Grady NP, Bade PS, Bartlett J, et al.** Practice parameters for evaluating new fever in critically ill adult patients. Task Force of the American College of Critical Care Medicine of the Society of Critical Care Medicine in collaboration with the Infectious Disease Society of America. *Crit Care Med.* 1998;26:392–408.

229. **Hughes WT, Armstrong D, Bodry GP.** 2002 guidelines for the use of antimicrobial agents in neutropenic patients with cancer. *Clin Infect Dis.* 2002;34:730–751.

230. **Bucaneve G, Micozzi A, Menichetti F, et al.** for the Gruppo Italiano Malattie Ematologiche dell'Adulto (GIMEMA) Infection Program. Levofloxacin to prevent bacterial infection in patients with cancer and neutropenia. *N Engl J Med.* 2005;353:977–987.

231. **Cullen M, Steven N, Billingham L, et al.** for the Simple Investigation in Neutropenic Individuals of the Frequency of Infection after Chemotherapy +/– Antibiotic in a Number of Tumours (SIGNIFICANT) Trial Group. Antibiotic prophylaxis after chemotherapy for solid cell tumors and lymphomas. *N Eng J Med.* 2005;353:988–998.

232. **Gafter-Gvili A, Fraser A, Paul M, et al.** Meta-analysis: Antibiotic prophylaxis reduces mortality in neutropenic patients. *Ann Int Med.* 2005;142:979–995.

233. **Eleutherakis-Papaiakovou E, Kostis E, Migkou M, et al.** Prophylactic antibiotics for the prevention of neutropenic fever in patients undergoing autologous stem-cell transplantation: Results of a single institution, randomized phase 2 trial. *Am J Hematol.* 2010;85(11):863–867.

234. **Slavin MA, Lingaratnam S, Mileshkin L, et al.; Australian Consensus Guidelines 2011 Steering Committee.** Use of antibacterial prophylaxis for patients with neutropenia. *Intern Med J.* 2011;41:102–109.

235. **Neumann S, Krause SW, Maschmeyer G, et al.** Primary prophylaxis of bacterial infections and Pneumocystis jirovecii pneumonia in patients with hematological malignancies and solid tumors, Guidelines of the Infectious Disease Working Party (AGIHO) of the German Society of Hematology and Oncology (DGHO). *Ann Hematol.* 2013;92:433–442.

236. **Freifeld A, Marchigiani D, Walsh T, et al.** A double-blind comparison of empirical oral and intravenous antibiotic therapy for low-risk febrile patients with neutropenia during cancer chemotherapy. *N Engl J Med.* 1999;341:305–311.

237. **Kern WV, Cometta A, de Bock R, et al.** Oral versus intravenous empirical antimicrobial therapy for fever in patients with granulocytopenia who are receiving cancer chemotherapy. International Antimicrobial Therapy Cooperative Group of the European Organization for the Research and Treatment of Cancer. *N Engl J Med.* 1999;341:312–318.

238. **Ozer H, Armitage JO, Bennett CL, et al. for the American Society of Clinical Oncology.** 2000 update of recommendations for the use of hematopoietic colony-stimulating factors: Evidence based, clinical practice guidelines. American Society of Clinical Oncology Growth Factors Expert Panel. *J Clin Oncol.* 2002;18:3558–3585.

239. **Lyman G.** Guidelines of the National Comprehensive Cancer Network on the use of myeloid growth factors with cancer chemotherapy: A review of the evidence. *J Natl Compr Canc Netw.* 2005;3: 557–571.

240. **Wey SB, Mori M, Pfaller MA, et al.** Risk factors for hospital-acquired candidemia: A matched case-control study. *Arch Intern Med.* 1989;149:2349–2353.

241. **Faser VJ, Jones M, Dunkel J, et al.** Candidemia in a tertiary care hospital: Epidemiology, risk factors, and predictors of mortality. *Clin Infect Dis.* 1992;15:414–421.

242. **Pappas PG, Rex JH, Sobel JD, et al.; for the Infectious Diseases Society of America.** Guidelines for treatment of candidiasis. *Clin Infect Dis.* 2004;38:161–189.

243. **Quigley EM, Quera R.** Small intestinal bacterial overgrowth: Roles of antibiotics, prebiotics, and probiotics. *Gastroenterology.* 2006;130: S78–S90.

244. **Quigley EM, Abu-Shanab A.** Small intestinal bacterial overgrowth. *Infec Dis Clin North Am.* 2010;24:943–59,viii–ix.

245. **Shah SC, Day LW, Somsouk M, et al.** Meta-analysis: Antibiotic therapy for small intestinal bacterial overgrowth. *Aliment Pharmacol Ther.* 2013;38:925–934.

246. **Lauritano EC, Gabrielli M, Scarpellini E, et al.** Small intestinal bacterial overgrowth recurrence after antibiotic therapy. *Am J Gastroenterol.* 2008;103:2031–2035.

247. **Vanderhoof JA, Young RJ, Murray N, et al.** Treatment strategies for small bowel bacterial overgrowth in short bowel syndrome. *J Pediatr Gastroenterol Nutr.* 1998;27:155–160.

248. **Stotzer PO, Blomberg L, Conway PL, et al.** Probiotic treatment of small intestinal bacterial overgrowth by Lactobacillus fermentum KLD. *Scand J Infect Dis.* 1996;28:615–619.

19 Nutritional Therapy

Paul M. Maggio
Norman W. Rizk

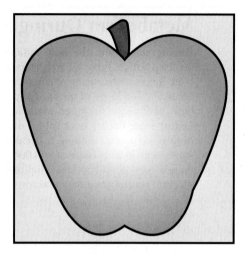

Traditionally, nutritional support has been viewed as an intervention to preserve lean body mass, maintain immune function, and avoid metabolic complications. As understanding of the biologic effects of nutrition has improved, the focus has shifted from nutrition as a supportive intervention to a therapy. **Delivering early and appropriate nutrition attenuates the metabolic stress response, prevents oxidative cellular injury, and modulates the immune response** (1). The beneficial impact of nutritional support on the outcome and quality of life of the gynecologic oncology patient has been widely recognized. To facilitate the appropriate institution of nutritional support, an understanding of the classification of malnutrition and its diagnosis is essential. Physicians should be familiar with enteral and parenteral nutrition, their means of delivery, and their associated complications. There should also be appropriate monitoring of the response to therapy. A team approach by physician, nutritionist, and pharmacist is ideal for achieving these goals.

Normal Body Metabolism

According to the first law of thermodynamics, the energy derived from ingested food must equal the energy expended or stored in the body at equilibrium. Although the quantity of energy intake and the amount expended and stored in any 24-hour period do not correspond exactly, **body weight eventually reflects the balance between energy intake and energy expenditure**.

Calories

The unit of energy exchange is the *calorie*, which is the amount of heat required to raise the temperature of 1 mL of water 1°C at 1 atmosphere of pressure.

Dietary Calories

The dietary calorie equals 1,000 calories. Thus, 1,500 dietary calories are equal to a 1,500-kilocalorie diet. This notation is used to describe body stores of energy and the quantity of food ingested.

Body Stores

Although diets are variable, all foods are broken down through digestion into monosaccharides, amino acids, fatty acids, and glycerol. These are redistributed to body stores or metabolized for energy.

The body stores of energy are very different from the composition of the diet. The average diet has from 30–50% fat calories, 40–60% carbohydrate calories, and 15–20% protein calories. **Roughly 1,200 carbohydrate calories are stored as glycogen in muscle and liver, whereas 130,000 to 160,000 calories are contained in fat;** one pound of fat represents 3,500 stored calories. The body also contains approximately 54,000 calories as protein in muscle and organs, but only 30–50% of this is available to be burned for energy. **Greater than a 50% depletion of total body protein is incompatible with life** (2).

Metabolism During Starvation

During starvation, the body adapts to spare vital protein stores. Carbohydrate stores are depleted within 3 days of total starvation at rest, or more rapidly if the metabolic effects of catabolic illnesses elevate the requirements. Many organs use glucose in large amounts, obligating the breakdown of 75 g/d of muscle early in starvation (3). If the muscle were to continue to be broken down at this rate, starvation would lead to death in 45 to 60 days, but **adaptation from a fed to a fasting state occurs over 2 to 3 days** (Fig. 19.1). **In this adaptation, peripheral tissues and organs use ketone bodies, a breakdown product of fat, in place of glucose.** Because the fat stores contain an average of 160,000 calories, survival can be extended to 140 to 160 days. Some muscle breakdown continues, limiting survival, because the brain and the red blood cells require glucose, necessitating the breakdown of 20 g/d of muscle even after full adaptation.

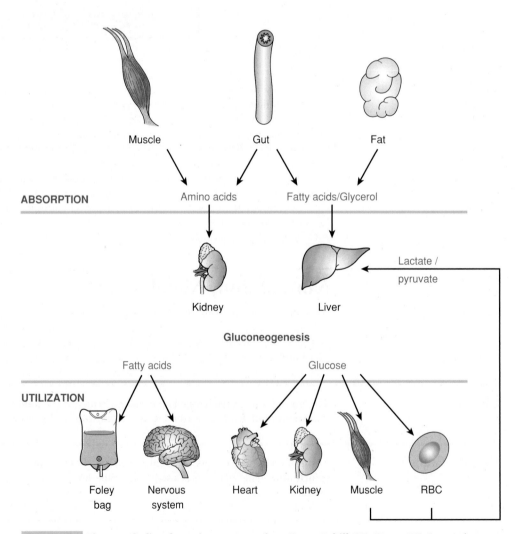

Figure 19.1 **The metabolic adaptation to starvation.** (From **Cahill GF, Owen OE.** Some observations on carbohydrate metabolism in man. In: **Dickens F, Randle PJ, Whelan WI, eds.** *Carbohydrate Metabolism and its Disorders.* New York, NY: Academic Press; 1968:497, with permission.)

Malnutrition

Malnutrition is caused by an imbalance of energy, protein, and other nutrients. It adversely affects body composition, function, and clinical outcome. If left untreated, it invariably leads to cachexia, a syndrome characterized by severe body weight, fat, and muscle loss (4). **About 40–55% of adult hospitalized patients in the United States are malnourished or at risk for malnutrition and 12% are severely malnourished** (5–8). Similar percentages of malnutrition have been documented in thousands of hospitalized patients throughout the world (9). Between 40% and 80% of cancer patients are malnourished (10,11) and **a study of gynecologic oncology patients found a prevalence of 54%** (95% confidence interval, 41–66%) (8). In 2004, the same investigators evaluated gynecologic oncology patients in a prospective cohort trial (12). Subjective assessment using the Subjective Global Assessment (SGA) and objective assessment using the Prognostic Nutrition Index (PNI) found the incidence of malnutrition in this population to be 61% and 70%, respectively.

Nutrition screening to identify patients at risk for malnutrition is an important component of caring for gynecologic oncology patients. Malnutrition is associated with decreased tolerance to cancer therapies, increased morbidity and mortality, decreased quality of life, and increased health care costs (13,14). Early recognition and treatment affords the best opportunity to prevent these complications. **The appropriate time to identify a patient as needing nutritional support is at the time the diagnosis of cancer is made** (6,15).

Risk Factors

Predisposing conditions frequently found in malnourished hospitalized patients include the following:

1. **Heart failure**
2. **Chronic obstructive pulmonary disease**
3. **Infection**
4. **Gastrointestinal (GI) disorders**
5. **Psychiatric disorders**
6. **Renal insufficiency**
7. **Malignancy**

It is typical for undernourished patients to have more than one predisposing condition (2).

Undernourished patients also commonly have vitamin and trace element deficiencies, particularly of vitamins A, D, E, B_{12}, and iron. Decreased stores of these vitamins can be detected in early malnutrition. Because vitamins are stored in small amounts, the provision of only dextrose and water intravenously leads to their rapid depletion, abnormal enzyme function, and clinical signs of vitamin deficiency.

Etiology of Malnutrition in the Cancer Patient

Many systemic illnesses, including cancer, predispose patients to malnutrition (Fig. 19.2). Although abnormalities of metabolism, digestion, absorption, and utilization of nutrients all contribute to malnutrition in such patients, **decreased nutrient intake is still an almost universal finding in malnourished patients,** with the exception of those with uncomplicated hyperthyroidism. Many changes that occur in cancer patients are similar to those seen in inflammatory diseases, such as autoimmune disorders, chronic heart failure, infections such as human immunodeficiency virus, and prolonged critical illness. In particular, **tumor necrosis factor (TNF), interleukins 1 and 6 (IL-1 and IL-6), and interferon-γ are etiologic agents of anorexia and cachexia** (16,17).

Anorexia

Anorexia, is the major factor contributing to decreased intake in many disease processes. During tumor growth, anorexia and reduced food intake markedly contribute to the development of malnutrition. **Serotonin plays a key role in the control of appetite** and there is evidence that administration of neutral amino acids can counteract anorexia mediated by the increased tryptophan concentrations observed in cancer patients with anorexia (18).

Although anorexia can be a feature of cancer, it can also be a side effect of many drugs, including antineoplastic drugs. A number of other commonly used drugs (e.g., anticholinergics, antihistamines, *methyldopa,* sympathomimetics, *clonidine,* and tricyclic antidepressants) may

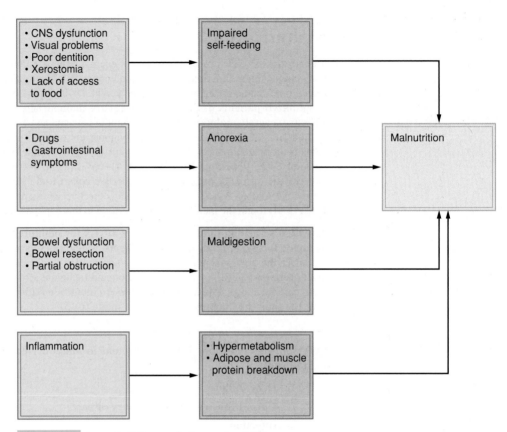

Figure 19.2 Impact of disease factors on nutrition.

cause a dry mouth, which decreases sensation and food palatability. **Another common type of anorexia is a learned aversion to food when it is known to cause adverse physical symptoms. GI diseases,** including reflux esophagitis, gastritis, and peptic ulcer, frequently cause dyspepsia. Irritable bowel syndrome, food allergies, lactose intolerance, diverticulae, and biliary disease **can cause diarrhea or flatulence that may contribute to anorexia**.

All of these GI problems cause patients to avoid foods altogether or to ingest an unbalanced diet. Improvements in the pharmacotherapy of nausea have lessened the anorexia associated with chemotherapy. **The pharmacologic classes for possible cancer cachexia treatment include appetite stimulants, metabolic inhibitors, anabolic agents, and anticytokine agents.** *Megestrol acetate, a progestational appetite stimulant, is an FDA-approved treatment for anorexia.* This progestational steroid increases appetite through the central nervous system and peripheral mechanisms, analogous to the increased appetite that women note during the luteal phase of the menstrual cycle. **Body weight gains are from fat alone** and may not improve survival. *Megestrol* dosing begins at 160 mg/d and may advance to 480 to 800 mg/d. There may be a trend toward an increased risk of thromboembolism or adrenal insufficiency. **American Society for Parenteral and Enteral Nutrition (ASPEN) guidelines recommend consideration of** *megestrol* **as a first-line agent. If this fails, a corticosteroid trial for several weeks may be warranted (19).**

Intestinal Dysfunction

Mechanical malfunction of the bowel is a particularly common problem among patients who have undergone abdominal radiation or extensive abdominal surgery. Postoperative or postirradiation adhesions can lead to partial or complete bowel obstruction. **In patients with a disseminated intra-abdominal malignancy such as ovarian cancer, an adynamic ileus, or intestinal pseudoobstruction can result in a nonfunctional GI tract.** Impaired capacity for self-feeding can markedly decrease food intake. Imaging or exploratory laparotomy may be indicated to define the nature, severity, and location of intestinal dysfunction.

Metabolic Disturbances

Cancer specifically affects nutrient metabolism. Patients with metastatic and localized cancer develop a chronic systemic inflammatory state that results in a hypermetabolism, including increased

Table 19.1 Metabolic Consequences of Cancer	
Host Metabolic Abnormality	*Consequence*
Increased glucose production	Rapid weight loss, muscle breakdown
Increased lipid mobilization	Hypertriglyceridemia, rapid wasting
Insulin resistance	Hyperglycemia, hypertriglyceridemia
Hypoglycemia secondary to tumor humoral factors	Syncope, fatigue
Diarrheal syndromes due to tumor humoral factors	Electrolyte disturbances

rates of hepatic glucose production, insulin resistance, whole-body glucose metabolism, lipolysis, and whole-body protein breakdown (20,21). These processes distinguish cancer associated weight loss from starvation, where weight loss is not accompanied by inflammatory and maladaptive metabolic changes. Improved nutrition often fails to correct such abnormalities when severe malnutrition is present, despite continuous parenteral or enteral alimentation with adequate nutrients (21–23). Specific metabolic disturbances and their consequences are presented in Table 19.1.

Clinical Features

Regardless of the metabolic features of malnutrition, weight loss is usually the presenting sign. **Severe malnutrition can be defined as >10% weight loss over 2 to 3 months or a history of inadequate oral intake longer than 7 days.** It is essential to know the patient's usual weight and ideal body weight (IBW).

Ideal Body Weight

For the purposes of assessment for malnutrition in gynecologic patients, a practical formula that can be used for determining the IBW is the following:

Hamwi equation for women: Ideal body weight = 100 lb for 5 ft + 5 lb/in > 5 ft

For example, a woman whose height is 5 ft, 4 in would have an IBW of 120 pounds. This equation has never been validated, but was compared to the body mass index (BMI) of 4.2 million people from life insurance tables in 1964. Overall it is equivalent to other predictive formulas of IBW (24). Some sources recommend that for small frames, 10 pounds should be subtracted and for large frames, 10 pounds should be added, although no definition of frame measurement has been made.

For many common cancers, loss of as little as 6% of usual body weight can have significant prognostic effects on survival (25), and **weight loss often mirrors declining performance status. Therefore, it's not only important to consider a patient's weight in terms of their IBW, but also to appreciate a change or loss in weight relative to their baseline.**

Weight Loss

Weight loss results from loss of body fat, body protein, or body water. Each liter of body water lost represents a weight loss of 2.2 pounds, but this weight loss can be corrected rapidly with rehydration. The degree to which losses of body protein or fat dominate the clinical picture is a reflection of the body's ability to adapt to a fat fuel economy in the face of inadequate nutrition (26). **There are three basic types of malnutrition: Kwashiorkor, marasmus, and a combination of the two, cachexia** (Fig. 19.3).

Kwashiorkor

This form of malnutrition is variously termed protein caloric malnutrition, hypoalbuminemic malnutrition, protein energy malnutrition, or kwashiorkor-like malnutrition of the adult. If malnutrition is rapid and occurs in the face of disease factors that affect nutrition, a rapid depletion of protein stores can occur out of proportion to the loss of body weight. Kwashiorkor originally referred to a tropical pediatric disease and meant "separation from the breast" in Swahili.

In hospitalized patients, the major signs of protein depletion are the following:

1. **Decrease in serum albumin** to less than 3.5 mg/dL
2. **Decrease in absolute lymphocyte count (ALC)** to less than 1,500/mm³

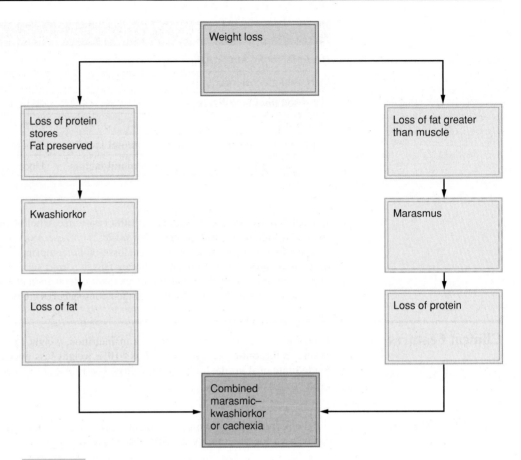

Figure 19.3 Classification of malnutrition.

3. **Decrease in serum transferrin** to less than 150 mg/dL
4. **Loss of reactivity to common skin test antigens**

It is possible for this form of malnutrition to occur in the absence of weight loss if the hypoalbuminemia leads to ascites or edema.

Marasmus

The other major form of malnutrition in adults is called marasmus, starvation, or chronic inanition. Primary malnutrition due to anorexia or dietary inadequacy is the most common form. **It is characterized by a depletion of fat stores and the obvious appearance of malnutrition with visible loss of muscle and fat in the arms and legs.** Although weight loss is often significant in these thin patients, protein stores can be remarkably preserved. It is not uncommon for the starved patient to have normal serum albumin and transferrin levels, a normal lymphocyte count and normal skin test responses.

Cachexia

When the two major forms of malnutrition occur together in patients with advanced malnutrition, the condition is called cachexia. Cachexia is a life-threatening condition and has also been termed **combined marasmic–kwashiorkor or mixed-form malnutrition of the adult**.

Cancer cachexia, also referred to as cancer cachexia syndrome (CCS), is related to proinflammatory cytokines such as IL-1, IL-2, IFNγ, and TNFα. Cytokines serve to decrease protein synthesis and increase proteolysis. Increased proteolysis releases amino acids to be utilized by the liver for energy production, and as precursors in the formation of C reactive protein and serum amyloid peptide. Cytokines also stimulate release of cortisol and catecholamines. Cachectic behavior further decreases a patient's activity (20). **In this advanced condition, there is depletion of body fat stores and body protein stores, which produce visible emaciation with loss of body muscle and fat, as well as decreased serum proteins.**

Table 19.2 Physical/Biochemical Markers of Malnutrition			
	Marasmus	*Kwashiorkor*	*Cachexia*
Albumin	Normal	↓	↓
Transferrin	Normal	↓	↓
White blood cell count	Normal	↓	↓
Skin tests	Normal	Negative	Negative
Body weight	↓	Normal	↓
Body fat	↓	Normal	↓

The exact contribution of malnutrition to mortality in hospitalized gynecologic oncology patients is difficult to quantify. The additive effects of malnutrition include impaired immunity, poor wound healing, and cardiorespiratory dysfunction, which all impact negatively on patient survival (27).

Diagnosis

To diagnose malnutrition, **all patients should be at least minimally screened or preferably assessed, for malnutrition upon diagnosis of cancer** (15). Low levels of circulating serum proteins can reflect impaired function of the liver and other organs, even in the absence of marked depletion of visceral and muscle protein (18). This usually occurs in the setting of excessive metabolic demands caused by specific illnesses that impair the body's ability to conserve protein. Similarly, protein and fat stores can be depleted markedly, while circulating proteins remain in the normal range. This in turn reflects a gradual adaptation to starvation in adults with anorexia and primary malnutrition.

A nutritionist can provide the nutritional assessment, which should include a history, physical examination, and laboratory evaluation. The assessment should include current medical problems/treatments; social support and functional status; anthropomorphic measurements; calculation of IBW; BMI; and visceral protein measurement. **The nutritional assessment can identify the current degree of malnutrition, determine the nutritional support required, and set the goals of therapy.** Assaying immune function also contributes to an understanding of the nutritional status.

Anthropometry, in which body stores are estimated by direct measurements, **and biochemical markers** that assess circulating proteins, **must be used in concert to determine the specific type of malnutrition** in any given patient (Table 19.2).

Anthropometric techniques include the measurement of body weight and height in adults. The patient's normal weight can be obtained from the history. The Hamwi formula described above is used to calculate the percentage of IBW. **The BMI is calculated by dividing weight in kg by height in meters squared (kg/m^2).** Normal BMI is 18.5 to 25, overweight is 25 to 29.9, with obesity being >30, and underweight being <18.5.

Fat stores can be measured by assessing skin-fold thickness. The most commonly used skin fold in practice is the triceps. For this measurement, the patient sits with the right arm hanging freely at the side. For bedridden patients, the right arm is flexed at the shoulder while the forearm crosses the chest. The midpoint between the acromion and the olecranon posteriorly over the triceps muscle is marked. The skin and subcutaneous tissue at the midpoint are then pinched and pressure-regulated calipers are applied for 3 seconds before a reading is taken (28). The calipers are designed to deliver a pressure of 10 g/mm^2 regardless of the fold thickness and can be used to compare the same patient's progress over time and to assess the severity of malnutrition.

There are a number of other means of body fat assessment such as bioelectrical impedance analysis and submersion measurements, but each institution should be capable of providing at least one type of assessment.

Protein Store Assessment

Midarm circumference and midarm muscle circumference can help to estimate lean body mass/protein stores. **Midarm muscle circumference (cm) = midarm circumference (cm) – (π × triceps skin-fold thickness (cm)).** It is an attempt to estimate lean body mass. Protein stores can also be assayed by a number of circulating proteins, most of which are secreted by the liver (29,30). Their synthesis and secretion are inhibited rapidly in the presence of protein malnutrition and they

Table 19.3 Serum Half-life of Circulating Proteins Decreased in Malnutrition

Protein	Half-life
Albumin	3–4 wk
Transferrin	1 wk
Thyroxine-binding prealbumin	2 d
Retinol-binding protein	10 hr

decrease to a variable extent in the circulation according to their metabolic half-lives. **The most widely used markers are albumin and transferrin.** Each has advantages and disadvantages (29).

Albumin

Albumin has a half-life of 21 days, so that significant decreases may not occur for up to 1 month after the onset of starvation. **Albumin may be decreased by rapid loss of serum proteins** (e.g., excessive losses from the GI tract), **by dilution by volume resuscitation, or by fluid shifts into ascites.** Restoration of the serum albumin to normal levels by nutritional means is slow and often lags behind clear improvement in nutritional status by other criteria.

Transferrin

Transferrin is synthesized in the liver and other sites, where it can act as a growth-promoting peptide. **In the liver, synthesis is modulated by the iron stores in the hepatocytes and by the overall protein status.** The half-life of the protein is 9 days and the body pool is only 5 g. The synthetic rate is the major factor determining serum levels and serum transferrin increases within 9 days of nutritional repletion. The problems with the interpretation of transferrin levels are that degradation rates increase during illness and iron deficiency falsely elevates the serum levels.

For these reasons transferrin and albumin must be interpreted within the context of anthropometric determinations of body weight and triceps skin-fold thickness.

Retinol- and Thyroxine-binding Proteins

Retinol-binding protein and thyroxine-binding prealbumin also are synthesized in the liver, with half-lives of 10 hours and 2 to 3 days, respectively. Their levels drop acutely with metabolic stress and retinol-binding protein is also filtered and broken down by the kidney. These factors complicate the interpretation of serum levels for the diagnosis of malnutrition, but **they can be used in a research setting to assess more quickly the response to nutritional support.**

Inflammation causes a ≥25% decrease in all of the aforementioned serum transport proteins (31). The serum half-lives of these circulating proteins are listed in Table 19.3.

Immune Function

The total lymphocyte count and delayed cutaneous hypersensitivity responses to skin test antigens are nonspecific markers of impaired immune function in malnourished patients (32):

1. Depressed levels of complement components, including C3
2. Reduced amounts of secretory immunoglobulin A in external body secretions
3. Abnormal T-cell function
4. Impairment of nonspecific defenses, including decreased epithelial integrity, decreased mucus production, and decreased ciliary motility.

Most patients with protein and caloric malnutrition have multiple deficiencies and **almost any single nutritional deficiency, if severe enough, can affect immune function** (33) (Figure 19.4). Correction of malnutrition improves immune function; this is especially true in the gynecologic oncology patient, whose immune function can be impaired by therapy as well as by the tumor itself.

Absolute Lymphocyte Count

The absolute lymphocyte count (ALC) is calculated by multiplying the percentage of lymphocytes by the total white blood cell count. The ALC and skin tests are the most widely used

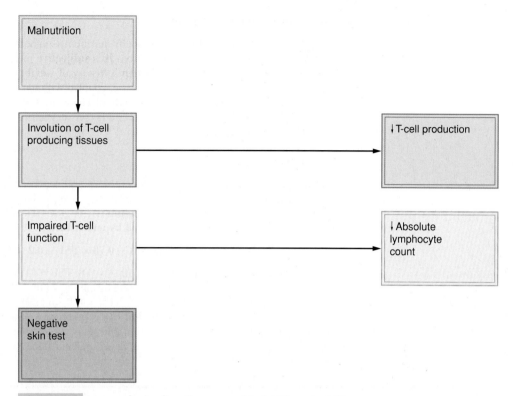

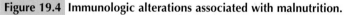

Figure 19.4 Immunologic alterations associated with malnutrition.

immune markers of nutritional status. The normal lymphocyte count is greater than 2,000/mm^3 in patients who are not receiving chemotherapy. **The ALC is not considered valid unless the white blood cell count is normal.**

Most circulating lymphocytes are T cells and involution of the tissues producing T cells occurs early in the course of malnutrition. **The delayed hypersensitivity skin test response reflects three processes:**

1. **Processing of the antigen by macrophages resulting in the generation of both effector and memory T cells**
2. **Recognition of antigen rechallenge** resulting in blast transformation, cellular proliferation, and generation of lymphokine-producing effector cells
3. **Production of a local wheal and flare,** secondary to the actions of lymphokines and chemotactic factors at the skin site.

Antigens that are frequently tested include purified protein derivative, streptokinase-streptodornase, mumps, *Candida, Trichophyton,* and coccidioidin. The prevalence of nonreactivity to skin test antigens is approximately 50% in patients whose serum albumin level is less than 3 g/dL, but it can be as high as 30% in patients whose serum albumin level exceeds 3 g/dL. Other problems with interpretation of skin tests include the following:

1. **Only about 60% of healthy patients respond to most of the antigens,** so that failure to respond to one or two antigens may not be predictive
2. **Primary illnesses, including sarcoidosis and lymphoma,** as well as immunosuppressive drugs, **produce energy.**

The delayed hypersensitivity (DH) and ALC are useful in uncomplicated nutritional deficiencies, but are not typically considered useful in this patient population.

The assessment of malnutrition by means of clinical examination in combination with routinely available laboratory tests provides an accurate estimation in more than 70% of patients (17). Difficulties with each of these tests have kept the nutritional assessment from becoming part of the routine database for every hospitalized patient.

Subjective Global Assessment

This is the most commonly utilized tool by nutritionists in both surgical and medical hospitalized patients to assess the risk for malnutrition. **It is subjective** in that it does not rely on calipers or laboratory values, but rather on the patient's history of weight change, dietary change, GI symptoms, functional status, and primary disease, coupled with the nutritionist's physical examination and global rating. A variant of this, the **Patient Generated SGA** (PGSGA**) has been developed for assessment of the oncology patient, and is considered highly sensitive (>90%) and specific for detection of malnutrition** (34,35).

Prognostic Nutritional Index

The Prognostic Nutritional Index (PNI) **combines anthropometric and laboratory tests to calculate a single index number**. It is a linear predictive model of increased morbidity and mortality after surgical procedures and **uses serum albumin** (A) in g/dL; **triceps skin fold** (TSF) in mm; **serum transferrin** (TFN) in mg/dL; and **delayed hypersensitivity** (DH) response (0–2). The formula is:

$$\text{PNI\%} = 158 - 16.6 \times A - 0.78 \times TSF - 0.2 \times TFN - 5.8 \times DH$$

For example, a well-nourished patient with A = 4.8, TSF = 14, TFN = 250, and DH = 2 has a PNI of 158 to 152.2, or a 5.8% chance of complications. On the other hand, a malnourished patient with abnormal indexes (A = 2.8, TSF = 9, TFN = 180, and DH = 1) has a PNI of 158 to 95.3, or a 62.7% chance of complications. **A PNI of <40 is taken as well nourished, whereas a PNI of >40 is taken as evidence of malnutrition.** In one study of 76 gynecologic oncology patients, serum albumin could be substituted for PNI to detect malnutrition (8). The PNI describes surgical risk reliably based on nutritional status.

Nutritional Support

Nutritional support is an adjunct to primary therapy for the gynecologic oncology patient. The aim is to prevent deterioration of nutritional status during planned primary therapy, such as radiation, surgery, and chemotherapy. **Early initiation of nutritional support is desirable.** This goal necessitates early evaluation, the proper choice of nutritional therapeutic modalities, and an accurate assessment of requirements.

After protein deficiency occurs, it is difficult to reverse, because less than 5% of the protein is replaced per day, regardless of the amount of substrate provided. Vitamins and minerals are replaced more easily, but there is no substitute for adequate planning to meet caloric and protein requirements essential for nutritional maintenance of vital functions.

The first intervention is dietary counseling. Modification of a patient's diet to small and frequent meals with liquids taken only between meals may help address early satiety and anorexia. Commercially prepared fortified foods can improve the intake of energy and nutrients. For those who remain malnourished after these interventions, other means of support may be considered (36).

Caloric Requirements

The protein and caloric requirements can be estimated at 0.8 g/kg/d and 20 to 35 kcal/kg/d for healthy adults, respectively (12). If malnutrition exists or if the patient's metabolism is elevated by infection or other metabolic stresses, then 1.5 to 2.5 g/kg/d of protein and 35 to 45 kcal/kg/d should be supplied. More exact formulas are available for pediatric patients and patients at the extremes of height and weight.

Need for Nutritional Therapy

Prior to initiating nutritional therapy, it is important to consider the overall treatment goals (palliative or curative) and the associated risks of each intervention. The decision to initiate nutritional therapy in patients with advanced cancer must take into account the patient's wishes. The palliative use of nutritional therapy in terminally ill cancer patients is rarely indicated (37).

There are two key aspects of the patient's nutritional status that affect decisions about nutritional therapy:

1. **The degree of prior malnutrition** at the time of assessment
2. **The degree of hypermetabolism** or metabolic abnormality expected to interfere with nutritional rehabilitation.

If the degree of prior malnutrition is minimal and the patient has only mild hypermetabolism after elective surgery, a temporary form of nutritional support can be used. On the other hand, if the patient requires additional calories to restore pre-existing severe malnutrition, forced intake of calories by an enteral or parenteral route can be used. The following guidelines should be applied:

1. **If a patient is to be without nutrition for a period of 7 days, some form of nutritional therapy should be used.**

2. **If nutritional therapy is to be continued enterally for more than 4 weeks, a permanent intestinal access should be considered.** If more than 2 weeks of parenteral nutritional support is required, long-term central access should be placed. Arrangements should be made for home enteral or parenteral nutrition (38).

Method of Support

The choice between parenteral and enteral therapy should be made on the basis of the availability and functional status of the GI tract (Fig. 19.5). **If the GI tract is functioning normally, the expense and complications of parenteral nutrition are not warranted.** Swallowing evaluation and nutritional assessment are useful in determining whether the enteral route is the best choice. Intake may also be improved by the pharmacologic therapies described previously. **If the GI tract is functional, but oral intake remains inadequate, a feeding device should be placed to assist intake.** Patients complaining of depression or pain should have these symptoms addressed concurrently.

Enteral Feeding

In view of the difficulties inherent in the use of parenteral nutritional support, every effort should be made to use the enteral route. Enteral access may be obtained at the bedside by placement of a nasal feeding tube, endoscopically by a gastroenterologic consultant, by an interventional radiologist under fluoroscopic or ultrasonic guidance, or by a surgeon in the operating room, depending upon the anticipated complexity of placement. **If a long-term nasal feeding tube is required, it should be changed to alternating nostrils every 4 to 6 weeks** (39). If enteral access is required beyond 4 weeks, consideration should be given to a gastrostomy or jejunostomy.

A gastrostomy port can be used at night for enteral support therapy by continuous infusion of isotonic enteral supplements at a rate no greater than 100 kcal/hr. The next day, the patient can cover the port with a dressing and go through her usual daily activities. This approach is often more acceptable to patients than a nasogastric tube, which is visible and irritating.

In some patients, the gastrostomy port has the added advantage that the stomach can be used as a reservoir for bolus feeding, which is more convenient. In cases of abnormal gastric motility,

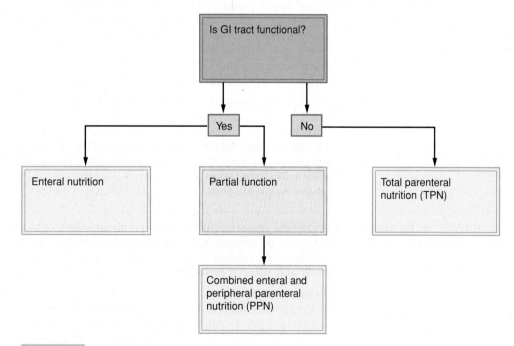

Figure 19.5 Parenteral versus enteral nutrition.

esophageal reflux, or possible aspiration of gastric contents, continuous slow infusion of supplement should be used, or a tube passed beyond the pylorus into the jejunum. **The gastrostomy tube may also be used as a venting port should nausea and vomiting develop.**

If the GI tract is atrophied from prior malnutrition, a period of rehabilitation with special formula diets can be used to renourish the patient gradually, so that routine formula diets can be used (40). The epithelium of the GI tract is directly nourished by the infused nutrients in the formula diet bathing these cells, and ultimately a complete formula diet can be used.

If the patient is already severely malnourished and hypermetabolic, with a nonfunctional GI tract, careful consideration should be given to initiation of concurrent parenteral nutrition during the period of nutritional rehabilitation of the GI tract. Tapering of parenteral nutrition may begin after tube feeds are between 33% and 50% of the goal for enteral feeds, and may be discontinued when tube feeds are between 50% and 75% of the goal (41).

The transition from tube feeding to oral feeding may require swallowing evaluation, holding tube feeding prior to meals, giving a bolus down the tube after each oral meal, or giving nighttime feeds. When oral intake is approximately 50% for 2 days, tube feeding may be tapered by time and volume.

Parenteral Feeding

Total parenteral nutrition (TPN) is the provision of all required calories in an intravenous solution of dextrose, amino acids, and emulsified lipids via a centrally located catheter. **Parenteral nutrition, although appearing more definitive, should not be used in the malnourished patient with a functional GI tract.** In some patients receiving chemotherapy or radiation therapy, mucosal inflammation, nausea, and vomiting impair normal intake. In such patients, TPN may be needed as an adjunct to restore functional status and allow continuation of therapy. Patients with a mid- to distal GI fistula often require avoidance of enteral feeding.

Moderate to severely malnourished patients should receive more than 7 days of parenteral nutrition before surgery for the therapy to be of benefit. In addition, life expectancy should be evaluated for those with advanced cancer. As per ASPEN guidelines, **only those with a life expectancy of greater than 3 months should be considered for specialized nutritional support** (42).

Peripheral parenteral nutrition (PPN) is composed of similar elements to TPN, but combined in lesser concentrations so that infusion of the less hyperosmolar (<900 to 1,000 mOsm/L) **solution may be tolerated by peripheral veins.** If PPN is needed for not more than 5 days, parenteral support probably is not warranted. Alternatively, if PPN is needed for 14 days or more, TPN should be given (42). Criteria for PPN administration include good peripheral access and ability to tolerate 2.5 to 3 L of fluid daily. Over time, PPNs 10% glucose solution may cause a chemical phlebitis, limiting the use of any single peripheral vein to a period of about 10 days. In patients receiving chemotherapy, peripheral veins are often sclerosed and a central venous route for nutrition and medications must be used.

TPN is usually administered through a central venous catheter (CVC) surgically placed in the subclavian vein, although other sites can be used, as described in Chapter 20. A large central vein is required for the ≥20% glucose solution plus added amino acids required for TPN. **The patient must be given special training in aseptic handling of the catheter site and use of the infusion equipment required.** Many medical centers have special home parenteral nutritional support teams and in some regions, private firms provide this service. Potential medical problems for these patients depend to a great extent on the experience of the team providing home parenteral support.

Evaluation of Response to Nutritional Support

Because the goal of nutritional support is the attainment of an anabolic state or reduction of nitrogen losses, **assessment of nitrogen balance is the most useful clinical tool to determine the effectiveness of therapy. Nitrogen balance is defined as the difference between nitrogen intake and nitrogen excretion.**

Because 1 g of nitrogen is equivalent to 6.25 g of protein, **nitrogen intake** can be determined by dividing protein intake, as determined from dietary records, by 6.25. **Nitrogen excretion** is defined as the urinary nitrogen excreted per 24 hours, plus a fixed estimate of 4 g per 24 hours for unmeasured nitrogen losses from cellular sloughing into the feces (1 g); losses from the skin (0.2 g); and nonurea nitrogen losses in the urine (2 g) (43). Because nitrogen balance is most usefully applied in a serial fashion in the same patient, the particular constants used to estimate unmeasured excretion are important only for comparison of published results.

At any given level of nitrogen intake, nitrogen balance improves with increased administration of nonprotein calories. The maximum benefit is achieved when the ratio of nonprotein calories to grams of nitrogen is 150:1 (44).

To assess adequacy of protein intake, patients with stable renal function, consistent protein intake, and the ability to collect a 24-hour urine sample, may benefit from a nitrogen balance study. Nitrogen balance reflects the balance between protein breakdown and synthesis, where nitrogen intake is measured as grams of protein over 24 hours divided by 6.25, and nitrogen excretion is measured by a 24-hour urinary urea nitrogen (UUN) assay. Nitrogen balance = protein intake (g/day)/6.25 − (UUN (g/day) + 4 g). The goal is +2 to +4, or the least negative balance attainable. If the UUN is negative, increasing the protein delivered, assisting its absorption, and increasing the total calories given should be considered.

Proteins vary in their biologic value, according to their mixture of essential and nonessential amino acids. Albumin has the ideal mixture of amino acids for optimal use of protein, and is assigned a biologic value of 100. Casein is close to albumin in its biologic quality, whereas meat proteins, such as those found in steak or tuna, have a biologic value of 80. Corns and beans, each with biologic values of 40 or less, can be combined in a protein mixture with a biologic value of 80, because the amino acid mixtures of the two proteins are complementary. **The protein requirement for normal people is 0.55 g/kg for protein with a high biologic value, such as milk or albumin, but 0.8 g/kg for the mixture of proteins found in the average American diet** (45).

Effect of Nutritional Support on Prognosis

Although it is easy to demonstrate the impact of nutrition in simple starvation, it is much more difficult to demonstrate the beneficial effect of nutritional support in a patient with a chronic illness such as cancer (46). Often the course of the underlying illness masks the beneficial effects of nutritional therapy.

In patients with mild disease or elective surgery, malnutrition is relatively well tolerated from a clinical standpoint. In such cases, nutritional rehabilitation usually occurs without any special effort as the underlying medical or surgical condition runs its course. **In patients with severe disease, nutrition is often relegated to the secondary list of problems, because the progress of the primary illness dictates therapeutic decisions.** In both of these instances, however, nutritional therapy may play a beneficial role in either preventing or retarding malnutrition in individual patients (47). **An extensive meta-analysis of 53 published studies of parenteral and enteral nutrition showed that survival was improved in 6 studies, unchanged in 43 and worse in 2 (48). Nonetheless, the judicious application of nutritional support for gynecologic oncology patients may lead to an improvement in the quality of life and prognosis** (49).

Nutrition usually is an adjunct to primary medical and surgical therapy. Broaching end-of-life topics should be done openly and early. According to the American Medical Association's Web site, **the decision to use any medical therapy "should be based on the best interests of the patient (what outcome would most likely promote the patient's well-being)".** Given the social and emotional value of nutrition, ultimately the autonomy of the patient should be guided by sound advice on what benefits, potential complications, and responsibilities come with specialized nutritional support. If there is any doubt as to whether nutrition should be provided, consultation with an ethicist may be of value.

Complications

Complications can occur after either enteral or parenteral nutrition. Complications can be mechanical, infectious, or metabolic (50).

Enteral Feeding

Tubes placed via the nares may cause nasal mucosal damage, septal necrosis, sinusitis, otitis, vocal cord dysfunction, and ulceration. Use of a smaller size (i.e., 5 to 12 F) tube helps minimize complications. **Overall complication rates approach 10% and include epistaxis, aspiration, and respiratory distress** (51). Inadvertent malplacement into the tracheobronchial tree occurs in less than 2% of patients, but may result in pneumothorax, pneumonia, empyema, or mediastinitis. Malpositioning is most likely to occur in patients with a depressed sensorium and a depressed cough reflex. It is not prevented by the use of a cuffed endotracheal tube. Placement should therefore be confirmed radiographically prior to beginning enteral feeding (52).

Dislodgement of nasoenteral tubes has been documented in 16–41% of placements. A nasal bridle may be useful (e.g., AMT, Brecksville, OH) to help prevent this occurrence. **Tubal occlusion occurs in up to 20% of cases.** Flushing regularly and using center specific protocols for declogging (e.g., *viokase* and *sodium bicarbonate*) may decrease the risk of occlusion. **Finally, up to 20% of patients with enteric tubes will experience dysphagia.**

The alternative approach of enterostomies may be associated with hemorrhage, bowel perforation, and bowel obstruction. Aspiration risk may increase as a result of sedation and ileus associated with the placement procedure itself. **Pneumoperitoneum occurs in up to 50% of tube placements** and may delay diagnosis of any perforation. Inadvertent ostomy removal may occur and must be urgently addressed.

Because **enteral feeding increases the risk of aspiration,** identifying patients with gastroesophageal reflux, gastric dysmotility, or progressive obstruction and intolerance can help minimize the risk. Other ways to decrease aspiration risk include head of bed elevation, evaluation of swallowing, assessment of tolerance to tube feeding, and frequent monitoring of the airway. The ASPEN guidelines for gastric residual volumes are to check every 4 to 5 hours until at goal, and to hold feeds if residual volumes are greater than 200 mL. **Nausea and/or vomiting develop in 12–20% of patients receiving enteral nutrition** (42).

Diarrhea is the most common complication associated with tube feeding (53) **and should be assessed and treated in the following ways:**

1. **Infectious diarrhea should first be excluded,** including *C. difficile* pseudomembranous colitis secondary to antibiotics.

2. **The rate of infusion can be decreased.** If the GI tract dysfunction is caused by atrophy of the epithelial cells, a gradual increase in infusion rate is often tolerated, starting with an initial rate of 25 mL/hr and increasing by twofold increments every 48 hours.

3. **The type of enteral formula can be changed to an isosmolar formula.** Many of the high-calorie or high-nitrogen supplements are hyperosmolar. Changing to an isotonic formula often decreases intestinal hypermotility. It is important to review medication lists to rule out any medications with a laxative effect. Stool anion gap may be sent to rule in osmotic rather than secretory diarrhea. Fecal fat should be checked if fat malabsorption is suspected. The patient's medical history should be reviewed for lactose and gluten intolerance.

4. **A number of specific medications can be used to decrease intestinal motility.** The presence of an obstruction or infectious diarrhea should be determined first, since these are contraindications to hypomotility agents.

5. **The level of enteral support can be decreased and temporarily combined with peripheral parenteral alimentation** until intestinal motility problems respond to the maneuvers discussed previously.

While evaluation of diarrhea is ongoing, attention should be kept on the clinical status of the patient as **dehydration may rapidly occur.** Dehydration with hypernatremia can be a problem in the elderly, in whom inadequate fluid intake can occur during the administration of a hypertonic enteral formula. When high-carbohydrate enteral formulas are used, glucosuria can occur even in patients without a prior history of diabetes.

Parenteral Feeding

The complications of parenteral nutrition are often more serious than those associated with enteral nutrition (54). **Pneumothorax and subclavian venous thrombosis are the most common catheter-related complications for temporary and permanent CVCs.** Pneumothorax should occur in only 1–2% of CVC insertions, but this rate is higher when transthoracic puncture is used rather than open surgical placement, or when less experienced personnel insert the catheter (55). A chest radiograph to confirm proper catheter placement and to exclude a pneumothorax is essential. A pneumothorax often resolves spontaneously, but a chest tube or pigtail catheter may be required in some cases. **Peripherally inserted central catheters (PICC) are another option for TPN. The lumen for TPN should be dedicated for TPN only,** to minimize the risk of infection. Femoral CVCs should be avoided because of an increased risk of infection and thrombosis.

Permanent catheters, such as Hickman or Port catheters provide ready access for parenteral nutrition, blood products, and chemotherapy, but can also be malpositioned, cause thrombosis, or become infected. Thrombosis of the catheter in the central veins has been reported in 5–10% of patients receiving parenteral nutrition, especially with the hypercoagulable states of sepsis or cancer (56). In most patients, the catheter should be flushed with *heparin* solution (300 unit/mL) to prevent this complication, predisposing the patient to the risk of *heparin*-induced thrombocytopenia (HIT). **When venous thrombosis occurs, the catheter must be removed.** PPN may be used, while a course of full intensity anticoagulation is given to treat the thrombosis and a new site for a CVC is selected. A minimum of a 3-month course of full-dose anticoagulation should be prescribed and that access site should be avoided in the future.

In patients committed to lifelong parenteral nutrition, the CVC site choice must be made carefully because only nine external sites are available for CVC placement: Internal jugular veins, subclavian veins, femoral veins, and in some centers, the inferior vena cava.

Infections occur in association with 2–5% of central catheters placed for parenteral nutrition. Mortality for catheter related blood stream infections is 12–25% (57). When the patient is febrile and a peripheral source of infection is not found within 96 hours, the catheter should be removed and cultured for evidence of catheter-related infection. **Infections most commonly occur from skin contaminants, such as gram-positive organisms, but can include fungi and unusual bacteria, especially if acquired during hospitalization. Fevers in patients requiring TPN should always prompt investigation of potential blood stream infection.**

Infected catheters can be a source of life-threatening septic phlebitis. Blood-borne infections from sources other than the catheter can be treated with intravenous antibiotics without removal of the catheter, but the patient should be observed carefully because the catheter may become seeded with bacteria. The subcutaneous tunnel of a permanent catheter may be a source of infection as well.

In patients treated with broad-spectrum antibiotics, systemic candidiasis can occur. The retina should be examined by an ophthalmologist for the presence of cotton-wool exudates that are pathognomonic, and blood cultures should be sent for special fungal isolation procedures if candidiasis is suspected. *Caspofungin* **(70 mg IV first day, then 50 mg IV daily) is a reasonable first-line agent in patients with suspected candidemia.** In addition to holding TPN, the CVC should be removed and consideration given to evaluation for endocarditis (58).

A variety of metabolic complications can occur during parenteral nutrition. **The most common is overfeeding, which results in excess CO_2 production, and occasionally hypercapnia** in patients with pulmonary disease (59). Blood sugars must be checked regularly, as hyperglycemia or even hyperosmolar nonketotic coma can occur as a result of transient insulin resistance, relative insulin deficiency, or more rarely, chromium deficiency. Sliding scale subcutaneous insulin, an insulin drip, or insulin added to the parenteral solutions are appropriate measures (60).

Hypoglycemia sometimes occurs with abrupt cessation of TPN. To avoid this, TPN should be tapered to half the standing infusion rate for 1 hour, before discontinuing it completely. Alternatively a D10W infusion can be substituted for the TPN at the same rate for 1 hour. Basic metabolic panels should be monitored for **metabolic acidosis, a less common problem** since acetate buffers have been used in parenteral solutions. **Abnormalities of phosphate, potassium, calcium, and magnesium can occur** because of excessive or inadequate administration, particularly in the presence of underlying disorders, such as renal failure or GI fistulae, which themselves predispose to electrolyte abnormalities (61,62).

Deficiencies of trace minerals such as zinc, copper, and chromium used to occur but are now rare, because these are now added routinely to parenteral solutions. Because multivitamin solutions are the same source for vitamin K, **the prothrombin time and partial prothrombin time should be monitored weekly**.

The most serious metabolic complication of TPN is refeeding syndrome, an acute state of electrolyte imbalance resulting from initiation of nutritional support. It is most likely to occur when TPN is commenced in the severely malnourished patient. Concern for this syndrome requires daily serum electrolytes initially and often electrolyte supplementation (63).

Renal abnormalities are sometimes troubling. Azotemia may worsen in patients with renal failure or when there is excessive administration of amino acids relative to nonprotein calories and this may be treated by reduction of the amino acid load. However amino acid requirements may be higher in patients on hemodialysis. Daily weights and a strict fluid balance chart are mandatory for volume monitoring.

Hepatobiliary complications occur as well. Steatosis is associated with dextrose overfeeding and a mild transaminitis may occur that typically resolves in 2 weeks. The latter can also reflect sepsis. **Cholestasis** manifests as a nonjaundiced patient (with bilirubin <2), with a mild increase in alkaline phosphatase, gamma-glutamyltransferase (GGT), and direct bilirubin. Finally, **gall-bladder stasis occurs in almost all TPN patients,** but consideration should be given to the possible development of cholangitis or cholecystitis.

Essential fatty acid (EFA) deficiency rarely occurs because of the use of intravenous lipid emulsions (64). In animal studies, EFA deficiency occurs after 12 days without lipid supplementation. In humans this complication can be avoided by providing 1 to 3 days per week of lipid infusion. **EFA deficiency clinically manifests as scaly skin, alopecia, hepatomegaly, or thrombocytopenia.** To avoid hypertriglyceridemia caused by lipid administration or dextrose overfeeding, **weekly triglyceride levels should be checked.** Rarely patients with egg allergy will react to the lipid infusion.

In most cases, the metabolic complications associated with parenteral nutrition respond to careful fluid and electrolyte management with daily monitoring of input and output. Complications can be avoided with effective communication between the physician, nutritionist, pharmacist, and patient.

Nutritional Support in Multiple Organ Failure Syndrome

Multiple organ failure syndrome (MOSF) can develop in critically ill patients secondary to a decline in cellular oxygen consumption, inflammatory cytokines, or sepsis (65). Cascading events, including at different times hypoperfusion/hypoxia, immunodysfunction, endocrine dysfunction, acute starvation, and metabolic derangements, may lead to early organ failure within 5 to 7 days after the initial insult, but can occur as late as 21 days.

The nutritional therapy provided for such patients has been called metabolic support, to differentiate it from the nutritional support given to more stable patients with chronic anorexia and starvation. In nutritional support, the goals are simply to provide adequate calories and nutrients to restore nutritional deficiencies and to maintain protein synthesis, positive nitrogen balance, and lean body mass (66). **Metabolic support of the critically ill patient at risk of MOSF is directed at partial caloric replacement, sustenance of important cellular and organ metabolism, and the avoidance of overfeeding.** Metabolic costs of overfeeding include lipogenesis, gluconeogenesis, thermogenesis, electrolyte imbalance, metabolic alkalosis, and hypervolemia. Excessive infusion rates and choice of the wrong mixture of macronutrients can be harmful in the critically ill patient (67).

A breakdown in the physical and immunologic barriers of the GI tract can promote MOSF. The GI tract is particularly susceptible to ischemic and reperfusion injury. Glutamine, a preferred fuel for the gut epithelium, may promote healing of the GI tract epithelium after an injury (68). In animal studies, an enteral formula containing glutamine has been shown to maintain muscle glutamine metabolism without stimulating tumor growth, while also improving GI mucosal integrity and nitrogen balance (69). Currently there are no recommendations for glutamine outside of burn or trauma patients (70). **The critical therapeutic difference between MOSF and chronic malnutrition is the need to avoid overfeeding by providing a hypocaloric protein-sparing nutritional regimen in the former.**

Provision of Nutritional Support

There are many methods of estimating basal energy requirements. The following are guidelines:

1. **Obese patients maintain their body weight when given between 15 to 25 kcal/kg of actual body weight (ABW) per day.**

2. **Normal weight patients maintain their weight when given 35 kcal/kg of ABW per day.**

3. In patients with malnutrition, there is a cost of anabolism that involves the calories necessary for new protein synthesis. **For patients with very severe illnesses and in whom malnutrition may be combined with sepsis or trauma to elevate energy requirements, ≤45 kcal/kg/d may be required.**

There are many other formulas for estimating energy requirements that take the patient's height into consideration. Taller patients have a higher resting energy expenditure at the same weight than shorter patients, because they have larger livers and other vital organs. In older people, metabolic rates tend to fall, in part because of a decrease in lean body mass. Although these equations are useful for clinical nutritional research, they are generally unnecessary for clinical management. A more practical set of guidelines is given in the following sections.

Estimation of Total Caloric Requirement

Severity of Illness	Daily Caloric Requirement
Mild	35 kcal/kg
Moderate	40 kcal/kg
Severe	45 kcal/kg

Estimation of Protein Requirement

The protein requirement can be estimated at approximately 1 g/kg of actual body weight (ABW) per day for normal individuals or 1 g/kg of IBW per day for obese patients. Stressed normal weight patients require 1.5 to 2.5 g/kg of ABW per day while stressed obese patients require 1.5 to 2 g/kg of IBW per day (41).

Estimation of Nonprotein Calories

One simple method of estimating nonprotein calories is to subtract the protein calories from the total number of calories required daily. **1 g of protein = 4 calories.** The nonprotein caloric requirement may be estimated by initially estimating the amount of nitrogen administered according to the following formula: **1 g nitrogen = 6.25 g protein.** By either the parenteral or the enteral route, **150 nonprotein calories must be provided for each gram of nitrogen administered**. Therefore, estimation of nonprotein calories can be achieved as follows:

$$\text{Nonprotein calories} = \frac{\text{Protein requirement} \times 150}{6.25}$$

Determination of Carbohydrate Requirement

It is usual to give approximately half the total calories as carbohydrates. Most nutritional solutions are premixed and the precise formulas available vary in different hospitals. **Custom TPN solutions are possible and may be useful to decrease hyperglycemia.** It is best to discuss custom solutions with a nutritionist and a pharmacist, as solution stability must be maintained, which limits the proportions of protein, fat, and carbohydrate that can be mixed.

Determination of Fat Requirement

The absolute fat requirement for EFAs (i.e., linoleic acid and linolenic acid) is only 4% of the total calories. The amount of fat usually administered either enterally or parenterally exceeds this amount. The balance of the calories necessary to fulfill the total caloric requirement after the protein and carbohydrate calories have been calculated is often given as fat. In all cases, the number of calories given as fat should be far less than 60% of the total calories, which is the maximal fat allowance.

Sample Calculations

Sample calculations for both enteral and parenteral formulations are presented.

Enteral

A 50-year-old woman who weighs 45 kg has a usual body weight of 70 kg and is severely ill with sepsis and postsurgical stress. Her GI tract is functional and enteral formulation must be prescribed. The following steps allow calculation of the specific requirements:

1. **The total daily caloric requirement** is estimated by multiplying the caloric requirement based on severity (in this case, 45 kcal/kg/d) by the patient's weight (i.e., 45 kg). Therefore, the caloric requirement is 45 kcal/kg × 45 kg = 2,025 kcal.
2. **The minimum protein requirement** is determined by multiplying the IBW by 1 g/kg (e.g., in this case 70 kg), and 1 g/kg = 70 g. Because protein = 4 kcal/g, the protein caloric need is 280 kcal.
3. **The estimation of nonprotein calories** is determined by multiplying the protein requirement (70 g) by 150 and this figure is divided by 6.25. Therefore, the minimum nonprotein calories required = (70 g × 150)/6.25 = 1,680 kcal.
4. **The determination of specific carbohydrate and fat needs** is empiric; that is, if approximately one-half the total caloric need is given in carbohydrates (in this case, 1,010 kcal), the remainder of the calories may be given as fat. Therefore, fat calories = 2,025 − (1,010 + 280) = 735 kcal.

5. **An enteral formula that approximates these caloric requirements should be used.** A standard formula containing 1 kcal/mL, 15% protein, 34% fat, and 51% carbohydrate would provide approximately 150 kcal of protein, 340 kcal of fat, and 510 kcal of carbohydrate for every liter of formula given to the patient. Therefore, this patient's caloric requirements would be met by giving her approximately 2 L of formula per day.

Parenteral

A 45-kg, 70-year-old woman has lost 15 kg as a result of postirradiation changes to the bowel. In view of her poor GI function, parenteral alimentation is appropriate. The estimation of her nutritional requirements is as follows:

1. **The total daily caloric requirement** is estimated by multiplying the caloric requirement based on severity by the patient's weight (i.e., 45 kcal/kg × 45 kg = 2,025 kcal).

2. **The minimum protein requirement** is determined by multiplying the usual body weight (60 kg) by 1 g/kg = 60 g. At 4 kcal/g, the protein caloric need is 240 kcal.

3. **The nonprotein caloric requirement** thus equals approximately 1,785 kcal, which should include approximately 775 kcal fat and 1,010 kcal carbohydrate.

4. **A standard TPN formula** containing 20% dextrose and 3.5% protein (e.g., *Travasol*) would provide 680 kcal of dextrose per liter and 35 g (140 kcal) of protein per liter. Therefore, 1.7 L of this formula would approximate the carbohydrate and protein needs of the patient. The parenteral solution is administered at a rate of 75 mL/hr.

5. **A single unit of 10% intravenous fat emulsion provides 550 kcal/unit.** Therefore, the usual amount of fat given would be provided by 1.4 units (or 700 mL). Because fat emulsions are available in single units, it is preferable to give this patient 2 units of fat emulsion per day or 1 unit of 20% lipid.

In this example, the intravenous fat emulsion provides needed additional calories, allowing for the more complete utilization of the administered protein. An additional reason to provide fat emulsions parenterally is the need to provide **EFA**s at a minimum level of 4% of total calories. For example, 4% × 2,000 kcal = 80 kcal/d. One 550 kcal unit of intravenous fat emulsion per week can meet this requirement. **In the absence of any fat administration, EFA deficiency develops in 4 to 6 weeks in most people, when endogenous stores of EFAs are depleted.** Because the cost of lipid emulsions has decreased considerably, fat is being used as a parenteral caloric source in amounts exceeding those needed to meet the minimal **EFA** requirements, as outlined in the previous example.

Standard mixtures of electrolytes per liter of solution are provided by most pharmacies and they are designed together with acetate buffers to deliver a nonacid solution with a pH of between 5.3 and 6.8. In unusual fluid and electrolyte situations, the composition of the solution can be custom designed, but this significantly increases the cost of parenteral nutrition and increases the possibility of the solution becoming insoluble or "cracking." The use of standard fluid and electrolyte solutions with supplements as necessary is preferable. Typical parenteral nutritional solutions are shown in Table 19.4.

Osmolarity and caloric content of the parenteral solution are related to the glucose and protein concentrations. For lipid preparations, the osmolarity and caloric content are also related to the percentage of lipid in the solution (Table 19.5).

Table 19.4 Typical Parenteral Nutrition Solutions							
Solution	*Na+ (mEq/L)*	*K+ (mEq/L)*	*Mg2+ (mEq/L)*	*Acetate (mEq/L)*	*Cl− (mEq/L)*	*Protein (g/L)*	*Calories/L (D 20)[a]*
FreAmine III 3%	35	24.5	5	44	40	29	800
Aminosyn 4.25%	70	66	10	142	98	85	850
Travasol 4.25%	70	60	10	135	70	89	850
Travasol 3.5%	25	15	5	54	25	37	820

[a]If admixed with a solution of 20% dextrose.

Table 19.5 Osmolarity and Caloric Content of Glucose and Lipids in Parenteral Nutritional Solutions		
Glucose Concentration (wt/vol)	**Osmolarity (mOsm/L)**	**Calories (kcal/dL)**
5%	250	17
10%	500	34
20%	1,000	68
50%	2,500	170
70%	3,500	237
Lipid Concentration (wt/vol)		
10%	280	110
20%	340	200

Recommended vitamins that should be provided on a daily basis in parenteral solutions are listed in Table 19.6. These substances are available in preformulated ampules and 1 ampule per day added directly to the parenteral solution meets all the requirements in most patients. In patients who are especially stressed (e.g., septic wounds), 500 mg of vitamin C should be given. Patients receiving common medications such as *phenytoin (Dilantin)* may require additional specific vitamin supplements (e.g., vitamin D). The amount of vitamin K provided in daily parenteral nutrition should be routinely reviewed by a pharmacist.

Major mineral requirements are listed in Table 19.7. The daily requirement has a wide range that depends largely on the extent of GI and renal losses. In patients with an abnormally high excretion, the losses must be replaced aggressively.

Supplementation with zinc, copper, chromium, and selenium is essential in parenteral nutrition (Table 19.8). Deficiency states of these trace elements have been described in patients who have been receiving parenteral nutrition without supplementation. These patients respond to the

Table 19.6 Guidelines for Daily Adult Parenteral Vitamin Supplementation	
Vitamin	**Daily Intravenous Dose**
A	3,300 International Unit
D	200 International Unit
E	10 International Unit
B_1 (thiamin)	3 mg
B_2 (riboflavin)	3.6 mg
B_3 (pantothenic acid)	15 mg
B_5 (niacin)	40 mg
B_6 (pyridoxine)	4 mg
B_7 (biotin)	60 mg
B_9 (folic acid)	400 mg
B_{12} (cobalamin)	5 mg
C (ascorbic acid)	100 mg
K	5 mg/wk[a]

[a]Parenteral vitamin K supplementation is not included in the official recommendation because some patients are receiving anticoagulants.

From **American Medical Association/Nutrition Advisory Group Guidelines.** *JPEN J Parenter Enteral Nutr.* 1979;3:258, with permission.

| Table 19.7 Range of Daily Requirements of Major Minerals and Electrolytes in Parenteral Solutions ||
Electrolyte	Daily Requirement Range
Sodium	50–250 mEq
Potassium	30–200 mEq
Chloride	50–250 mEq
Magnesium	10–30 mEq
Calcium	10–20 mEq
Phosphorus	10–40 mmol

Modified from **Alpers DH, Clouse RE, Stenson WF**. Manual of nutritional therapeutics. Boston: Little, Brown; 1983:238.

specific replacement of deficient trace elements. **Patients who require home TPN should have trace element levels measured prior to discharge.**

Iron supplementation is not recommended in the acutely ill patient. Iron levels should be documented. **Manganese has not been clearly established as an essential component of TPN solutions,** but it has been included in some recommended regimens. **Iodine is not normally supplemented,** because the transdermal absorption of iodine-containing solutions that are used to clean catheter sites permits intake of the required amount of iodine. Iodine deficiency is associated with a high TSH. **Chromium levels may be useful in the diabetic patient,** as chromium is an insulin receptor cofactor, and deficiency may cause hypo- or hyperglycemia.

In the presence of excessive GI losses (e.g., small bowel fistula), additional zinc should be given for replacement. It is recommended that 12.2 mg of additional zinc per liter of small bowel loss should be given.

In patients who are being given enteral supplementation, 2 L of formula per day includes all the recommended dietary allowance for vitamins, minerals, and trace elements.

Further information regarding nutritional support may be obtained from the American Society for Parenteral and Enteral Nutrition (ASPEN) at http://www.nutritioncare.org.

Table 19.8 Suggested Daily Adult Intravenous Requirements of Essential Trace Elements and Associated Deficiency Syndromes		
Trace Element	Requirement	Deficiency Syndrome
Iron	10–18 mg/d	Anemia
Copper[a]	30 µg/kg/d	Rare hemolysis
Zinc[a]	15 mg/d	Blepharitis, conjunctivitis, growth retardation, dermatitis, diarrhea
Selenium[a]	50–200 µg/d	Cardiomyopathy
Chromium[a]	20 µg/d	Glucose intolerance, hypercholesterolemia, hyper-aminoacidemia
Manganese	3–5 mg/d	Dermatitis, hypocholesterolemia, hair color change, decreased hair, and nail growth
Iodine	100 µg/d	Hypothyroidism
Fluoride	1.5–4 mg/d	Anemia, growth retardation
Molybdenum[b]	200–500 µg/d	Muscle cramps

[a]Required in total parenteral nutrition solutions.

[b]Not absolutely required but included in most formulations.

Adapted from **AMA Department of Foods and Nutrition**. Guidelines for essential trace element preparations for parenteral use: A statement by an expert panel. *JAMA*. 1979;241:2051–2054, with permission.

References

1. **McClave SA, Martindale RG, Vanek VW, et al.** Guidelines for the Provision and Assessment of Nutrition Support Therapy in the Adult Critically Ill Patient: Society of Critical Care Medicine (SCCM) and American Society for Parenteral and Enteral Nutrition (A.S.P.E.N.). *JPEN J Parenter Enteral Nutr.* 2009;33(3):277–316.

2. **Mcwhirter JP, Pennington CR.** Incidence and recognition of malnutrition in-hospital. *Brit Med J.* 1994;308(6934):945–948.

3. **Moore FD BM.** *Manual of Surgical Nutrition.* In: **Ballinger WF, Drucker WR, eds.** Philadelphia, PA: WB Saunders; 1975, 169–222.

4. **Santarpia L, Contaldo F, Pasanisi F.** Nutritional screening and early treatment of malnutrition in cancer patients. *J Cachexia Sarcopenia Muscle.* 2011;2(1):27–35.

5. **Gallagher-Allred CR, Voss AC, Finn SC, et al.** Malnutrition and clinical outcomes: The case for medical nutrition therapy. *J Am Diet Assoc.* 1996;96(4):361–366, 369; quiz 7–8.

6. **Caro MM, Laviano A, Pichard C, et al.** Relationship between nutritional intervention and quality of life in cancer patients. *Nutr Hosp.* 2007;22(3):337–350.

7. **Naber TH, Schermer T, de Bree A, et al.** Prevalence of malnutrition in nonsurgical hospitalized patients and its association with disease complications. *Am J Clin Nutr.* 1997;66(5):1232–1239.

8. **Santoso JT, Canada T, Latson B, et al.** Prognostic nutritional index in relation to hospital stay in women with gynecologic cancer. *Obstet Gynecol.* 2000;95(6):844–846.

9. **Baccaro F, Moreno JB, Borlenghi C, et al.** Subjective global assessment in the clinical setting. *JPEN J Parenter Enter Nutr.* 2007;31(5):406–409.

10. **Nitenberg G, Raynard B.** Nutritional support of the cancer patient: Issues and dilemmas. *Crit Rev Oncol Hematol.* 2000;34(3):137–168.

11. **Sarhill N, Mahmoud F, Walsh D, et al.** Evaluation of nutritional status in advanced metastatic cancer. *Support Care Cancer.* 2003;11(10):652–659.

12. **Santoso JT, Cannada T, O'Farrel B, et al.** Subjective versus objective nutritional assessment study in women with gynecological cancer: A prospective cohort trial. *Int J Gynecol Cancer.* 2004;14(2):220–223.

13. **Capra S, Ferguson M, Ried K.** Cancer: Impact of nutrition intervention outcome–nutrition issues for patients. *Nutrition.* 2001;17(9):769–772.

14. **van Bokhorst-de van der Schueren MA.** Nutritional support strategies for malnourished cancer patients. *Eur J Oncol Nurs.* 2005;9(suppl 2):S74–S83.

15. **Huhmann MB, August DA.** Review of American Society for Parenteral and Enteral Nutrition (ASPEN) Clinical Guidelines for Nutrition Support in Cancer Patients: Nutrition screening and assessment. *Nutr Clin Pract.* 2008;23(2):182–188.

16. **Nicolini A, Ferrari P, Masoni MC, et al.** Malnutrition, anorexia and cachexia in cancer patients: A mini-review on pathogenesis and treatment. *Biomed Pharmacother.* 2013;67(8):807–817.

17. **McNamara MJ, Alexander HR, Norton JA.** Cytokines and their role in the pathophysiology of cancer cachexia. *JPEN J Parenter Enteral Nutr.* 1992;16(6 suppl):50S–55S.

18. **Gough DB, Heys SD, Eremin O.** Cancer cachexia: Pathophysiological mechanisms. *Eur J Surg Oncol.* 1996;22(2):192–196.

19. **Inui A.** Cancer anorexia-cachexia syndrome: Current issues in research and management. *CA Cancer J Clin.* 2002;52(2):72–91.

20. **Morley JE, Thomas DR, Wilson MM.** Cachexia: Pathophysiology and clinical relevance. *Am J Clin Nutr.* 2006;83(4):735–743.

21. **Heber D, Byerley LO, Chi J, et al.** Pathophysiology of malnutrition in the adult cancer patient. *Cancer.* 1986;58(8 suppl):1867–1873.

22. **Gianotti L, Braga M, Vignali A, et al.** Effect of route of delivery and formulation of postoperative nutritional support in patients undergoing major operations for malignant neoplasms. *Arch Surg.* 1997;132(11):1222–1229; discussion 9–30.

23. **Laughlin EH, Dorosin NN, Phillips YY.** Total parenteral nutrition: A guide to therapy in the adult. *J Fam Pract.* 1977;5(6):947–957.

24. **Shah B, Sucher K, Hollenbeck CB.** Comparison of ideal body weight equations and published height-weight tables with body mass index tables for healthy adults in the United States. *Nutr Clin Pract.* 2006;21(3):312–319.

25. **Chlebowski RT, Palomares MR, Lillington L, et al.** Recent implications of weight loss in lung cancer management. *Nutrition.* 1996;12(1 suppl):S43–S47.

26. **Tisdale MJ.** Cancer cachexia: Metabolic alterations and clinical manifestations. *Nutrition.* 1997;13(1):1–7.

27. **Alexander JW, Ogle CK, Nelson JL.** Diets and infection: Composition and consequences. *World J Surg.* 1998;22(2):209–212.

28. **Jensen TG, Dudrick SJ, Johnston DA.** A comparison of triceps skinfold and upper arm circumference measurements taken in standard and supine positions. *JPEN J Parenter Enteral Nutr.* 1981;5(6):519–521.

29. **Ottery FD.** Definition of standardized nutritional assessment and interventional pathways in oncology. *Nutrition.* 1996;12(1 suppl):S15–S19.

30. **Tchekmedyian NS, Zahyna D, Halpert C, et al.** Assessment and maintenance of nutrition in older cancer patients. *Oncology.* 1992;6(2 suppl):105–111.

31. **Gabay C, Kushner I.** Acute-phase proteins and other systemic responses to inflammation. *N Engl J Med.* 1999;340(6):448–454.

32. **Chen MK, Souba WW, Copeland EM, 3rd.** Nutritional support of the surgical oncology patient. *Hematol Oncol Clin North Am.* 1991;5(1):125–145.

33. **Buzby GP, Mullen JL, Matthews DC, et al.** Prognostic nutritional index in gastrointestinal surgery. *Am J Surg.* 1980;139(1):160–167.

34. **Kubrak C, Jensen L.** Critical evaluation of nutrition screening tools recommended for oncology patients. *Cancer Nurs.* 2007;30(5):E1–E6.

35. **Barbosa-Silva MC, Barros AJ.** Indications and limitations of the use of subjective global assessment in clinical practice: An update. *Curr Opin Clin Nutr Metab Care.* 2006;9(3):263–269.

36. **Rock CL, Doyle C, Demark-Wahnefried W, et al.** Nutrition and physical activity guidelines for cancer survivors. *CA Cancer J Clin.* 2012;62(4):243–274.

37. **August DA, Huhmann MB; American Society for Parenteral and Enteral Nutrition (A.S.P.E.N.) Board of Directors.** clinical guidelines: Nutrition support therapy during adult anticancer treatment and in hematopoietic cell transplantation. *JPEN J Parenter Enteral Nutr.* 2009;33(5):472–500.

38. **ASPEN Board of Directors and the Clinical Guidelines Task Force.** Guidelines for the use of parenteral and enteral nutrition in adult and pediatric patients. *JPEN J Parenter Enteral Nutr.* 2002;26(1 suppl):1SA–138SA.

39. **Stroud M, Duncan H, Nightingale J; British Society of Gastroenterology.** Guidelines for enteral feeding in adult hospital patients. *Gut.* 2003;52(suppl 7):vii1–vii12.

40. **Sirbu ER, Margen S, Calloway DH.** Effect of reduced protein intake on nitrogen loss from the human integument. *Am J Clin Nutr.* 1967;20(11):1158–1165.

41. **Russell M.** *ASPEN Nutrition Support Practice Manual.* 2nd ed. American Society for Parenteral & Enteral Nutrition; 2005.

42. **Gottschlich MM.** *The American Society for Parenteral and Enteral Nutrition's Nutrition support core Curriculum: A Case-Based Approach-the Adult Patient.* Silver Spring, MD; 2007.

43. **Calloway DH, Spector H.** Nitrogen balance as related to caloric and protein intake in active young men. *Am J Clin Nutr.* 1954;2(6):405–412.

44. **Dietary reference Intakes for Energy, Carbohydrate, Fat, Fatty Acids, Cholesterol, Protein, and Amino Acids 2002.** Available from: http://www.nap.edu.

45. **Pillar B, Perry S.** Evaluating total parenteral nutrition: Final report and statement of the Technology Assessment and Practice Guidelines Forum. *Nutrition.* 1990;6(4):314–318.

46. **Klein S, Simes J, Blackburn GL.** Total parenteral nutrition and cancer clinical trials. *Cancer.* 1986;58(6):1378–1386.

47. **Klein S, Koretz RL.** Nutrition support in patients with cancer: What do the data really show? *Nutr Clin Pract.* 1994;9(3):91–100.

48. **Bethel RA, Jansen RD, Heymsfield SB, et al.** Nasogastric hyperalimentation through a polyethylene catheter: An alternative to central venous hyperalimentation. *Am J Clin Nutr.* 1979;32(5):1112–1120.

49. **Lis CG, Gupta D, Lammersfeld CA, et al.** Role of nutritional status in predicting quality of life outcomes in cancer-a systematic review of the epidemiological literature. *Nutr J.* 2012;11:27.

50. **Voitk AJ, Echave V, Brown RA, et al.** Use of elemental diet during the adaptive stage of short gut syndrome. *Gastroenterology.* 1973;65(3):419–426.

51. **Iyer KR, Crawley TC.** Complications of enteral access. *Gastrointest Endosc Clin N Am.* 2007;17(4):717–729.

52. **Baskin WN.** Acute complications associated with bedside placement of feeding tubes. *Nutr Clin Pract.* 2006;21(1):40–55.

53. **Heymsfield SB, Bethel RA, Ansley JD, et al.** Enteral hyperalimentation: An alternative to central venous hyperalimentation. *Ann Intern Med.* 1979;90(1):63–71.

54. **Feliciano DV, Mattox KL, Graham JM, et al.** Major complications of percutaneous subclavian vein catheters. *Am J Surg.* 1979; 138(6):869–874.

55. **Ryan JA, Jr., Abel RM, Abbott WM, et al.** Catheter complications in total parenteral nutrition. A prospective study of 200 consecutive patients. *N Engl J Med.* 1974;290(14):757–761.

56. **Covelli HD, Black JW, Olsen MS, et al.** Respiratory failure precipitated by high carbohydrate loads. *Ann Intern Med.* 1981;95(5):579–581.

57. **O'Grady NP, Alexander M, Dellinger EP, et al.** Guidelines for the prevention of intravascular catheter-related infections. *Infec Control Hosp Epidemiol.* 2002;23(12):759–769.

58. **Pappas PG, Rex JH, Sobel JD, et al.** Guidelines for treatment of candidiasis. *Clin Infect Dis.* 2004;38(2):161–189.

59. **Ryan JA, Jr.** Complications of total parenteral nutrition. **Fischer JE, ed.** Boston, MA: Little Brown; 1976:55.

60. **Ruberg RL, Allen TR, Goodman MJ, et al.** Hypophosphatemia with hypophosphaturia in hyperalimentation. *Surg Forum.* 1971;22:87–88.

61. **Fleming CR, Hodges RE, Hurley LS.** A prospective study of serum copper and zinc levels in patients receiving total parenteral nutrition. *Am J Clin Nutr.* 1976;29(1):70–77.

62. **Fleming CR, McGill DB, Hoffman HN, 2nd, et al.** Total parenteral nutrition. *Mayo Clin Proc.* 1976;51(3):187–199.

63. **Marinella MA.** Refeeding syndrome in cancer patients. *Int J Clin Pract.* 2008;62(3):460–465.

64. **Blackburn GL, Wan JM, Teo TC, et al.** *Metabolic Support in Organ Failure.* **Behari DJ, ed.** Fullerton, CA: Society of Critical Care Medicine; 1989.

65. **Cerra FB.** Hypermetabolism, organ failure, and metabolic support. *Surgery.* 1987;101(1):1–14.

66. **Windmueller HG.** Glutamine utilization by the small intestine. *Adv Enzymol Relat Areas Mol Biol.* 1982;53:201–237.

67. **Fox AD, Kripke SA, De Paula J, et al.** Effect of a glutamine-supplemented enteral diet on methotrexate-induced enterocolitis. *JPEN J Parenter Enteral Nutr.* 1988;12(4):325–331.

68. **Klimberg VS, Souba WW, Salloum RM, et al.** Glutamine-enriched diets support muscle glutamine metabolism without stimulating tumor growth. *J Surg Res.* 1990;48(4):319–323.

69. **Nuutinen LS, Kauppila A, Ryhanen P, et al.** Intensified nutrition as an adjunct to cytotoxic chemotherapy in gynaecological cancer patients. *Clin Oncol.* 1982;8(2):107–112.

70. **Jones NE, Heyland DK.** Pharmaconutrition: A new emerging paradigm. *Curr Opin Gastroenterol.* 2008;24(2):215–222.

Surgical Techniques

Jonathan S. Berek
Amer Karam
David Cibula

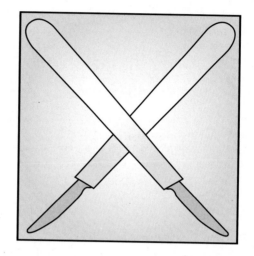

In order to surgically manage gynecologic malignancies, it is frequently necessary to perform surgical procedures beyond the genital tract. These include selected operations on the intestinal and urologic tracts, and plastic reconstructive operations such as the creation of a neovagina. In addition, central venous access is frequently required for hyperalimentation or chemotherapy. **In some centers, most of the operations are performed by the gynecologic oncologist, while in other centers, the emphasis is on the development of a multidisciplinary team** with involvement of urologists, colorectal, upper gastrointestinal and plastic surgeons for the surgical procedures, and anesthesiologists for the central lines. The techniques for these nongynecologic procedures are presented in this chapter.

Central Lines

Central venous-access catheters are often necessary in the critically ill gynecologic oncology patient for either central venous pressure monitoring, centrally administered hyperalimentation, or chemotherapy (1–3). The most frequently used veins are the subclavian and the jugular. **The brachial veins are used for peripherally inserted central catheters (PICC lines)** (4). The results of three-pooled meta-analyses have shown that ultrasound-guided placement of central venous access devices reduces the number of complications, failures, and the insertion time (4–6). Static ultrasonic images can help localize the veins using the traditional anatomic landmark techniques, but dynamic images can also be used to guide the needle into the vein in real-time.

Subclavian Venous Catheter

Infraclavicular Technique

Although there are many different techniques for the insertion of a central venous catheter into the subclavian vein, the **infraclavicular technique** remains the one most commonly employed and the simplest. The subclavian vein lies immediately deep to the clavicle within the costoclavicular triangle, where the vein is more commonly approached from the right side (Fig. 20.1A). The **costoclavicular-scalene triangle** is bounded by the medial end of the clavicle anteriorly, the upper surface of the first rib posteriorly, and the anterior scalene muscle laterally (1). The anterior

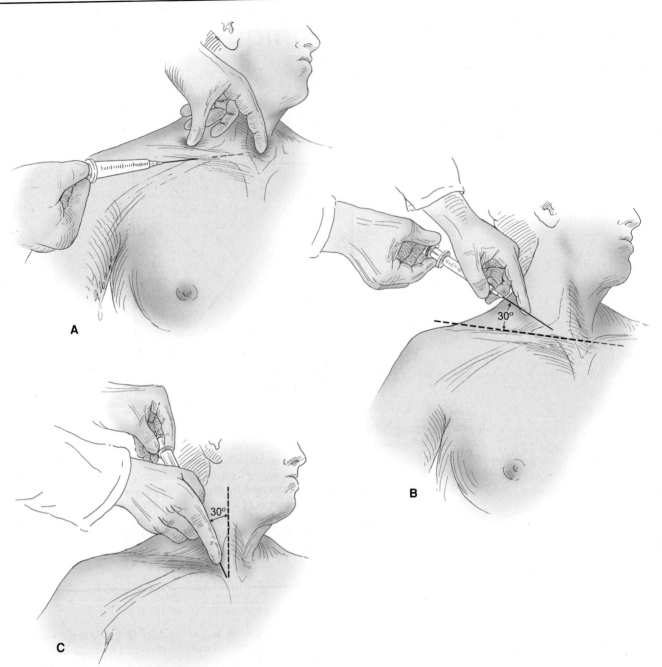

Figure 20.1 Central venous catheter insertion sites. The right subclavian and right internal jugular venous insertion sites are illustrated. The insertion sites for the subclavian venous catheter: **(A)** via the infraclavicular technique; **(B)** via the supraclavicular technique; **(C)** the site of insertion for the internal jugular vein. The needle is directed toward the suprasternal notch.

scalene muscle separates the subclavian vein anteriorly from the subclavian artery posteriorly. Just deep to the subclavian artery are the nerves of the brachial plexus. The subclavian vein is covered by the medial 5 cm of the clavicle. Just deep to the medial head of the clavicle, the right internal jugular vein joins the right subclavian vein to form the innominate vein, which then descends into the chest, where it joins the left innominate vein to form the superior vena cava in the retrosternal space.

There are several other vital structures in the scalene triangle. The phrenic nerve courses anterior to the anterior scalene muscle and therefore lies immediately deep to the subclavian vein. If the deep wall of the vein is penetrated, the phrenic nerve can be injured. **If the subclavian artery is penetrated, the brachial plexus, lying just deep to the vessel, can be injured. The**

right lymphatic duct and the thoracic duct on the left enter their respective subclavian veins near the junction with the internal jugular veins and therefore may be injured by a misplaced needle. **The most common injury is to the pleura,** the apex of which is just beneath the subclavian vein at the junction of the internal jugular vein.

The technique for infraclavicular insertion of a catheter into the right subclavian vein is as follows:

1. The patient is placed in the supine position, with the foot of the bed elevated about 1 foot so that **the patient is in the Trendelenburg position.** If possible, a bed that can be tilted into this position should be used. This position creates venous distention and increases the intraluminal pressure within the subclavian vein. The patient's head should be tilted away from the site of insertion so that the landmarks can be identified easily.

2. After careful skin preparation with *chlorhexidine gluconate* solution, **the skin and subjacent tissues are anesthetized** by means of *lidocaine* without *epinephrine.*

3. **The site of insertion is located at the junction of the middle and medial thirds of the clavicle,** approximately 1 cm below the bone's inferior margin.

4. Before insertion of the catheter needle, **a probe needle is used to localize the subclavian vein** and to identify the presence of dark venous blood. An 18-gauge needle attached to a 10-mL syringe filled with normal saline solution is used.

5. **A 14-gauge Intracath needle is used to insert the catheter** (Fig. 20.1A). The needle attached to the syringe is inserted into the skin with the bevel directed toward the heart. The needle should be held and directed parallel to the anterior chest wall.

6. **After insertion through the skin, the needle is directed medially and advanced along the undersurface of the clavicle** in the direction of the suprasternal notch.

7. The syringe is pulled gently to apply suction as the needle is inserted. **The patient should exhale during insertion to avoid an air embolus.**

8. After a free flow of blood has been obtained, the needle is held carefully in place, the syringe is detached, and the central venous catheter is advanced inside the lumen of the needle. The catheter should advance freely, and there should be blood returning through the catheter. **The catheter is advanced into the innominate vein and then into the superior vena cava.** The catheter should be aspirated, and if blood is easily withdrawn, the needle is removed.

9. **While the needle is in place, the catheter should not be withdrawn** because the tip can be sheared off and embolize.

10. **The end of the catheter is connected to an intravenous set,** and the catheter is sutured to the skin.

11. **The position of the catheter is verified by a chest radiograph.** It should be located in the superior vena cava, not in the right atrium or ventricle, as this can result in trauma to the heart.

If central venous pressure readings are to be determined, the intravenous line is attached to a manometer, and the base of the water column is positioned at the level of the right atrium, which is about 5 cm posterior to the fourth costochondral junction when the patient is in the supine position. **The normal central venous pressure should be between 5 and 12 cm of water.**

The complication rate for central venous catheter insertion through the subclavian route is about 1–2% (1). Most serious complications are related to puncture of the pleura and lung or perforation and laceration of vessels, resulting in a pneumothorax or hemothorax. **Catheter-related infection is seen in about 0.5% of patients, and the catheter should be removed if this source of infection is suspected.**

Supraclavicular Insertion

An alternative route of insertion into the subclavian vein is the supraclavicular route (Fig. 20.1B). Some prefer this to the infraclavicular route, but the morbidity of insertion is comparable with the two methods, and the preference is related to the technique that is most comfortable for the operator.

The technique for insertion is identical to that of the infraclavicular route, except that the needle is inserted above the clavicle, approximately 5 cm lateral to the midsternal notch. The angle of insertion is about 30 degrees from a line drawn between the two shoulders and directed caudally. The needle is aimed at the suprasternal notch.

Jugular Venous Catheterization

Another alternative for central venous access is the use of the jugular veins, either the internal or external vein. **Jugular venous catheterization is frequently the method of choice when the catheter is inserted intraoperatively and the catheter is to be used primarily for acute monitoring.** The advantage is that there is relatively easy access while the patient is anesthetized and draped for surgery, whereas the disadvantage is that it is more difficult to anchor the catheter because the neck is more mobile than the anterior chest wall. The location for the insertion site is illustrated in Figure 20.1C.

The technique for insertion is as follows:

1. **The patient is placed in the Trendelenburg position.** With the patient's head turned away from the side of insertion, the needle is inserted just above the medial head of the clavicle between the medial and middle heads of the sternocleidomastoid muscle, where a small pocket is readily apparent and helps to localize the site for insertion.

2. **The angle of insertion is about 20 to 30 degrees from the sagittal median of the patient, and the direction is toward the heart.**

3. **As with subclavian catheterization, the use of a probe needle will help to localize the appropriate vessel.**

4. **The technique of catheter placement is the same as described above for the subclavian catheter.** However, the length of catheter that must be inserted is less, as the distance to the proper location in the superior vena cava is less.

5. **The position of the line inserted intraoperatively is checked with a chest radiograph** obtained in the recovery room if the catheter is to be left in place.

External jugular catheters may also be used in patients who are under general anesthesia. Some patients have relatively prominent external jugular veins, and they are very easily catheterized. **The external jugular is not durable,** however, **and this route is not useful for central hyperalimentation.** The complication rate for jugular venous catheterization is essentially the same as that for the subclavian route.

Dynamic Ultrasonic Technique

When using dynamic images to guide the needle, several additional steps are necessary to ensure successful placement:

- Steps should be taken to ensure the sterility of the probe using a sterile probe cover.
- Ultrasonic gel should be applied to the head of the probe and any air bubbles forced out.
- Sterile ultrasonic/conductive gel should be applied between the skin and the probe cover.

When the ultrasonic probe is ready:

- The target vein should be centered on the ultrasonic picture.
- The focus should be focused on the needle tip rather than the shaft, which can be accomplished by moving the needle up and down within the tissue to better see it, or by rocking the probe back and forth.
- When in the vein, the probe can be removed and the remaining steps accomplished according to the traditional techniques.

Semipermanent Lines

The placement of semipermanent lines is useful in patients who require prolonged access to the central venous system, such as those with a chronic intestinal obstruction or fistula who are to receive hyperalimentation after discharge from hospital (1).

Broviac, Hickman, and Quinton Catheters

The most common types of lines are catheters made of flexible, synthetic rubber (e.g., Broviac, Hickman, or Quinton catheters). The catheters are available in several sizes, although the adult type is used for most patients; the length is adapted by cutting the catheters as necessary. The catheters are available with either a single or double lumen. **The single-lumen catheters usually are sufficient for parenteral nutrition, whereas the double-lumen ones may be necessary for patients requiring frequent bolus medication, such as intravenous pain or antibiotic medications** (2,3).

The most common site for insertion of a semipermanent catheter is the right subclavian vein. The method of insertion is initially identical to the technique employed for the insertion of a temporary catheter, but an insertion cannula, called a Cook introducer, can simplify and facilitate insertion of the catheter (Fig. 20.2). It is preferable to insert the catheter under fluoroscopic guidance.

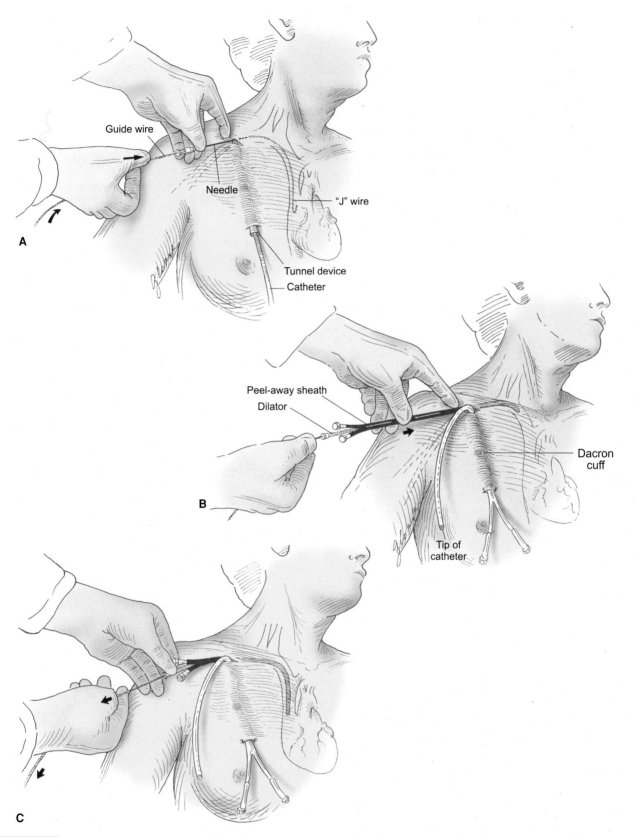

Figure 20.2 Semipermanent catheter insertion. The technique for insertion of the semipermanent (e.g., Hickman) catheter. **A:** After the catheter is tunneled in the subcutaneous tissue, a needle is inserted into the right subclavian vein, a guide wire is inserted through the needle, and the needle is withdrawn. **B:** The Cook introducer then is inserted over the guide wire. **C:** After the introducer with its outer sheath is in place in the right subclavian vein, the wire is withdrawn. (*continued*)

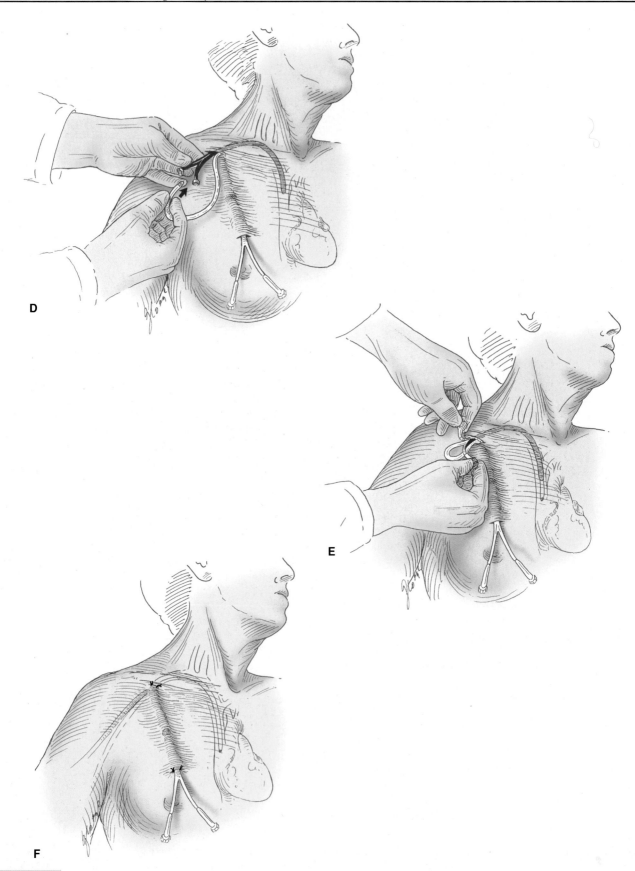

Figure 20.2 *Continued.* **D:** The central catheter of the Cook introducer is withdrawn, and the free end of the semipermanent catheter is inserted through the outer sheath. **E:** The outer sheath of the Cook introducer is peeled away. **F:** The semipermanent catheter is tunneled in the subcutaneous tissue under the skin of the right side of the chest, and the free end is exteriorized.

The technique is as follows:

1. After the patient has been properly positioned and the anterior chest and clavicular areas prepared, **the subclavian vein is identified in the manner described above**.

2. A premade kit is available for the Cook introducer. **An 18-gauge needle is used to introduce a guide wire into the subclavian vein, and the guide wire is passed into the superior vena cava** under fluoroscopy (Fig. 20.2A).

3. The proper position of the guide wire is documented, and **the Cook introducer is fed over the guide wire** and advanced into the subclavian vein (Fig. 20.2B).

4. The introducer has an inner catheter and an outer sheath. After insertion of the entire apparatus, the central cannula is removed (Fig. 20.2C) and **the semipermanent catheter is threaded through the outer sheath,** which remains in the subclavian vein (Fig. 20.2D).

5. After the semipermanent catheter has been inserted, **the outer sheath is peeled away,** leaving the catheter in place (Fig. 20.2E).

6. **The proximal end of the semipermanent catheter is tunneled under the skin** of the anterior chest wall **and exteriorized through a stab incision in the skin** as illustrated (Fig. 20.2F).

7. **An intravenous line is connected to the catheter's adapter,** and fluid is run into the line to establish its patency. The catheter is sutured into place.

Peripherally Inserted Central Catheter Lines

Another type of semipermanent line is inserted through a peripheral access site and is called the peripherally inserted central catheter or PICC line. The PICC line is inserted into the brachial vein in the antecubital fossa. The catheter is passed cephalad until it reaches the central subclavian vein. This line is suitable for the infusion of parenteral nutrition as well as chemotherapy. **The PICC line may be more desirable than a totally implantable line when short-term use is contemplated, for example, 3 to 4 months.**

This approach is less durable than the centrally inserted catheters and somewhat more cumbersome because of the location of the insertion site. However, **its main advantage is that it can be easily inserted at the bedside** (7). Furthermore, it can be placed by a certified nurse or an intravenous technician trained in the insertion technique. Alternately, an implantable port can be inserted in the antecubital fossa by a physician.

Peritoneal Catheters

Peritoneal catheters are used in gynecologic oncology for the instillation of intraperitoneal chemotherapy. **A commonly used catheter is a completely implantable single lumen 9.6-Fr MRI safe Port-a-Cath.** This catheter has not been associated with an increased risk of complications or treatment discontinuation (8,9). Alternatively, a Hickman venous access catheter can be used.

The catheter is implanted into the peritoneal cavity lateral to the midline laparotomy incision (Fig. 20.3). The catheter is tunneled in the subcutaneous tissue and brought out through a stab incision lateral to the fascial incision. The tip of the catheter in the peritoneal cavity is directed toward the pelvic cul-de-sac.

An alternative approach is the use of a completely implantable port, which is attached directly to a fenestrated peritoneal catheter or venous access catheter. The port is inserted into the subcutaneous tissue and positioned in the left or right lower quadrant of the anterior abdomen, or over the lower anterior rib cage for ready access (Fig. 20.4). Both laparotomy and laparoscopy can be utilized for port placement. Postprocedure, the port is entered percutaneously with a 21-gauge needle.

The reported rate of catheter-related complications ranges from 3–34% (8,10–14). In the most recent phase III study of IP versus IV chemotherapy for the treatment of ovarian cancer, Walker et al. reported that **40 (19.5%) of 205 patients randomized to the IP arm had complications,** including infection ($n = 21$); blockage ($n = 10$); leakage ($n = 3$); access problems ($n = 5$); and vaginal leakage of fluid ($n = 1$) (10). Of the 119 patients (58%) discontinuing IP therapy, catheter-related complications accounted for 34% of cases (40 of 119). Both Tenckhoff or implantable ports with attached fenestrated or venous (Hickman) catheters were used.

Minor infections can be treated with antibiotics, and low-grade peritonitis can be treated by the instillation of antibiotics directly via the catheter. **For persistent and severe infections, the**

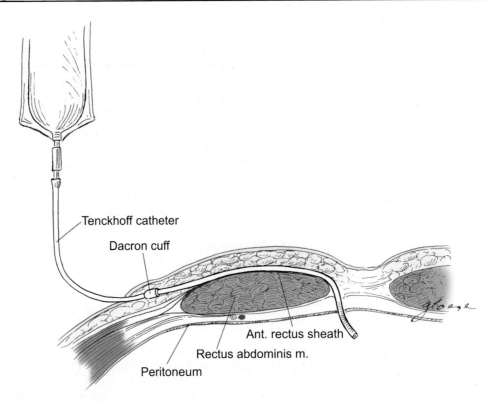

Tenckhoff catheter

Dacron cuff

Ant. rectus sheath

Rectus abdominis m.

Peritoneum

Figure 20.3 Tenckhoff peritoneal catheter. The placement of the Tenckhoff catheter into the peritoneal cavity is illustrated.

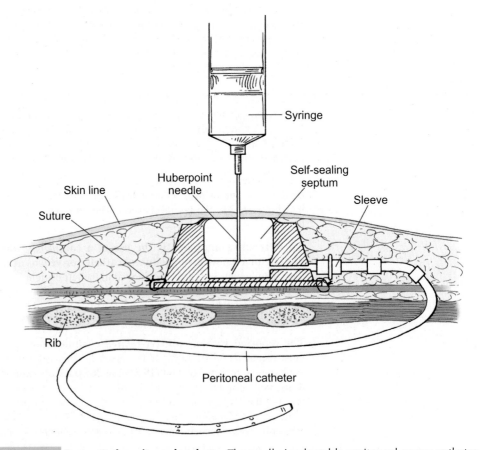

Syringe

Self-sealing septum

Sleeve

Skin line

Huberpoint needle

Suture

Rib

Peritoneal catheter

Figure 20.4 Port-a-Cath peritoneal catheter. The totally implantable peritoneal access catheter is tunneled through the subcutaneous tissues into the peritoneal cavity.

peritoneal catheter may require removal. **In other studies, the most common problem associated with the catheters has been blockage** (14), as there is no effective way to prevent deposition of fibrin around the catheter. Occasionally, this produces a "ball valve" effect; that is, fluid will flow in but will not flow out. While some authors report higher fibrin sheath formation and adhesions in association with fenestrated catheters and dacron cuffs, a recent retrospective study of fenestrated peritoneal catheters reported that only 9 of 342 patients (3%) required discontinuation secondary to catheter complications (8).

Incisions

Particularly important in the operative plan for any patient is the determination of the type of incision to be made. The surgeon should have a general philosophy and *modus operandi* when planning the surgical procedure. There are certain incisions that are more appropriate in patients who are undergoing surgery for cancer rather than for benign conditions. In addition, special guidelines for the closure of incisions should be followed.

Vertical Incisions

Abdominal incisions used in the gynecologic oncology patient are most commonly vertical. Transverse incisions are also appropriate in certain circumstances. The indications and techniques for these incisions and their modifications are discussed.

Patients with suspected malignancies of the ovary or fallopian tube are best explored through a vertical abdominal incision. With a vertical incision, the patient's disease can be staged properly. Also, this approach permits the removal of any upper abdominal metastases, which cannot always be appreciated preoperatively. The most likely site of resectable upper abdominal disease is the omentum. For an omentectomy, access to the region of the splenic and hepatic flexures is required.

A vertical incision is also necessary in patients being explored for intestinal obstruction or fistulae. The performance of a para-aortic lymphadenectomy is facilitated by a vertical incision. Patients being explored for recurrent malignancies or for possible pelvic exenteration also require a vertical abdominal incision.

The most commonly used vertical incision is in the midline. This incision has the advantage of being easy to perform; it can be accomplished quickly, because the midline is the least vascular area of the abdominal wall, and the smallest depth of tissue must be divided. The principal blood supply to the anterior abdominal wall is from the inferior epigastric vessels, which are located laterally in the rectus sheath posterior to the rectus abdominis muscles, and these vessels are avoided by the midline incision.

The principal problem associated with the midline incision is that it has the highest rate of wound dehiscence when compared with all other incisions. The wound disruption rate is about 0.1–0.65% (15,16), although this rate may be higher in patients with cancer, particularly those with ascites and malnutrition, or those needing postoperative radiation.

Dehiscence rates as high as 2–3% have been reported in obese, diabetic patients with cancer (16). The majority of wound dehiscences are associated with wound infection or poor closure technique. **The occurrence of a ventral hernia is associated with wound disruption secondary to infection and is more common in patients with malignancy** (17).

Transverse Incisions

In patients with a probable benign condition who are undergoing abdominal exploration for the first time, a lower transverse abdominal incision is frequently employed. **The advantage of this incision is that it is more cosmetic, generally less painful, and associated with fewer incisional hernias** (18). The disadvantage is the relative problem of upper abdominal exposure and the more frequent occurrence of wound hematomas.

If exposure to the upper abdomen is required, the surgeon has several choices. The incision can be modified by division of the rectus abdominis muscles in a transverse direction at the level of the incision (i.e., **a Maylard incision**), or the rectus abdominis muscles may be detached from the symphysis pubis (i.e., **the Cherney incision**). After division or mobilization of the rectus muscles, the inferior epigastric vessels are ligated bilaterally and, if necessary, the incision is further extended laterally by incising (with the diathermy) the "strap" muscles of the anterior abdominal wall. The conversion of the incision to a Maylard or a Cherney incision always provides considerably more exposure in the pelvis and low para-aortic area.

If better access to the upper abdomen is required, the incision can be modified further by extending the incision cephalad to form a **"J,"** a reverse **"J,"** or **a "hockey stick" incision**. In general, any of these techniques is preferable to the making of a second incision, that is, a midline incision coincident with the transverse incision, a so-called **"T"** incision. The principal difficulty with the latter approach is the weakness of the incision at the point of intersection of the two incisions.

In patients undergoing radical hysterectomy and pelvic lymphadenectomy for early-stage cervical cancer, a lower abdominal transverse incision is adequate.

Incisional Closure

Of primary importance is the technique of incisional closure. The closure can be accomplished by closing the peritoneum, fascia, subcutaneous tissue, and skin individually, or a bulk closure can be performed that incorporates the peritoneum and the fascia together. **This bulk closure or internal retention suture, the "Smead–Jones" closure, is the strongest closure technique** (16). Mass closure with a continuous, single strand of polyglyconate monofilament absorbable suture (*Maxon*) or polydioxanone (*PDS*) has been shown to be an effective, safe alternative to the use of interrupted sutures, even in vertical midline incisions (17,19,20).

Internal Retention Suture

The Smead–Jones, or internal retention, technique uses interrupted sutures that are placed as illustrated in Figure 20.5. The sutures are placed in a far-far, near-near distribution, which is a modified figure-of-eight. The first suture is placed through the anterior fascia, rectus muscle, posterior fascia, and peritoneum and the second through the anterior fascial layer only. The key is to place the sutures at least 1.5 to 2 cm from the fascial edge and not more than 1 cm apart (19). **The disruption rate for midline incisions closed with this technique should be less than 0.2%.**

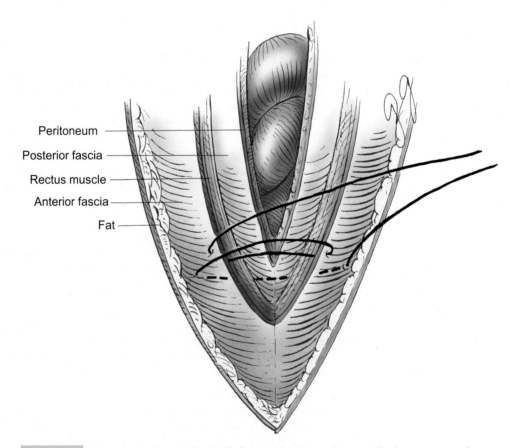

Peritoneum
Posterior fascia
Rectus muscle
Anterior fascia
Fat

Figure 20.5 Internal retention abdominal closure. The "Smead–Jones" far-far, near-near closure.

Suture Material

The choice of suture should be dictated by the circumstances (20). If there is evidence of significant infection, as with an abscess or an intestinal injury, a monofilament, nonabsorbable suture is most appropriate. The most frequently used substances are nylon sutures, such as *Prolene*. **For vertical incisions, an absorbable, long-lasting synthetic suture offers the best combination of strength, durability, and ease of use.** Most suitable is either monofilament polyglyconate suture (*Maxon*) or monofilament polydioxanone (*PDS*). Braided, polyglycolic acid (*PGA*) suture, such as *Vicryl* or *Dexon,* is suitable for transverse incisions (20,21). A grade 0 or 1 suture is necessary to provide a suitably strong closure. The tissue reactivity to these synthetic materials is less than that of chromic catgut. Nonabsorbable polyfilament materials, such as cotton and silk, should not be used for closure of incisions because of the higher potential for "stitch abscess" formation (17).

External Retention Suture

Retention sutures that are external can be used to prevent evisceration in patients who are at high risk of this potentially catastrophic occurrence. **The routine use of internal retention sutures has reduced the need for the external retention sutures.** However, in patients who are morbidly obese, have a major wound infection, or whose incisions have eviscerated in the past, the addition of external retention sutures may be indicated. These sutures should be placed in a manner similar to internal retention sutures, that is, far-far, near-near, with the far sutures also placed through the skin so that the retention sutures are knotted externally. **The preferable suture material for this closure is nylon.** The external retention sutures are inserted through a rubber "bolster" that helps to protect the skin from injury from the suture. Sutures are placed at approximately 2- to 3-cm intervals, and interrupted fascial sutures are placed between them.

Skin Closure

Primary Closure

Skin closure of vertical incisions in cancer patients generally should be interrupted, preferably with metal skin clips. Subcuticular closures are not appropriate in most circumstances for vertical incisions, but they are quite cosmetic and acceptable for small transverse incisions where the risk of wound infection is low (22).

Secondary Closure

A delayed or secondary skin closure is useful in patients whose incisions are infected, that is, after the drainage of an intra-abdominal abscess or repair of an intestinal fistula. This is achieved by placement of interrupted mattress sutures in the skin, which are not tied, so that the skin remains unapproximated. Thus the skin can be closed later, usually after 3 to 4 days, when the infection is under control. Negative pressure wound therapy may help in accelerating the healing process but definitive evidence is lacking (23).

Intestinal Operations

Preoperative Intestinal Preparation

If bowel resection is planned or contemplated, a mechanical and antibiotic "bowel preparation" may be undertaken preoperatively. **If the intestine is prepared properly, the segment is well vascularized, and there is no sepsis, prior irradiation, or evidence of tumor at the site of anastomosis, colonic reanastomosis can be accomplished without leakage in 98% of the cases** (24). More proximal resection of the small intestine can be performed without a bowel preparation, because this portion of the intestine does not contain bacteria.

An effective protocol for bowel preparation is presented in Table 20.1. **Recently, the FDA issued a Safety Alert discussing the risk of acute phosphate nephropathy, a rare type of renal failure associated with oral sodium phosphate bowel cleansing that may lead to permanent renal impairment.** Increased risk has been associated with multiple factors including advanced age, kidney disease, and use of medications affecting renal perfusion and function. In response, over-the-counter oral sodium phosphate preparations such as *Fleet Phospho-soda* have been recalled. Bowel preparation regimens should be individualized for patients after assessment of risk factors. Alternative bowel preparation regimens include magnesium citrate and *Golytely.*

There is controversy regarding the use of bowel preparations in general as well as the optimal "bowel prep," as it is uncertain whether, in addition to the mechanical preparation, the

Table 20.1 Intestinal Preparation	
Preoperative Day 2	Clear liquid diet
Preoperative Day 1	Clear liquid diet
	Mechanical Prep
	Magnesium Citrate (one bottle of laxative 4 PM.)
	Fleet enemas until no solid stool in PM (Optional)
Day of Surgery	Fleet enemas until clear (Optional)

antibiotic preparation is necessary (25,26). Several meta-analyses of patients undergoing elective colorectal procedures have found either no difference or increased rates of anastomotic leakage and wound infection when prophylactic mechanical bowel preparation is used (26,27). However, bowel resections for gynecologic malignancies are performed in a different patient population, often in the presence of ascites, extensive carcinomatosis, and multiple sites of bowel involvement.

Lacking studies in the gynecologic oncology population, the use of mechanical bowel preparation and antibiotics is predominantly determined by surgeon preference. Before laparotomy for small intestinal obstruction caused by ovarian cancer, in selected cases, it may be useful to insert a nasogastric (NG) tube for 24 to 48 hours preoperatively to avoid the possibility of vomiting and aspiration (28).

Minor Intestinal Operations

The most common intestinal operations are lysis of adhesions, repair of an enterotomy, and creation of an intestinal stoma.

Repair of Enterotomy

Intestinal enterotomy is a common inadvertent occurrence in abdominal surgery, and it can occur in the most experienced hands. Factors that predispose to serosal and mucosal injury include extensive adhesions, intra-abdominal carcinomatosis, radiation therapy, chemotherapy, prior abdominal surgery, and peritonitis.

An enterotomy usually does not cause any problems, provided it is identified and repaired. **Any defect should be repaired when it occurs or marked with a long stitch so that it will not be overlooked later.** At the completion of any intra-abdominal exploration necessitating significant lysis of adhesions, the surgeon must "run the bowel," carefully inspecting it to exclude either a serosal injury or an enterotomy.

Serosal defects through which the intestinal mucosa can be seen must be repaired. Less complete defects must be repaired in all patients who have had radiation treatment to the abdomen. When in doubt, the defect should be repaired to minimize the risk of intestinal breakdown, peritonitis, abscess, and fistula.

When there is an enterotomy, the repair should be made with interrupted 3-0 or 4-0 sutures on a gastrointestinal needle, placed at 2- to 3-mm intervals along the defect. The suture materials most commonly employed are PGA (*Vicryl* or *Dexon*). **The direction of closure should be perpendicular to the lumen of the bowel to minimize the potential for lumenal stricture** (Fig. 20.6).

With small defects (i.e., <5 to 6 mm), the closure can be accomplished with a single layer of sutures passed through both the serosa and the mucosa. However, it is preferable to close more extensive defects in two layers: an inner full-thickness layer covered with an outer seromuscular layer. Care should be taken to approximate the tissues carefully without cutting through the fragile serosa.

Gastrostomy

A gastrostomy may be necessary in patients with chronic intestinal obstruction, usually from terminal ovarian cancer. It is particularly useful in those who require prolonged intestinal intubation, and in whom the underlying intestinal blockage cannot be relieved adequately. This procedure may permit the removal of an uncomfortable NG tube that is irritating to the nasopharynx. **While**

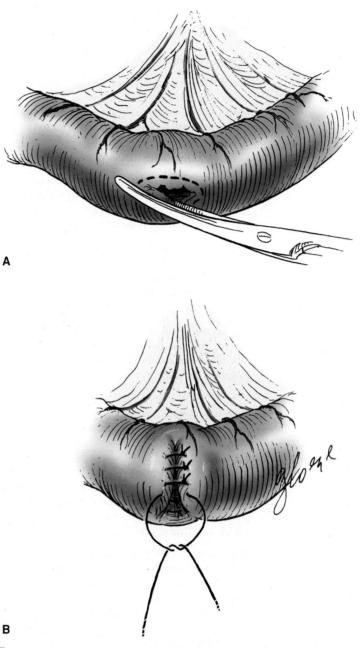

A

B

Figure 20.6 **Closure of an intestinal enterotomy. A:** The edges of the enterotomy are trimmed. **B:** The enterotomy is closed perpendicular to the lumen in two layers.

surgically placed gastrostomy tubes have been the norm for many years, percutaneously or endoscopically placed gastrostomy tubes have more recently gained wide acceptance, since they tend to be less costly and faster to perform, with similar complication rates (29). Open gastrostomies are still useful when the tubes cannot be placed endoscopically or radiologically, or in patients undergoing a separate procedure. The two most common surgical approaches are the Witzel and the Stamm gastrostomies (30–32).

Stamm Gastrostomy

The simplest technique is the Stamm gastrostomy, in which a small incision is made in the inferior anterior gastric wall. A Foley catheter with a 30-mL balloon is brought into the peritoneal cavity through a separate stab incision in the left upper outer quadrant of the abdomen. Two or three successive purse-string sutures with 2-0 absorbable suture material are used to invert the stomach around the tube. Interrupted 2-0 silk or PGA sutures are placed in the serosa, and the same material is used to suture the serosa to the peritoneum, approximating the gastric wall to the anterior abdominal wall in an effort to prevent leakage.

Witzel Gastrostomy

The Witzel technique is similar, but the catheter is tunneled within the gastric wall for several centimeters with Lembert sutures of 2-0 PGA. This technique results in a serosal tunnel that may further reduce the risk of leakage. **The most important step in preventing gastrostomy leakage is approximation of the gastric serosa to the anterior abdominal wall.**

Percutaneous Gastrostomy

Another technique for gastrostomy in patients not otherwise undergoing laparotomy is the percutaneous placement of a catheter into the stomach. This method involves the initial passage of a gastroscope. The site for catheter insertion is illuminated by a fiberoptic light source through the gastroscope, and the catheter is introduced into the stomach percutaneously.

Cecostomy

The performance of a cecostomy may be useful in the occasional patient who has an obstruction of the colon and a grossly dilated cecum and in whom a simple palliative measure to relieve the obstruction is indicated. A more definitive procedure for relief of the obstruction may be appropriate when the patient's condition is more stable.

The cecostomy is performed by placement of a Foley catheter into the dilated portion of the cecum. The tube is sutured into place by the technique employed for a Stamm gastrostomy. The tube is exteriorized through a stab incision in the right lower quadrant of the abdomen and attached to gravity drainage.

Colostomy

Colostomies may be temporary or permanent. **A temporary colostomy may be indicated for "protection" of a colonic reanastomosis** in patients who have had prior radiation therapy or to palliate severe radiation proctitis and bleeding. It is indicated also in patients who have a large bowel fistula (e.g., rectovaginal fistula) to allow the inflammation to subside before definitive repair. **A permanent colostomy is indicated in patients who have an irreparable fistula or a colonic obstruction from a pelvic tumor that cannot be resected. A permanent colostomy is also indicated in patients undergoing total pelvic exenteration,** unless the distal rectum can be preserved and the colon reanastomosed, and in those who require anoproctectomy because of advanced vulvar cancer.

The site of the colostomy should be selected so that the stomal appliance and bag can be applied to the skin of the anterior abdominal wall without difficulty. The best site is approximately midway between the umbilicus and the anterior iliac crest. The most distal site possible should be employed in the large intestine. After selection of the stomal site, a circular skin incision is made to accommodate two fingers. The subcutaneous tissue is removed, and the fascia of the rectus sheath is incised similarly (Fig. 20.7). The end of the colon is brought through the stoma and sutured to fascia with interrupted 2-0 silk or PGA suture, and the stoma is everted to the skin to form a "rosebud" with the use of interrupted 2-0 or 3-0 absorbable braided suture.

Temporary

For patients who require temporary diversion, a transverse or sigmoid colostomy is usually created. The most distal portion of the colon should be used to allow the most formed stool possible. **A loop colostomy is usually created:** A loop of the colon is brought out through an appropriately placed separate incision in the abdominal wall. The loop is maintained by suturing it to the fascia beneath it. It can be reinforced with a rod of glass or plastic passed through a hole in the mesentery. The stoma can be opened immediately by means of an incision along the taenia coli in the longitudinal direction. Alternatively, the loop may be "matured" 1 to 2 days later to minimize the risk of sepsis if the bowel is unprepared.

The colon can be brought out as an end colostomy, which requires transection of the colon. This can be readily accomplished by means of a gastrointestinal anastomosis (GIA) stapler, which closes and transects the colon simultaneously. The distal end is sutured to the fascia, and the proximal end is brought out as the colostomy. If the distal colon must also be diverted (because of distal obstruction), a double-barrel colostomy can be created.

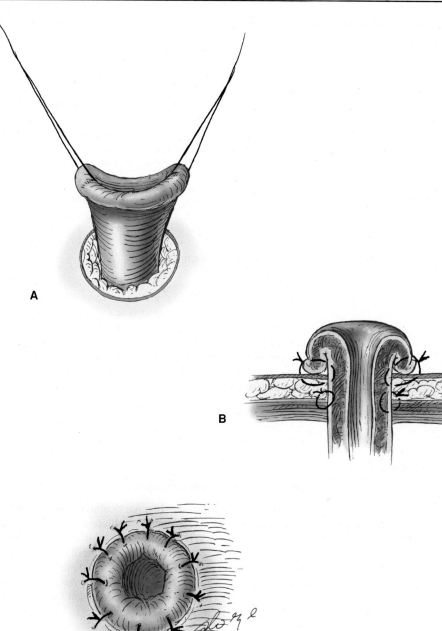

Figure 20.7 **The formation of a colostomy. A:** The end of the colon is brought through the abdominal wall. **B:** It is sutured to the fascia and skin. **C:** The "rosebud" stoma is formed.

Permanent

A permanent colostomy is an end or terminal colostomy, performed as far distally as possible. The distal loop of the transected colon may be oversewn to create a **Hartman's pouch** if there is no distal obstruction. In patients in whom there is complete distal obstruction, a **mucous fistula** should be created.

Enterostomy

If the colon is surgically inaccessible because of extensive carcinomatosis or radiation-induced adhesions, it may become necessary to palliate the bowel obstruction by the creation of a small intestinal stoma. Because the small-bowel contents are loose and irritating compared with colonic contents, **an ileostomy or a jejunostomy should be undertaken only when absolutely necessary**.

Major Intestinal Operations

Intestinal Resection and Reanastomosis

After a segment of bowel, along with its wedge-shaped section of mesentery, has been resected, a reanastomosis may be performed. The most commonly used technique for reanastomosis is the **end-to-end anastomosis (EEA)**, which is performed as either an open two-layered closure or a closed one-layered anastomosis. An **end-to-side anastomosis** may be used to create a J-pouch, that is, a segment of bowel created to improve low colonic continence (24). A **side-to-side anastomosis** may be useful to increase the size of the lumen at the site of anastomosis.

Increasingly, the use of surgical stapling devices has permitted more rapid performance of the reanastomosis, which is particularly useful when more than one resection is being carried out or when the duration of the procedure is of major concern.

Hand-sewn Anastomosis

End-to-end Enteroenterostomy

When the reanastomosis is to be hand sewn, the proximal and distal ends are clamped with Bainbridge clamps (Fig. 20.8A), and the posterior interrupted, seromuscular **Lembert stitches** are placed with 3-0 PGA sutures (*Vicryl* or *Dexon*) (Fig. 20.8B). The clamps are removed, the devitalized ends are trimmed, and an inner continuous full-thickness layer of 3-0 PGA suture is placed to complete the posterior portion of the anastomosis. After the corner is reached, the needle is brought through the wall to the outside, and the continuous layer is completed anteriorly with a **Connell stitch** (outside-in, inside-out) to complete the inner layer (Fig. 20.8C). The anterior seromuscular layer is then placed with interrupted 3-0 PGA sutures (Fig. 20.8D). The defect in the intestinal mesentery is repaired.

A single-layered closed technique is occasionally used for colonic reanastomosis in obstructed, unprepared bowel in an effort to minimize peritoneal contamination (33–35). In these circumstances, however, the use of the surgical staplers is now recommended (36).

Side-to-side Enteroenterostomy

The side-to-side anastomosis is particularly useful in patients who are undergoing intestinal bypass rather than resection to palliate bowel obstruction, for example, in patients with unresectable or recurrent tumor. The loops of intestine are aligned side to side, and linen-shod clamps are applied to prevent spillage of intestinal contents. A posterior row of 3-0 PGA sutures is placed with interrupted Lembert sutures, and the lumina are created. An inner layer of continuous, full-thickness 3-0 PGA sutures is placed and continued anteriorly to complete the layer with a Connell stitch. The anastomosis is completed by placement of an anterior seromuscular layer with the use of interrupted 3-0 PGA sutures.

Intestinal Staplers

The principal advantage of the gastrointestinal staplers is the speed with which they can be employed. There is no increase in the complication rate with the use of staplers as compared with hand-sewn anastomoses (24,36,37). The staplers are especially useful in facilitating reanastomosis after low resection of the rectosigmoid colon, because a hand-sewn anastomosis is technically difficult when performed deep in the pelvis. A disadvantage of the staplers is their increased cost, and staplers are difficult to use when the intestinal tissues are very edematous.

Types of Stapling Devices

The staplers are available in either reusable metal devices or in single-use disposable devices (Fig. 20.9A–C).

Thoracoabdominal Stapler

The thoracoabdominal (TA) stapler comes in several sizes, the TA-30, TA-55, TA-60, and TA-90, corresponding to the length, in millimeters, of the row of staples. Individual staples are either 3.5 or 4.8 mm long. The TA closes the lumen in an everting fashion. A TA device is available with a flexible, rotating end, called a Roticulator 55 that can be adjusted for placement into narrow areas (e.g., the deep pelvis).

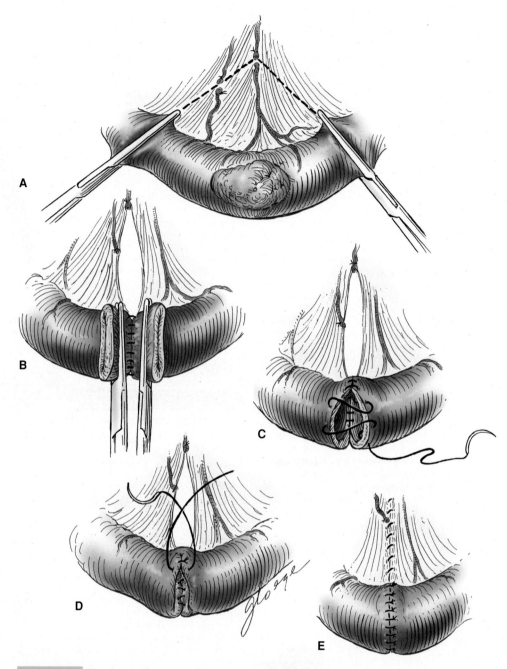

Figure 20.8 **Hand-sewn end-to-end enteroenterostomy. A:** The tumor and bowel are resected along with the mesentery. **B:** The posterior seromuscular layer is sutured. **C:** The Connell stitch is placed. **D:** The anterior seromuscular layer is placed. **E:** The completed anastomosis.

Gastrointestinal Anastomosis Stapler

The gastrointestinal anastomosis device places two double rows of staples and then cuts the tissue between the two rows.

End-to-end Anastomosis Stapler

The end-to-end anastomosis stapler is used primarily to approximate two ends of the colon, especially to facilitate the reanastomosis of the lower colon after pelvic exenteration or resection of pelvic disease in patients with ovarian cancer. The stapler places a double row of staples, approximates the two ends of the intestine, and cuts the devitalized tissue inside the staple line. It is available in diameters of 21, 25, 28, 31, and 35 mm, and a metal sizing device is used to measure the diameter of the intestinal lumen.

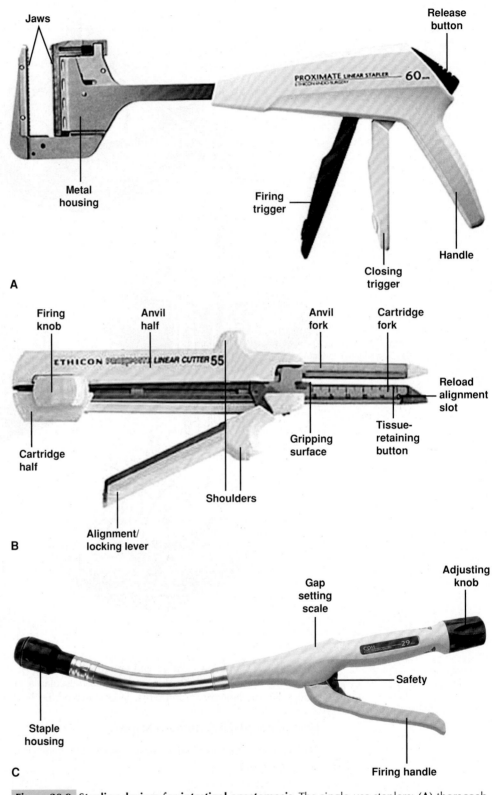

Figure 20.9 **Stapling devices for intestinal anastomosis.** The single-use staplers: **(A)** thoracoabdominal (TA); **(B)** gastrointestinal anastomosis (GIA); **(C)** end-to-end anastomosis (EEA).

Intraluminal Stapler

The intraluminal stapler (ILS) is a disposable EEA stapler that has a detachable anvil. This removable feature can facilitate the placement of the anvil into a portion of one intestine that is difficult to mobilize. The anvil can be reattached to the rod of the ILS device after it has been placed in the anastomosis.

Stapling Technique

Functional End-to-end Enteroenterostomy Anastomosis	This operation is illustrated in Fig. 20.10. The GIA stapler is used to staple and divide each end of the bowel segment to be resected. The antimesenteric borders of the bowel loops are approximated, and the corners are resected. A fork of the GIA device is inserted into each bowel lumen, and after alignment, the stapler is fired. The defect where the stapler was introduced then is closed with a TA stapler.
Side-to-side Enteroenterostomy Anastomosis	When a bypass enteroenterostomy is performed, the two loops of bowel to be anastomosed side to side are aligned, an enterotomy is created in each loop, and a fork of the GIA stapler is slid into each lumen, fired, and removed. This creates the lumen between the two bowel segments, and the enterotomy that is left when the instrument is withdrawn is then approximated with a TA stapler.
Low Colonic End-to-end Anastomosis	A low colonic resection is performed by isolating and removing the portion of the rectosigmoid colon involved with disease. The Roticulator 55 is commonly used to staple the distal bowel prior to resection. The descending colon is mobilized, a purse-string suture is placed around the distal end, the anvil is inserted, and the purse-string suture is tightened (Fig 20.11). The open end of the EEA stapler is inserted through the anus and the trocar is pushed through, or adjacent to, the staple line. The anvil is attached to the trocar, and the EEA is then closed, approximating the two ends of the colon. The instrument is fired and removed. A reinforcing layer of interrupted 3-0 *Vicryl* Lembert sutures is placed anteriorly, and the anastomosis is palpated to confirm that it is intact. The pelvis should also be filled with saline solution, and air insufflated through the rectum to search for bubbles, which would indicate a defect in the anastomosis (33).
Low Colonic End-to-side Anastomosis: J-pouch	An alternative end-to-side (functional end-to-end) low colonic anastomosis can be performed with the use of one of the disposable stapling devices, which has a removable distal one-piece anvil: the ILS. In this manner, a J-pouch can be created, which has the potential to improve the continence of patients (Fig. 20.12A–D). **Studies comparing the colonic J-pouch with the direct end-to-end anastomosis have suggested that there is a lower leak rate, better continence rate, fewer stools per day, and better control of urgency and flatus** (38–41). The problem with this approach is that some patients have more difficulty emptying the pouch, a problem that can be minimized by limiting the size of the pouch to about 5 cm in length (42). The J-pouch is created by first folding the distal colon onto itself and stapling side to side with a GIA stapler (Fig. 20.12A). The pouch is then anastomosed to the rectal stump using an end-to-side technique with an EEA stapler (Fig. 20.12B) and by detaching the anvil, which is inserted in the proximal colon segment. The approach shown is the typical one used when the patient is in the supine position. Alternatively, when the patient is in a lithotomy position, the EEA device can be inserted retrograde through the anus with the devise cap inserted into the J-pouch as illustrated above in Fig. 21.11A and below in Fig 21.13A. The center rod of the open EEA instrument without the anvil is inserted through an opening in the bowel or through the anus (Fig. 20.12C). Then the rod is inserted through or near the staple line. In the other segment of bowel, a purse-string suture is placed, and the free anvil is inserted within the lumen of the bowel within the purse-string suture. The anvil is then screwed onto the rod, the device is closed, and the anastomosis is created (Fig. 20.12D).
Low Colonic Side-to-side Anastomosis	An alternative side-to-side technique (functional end-to-end) anastomosis of the distal colon can be used when the portion of removed bowel is proximal enough to permit this operation (i.e., fully preserved rectum). The GIA instrument is used to perform the colorectal anastomosis. After the segment of colon to be resected is mobilized, the proximal colon to be reanastomosed is closed with either the GIA or the TA-55 instrument. A stab wound is made in the antimesenteric border

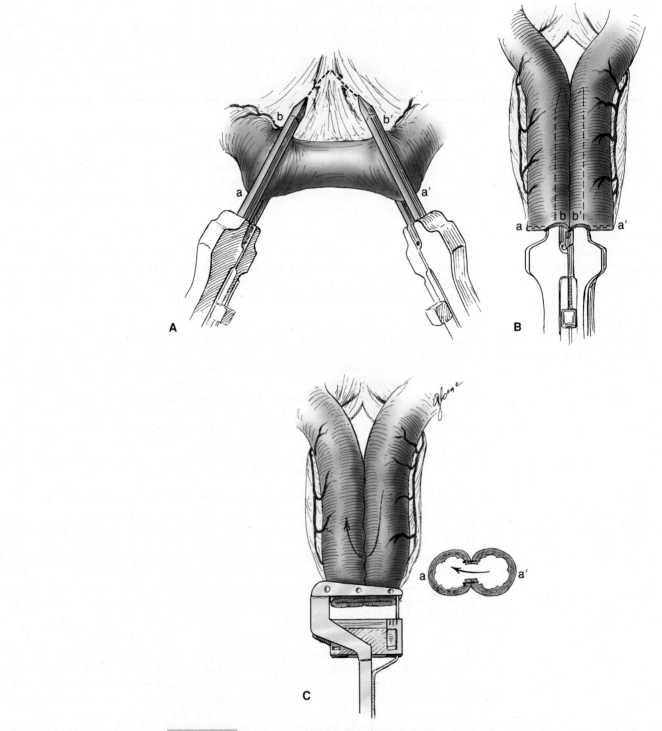

Figure 20.10 Functional end-to-end anastomosis using the stapling technique. A: The gastrointestinal anastomosis (GIA) stapler is used to resect the intestine. **B:** The segments of the transected intestine are placed side to side, and each antimesenteric corner is incised to create two holes into which the two forks of a second GIA stapler are placed (b-b'). The GIA stapler is fired to create the new intestinal lumen. **C:** The thoracoabdominal (TA) stapler is placed over the end and "fired" to close the remaining defect. Note the cross section at a-á.

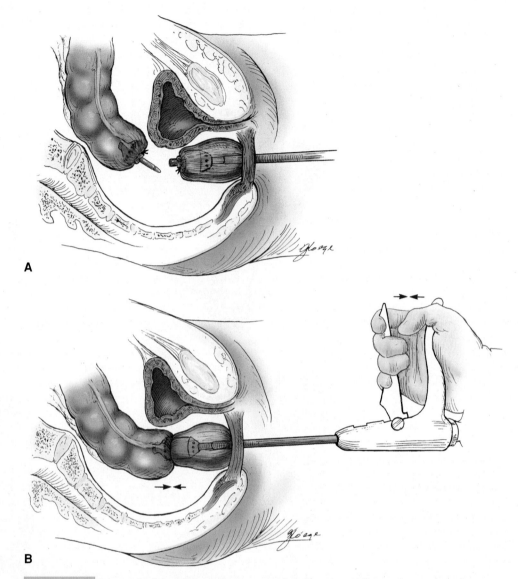

A

B

Figure 20.11 **Low colonic end-to-end anastomosis using the end-to-end anastomosis (EEA) stapler. A:** After resection of the rectosigmoid colon, the distal end of the descending colon is mobilized and a purse-string suture is placed by hand or with a special instrument. The anvil is inserted into the distal end of the descending colon and the purse-string suture is tied around it. The open end of the EEA stapler is inserted through the anus, and the trocar is pushed through the staple line. The anvil is attached to the trocar. **B:** The EEA device is closed and "fired."

of the colon about 5 cm proximal to the staple line closure. A corresponding stab wound is made in the left anterolateral wall of the rectum at the proximal point of the planned site of anastomosis. The proximal colon is placed into the retrorectal space, side to side along the rectum; the GIA device is placed into the proximal and distal segments; and the instrument is closed and fired. The remaining single defect is closed with either a hand-sewn, double layer of 3-0 sutures or the rotating TA-55 device (Roticulator 55).

Low Colonic Coloplasty

A newer form of colorectal anastomosis is the coloplasty (see Chapter 22), which may have advantages over the colonic J-pouch for patients undergoing pelvic exenteration. The principal advantage is that this technique may be easier to perform in a narrow pelvis, such as in those patients undergoing a pelvic exenteration and simultaneous creation of a neovagina. In a randomized study of the three techniques, patients undergoing the coloplasty and colonic J-pouch had significantly more favorable compliance, reservoir volume, and fewer bowel movements per day than those having a straight anastomosis (43).

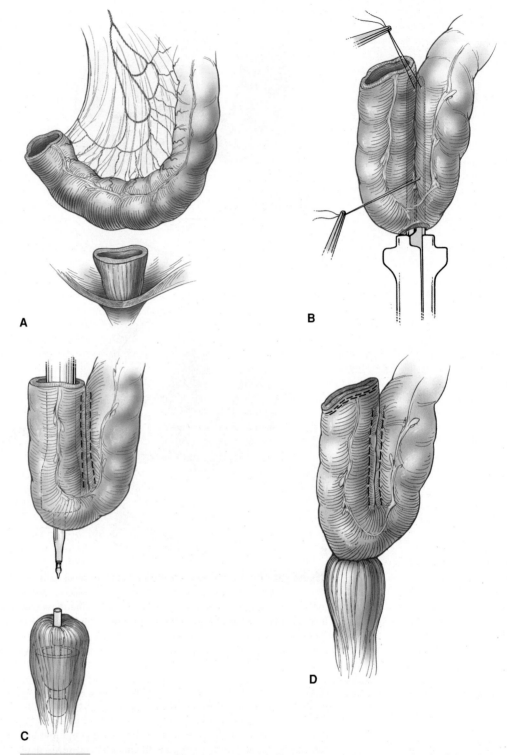

Figure 20.12 Low colonic end-to-side anastomosis (EEA) to create a J-pouch. A: The end-to-side anastomosis allows the mesocolon to be preserved and to cover the sacral hollow. **B:** The terminal end of the colon has the J-pouch created by stapling a loop side-to-side using a gastro-intestinal anastomosis (GIA) stapler. **C:** The EEA device is then used to anastomose the rectal stump end-to-side with the pouch. Alternatively, the EEA device can be inserted retrograde through the anus with the devise cap inserted into the J-pouch as illustrated above in Fig. 21.11A and below in Fig. 21.13A. **D:** The end of the pouch is stapled closed with a GIA or thoracoab-dominal (TA) stapler.

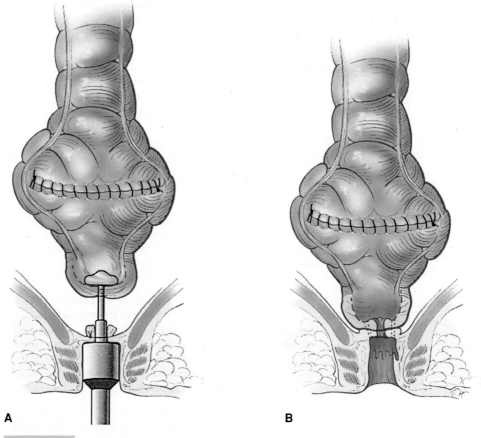

A   B

Figure 20.13 **Low colonic coloplasty. A:** The distal colon is incised in the longitudinal direction and resutured in the transverse direction to create a widening of the portion of the colon to be anastomosed to the rectum. **B:** The rectum is anastomosed to the distal colon using the end-to-end anastomosis (EEA) stapler.

The technique of coloplasty (Fig. 20.13) is illustrated. The lower part of the proximal colon is incised longitudinally and then reapproximated in the transverse direction (Fig. 20.13A). In this manner, a small, simple reservoir is created. The EEA stapler is used and then closed to create the anastomosis just as with the other techniques outlined above (Fig. 20.13B).

Postoperative Care

Historically, after resection of the small bowel, an NG tube has been placed for 24 to 48 hours to reduce the volume of intestinal secretions that must pass through the site of anastomosis. However, numerous studies including a recent meta-analysis of 33 studies with 5,240 patients undergoing open abdominal procedures (including 14 studies of gastroduodenal or colorectal procedures) have demonstrated that **prophylactic nasogastric decompression is associated with a slower return to bowel function and increased pulmonary complications, with no difference in anastomotic leaks** (44,45).

Nasogastric decompression remains integral to the management of small bowel obstruction.

Postoperative use is individualized based on preoperative diagnosis and intraoperative assessment. In patients who have received pelvic or abdominal irradiation, the upper intestinal tract may remain intubated until bowel function has returned, as signified by the passage of flatus or stool. Oral feeding can begin as patients develop an appetite, and **early feeding has been shown to be safe following both small and large bowel resection** (46–48).

In patients who have undergone colonic resection and reanastomosis, enemas and cathartics should be avoided.

Intravenous fluids must be continued while the patient is receiving nil by mouth. In patients whose recovery is likely to be prolonged beyond 7 days, such as those who have previously received whole-abdominal irradiation, consideration should be given to the use of parenteral nutrition, as discussed in Chapter 19. In such patients, a gastrostomy tube may be useful to avoid prolonged nasogastric intubation.

Upper Abdominal Cytoreduction

Advanced ovarian cancer is typically spread by implantation in the peritoneal cavity. Due to circulation of the peritoneal fluid, disease is typically disseminated beyond the pelvis into the upper abdomen, infiltrating the omentum, often up to the splenic hilum, diaphragm, mostly on the right side, and liver capsule. Maximal surgical effort to achieve complete tumor removal should be the goal of the primary debulking surgery, and any surgery for recurrent disease (49–54).

Omentectomy

Although omentectomy is a regular part of both staging and debulking operations in ovarian cancer patients, the extent and completeness of the procedure differs. Microscopic metastatic disease is detected in about 10% of patients with seemingly early stage disease, but the risk of separate supra and infracolic involvement is unknown. In many advanced cases, metastases are noted in the supracolic omentum and a complete omentectomy should be performed for debulking purposes (55,56).

The greater omentum is composed of a double layer of peritoneum attached to the greater curvature of the stomach and to the transverse colon. Its descending and ascending portions fuse below the colon to form a four-layered structure. Total omentectomy includes resection of both the infracolic and supracolic portions, up to the greater curvature of the stomach and lower pole of the spleen. During the procedure, the omentum is reflected off the transverse colon, and its supracolic portion is carefully separated from the transverse mesocolon, which must be spared. Finally it is resected from the greater curvature of the stomach, after securing the short gastric vessels.

The lesser omentum connects the lesser curvature of the stomach and proximal duodenum with the liver, and contains the gastrohepatic and hepatoduodenal ligaments. While the central gastrohepatic ligament can be resected if infiltrated by metastases, its right portion contains the hepatoduodenal ligament, which must be carefully preserved, since it contains the portal vein, hepatic artery, and extrahepatic bile duct.

Splenectomy

The spleen is a fragile organ, which is localized in the left upper quadrant. In the event of significant metastatic involvement of the splenic surface, or less commonly of its hilum or parenchyma, the spleen must be removed, since it cannot be partially resected. A splenectomy may also be indicated in the event of significant bleeding as a result of an injury sustained during the omentectomy.

A splenectomy can be approached in an antegrade or retrograde fashion (Fig. 20.14). The splenic flexure of the colon must first be freed by detaching the phrenicocolic ligament. The two layers of the gastrosplenic ligament, containing short gastric vessels and left gastroepiploic branches of the splenic artery, are dissected from the stomach. In a retrograde approach, the phrenicosplenic ligament, which forms the dorsal attachment of the spleen to the diaphragm is released, allowing the spleen to be mobilized and the splenic hilum to be exposed. The tail of the pancreas is then separated from the pancreatic impression on the spleen along the avascular space between the two organs. The splenic vessels, usually multiple veins and the splenic artery, can be separately ligated while minimizing the risk of pancreatic injury.

The **anterograde approach** is associated with a higher risk of injury to the pancreatic tail, since the splenic vessels are divided first, followed by the resection of the phrenicosplenic ligament. The anterograde approach may be useful in the event of significant adhesions or tumor burden between the spleen and the diaphragm, and it allows for concurrent left diaphragmatic stripping.

Liver Mobilization, Diaphragm Stripping, and Resection

Many cases of advanced ovarian cancer include metastatic diaphragmatic involvement (7) with the right diaphragm being more frequently involved. **The key to a complete and safe debulking of the right upper quadrant and diaphragm is an adequate liver mobilization. During the liver mobilization, the following peritoneal folds must be mobilized: the round ligament,** which forms the lower edge of the falciform ligament and contains the obliterated umbilical vein remnant; **the falciform ligament,** which is a thin anteroposterior layer of the coronary ligament; the

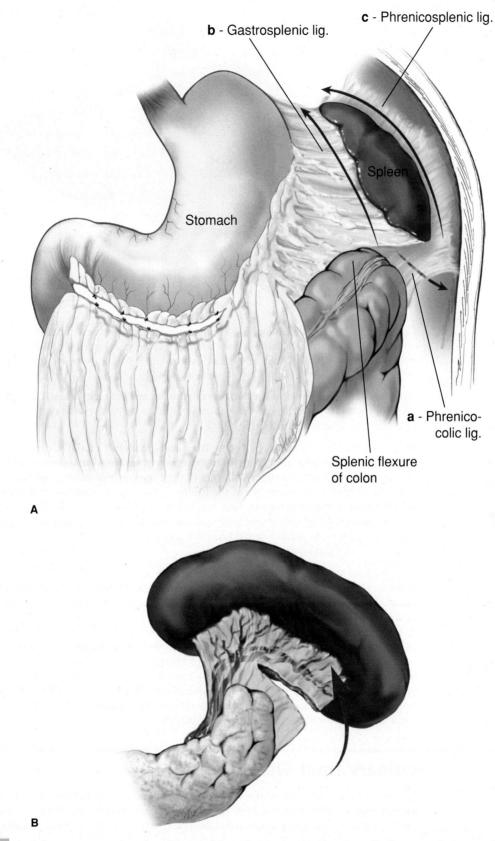

b - Gastrosplenic lig.

c - Phrenicosplenic lig.

Spleen

Stomach

a - Phrenico-
colic lig.

Splenic flexure
of colon

A

B

Figure 20.14 **A:** Splenectomy requires detachment of three ligaments: (a) phrenicocolic ligament, (b) gastrosplenic ligament and (c) phrenicosplenic ligament. **B:** Retrograde approach allows safer separation of the spleen from the pancreas. After all three ligaments are detached and spleen is fully mobilized, dorsal avascular part of the splenic hilus is disected, spleen is lifted up and splenic vessels are exposed between spleen and pancreas, so they can be safely ligated avoiding risk of pancreatic tail injury.

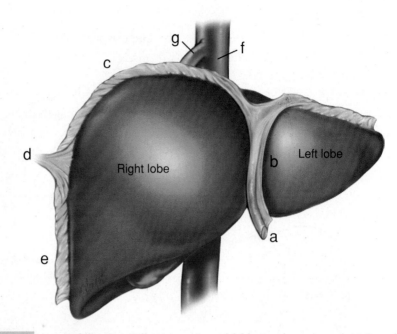

Figure 20.15 Liver Mobilization. Following peritoneal folds must be separated: (a) Round ligament; (b) Falciform ligament; (c) Superior layer of coronary ligament; (d) Right triangular ligament; (e) Inferior layer of coronary ligament. Large vessels are exposed: (f) Vena cava superior; (g) Right hepatic vein.

superior and inferior layers of **the coronary ligament,** and the **right triangular ligament,** a small fold that passes from the liver to the diaphragm, formed by the apposition of the upper and lower layers of the coronary ligament (Fig. 20.15).

There are the two critical steps during liver mobilization. Cranially, care must be taken to avoid injuring the vena cava and two hepatic veins once the two layers of the falciform ligament separate to form the superior layers of the coronary ligaments. Caudally, care must be taken to avoid venous injury when the inferior vena cava is exposed with dissection of the inferior right coronary ligament. After the peritoneal folds have been divided, the right liver lobe may be mobilized and pulled medially and caudally, allowing the right diaphragm to be fully exposed. Care must be taken to avoid excessive spot pressure on the liver capsule, which may lead to deep parenchymal injury.

Once the liver has been adequately mobilized and the major vessels identified, the affected peritoneum may be dissected from the diaphragm. **"Diaphragmatic stripping" is straightforward and can usually be accomplished quickly along the peripheral muscular part. It begins to be more demanding toward the central tendinous area,** where the diaphragm is reduced to a thin aponeurosis, often requiring a full thickness resection. Once the resection and stripping of the diaphragm have been completed, any defect into the pleura can be reapproximated using two continuous one-layer sutures running from the opposing edges toward the center. A drain or Foley catheter should be inserted into the thoracic cavity before both sutures are tied. The anesthesiologist is then asked to provide maximum inspiration, which helps to force out any residual air from the thoracic cavity before the drain is removed and the sutures are tied. The distal end of the drain is placed under water so that any air in the pleural cavity bubbles out.

Urinary Tract Operations

The preoperative evaluation of the urinary tract is important in patients with gynecologic malignancies because of the frequent involvement of the urinary organs, especially the bladder and the distal ureters (57,58). Renal function and ureteric patency must be assessed preoperatively.

Cystoscopy

Cystoscopy may be performed as part of the staging for cervical and vaginal cancers, unless the disease has been diagnosed early (57), or an MRI has clearly defined the primary tumor. Cystoscopy is also indicated in patients with a lower urinary tract fistula or unexplained hematuria.

Cystoscopic examination may demonstrate external compression of the bladder by a tumor, bullous edema produced by the blockage of lymphatic vessels from adjacent tumor growth, or mucosal involvement with tumor. When a mucosal lesion is seen, a biopsy can confirm the diagnosis.

Technique

Cystoscopy is performed with the patient in the dorsal lithotomy position. After preparation and draping of the area, the cystoscopic obturator and sheath are inserted into the urethra and carefully advanced into the bladder, after which the obturator is removed. The cystoscope is inserted into the sheath. About 250 to 400 mL of normal saline solution are instilled into the bladder to permit a thorough inspection of the entire mucosa.

Cystostomy

A suprapubic cystostomy catheter is useful in patients who require prolonged bladder drainage. This catheter may be useful in patients undergoing radical hysterectomy for cervical cancer or extensive resection of pelvic tumor because of the temporary disruption of bladder innervation that occurs with these dissections. The suprapubic catheter can be easier for the patient to manage than a transurethral Foley catheter, and the rate of bladder infection is lower (59). The other convenient aspect of this catheter is that it can facilitate trials of voiding. The patient can clamp the catheter for a specified interval, void, and then unclamp to check for residual urine. When the residual urine is less than 75 to 100 mL, the catheter can be removed. However, many patients can be managed successfully after radical hysterectomy with a period of continuous transurethral catheterization followed by intermittent self-catheterization (59–61).

Technique

The catheter used is an 18-Fr Silastic Foley catheter with a 5- to 10-mL balloon. This catheter is well tolerated by patients, produces minimal local tissue irritation, and is of sufficient caliber that blockage of the catheter lumen is not a major problem.

The placement of a suprapubic catheter involves the following steps:

1. **The catheter is inserted through a stab incision** in the skin, subcutaneous tissue, and fascia, and a small hole is made in the dome of the bladder.
2. **The tip of the catheter is inserted into the bladder,** and a seromuscular purse-string suture is placed around the defect with 3-0 PGA sutures.
3. **A second reinforcing layer** consisting of either 2-0 absorbable braided PGA suture is placed in the bladder.
4. **With the Foley balloon distended, the catheter is pulled up so that the bladder is applied snugly to the anterior abdominal wall.**
5. **The catheter can be attached to a urinary drainage bag,** and it can also be attached to a smaller "leg bag," which is more portable and therefore easier for the patient to manage after discharge from the hospital.

Ureteral Obstruction

Ureteral obstruction is the most common urinary complication in patients with gynecologic malignancies. This problem is seen particularly in patients with cervical or vaginal cancer, either at the time of diagnosis or with recurrent disease. It may result from direct tumor extension into the bladder or distal ureters, or from compression by lymph node metastases. In patients with intra-abdominal carcinomatosis, most often from ovarian cancer, extensive pelvic tumor may cause significant progressive ureteral obstruction. **The most frequent site of lower urinary tract obstruction in gynecologic patients is the ureterovesical junction** (58).

Postoperative obstruction is usually incomplete and results from edema, possible infection, and partial devascularization of the distal ureter. However, the obstruction may be complete, and when it is, it most often results from inadvertent suture ligature of the distal ureter when the surgeon has been attempting to ligate the blood vessels of the cardinal ligament (62). Chronic obstruction can result from stenosis after pelvic irradiation, particularly if pelvic surgery has also been performed.

In patients who have a partial ureteral obstruction, the passage of a retrograde stent at the time of cystoscopy might bypass the site of blockage. The retrograde stent used is a 7- to 9-Fr flexible, double "J" retrograde ureteral stent; it is inserted with the aid of a stent-placement apparatus that has an elevator attachment to the cystoscope. Great care must be taken, as **this procedure has**

the risk of ureteral perforation. When the stent does not pass readily, the performance of a **percutaneous nephrostomy** is preferable.

In patients in whom complete ureteral obstruction is suspected (i.e., because of a rising serum creatinine level or the development of an acute unilateral hydronephrosis), a computed tomographic urogram should be performed if the serum creatinine value is less than 2 mg/dL; an ultrasonogram should be obtained if the level is higher. In patients with complete ureteral obstruction, the problem must be corrected immediately, either by temporary urinary diversion by means of a percutaneous nephrostomy, or by re-exploration and repair of the ureter. **Repair may be by either reanastomosis or reimplantation.**

Mild degrees of hydroureter are managed by bladder drainage alone in most patients, as these problems are usually temporary and resolve gradually as the edema subsides. Infection should be treated with appropriate antibiotics.

In patients undergoing radical hysterectomy and bilateral pelvic lymphadenectomy, postoperative ureteral damage from devascularization can be decreased by minimizing the collection of fluid in the retroperitoneal space by leaving the pelvic peritoneum open.

Retrograde Pyelography

If an excretory urogram cannot be performed (e.g., because of dye sensitivity) or if the study is inconclusive, retrograde pyelography may be necessary. This procedure is potentially morbid and should be performed only if the information to be gained is critical to the decision regarding diversion of the affected kidney (63,64). Contrast injected beyond a high-grade obstruction can produce pyelonephritis and sepsis, and may require urgent drainage through a percutaneous nephrostomy. The attempted passage of a retrograde ureteral catheter or stent may be useful for diagnosis, and it will stent the ureter if the obstruction has not resulted from a misplaced suture ligature.

Percutaneous Nephrostomy

In patients with an obstructed ureter that cannot be decompressed by means of a retrograde ureteral stent, a percutaneous nephrostomy tube can be placed under fluoroscopic guidance (65). This procedure is relatively easy to perform, and the tube can be changed or replaced as necessary. In addition, an antegrade ureteral catheter or stent may be passed through a nephrostomy to allow removal of the percutaneous stent in patients in whom a retrograde catheter could be passed.

Ureteral Reanastomosis (Ureteroureterostomy)

When the ureter has been transected or damaged beyond repair, it will have to be revised and reanastomosed or reimplanted into the urinary bladder. If the ureteral injury is above the level of the pelvic brim, a simple reanastomosis is the procedure of choice. The two ends of the ureters are trimmed at a 45-degree angle. A double "J" ureteral stent is passed into the distal ureter with one "memory" end inserted into the bladder. The proximal end of the ureter is placed over the stent and sutured to its distal counterpart (65,66). Interrupted 4-0 absorbable PGA sutures are placed at close intervals in a circumferential fashion (Fig. 20.16). After several weeks, the absence of leakage can be established by means of intravenous pyelography, and the stent can be removed through a cystoscope.

Ureteroneocystostomy

The reimplantation of the distal ureter into the bladder is known as the **Leadbetter procedure, or ureteroneocystostomy** (67). This operation is preferred for the ureter that has been disrupted distal to the pelvic brim, as long as the bladder can be sufficiently mobilized on the side of reimplantation. Integral to successful ureteral reimplantation is the creation of a submucosal tunnel (Fig. 20.17). The tunnel minimizes the risk of vesicoureteral reflux and chronic, recurrent pyelonephritis (68,69).

The technique is as follows:

1. **The distal ureter is prepared by careful resection of any devitalized tissue** while the maximum length is preserved.

2. **The bladder base is mobilized, and the dome of the bladder is affixed laterally to the psoas muscle by means of a lateral cystopexy, a "psoas hitch"** (70,71). This permits stabilization of the bladder as well as extension of the bladder toward the end of the resected ureter, and it is especially important if the ureter is somewhat foreshortened.

3. **A cystotomy is made, and a tunnel is initiated by injection of the submucosal plane with saline solution to raise the mucosa.** The mucosa is incised, and a tonsil forceps

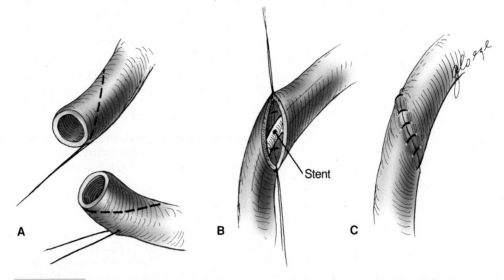

Figure 20.16 Ureteroureterostomy. A: The two ends of the ureters are cut diagonally. **B:** A ureteral stent is inserted into the proximal and distal ureter, and interrupted full-thickness sutures are placed. **C:** The completed anastomosis.

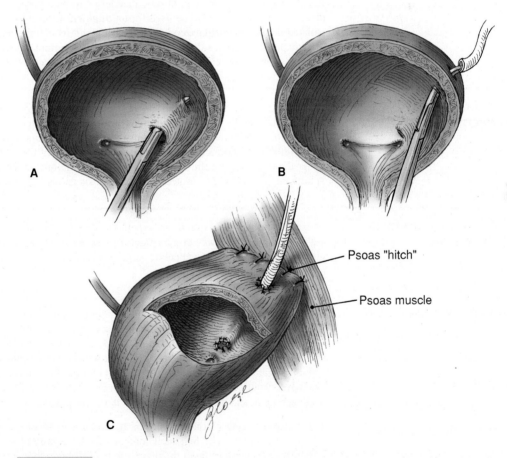

Figure 20.17 Ureteroneocystostomy. A: A submucosal tunnel is created. **B:** The ureter is brought into the bladder. **C:** The ureter is passed through the tunnel and sutured to the bladder serosa and mucosa. The serosa of the bladder is sutured to the psoas muscle to stabilize the anastomosis.

is inserted submucosally for a length of 1 to 1.5 cm to the site where the serosa is to be incised. An incision in the serosa is made over the pointed tip of the clamp to create an opening to the tunnel that passes through the muscularis and mucosa of the bladder wall.

4. **The ureter is gently pulled through the submucosal tunnel, and mucosa-to-mucosa stitches are placed with interrupted 4-0 PGA suture material.** A ureteric stent, preferably a soft plastic double "J," is passed up the ureter into the renal calyx, and the other end is placed in the bladder lumen. The site of entrance of the ureter is sutured to the bladder serosa with 4-0 PGA.

5. **A suprapubic cystostomy is performed, and the cystotomy is closed with two layers of interrupted 2-0 absorbable suture.** The retroperitoneum is drained with a Jackson-Pratt drain. The ureteral stent is left in place 10 to 14 days and then removed through a cystoscope.

In cases where there is inadequate length of viable ureter, additional techniques can be utilized. The **Boari flap** utilizes a segment of bladder to bridge the defect to the remaining ureter (72,73). A U-shaped flap is created, turned superiorly and tubularized to create the additional length required. It should not be performed in patients with a history of prior radiation because of the increased risk of flap ischemia and failure. **Ileal interposition** can also be used to replace a portion of the ureter (74–76). First the required length of ileum is isolated and the ureter is anastomosed to the proximal end of the ileal segment in an end-to-side fashion with 4-0 delayed absorbable sutures. The ileum is then anastomosed in a tension-free fashion to the dome of the mobilized bladder.

In patients with a contracted, fibrotic bladder or when a portion of bladder requires resection for disease, the ileum can also be used for an **augmentation ileocystoplasty**. In this procedure, the isolated ileum is detubularized by opening it along its antimesenteric border and folding it into a "U" shape. The medial sides are sewn together using a running delayed absorbable suture, creating an **ileal** segment, which can be anastomosed to the bladder (69,76).

Transureteroureterostomy

Another procedure that can be useful in the carefully selected patient is the transureteroureterostomy (TUU) (66). When the distal ureter must be resected on one side, and the proximal ureter is too short to permit ureteroneocystostomy, it is possible to anastomose the distal end of the resected ureter into the contralateral side (66,77). The distal end of the partially resected ureter is tunneled under the mesentery of the sigmoid colon and approximated, end to side, to the recipient ureter. A ureteral stent is used to protect the anastomosis and is left in place for at least 7 to 10 days.

Permanent Urinary Diversion

Permanent urinary diversion must be performed after cystectomy or in patients who have an irreparable fistula of the lower urinary tract. Lower urinary tract fistulae can result from progressive tumor growth or from radical pelvic surgery and/or pelvic irradiation. The most common fistula is ureterovaginal.

Urinary Conduit

The most frequently employed techniques for urinary diversion are the creation of an **ileal conduit** (the **"Bricker procedure"**), the creation of a **transverse colon conduit** (78), and the creation of a **"continent" urinary conduit** (e.g., the Kock, Miami, Indiana, Mainz, and Rome pouches) (79–82). The ileal conduit has been the most widely used means of permanent urinary diversion, and it is suitable for most patients. A segment of transverse colon can be used if the ileum has been extensively injured (e.g., by radiation therapy). The transverse colon is usually away from the irradiated field, and thus its vascularity is not compromised.

The continent urinary conduit may be helpful for gynecologic oncology patients who require exenterative surgery. The first such conduit was the **continent ileal conduit (or "Kock pouch")**. It requires a longer portion of the ileum (up to 100 cm), a longer operative time (4 to 6 hours), and greater technical skills for the creation of the continence mechanism. It is now rarely performed (79,83).

The continent colon conduit utilizes the intestine from the terminal ileum to the midportion of the transverse colon and has been popularized in Indiana, Miami, and Mainz. These pouches are technically somewhat easier to perform than the Kock pouch. The type of continent conduit created is generally determined by the training and preference of the surgeon (80,81,83–87).

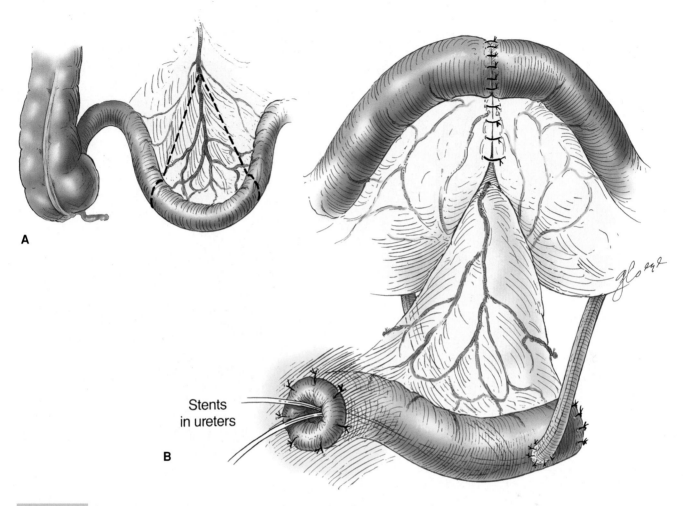

Figure 20.18 **Ileal urinary conduit. A:** A segment of nonirradiated ileum is used for the conduit. **B:** The ileum is reanastomosed, and the ureters are sewn into the "butt" end of the conduit. Note that ureters are stented individually.

Technique

The technique for the creation of an ileal conduit involves the isolation of a segment of ileum at a site where the intestine appears healthy and nonirradiated. This is typically about 30 to 40 cm proximal to the ileocecal junction. The conduit requires a segment of ileum measuring approximately 20 cm and its associated mesentery. After isolation of the segment, the ileum is reanastomosed (Fig. 20.18). The ureters are implanted into the closed proximal end of the ileal segment, and double "J" ureteric stents are placed into both ureters. A no. 8 pediatric feeding tube made of soft flexible plastic can also be employed for the ureteric stent, as it is relatively atraumatic. The "butt" end of the conduit is sutured to the area of the sacral promontory.

The distal end of the conduit is brought through the anterior abdominal wall of the right lower quadrant, approximately midway between the umbilicus and the anterior superior iliac crest. The ureteral stents should be left in place for about 10 days.

When a **transverse-colon conduit** is selected, the technique is essentially the same. Care must be taken in both techniques to ensure that the vascularity of the intestinal mesentery is not interrupted. The mesentery of the reanastomosed bowel must be reapproximated to prevent herniation of intestinal loops through the defect (78).

The technique for creation of a continent Miami or Indiana pouch (80,88,89) **involves resection of the intestine from the last 10 to 15 cm of ileum to the midportion of the transverse colon.** The colon is opened along the antimesenteric border through the teniae coli (Fig. 20.19A). The ileum is used to create the continence mechanism (Fig. 20.19B). The ileal–cecal valve serves as the principal portion of the mechanism; the terminal ileum is narrowed, and several purse-string sutures are placed near the valve to reinforce the continence portion of the conduit (Fig. 20.19C).

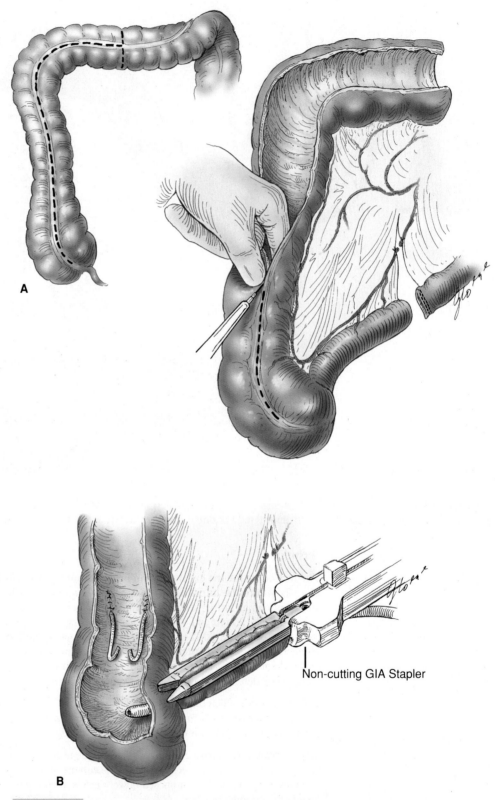

Non-cutting GIA Stapler

Figure 20.19 **Colon continent urinary conduit: the "Miami" pouch. A:** The segment of distal ileum and ascending and transverse colon is isolated, and the segment is opened on its antimesenteric border along the teniae coli. **B:** The ureters are reimplanted into the mesenteric side of the ascending colon, a continence mechanism is created with purse-string sutures near the ileal–cecal junction, and a noncutting double staple line is performed with a gastrointestinal anastomosis (GIA) stapler.

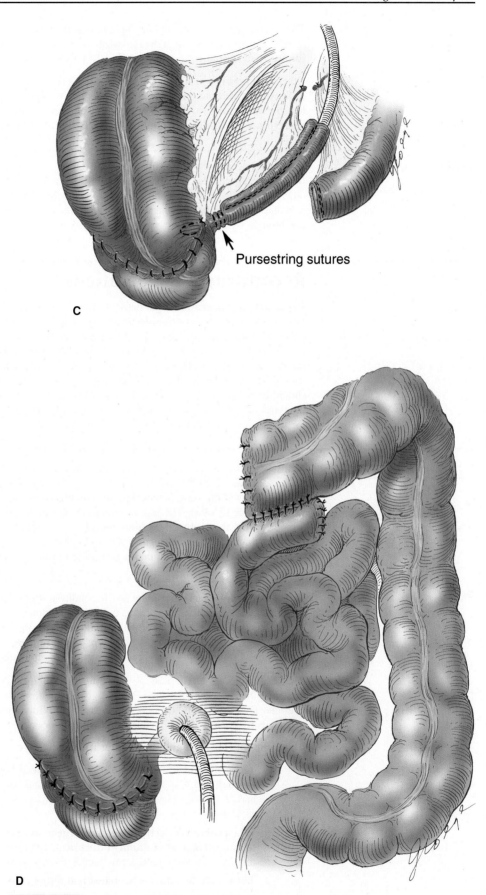

Pursestring sutures

C

D

Figure 20.19 *Continued.* **C:** The conduit is closed with sutures, and the ileal stoma is created. **D:** The intestines are reconstituted with an ileal–transverse colon anastomosis.

The ascending colon is sutured or stapled to the proximal transverse colon to create a low-pressure pouch. This process is called detubularization of the bowel. An ileotransverse anastomosis is performed to reconstitute the intestine (Fig. 20.19D).

Other modifications of the ileocolonic continent reservoir have been described. The **Rome pouch** utilizes multiple transverse teniamyotomies of the cecum instead of detubularization to create a low-pressure reservoir (82,86). Bochner et al. describe the use of a **modified ureteroileocecal reservoir,** which **utilizes the appendix to create the cutaneous stoma** (84).

Skin Ureterostomy

In rare instances, a terminally ill patient undergoing exploratory surgery will have a bladder fistula. In such circumstances, one ureter can be ligated, and a skin ureterostomy can be created with the other ureter. The ureter is mobilized from its attachments and brought laterally through the retroperitoneal space to the lateral and anterior abdominal wall. The ureter is tunneled through the fascia and brought out through a stab incision in the skin, where it is affixed to create a small stoma (90).

Reconstructive Operations

Reconstructive operations, particularly pelvic floor reconstruction and creation of a neovagina, are important in patients who are undergoing extensive extirpative procedures, such as pelvic exenteration (see Chapter 23). Vaginal reconstruction helps to provide support to the pelvic floor, thereby reducing the prospect of perineal herniation. By helping to fill the pelvis, vaginal reconstruction also decreases the incidence of enteroperineal fistulae. Pelvic floor reconstruction should be performed in all patients undergoing a pelvic exenteration, and vaginal reconstruction should be performed simultaneously in most patients. The surgeon must be well acquainted with the types of graft that can be employed in the performance of these reconstructive operations and the techniques necessary to accomplish them (91).

Grafts

Grafts used for reconstructive operations in the pelvis are either skin grafts, which can be full or partial (split) thickness (92–94), or myocutaneous grafts, which are composed of the full thickness of the skin, its contiguous subcutaneous tissues, and a portion of a closely associated muscle (95–98). The most frequently used myocutaneous pedicle grafts contain muscle segments from the **rectus abdominis muscle** of the anterior abdominal wall, **gracilis muscle** of the inner thigh, the **bulbocavernosus muscle** of the vulva, the **tensor fascia lata muscle** of the lateral thigh, and the **gluteus maximus muscle of the buttocks.**

Skin Grafts

Skin grafts must be harvested under sterile conditions (92,94). The donor site most frequently used to obtain a split-thickness skin graft is either the anterior and medial thigh or the buttock. Although the thigh may be more readily accessible to the surgeon, the buttock donor site has cosmetic advantages; however, this latter site may be more uncomfortable in the postoperative recovery period. The selection of the donor site should be made preoperatively after discussion with the patient.

A dermatome is used to harvest the skin graft. Several different types of dermatome are available, including the Brown air-powered, electrically driven dermatome and the Padgett hand-driven dermatome. The surgeon should select the instrument with which he or she has the greatest facility, as an equally good graft can be harvested with either one.

The technique for obtaining the skin graft is as follows:

1. **The graft width and thickness can be determined by adjusting the settings of the dermatome.** A split-thickness graft can be obtained by setting the thickness between 14 and 16 one-thousandths of an inch. Full-thickness grafts are 20 to 24 one-thousandths of an inch.

2. **When using the dermatome, the surgeon must apply firm, steady pressure in order to harvest a graft of uniform thickness.** To minimize friction, mineral oil is applied to the skin over which the dermatome is to be passed.

3. **The skin to be taken is stretched and flattened by the surgical assistant with the use of a tongue depressor.** A second assistant picks up the leading edge of the graft as it is being harvested.

4. The harvested graft is kept moist in saline solution while the recipient site is being prepared.

5. The graft may be "pie crusted" by making small incisions in the surface. This technique maximizes the dimension of the graft while permitting the escape of fluid that might otherwise accumulate between the graft and the recipient site. Extensive pie crusting may result in contracture when the graft is used to create a neovagina.

Pedicle Grafts

The purpose of the pedicle graft is to provide a substantial amount of tissue along with its blood supply, either to repair an anatomic defect or to create a new structure, such as a neovagina. The pedicle graft can be either a full-thickness skin and subcutaneous tissue graft, as is used frequently for closure of a vulvar defect, for example, a "Z-plasty" (a "rhomboid flap"), or a myocutaneous graft, for example, a rectus abdominis or gracilis (91,96,99).

Before harvesting a pedicle graft, the surgeon should carefully outline the incisions on the skin with a marker pen. During the mobilization of the myocutaneous pedicle, the surgeon must carefully isolate and preserve the neurovascular bundle that supplies the muscle.

Vaginal Reconstruction

Vaginal reconstruction in the gynecologic oncology patient is performed either to revise or replace a vagina that has stenosed as a result of prior vaginal surgery and/or radiation, or to create a neovagina when the vagina has been removed.

Split-thickness Graft

When the vagina is fibrotic after irradiation, the scarred vaginal tissue first must be resected before placement of the split-thickness skin graft (92–94). The skin graft is placed over a vaginal stent that is then inserted into the space created by resection of the old, scarred vagina (Fig. 20.20A). The **Heyer–Schulte stent** is the vaginal stent preferred for this purpose, because it is inflatable, can be easily removed and replaced by the patient, and has its own drainage tube (Fig. 20.20B).

Split-thickness skin grafts can also be used in patients undergoing exenteration, but this approach is less satisfactory than the use of myocutaneous pedicle grafts. When an anterior exenteration is performed, or when a portion of the rectosigmoid colon is resected but primarily reanastomosed, a neovagina can be created with the use of skin grafts. The omentum is mobilized by ligating and dividing the short gastric vessels along the greater curvature of the stomach, preserving the left gastroepiploic pedicle (Fig. 20.21A). The omentum is then placed into the pelvis and sutured to the rectosigmoid posteriorly and laterally to create a pocket for the neovagina. Split-thickness skin graft(s) must be harvested, sewn over a vaginal stent, and inserted into the newly created pelvic space (Fig. 20.21B).

Transverse Rectus Abdominis Myocutaneous (TRAM) and Vertical Rectus Abdominis Myocutaneous (VRAM) Pedicle Grafts

A single rectus abdominis pedicle graft can be used to create a neovagina (91,93–98,100–104), or to repair a pelvic or perineal defect (97,98). This is our preferred technique for creation of a neovagina performed simultaneously with a pelvic exenteration (Fig. 20.22). The technique is relatively straightforward and has the advantage of a single pedicle harvested from the same site of the abdominal incision used to perform the exploratory surgery. This approach avoids the use of separate incisions on the inner aspects of the thigh, as needed for the gracilis myocutaneous pedicle graft. The disadvantage is that the amount of tissue mobilized from the anterior abdominal is limited, and thus, the ability to adjust the size of the neovagina is somewhat limited. If too large a pedicle is created, there will be too much tension for the abdominal closure, and this can also create distortion of the anterior abdominal wall skin.

The pedicle location is shown in Figure 20.22A. The oval-shaped pedicle should measure approximately 6 to 8 by 10 cm. The skin of the pedicle is incised, and the cephalad portion of the rectus abdominis muscle and attached myofascial tissues are transected (Fig. 20.22B). The tubular neovagina is created by suturing together the sides of the pedicle. One end is left open, and this becomes the distal neovagina. The pedicle is harvested, mobilized, and brought into the pelvis (Fig. 20.22C). The pedicle graft is then sutured to the preserved vaginal introitus to complete the procedure (Fig. 20.22D).

Gracilis Myocutaneous Pedicle Grafts

Bilateral gracilis myocutaneous pedicle grafts can be used to construct a neovagina (91,105–107). In addition, the grafts provide excellent support for the pelvic viscera. The gracilis myocutaneous graft is harvested (Fig. 20.23A) from the inner aspect of the thigh.

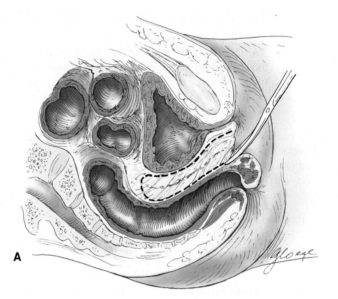

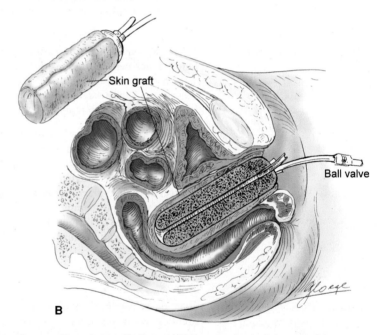

Figure 20.20 Creation of neovagina after radiation. **A:** The vaginal scar is resected in preparation for vaginal reconstruction with split-thickness skin grafts. **B:** A Heyer–Schulte vaginal stent has the skin graft placed around it, and this is inserted into the pelvic space to create a neovagina.

A line is drawn from the pubic tubercle to the medial epicondyle, and this delineates the anterior margin of the graft. The graft should be about 5 cm wide and about 10 cm long. A skin bridge is preserved between the vulva and the pedicle. The myocutaneous pedicle graft is mobilized by transecting the gracilis muscle distally in continuity with the skin and subcutaneous tissue (Fig. 20.23B). **The vascular pedicle is proximal, and it must be carefully identified and preserved.**

The pedicle is "harvested," brought under the skin bridge of the vulva, and exteriorized through the introitus (Fig. 20.23C). The two grafts are sutured together to create a hollow neovagina (Fig. 20.23D,E). The entire neovagina is placed into the pelvis by posterior and upward rotation and sutured to the introitus (Fig. 20.23F). The apex is sutured to the symphysis pubis and/or the anterior sacrum. At the completion of the procedure, an omental pedicle is brought down over the graft to reconstruct the pelvic floor (Fig. 20.23G).

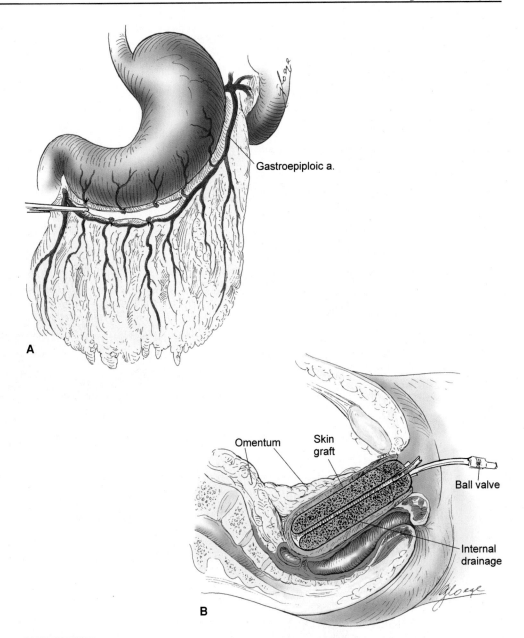

Figure 20.21 **Creation of a neovagina after a modified pelvic exenteration. A:** Mobilization of the omentum. This is accomplished by ligating and dividing the right gastroepiploic artery and the short gastric arteries along the greater curvature of the stomach. **B:** The omentum is used to create a "pocket" for the placement of a split-thickness skin graft.

Bulbocavernosus Pedicle Grafts	The bulbocavernosus myocutaneous pedicle graft has been used for repair of radiation-induced rectovaginal fistulae (**Martius procedure**), but the procedure has been adopted for the creation of a neovagina (108–110). The procedure is performed by making an incision over the labium majus, isolating the bulbocavernosus muscle superiorly and anteriorly, and mobilizing it on a posterior vulvar pedicle. The graft is tunneled under a skin bridge at the posterior introitus and sutured to the pedicle of the other side.
Colonic Segment	Some authors have preferred to use a segment of colon to create a neovagina (111–113). This technique has had mixed success in the past, but an approach using a portion of the ascending colon may be an improvement over earlier procedures.

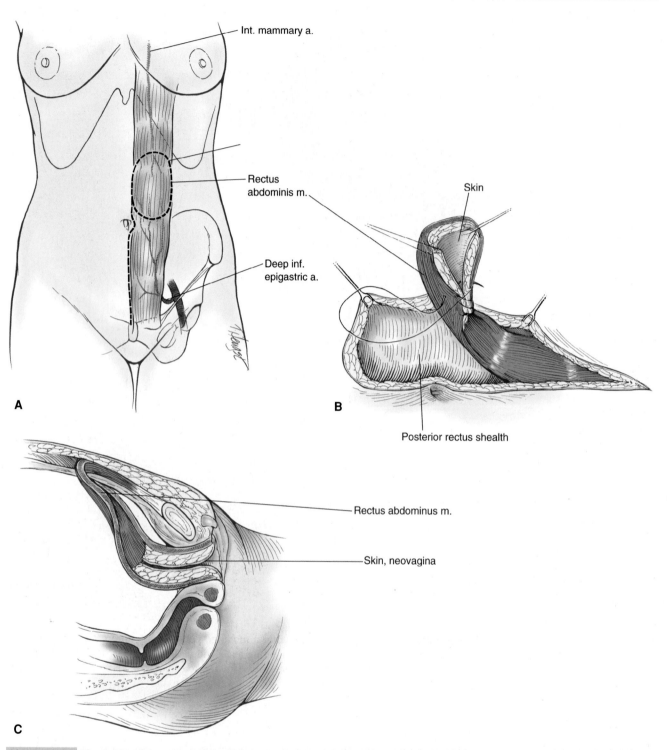

Figure 20.22 **The transpelvic rectus abdominis myocutaneous (TRAM flap) pedicle graft. A:** The location of the myocutaneous pedicle flap of the rectus abdominis muscle. **B:** The pedicle is harvested, and the tubular neovagina is created by suturing the full-thickness of the muscle, subcutaneous tissue, and skin of the anterior abdominal wall. **C:** The pedicle graft is brought down into the pelvis, and the leading edge is sutured to the preserved vaginal introitus.

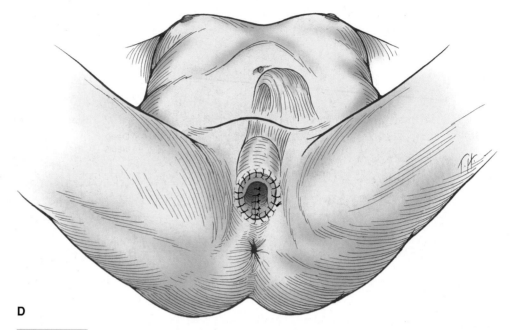

D

Figure 20.22 *Continued.* **D:** The final result is a neovagina that also helps to protect the pelvic floor from intestinal adhesions.

Vulvar and Perineal Reconstruction

Whenever feasible, the vulva should be closed primarily after radical vulvectomy. With radical local excision or a separate incision approach for the groin dissection, primary closure of the vulvar skin can be accomplished in almost all patients.

Rhomboid Pedicle Graft

If there is any tension on the skin edges, the skin can be mobilized by means of a Z-plasty using the adjacent skin and subcutaneous tissue. This is called a rhomboid flap (91,114). The technique (Fig. 20.24) involves the repositioning of a rhomboid flap of full-thickness skin and subcutaneous tissue. Use of these pedicle grafts will usually allow for the primary closure of vulvar defects after radical vulvar surgery, but if necessary, a split-thickness skin graft can be used. Myocutaneous pedicle grafts, such as a unilateral gracilis graft, can also be used to cover a large vulvar defect. A refinement of this procedure involves fasciocutaneous flaps raised from the gluteal folds, the so-called Lotus Petal Flap (115,116).

Tensor Fascia Lata Pedicle Graft

The tensor fascia lata pedicle graft, harvested from the lateral aspect of the thigh, can be useful in covering large defects of the lower abdomen, groin, and anterior vulva. The flap is particularly useful in patients who require extensive resection of a large groin recurrence or large, fixed groin nodes (100).

The graft is obtained by harvesting a myocutaneous pedicle from its proximal origin at the anterosuperior aspect of the iliac bone to its distal insertion on the lateral condyle of the tibia. The length of the proposed flap is determined by measuring the distance from the muscle's vascular supply, located 6 to 8 cm distal to the anterior superior iliac spine, to the most inferior or distal point of the recipient site (e.g., the posterior vulva). The blood supply is from the lateral circumflex femoral artery located deep to the fascia lata, between the rectus femoris and the vastus lateralis. The posterior border of the graft is defined as a line from the greater trochanter of the hip down to the knee, and the distal border is located about 5 cm proximal to the knee. The width of the flap is determined by the width of the defect to be covered, but typically it is 6 to 8 cm, with a length of up to 40 cm.

The pedicle graft is harvested after the defect has been created in order to permit a more accurate measurement of the flap. The flap is first incised distally, and care is taken to avoid injury to the proximal blood supply. Once the flap is elevated, it is rotated into place, and sutured from its most distal point proximally. The donor site is closed primarily.

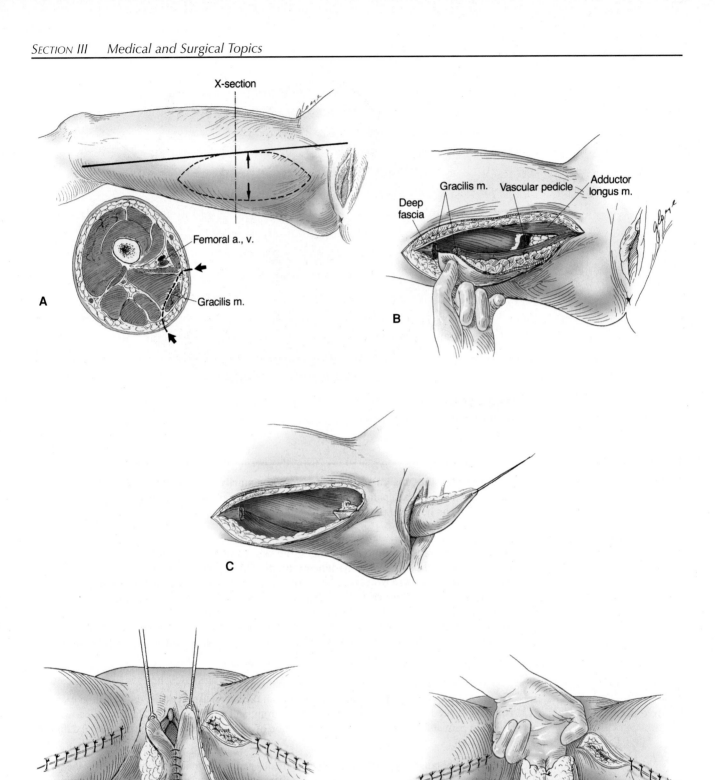

Figure 20.23 **The gracilis myocutaneous pedicle graft. A:** The pedicle graft is outlined on the inner thigh overlying the gracilis muscle. **B:** The myocutaneous pedicle graft is mobilized. **C:** The pedicle is brought under the skin bridge of the vulva. **D, E:** The two grafts are sutured together. **F:** The neovagina is placed into the pelvis and sutured to the introitus. **G:** An omental pedicle is used to cover the graft. (Reproduced from **Berek JS, Hacker NF, Lagasse LD.** Vaginal reconstruction performed simultaneously with pelvic exenteration. *Obstet Gynecol.* 1984;63:318, with permission from the American College of Obstetricians and Gynecologists.)

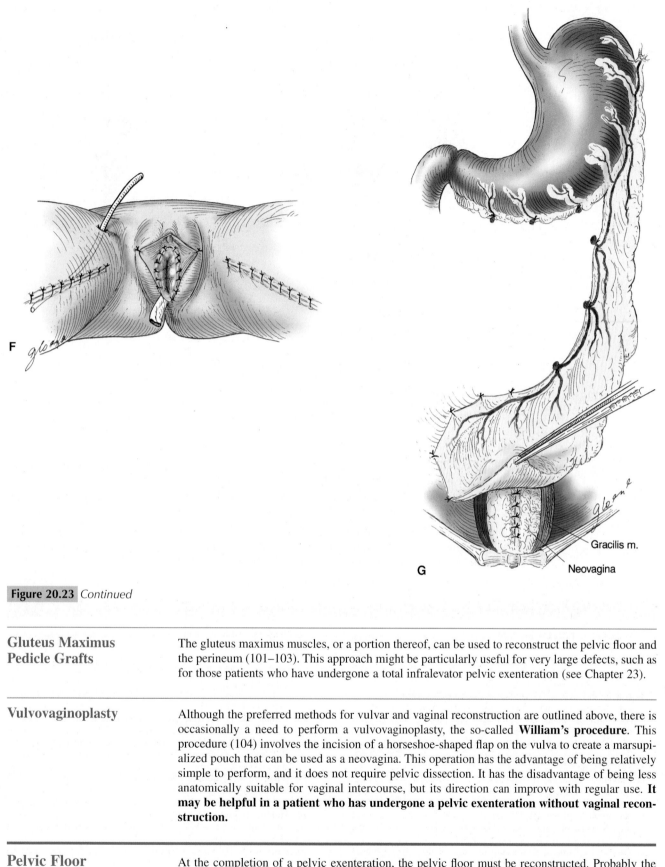

F

G

Gracilis m.

Neovagina

Figure 20.23 *Continued*

Gluteus Maximus Pedicle Grafts

The gluteus maximus muscles, or a portion thereof, can be used to reconstruct the pelvic floor and the perineum (101–103). This approach might be particularly useful for very large defects, such as for those patients who have undergone a total infralevator pelvic exenteration (see Chapter 23).

Vulvovaginoplasty

Although the preferred methods for vulvar and vaginal reconstruction are outlined above, there is occasionally a need to perform a vulvovaginoplasty, the so-called **William's procedure**. This procedure (104) involves the incision of a horseshoe-shaped flap on the vulva to create a marsupialized pouch that can be used as a neovagina. This operation has the advantage of being relatively simple to perform, and it does not require pelvic dissection. It has the disadvantage of being less anatomically suitable for vaginal intercourse, but its direction can improve with regular use. **It may be helpful in a patient who has undergone a pelvic exenteration without vaginal reconstruction.**

Pelvic Floor Reconstruction

At the completion of a pelvic exenteration, the pelvic floor must be reconstructed. Probably the most effective procedure is to perform an **omental pedicle graft** (provided there is sufficient omentum) and to use myocutaneous pedicle grafts whenever possible to reconstruct the vagina. In

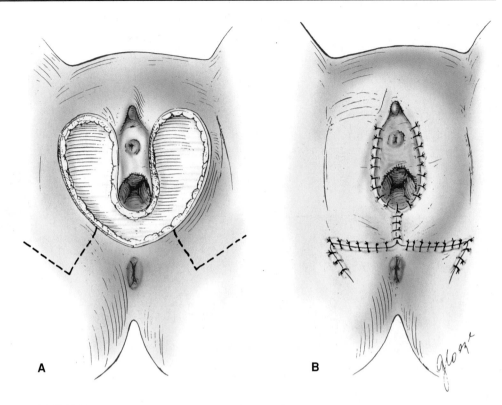

Figure 20.24 **A:** The "rhomboid flap" is used to close a posterior vulvar defect. **B:** The pedicle grafts are bilateral "Z-plasties" that are sutured together in the midline.

patients in whom this is not possible, alternatives include the use of **a variety of graft materials, either natural or synthetic** (117). A natural material that has been used is dura mater, but this is often unavailable (89). All areas that can be directly peritonealized should be carefully covered with peritoneal pedicle grafts.

Synthetic grafts using **Marlex** have been associated with a high incidence (more than 20%) of infectious morbidity and are therefore less desirable. However, if a pedicle graft is not feasible, the synthetic material Gore-Tex may be the best alternative (118–120).

References

1. **Gallieni M, Pittiruti M, Biffi R.** Vascular access in oncology patients. *CA Cancer J Clin.* 2008;58(6):323–346.
2. **Volkow P, Vazquez C, Tellez O, et al.** Polyurethane II catheter as long-indwelling intravenous catheter in patients with cancer. *Am J Infect Control.* 2003;31(7):392–396.
3. **Kuizon D, Gordon SM, Dolmatch BL.** Single-lumen subcutaneous ports inserted by interventional radiologists in patients undergoing chemotherapy: Incidence of infection and outcome of attempted catheter salvage. *Arch Intern Med.* 2001;161(3):406–410.
4. **Hind D, Calvert N, McWilliams R, et al.** Ultrasonic locating devices for central venous cannulation: Meta-analysis. *BMJ.* 2003; 327(7411):361.
5. **Calvert N, Hind D, McWilliams R, et al.** Ultrasound for central venous cannulation: Economic evaluation of cost-effectiveness. *Anaesthesia.* 2004;59(11):1116–1120.
6. **Randolph AG, Cook DJ, Gonzales CA, et al.** Ultrasound guidance for placement of central venous catheters: A meta-analysis of the literature. *Crit Care Med.* 1996;24(12):2053–2058.
7. **Turcotte S, Dube S, Beauchamp G.** Peripherally inserted central venous catheters are not superior to central venous catheters in the acute care of surgical patients on the ward. *World J Surg.* 2006; 30(8):1605–1619.
8. **Black D, Levine DA, Nicoll L, et al.** Low risk of complications associated with the fenestrated peritoneal catheter used for intraperitoneal chemotherapy in ovarian cancer. *Gynecol Oncol.* 2008;109(1):39–42.
9. **Ivy JJ, Geller M, Pierson SM, et al.** Outcomes associated with different intraperitoneal chemotherapy delivery systems in advanced ovarian carcinoma: A single institution's experience. *Gynecol Oncol.* 2009;114(3):420–423.
10. **Walker JL, Armstrong DK, Huang HQ, et al.** Intraperitoneal catheter outcomes in a phase III trial of intravenous versus intraperitoneal chemotherapy in optimal stage III ovarian and primary peritoneal cancer: A Gynecologic Oncology Group Study. *Gynecol Oncol.* 2006;100(1):27–32.
11. **Davidson SA, Rubin SC, Markman M, et al.** Intraperitoneal chemotherapy: Analysis of complications with an implanted subcutaneous port and catheter system. *Gynecol Oncol.* 1991;41(2):101–106.
12. **Makhija S, Leitao M, Sabbatini P, et al.** Complications associated with intraperitoneal chemotherapy catheters. *Gynecol Oncol.* 2001; 81(1):77–81.
13. **Fujiwara K, Sakuragi N, Suzuki S, et al.** First-line intraperitoneal carboplatin-based chemotherapy for 165 patients with epithelial ovarian carcinoma: Results of long-term follow-up. *Gynecol Oncol.* 2003;90(3):637–43.

14. **Helm CW.** Ports and complications for intraperitoneal chemotherapy delivery. *BJOG.* 2012;119(2):150–159.

15. **Le Huu Nho R, Mege D, Ouaissi M, et al.** Incidence and prevention of ventral incisional hernia. *J Visc Surg.* 2012;149(5 suppl):e3–e14.

16. **van 't Riet M, Steyerberg EW, Nellensteyn J, et al.** Meta-analysis of techniques for closure of midline abdominal incisions. *Br J Surg.* 2002;89(11):1350–1356.

17. **Israelsson LA, Millbourn D.** Prevention of incisional hernias: How to close a midline incision. *Surg Clin North Am.* 2013;93(5):1027–1040.

18. **Seiler CM, Deckert A, Diener MK, et al.** Midline versus transverse incision in major abdominal surgery: A randomized, double-blind equivalence trial (POVATI: ISRCTN60734227). *Ann Surg.* 2009; 249(6):913–920.

19. **Israelsson LA, Millbourn D.** Closing midline abdominal incisions. *Langenbecks Arch Surg.* 2012;397(8):1201–1207.

20. **Sajid MS, Parampalli U, Baig MK, et al.** A systematic review on the effectiveness of slowly-absorbable versus non-absorbable sutures for abdominal fascial closure following laparotomy. *Int J Surg.* 2011;9(8):615–625.

21. **O'Dwyer PJ, Courtney CA.** Factors involved in abdominal wall closure and subsequent incisional hernia. *Surgeon.* 2003;1(1):17–22.

22. **Mackeen AD, Berghella V, Larsen M-L.** Techniques and materials for skin closure in caesarean section. *Cochrane Database Syst Rev.* 2012;11:CD003577.

23. **Gregor S, Maegele M, Sauerland S, et al.** Negative pressure wound therapy: A vacuum of evidence? *Arch Surg.* 2008 Feb; 143(2):189–96.

24. **Slieker JC, Daams F, Mulder IM, et al.** Systematic review of the technique of colorectal anastomosis. *JAMA Surg.* 2013;148(2):190–201.

25. **Zmora O, Pikarsky AJ, Wexner SD.** Bowel preparation for colorectal surgery. *Dis Colon Rectum.* 2001;44(10):1537–1549.

26. **Pineda CE, Shelton AA, Hernandez-Boussard T, et al.** Mechanical bowel preparation in intestinal surgery: A meta-analysis and review of the literature. *J Gastrointest Surg.* 2008;12(11):2037–2044.

27. **Guenaga KF, Matos D, Wille-Jorgensen P.** Mechanical bowel preparation for elective colorectal surgery. *Cochrane Database Syst Rev.* 2011;(9):CD001544.

28. **Soriano A, Davis MP.** Malignant bowel obstruction: Individualized treatment near the end of life. *Cleve Clin J Med.* 2011;78(3):197–206.

29. **Stiegmann GV, Goff JS, Silas D, et al.** Endoscopic versus operative gastrostomy: Final results of a prospective randomized trial. *Gastrointest Endosc.* 1990;36(1):1–5.

30. **Bankhead RR, Fisher CA, Rolandelli RH.** Gastrostomy Tube Placement Outcomes: Comparison of Surgical, Endoscopic, and Laparoscopic Methods. *Nutr Clin Pract.* 2005;20(6):607–612.

31. **Helmkamp BF, Krebs HB, Kiley LA.** Witzel gastrostomy in gynecologic surgery. *Gynecol Oncol.* 1997;67(3):291–294.

32. **Dolan EA.** Malignant bowel obstruction: A review of current treatment strategies. *Am J Hosp Palliat Care.* 2011;28(8):576–582.

33. **Burch JM, Franciose RJ, Moore EE, et al.** Single-layer continuous versus two-layer interrupted intestinal anastomosis: A prospective randomized trial. *Ann Surg.* 2000;231(6):832–837.

34. **Everett WG.** A comparison of one layer and two layer techniques for colorectal anastomosis. *Br J Surg.* 1975;62(2):135–140.

35. **Flyger HL, Hakansson TU, Jensen LP.** Single layer colonic anastomosis with a continuous absorbable monofilament polyglyconate suture. *Eur J Surg.* 1995;161(12):911–913.

36. **Neutzling CB, Lustosa SAS, Proenca IM, et al.** Stapled versus handsewn methods for colorectal anastomosis surgery. *Cochrane Database Syst Rev.* 2012;2:CD003144.

37. **Schmidt O, Merkel S, Hohenberger W.** Anastomotic leakage after low rectal stapler anastomosis: Significance of intraoperative anastomotic testing. *Eur J Surg Oncol.* 2003;29(3):239–243.

38. **Michelassi F, Block GE.** A simplified technique for ileal J-pouch construction. *Surg Gynecol Obstet.* 1993;176(3):290–294.

39. **Ho YH, Foo CL, Seow-Choen F, et al.** Prospective randomized controlled trial of a micronized flavonidic fraction to reduce bleeding after haemorrhoidectomy. *Br J Surg.* 1995;82(8):1034–1035.

40. **Hallbook O, Pahlman L, Krog M, et al.** Randomized comparison of straight and colonic J pouch anastomosis after low anterior resection. *Ann Surg.* 1996;224(1):58–65.

41. **Mathur P, Hallan RI.** The colonic J-pouch in colo-anal anastomosis. *Colorectal Dis.* 2002;4(5):304–312.

42. **Hida J, Yasutomi M, Fujimoto K, et al.** Functional outcome after low anterior resection with low anastomosis for rectal cancer using the colonic J-pouch. Prospective randomized study for determination of optimum pouch size. *Dis Colon Rectum.* 1996;39(9):986–991.

43. **Furst A, Suttner S, Agha A, et al.** Colonic J-pouch vs. coloplasty following resection of distal rectal cancer: Early results of a prospective, randomized, pilot study. *Dis Colon Rectum.* 2003;46(9):1161–1166.

44. **Nelson R, Edwards S, Tse B.** Prophylactic nasogastric decompression after abdominal surgery. *Cochrane Database Syst Rev.* 2007; CD004929.

45. **Yang Z, Zheng Q, Wang Z.** Meta-analysis of the need for nasogastric or nasojejunal decompression after gastrectomy for gastric cancer. *Br J Surg.* 2008;95(7):809–816.

46. **Mangesi L, Hofmeyr GJ.** Early compared with delayed oral fluids and food after caesarean section. *Cochrane Database Syst Rev.* 2002; (3):CD003516.

47. **Lewis SJ, Egger M, Sylvester PA, et al.** Early enteral feeding versus "nil by mouth" after gastrointestinal surgery: Systematic review and meta-analysis of controlled trials. *BMJ.* 2001;323(7316):773–776.

48. **Petrelli NJ, Cheng C, Driscoll D, et al.** Early postoperative oral feeding after colectomy: An analysis of factors that may predict failure. *Ann Surg Oncol.* 2001;8(10):796–800.

49. **Ang C, Chan KKL, Bryant A, et al.** Ultra-radical (extensive) surgery versus standard surgery for the primary cytoreduction of advanced epithelial ovarian cancer. *Cochrane Database Syst Rev.* 2011;CD007697.

50. **Elattar A, Bryant A, Winter-Roach BA, et al.** Optimal primary surgical treatment for advanced epithelial ovarian cancer. *Cochrane Database Syst Rev.* 2011;CD007565.

51. **Harter P, Bois du A, Hahmann M, et al.** Surgery in recurrent ovarian cancer: The Arbeitsgemeinschaft Gynaekologische Onkologie (AGO) DESKTOP OVAR trial. *Ann Surg Oncol.* 2006;13(12):1702–1710.

52. **Bois du A, Reuss A, Pujade-Lauraine E, et al.** Role of surgical outcome as prognostic factor in advanced epithelial ovarian cancer: A combined exploratory analysis of 3 prospectively randomized phase 3 multicenter trials: By the Arbeitsgemeinschaft Gynaekologische Onkologie Studiengruppe Ovarialkarzinom (AGO-OVAR) and the Groupe d"Investigateurs Nationaux Pour les Etudes des Cancers de l"Ovaire (GINECO). *Cancer.* 2009;115(6):1234–1244.

53. **Chi DS, Franklin CC, Levine DA, et al.** Improved optimal cytoreduction rates for stages IIIC and IV epithelial ovarian, fallopian tube, and primary peritoneal cancer: A change in surgical approach. *Gynecol Oncol.* 2004;94(3):650–654.

54. **Bristow RE, Tomacruz RS, Armstrong DK, et al.** Survival effect of maximal cytoreductive surgery for advanced ovarian carcinoma during the platinum era: A meta-analysis. *J Clin Oncol.* 2002;20(5):1248–1259.

55. **Pomel C, Jeyarajah A, Oram D, et al.** Cytoreductive surgery in ovarian cancer. *Cancer Imaging.* 2007;7:210–215.

56. **Trimbos JB, Vergote I, Bolis G, et al.** Impact of adjuvant chemotherapy and surgical staging in early-stage ovarian carcinoma: European Organisation for Research and Treatment of Cancer-Adjuvant ChemoTherapy in Ovarian Neoplasm trial. *J Natl Cancer Inst.* 2003; 95(2):113–125.

57. **American College of Obstetricians and Gynecologists.** ACOG Committee Opinion. Number 372. July 2007. The Role of cystourethroscopy in the generalist obstetrician-gynecologist practice. *Obstet Gynecol.* 2007;110(1):221–224.

58. **Gilmour DT, Das S, Flowerdew G.** Rates of urinary tract injury from gynecologic surgery and the role of intraoperative cystoscopy. *Obstet Gynecol.* 2006;107(6):1366–1372.

59. **Naik R, Maughan K, Nordin A, et al.** A prospective randomised controlled trial of intermittent self-catheterisation vs. supra-pubic catheterisation for post-operative bladder care following radical hysterectomy. *Gynecol Oncol.* 2005;99(2):437–442.

60. **Hooton TM, Bradley SF, Cardenas DD, et al.** Diagnosis, prevention, and treatment of catheter-associated urinary tract infection in adults: 2009 International Clinical Practice Guidelines from the Infectious Diseases Society of America. *Clin Infect Dis.* 2010;50(5):625–663.

61. **Niel-Weise BS, van den Broek PJ.** Urinary catheter policies for short-term bladder drainage in adults. *Cochrane Database Syst Rev.* 2005;(3):CD004203.

62. **Ibeanu OA, Chesson RR, Echols KT, et al.** Urinary tract injury during hysterectomy based on universal cystoscopy. *Obstet Gynecol.* 2009;113(1):6–10.

63. **Webb JA.** Ultrasonography in the diagnosis of renal obstruction. *BMJ.* 1990;301(6758):944–946.

64. **Dayal M, Gamanagatti S, Kumar A.** Imaging in renal trauma. *World J Radiol.* 2013;5(8):275–284.

65. **Abboudi H, Ahmed K, Royle J, et al.** Ureteric injury: A challenging condition to diagnose and manage. *Nat Rev Urol.* 2013;10(2):108–115.

66. **Brandes S, Coburn M, Armenakas N, et al.** Diagnosis and management of ureteric injury: An evidence-based analysis. *BJU Int.* 2004;94(3):277–289.

67. **Brueziere J.** [Leadbetter-Politano operation in the treatment of vesico-ureteral reflux in children. Indications, technic and outcome]. *Ann Chir Infant.* 1966;7(1):67–76.

68. **Thrasher JB, Temple DR, Spees EK.** Extravesical versus Leadbetter-Politano ureteroneocystostomy: A comparison of urological complications in 320 renal transplants. *J Urol.* 1990;144(5):1105–1109.

69. **Kayler L, Kang D, Molmenti E, et al.** Kidney transplant ureteroneocystostomy techniques and complications: Review of the literature. *Transplant Proc.* 2010;42(5):1413–1420.

70. **Ahn M, Loughlin KR.** Psoas hitch ureteral reimplantation in adults–analysis of a modified technique and timing of repair. *Urology.* 2001;58(2):184–187.

71. **Ehrlich RM, Melman A, Skinner DG.** The use of vesico-psoas hitch in urologic surgery. *J Urol.* 1978;119(3):322–325.

72. **Simmons MN, Gill IS, Fergany AF, et al.** Technical modifications to laparoscopic Boari flap. *Urology.* 2007;69(1):175–180.

73. **Konigsberg H, Blunt KJ, Muecke EC.** Use of Boari flap in lower ureteral injuries. *Urology.* 1975;5(6):751–755.

74. **Bonfig R, Gerharz EW, Riedmiller H.** Ileal ureteric replacement in complex reconstruction of the urinary tract. *BJU Int.* 2004;93(4):575–580.

75. **Verduyckt FJH, Heesakkers JPFA, Debruyne FMJ.** Long-term results of ileum interposition for ureteral obstruction. *Eur Urol.* 2002;42(2):181–187.

76. **Elkas JC, Berek JS, Leuchter R, et al.** Lower urinary tract reconstruction with ileum in the treatment of gynecologic malignancies. *Gynecol Oncol.* 2005;97(2):685–692.

77. **Joung JY, Jeong IG, Seo HK, et al.** The efficacy of transureteroureterostomy for ureteral reconstruction during surgery for a non-urologic pelvic malignancy. *J Surg Oncol.* 2008;98(1):49–53.

78. **Ravi R, Dewan AK, Pandey KK.** Transverse colon conduit urinary diversion in patients treated with very high dose pelvic irradiation. *Br J Urol.* 1994;73(1):51–54.

79. **Hart S, Skinner EC, Meyerowitz BE, et al.** Quality of life after radical cystectomy for bladder cancer in patients with an ileal conduit, cutaneous or urethral kock pouch. *J Urol.* 1999;162(1):77–81.

80. **Salom EM, Mendez LE, Schey D, et al.** Continent ileocolonic urinary reservoir (Miami pouch): The University of Miami experience over 15 years. *Am J Obstet Gynecol.* 2004;190(4):994–1003.

81. **Leissner J, Black P, Fisch M, et al.** Colon pouch (Mainz pouch III) for continent urinary diversion after pelvic irradiation. *Urology.* 2000 Nov 1;56(5):798–802.

82. **Panici PB, Angioli R, Plotti F, et al.** Continent ileocolonic urinary diversion (Rome pouch) for gynecologic malignancies: Technique and feasibility. *Gynecol Oncol.* 2007;107(2):194–199.

83. **Houvenaeghel G, Moutardier V, Karsenty G, et al.** Major complications of urinary diversion after pelvic exenteration for gynecologic malignancies: A 23-year mono-institutional experience in 124 patients. *Gynecol Oncol.* 2004;92(2):680–683.

84. **Bochner BH, McCreath WA, Aubey JJ, et al.** Use of an ureteroileocecal appendicostomy urinary reservoir in patients with recurrent pelvic malignancies treated with radiation. *Gynecol Oncol.* 2004; 94(1):140–146.

85. **Karsenty G, Moutardier V, Lelong B, et al.** Long-term follow-up of continent urinary diversion after pelvic exenteration for gynecologic malignancies. *Gynecol Oncol.* 2005;97(2):524–528.

86. **Angioli R, Zullo MA, Plotti F, et al.** Urologic function and urodynamic evaluation of urinary diversion (Rome pouch) over time in gynecologic cancers patients. *Gynecol Oncol.* 2007;107(2):200–204.

87. **El-Lamie IK.** Preliminary experience with Mainz type II pouch in gynecologic oncology patients. *Eur J Gynaecol Oncol.* 2001;22(1):77–80.

88. **Penalver MA, Bejany DE, Averette HE, et al.** Continent urinary diversion in gynecologic oncology. *Gynecol Oncol.* 1989;34(3):274–88.

89. **Donato D, Jarrell M, Averette H, et al.** Reconstructive techniques in gynecologic oncology: The use of human dura mater allografts. *Eur J Gynaecol Oncol.* 1988;9(2):135–139.

90. **Chitale SV, Chitale VR.** Bilateral ureterocutaneostomy with modified stoma: Long-term follow-up. *World J Urol.* 2006;24(2):220–223.

91. **Pusic AL, Mehrara BJ.** Vaginal reconstruction: An algorithm approach to defect classification and flap reconstruction. *J Surg Oncol.* 2006;94(6):515–521.

92. **Seccia A, Salgarello M, Sturla M, et al.** Neovaginal reconstruction with the modified McIndoe technique: A review of 32 cases. *Ann Plast Surg.* 2002;49(4):379–384.

93. **Hyde SE, Hacker NF.** Vaginal reconstruction in the fibrotic pelvis. *Aust N Z J Obstet Gynaecol.* 1999;39(4):448–453.

94. **Bekerecioglu M, Balat O, Tercan M, et al.** Adaptation process of the skin graft to vaginal mucosa after McIndoe vaginoplasty. *Arch Gynecol Obstet.* 2008;277(6):551–554.

95. **Horch RE, Gitsch G, Schultze-Seemann W.** Bilateral pedicled myocutaneous vertical rectus abdominus muscle flaps to close vesicovaginal and pouch-vaginal fistulas with simultaneous vaginal and perineal reconstruction in irradiated pelvic wounds. *Urology.* 2002; 60(3):502–507.

96. **Soper JT, Secord AA, Havrilesky LJ, et al.** Comparison of gracilis and rectus abdominis myocutaneous flap neovaginal reconstruction performed during radical pelvic surgery: Flap-specific morbidity. *Int J Gynecol Cancer.* 2007;17(1):298–303.

97. **Sood AK, Cooper BC, Sorosky JI, et al.** Novel modification of the vertical rectus abdominis myocutaneous flap for neovagina creation. *Obstet Gynecol.* 2005;105(3):514–518.

98. **Soper JT, Secord AA, Havrilesky LJ, et al.** Rectus abdominis myocutaneous and myoperitoneal flaps for neovaginal reconstruction after radical pelvic surgery: Comparison of flap-related morbidity. *Gynecol Oncol.* 2005;97(2):596–601.

99. **O'Connell C, Mirhashemi R, Kassira N, et al.** Formation of functional neovagina with vertical rectus abdominis musculocutaneous (VRAM) flap after total pelvic exenteration. *Ann Plast Surg.* 2005; 55(5):470–473.

100. **Huang LY, Lin H, Liu YT, et al.** Anterolateral thigh vastus lateralis myocutaneous flap for vulvar reconstruction after radical vulvectomy: A preliminary experience. *Gynecol Oncol.* 2000;78(3Pt 1):391–393.

101. **Arkoulakis NS, Angel CL, DuBeshter B, et al.** Reconstruction of an extensive vulvectomy defect using the gluteus maximus fasciocutaneous V-Y advancement flap. *Ann Plast Surg.* 2002;49(1):50–54.

102. **Germann G, Cedidi C, Petracic A, et al.** The partial gluteus maximus musculocutaneous turnover flap. An alternative concept for simultaneous reconstruction of combined defects of the posterior perineum/sacrum and the posterior vaginal wall. *Br J Plast Surg.* 1998;51(8):620–623.

103. **Salgarello M, Farallo E, Barone-Adesi L, et al.** Flap algorithm in vulvar reconstruction after radical, extensive vulvectomy. *Ann Plast Surg.* 2005;54(2):184–190.

104. **Hoffman MS, Fiorica JV, Roberts WS, et al.** Williams' vulvovaginoplasty after supralevator total pelvic exenteration. *South Med J.* 1991;84(1):43–45.

105. **Copeland LJ, Hancock KC, Gershenson DM, et al.** Gracilis myocutaneous vaginal reconstruction concurrent with total pelvic exenteration. *Am J Obstet Gynecol.* 1989;160(5 Pt 1):1095–1101.

106. **Lacey CG, Stern JL, Feigenbaum S, et al.** Vaginal reconstruction after exenteration with use of gracilis myocutaneous flaps: The University of California, San Francisco experience. *Am J Obstet Gynecol.* 1988;158(6Pt 1):1278–1284.

107. **Jurado M, Bazan A, Elejabeitia J, et al.** Primary vaginal and pelvic floor reconstruction at the time of pelvic exenteration: A study of morbidity. *Gynecol Oncol.* 2000;77(2):293–297.

108. **Green AE, Escobar PF, Neubaurer N, et al.** The Martius flap neovagina revisited. *Int J Gynecol Cancer.* 2005;15(5):964–966.

109. **Lee D, Dillon BE, Zimmern PE.** Long-term Morbidity of Martius Labial Fat Pad Graft in Vaginal Reconstruction Surgery. *Urology.* 2013 82(6):1261–1266.

110. **Wierrani F, Grunberger W.** Vaginoplasty using deepithelialized vulvar transposition flaps: The Grunberger method. *J Am Coll Surg.* 2003;196(1):159–162.

111. **Parsons JK, Gearhart SL, Gearhart JP.** Vaginal reconstruction utilizing sigmoid colon: Complications and long-term results. *J Pediatr Surg.* 2002;37(4):629–633.

112. **Kapoor R, Sharma DK, Singh KJ, et al.** Sigmoid vaginoplasty: Long-term results. *Urology.* 2006;67(6):1212–1215.

113. **Ferrari JP, Hemphill AF, Xu J, et al.** Modified rotational bowel vaginoplasty after total pelvic exenteration. *Ann Plast Surg.* 2013; 70(3):335–336.

114. **Ayhan A, Tuncer ZS, Dogan L, et al.** Skinning vulvectomy for the treatment of vulvar intraepithelial neoplasia 2-3: A study of 21 cases. *Eur J Gynaecol Oncol.* 1998;19(5):508–510.

115. **Buda A, Confalonieri PL, Rovati LCV, et al.** Better anatomical and cosmetic results using tunneled lotus petal flap for plastic reconstruction after demolitive surgery for vulvar malignancy. *Int J Gynecol Cancer.* 2012;22(5):860–864.

116. **Sawada M, Kimata Y, Kasamatsu T, et al.** Versatile lotus petal flap for vulvoperineal reconstruction after gynecological ablative surgery. *Gynecol Oncol.* 2004;95(2):330–335.

117. **Elaffandi AH, Khalil HH, Aboul Kassem HA, et al.** Vaginal reconstruction with a greater omentum-pedicled graft combined with a vicryl mesh after anterior pelvic exenteration. Surgical approach with long-term follow-up. *Int J Gynecol Cancer.* 2007;17(2):536–542.

118. **Kohli N, Miklos JR.** Use of synthetic mesh and donor grafts in gynecologic surgery. *Curr Womens Health Rep.* 2001;1(1):53–60.

119. **Birch C, Fynes MM.** The role of synthetic and biological prostheses in reconstructive pelvic floor surgery. *Curr Opin Obstet Gynecol.* 2002;14(5):527–535.

120. **Chen CCG, Ridgeway B, Paraiso MFR.** Biologic grafts and synthetic meshes in pelvic reconstructive surgery. *Clin Obstet Gynecol.* 2007;50(2):383–411.

21 Laparoscopy

Kenneth D. Hatch
Jonathan S. Berek

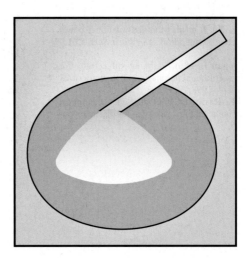

Laparoscopy is widely accepted for numerous gynecologic oncology operative procedures. These operations have been associated with short hospital stays, quick recovery times, and rapid return to full activity. The assistance of video monitors makes laparoscopy a preferred technique because the surgeon can view the operation in real time. Laparoscopy continues to undergo evaluation of its feasibility, morbidity, cost-effectiveness, and long-term outcome for patients compared with the standard laparotomy.

Gynecologic oncology care provided the unique opportunity for prospective study of the use of operative laparoscopy because of the limited number of specialists performing the procedures and the need to perform pelvic and para-aortic lymphadenectomy to stage several gynecologic malignancies. As surgeons have adopted minimally invasive technologies, innovations in instrumentation from bipolar coagulation devices to large-scale robotically-assisted devices have been developed to facilitate laparoscopic approaches for increasingly complex surgical procedures (see Chapter 22).

The skills to manage gynecologic malignancies by laparoscopic techniques are acquired through a commitment on the surgeon's part to learn the technique. It requires up-to-date equipment and a team familiar with the procedures. Hands-on experience in an animal laboratory and proctored learning in the operating suite are highly recommended. In the hands of experienced laparoscopic surgeons and with properly selected patients, laparoscopic surgery appears to result in outcomes comparable with laparotomy. Innovative technologies such as robotic-assisted surgical units may further expand the scope and use of minimally invasive techniques in the field of gynecologic oncology.

Laparoscopic Pelvic and Para-aortic Lymphadenectomy

The performance of a pelvic and para-aortic lymphadenectomy, either a partial lymphadenectomy (lymph node sampling) or complete lymphadenectomy, is the key procedure for the staging of gynecologic malignancies. Dargent and Salvat (1) used the laparoscope to perform limited pelvic lymphadenectomy in women with cervical cancer. This was not widely accepted because of its limited access to the pelvic lymph nodes and the inability to evaluate the lymph nodes in the common iliac and para-aortic chains. **Childers and Surwit (2) described pelvic and para-aortic lymphadenectomy performed in conjunction with a laparoscopically assisted**

vaginal hysterectomy and bilateral salpingo-oophorectomy in two women with endometrial cancer. Nezhat et al. (3) published a case of laparoscopic radical hysterectomy and pelvic and para-aortic lymphadenectomy, although the dissection went only 2 cm above the aortic bifurcation, an inadequate evaluation. These early publications were limited case reports that gave no information on morbidity, mortality, or complications.

Querleu et al. (4) performed transperitoneal laparoscopic pelvic lymphadenectomy on 39 patients with cervical cancer. Five patients had metastatic lymph nodes and were treated with radiation therapy. Thirty-two patients underwent abdominal radical hysterectomy and evaluation of the completeness of the laparoscopic lymphadenectomy. The sensitivity for lymph node-positivity by laparoscopy was 100%. However, the number of additional lymph nodes found at laparotomy was not stated. Childers et al. (5) reported 59 patients with endometrial cancer who were staged laparoscopically, followed by vaginal hysterectomy and bilateral salpingo-oophorectomy. Of the 31 patients deemed candidates for staging based on criteria including high-grade or deep myometrial invasion, lymphadenectomy was completed in 29 patients (obesity precluded it in two patients), for a feasibility rate of 93%. Three major and three minor complications were reported. The surgical complications were experienced early in the series and led to alternative techniques as the series progressed. The average hospital stay was 2.9 days, but the operative time, lymph node counts, and cost analysis were lacking.

These early series emphasized pelvic lymphadenectomy, but it remained necessary to do para-aortic lymphadenectomy for laparoscopy to be fully accepted as a technique to stage all gynecologic malignancies. Childers et al. (6) reported their initial experience with pelvic and para-aortic lymphadenectomy extending from the duodenum to the bifurcation in 18 patients with cervical cancer. They subsequently summarized their experience in para-aortic lymphadenectomy with a report of 61 women with cervical, endometrial, or ovarian cancer (7). In three patients (5%), obesity prevented the completion of the surgery, and in one patient (0.8%), adhesions were responsible for failure. Lymph node counts were available in 23 patients: For the right-sided lymphadenectomy, there was an average lymph node count of three. The operating time for the six patients, who underwent a bilateral para-aortic lymphadenectomy ranged from 25 to 70 minutes, depending on whether or not a unilateral or bilateral procedure was performed (these times included only the time to complete the lymphadenectomy). The hospital stay for the 33 patients undergoing laparoscopic lymphadenectomy was 1.3 days. There was one vena caval injury that required transfusion and laparotomy, a complication rate comparable with that of open surgery. Spirtos et al. (8) reported 40 patients who underwent bilateral limited para-aortic lymphadenectomy (sampling). Five laparotomies were performed: Two to remove unsuspected metastases, two for control of hemorrhage, and one because of equipment failure. In two patients, the left-sided lymphadenectomy was judged to be inadequate, which was an overall failure rate of 12.5%. An average of eight para-aortic lymph nodes were removed: Four from the right side and four from the left side. Most of the patients also underwent a pelvic lymphadenectomy and hysterectomy. The mean operative time was 3 hours, 13 minutes, and the average hospital stay was 2.9 days. In these series (4–6,9), laparotomy was used to confirm the accuracy of the lymphadenectomy and in each report, all positive lymph nodes were identified.

Possover et al. (10) reported 84 patients who underwent laparoscopic pelvic and para-aortic lymphadenectomy for cervical cancer. The surgeon visually classified the lymph nodes as positive or negative. The sensitivity and specificity of visualization was 92.3%. When frozen-section analysis was combined with laparoscopic assessment, 100% of the positive lymph nodes were identified. Based on these findings, in 13 of the 84 patients (15.5%), the treatment plan was altered during surgery. Possover et al. (11) analyzed videotapes of 112 para-aortic lymphadenectomies and detailed the ventral tributaries of the infrarenal vena cava (Fig. 21.1). They divided the vena cava into three levels based on the distribution of venous tributaries. This is a significant contribution to anatomic knowledge and is an important guide for beginning laparoscopic surgeons. A perforator of the inferior vena cava at the level of the bifurcation of the aorta is shown in Figure 21.1A. A diagram of the most common sites where perforators are encountered during a para-aortic lymphadenectomy is shown in Figure 21.1B.

Multiple studies report the adequacy and safety of laparoscopic pelvic and para-aortic lymphadenectomy in gynecologic cancer (12–19). In the experience by Kohler et al. reporting the laparoscopic para-aortic left-sided transperitoneal infrarenal lymphadenectomy, the number of lymph nodes removed could be doubled compared with an inframesenteric lymphadenectomy (12). In one of the largest series to date, they reported on 650 patients undergoing laparoscopic transperitoneal pelvic ($n = 499$) or para-aortic ($n = 468$) (combined pelvic and para-aortic $n = 362$) lymphadenectomies (19). The mean number of pelvic lymph nodes removed

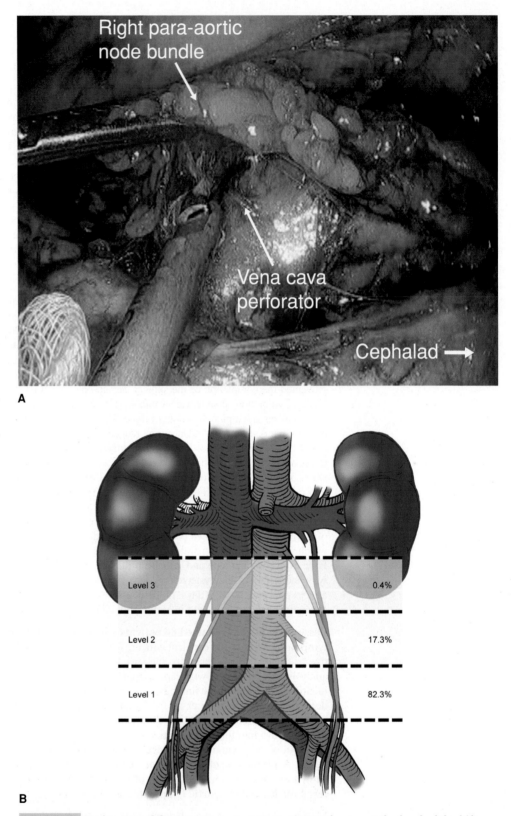

Figure 21.1 Perforators of the vena cava. **A: A vena cava perforator at the level of the bifurcation of the aorta. B: Diagram of the most common sites where perforators are encountered during the performance of a para-aortic lymphadenectomy.** The figure shows the anatomic distribution of 237 venous tributaries in 112 patients undergoing laparoscopic lymphadenectomy according to different levels of the inferior vena cava. (From **Possover M, Plaul K, Krause N, et al.** Left-sided laparoscopic para-aortic lymphadenectomy: Anatomy of the ventral tributaries of the infrarenal vena cava. *Am J Obstet Gynecol.* 1998;179:1295–1297, with permission.)

from 1994 to 2003 remained fairly constant (16.9 to 21.9). However, the mean number of para-aortic lymph nodes increased from 5.5 in 1994 to 18.5 in 2003, reflecting improvements in technique and extensive training. **Intraoperative complications (bowel or vessel injury) occurred in 2.9% of patients while 5.8% had postoperative complications for an overall complication rate of 8.7%.** The authors reported that no major intraoperative complications were encountered during the last 5 years of the study.

Querleu et al. subsequently reported on their experience with transperitoneal and extraperitoneal lymphadenectomy in 1,000 gynecologic cancer patients (18). This study included 777 pelvic (757 transperitoneal, 20 extraperitoneal) and 415 aortic lymphadenectomies (155 transperitoneal, 260 extraperitoneal) in patients with early cervical carcinoma ($n = 456$); advanced cervical carcinoma ($n = 219$); vaginal carcinoma ($n = 4$); endometrial carcinoma ($n = 182$); and ovarian carcinoma ($n = 139$). The mean number of pelvic lymph nodes removed was 18 via a transperitoneal approach; the mean number of para-aortic lymph nodes removed was 17 via a transperitoneal approach versus 21 via an extraperitoneal approach. **The authors reported an increase in the number of lymph nodes removed with increasing experience,** yielding an average of 24 pelvic and 22 aortic lymph nodes in 2003. **Intraoperative complications occurred in 2% of patients** including injury to vascular structures (1.1%); bowel (0.3%); ureter (0.3%); and nerves (0.3%). Five patients underwent conversion to laparotomy for completion of the lymphadenectomy, secondary to fixed lymph nodes or extensive adhesions. Conversion to laparotomy occurred in an additional two patients secondary to bowel or ureteric injury. Five patients required a second surgical intervention as a result of postoperative complications, most commonly bowel obstruction ($n = 4$).

Infrarenal Para-aortic Lymphadenectomy

Most of the early studies of para-aortic lymphadenectomy described dissection and removal of the right para-aortic lymph nodes to the duodenum and left-sided lymph nodes to the inferior mesenteric artery (IMA). Kohler et al. (12) were the first to report a transperitoneal technique for left infrarenal lymph nodes. Querleu et al. (18) staged patients for ovarian cancer, performing a left infrarenal lymphadenectomy and developing the left extraperitoneal para-aortic lymphadenectomy to surgically stage advanced cervical cancer prior to radiation treatment. Mariani et al. (20) at the Mayo Clinic reported their experience in the staging of endometrial cancer using either laparotomy or laparoscopic staging of the para-aortic lymph nodes including the infrarenal lymph nodes. They found that 63 (22%) of 281 patients had lymph node metastasis; 33% of these were in the pelvis alone; 51% had both pelvis and para-aortic; and 16% had para-aortic only. Most importantly, 77% of the patients with positive para-aortic lymph nodes had metastasis to the infrarenal lymph nodes. Those patients who were laparoscopically staged had left extraperitoneal lymphadenectomies. This report has stimulated gynecologic oncologists to remove the infrarenal lymph nodes when indicated by level of risk. **The extraperitoneal approach has been the preferred method, because it can be used in obese patients or those with extensive intraperitoneal adhesions.**

Extraperitoneal para-aortic lymphadenectomy for gynecologic cancer was first reported by Vasilev et al. (21) and Dargent et al. (22). The original goal of the retroperitoneal approach was to surgically stage cervical cancers so that radiotherapy could be directed to the appropriate fields without the risk of adhesion formation that accompanies transperitoneal surgery. The peritoneum forms a barrier between the lymphadenectomy and the bowel allowing for better visualization for laparoscopic removal of infrarenal lymph nodes especially in obese women. **Querleu et al. (23) described the detailed technique in 42 patients with advanced cervical cancer where the positive lymph node rate was 32% and the mean number of lymph nodes removed was 20.7. Sonoda et al. (24) further characterized the results and complications in 111 women with cervical cancer**—the mean age was 46 and the mean BMI was 24. The operative time was 157 minutes, the hospital stay was 2 days and the lymph node count was 19. The most common complication was lymphocele and the procedure was modified to include a peritoneal window at the end of the procedure to allow lymph to be absorbed by the peritoneum. **They recommended this procedure in cervical cancer patients who would be candidates for extended-field radiation if positive lymph nodes were found.** Twenty-seven women had positive lymph nodes and 21 patients underwent extended-field radiation with chemotherapy. Nine women underwent extended-field radiation alone. Mean survival was 38.6 months in the lymph node-negative group and 26.5 months in the lymph node-positive. **The laparoscopic extraperitoneal lymphadenectomy has been reported by a number of authors and the results will be discussed below in the sections on cervical cancer and endometrial cancer (25–28).**

Table 21.1 Recurrence Rates for Laparoscopic Surgery versus Laparotomy for Endometrial Cancer

	Laparoscopy			Laparotomy		
	n	Months Follow-up	% Recurrence	*n*	Months Follow-up	% Recurrence
Gemignani et al., 1999 (15)	59	18	6	235	30	7
Eltabbakh, 2002 (44)	100	27	7	86	48	10
Malur et al., 2001 (45)	37	16	3	33	16	3
Holub et al., 2002 (39)	177	33	6	44	45	7
Hatch, 2003 (46)	111	33	7	55	33	14
Obermair et al., 2004 (47)	226	29[a]	4	284	29	14
Zapico et al., 2005 (48)	38	36	5	37	53	5
Kim et al., 2005 (49)	74	31	1	168	37	1
Frigerio et al., 2006 (50)	55	27	0	55	33	5
Kalogiannidis et al., 2007 (51)	69	51	9	100	52	16
Walker et al., 2012 (34)	1,696	59	12	920	59	11

[a]Median follow-up for total study population.

Indications for Laparoscopic Surgery

Endometrial Cancer

Most women with endometrial cancer present with disease confined to the uterus. The treatment consists of total hysterectomy, bilateral salpingo-oophorectomy, and surgical staging, which includes peritoneal washings, inspection of the abdomen, and retroperitoneal lymphadenectomy. **The early studies showed an advantage for laparoscopic staging compared with historical or matched controls in postoperative pain, blood loss, length of hospital stay, and postoperative complications** (2,12–15,36,37). **Long-term survival of patients reported in these studies is presented in** Table 21.1 (15,39,44–51).

Surgical staging by pelvic and para-aortic lymphadenectomy followed by laparoscopically assisted vaginal hysterectomy or laparoscopic total hysterectomy has been established by randomized controlled trials comparing laparoscopy to laparotomy. Palomba et al. (29) summarized the first four of these trials. Two of these studies (30,31) had long-term follow-up of 202 patients with no difference in disease-free survival (87.3% in laparoscopy and 80% in laparotomy). The operative times were longer for laparoscopy; but the blood loss, transfusion, and postoperative complications were less. The lymph node count for both pelvic and para-aortic was the same. Malzoni et al. (32) reported 159 patients followed for a median of 38 months. He included patients with BMI up to 39. The operative times were 139 minutes for laparoscopy and 123 for laparotomy. The blood loss was 50 mL versus 145 mL and the mean length of stay was 2.1 days versus 5.1 days. There were 8.6% recurrences in the laparoscopy group, and 11.5% in the laparotomy group. Janda et al. (33) published the results of a multi-institutional trial in Australia, New Zealand, and Hong Kong. A total of 332 patients were randomized and filled out quality-of-life questionnaires for up to 6 months to identify early and late complications. There were no restrictions on weight: 40% of the total laparoscopic hysterectomy and 36% of the total abdominal hysterectomy patients were above BMI 35. Operating times were longer in the total laparoscopic hysterectomy group (138 minutes vs. 109 minutes). Lymphadenectomy was not required and 40.5% of the total laparoscopic hysterectomy and 67.6% of the total abdominal hysterectomy patients had lymph nodes removed. Hospital stay was longer than 2 days in all but 2% of the total abdominal hysterectomy patients and 37% of the total laparoscopic hysterectomy. The number of intraoperative adverse events was the same in both groups, but the late adverse events were doubled in the total abdominal hysterectomy group. These included wound dehiscence, bleeding, and infection. **The QOL analysis favored the total laparoscopic hysterectomy from baseline through the 6-month period.**

The Gynecologic Oncology Group (GOG) conducted the LAP 2 trial, a large, prospective, randomized trial designed to determine equivalency in early-stage endometrial cancer outcomes in laparoscopically assisted vaginal hysterectomy and bilateral salpingo-oophorectomy

with surgical staging, when compared with traditional open surgery (34). **It is the only randomized controlled trial that required pelvic and para-aortic lymphadenectomy. Results of this important study help answer many questions regarding feasibility, appropriate patient selection, and short-term and long-term oncologic outcomes of laparoscopy in the management of endometrial cancer.** This study enrolled 2,616 patients and there were 1,696 patients randomized to laparoscopy and 920 to laparotomy in a two-to-one randomization ratio. **Length of stay was shorter in the laparoscopic arm (median 3 days, range 0 to 95) versus laparotomy arm (median 4 days, range 1 to 49). Operative time was increased with laparoscopic procedures (3.3 hours vs. 2.2 hours) and approximately 23% of patients who were randomized to laparoscopy required laparotomy to complete staging.** The BMI initially was limited to 34 and below; however, 388 patients were enrolled with BMI greater than 35. There were 434 (23%) women in the laparoscopy group who were converted to laparotomy for the following reasons: poor exposure 14.6%, resection of metastatic disease 4.1%, bleeding and other 4.3%. Laparoscopic operative times were significantly longer—204 minutes versus 130 minutes. Pelvic and para-aortic lymphadenectomy was accomplished in 92% of the laparoscopic group and 96% of the laparotomy group. Detection of advanced stage was the same in both groups—17%. There was no difference in initial blood loss.

With a median follow-up of 59 months, the recurrence and survival results from GOG LAP2 were reported. The estimated recurrence rate was 11.4% in the laparoscopy group and 10.2% in the laparotomy group. The estimated 5-year survival was 89.9% in both arms. There was no difference in the postoperative treatments or the site of first recurrence, which would seem to dispel the concern that laparoscopy did not detect disease in the infrarenal lymph nodes or caused more intra-abdominal recurrence by spreading malignant cells via the intrauterine manipulator. There were four port site recurrences (0.24%) unique to the laparoscopic arm and three of these patients had advanced disease at the time of surgery. **Therefore, surgical staging with operative laparoscopy followed by vaginal hysterectomy or laparoscopic total hysterectomy has been proposed as an alternative to laparotomy** (2,12–15,36–38).

The other randomized trials showed less blood loss in the laparoscopic group, but they did not require lymphadenectomy in all patients. Only one study by Tozzi et al. had more than 50% of patients who had para-aortic lymphadenectomy (29). **The quality of life in this trial reported by Kornblith et al. (35) noted less pain, earlier resumption of normal activities, earlier return to work, and better body image, which was sustained for 6 months.**

Women with endometrial cancer are often obese with BMI greater than 35 (40–42,44). This was thought to be a limiting factor in using laparoscopy to stage and treat endometrial cancer. As surgical skills have grown, **laparoscopy has been used successfully in these women.** Holub et al. (41) completed staging and hysterectomies successfully in 94.4% of 33 patients with BMIs of 30 to 40. After hysterectomy, the pelvic and para-aortic lymphadenectomy was performed based on grade and depth of invasion. Women who had BMI from 30 to 40 were compared to those who were under 30. Two women in the obese group were converted to laparotomy to complete staging. Lymph node staging was completed in 94.4% of the women in whom it was indicated. Scribner et al. (43) reported 55 patients who had planned laparoscopic staging for endometrial cancer. The BMI ranged from 28 to 60. Those women with BMI greater than 35 had a decreased success rate (44%) versus those under 35 (82.1%). **In the GOG LAP2 trial, 322 patients had a BMI of greater than 35** (34): **The number of patients converted to laparotomy was 17.5% in patients with BMI 25 to 30; 26.5% from 30 to 35; and 57.1% in patients with BMI over 40. Failure to complete laparoscopic staging was greater with increasing BMI, metastatic disease, and age.**

The concept of sentinel node removal has been studied in endometrial cancer in several small studies. Techniques utilized for the detection of sentinel lymph nodes include injection of blue dye, injection of a radiocolloid, or both. Studies in endometrial cancer have focused on injection of the tracer into the uterine corpus (subserosal or myometrial), the cervix, the endometrium using hysteroscopy, or combined sites (52). The sentinel lymph node detection rates using injection of the subserosal myometrium alone ranged from 0–92% (53–58). Altgassen reported the highest detection rate (92%) utilizing eight injection sites, in contrast to the one to three sites reported by several other authors. Similarly, Li et al. (55) reported a 75% detection rate using three subserosal myometrial sites and two subserosal isthmic sites. Reported detection rates using cervical injection alone ranged from 80–100% (59–62). Holub et al. reported a detection rate using cervical and subserosal myometrial injections of 84% (63). Hysteroscopic injection of the endometrium has yielded detection rates of 50–100% (64–67). **While the possibility of laparoscopic assessment of sentinel lymph nodes and targeted sampling is interesting, sentinel lymph node detection in endometrial cancer remains investigational.**

Cervical Cancer

The use of laparoscopy in the treatment of cervical cancer was initially limited by the fact that there was no apparent advantage to laparoscopic lymphadenectomy, because the standard operation for the primary cervical tumor was radical abdominal hysterectomy. **Dargent (68) first suggested that laparoscopic pelvic lymphadenectomy could be followed by a Schauta radical vaginal hysterectomy** and has published long-term results, reporting a 95.5% 3-year survival rate in 51 patients with negative pelvic lymph nodes. Querleu (69) reported on eight patients and demonstrated an average blood loss of less than 300 mL, an average hospital stay of 4.2 days, and decreased pain from the elimination of an abdominal incision.

Hatch et al. (70) reported 37 patients treated by laparoscopic pelvic and para-aortic lymphadenectomy followed by radical vaginal hysterectomy. The mean operative time was 225 minutes, the mean blood loss was 525 mL and the average hospital stay was 3 days. Blood transfusion was required in 11% of the patients, compared with the range of 35–95% reported in the literature for radical abdominal hysterectomy. Complications occurred early in the series and included two cystotomies repaired at surgery without an increase in hospital stay. In two patients (5.4%), ureterovaginal fistulae developed that were treated by ureteral stents. These were removed 6 weeks later without further operative intervention.

Schneider et al. (71) reported 33 patients in whom bipolar techniques were used for lymphadenectomy and to transect the cardinal ligaments and uterine vessels. Hysterectomy was completed by the Schauta–Stoeckel technique. There were five (15%) intraoperative injuries managed successfully without sequelae. Four patients required transfusion. Numerous retrospective studies comparing laparoscopically assisted radical hysterectomy versus radical abdominal hysterectomy have reported increased operative time but decreased blood loss, decreased transfusion rates and hospital length of stay in patients undergoing the minimally invasive procedures (72–76).

Studies have shown that the complication rates decrease as the operator's experience increases (77,78). Long-term survival has been reported by Hertel et al. (14) for 200 patients, with a mean follow-up of 40 months. The projected 5-year survival was 83%. For the 100 patients who were stage I, lymphovascular space-negative and lymph node-negative, the survival was 98%.

Laparoscopic Radical Hysterectomy

Although most initial reports in the literature detailed some form of laparoscopically assisted radical vaginal hysterectomy, there are increasing reports of laparoscopic radical hysterectomy. **Spirtos et al. (13) reported laparoscopic radical hysterectomy (type III) with aortic and pelvic lymphadenectomy in 78 patients.** The average operative time was 205 minutes, length of hospitalization was 3.2 days, and blood loss was 225 mL; one transfusion was necessary. There were acceptable intraoperative and postoperative complications. With a minimum of 3 years follow-up, the disease-free survival was 95%. Numerous authors have reported similar findings (57,79–83). In one of the largest series, Puntambekar et al. (81) reported on 248 patients with early stage cervical cancer, noting a median operative time of 292 minutes, median number of resected pelvic lymph nodes of 18, median blood loss of 165 mL, and a median length of stay of 3 days. Other studies have reported longer operating times ranging from 196 to 344 minutes (57,76,83,84).

The issue of blood loss and transfusion has become very important to patients and surgeons since the identification of the human immunodeficiency virus and other blood-borne pathogens. **Every report on laparoscopic lymphadenectomy and radical hysterectomy has noted a significant decrease in blood loss and transfusion rates. Other societal advantages are the decreased hospital stay and rapid return to normal function, even with radical surgery.**

Laparoscopic Nerve-sparing Radical Hysterectomy

Preservation of the superior hypogastric nerve plexus, the hypogastric nerve, and the inferior hypogastric plexus is important for function of the bladder and rectum. The superior hypogastric plexus is composed of sympathetic nerves that allow the bladder to store urine. If this is damaged, the bladder will have a small-volume and high pressure under parasympathetic control. The inferior hypogastric plexus is composed of parasympathetic nerves that initiate urination. If the inferior hypogastric plexus is damaged, the patient will have lack of sensation and be unable to initiate urination. The hypogastric nerve connects the two plexuses. If it is severed, the patient will have a mixed pattern, consisting of an initial small-volume, high-pressure phase followed by a hypotonic high-residual state. This may lead to the need for chronic self-catheterization.

Damage to the superior hypogastric plexus can occur at the time of para-aortic lymphadenectomy or presacral lymphadenectomy. Injury to the hypogastric nerve may occur when

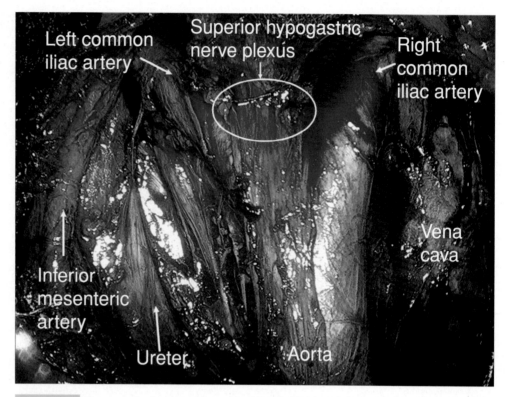

Figure 21.2 The superior hypogastric nerve plexus is preserved during the para-aortic lymphadenectomy.

clamping the cardinal or uterosacral ligaments. Injury to the inferior hypogastric plexus may occur with lateral dissection of the cardinal ligaments, dissection of the posterior vesicouterine ligament, or with removal of paravaginal tissue.

Recent description of the anatomy of these nerves and the surrounding blood vessels has established the role of nerve-sparing techniques when performing radical hysterectomy (85). **The laparoscope is an excellent tool to identify and preserve the nerves, because it magnifies small vessels and nerves so that the surgeon can more easily identify them.**

The technique performed is described below (Figs. 21.2–21.8):

1. **The patient is placed in the lithotomy position with Trendelenburg tilt to the table. A nasogastric tube is placed** to reduce the distention of the stomach. The four trocars are placed in the lower abdomen in a diamond shape.

2. **The para-aortic lymphadenectomy is performed first when the tumor is 2 cm or greater in size.** This allows for exposure of the superior hypogastric plexus (Fig. 21.2).

3. **The hypogastric nerve is located by opening the peritoneum between the ureter and the sigmoid colon mesentery** (Fig. 21.3). The hypogastric nerve is dissected down into the pelvis and its location dorsal to the uterine artery is shown (Fig. 21.4).

4. **The uterine artery is divided and the hypogastric nerve is dissected lateral and dorsal to the ureter** (Fig. 21.5).

5. **The anterior vesicouterine ligament with its vessels and connective tissue is divided and the ureter dissected laterally** (Fig. 21.6). The branch of the nerve following the ureter into the base of the bladder is preserved in the posterior vesicouterine ligament (Fig. 21.7).

6. **The cardinal ligament can be divided medial to the nerve and ligament** (Fig. 21.8).

The operation can be completed by the vaginal route or with further dissection through the laparoscope. The vaginal route allows more precise removal of the vaginal margin.

The urethral catheter is left in place for 48 hours. Then the patient is allowed to void and a postvoid residual is obtained. If she had good sensation of bladder fullness and a residual urine amount less than 60 cc, the catheter is left out. If she is unable to void, has no sensation of filling, or if the residual urine

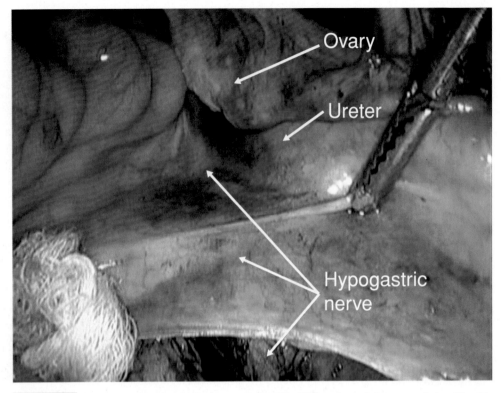

Figure 21.3 Traction on the peritoneum overlying the bifurcation of the aorta helps identify the course of the hypogastric nerve 2 to 3 cm medial to the ureter at the pelvic brim.

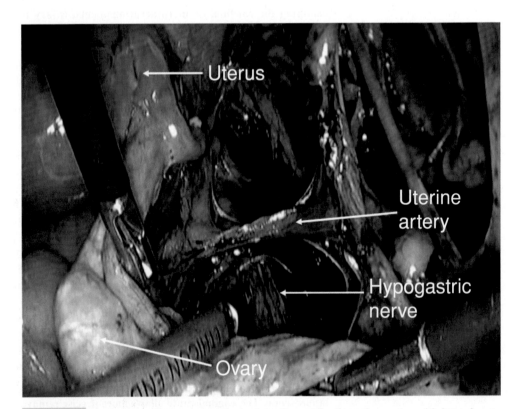

Figure 21.4 The hypogastric nerve continues into the pelvis along the ureter with branches to the rectum, uterus, and inferior hypogastric plexus.

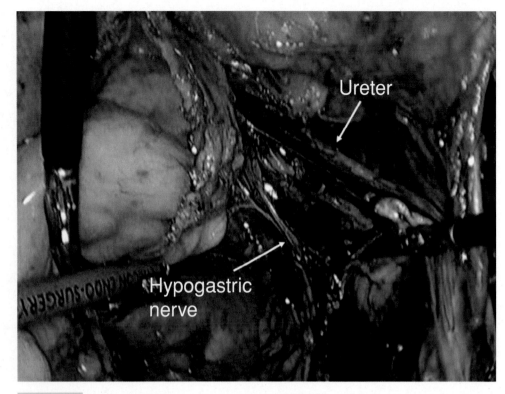

Figure 21.5 The hypogastric nerve is 1 to 2 cm dorsal to the uterine artery and can be preserved if mass ligature of the cardinal ligament is avoided.

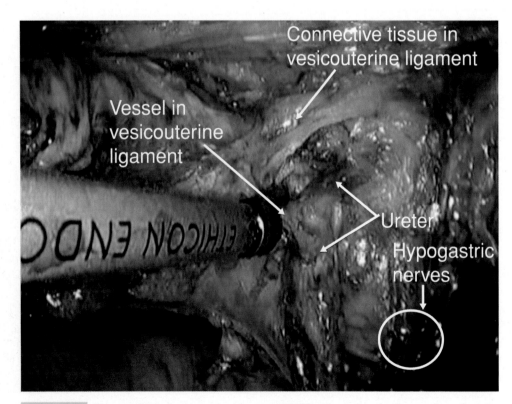

Figure 21.6 The vessels and connective tissue medial to the ureter is dissected so that the ureter can be retracted laterally out of the cardinal ligament tunnel.

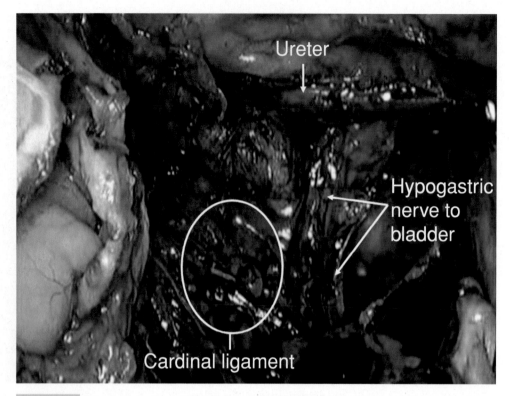

Figure 21.7 **The ureter is now retracted laterally with the hypogastric nerve.** The cardinal ligament can now be divided.

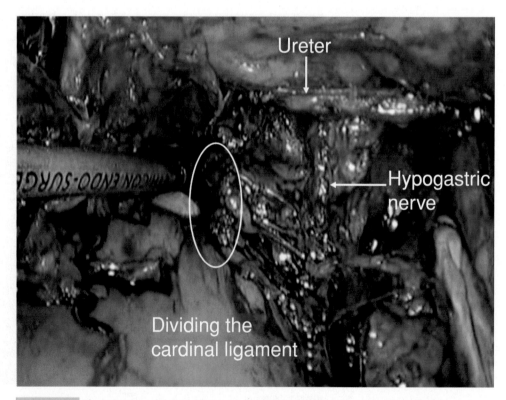

Figure 21.8 The anterior vesicouterine vessels and connective tissue are transected.

is over 60 cc, the catheter is left in place for 7 days. The nerve-sparing operation has been performed in a total of 33 patients. Twenty-one of these patients had a laparoscopic lymphadenectomy and radical vaginal trachelectomy. Twelve had a laparoscopic lymphadenectomy and radical hysterectomy completed by laparoscopy or by vaginal assistance. Eight of the patients were unable to void with residual of less than 60 cc at 7 days. All of the patients were able to void at 21 days.

Surgical Staging of Locally Advanced Cervical Cancer

Vidaurreta et al. (86) staged 91 patients, stages IIB, IIIA, IIIB, and IVA. Computed tomography (CT) was performed in 49 patients, with 38 (78%) read as normal and 11 (22%) as positive. Histologic evaluation revealed metastases in 18 of the 38 (47.4%) patients with negative scans and no metastases were found in 5 of the 11 (45.5%) with positive scans. Hertel et al. (87) compared laparoscopic surgical staging with magnetic resonance imaging (MRI) and CT scan in 101 patients, 91 of whom had a CT scan, 67 of whom had an MRI scan and 49 of whom had both. False-positive or false-negative results were found in 22% of patients. Ten patients had false-positive para-aortic lymph node metastases. These studies used transperitoneal para-aortic lymphadenectomy. Extra-peritoneal lymphadenectomy for locally advanced cervical cancer (LACC) was developed by Dargent and Querleu, because of the ability to remove the infrarenal lymph nodes without encountering the problems of adhesions. Leblanc (25) updated this series to include 184 patients.

Le Blanche et al. (25) performed preoperative MRI on 129 patients and reported a sensitivity of 29% and specificity of 73%. A CT was performed on 18 patients with a sensitivity of 33% and specificity of 71%. Patients with positive para-aortic lymph nodes underwent extended-field radiotherapy and most had chemotherapy. The disease-free survival for the lymph node-positive patients was 63.9% at 3 years and 56.3% at 5 years. Patients with microscopic (5 mm or less) lymph node disease had the same survival as lymph node-negative patients at 5 years (58%).

Ramirez (27) reported 60 patients with Stage IB2 to Stage IVA who had preoperative PET/CT prior to extraperitoneal lymphadenectomy. Of 26 patients with negative pelvic and para-aortic lymph nodes on PET, there were 3 (12%) positive para-aortic lymph nodes. Of 27 patients with PET-positive pelvic lymph nodes and negative para-aortic lymph nodes, there were 6 (22%) that had positive para-aortic lymph nodes. Seven patients had positive para-aortic lymph nodes on PET and 5 (71.4%) had positive para-aortic lymph nodes. **The sensitivity of PET/CT was 36% and the specificity was 96%.**

Sentinel Lymph Nodes

The initial studies of sentinel lymph node detection showed excellent sensitivity, negative predictive value, and accuracy (88,89). Subsequent studies have used both blue dye and Technetium 99m detection methods with varying levels of success (Table 21.2) (90–102,103).

Radical Vaginal Trachelectomy with Laparoscopic Lymphadenectomy

Radical hysterectomy, with or without adjuvant therapy for patients with early cervical cancer, is associated with high cure rates. However, in young patients desiring fertility, alternative surgical options have been increasingly explored. **Dargent et al. (104) first presented a series of 28 patients who underwent laparoscopic pelvic lymphadenectomy followed by radical vaginal trachelectomy.** After a median follow-up of 36 months, there was only one recurrence in the para-aortic lymph nodes of a 27-year-old patient with stage IB adenocarcinoma. The pelvic lymph nodes were negative and the margins were free. Among the eight patients who attempted pregnancy, three had cesarean section at 36 weeks' gestation and three had a spontaneous abortion. **The second report on radical vaginal trachelectomy was published by Roy and Plante** (105). Thirty patients underwent laparoscopic pelvic lymphadenectomy and radical vaginal trachelectomy; only six women had attempted pregnancy at the time of reporting and four had healthy infants delivered by cesarean section.

Since these initial reports, several authors have reported their experience with radical trachelectomy (Table 21.3) (106–115,117,118). Excellent reviews of radical trachelectomy have been presented by Shepherd (119) and Plant (120).

The indications for radical trachelectomy most commonly employed are the following:

1. **Desire for future childbearing**
2. **Stage IA1 disease with extensive lymph-vascular space invasion**
3. **Stage IA2 disease**
4. **Stage IB1 ≤2 cm diameter with no involvement of the upper endocervix on MRI or intraoperative frozen section**

Table 21.2 Sentinel Node Detection for Patients with Cervical Cancer (Series with ≥50 Patients)

Reference	Number of Patients	Percent with Sentinel Lymph Nodes	Sensitivity	Negative Predictive Value	Detection Method
Malur et al., 2001 (90)[a]	50	78	83	97	BD, RC, or both
Plante, 2003 (92)	70	87		100	BD
Dargent, Enria, 2003 (93)	70	NR[b]	100	NR	BD
Silva et al., 2005 (94)	56	93	82	92	RC
Rob et al., 2005 (95)	100	80	100	99	BD
Rob et al., 2005 (95)	83	96	100	100	BD + RC
Di Stefano et al., 2005 (96)	50	90	90	97	BD
Angioli et al., 2005 (97)	37	70	100	100	RC
Lin et al., 2005 (98)	30	100	100	100	RC
Schwendinger et al., 2006 (99)	47	83	90	97	BD
Wydra et al., 2006 (100)	100	100	100	100	BD + RC
Yuan et al., 2007 (102)	81	94[c]	NR	95	BD
Devaja et al., 2012 (103)	86	98[d]	98	100	BD + RC

[a]Total reported included BD alone (*n* = 9), RC alone (*n* = 21), and combined (*n* = 20). For combined technique, sensitivity = 100, NPV = 100.

[b]90% rate of sentinel nodes found in 14 of 139 attempted dissections in 70 patients.

[c]Reported for subgroup of 49 patients with 4 mL of methylene blue. Subgroup of 28 patients with 2- to 3-mL injection = 66% detection.

[d]Subgroup using combined BD + RC technique.

BD, Blue dye; RC, Radiolabeled colloid; NR, not reported.

5. **Histology: Squamous, adenocarcinoma, or adenosquamous**

6. **No metastases to regional lymph nodes**

Risk factors for recurrence include lesion size greater than 2 cm, depth of invasion greater than 1 cm, and lymphovascular space invasion (92). However, some authors suggest that conservative fertility-sparing surgery may be appropriate for select patients with larger lesions that are clearly exophytic (116).

Lanowska et al. (117) published the largest series with the longest follow-up of recurrence and survival in women who had radical vaginal trachelectomy after laparoscopic lymphadenectomy. Two hundred and twenty-five patients were treated and the median follow-up was 37 months. The 5-year disease-free survival and overall survival was 94.4% and 97.4%. Plante et al. (118) reported the outcome of 125 patients who underwent vaginal radical trachelectomy. In their study, tumor size larger than 2 cm was associated with a significantly increased risk of recurrence and a higher chance of abandoning the operation. Regarding the obstetrical outcome, 58 women conceived a total of 106 pregnancies; 77 (73%) reached the third trimester and 58 of these (75%) delivered at term.

A systematic review of 504 women undergoing radical trachelectomy described the gestational outcomes of 200 pregnancies resulting in 133 third trimester deliveries. The first trimester abortion rate was 19%, which is similar to the general population. **The second trimester spontaneous abortion rate was 9.5% (19 of 200) when defined as earlier than 24 weeks. Overall, 84 of 200 pregnancies (42%) resulted in term deliveries of viable infants, but 25% (49 of 200) of total pregnancies or 37% of third-term deliveries were preterm. Moreover, 13 of 133 patients (9.8%) delivered from 24 to 28 weeks, and 14 (10.5%) delivered from 24 to 34 weeks** (121). **These pregnancies should be managed by maternal-fetal medicine specialists.**

Ovarian Cancer

Laparoscopy has been used for several decades to manage adnexal masses and as a second-look procedure to avoid laparotomy in patients with persistent disease after primary chemotherapy. More recently, it has been reported to be useful for staging apparently early cancer of the ovary.

Table 21.3 Radical Trachelectomy for Fertility Preservation in Patients with Early-Stage Cervical Cancer: Oncologic Outcomes

| Authors | Cases | Size | | | Histology | | | | | | |
		<2 cm n (%)	>2 cm n (%)	Squamous n (%)	Adeno n (%)	Intraop Complications n (%)	Aborted Procedure n/Total[a] (%)	Follow-up (median, range)	Recurrences n (%)	Deaths n (%)
Steed and Covens, 2003 (111)	93	85 (91)	8 (9)	42 (48)	44 (52)		0/93 (0)	30 (1–103)	7 (7)	4 (4.2)
Burnett et al., 2003 (112)	19	19 (100)	0 (0)	10 (53)	9 (47)	0 (0)	2/21 (10)	31 (22–44)	0 (0)	0 (0)
Schlaerth et al., 2003 (113)	10	8 (80)	2 (20)	4 (40)	6 (60)	2 (17)	0 (0)	47 (28–84)	0 (0)	0 (0)
Plante et al., 2004 (109)	72	64 (89)	8 (11)	42 (58)	30 (42)	5 (6)	10/82 (12)	(6)	2 (3)	1 (1)
Shepherd et al., 2006 (110)	123[a]	NR	NR	83 (66)	33 (27)	6 (5)	NR	45	5 (4)	4 (3)
Marchiole et al., 2007 (108)	118	91 (81)[b]	21 (19)	90 (76)	25 (21)	3 (2.5)	17/135 (13)	95 (31–234)	7 (6)	4 (4)
Sonoda et al., 2008 (114)	43[c]	43 (100)	0 (0)	24 (55)	19 (44)	0 (0)	2/43	21 (3–60)[d]	1 (3)	0 (0)
Chen et al., 2008 (115)	16	9 (56)	7 (44)	14 (88)	2 (13)	0 (0)	0 (0)	28 (8–50)	0 (0)	0 (0)
Lanowska et al., 2011 (117)	212	131 (62)	81 (38)	154 (73)	58 (27)	6 (3)	0 (0)	37 (0–171)	8 (5.7)	4 (1.9)
Plante et al., 2011 (118)	125	111 (89)	14 (11)	69 (56)	56 (44)	7 (5.6)	15/140[a] (9.3)	95 (4–25)	6 (4.8)	2 (1.6)

[a]Total number of cases selected for radical trachelectomy.

[b]Aborted cases/total number of cases attempted.

[c]Excluding 6 patients with stage IIa disease (size not given).

[d]Follow-up data for 36 patients without aborted procedure (2) or post-op treatment (5).

NR, not reported.

Evaluation of the Suspicious Adnexal Mass

Laparotomy is accepted as the standard of care for management of the suspicious adnexal mass. However, it is possible to mismanage adnexal masses regardless of whether laparotomy or laparoscopy is used. The incidence with which an unexpected malignancy is encountered when managing an adnexal mass is reported to be between 0.4% and 2.9% (122–124). Childers et al. (125) and Canis et al. (126) used laparoscopy for management of suspicious adnexal masses and reported malignancy rates of 14% and 15%, respectively. More than 80% of the masses were managed by laparoscopy. All of the malignancies were properly diagnosed and treated, including 13 staged by laparoscopy. **A frozen section should be obtained so that surgical staging and appropriate treatment are not delayed.**

Staging requires an infracolic omentectomy, peritoneal washings, multiple biopsies from the peritoneal surfaces, hemidiaphragms, and pelvic and para-aortic lymph node biopsies. Laparoscopic omentectomy has been described using a stapling technique (127), but has been simplified further with the advent of laparoscopic bipolar vessel sealing devices, which incorporate both bipolar cautery and cutting functions.

Several investigators have reported their experiences with staging of early ovarian, fallopian tube, or primary peritoneal cancers. Querleu and LeBlanc (128) described the first adequate laparoscopic surgical staging for ovarian carcinoma in eight patients undergoing pelvic and para-aortic lymph node sampling up to the level of the renal veins. An average of nine lymph nodes (range 6 to 17) were removed, with an average operative time of 111 minutes, postoperative stay of 2.8 days, and blood loss of less than 300 mL. None of the lymph nodes were positive.

Childers et al. (129) reported 14 patients undergoing staging for presumed early ovarian cancer. Metastatic disease was discovered in eight patients (57%) and the appropriate treatment instituted.

Subsequent series by Pomel ($n = 10$) (130); Tozzi ($n = 24$) (131); Chi ($n = 20$) (132); Spirtos ($n = 73$) (133); and Leblanc ($n = 44$; 36 epithelial, 8 germ cell or granulosa cell) (134) have confirmed similar feasibility. Brockbank et al. (135) published a prospective series of 35 women with early stage ovarian or tubal carcinoma who had undergone a prior surgical procedure where the diagnosis had been made. The cancer was upstaged in 8 (23%); omental metastasis in four, pelvic lymph node positive in two, para-aortic lymph node positive in one, and contralateral ovary positive in one patient. Sixty-three percent received chemotherapy. The disease-free survival was 94% at median follow-up of 18 months.

Results of these small series are encouraging and support the development of studies with larger sample sizes and long-term follow-up. However, the low incidence of early stage disease underscores the difficulty of clinical trial development in this patient group. **At this time, laparoscopy for the staging of ovarian cancer remains investigational. It may be considered for patients with apparent early stage disease at presentation, for staging of unstaged patients, or for patients who are candidates for fertility-sparing oophorectomy and staging alone.**

The two major concerns over the use of laparoscopy for adnexal masses are (i) delay in diagnosis and thus treatment; and (ii) rupture of the adnexal mass that is subsequently found to be malignant, which converts the stage from a possible IA to IC. Studies on laparotomy show that if the tumor is removed and proper treatment instituted, rupture does not affect the outcome (136–138), but it is prudent to avoid rupture in order to minimize any theoretical increase in the risk. If the tumor is ruptured and the treatment is delayed, the prognosis is worsened (139). Thus, **the use of laparoscopy should be limited to suspicious masses that are small enough to be removed intact or utilizing endoscopic bags to allow for cyst aspiration without the leakage of cyst contents into the peritoneal cavity.**

Second-look Laparoscopy

Laparoscopy was initially used before planned second-look laparotomy to identify residual disease and thus avoid the laparotomy. This strategy resulted in a reduction in the need for laparotomy in 50% of patients (140). Improvements in laparoscopic equipment encouraged some investigators to perform the entire second-look procedure by laparoscopy. Childers et al. (129) reported 44 reassessment laparoscopies in 40 women. Twenty-four of the procedures were positive, including five that were only microscopically positive. Five patients (11%) had inadequate laparoscopies because of adhesions; recurrent disease developed in all of them. Eight of the 20 patients (40%) who were negative later developed recurrent disease. All of these data were similar to those obtained with second-look laparotomy. Abu-Rustum et al. (141) reported 31 women having second-look laparoscopy and compared them with 70 patients who had laparotomy and 8 who had both. The rates of positivity were 54.8%, 61.4%, and 62.5%, respectively. The recurrence rates after a negative second-look were 14.8% for laparoscopy versus 14.3% for laparotomy. Clough et al. (142) reported 20 patients who had laparoscopy followed by laparotomy at the same surgery, with a positive predictive value for laparoscopy of 86% (12 of 14 patients).

The effects of the CO_2 pneumoperitoneum and laparoscopy on the long-term survival of women undergoing second-look operations have been reported by Abu-Rustum and associates (143). Over an 11-year period, 289 patients had positive second-look operations. There were 131 laparoscopies using CO_2, 139 laparotomies and 19 laparoscopies converted to laparotomy. The groups were controlled for age, stage, histology, grade, and size of disease found at second look. The median survival for patients who had laparoscopy was 41.1 months and for laparotomy 38.9 months ($p = 0.742$). Thus, **the overall survival was independent of the surgical approach.**

Second-look assessment has generally declined in practice, because approximately 50% of patients with negative second-look surgeries eventually recur (144). However, minimally invasive techniques continue to play a role in the management of patients with advanced ovarian cancer, including the placement of ports for intraperitoneal chemotherapy, if not performed at the initial surgery.

Complications

Complication rates of laparoscopy for malignant disease are higher than for benign disease (145). The rate depends on the type of case and the experience of the surgeon. Laparoscopic second look surgeries have the highest rate of injury to bowel because of the adhesions from previous surgery. Vascular injuries from trocars or the performance of lymphadenectomy can occur in any procedure.

Postoperative wound infection, ileus, and fever occur at lower rates than after laparotomy. Herniation of omentum or bowel into the trocar sites is a complication unique to laparoscopy. Boike et al. (146) reported 19 cases from 11 institutions. No patient had a hernia through a port smaller than 10 cm and therefore it is recommended that all port sites greater than 10 mm be closed. Kadar et al. (147) reported a 0.17% rate of herniation among 3,560 laparoscopic operations.

Abdominal wall port-site implantations have been reported with nearly every tumor type, particularly ovarian cancer. However, in a review of 1,335 transperitoneal laparoscopies in 1,288 women with malignant disease, Abu-Rustum et al. reported that laparoscopy-related subcutaneous tumor implantation is rare, occurring in only 13 (0.97%) cases (148). **Because the presence of ascites predisposes to port-site recurrences, laparoscopy is contraindicated in the presence of ascites.**

Technique

Preoperative Preparation

Patient preparation begins with a clear liquid diet the day before the surgical procedure. Evacuation of the bowel may be accomplished with a laxative or an oral gastrointestinal lavage solution. It is important for the bowel to be collapsed during the laparoscopic lymphadenectomy so that proper exposure can be obtained. This is particularly important if the patient is somewhat obese and para-aortic lymphadenectomy is planned.

Operative Approach

The recommended technique of laparoscopy is as follows:

1. **The patient is positioned in a dorsal lithotomy position with legs in stirrups that give good support to the legs and decrease the tension on the femoral and peroneal nerves** (Fig. 21.9). It is helpful to have adjustable stirrups that allow for conversion from the low lithotomy to a leg-flexed position for vaginal surgery. The arms are tucked

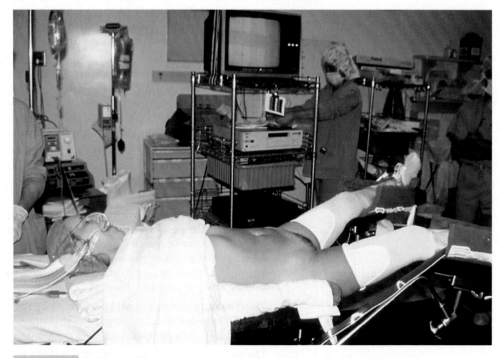

Figure 21.9 Patient position for laparoscopically assisted radical hysterectomy.

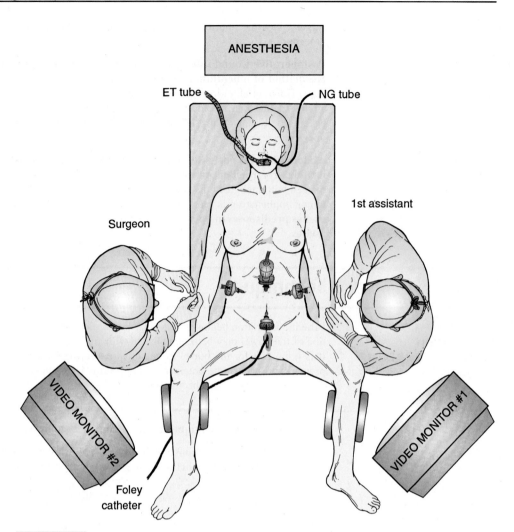

ANESTHESIA

ET tube

NG tube

1st assistant

Surgeon

VIDEO MONITOR #2

VIDEO MONITOR #1

Foley
catheter

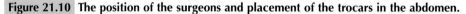

Figure 21.10 The position of the surgeons and placement of the trocars in the abdomen.

at the side, an endotracheal tube is positioned, and a Foley catheter is placed in the bladder.

2. **The first trocar is inserted into the umbilicus if the patient does not have a midline incision. If there is a midline incision,** then a left upper quadrant insufflation and 5-mm trocar are used. The left upper quadrant approach for patients with previous midline incisions allows the laparoscope to be placed away from possible adhesions that can be dissected from the umbilicus before placing the 10-mm trocar.

3. **Additional trocars are placed in the right and left lower quadrants and in the suprapubic site.** Typically, a 10-mm trocar is placed in the suprapubic site so that the laparoscope can be placed in that port to help with packing the bowel or in dissecting adhesions from around the umbilical port (Fig. 21.9, Fig. 21.10).

4. **The bowel should be carefully packed into the upper abdomen so that adequate exposure of the para-aortic area and pelvis can be obtained.** Sponges or minilaparotomy packs can be placed around loops of bowel to aid in exposure and to blot small amounts of blood. The principles of laparoscopic surgery are the same as those of laparotomy. There must be adequate exposure, identification of the anatomy and removal of the appropriate tissue.

5. **The lymphadenectomy is best performed by the surgeon on the side opposite the side of dissection** (i.e., the surgeon on the patient's right side dissects the left pelvic lymph nodes). The peritoneal incisions are left open and drains are not placed.

6. **The para-aortic lymphadenectomy is usually performed first.** The anatomic location of the para-aortic lymphadenectomy is presented in Fig. 21.11, noting the sites of

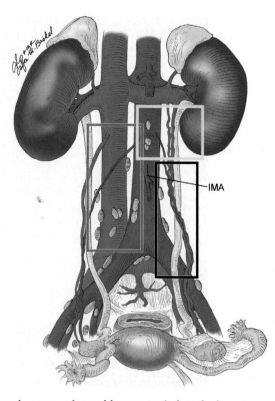

Figure 21.11 Para-aortic transperitoneal laparoscopic lymphadenectomy. The area of the right-sided para-aortic lymphadenectomy is marked by a *red line,* the area of the left-sided inframesenteric lymphadenectomy is marked by a *yellow line,* and the area of the infrarenal lymphadenectomy is marked by a *black line.* (From **Köhler C, Tozzi R, Klemm P, et al.** Laparoscopic para-aortic left-sided transperitoneal infrarenal lymphadenectomy in patients with gynecologic malignancies: Technique and results. *Gynecol Oncol.* 2003;91:139–148.) (12)

the right-sided para-aortic lymphadenectomy (red line), the left-sided inframesenteric lymphadenectomy (yellow line), and the infrarenal lymphadenectomy (black line). Both the right- and left-sided aortic lymph nodes are dissected. The peritoneum is incised between the sigmoid mesentery and the mesentery of the cecum. The right paraaortic nodes are usually dissected first. The lymph node chain is isolated, and dissection is carried out. Monopolar surgery, bipolar surgery, harmonic scalpel, and the argon beam coagulator have all been used successfully. The landmarks are usually the reflection of the duodenum and inferior mesenteric vessel superiorly and the psoas muscles laterally. The ureter must be identified and placed on traction by the assistant to keep it out of the operative field (Fig. 21.11). The lymph node bundle ventral to the vena cava is grasped and ventral traction is applied. The connective tissue between the nodes and the common iliac artery is dissected exposing the vena cava. The dissection is carried cephalad until the duodenum is reached. The upper extent is the right ovarian vein emptying into the vena cava. The left inframesenteric dissection is performed by lifting the sigmoid mesentery ventrally and finding the window under the inferior mesenteric artery IMA. The left ureter is identified. The lymph nodes on the left side are lateral and slightly dorsal to the aorta. The infrarenal left-sided para-aortic lymphadenectomy is initiated by mobilizing and elevating the duodenum and the pancreas. The confluence of the left renal vein and the vena cava is identified, and the upper border of the renal vein is the cranial limit of the lymphadenectomy. The dissection is carried out laterally following the left renal vein. The left ovarian vein is identified underneath the mesocolon. The left ureter is identified and pushed laterally by placing it on traction to keep it out of the operative field. The ureter and the left ovarian vein form the lateral border of the lymph node dissection. The lymph node tissue is dissected away from the **IMA,** which is isolated and preserved. The lymph node and fatty tissue are dissected away from the anterior and lateral aspect of the aorta up to the level of the renal vein and remove *en bloc.* The obese patient will require steeper Trandelenburg postioning and an additional laparoscopic port.

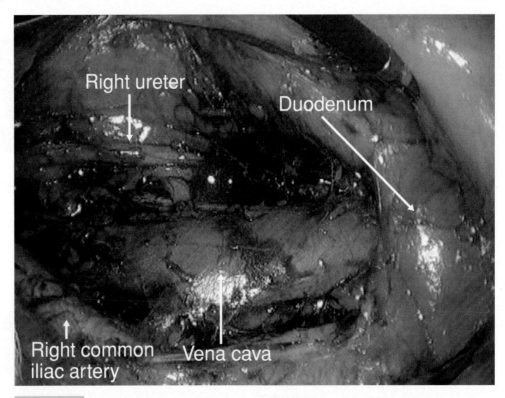

Figure 21.12 Completed right common iliac and lower para-aortic lymphadenectomy.

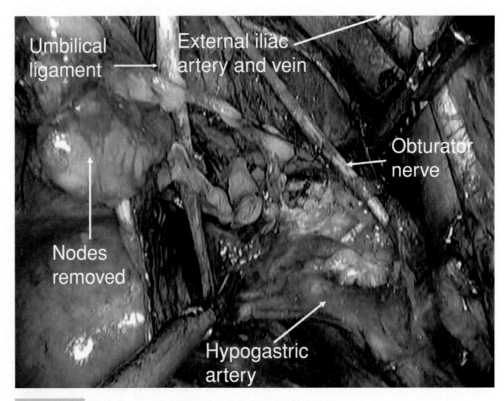

Figure 21.13 Partially completed right pelvic lymphadenectomy.

7. **The proximal common iliac lymph nodes are dissected and removed through the retroperitoneal incision made from the para-aortic lymph nodes down to the middle common iliac lymph nodes.** The remaining common iliac lymph nodes are dissected and removed through the incision for the pelvic lymphadenectomy (Fig. 21.12).

8. **Dividing the round ligaments and finding the lateral pelvic space exposes the pelvic lymph nodes.** The obliterated umbilical artery is retracted medially, which opens the entire lateral pelvic space.

9. **The disease and clinical circumstances, as outlined previously, determine the extent of the pelvic lymphadenectomy.** To perform a **pelvic lymph node sampling,** the lymph nodes are removed medial to the external iliac and anterior to the obturator nerve (Fig. 21.13). For a **complete lymphadenectomy,** the lymph nodes are also removed from between the iliac vessels and the psoas muscle and from the obturator fossa.

10. **All port sites 10 mm or larger should have the fascia and peritoneal layers closed to prevent herniation of bowel.** Several instruments are available to pass the suture through the skin incision lateral to the port and back up on the opposite side. The skin is closed and a local anesthetic is injected around the port site to decrease postoperative pain.

Detailed step-by-step images and details of the operation can be found on this book's website and video of the surgical procedure is available in *LWW Laparoscopy for Gynecology and Oncology* (Kenneth Hatch, MD).

Postoperative Management

Patients are given liquids on the day of surgery and the diet is advanced expeditiously. Early ambulation is encouraged. The patient's progress is usually rapid. **Adynamic ileus is unusual after laparoscopic surgery, but any abdominal distention, worsening of pain, or vomiting must be taken seriously. Unsuspected bowel injuries manifest themselves by abdominal distention, pain, and free air in the peritoneal cavity.** The CO_2 should be absorbed within hours, so any free air in the abdomen is highly suspicious.

References

1. **Dargent D, Salvat J.** *Envahissenent Ganglionnaire Pelvien: Place De La Pelviscopie Retroperitoneale.* Paris: Medsi, McGraw-Hill; 1989.
2. **Childers J, Surwit E.** A combined laparoscopic vaginal approach in the management of stage I endometrial cancer. *Gynecol Oncol.* 1991; 45:46–51.
3. **Nezhat C, Burrell M, Nezhat F.** Laparoscopic radical hysterectomy with para aortic and pelvic node dissection. *Am J Obstet Gynecol.* 1992;166:864–865.
4. **Querleu D, LeBlanc E, Castelain B.** Laparoscopic pelvic lymphaddenectomy in the staging of early carcinoma of the cervix. *Am J Obstet Gynecol.* 1991;164:579–581.
5. **Childers J, Brzechffa P, Hatch K, et al.** Laparoscopically assisted surgical staging (LASS) of endometrial cancer. *Gynecol Oncol.* 1992;51:33–38.
6. **Childers J, Hatch K, Surwit E.** The role of laparoscopic lymphadenectomy in the management of cervical carcinoma. *Gynecol Oncol.* 1992;47:38–43.
7. **Childers J, Hatch K, Tran A-H, et al.** Laparoscopic paraaortic lymphadenectomy in gynecologic malignancies. *Obstet Gynecol.* 1993; 82:741–747.
8. **Spirtos NM, Schlaerth JB, Spirtos TW, et al.** Laparoscopic bilateral pelvic and paraaortic lymph node sampling: An evolving technique. *Am J Obstet Gynecol.* 1995;173:105–111.
9. **Fowler J, Carter J, Carlson JW, et al.** Lymph node yield from laparoscopic lymphadenectomy in cervical cancer: A comparative study. *Gynecol Oncol.* 1993;51:187–192.
10. **Possover M, Krause N, Kuhne-Heid R, et al.** Value of laparoscopic evaluation of paraaortic and pelvic lymph nodes for treatment of cervical cancer. *Am J Obstet Gynecol.* 1998;178: 806–810.
11. **Possover M, Plaul K, Krause N, et al.** Left-sided laparoscopic para-aortic lymphadenectomy: Anatomy of the ventral tributaries of the infrarenal vena cava. *Am J Obstet Gynecol.* 1998;179: 1295–1297.
12. **Köhler C, Tozzi R, Klemm P, et al.** Laparoscopic paraaortic left-sided transperitoneal infrarenal lymphadenectomy in patients with gynecologic malignancies: Technique and results. *Gynecol Oncol.* 2003;91:139–148.
13. **Spirtos NM, Eisenkop SM, Schlaerth JB, et al.** Laparoscopic radical hysterectomy (type III) with aortic and pelvic lymphadenectomy in patients with stage I cervical cancer: Surgical morbidity and inter-mediate follow-up. *Am J Obstet Gynecol.* 2002;187:340–348.
14. **Hertel H, Kohler C, Michels W, et al.** Laparoscopic-assisted radical vaginal hysterectomy (LARVH): Prospective evaluation of 200 patients with cervical cancer. *Gynecol Oncol.* 2003;90:505–511.
15. **Gemignani ML, Curtin JP, Zelmanovich J, et al.** Laparoscopic-assisted vaginal hysterectomy for endometrial cancer: Clinical outcomes and hospital charges. *Gynecol Oncol.* 1999;73:5–11.
16. **Scribner, DR Jr, Walker JL, et al.** Laparoscopic pelvic and para-aortic lymph node dissection: Analysis of the first 100 cases. *Gynecol Oncol.* 2001;82:498–503.
17. **Abu-Rustum NR, Chi DS, Sonoda Y, et al.** Transperitoneal laparoscopic pelvic and para-aortic lymph node dissection using the argon-beam coagulator and monopolar instruments: An 8-year study and description of technique. *Gynecol Oncol.* 2003;89:504–513.
18. **Querleu D, Leblanc E, Cartron G, et al.** Audit of preoperative and early complications of laparoscopic lymph node dissection in 1000 gynecologic cancer patients. *Am J Obstet Gynecol.* 2006;195:1287–1292.
19. **Köhler C, Klemm P, Schau A, et al.** Introduction of transperitoneal lymphadenectomy in a gynecologic oncology center: Analysis of 650 laparoscopic pelvic and/or paraaortic transperitoneal lymphadenectomies. *Gynecol Oncol.* 2004;95:52–61.

20. **Mariani A, Dowdy SC, Cliby WA, et al.** Prospective assessment of lymphatic dissemination in endometrial cancer: A paradigm shift in surgical staging. *Gynecol Oncol.* 2008;109:11–18.

21. **Vasilev SA, McGonigle KF.** Extraperitoneal laparoscopic para-aortic lymph node dissection. *Gynecol Oncol.* 1996;61:315–320.

22. **Dargent D, Ansquer Y, Mathevet P.** Technical development and results of left extraperitoneal laparoscopic paraaortic lymphadenectomy for cervical cancer. *Gynecol Oncol.* 2000;77:87–92.

23. **Querleu D, Dargent D, Ansquer Y, et al.** Extraperitoneal endosurgical aortic and common iliac dissection in the staging of bulky or advanced cervical carcinomas. *Cancer.* 2000;88:1883–1891.

24. **Sonoda Y, Leblanc E, Querleu D, et al.** Prospective evaluation of surgical staging of advanced cervical cancer via a laparoscopic extraperitoneal approach. *Gynecol Oncol.* 2003;91:326–331.

25. **Leblanc E, Narducci F, Frumovitz M, et al.** Therapeutic value of pretherapeutic extraperitoneal laparoscopic staging of locally advanced cervical carcinoma. *Gynecol Oncol.* 2007;105:304–311.

26. **Dowdy SC, Aletti G, Cliby WA, et al.** Extra-peritoneal laparoscopic para-aortic lymphadenectomy–a prospective cohort study of 293 patients with endometrial cancer. *Gynecol Oncol.* 2008;111:418–424.

27. **Ramirez PT, Jhingran A, Macapinlac HA.** Laparoscopic extraperitoneal para-aortic lymphadenectomy in locally advanced cervical cancer: A prospective correlation of surgical findings with positron emission tomography/computed tomography findings. *Cancer.* 2011; 117:1928–1934.

28. **Gil-Moreno A, Magrina JF, Pérez-Benavente A, et al.** Location of aortic node metastases in locally advanced cervical cancer. *Gynecol Oncol.* 2012;125:312–314.

29. **Palomba S, Falbo A, Mocciaro R, et al.** Laparoscopic treatment for endometrial cancer: A meta-analysis of randomized controlled trials (RCTs). *Gynecol Oncol.* 2009;112:415–421.

30. **Tozzi R, Malur S, Köhler C, et al.** Laparoscopy versus laparotomy in endometrial cancer: First analysis of survival of a randomized prospective study. *J Min Invasive Gynecol.* 2005;12:130–136.

31. **Zullo F, Palomba S, Russo T, et al.** A prospective randomized comparison between laparoscopic and laparotomic approaches in women with early stage endometrial cancer: A focus on quality of life. *Am J Obstet Gynecol.* 2005;193:1344–1355.

32. **Malzoni M, Tinelli R, Cosentino F, et al.** Total laparoscopic hysterectomy versus abdominal hysterectomy with lymphadenectomy for early-stage endometrial cancer: A prospective randomized study. *Gynecol Oncol.* 2009;112:126–133.

33. **Janda M, Gebski V, Brand A, et al.** Quality of life after total laparoscopic hysterectomy versus total abdominal hysterectomy for stage I endometrial cancer (LACE): A randomized clinical trial. *Lancet Oncol.* 2010;11:772–780.

34. **Walker JL, Piedmonte MR, Spirtos NM, et al.** Recurrence and survival after random assignment to laparoscopy versus laparotomy for comprehensive surgical staging of uterine cancer: Gynecologic Oncology Group LAP2 study. *J Clin Oncol.* 2012;30: 695–700.

35. **Kornblith AB, Huang HQ, Walker JL, et al.** Quality of Life of Patients With Endometrial Cancer Undergoing Laparoscopic International Federation of Gynecology and Obstetrics Staging Compared With Laparotomy: A Gynecologic Oncology Group Study. *J Clin Oncol.* 2009;27:5337–5342.

36. **Spirtos N, Schlaerth J, Gross GM, et al.** Cost and quality of life analyses of surgery for early endometrial cancer: Laparotomy versus laparoscopy. *Am J Obstet Gynecol.* 1996;174:1795–1799.

37. **Melendez TD, Childers JM, Nour M, et al.** Laparoscopic staging of endometrial cancer: The learning experience. *J Soc Laparoendosc Surg.* 1997;1:45–49.

38. **Scribner DR Jr, Mannel RS, Walker JL, et al.** Cost analysis of laparoscopy versus laparotomy for early endometrial cancer. *Gynecol Oncol.* 1999;75:460–463.

39. **Holub Z, Jabor A, Bartos P, et al.** Laparoscopic surgery for endometrial cancer: Long-term results of a multicentric study. *Eur J Gynaecol Oncol.* 2002;23:305–310.

40. **Khosia I, Lowe C.** Indices of obesity derived from body weight and height. *Br J Prev Med Soc.* 1967;21:122–124.

41. **Holub Z, Bartos P, Jabor A, et al.** Laparoscopic surgery in obese women with endometrial cancer. *J Am Assoc Gynecol Laparosc.* 2000;7:83–88.

42. **Eltabbakh GH, Shamonki MI, Moody JM, et al.** Hysterectomy for obese women with endometrial cancer: Laparoscopy or laparotomy? *Gynecol Oncol.* 2000;78:329–335.

43. **Scribner DR Jr, Walker JL, Johnson GA, et al.** Laparoscopic pelvic and paraaortic lymph node dissection in the obese. *Gynecol Oncol.* 2002;84(3):426–430.

44. **Eltabbakh GH.** Analysis of survival after laparoscopy in women with endometrial carcinoma. *Cancer.* 2002;95:1894–1901.

45. **Malur S, Possover M, Michels W, et al.** Laparoscopic-assisted vaginal versus abdominal surgery in patients with endometrial cancer-a prospective randomized trial. *Gynecol Oncol.* 2001;80: 239–244.

46. **Hatch KD.** Clinical outcomes and long-term survival after laparoscopic staging and hysterectomy for endometrial cancer. *Proc Soc Gynecol Oncol.* 2003;35(abst).

47. **Obermair A, Manolitsas TP, Leung Y, et al.** Total laparoscopic hysterectomy for endometrial cancer: Patterns of recurrence and survival. *Gynecol Oncol.* 2004;92:789–793.

48. **Zapico A, Fuentes P, Grassa A, et al.** Laparoscopic-assisted vaginal hysterectomy versus abdominal hysterectomy in stages I and II endometrial cancer. Operating data, follow up and survival. *Gynecol Oncol.* 2005;98:222–227.

49. **Kim DY, Kim MK, Kim JH, et al.** Laparoscopic-assisted vaginal hysterectomy versus abdominal hysterectomy in patients with stage I and II endometrial cancer. *Int J Gynecol Cancer.* 2005;15:932–937.

50. **Frigerio L, Gallo A, Ghezzi F, et al.** Laparoscopic-assisted vaginal hysterectomy versus abdominal hysterectomy in endometrial cancer. *Int J Gynaecol Obstet.* 2006;93:209–213.

51. **Kalogiannidis I, Lambrechts S, Amant F, et al.** Laparoscopy-assisted vaginal hysterectomy compared with abdominal hysterectomy in clinical stage I endometrial cancer: Safety, recurrence, and long-term outcome. *Am J Obstet Gynecol.* 2007;196:248.e1–e8.

52. **Khoury-Collado F, Abu-Rustum NR.** Lymphatic mapping in endometrial cancer: A literature review of current techniques and results. *Int J Gynecol Cancer.* 2008;18(6):1163–1168.

53. **Burke TW, Levenback C, Tornos C, et al.** Intraabdominal lymphatic mapping to direct selective pelvic and paraaortic lymphadenectomy in women with high-risk endometrial cancer: Results of a pilot study. *Gynecol Oncol.* 1996;62:169–173.

54. **Echt ML, Finan MA, Hoffman MS, et al.** Detection of sentinel lymph nodes with lymphazurin in cervical, uterine, and vulvar malignancies. *South Med J.* 1999;92:204–208.

55. **Li B, Li XG, Wu LY, et al.** A pilot study of sentinel lymph nodes identification in patients with endometrial cancer. *Bull Cancer.* 2007;94:E1–E4.

56. **Frumovitz M, Bodurka DC, Broaddus RR, et al.** Lymphatic mapping and sentinel node biopsy in women with high-risk endometrial cancer. *Gynecol Oncol.* 2007;104:100–103.

57. **Frumovitz M, dos Reis R, Sun CC, et al.** Comparison of total laparoscopic and abdominal radical hysterectomy for patients with early-stage cervical cancer. *Obstet Gynecol.* 2007;110:96–102.

58. **Altgassen C, Pagenstecher J, Hornung D, et al.** A new approach to label sentinel nodes in endometrial cancer. *Gynecol Oncol.* 2007; 105:457–461.

59. **Gargiulo T, Giusti M, Bottero A, et al.** Sentinel lymph node (SLN) laparoscopic assessment in early stage endometrial cancer. *Minerva Ginecol.* 2003;55:259–262.

60. **Pelosi E, Arena V, Baudino B, et al.** Pre-operative lymphatic mapping and intra-operative sentinel lymph node detection in early stage endometrial cancer. *Nucl Med Commun.* 2003;24:971–975.

61. **Barranger E, Cortez A, Grahek D, et al.** Laparoscopic sentinel node procedure using a combination of patent blue and radiocolloid in women with endometrial cancer. *Ann Surg Oncol.* 2004;11:344–349.

62. **Lelievre L, Camatte S, Le Frere-belda MA, et al.** Sentinel lymph node biopsy in cervix and corpus uteri cancers. *Int J Gynecol Cancer.* 2004;14:271–278.

63. **Holub Z, Jabor A, Lukac J, et al.** Laparoscopic detection of sentinel lymph nodes using blue dye in women with cervical and endometrial cancer. *Med Sci Monit.* 2004;10:CR587–CR591.

64. **Niikura H, Okamura C, Utsonomiya H, et al.** Sentinel lymph node detection in patients with endometrial cancer. *Gynecol Oncol.* 2004; 92:669–674.

65. Fersis N, Gruber I, Relakis K, et al. Sentinel node identification and intraoperative lymphatic mapping. First results of a pilot study in patients with endometrial cancer. *Eur J Gynaecol Oncol.* 2004;25:339–342.

66. Raspagliesi F, Ditto A, Kusamura S, et al. Hysteroscopic injection of tracers in sentinel node detection of endometrial cancer: A feasibility study. *Am J Obstet Gynecol.* 2004;191:435–439.

67. Maccauro M, Lucignani G, Aliberti G, et al. Sentinel lymph node detection following the hysteroscopic peritumoural injection of 99mTc-labelled albumin nanocolloid in endometrial cancer. *Eur J Nucl Med Mol Imaging.* 2005;32:569–574.

68. Dargent D. A new future for Schauta's operation through a presurgical retroperitoneal pelviscopy. *Eur J Gynaecol Oncol.* 1987;8:292–296.

69. Querleu D. Laparoscopically assisted radical vaginal hysterectomy. *Gynecol Oncol.* 1993;51:248–254.

70. Hatch KD, Hallum AV III, Nour M. New surgical approaches to treatment of cervical cancer. *J Natl Cancer Inst Monogr.* 1996;21:71–75.

71. Schneider A, Possover M, Kamprath S, et al. Laparoscopy-assisted radical vaginal hysterectomy modified according to Schauta-Stoeckel. *Obstet Gynecol.* 1996;88:1057–1060.

72. Morgan DJ, Hunter DC, McCracken G, et al. Is laparoscopically assisted radical vaginal hysterectomy for cervical carcinoma safe? A case control study with follow up. *BJOG.* 2007;114:537–542.

73. Jackson KS, Das N, Naik R, et al. Laparoscopically assisted radical vaginal hysterectomy vs. radical abdominal hysterectomy for cervical cancer: A match controlled study. *Gynecol Oncol.* 2004;95:655–661.

74. Steed H, Rosen B, Murphy J, et al. A comparison of laparoscopic-assisted radical vaginal hysterectomy and radical abdominal hysterectomy in the treatment of cervical cancer. *Gynecol Oncol.* 2004;93:588–593.

75. Sharma R, Bailey J, Anderson R, et al. Laparoscopically assisted radical vaginal hysterectomy (Coelio-Schauta): A comparison with open Wertheim/Meigs hysterectomy. *Int J Gynecol Cancer.* 2006;16:1927–1932.

76. Malur S, Possover M, Schneider A. Laparoscopically assisted radical vaginal versus radical abdominal hysterectomy type II in patients with cervical cancer. *Surg Endosc.* 2001;15:289–292.

77. Renaud MC, Plante M, Roy M. Combined laparoscopic and vaginal radical surgery in cervical cancer. *Gynecol Oncol.* 2000;79:59–63.

78. Querleu D, Narducci F, Poulard V, et al. Modified radical vaginal hysterectomy with or without laparoscopic nerve-sparing dissection: A comparative study. *Gynecol Oncol.* 2002;85:154–158.

79. Nezhat C, Nezhat F, Burrell MO, et al. Laparoscopic radical hysterectomy with paraaortic and pelvic node dissection. *Am J Obstet Gynecol.* 1994;170:699.

80. Canis M, Mage G, Wattiez A, et al. Vaginally assisted laparoscopic radical hysterectomy. *J Gynecol Surg.* 1992;8:103–104.

81. Puntambekar SP, Palep RJ, Puntambekar SS, et al. Laparoscopic total radical hysterectomy by the Pune technique: Our experience of 248 cases. *J Minim Invasive Gynecol.* 2007;14:682–689.

82. Gil-Moreno A, Puig O, Pérez-Benavente MA, et al. Total laparoscopic radical hysterectomy (type II-III) with pelvic lymphadenectomy in early invasive cervical cancer. *J Minim Invasive Gynecol.* 2005;12:113–120.

83. Malzoni M, Tinelli R, Cosentino F, et al. Feasibility, morbidity, and safety of total laparoscopic radical hysterectomy with lymphadenectomy: Our experience. *J Minim Invasive Gynecol.* 2007;14:584–590.

84. Pomel C, Atallah D, Le Bouedec G, et al. Laparoscopic radical hysterectomy for invasive cervical cancer: 8-year experience of a pilot study. *Gynecol Oncol.* 2003;91:534–539.

85. Fujii S, Takakura K, Matsumura N, et al. Anatomic identification and functional outcomes of the nerve sparing okabayashi radical hysterectomy. *Gynecol Oncol.* 2007;107:4–13.

86. Vidaurreta J, Bermudez A, di Paola G, et al. Laparoscopic staging in locally advanced cervical carcinoma: A new possible philosophy? *Gynecol Oncol.* 1999;75:366–371.

87. Hertel H, Kohler C, Elhawary T, et al. Laparoscopic staging compared with imaging techniques in the staging of advanced cervical cancer. *Gynecol Oncol.* 2002;87:46–51.

88. Dargent D, Martin X, Mathevet P. Laparoscopic assessment of the sentinel lymph nodes in early stage cervical cancer. *Gynecol Oncol.* 2000;79:411–415.

89. Lantzsch T, Wolters M, Grimm J, et al. Sentinel node procedure in Ib cervical cancer: A preliminary series. *Br J Cancer.* 2001;85:791–794.

90. Malur S, Krause N, Kohler C, et al. Sentinel lymph node detection in patients with cervical cancer. *Gynecol Oncol.* 2001;80:254–257.

91. Levenback C, Coleman RL, Burke TW, et al. Lymphatic mapping and sentinel node identification in patients with cervix cancer undergoing radical hysterectomy and pelvic lymphadenectomy. *J Clin Oncol.* 2002;20:688–693.

92. Plante M. Fertility preservation in the management of cervical cancer. *CME J Gynecol Oncol.* 2003;8:128–138.

93. Dargent D, Enria R. Laparoscopic assessment of the sentinel lymph nodes in early cervical cancer. Technique—preliminary results and future developments. *Crit Rev Oncol Hematol.* 2003;48:305–310.

94. Silva LB, Silva-Filho AL, Traiman P, et al. Sentinel node detection in cervical cancer with (99 m)Tc-phytate. *Gynecol Oncol.* 2005;97:588–595.

95. Rob L, Strnad P, Robova H, et al. Study of lymphatic mapping and sentinel node identification in early stage cervical cancer. *Gynecol Oncol.* 2005;98:281–288.

96. Di Stefano AB, Acquaviva G, Garozzo G, et al. Lymph node mapping and sentinel node detection in patients with cervical carcinoma: A 2-year experience. *Gynecol Oncol.* 2005;99:671–679.

97. Angioli R, Palaia I, Cipriani C, et al. Role of sentinel lymph node biopsy procedure in cervical cancer: A critical point of view. *Gynecol Oncol.* 2005;96:504–509.

98. Lin YS, Tzeng CC, Huang KF, et al. Sentinel node detection with radiocolloid lymphatic mapping in early invasive cervical cancer. *Int J Gynecol Cancer.* 2005;15:273–277.

99. Schwendinger V, Müller-Holzner E, Zeimet AG, et al. Sentinel node detection with the blue dye technique in early cervical cancer. *Eur J Gynaecol Oncol.* 2006;27:359–362.

100. Wydra D, Sawicki S, Wojtylak S, et al. Sentinel node identification in cervical cancer patients undergoing transperitoneal radical hysterectomy: A study of 100 cases. *Int J Gynecol Cancer.* 2006;16:649–654.

101. Hauspy J, Beiner M, Harley I, et al. Sentinel lymph nodes in early stage cervical cancer. *Gynecol Oncol.* 2007;105:285–290.

102. Yuan SH, Xiong Y, Wei M, et al. Sentinel lymph node detection using methylene blue in patients with early stage cervical cancer. *Gynecol Oncol.* 2007;106:147–152.

103. Devaja O, Mehra G, Coutts M, et al. A prospective single-center study of sentinel lymph node detection in cervical carcinoma: Is there a place in clinical practice? *Int J Gynecol Cancer.* 2012;22:1044–1049.

104. Dargent D, Brun J, Roy M, et al. Pregnancies following radical trachelectomy for invasive cervical cancer. *Gynecol Oncol.* 1994;52:105(abst).

105. Roy M, Plante M. Pregnancies after radical vaginal trachelectomy for early stage cervical cancer. *Am J Obstet Gynecol.* 1998;179:1491–1496.

106. Dargent D. Radical trachelectomy: An operation that preserves the fertility of young women with invasive cervical cancer. *Bull Acad Natl Med.* 2001;185:1295–1304.

107. Dargent D, Franzosi F, Ansquer Y, et al. Extended trachelectomy relapse: Plea for patient involvement in the medical decision. *Bull Cancer.* 2002;89:1027–1030.

108. Marchiole P, Benchaib M, Buenerd A, et al. Oncological safety of laparoscopic-assisted vaginal radical trachelectomy (LARVT or Dargent's operation): A comparative study with laparoscopic-assisted vaginal radical hysterectomy (LARVH). *Gynecol Oncol.* 2007;106:132–141.

109. Plante M, Renaud MC, François H, et al. Vaginal radical trachelectomy: An oncologically safe fertility-preserving surgery. An updated series of 72 cases and review of the literature. *Gynecol Oncol.* 2004;94:614–623.

110. Shepherd JH, Spencer C, Herod J, et al. Radical vaginal trachelectomy as a fertility-sparing procedure in women with early-stage

cervical cancer-cumulative pregnancy rate in a series of 123 women. *BJOG.* 2006;113:719–724.

111. **Steed H, Covens A.** Radical vaginal trachelectomy and laparoscopic pelvic lymphadenectomy for preservation of fertility. *Postgrad Obstet Gynecol.* 2003;23:1–7.

112. **Burnett AF, Roman LD, O'Meara AT, et al.** Radical vaginal trachelectomy and pelvic lymphadenectomy for preservation of fertility in early cervical carcinoma. *Gynecol Oncol.* 2003;88:419–423.

113. **Schlaerth JB, Spirtos NM, Schlaerth AC.** Radical trachelectomy and pelvic lymphadenectomy with uterine preservation in the treatment of cervical cancer. *Am J Obstet Gynecol.* 2003;188:29–34.

114. **Sonoda Y, Chi DS, Carter J, et al.** Initial experience with Dargent's operation: The radical vaginal trachelectomy. *Gynecol Oncol.* 2008;108:214–219.

115. **Chen Y, Xu H, Zhang Q, et al.** A fertility-preserving option in early cervical carcinoma: Laparoscopy-assisted vaginal radical trachelectomy and pelvic lymphadenectomy. *Eur J Obstet Gynecol Reprod Biol.* 2008;136:90–93.

116. **Plante M, Roy R.** Fertility-preserving options for cervical cancer. *Oncology (Williston Park).* 2006;20:479–488; discussion 491–493.

117. **Lanowska M, Mangler M, Spek A, et al.** Radical vaginal trachelectomy (RVT) combined with laparoscopic lymphadenectomy: Prospective study of 225 patients with early-stage cervical cancer. *Int J Gynecol Cancer.* 2011;21:1458–1464.

118. **Plante M, Gregoire J, Renard MC, et al.** The vaginal radical trachelectomy: An update of a series of 125 cases and 106 pregnancies. *Gynecol Oncol.* 2011;121:290–297.

119. **Shepherd J.** Cervical cancer. *Best Prac Res Clin Obstet Gynaecol.* 2012;26:293–309.

120. **Plante M.** Evolution in fertility-preserving options for early-stage cervical cancer: Radical trachelectomy, simple trachelectomy, neoadjuvant chemotherapy. *Int J Gynecol Cancer.* 2013;23:982–989.

121. **Jolley JA, Battista L, Wing DA.** Management of pregnancy after radical trachelectomy: Case reports and systematic review of the literature. *Am J Perinatol.* 2007;24:531–539.

122. **Nezhat F, Nezhat C, Welander CE, et al.** Four ovarian cancers diagnosed during laparoscopic management of 1011 women with adnexal masses. *Am J Obstet Gynecol.* 1992;167:790–796.

123. **Canis M, Mage G, Pouly JL, et al.** Laparoscopic diagnosis of adnexal cystic masses: A 12-year experience with long-term follow-up. *Obstet Gynecol.* 1994;83:707–712.

124. **Lehner R, Wenzl R, Heinzl H, et al.** Influence of delayed staging laparotomy after laparoscopic removal of ovarian masses later found malignant. *Obstet Gynecol.* 1998;92:967–971.

125. **Childers JM, Nasseri A, Surwit EA.** Laparoscopic management of suspicious adnexal masses. *Am J Obstet Gynecol.* 1996;175:1451–1459.

126. **Canis M, Pouly JL, Wattiez A, et al.** Laparoscopic management of adnexal masses suspicious at ultrasound. *Obstet Gynecol.* 1997;89:679–683.

127. **Boike GM, Graham JE Jr.** Laparoscopic omentectomy in staging and treating gynecologic cancers. *J Am Assoc Gynecol Laparosc.* 1995;2–4(suppl):S4.

128. **Querleu D, LeBlanc E.** Laparoscopic infrarenal paraaortic lymph node dissection for restaging of carcinoma of the ovary or fallopian tube. *Cancer.* 1994;73:1467–1471.

129. **Childers J, Lang J, Surwit E, et al.** Laparoscopic surgical staging of ovarian cancer. *Gynecol Oncol.* 1995;59:25–33.

130. **Pomel C, Provencher D, Dauplat J, et al.** Laparoscopic staging of early ovarian cancer. *Gynecol Oncol.* 1995;58:301–306.

131. **Tozzi R, Köhler C, Ferrara A, et al.** Laparoscopic treatment of early ovarian cancer: Surgical and survival outcomes. *Gynecol Oncol.* 2004;93:199–203.

132. **Chi DS, Abu-Rustum NR, Sonoda Y, et al.** The safety and efficacy of laparoscopic surgical staging of apparent stage I ovarian and fallopian tube cancers. *Am J Obstet Gynecol.* 2005;192:1614–1619.

133. **Spirtos NM, Eisekop SM, Boike G, et al.** Laparoscopic staging in patients with incompletely staged cancers of the uterus, ovary, fallopian tube, and primary peritoneum: A Gynecologic Oncology Group (GOG) study. *Am J Obstet Gynecol.* 2005;193:1645–1649.

134. **Leblanc E, Sonoda Y, Narducci F, et al.** Laparoscopic staging of early ovarian carcinoma. *Curr Opin Obstet Gynecol.* 2006;18:407–412.

135. **Brockbank EC, Harry V, Kolomainen D, et al.** Laparoscopic staging for apparent early stage ovarian or fallopian tube cancer. First case series from a UK cancer centre and systematic literature review. *Eur J Surg Oncol.* 2013;39:912–917.

136. **Dembo AJ, Davy M, Stenwig AE, et al.** Prognostic factors in patients with stage I epithelial ovarian cancer. *Obstet Gynecol.* 1990;75:263–273.

137. **Sevelda P, Vavra N, Schemper M, et al.** Prognostic factors for survival in stage I epithelial ovarian carcinoma. *Cancer.* 1990;65:2349–2352.

138. **Vergote IB, Kaern J, Abeler VM, et al.** Analysis of prognostic factors in stage I epithelial ovarian carcinoma: Importance of degree of differentiation and deoxyribonucleic acid ploidy in predicting relapse. *Am J Obstet Gynecol.* 1993;160:40–52.

139. **Maiman M, Seltzer V, Boyce J.** Laparoscopic excision of ovarian neoplasms subsequently found to be malignant. *Obstet Gynecol.* 1991;77:563–565.

140. **Ozols RF, Fisher RI, Anderson T, et al.** Peritoneoscopy in the management of ovarian cancer. *Am J Obstet Gynecol.* 1981;140:611–619.

141. **Abu-Rustum NR, Barakat RR, Siegel PL, et al.** Second-look operation for epithelial ovarian cancer: Laparoscopy or laparotomy? *Obstet Gynecol.* 1996;88:549–553.

142. **Clough KB, Ladonne JM, Nos C, et al.** Second look for ovarian cancer: Laparoscopy or laparotomy? A prospective comparative study. *Gynecol Oncol.* 1999;72:411–417.

143. **Abu-Rustum NR, Sonoda Y, Chi DS, et al.** The effects of CO_2 pneumoperitoneum on the survival of women with persistent metastatic ovarian cancer. *Gynecol Oncol.* 2003;90:431–434.

144. **Rubin SC, Randall TC, Armstrong KA, et al.** Ten-year follow-up of ovarian cancer patients after second-look laparotomy with negative findings. *Obstet Gynecol.* 1999;93:21–24.

145. **Abu-Rustum N, Barakat R, Curtin J.** Laparoscopic complications in gynecologic surgery for benign or malignant disease. *Gynecol Oncol.* 1998;68:107(abst).

146. **Boike GM, Miller CE, Spirtos NM, et al.** Incisional bowel herniations after operative laparoscopy: A series of nineteen cases and review of the literature. *Am J Obstet Gynecol.* 1995;172:1726–1733.

147. **Kadar N, Reich H, Liu CY, et al.** Incisional hernias after major laparoscopic gynecologic procedures. *Am J Obstet Gynecol.* 1993;168:1493–1495.

148. **Abu-Rustum NR, Rhee EH, Chi DS, et al.** Subcutaneous tumor implantation after laparoscopic procedures in women with malignant disease. *Obstet Gynecol.* 2004;103:480–487.

22 Robotic Surgery

Joshua Z. Press
Walter H. Gotlieb

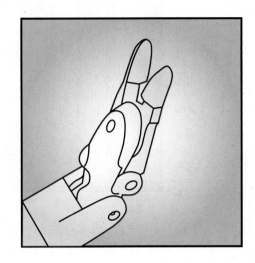

The focus of health care delivery is shifting toward modalities that provide the best value for patients, which requires optimization of the physical, emotional, and economic aspects of care. **Se Assuming oncologic outcomes are maintained, the adoption of minimally invasive surgery (MIS) appears to provide maximum value for patients requiring surgery for gynecologic cancers.** Since the first reports of laparoscopic pelvic and para-aortic lymphadenectomy in the early 1990s (1,2), MIS techniques have been successfully applied to the surgical treatment of most gynecologic cancers. Laparoscopic approaches have been described for endometrial cancer (3), cervical cancer (4), and ovarian cancer (5,6), involving complex procedures such as radical hysterectomy (7), pelvic and para-aortic lymphadenectomy and, less successfully, ovarian cancer debulking (8,9). Numerous retrospective series have highlighted the advantages of laparoscopy over laparotomy for both endometrial cancer (10,11) and cervical cancer (12). **Several prospective randomized studies have demonstrated that treatment of endometrial cancer by laparoscopy significantly reduces morbidity without sacrificing oncologic outcome** (13–15). Benefits include shorter hospitalization, reduced postoperative complications, improved quality of life, and reduced risk of major surgical adverse events (16–18).

Surgeons have encountered a long and steep learning curve for laparoscopy as a result of the limited degree of motion and dexterity offered by the rigid instruments, and the dependence, until very recently, on two-dimensional video images. This has resulted in longer operative times, leading to significant surgeon fatigue, physical strain, and even injury (19). Although experienced, highly skilled laparoscopic surgeons have challenged the limits of laparoscopy for gynecologic malignancies over the past 20 years, until recently adoption of MIS has been limited. **Members of the Society of Gynecologic Oncology (SGO) were surveyed in 2002 and although 84% performed some laparoscopic surgery, 80% of these cases were either for diagnosis of adnexal mass or prophylactic bilateral salpingo-oophorectomy for women at high risk.** Only 56% considered laparoscopy appropriate for endometrial cancer staging, and only 3% of respondents used laparoscopy for more than 50% of their surgeries (20). The broad application of laparoscopy for gynecologic oncology has been hindered by the heterogeneity of gynecologic cancer patients, who are often elderly, obese, and have multiple comorbidities. The largest randomized trial comparing laparoscopy to laparotomy for endometrial cancer staging (LAP2) showed that the rate of conversion to laparotomy for women with body mass index (BMI) >40 kg/m^2 was 57%, and for each 10-year increase in age, the chance of conversion increased by 30% (13). Overall, **the complexity of oncologic procedures and the resulting long learning curve have made it difficult to safely transition to MIS.**

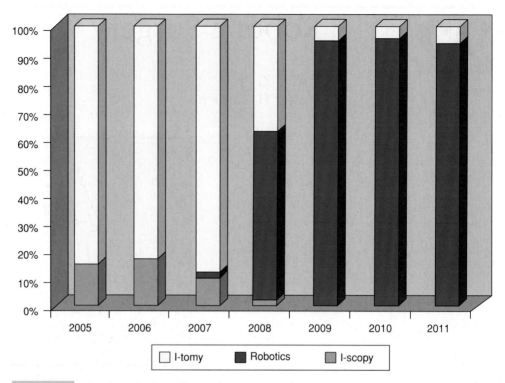

Figure 22.1 **Adoption of minimally invasive surgical techniques for endometrial and cervical cancer surgery.** Introduction of a robotics program in 2007 increased use of MIS from 17% to 66% within 12 months and to over 95% thereafter. (McGill University, Jewish General Hospital, Montreal, Canada) (36).

For many years, laparoscopy appeared to represent an alternative approach offered by expert surgeons with special skills that benefitted only a small number of patients. With the development of new techniques and technologies, it has been possible for a greater number of surgeons to apply MIS to more complex surgery, and to extend the associated benefits to a greater proportion of patients. Examples include the development improved optics, enhanced laparoscopic instrumentation such as bipolar coagulators (e.g., harmonic scalpel, Ligasure, and Plasma Kinetic) (21), and strong endoscopic bags, which allow complex masses and bulky uteri to be removed without spillage of tumor tissue (22). A major advancement leading to increased application of MIS in gynecologic oncology has been the development and implementation of robotic surgical technology. **Since the advent of robotics, there has been a very rapid increase in the use of MIS for women with gynecologic malignancies** (Fig. 22.1). The aim of this chapter is to evaluate how robotics can complement laparoscopy, and further decrease the use of laparotomy for the treatment of gynecologic malignancies.

Robotic Surgery: A Novel MIS Technology

The term "robotics" refers to the introduction of a computer interface and the integration of mechanical arms between the surgeon and the patient. This technology provides increased 7-degree freedom in instrumental range of motion, three-dimensional stereoscopic immersion optics, and wristed instrumentation that allows increased dexterity and tremor reduction, while improving surgeon comfort and reducing surgeon fatigue (23). **Robotics has permitted surgeons to apply open surgical techniques to the MIS setting, thereby increasing adoption of MIS, with a lower rate of conversion to laparotomy even in complicated, elderly, and obese patients** (24,25).

Robotic surgical systems were originally developed by NASA (US National Aeronautics and Space Administration) to permit surgery in space. They were adopted by the United States military to allow field surgery from a distance (26). After this prototype robotic system was acquired by the surgeon and entrepreneur **Frederic H. Moll in 1995,** it was incorporated into a new company called **Intuitive Surgical Devices, Inc. (Sunnyvale, California),** and by the turn of the century, it had been transformed into the first commercially available surgical robot, named the *da Vinci* **Surgical System**.

The first series of robotic hysterectomies was reported in 2002 using the *da Vinci* system, which included one hysterectomy for endometrial cancer (27). **In 2005,** several robotic surgical series for gynecologic cancer were reported (28,29), and **the *da Vinci* system was approved by the FDA (U.S. Food and Drug Administration) for MIS in gynecologic surgery.** By 2008, the feasibility of robotic surgery for endometrial cancer staging was well established, and was shown to have significantly less postoperative morbidity than laparotomy (30).

The introduction of robotics has corresponded with a rapid increase in the application of MIS to endometrial and cervical cancer in particular (31–33). A role has been reported for the staging of early ovarian cancer, and for the treatment of advanced and recurrent disease (34). **The use of robotics has helped increase the proportion of women who are able to benefit from the advantages of MIS, particularly for a certain subset of patients, including the elderly and those with an elevated BMI** (25,35,36). The improved ergonomics afforded by the seated position of the surgeon may decrease surgeon fatigue and injury (37). While many groups report rapid utilization after acquisition of robotic systems, with increases in some centers from 17% to 98% within 2 years (Fig. 22.1) (32), others have questioned whether the technology has been implemented without adequate scientific support (38). As with many innovations, **the adoption of robotics for gynecologic cancer surgery has stimulated controversy, particularly regarding the economics of this expensive technology** (39).

Robotic System: *da Vinci* Surgical System

Although there are several robotic systems in development, the only commercially available system is the *da Vinci* Surgical System (Intuitive Surgical, Inc., Sunnyvale, California, USA), and all publications regarding robotic surgery for gynecologic cancers have utilized this system. **The *da Vinci* surgical system comprises three major components** (Fig. 22.2):

1. **Patient-side Cart**
2. **Computer stand-interface**
3. **Surgeon console**

The surgeon's movements are transmitted from the Surgeon Console through the Computer Interface, and result in movement of the instrument arms on the Patient-side Cart. The camera images are relayed from the camera arm on the Patient-side Cart, through the Computer Interface, and are displayed on the image visor of the Surgeon Console.

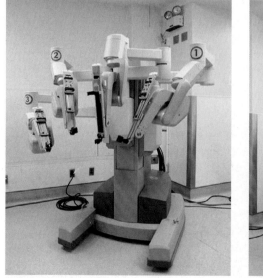

A Patient-side cart

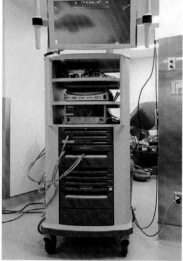

B Computer stand/interface

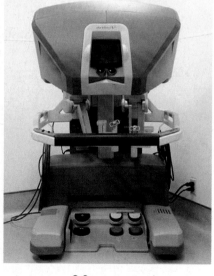

C Surgeon console

Figure 22.2 **Components of the latest generation *da Vinci* Robot, the Si Model: (A) Patient-side Cart (B) Computer Stand/interface (C) Surgeon Console.** Arm *3* can be placed on the right (as presented here) or to the left of the column depending on the surgeon's preference.

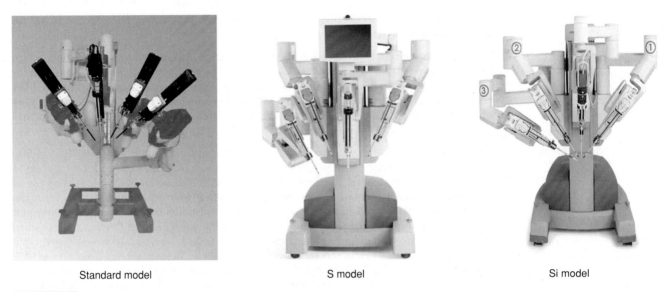

Standard model   S model   Si model

Figure 22.3 **Three generations of the *da Vinci* robot:** Standard Model (2000), S Model (2006), and Si Model (2009).

There have been four generations of the *da Vinci* Surgical System, named the Standard, S, Si, and Xi (Fig. 22.3–Xi not shown). Each generation has incorporated a variety of improvements, including more efficient docking clamps, improved ergonomics at the surgeon console, and finger clutching to allow more efficient master control adjustments. Although the current *da Vinci* systems lack haptic/tactile feedback, surgeons report that the 3D stereoscopic vision system allows for adequate assessment of tissue consistency and control of instrument tension. The new da Vinci Xi version, just introduced in 2014, has a similar console; but the interface and the patient-side cart have been significantly upgraded, with new trocars, camera, and docking mechanisms.

Robotic System Components

Patient-side Cart

This mobile unit (Fig. 22.2A) is positioned beside the patient (Fig. 22.4), and supports the central camera arm and three instrument arms, which are numbered 1, 2, and 3. The Patient-side Cart is

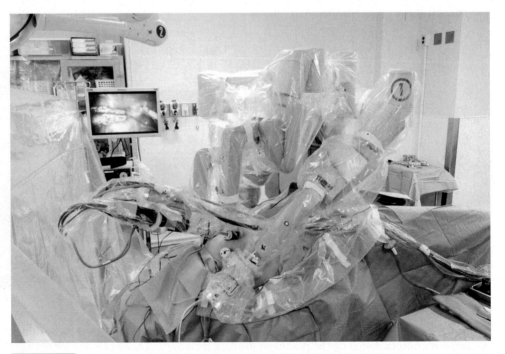

Figure 22.4 **Operating room with robotic system set-up (left-sided docking).**

"docked" to the patient by latching each of these arms to special robotic trocars, which are inserted into the patient's abdomen, similar to laparoscopy. The third instrument arm can be moved to either the right or left side of the Patient-side Cart, depending on the planned procedure. The camera is inserted into the central camera arm, and selected operative instruments can be inserted through instrument arms 1 and 3.

Computer Stand-interface

A computer interface is placed between the Surgeon Console and the Patient-side Cart (Fig. 22.2B). It integrates and transmits information between the surgeon and the Patient-side Cart. This tower includes the gas insufflator and energy source controls.

Surgeon Console

The surgeon sits at the Surgeon Console (Fig. 22.2C) and views the operative field through a high definition, three-dimensional immersion image visor (Fig. 22.5A). None of the robotic arms can move until the surgeon's face is placed against the image visor. Switches on the left side of the Surgeon Console control ergonomic adjustments of the image visor, arm board, and foot pedals to maximize surgeon comfort, allowing the surgeon to maintain a comfortable position throughout the procedure (Fig. 22.5C). A selection screen on the arm board allows for adjustments to a variety of system parameters (e.g., audio, video, and mechanical) and allows for designation of instrument control if using a Dual-Console for teaching (Fig. 22.5E). The Surgeon Console includes hand controls (Fig. 22.5F) and foot pedals (Fig. 22.6), which give the surgeon complete control over the camera and instruments while performing surgical tasks. A clutching mechanism allows the surgeon to adjust the arms and hands to a comfortable position without moving the robotic instruments,

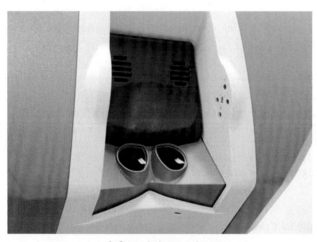

A Console image visor

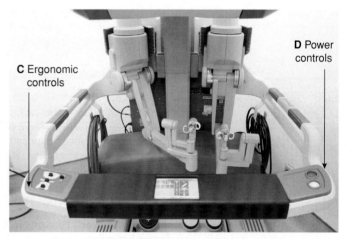

B Surgeon console arm board

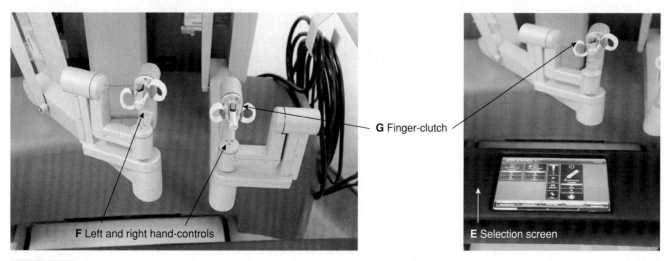

F Left and right hand-controls

G Finger-clutch

E Selection screen

Figure 22.5 *da Vinci* **Robot Si Model surgeon console components.**

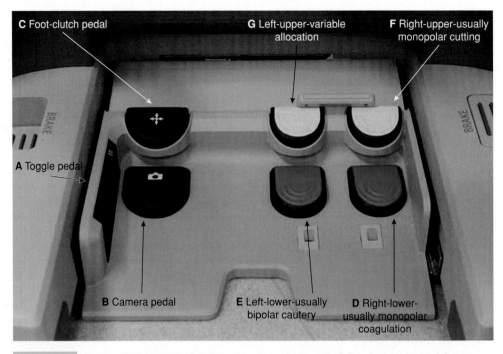

Figure 22.6 *da Vinci* **Robot Si Model: Surgeon Console Foot Pedal components and functions.**

allowing the surgeon to continuously operate "in front of her/him," irrespective of how the robotic arms are oriented in the patient's abdomen.

Surgeon Console—Hand Controls

There are master control handles into which fingers from each of the surgeon's hands fit into one of two master handles to control the movement of the robotic arms and instrument's tips (Fig. 22.5F). In conjunction with the camera pedals, they control camera functions. Twisting the control handles causes the tips of the instruments to rotate, while squeezing the control handles results in opening/ closing of the instrument tips. With the newest Si model, pulling on the finger-clutch levers allows for comfortable adjustment of the surgeon's arms and hands, similar to the foot clutch.

Surgeon Console—Foot Pedals

The ground board contains multiple foot pedals that activate functions associated with different instrument arms (Fig. 22.6):

(a) **Toggle pedal**—this side pedal toggles control of the three instrument arms, such that at any time two arms can be moved. The third inactivated arm is maintained in the position it was last located, including any grasps.

(b) **Camera pedal**—when this foot pedal is activated and held, the robotic arms are immobilized and the hand movements control the camera, including focus, zoom, and camera movements.

(c) **Instrument Foot-clutch pedal**—when the instrument clutch is activated, the arms can be moved without the instrument arms moving, allowing the surgeon to place arms back into a comfortable position wherever operating in the abdomen. On the newer Si model, the clutch is available as a hand clutch (Fig. 22.5G) or a foot clutch, while on the S mode, it is only available as a foot clutch (Fig. 22.6C).

(d) **Right-sided foot pedal lower**—usually allocated to monopolar coagulation (e.g., Curved scissors, Fig. 22.7A).

(e) **Left-sided foot pedal lower**—usually allocated to bipolar cautery (e.g., Maryland grasper, or Fenestrated Grasper, Fig. 22.7B).

(f) **Right-sided foot pedal upper**—usually allocated to monopolar cutting.

(g) **Left-sided foot pedal upper**—multiple use pedal—for additional allocations.

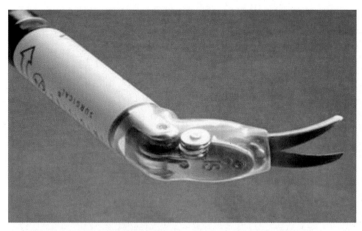

A Curved scissors – monopolar

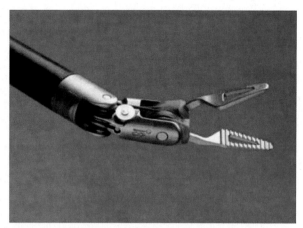

B Maryland dissector – bipolar

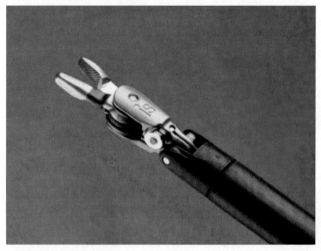

C Suture-cut needle driver

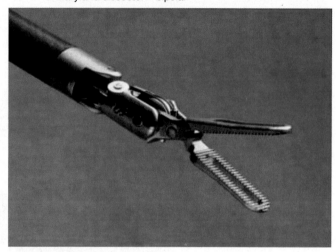

D Prograsp

Figure 22.7 **Commonly used instruments in gynecologic cancer surgeries.**

Patient Positioning, Docking, and Instrumentation

Preparation and positioning is particularly important for robotic surgery because after the robot is docked, the Patient-side Cart and operative table cannot be moved without undocking. Successful application of robotics requires a well-trained operating room team to ensure that preparation and docking occurs efficiently. For most gynecologic oncologic procedures, the patient is placed in the lithotomy position with legs in adjustable stirrups, and is secured to the bed with gel pads or shoulder bolsters to prevent movement after placement into steep Trendelenburg position.

The procedure is initiated in a similar fashion to traditional laparoscopy by insufflating the abdomen with carbon dioxide gas, using a Veress needle, blunt trocar entry, or by inserting a trocar under direct vision via an open laparoscopic technique, or using transparent trocars and a camera. The exact location for port placement will depend on the planned procedure. **A general position of trocars needed to complete a hysterectomy or radical hysterectomy with pelvic and para-aortic lymphadenectomy is shown in** Figure 22.8A. This includes a 12-mm port for the camera (Fig. 22.8B) and three 8-mm ports for the robotic instrument arms (Fig. 22.8C). Most surgeons will also place one 12-mm accessory port for a bedside assistant, who can use suction, pass sutures or surgical clips, or remove specimens.

Docking technique and trocar placement are particularly important components of robotic surgery, because the arms are set in place after docking. Although the original technique for hysterectomy involved docking the Patient-side Cart between the patient's legs (front-docking), many surgeons

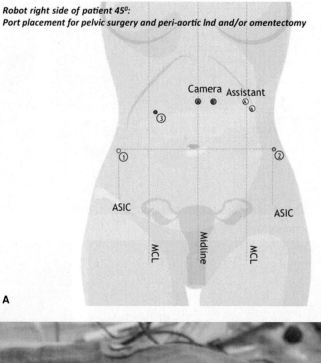

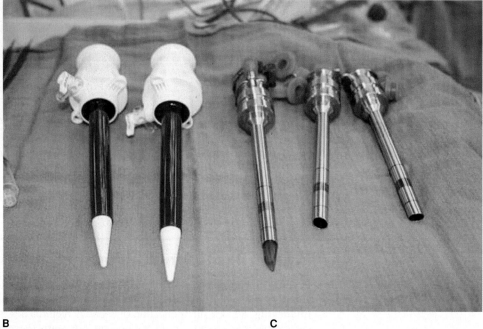

Figure 22.8 A: Typical trocar placement sites for robotic hysterectomy and lymphadenectomy: Camera can be placed at either *blue* markings, avoiding the falciform ligament. The assistant port moves in accordance. Robotic trocar sites are indicated by numbers. For left-sided docking, the port site locations are reversed. **B: 12-mm and accessory trocars, C: 8-mm robotic trocars.**

now use side docking or parallel docking because this permits access to the vagina for uterine manipulation or the removal of specimens (22). Side docking and parallel docking can be performed from either the right or left side of the patient depending on which side the surgeon would prefer to swing the third arm (Fig. 22.9A,B). **One challenge for robotic gynecologic oncologic surgery has been accessing multiple quadrants to permit resection of more advanced disease, mainly in the upper abdomen. Surgeons have found that by undocking, rotating the patient and/or the patient cart during the surgery and redocking over the patient's shoulder (Fig. 22.9C), it is possible to access the upper abdominal quadrants for dissection of organs such as the diaphragm, liver, and spleen.**

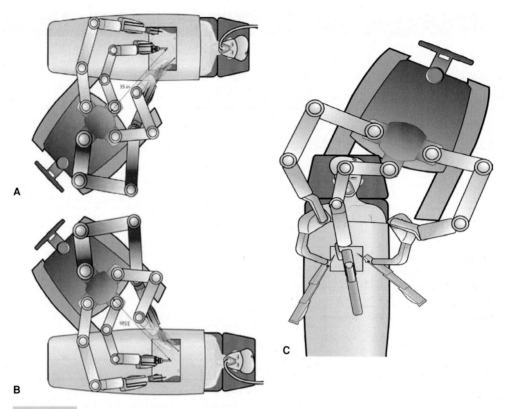

Figure 22.9 Docking Techniques: A: Left-Side docking, **B:** Right-Side docking, **C:** Over shoulder/head docking for upper abdominal resection.

After the instrument arms have been docked to the trocars, the camera and surgical instruments can be introduced through the trocars and secured to the robotic arms. The camera arm can be fitted with either an 8.5-mm or 12-mm high-definition endoscope (0° or 30°). A variety of instruments have been developed including those for grasping, dissecting, and suturing (examples shown in Fig. 22.7). In addition to these standard instruments, a variety of specialty instruments have been adapted for use with the robotic platform, such as Clip Appliers, Vessel Sealers, Harmonic ACE, PK Dissecting Forceps, and bowel stapling devices. Many surgeons will also use a uterine manipulator to assist with positioning of the uterus during the dissection, and to facilitate the colpotomy. **Commonly used uterine manipulators include the RUMI** (Cooper Surgical, Turnbull, CT, USA), **V-CARE** (ConMed, Utica, NY, USA), **and HOHL manipulator** (Karl Storz, Tuttlingen, GE). Although some have hypothesized that placing a manipulation tool into the uterine cavity could result in dissemination of cancer cells into the peritoneal cavity, published data indicate this has no clinical significance (40–42). Alternatives without intrauterine components have been proposed to alleviate this potential issue (22).

Robotic Applications in Gynecologic Oncology

Robotic surgery has been used to treat uterine cancer, cervical cancer, and ovarian cancer. Robotic techniques have been described for most components of gynecologic cancer surgery, including extrafascial hysterectomy, radical hysterectomy, radical trachelectomy, staging with pelvic and para-aortic lymphadenectomy, debulking procedures, and pelvic exenteration. Although there have been numerous publications demonstrating the feasibility and advantages of robotic techniques, **there have been no randomized trials comparing robotic surgery with either laparotomy or laparoscopy**. Most publications compare a series of robotic cases to a contemporary cohort of cases done by laparoscopy and/or laparotomy, or to a group of historical controls. Despite being very encouraging, interpreting these studies can be difficult, as they are limited by weaknesses such as selection bias, reporting bias, and learning curve differences.

Table 22.1 Studies of Robotics for Unselected Patients with Endometrial Cancer

Author	Year	Technique	N	BMI	Age	OR Time (min)	EBL (mL)	Transfusion (%)	Hospital Stay (days)	Overall Complications (%)	Conversion Rate (%)
Bell et al. (46)	2008	Robotic	40	33	63	184	166	5	2.3	7.5	N/A
		Laparotomy	40	32	72	109	317	10	4	28	N/A
		Laparoscopy	30	32	68	171	253	15	2	20	
Boggess et al. (30)	2008	Robotic	103	33	62	191	75	1	1	5.8	2.9
		Laparotomy	138	35	64	147	266	1.5	4.4	29.7	—
		Laparoscopy	81	29	62	213	146	2.5	1.2	13.6	4.9
DeNardis et al. (49)	2008	Robotic	56	29	59	177	105	0	1	21	5.4
		laparotomy	106	34	63	79	241	8.5	3.2	61	—
Seamon et al. (53)	2009	Robotic	105	34	59	242	88	3	1	13	12
		Laparoscopy	76	29	57	287	200	18	2	14	26
Holloway et al. (54)	2009	Robotic	100	29	60	171	103	0	1.1	20	4
Peiretti et al. (55)	2009	Robotic	80	25	58	181	44	1.3	2.5	24	3.8
Lowe et al. (56) (Database)	2009	Robotic	405	32	62	171	88	0	1.8	18	6.7
Cardenas-Goicoechea et al. (51)	2010	Robotic	102	32	62	237	109	2.9	1.9	9.8	1
		Laparoscopy	173	33	60	178	187	1.7	2.3	7.5	5.2
Paley et al. (31)	2011	Robotic	377	31	62	184	47	0.5	1.4	6.4	2.9
		Laparotomy	131	32	63	139	198	0.8	5.3	20.6	—
Coronado et al. (47)	2012	Robotic	71	29	67	189	99	4.2	3.5	21	2.4
		Laparotomy	192	30	65	157	232	14	8.1	35	—
		Laparoscopy	84	27	66	218	190	7.1	4.6	29	8.3
Backes et al. (48)	2012	Robotic	471	32	60	N/A	90	3	1	7.2	6.4
		laparotomy	32[a]	—	—	—	—	—	—	12.5	—
ElSahwi et al. (50)	2012	Robotic	155	35	62	127	119	1.3	1.5	20	0
		Laparotomy	150	33	65	141	185	7.7	4	69	—
Lau et al. (32)[b]	2012	Robotic	143	32	65	241	74	1.4	2.2	13	4.2
		Laparotomy	160	29	66	207	266	6.3	5.5	42	—
Leitao et al. (52)	2012	Robotic	347	29	60	184	100	0.3	2	14	11
		Laparoscopy	302	28	62	213	50	0.4	1	10	13
Fader et al. (11) (Mixed MIS)	2012	MIS[d]	191	30	65	193	N/A	N/A	1	8.4	9.9
		Laparotomy	192	32	67	135			4	31	—
OVERALL (Means)[c]		**Robotic**	**2555**	**31**	**61**	**186**	**86**	**1**	**1.6**	**13**	**5.7**
		Laparotomy	**949**	**31**	**63**	**142**	**227**	**7**	**5.1**	**40**	**—**
		Laparoscopy	**746**	**29**	**62**	**211**	**131**	**4**	**1.9**	**13**	**11**

[a]Comparison group consisted of the robotic surgeries converted to laparotomy.

[b]Control group included 133 laparotomies and 27 laparoscopies.

[c]Summarized data from all listed studies were weighted by number of patients in each study to create the overall mean.

[d]MIS cases included 65% robotic and 35% laparoscopic cases.

N/A = data not available in the manuscript.

Endometrial Cancer

Most of the first reports of robotic gynecologic oncologic surgery involved hysterectomy and staging of endometrial cancer. Numerous series have reported the success of robotics for endometrial cancer staging, and have shown decreased morbidity compared to laparotomy, with low rates of conversion (Table 22.1). In addition, there have been two systematic reviews of the safety and effectiveness of robotic surgery for endometrial cancer (43,44). Both of these reviews have demonstrated that **compared to laparotomy, robotic or laparoscopic surgery for endometrial cancer is associated with increased operative time, but significantly decreased blood loss, need for transfusion, hospital stay, and postoperative complications.** Although the accuracy, reproducibility, and comparison between pathology laboratories is questionable, pelvic and para-aortic lymph node counts with robotics is at least equivalent and possibly better than laparotomy. A comparison between robotics and standard laparoscopy has demonstrated lower postoperative pain and pain medication requirements when robotic surgery has been used for endometrial cancer staging (45). **One important observation from robotic studies is the low rate of conversion to laparotomy, which ranges from 1–12%,** even among subgroups known to be technically challenging for MIS approaches, such as the obese and elderly populations (Table 22.1).

Robotics in Obese Patients

Endometrial cancer frequently affects women with high BMI, who are also at increased surgical risk as a result of associated comorbidities such as diabetes, hypertension, and atherosclerosis. Although the elevated surgical risk in these patients makes them ideal candidates for MIS, conversion rates with laparoscopy have been high in these women. In the LAP2 study, the overall conversion rate from laparoscopy to laparotomy was 25%, but increased to 57% in patients with BMI > 40 (17). **Robotic surgery has been particularly useful in facilitating MIS for women with increased BMI** (Table 22.2). Lau et al. compared endometrial cancer staging procedures for women with BMI < 30, 30 to 39, and 40 to 59 and demonstrated that, despite more frequent comorbidities in the more obese subgroup, there were no significant differences in surgical console time, major postoperative complications, overall wound complications, or length of hospitalization (25). The conversion rate was only 10% in those with BMI 40 to 59, and all the conversions were by mini laparotomy to remove an enlarged uterus that could not be removed intact through the vagina. **When compared to laparotomy, the use of robotic endometrial cancer staging for women with an elevated BMI is associated with fewer complications, shorter hospital stay, and equivalent lymph node counts, with a conversion rate around 15%** (24,35). **A retrospective**

Table 22.2 Studies of Robotics for Obese and Elderly Patients with Endometrial Cancer

Author	Year	Technique	N	BMI	Age	OR Time (min)	EBL (mL)	Transfusion (%)	Hospital Stay (days)	Overall Complications (%)	Conversion Rate (%)
Obese Patients											
Gehrig et al. (57) (BMI > 30)	2008	Robotic	49	38	61	189	50	—	1	6.5	0
		Laparoscopy	32	35	61	215	250	—	1.3	17	9.4
Seamon et al. (24) (BMI > 30)	2009	Robotic	109	40	58	228	109	2	1	11	15.6
		Laparotomy	191	40	62	143	394	9	3	27	—
Lau et al. (25) (All Robotic)	2011	(BMI < 30)	52	46	69	237	64	1.9	1	15	5.7
		(BMI 30–40)	33	34	67	255	96	6	2	36	3
		(BMI > 40)	23	25	55	257	94	0	2	17	8.7
Bernardini et al. (35) (BMI > 35)	2012	Robotic	45	40	61	270	200	2.2	2	16	4.4
		Laparotomy	41	42	62	165	300	7.3	4	44	—
Elderly Patients											
Lowe et al. (58) (All Robotic)	2010	(All ages)	395	32	62	167	50	0	1	19	7
		(Age 80–95)	27	28	84	192	50	0	1	37	3.7
Vaknin et al. (36) (All Robotic)	2010	(Age < 70)	59	29	57	243	81	2	1	20	7
		(Age > 70)	41	33	78	253	83	0	2	17	5

comparison of robotic and laparoscopic endometrial cancer surgery for obese women showed shorter operative times, less blood loss, increased lymph node counts, and shorter hospital stay with the robotic approach (57).

Robotics in Elderly Patients

Another group who may particularly benefit from robotic surgery is elderly women (Table 22.2). The endometrial cancers diagnosed in elderly women are frequently of high-grade aggressive histology, and optimal surgery may require extensive lymphadenectomy in patients with additional complex comorbidities. In the LAP2 study, the conversion rate increased by 30% for every additional decade of age (13). In contrast, **a comparison of robotic surgery for women younger than 70 years of age to women greater than 70 demonstrated similar operative times, blood loss, and overall perioperative morbidity, with a conversion rate of only 5% in women older than 70 years** (36) and 3.7% in women over the age of 80 (58). Overall, robotic surgery can help facilitate thorough surgery in fragile, elderly patients with aggressive endometrial cancers.

In summary, although randomized clinical trials are lacking, multiple studies have shown decreased morbidity compared to laparotomy, with low rates of conversion. Two studies have shown equivalent recurrence-free survival (32,59), and one has shown equivalent 5-year survival following robotic surgery for endometrial cancer (60).

Cervical Cancer

Radical Hysterectomy

Compared to endometrial cancer, the transition to MIS for treatment of cervical cancer has been slower, which is likely related to the technical complexity and steep learning curve of conventional laparoscopic radical hysterectomy. However, since the introduction of robotics, there has been a rapid increase in the use of MIS for radical hysterectomy and treatment of cervical cancer. **Based on the small retrospective series published, it appears that robotic radical hysterectomy is feasible, associated with less morbidity than laparotomy, and seems to be easier to implement than traditional laparoscopy** (Table 22.3). A systematic review comparing 327 robotic, 1,339 laparoscopic, and 1,552 open radical hysterectomies showed that the MIS approaches had significantly less blood loss, transfusion requirements, and postoperative infectious morbidity, with similar oncologic outcomes (12). Robotic surgery was also associated with less postoperative narcotic pain medication, quicker resumption of regular diet, and shorter hospitalization (61).

The pathologic features of radical hysterectomy specimens are similar between robotic, laparoscopy, and laparotomy, including parametrial and vaginal resection margin lengths, lymph node counts, and risk of positive surgical margins (64,68). Thus, there is no difference in the proportion of patients requiring adjuvant therapy after robotic radical hysterectomy. Based on available data, progression-free and overall survival after robotic radical hysterectomy for cervical cancer appears to be at least equivalent to laparotomy (66). A multicenter Phase III randomized clinical trial is currently accruing patients, comparing MIS radical hysterectomy (total laparoscopic or robotic) with open radical hysterectomy for Stage IA1 to IB1 cervical cancer (NCT00614211) with an estimated completion date in 2017 (74).

In summary, evidence from available retrospective series for cervical cancer reveals decreased morbidity with robotics and similar recurrence rates, progression-free survival, and disease-specific survival, when compared to open laparotomy (66).

Radical Trachelectomy

Women with cervical cancer are frequently diagnosed in the reproductive age group, so fertility preservation can be an important issue. The use of radical trachelectomy for early cervical cancer has been shown to have similar efficacy and safety compared with radical hysterectomy (75). Plante et al. showed that vaginal radical trachelectomy with laparoscopic lymphadenectomy is oncologically safe for women with cervical tumors less than 2 cm in size, and has good fertility and obstetrical outcomes (76). The feasibility of robotic radical trachelectomy with sparing of the main branches of the uterine artery was described in 2008 (77), and the possible benefits of the robotic technique have been elucidated in several small series (78–81). Persson et al. compared robotic radical trachelectomy in 13 patients with vaginal radical trachelectomy in 12 patients and found that the cervical length was equal, but there was a more accurate placement of the cervical cerclage with the robotic approach (78). Nick et al. reported on 37 patients who underwent attempted radical trachelectomy

Table 22.3 Studies of Robotic Radical Hysterectomy for Cervical Cancer

Author	Year	Technique	N	BMI	Age	OR Time (min)	Blood Loss (mL)	Trans-fusion (%)	Conver-sions (%)	Complica-tions (%)	Hospital Stay (days)	Positive Margins (%)	Recurrences (%)
Magrina et al. (63)	2008	Robotic	27	27	50	190	133	3.7	0	22	1.7	N/A	0
		Laparotomy	31	27	51	167	444	9.7	—	23	3.6	—	0
		Laparoscopy	35	27	55	220	208	0	0	19	2.4	—	0
Boggess et al. (65)	2008	Robotic	51	29	47	211	96	0	0	7.8	1	N/A	1.9
		Laparotomy	42	26	42	248	417	8	—	16	3.2	—	—
Ko et al. (67)	2008	Robotic	16	28	42	290	82	6.3	0	18	1.7	0	0
		Laparotomy	32	27	42	219	660	31	—	25	4.9	6.2	0
Nezhat et al. (71)	2008	Robotic	13	N/A	55	323	157	00	0	46	2.7	0	0
		Laparoscopy	30		47	318	200	—	0	27	3.8	3.3	0
Estape et al. (62)	2009	Robotic	32	30	55	144	130	3.1	0	22	2.6	16	3.2
		Laparotomy	14	30	42	114	621	36	—	35	4	18	14.3
		Laparoscopy	17	28	53	132	209	0	0	29	2.3	21	0
Maggioni et al. (68)	2009	Robotic	40	24	44	272	78	7.5	0	48	3.7	0	13
		Laparotomy	40	24	50	200	222	23	—	—	5	7.5	13
Lowe et al. (72)	2009	Robotic	42	25	41	215	50	0	2.4	17	1	0	0
Persson et al. (73)	2009	Robotic	80	24	48	262	150	0	3.8	59	3	19[a]	3.8
Cantrell et al. (66)	2010	Robotic	63	28	43	213	50	N/A	0	4.8	1	2	1.6
		Laparotomy	64	25	42	240	400	—	—	13	4	4	12.5
Halliday et al. (61)	2010	Robotic	16	26	49	351	106	0	0	19	1.9	0	0
		Laparotomy	24	25	47	283	546	13	—	41	7.2	0	0
Nam et al. (69)	2010	Robotic	32	22	45	219	220	3.1	0	75	12	N/A	6.3
		Laparotomy	32	22	46	210	532	64	—	56	17	—	—
Schreuder et al. (70)	2010	Robotic	13	N/A	43	434	300	N/A	0	7.6	4	N/A	15
		Laparotomy	14		46	225	2,000	—	—	21	9	—	7.1
Sert and Abeler (64)	2011	Robotic	35	25	44	263	82	N/A	0	20	3.8	0	14
		Laparotomy	26	23	45	163	595	—	—	86	9.2	0	0
		Laparoscopy	6	25	45	364	164	—	0	46	8.4	0	0
OVERALL (Means)		**Robotic**	460	26	46	242	113	2	1	30	2.9	6	4
		Laparotomy	319	25	45	215	530	25	—	40	6.3	5	5
		Laparoscopy	88	27	51	246	202	0	0	26	3.3	9	0

[a]Less than 8-mm of free margin as per institutional protocol; N/A = data not available in the manuscript.

(12 robotic and 25 laparotomy) and found that 5 required conversion to complete hysterectomy as a result of close endocervical margins (4 robotic, 1 open). The robotic cases had less blood loss and decreased hospitalization, with no difference in surgical time or serious morbidity (82).

Specialized Techniques

Nerve-sparing techniques for radical hysterectomy and radical trachelectomy require meticulous dissection to preserve the hypogastric nerve plexus in an attempt to reduce postoperative bladder and rectal dysfunction (83). Authors have speculated that the precision and stereotactic vision of robotics may help facilitate these nerve-sparing approaches (84). **Although reports are limited, feasibility has been reported for nerve-sparing radical hysterectomy** (84),

nerve-sparing radical trachelectomy (85), **and nerve-sparing parametrectomy** (86). Hong et al. compared one surgeon's experience with their first 50 robotic nerve-sparing radical hysterectomies and first 50 laparoscopic nerve-sparing radical hysterectomies and reported less blood loss and a lower intraoperative complication rate with the robotic approach. **Other advanced procedures that have been performed robotically include extraperitoneal para-aortic lymphadenectomy up to the left renal vein** (87,88) **and transperitoneal infrarenal aortic lymphadenectomy** (89).

Ovarian Cancer

Adoption of laparoscopy for the management of ovarian cancer remains limited (90) and has mainly focused on early stage disease (6,91). A consensus statement released by the SGO in 2012 suggested that as a result of limited upper abdominal access, "early-stage or small-volume disease may be more amendable than more advanced disease to robotic surgery" (33). This limitation has been challenged by the development of novel multiquadrant docking and positioning techniques that facilitate access to upper abdominal disease. **Although there continues to be controversy regarding oncologic outcome, robotics has been successfully applied to the treatment of advanced ovarian cancer, including primary debulking surgery with radical dissection such as supracolic omentectomy, diaphragmatic stripping, and splenectomy.** Magrina et al. reported a series of 25 patients with epithelial ovarian cancer undergoing primary surgical debulking using robotics, with comparison to a similar historical group undergoing laparoscopy and laparotomy (34). The robotic approach resulted in less blood loss and decreased hospital stay, with similar overall survival. However, **the benefits of robotics were not seen in patients requiring major procedures, such as bowel resection, full thickness diaphragmatic resection, liver resection, or splenectomy** (34).

Robotics may serve as a tool for interval debulking surgery after neoadjuvant chemotherapy for advanced disease. Complete surgical cytoreduction results in a significant improvement in survival, motivating many surgeons to perform aggressive radical primary debulking surgeries (92). However, others have advocated the use of neoadjuvant chemotherapy to decrease tumor burden prior to attempting complete cytoreduction, followed by additional chemotherapy. A multicenter randomized controlled trial has demonstrated equivalent oncologic outcomes between these two approaches, but with significantly less surgical morbidity in the neoadjuvant chemotherapy and interval debulking arm (93). The impressive reduction in tumor burden sometimes seen after neoadjuvant chemotherapy has inspired some surgeons to perform the interval debulking surgery robotically, with the intention of decreasing perioperative morbidity, and allowing additional chemotherapy to be started earlier. **Encouraging results from robotic interval debulking surgeries have been presented at meetings and peer reviewed manuscripts are expected shortly.**

Another application of robotics in ovarian cancer has been for secondary cytoreduction. The goal may be complete cytoreduction after a patient has achieved a prolonged disease-free interval following chemotherapy, or it may be to excise disease that is causing symptoms. The feasibility of robotic secondary cytoreduction has been reported in a selected series of patients with recurrent ovarian cancer and compared with laparotomy (94). In this series, robotic surgery was associated with reduced blood loss and shorter hospital stay, but had similar operating time, complications, and complete debulking compared to laparotomy (94). Components of robotic secondary cytoreduction have included resection of isolated liver and full thickness diaphragmatic recurrence, and this required docking over the right shoulder (95). At present, **the use of robotics in advanced ovarian cancer is still investigational and its widespread implementation will likely be linked to the development of improved systemic treatments.**

In summary, the role of robotics for advanced and recurrent ovarian cancer is being investigated. **The most appropriate use of robotics in ovarian cancer is for the comprehensive staging of apparent early-stage disease.**

Pelvic Exenteration

The use of robotics for recurrent cervical cancer has been reported in several small case series, including total pelvic exenteration (96,97) and anterior pelvic exenteration (98). Although these reports are limited, authors have suggested that use of the robotic technique is associated with less blood loss and shorter hospitalization compared with laparotomy.

Sentinel Lymph Nodes

Sentinel lymph nodes have found a role in a variety of cancers, including breast cancer, melanoma, and vulvar cancer, allowing for assessment of lymphatic metastases while minimizing surgical morbidity. The utility of sentinel lymph node assessment has also been suggested for cervical cancer (99) and endometrial cancer (100), potentially allowing identification of patients requiring adjuvant treatment without the morbidity of complete lymphadenectomy.

A variety of techniques have been developed, usually involving cervical injection of technetium-99 (Tc-99), combined with colored dye, such as isosulfan blue or methylene blue. The enhanced visual system and instrumental dexterity of the robotic platform has been applied to locating and removing sentinel lymph nodes in endometrial cancer using these traditional techniques (101). In addition, **the visual system of the *da Vinci* Si model includes near-infrared fluorescent imaging capabilities, which facilitates newer techniques for sentinel nodes detection using Indocyanine Green (ICG) fluorescent dye.** It is possible for the surgeon to toggle the camera between the regular color mode and a special near-infrared mode, which highlights lymphatic channels and lymph nodes containing the ICG dye (Fig. 22.10). The use of the *da Vinci* near-infrared system with ICG dye has been associated with an increased sentinel lymph node detection rate in endometrial cancer, with the bilateral detection rate being reported from 80–100% (102,103).

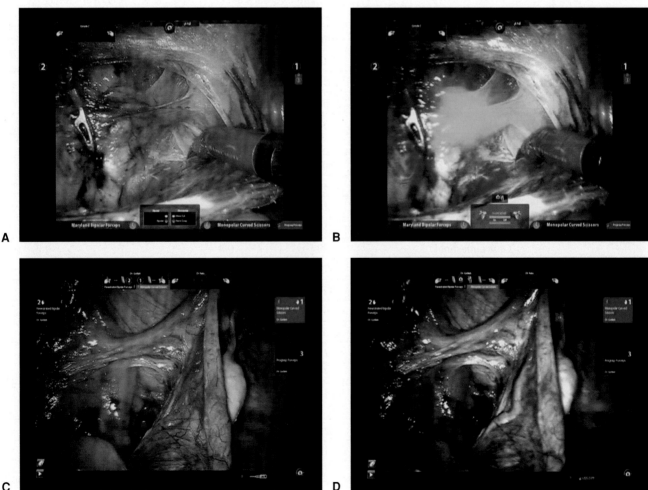

Figure 22.10 Sentinel lymph node visualization following cervical injection. A: Sentinel pelvic node visualized with methylene blue dye, **B:** Same sentinel node visualized with ICG dye, **C:** Lymphatic channel in IP ligament visualized with methylene blue dye, **D:** Same lymphatic channel visualized with ICG dye.

Complications

The use of MIS techniques has significantly decreased hospital stay and morbidity for gynecologic oncologic surgery (34), particularly with respect to intraoperative blood loss, transfusion requirements, and postoperative wound complications for endometrial cancer staging (48,104) and for radical hysterectomy (105). As with laparoscopy, patients undergoing robotic surgery must tolerate a pneumoperitoneum while in steep Trendelenburg for prolonged periods of time. Particular attention must be directed to patient positioning, and protection with padding to avoid injury. Despite requiring extended periods of time in this potentially compromised position, anesthetic complications are rare (106), even in patients with high (ASA 3–4) anesthetic risk (107).

Overall complication rates for endometrial cancer staging procedures are similar between robotics (8.1%) and laparoscopy (9.8%), and are less than with laparotomy (104). Reports regarding specific complications with robotic surgery vary widely, depending on how complications are defined, and the strategy used for investigation and documentation (108). A summary of the incidence of specific intraoperative and postoperative complications reported in studies of robotic surgery for endometrial and cervical cancer is shown in Table 22.4.

Table 22.4 Complications Associated with Robotic Surgery. Pooled Data from the Studies Listed in Tables 22.1 and 22.3

		Endometrial Cancer (N = 2,145)		Cervical Cancer (N = 448)	
		Number	**Percentage (%)**	**Number**	**Percentage (%)**
Conversions		116	5.4	4	0.9
Transfusion		35	1.6	7	1.6
Readmission		68	3.2	19	4.2
Reoperation		32	1.5	11	2.5
Perioperative Deaths		4	0.2	0	0
Total Complications		349	16.3	142	32
Intraoperative		35	1.6	11	2.5
	Vascular	14	0.7	0	0
	Genitourinary	11	0.5	9	2
	Gastrointestinal	9	0.4	1	0.2
	Nerve	2	0.1	2	0.5
Postoperative		322	15	131	29
	Infection	56	2.6	33	7.4
	Lymphedema	65	2	18	4
	Cuff dehiscence	28	1.3	11	2.5
	Wound/Port Site	26	1.2	9	2
	Lymphocyst/Lymphocele/Pelvic Abscess	23	1.1	11	2
	Renal/genitourinary	22	1	17	3.8
	Venous thromboembolism	17	0.8	4	0.9
	GI/Ileus	15	0.7	10	2.2
	Pulmonary	15	0.7	5	1.1
	Cardiac	9.5	0.4	2	0.5
	Other	45	2.1	13	2.9

Although the low overall complication rate associated with robotic surgery is encouraging, some unique complications have been observed with this new technology. Vaginal vault dehiscence is a rare complication of hysterectomy performed by any technique, but initial reports of robotic hysterectomy have noted an increased risk of this particular complication, with rates reported from 2–3%. Proposed causes have included increased use of electrocautery when performing colpotomy, incorporation of less vaginal tissue in closure resulting from increased magnification, increased knot tension, and earlier resumption of physical and sexual activity. Vaginal vault dehiscence has also been associated with the use of adjuvant brachytherapy and chemotherapy for gynecologic cancers (109,110). Strategies shown to reduce the risk of vaginal vault dehiscence include the use of delayed absorbable suture such as Maxon or PDS, or use of delayed absorbable barbed suture (e.g., V-lock) (110). Others have recommended using cutting current when performing colpotomy to reduce tissue damage, and delaying resumption of sexual activity for up to 12 weeks.

Another complication reported with robotics results from collisions between the arms, inducing a small tear in the insulating sheath that covers the monopolar scissor tip. This can lead to cautery injury from an unintended electrosurgical arc to surrounding structures (111). Often intraoperative complications can be repaired robotically without conversion to laparotomy, including significant vascular injuries, taking advantage of the improved stable vision, hand dexterity, and the third arm. The latter can be used to apply pressure while the repair is performed with the other two operative arms. A variety of repairs have been reported, including bladder laceration and aortic injury (34), ureteric injury and enterotomy (48), and repair of the obturator nerve (112).

Although lymphedema can be a major long-term morbidity after lymphadenectomy, many reports of robotic surgery do not specifically comment on this potential complication. One report that focused on this issue identified lymphedema in 13% of women after robotic endometrial cancer staging (48). Persson et al. followed patients for 1 year after robotic radical hysterectomy and lymphadenectomy and found that 10 out of 43 (23%) had some degree of lymphedema, and 5% suffered from severe distal involvement (73).

Robotic Utilization

Cost-effectiveness

One of the major concerns voiced against robotic surgery relates to the high acquisition and maintenance costs. The proprietary disposable instruments are also expensive, and must be replaced after 10 uses. Robotics requires a large team of dedicated, well-trained operating room staff to ensure that the system is setup correctly and efficiently. Furthermore, operative time for complex procedures is generally longer than laparotomy, which translates into increased operating room expense. However, when compared to laparotomy, patients treated for endometrial cancer using robotics can be discharged earlier from the hospital, return to normal activities sooner (24 days compared to 52 days), and require less treatment/hospitalization for postoperative complications. These decreased postoperative expenses may quickly offset the financial investment for robotics (46).

Several publications have attempted to quantify the comparative cost per case between laparotomy, laparoscopy, and robotics for endometrial cancer and cervical cancer, incorporating both in hospital and out-of-hospital costs (Table 22.5). Based on these data, the overall cost of robotic surgery for endometrial cancer treatment is significantly less than that for laparotomy, but appears more costly than traditional laparoscopy, while for cervical cancer treatment, robotic surgery may be less expensive than either laparotomy or laparoscopy.

A government-sponsored report created by the Canadian Agency for Drugs and Technology in Health has indicated that the impact of robotic gynecologic surgery on a hospital budget depends on the surgical volume. Assuming a robotic system purchased by the hospital can be used for 7 years, robotic surgery for gynecologic surgery becomes cost-effective in Canada after 250 cases, and this decreases to 75 cases if the robot is donated to the hospital, as has been the case at most facilities in Canada (115).

Training and Education

Pioneering robotic surgical techniques has required surgeons to apply their previous laparoscopic and open surgical skills to this novel technology. Surgeons have quickly observed that they could improve their robotic surgical skills at a rapid rate, with minimal intraoperative

Table 22.5 Studies Analyzing the Cost of Robotic Surgery						
				Average Cost Per Case		
	Authors	*Year*	*Analysis Model*	**Robotic**	**Laparotomy**	**Laparoscopy**
Endometrial Cancer	Bell et al. (46)	2008		$8,212	$12,943	$7,570
	Barnett et al. (113)	2010	Societal	$11,476	$12,847	$10,128
			Hospital with robot	$8,770	$7,009	$6,581
			Hospital without robot	$7,478	$7,009	$6,581
	Shah et al. (114)	2011		$54,062	$59,997	$41,339
	Lau et al. (32)	2012	With Amortization	$7,644	$10,368	—
			Without Amortization	$8,370	$10,368	—
	Coronado et al. (47)	2012	Surgical Cost	€3,018	€1,144	€2,335
			Hospitalization Cost	€2,045	€4,385	€2,694
			Global Cost	€5,048	€4,681	€4,594
	Wright et al. (104)	2012	Perspective Database	$10,681	—	$8,996
Cervical Cancer	Halliday et al. (61)	2010	Hospitalization Cost	$8,183	$11,764	—
	Wright et al. (105)	2012	Perspective Database	$10,176	$9,618	$11,774

Lau et al: Historical cohort: Included 133 laparotomies combined with 27 laparoscopies. With Amortization means incorporation of the initial cost and maintenance of the robotic system, divided over 10 years.

Barnett et al: Societal: Included costs associated with surgery, acquisition and maintenance of the robot, hospitalization, lost wages, and caregiver costs. Hospital with robot: Excluded the lost wages and caregiver costs. Hospital without robot: Excluded the lost wages, and assumed prior hospital ownership of the robot.

Coronado et al: Costs are in Euros. Surgical Cost: Technical resources, personnel, instruments, operating room cost, complications, and other surgical procedures. Hospitalization Cost: Days of hospital stay, complications, transfusions, and need for unit care. Global cost: All costs measured.

complications occurring during this learning period (116). Individual surgeons learning MIS techniques have noted significant improvement in operative time after only 20 robotic cases, which had not been achieved after their first 20 laparoscopic cases (116,117). At one center with three surgeons and two fellows, it was observed that after 100 robotic endometrial cancer staging surgeries, there was significant improvement in total lymph node counts and para-aortic lymph node counts, and decreased surgical time from 203 minutes to 160 minutes (54). **Proficiency with robotic endometrial cancer staging has been documented after completing 20 procedures, with limited additional improvement in operative time beyond 40 cases** (118,119).

Robotics has created new challenges for educators, whose traditional methods for open surgical training involved direct hands-on guidance between surgical mentors and learners. During robotic surgery, the primary surgeon is isolated from both the patient and the learner by the Surgeon Console. Guidance must be given verbally or using visual images, and surgeons have limited opportunity to directly intervene if students using the Surgeon Console are proceeding incorrectly. To help with some of these issues, **a Dual-Console System (*da Vinci Si*Dual Console) has been developed** where two surgeons can operate from two separate Consoles, and control of instruments can be toggled between the two, similar to automobiles used for driving lessons that have two steering wheels. When the learner has control of the operative instruments, the teaching surgeon has the capability to draw on the image screen using their master control handles. **This technology has helped surgeons incorporate residents and fellows into robotic surgeries without increasing complications** (120,121).

The presence of the Computer Interface provides opportunities for telementoring and has facilitated the development of a new technology for surgical simulation, including simulators, which interface directly with the Surgeon Console, such as the ***da Vinci* Skills Simulator** (Intuitive Surgical, Inc., Sunnyvale, California, USA). Simulated surgical exercises can be displayed on the image visor screen, while students control simulated instruments using the actual robotic Surgeon Console. In addition to surgical training, these simulators have been used to evaluate proficiency prior to allowing students to proceed with live surgery (122), and as a warm-up tool immediately before starting live surgery (123).

Technological Advances

Robotic systems have only recently been introduced in the armamentarium of the surgeon, and are constantly evolving. **Fluorescent Imaging with ICG dye represents one of the first technologies to be merged with the three-dimensional high-definition robotic imaging systems** (103). Future robotic platforms may provide more advanced imaging with **incorporation of radiologic images into the image visor** and possibly **layering of real-time radiologic images onto the live visual field**. Additional advantages of the Computer Interface might include **digital image analysis** (such as the evaluation of differences in color, movement and temperature of the tissues, spontaneously or after injection of vital dyes) with feedback to the surgeon, and **computer analysis of surgeon efficiency** that could lead to outcome analysis and improvement programs.

Another advancement in MIS has been the development of Single-Site systems, in which all of the operative arms are introduced through one single port. Laparoendoscopic single-site (LESS) is an adaptation of laparoscopy using a single multichannel port combined with unique articulating instruments, that has been used successfully for endometrial cancer staging (124), including pelvic and para-aortic lymphadenectomy (125). Single-site ports have also been incorporated into robotic surgical systems. The *da Vinci* Single-Site Instrumentation is a single-site system introduced through a 2- to 2.5-cm incision that accommodates 5-mm cannulas and an 8.5-mm endoscope, which are docked to the *da Vinci* Si System. Use of this system to treat low-risk endometrial cancer has been reported, but did not include lymphadenectomy (126). Although outcomes following single-site MIS are still unclear, and the role of robotics in facilitating these techniques requires further evaluation, these ultra-MIS techniques may find a role in treatment of gynecologic malignancies in the future.

While Intuitive Surgical currently produces the only commercially available system, **numerous other companies around the world have been working on alternatives, such as Titan Medical** (Toronto, Canada), **SOFAR** (Milan, Italy), **IBIS** (Tokyo, Japan), and the **ARAKNES project** (Europe). These efforts may eventually provide commercial alternatives, which could help reduce the cost of robotics, while contributing unique features that can further advance surgical performance. For example, while haptic or tactile feedback has traditionally been an important component of both open and laparoscopic surgery, robotic surgeons must rely entirely on visual feedback to assess the consistency of tissues, and to establish appropriate tissue tension during dissection. **The Telelap Alf-X (SOFAR) is a multiport system incorporating a mechanism for haptic sensation** (127). Titan Medical (Toronto, Canada) has focused on a prototype for a new single-port system called Single Port Orifice Robotic Technology (SPORT). The role for these alternative robotic systems in gynecologic oncology remains to be seen.

References

1. **Querleu D, Leblanc E, Castelain B.** Laparoscopic pelvic lymphadenectomy in the staging of early carcinoma of the cervix. *Am J Obstet Gynecol.* 1991;164:579–581.
2. **Childers JM, Hatch K, Surwit EA.** The role of laparoscopic lymphadenectomy in the management of cervical carcinoma. *Gynecol Oncol.* 1992;47:38–43.
3. **Leiserowitz GS, Xing G, Parikh-Patel A, et al.** Laparoscopic versus abdominal hysterectomy for endometrial cancer: Comparison of patient outcomes. *Int J Gynecol Cancer.* 2009;19:1370–1376.
4. **Ramirez PT, Soliman PT, Schmeler KM, et al.** Laparoscopic and robotic techniques for radical hysterectomy in patients with early-stage cervical cancer. *Gynecol Oncol.* 2008;110:S21–S24.
5. **Nezhat FR, Ezzati M, Chuang L, et al.** Laparoscopic management of early ovarian and fallopian tube cancers: Surgical and survival outcome. *Am J Obstet Gynecol.* 2009;200:83.e1–e6.
6. **Ghezzi F, Malzoni M, Vizza E, et al.** Laparoscopic staging of early ovarian cancer: Results of a multi-institutional cohort study. *Ann Surg Oncol.* 2012;19:1589–1594.
7. **Chen Y, Xu H, Li Y, et al.** The outcome of laparoscopic radical hysterectomy and lymphadenectomy for cervical cancer: A prospective analysis of 295 patients. *Ann Surg Oncol.* 2008;15:2847–2855.
8. **Nezhat FR, DeNoble SM, Liu CS, et al.** The safety and efficacy of laparoscopic surgical staging and debulking of apparent advanced stage ovarian, fallopian tube, and primary peritoneal cancers. *JSLS.* 2010;14:155–168.
9. **Nezhat FR, Denoble SM, Cho JE, et al.** Safety and efficacy of video laparoscopic surgical debulking of recurrent ovarian, fallopian tube, and primary peritoneal cancers. *JSLS.* 2012;16:511–518.
10. **He H, Zeng D, Ou H, et al.** Laparoscopic treatment of endometrial cancer: Systematic review. *J Minim Invasive Gynecol.* 2013;20:413–423.
11. **Fader AN, Seamon LG, Escobar PF, et al.** Minimally invasive surgery versus laparotomy in women with high grade endometrial cancer: A multi-site study performed at high volume cancer centers. *Gynecol Oncol.* 2012;126:180–185.
12. **Geetha P, Nair MK.** Laparoscopic, robotic and open method of radical hysterectomy for cervical cancer: A systematic review. *J Minim Access Surg.* 2012;8:67–73.
13. **Walker JL, Piedmonte MR, Spirtos NM, et al.** Laparoscopy compared with laparotomy for comprehensive surgical staging of uterine cancer: Gynecologic Oncology Group Study LAP2. *J Clin Oncol.* 2009;27:5331–5336.
14. **Walker JL, Piedmonte MR, Spirtos NM, et al.** Recurrence and survival after random assignment to laparoscopy versus laparotomy for comprehensive surgical staging of uterine cancer: Gynecologic Oncology Group LAP2 Study. *J Clin Oncol.* 2012;30:695–700.

15. **Obermair A, Janda M, Baker J, et al.** Improved surgical safety after laparoscopic compared to open surgery for apparent early stage endometrial cancer: Results from a randomised controlled trial. *Eur J Cancer.* 2012;48:1147–1153.

16. **Tozzi R, Malur S, Koehler C, et al.** Laparoscopy versus laparotomy in endometrial cancer: First analysis of survival of a randomized prospective study. *J Minim Invasive Gynecol.* 2005;12:130–136.

17. **Kornblith AB, Huang HQ, Walker JL, et al.** Quality of life of patients with endometrial cancer undergoing laparoscopic international federation of gynecology and obstetrics staging compared with laparotomy: A Gynecologic Oncology Group study. *J Clin Oncol.* 2009;27:5337–5342.

18. **Janda M, Gebski V, Brand A, et al.** Quality of life after total laparoscopic hysterectomy versus total abdominal hysterectomy for stage I endometrial cancer (LACE): A randomised trial. *Lancet Oncol.* 2010;11:772–780.

19. **Reyes DA, Tang B, Cuschieri A.** Minimal access surgery (MAS)-related surgeon morbidity syndromes. *Surg Endosc.* 2006;20:1–13.

20. **Frumovitz M, Ramirez PT, Greer M, et al.** Laparoscopic training and practice in gynecologic oncology among Society of Gynecologic Oncologists members and fellows-in-training. *Gynecol Oncol.* 2004; 94:746–753.

21. **Puntambekar SP, Palep RJ, Puntambekar SS, et al.** Laparoscopic total radical hysterectomy by the Pune technique: Our experience of 248 cases. *J Minim Invasive Gynecol.* 2007;14:682–689.

22. **Peeters FV, Zvi V, Lau S, et al.** Technical modifications in the robotic-assisted surgical approach for gynaecologic operations. *J Robotic Surg.* 2010;4:253–257.

23. **Cho JE, Nezhat FR.** Robotics and gynecologic oncology: Review of the literature. *J Minim Invasive Gynecol.* 2009;16:669–681.

24. **Seamon LG, Bryant SA, Rheaume PS, et al.** Comprehensive surgical staging for endometrial cancer in obese patients: Comparing robotics and laparotomy. *Obstet Gynecol.* 2009;114:16–21.

25. **Lau S, Buzaglo K, Vaknin Z, et al.** Relationship between body mass index and robotic surgery outcomes of women diagnosed with endometrial cancer. *Int J Gynecol Cancer.* 2011;21:722–729.

26. **Satava RM.** Robotic surgery: From past to future-a personal journey. *Surg Clin North Am.* 2003;83:1491–500, xii.

27. **Diaz-Arrastia C, Jurnalov C, Gomez G, et al.** Laparoscopic hysterectomy using a computer-enhanced surgical robot. *Surg Endosc* 2002;16:1271–1273.

28. **Marchal F, Rauch P, Vandromme J, et al.** Telerobotic-assisted laparoscopic hysterectomy for benign and oncologic pathologies: Initial clinical experience with 30 patients. *Surg Endosc.* 2005;19:826–831.

29. **Field JB, Benoit MF, Dinh TA, et al.** Computer-enhanced robotic surgery in gynecologic oncology. *Surg Endosc.* 2007;21:244–246.

30. **Boggess JF, Gehrig PA, Cantrell L, et al.** A comparative study of 3 surgical methods for hysterectomy with staging for endometrial cancer: Robotic assistance, laparoscopy, laparotomy. *Am J Obstet Gynecol.* 2008;199:360.e1–e9.

31. **Paley PJ, Veljovich DS, Shah CA, et al.** Surgical outcomes in gynecologic oncology in the era of robotics: Analysis of first 1000 cases. *Am J Obstet Gynecol.* 2011;204:551.e1–e9.

32. **Lau S, Vaknin Z, Ramana-Kumar AV, et al.** Outcomes and cost comparisons after introducing a robotics program for endometrial cancer surgery. *Obstet Gynecol.* 2012;119:717–724.

33. **Ramirez PT, Adams S, Boggess JF, et al.** Robotic-assisted surgery in gynecologic oncology: A Society of Gynecologic Oncology consensus statement. Developed by the Society of Gynecologic Oncology's Clinical Practice Robotics Task Force. *Gynecol Oncol.* 2012;124:180–184.

34. **Magrina JF, Zanagnolo V, Noble BN, et al.** Robotic approach for ovarian cancer: Perioperative and survival results and comparison with laparoscopy and laparotomy. *Gynecol Oncol.* 2011;121:100–105.

35. **Bernardini MQ, Gien LT, Tipping H, et al.** Surgical outcome of robotic surgery in morbidly obese patient with endometrial cancer compared to laparotomy. *Int J Gynecol Cancer.* 2012;22:76–81.

36. **Vaknin Z, Perri T, Lau S, et al.** Outcome and quality of life in a prospective cohort of the first 100 robotic surgeries for endometrial cancer, with focus on elderly patients. *Int J Gynecol Cancer.* 2010; 20:1367–1373.

37. **Butler KA, Kapetanakis VE, Smith BE, et al.** Surgeon fatigue and postural stability: Is robotic better than laparoscopic surgery? *J Laparoendosc Adv Surg Tech A.* 2013;23:343–346.

38. **Schiavone MB, Kuo EC, Naumann RW, et al.** The commercialization of robotic surgery: Unsubstantiated marketing of gynecologic surgery by hospitals. *Am J Obstet Gynecol.* 2012;207:174.e1–e7.

39. **Leitao MM, Jr.** Potential pitfalls of the rapid uptake of new technology in surgery: Can comparative effectiveness research help? *J Clin Oncol.* 2012;30:767–769.

40. **Eltabbakh GH, Mount SL.** Laparoscopic surgery does not increase the positive peritoneal cytology among women with endometrial carcinoma. *Gynecol Oncol.* 2006;100:361–364.

41. **Lim S, Kim HS, Lee KB, et al.** Does the use of a uterine manipulator with an intrauterine balloon in total laparoscopic hysterectomy facilitate tumor cell spillage into the peritoneal cavity in patients with endometrial cancer? *Int J Gynecol Cancer.* 2008;18:1145–1149.

42. **Polyzos NP, Mauri D, Tsioras S, et al.** Intraperitoneal dissemination of endometrial cancer cells after hysteroscopy: A systematic review and meta-analysis. *Int J Gynecol Cancer.* 2010;20:261–267.

43. **Reza M, Maeso S, Blasco JA, et al.** Meta-analysis of observational studies on the safety and effectiveness of robotic gynaecological surgery. *Br J Surg.* 2010;97:1772–1783.

44. **Gaia G, Holloway RW, Santoro L, et al.** Robotic-assisted hysterectomy for endometrial cancer compared with traditional laparoscopic and laparotomy approaches: A systematic review. *Obstet Gynecol.* 2010;116:1422–1431.

45. **Leitao MM, Jr., Malhotra V, Briscoe G, et al.** Postoperative pain medication requirements in patients undergoing computer-assisted ("Robotic") and standard laparoscopic procedures for newly diagnosed endometrial cancer. *Ann Surg Oncol.* 2013;20(11):3561–3567.

46. **Bell MC, Torgerson J, Seshadri-Kreaden U, et al.** Comparison of outcomes and cost for endometrial cancer staging via traditional laparotomy, standard laparoscopy and robotic techniques. *Gynecol Oncol.* 2008;111:407–411.

47. **Coronado PJ, Herraiz MA, Magrina JF, et al.** Comparison of perioperative outcomes and cost of robotic-assisted laparoscopy, laparoscopy and laparotomy for endometrial cancer. *Eur J Obstet Gynecol Reprod Biol.* 2012;165:289–294.

48. **Backes FJ, Brudie LA, Farrell MR, et al.** Short- and long-term morbidity and outcomes after robotic surgery for comprehensive endometrial cancer staging. *Gynecol Oncol.* 2012;125:546–551.

49. **DeNardis SA, Holloway RW, Bigsby GE 4th, et al.** Robotically assisted laparoscopic hysterectomy versus total abdominal hysterectomy and lymphadenectomy for endometrial cancer. *Gynecol Oncol.* 2008;111:412–417.

50. **ElSahwi KS, Hooper C, De Leon MC, et al.** Comparison between 155 cases of robotic vs. 150 cases of open surgical staging for endometrial cancer. *Gynecol Oncol.* 2012;124:260–264.

51. **Cardenas-Goicoechea J, Adams S, Bhat SB, et al.** Surgical outcomes of robotic-assisted surgical staging for endometrial cancer are equivalent to traditional laparoscopic staging at a minimally invasive surgical center. *Gynecol Oncol.* 2010;117:224–228.

52. **Leitao MM, Jr., Briscoe G, Santos K, et al.** Introduction of a computer-based surgical platform in the surgical care of patients with newly diagnosed uterine cancer: Outcomes and impact on approach. *Gynecol Oncol.* 2012;125:394–399.

53. **Seamon LG, Cohn DE, Henretta MS, et al.** Minimally invasive comprehensive surgical staging for endometrial cancer: Robotics or laparoscopy? *Gynecol Oncol.* 2009;113:36–41.

54. **Holloway RW, Ahmad S, DeNardis SA, et al.** Robotic-assisted laparoscopic hysterectomy and lymphadenectomy for endometrial cancer: Analysis of surgical performance. *Gynecol Oncol.* 2009;115: 447–452.

55. **Peiretti M, Zanagnolo V, Bocciolone L, et al.** Robotic surgery: Changing the surgical approach for endometrial cancer in a referral cancer center. *J Minim Invasive Gynecol.* 2009;16:427–431.

56. **Lowe MP, Johnson PR, Kamelle SA, et al.** A multiinstitutional experience with robotic-assisted hysterectomy with staging for endometrial cancer. *Obstet Gynecol.* 2009;114:236–243.

57. **Gehrig PA, Cantrell LA, Shafer A, et al.** What is the optimal minimally invasive surgical procedure for endometrial cancer staging in the obese and morbidly obese woman? *Gynecolo Oncol.* 2008; 111:41–45.

58. **Lowe MP, Johnson PR, Kamelle SA, et al.** Robotic surgical management of endometrial cancer in octogenarians and nonagenarians: Analysis of perioperative outcomes and review of literature. *J Robotic Surg.* 2010;4:109–115.

59. **Brudie LA, Backes FJ, Ahmad S, et al.** Analysis of disease recurrence and survival for women with uterine malignancies undergoing robotic surgery. *Gynecol Oncol.* 2013;128:309–315.

60. **Kilgore JE, Jackson AL, Ko EM, et al.** Recurrence-free and 5-year survival following robotic-assisted surgical staging for endometrial carcinoma. *Gynecol Oncol.* 2013;129:49–53.

61. **Halliday D LS, Vaknin Z, Deland C, et al.** Robotic radical hysterectomy: Comparison of outcomes and cost. *J Robotic Surg.* 2010; 4:211–216.

62. **Estape R, Lambrou N, Diaz R, et al.** A case matched analysis of robotic radical hysterectomy with lymphadenectomy compared with laparoscopy and laparotomy. *Gynecol Oncol.* 2009;113:357–361.

63. **Magrina JF, Kho RM, Weaver AL, et al.** Robotic radical hysterectomy: Comparison with laparoscopy and laparotomy. *Gynecol Oncol.* 2008;109:86–91.

64. **Sert MB, Abeler V.** Robot-assisted laparoscopic radical hysterectomy: Comparison with total laparoscopic hysterectomy and abdominal radical hysterectomy; one surgeon's experience at the Norwegian Radium Hospital. *Gynecol Oncol.* 2011;121:600–604.

65. **Boggess JF, Gehrig PA, Cantrell L, et al.** A case-control study of robot-assisted type III radical hysterectomy with pelvic lymph node dissection compared with open radical hysterectomy. *Am J Obstet Gynecol.* 2008;199:357.e1–e7.

66. **Cantrell LA, Mendivil A, Gehrig PA, et al.** Survival outcomes for women undergoing type III robotic radical hysterectomy for cervical cancer: A 3-year experience. *Gynecol Oncol.* 2010;117:260–265.

67. **Ko EM, Muto MG, Berkowitz RS, et al.** Robotic versus open radical hysterectomy: A comparative study at a single institution. *Gynecol Oncol.* 2008;111:425–430.

68. **Maggioni A, Minig L, Zanagnolo V, et al.** Robotic approach for cervical cancer: Comparison with laparotomy: A case control study. *Gynecol Oncol.* 2009;115:60–64.

69. **Nam EJ, Kim SW, Kim S, et al.** A case-control study of robotic radical hysterectomy and pelvic lymphadenectomy using 3 robotic arms compared with abdominal radical hysterectomy in cervical cancer. *Int J Gynecol Cancer.* 2010;20:1284–1289.

70. **Schreuder HW, Zweemer RP, van Baal WM, et al.** From open radical hysterectomy to robot-assisted laparoscopic radical hysterectomy for early stage cervical cancer: Aspects of a single institution learning curve. *Gynecol Surg.* 2010;7:253–258.

71. **Nezhat FR, Datta MS, Liu C, et al.** Robotic radical hysterectomy versus total laparoscopic radical hysterectomy with pelvic lymphadenectomy for treatment of early cervical cancer. *JSLS.* 2008;12: 227–237.

72. **Lowe MP, Chamberlain DH, Kamelle SA, et al.** A multi-institutional experience with robotic-assisted radical hysterectomy for early stage cervical cancer. *Gynecol Oncol.* 2009;113:191–194.

73. **Persson J, Reynisson P, Borgfeldt C, et al.** Robot assisted laparoscopic radical hysterectomy and pelvic lymphadenectomy with short and long term morbidity data. *Gynecol Oncol.* 2009;113:185–190.

74. **Obermair A, Gebski V, Frumovitz M, et al.** A phase III randomized clinical trial comparing laparoscopic or robotic radical hysterectomy with abdominal radical hysterectomy in patients with early stage cervical cancer. *J Minim Invasive Gynecol.* 2008;15:584–588.

75. **Xu L, Sun FQ, Wang ZH.** Radical trachelectomy versus radical hysterectomy for the treatment of early cervical cancer: A systematic review. *Acta Obstet Gynecol Scand.* 2011;90:1200–1209.

76. **Plante M, Gregoire J, Renaud MC, et al.** The vaginal radical trachelectomy: An update of a series of 125 cases and 106 pregnancies. *Gynecol Oncol.* 2011;121:290–297.

77. **Geisler JP, Orr CJ, Manahan KJ.** Robotically assisted total laparoscopic radical trachelectomy for fertility sparing in stage IB1 adenosarcoma of the cervix. *J Laparoendosc Adv Surg Tech A.* 2008; 18:727–729.

78. **Persson J, Kannisto P, Bossmar T.** Robot-assisted abdominal laparoscopic radical trachelectomy. *Gynecol Oncol.* 2008;111:564–567.

79. **Chuang LT, Lerner DL, Liu CS, et al.** Fertility-sparing robotic-assisted radical trachelectomy and bilateral pelvic lymphadenectomy in early-stage cervical cancer. *J Minim Invasive Gynecol.* 2008;15: 767–770.

80. **Burnett AF, Stone PJ, Duckworth LA, et al.** Robotic radical trachelectomy for preservation of fertility in early cervical cancer: Case series and description of technique. *J Minim Invasive Gynecol.* 2009; 16:569–572.

81. **Ramirez PT, Schmeler KM, Malpica A, et al.** Safety and feasibility of robotic radical trachelectomy in patients with early-stage cervical cancer. *Gynecol Oncol.* 2010;116:512–515.

82. **Nick AM, Frumovitz MM, Soliman PT, et al.** Fertility sparing surgery for treatment of early-stage cervical cancer: Open vs. robotic radical trachelectomy. *Gynecol Oncol.* 2012;124:276–280.

83. **Fujii S, Takakura K, Matsumura N, et al.** Anatomic identification and functional outcomes of the nerve sparing Okabayashi radical hysterectomy. *Gynecol Oncol.* 2007;107:4–13.

84. **Magrina JF, Pawlina W, Kho RM, et al.** Robotic nerve-sparing radical hysterectomy: Feasibility and technique. *Gynecol Oncol.* 2011; 121:605–609.

85. **Hong DG, Lee YS, Park NY, et al.** Robotic uterine artery preservation and nerve-sparing radical trachelectomy with bilateral pelvic lymphadenectomy in early-stage cervical cancer. *Int J Gynecol Cancer.* 2011;21:391–396.

86. **Magrina JF, Magtibay PM.** Robotic nerve-sparing radical parametrectomy: Feasibility and technique. *Int J Med Robot.* 2012;8:206–209.

87. **Narducci F, Lambaudie E, Houvenaeghel G, et al.** Early experience of robotic-assisted laparoscopy for extraperitoneal para-aortic lymphadenectomy up to the left renal vein. *Gynecol Oncol.* 2009; 115:172–174.

88. **Magrina JF, Kho R, Montero RP, et al.** Robotic extraperitoneal aortic lymphadenectomy: Development of a technique. *Gynecol Oncol.* 2009;113:32–35.

89. **Magrina JF, Long JB, Kho RM, et al.** Robotic transperitoneal infrarenal aortic lymphadenectomy: Technique and results. *Int J Gynecol Cancer.* 2010;20:184–187.

90. **Iglesias DA, Ramirez PT.** Role of minimally invasive surgery in staging of ovarian cancer. *Curr Treat Options Oncol.* 2011;12: 217–229.

91. **Ghezzi F, Cromi A, Uccella S, et al.** Laparoscopy versus laparotomy for the surgical management of apparent early stage ovarian cancer. *Gynecol Oncol.* 2007;105:409–413.

92. **Chang SJ, Hodeib M, Chang J, et al.** Survival impact of complete cytoreduction to no gross residual disease for advanced-stage ovarian cancer: A meta-analysis. *Gynecol Oncol.* 2013;130:493–498.

93. **Vergote I, Trope CG, Amant F, et al.** Neoadjuvant chemotherapy or primary surgery in stage IIIC or IV ovarian cancer. *N Engl J Med.* 2010;363:943–953.

94. **Magrina JF, Cetta RL, Chang YH, et al.** Analysis of secondary cytoreduction for recurrent ovarian cancer by robotics, laparoscopy and laparotomy. *Gynecol Oncol.* 2013;129(2):336–340.

95. **Holloway RW, Brudie LA, Rakowski JA, et al.** Robotic-assisted resection of liver and diaphragm recurrent ovarian carcinoma: Description of technique. *Gynecol Oncol.* 2011;120:419–422.

96. **Lim PC.** Robotic assisted total pelvic exenteration: A case report. *Gynecol Oncol.* 2009;115:310–311.

97. **Davis MA, Adams S, Eun D, et al.** Robotic-assisted laparoscopic exenteration in recurrent cervical cancer Robotics improved the surgical experience for 2 women with recurrent cervical cancer. *Am J Obstet Gynecol.* 2010;202:663 e1.

98. **Lambaudie E, Narducci F, Leblanc E, et al.** Robotically-assisted laparoscopic anterior pelvic exenteration for recurrent cervical cancer: Report of three first cases. *Gynecol Oncol.* 2010;116:582–583.

99. **Lecuru F, Mathevet P, Querleu D, et al.** Bilateral negative sentinel nodes accurately predict absence of lymph node metastasis in early cervical cancer: Results of the SENTICOL study. *J Clin Oncol.* 2011; 29:1686–1691.

100. **Abu-Rustum NR, Khoury-Collado F, Pandit-Taskar N, et al.** Sentinel lymph node mapping for grade 1 endometrial cancer: Is it the answer to the surgical staging dilemma? *Gynecol Oncol.* 2009; 113:163–169.

101. **How J, Lau S, Press J, et al.** Accuracy of sentinel lymph node detection following intra-operative cervical injection for endometrial cancer: A prospective study. *Gynecol Oncol.* 2012;127:332–337.

102. **Holloway RW, Bravo RA, Rakowski JA, et al.** Detection of sentinel lymph nodes in patients with endometrial cancer undergoing robotic-assisted staging: A comparison of colorimetric and fluorescence imaging. *Gynecol Oncol.* 2012;126:25–29.

103. **Rossi EC, Ivanova A, Boggess JF.** Robotically assisted fluorescence-guided lymph node mapping with ICG for gynecologic malignancies: A feasibility study. *Gynecol Oncol.* 2012;124:78–82.

104. **Wright JD, Burke WM, Wilde ET, et al.** Comparative effectiveness of robotic versus laparoscopic hysterectomy for endometrial cancer. *J Clin Oncol.* 2012;30:783–791.

105. **Wright JD, Herzog TJ, Neugut AI, et al.** Comparative effectiveness of minimally invasive and abdominal radical hysterectomy for cervical cancer. *Gynecol Oncol.* 2012;127:11–17.

106. **Badawy M BF, Al-Halal H, Azar T, et al.** Anesthesia considerations for robotic surgery in gynecologic oncology. *J Robotic Surg.* 2011;5:235–239.

107. **Siesto G, Ornaghi S, Ieda N, et al.** Robotic surgical staging for endometrial and cervical cancers in medically ill patients. *Gynecol Oncol.* 2013;129:593–597.

108. **Persson J, Imboden S, Reynisson P, et al.** Reproducibility and accuracy of robot-assisted laparoscopic fertility sparing radical trachelectomy. *Gynecol Oncol.* 2012;127:484–488.

109. **Wiebe E, Covens A, Thomas G.** Vaginal vault dehiscence and increased use of vaginal vault brachytherapy: What are the implications? *Int J Gynecol Cancer.* 2012;22:1611–1616.

110. **Drudi L, Press JZ, Lau S, et al.** Vaginal vault dehiscence after robotic hysterectomy for gynecologic cancers: Search for risk factors and literature review. *Int J Gynecol Cancer.* 2013;23:943–950.

111. **Cormier B, Nezhat F, Sternchos J, et al.** Electrocautery-associated vascular injury during robotic-assisted surgery. *Obstet Gynecol.* 2012;120:491–493.

112. **Nezhat FR, Chang-Jackson SC, Acholonu UC, Jr., et al.** Robotic-assisted laparoscopic transection and repair of an obturator nerve during pelvic lymphadenectomy for endometrial cancer. *Obstet Gynecol.* 2012;119:462–464.

113. **Barnett JC, Judd JP, Wu JM, et al.** Cost comparison among robotic, laparoscopic, and open hysterectomy for endometrial cancer. *Obstet Gynecol.* 2010;116:685–693.

114. **Shah NT, Wright KN, Jonsdottir GM, et al.** The Feasibility of Societal Cost Equivalence Between Robotic Hysterectomy and Alternate Hysterectomy Methods for Endometrial Cancer. *Obstet Gynecol Int.* 2011;2011:570464.

115. **Health Quality Ontario.** Robotic-assisted minimally invasive surgery for gynecologic and urologic oncology: An evidence-based analysis. *Ont Health Tech Assess Ser.* 2010;10:1–118.

116. **Lim PC, Kang E, Park do H.** A comparative detail analysis of the learning curve and surgical outcome for robotic hysterectomy with lymphadenectomy versus laparoscopic hysterectomy with lymphadenectomy in treatment of endometrial cancer: A case-matched controlled study of the first one hundred twenty two patients. *Gynecol Oncol.* 2011;120:413–418.

117. **Lim PC, Kang E, Park do H.** Learning curve and surgical outcome for robotic-assisted hysterectomy with lymphadenectomy: Case-matched controlled comparison with laparoscopy and laparotomy for treatment of endometrial cancer. *J Minim Invasive Gynecol.* 2010;17:739–748.

118. **Seamon LG, Cohn DE, Richardson DL, et al.** Robotic hysterectomy and pelvic-aortic lymphadenectomy for endometrial cancer. *Obstet Gynecol.* 2008;112:1207–1213.

119. **Seamon LG, Fowler JM, Richardson DL, et al.** A detailed analysis of the learning curve: Robotic hysterectomy and pelvic-aortic lymphadenectomy for endometrial cancer. *Gynecol Oncol.* 2009;114:162–167.

120. **Smith AL, Krivak TC, Scott EM, et al.** Dual-console robotic surgery compared to laparoscopic surgery with respect to surgical outcomes in a gynecologic oncology fellowship program. *Gynecol Oncol.* 2012;126:432–436.

121. **Marengo F, Larrain D, Babilonti L, et al.** Learning experience using the double-console da Vinci surgical system in gynecology: A prospective cohort study in a University hospital. *Arch Gynecol Obstet.* 2012;285:441–445.

122. **Liss MA, Abdelshehid C, Quach S, et al.** Validation, correlation, and comparison of the da Vinci trainer(™) and the daVinci surgical skills simulator(™) using the Mimic(™) software for urologic robotic surgical education. *J Endourol.* 2012;26:1629–1634.

123. **Lendvay TS, Brand TC, White L, et al.** Virtual reality robotic surgery warm-up improves task performance in a dry laboratory environment: A prospective randomized controlled study. *J Am Coll Surg.* 2013;216:1181–1192.

124. **Fanfani F, Rossitto C, Gagliardi ML, et al.** Total laparoendoscopic single-site surgery (LESS) hysterectomy in low-risk early endometrial cancer: A pilot study. *Surg Endosc.* 2012;26:41–46.

125. **Fagotti A, Boruta DM, 2nd, Scambia G, et al.** First 100 early endometrial cancer cases treated with laparoendoscopic single-site surgery: A multicentric retrospective study. *Am J Obstet Gynecol.* 2012;206:353.e1–e6.

126. **Vizza E, Corrado G, Mancini E, et al.** Robotic single-site hysterectomy in low risk endometrial cancer: A pilot study. *Ann Surg Oncol.* 2013;20:2759–2764.

127. **Gidaro S, Buscarini M, Ruiz E, et al.** Telelap Alf-X: A novel Tele-surgical System for the 21st Century. *Surg Technol Int.* 2012;22:20–25.

23 Pelvic Exenteration

Kenneth D. Hatch
Jonathan S. Berek

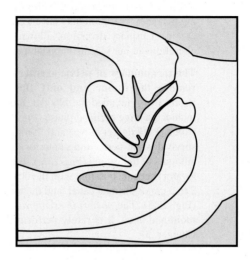

Pelvic exenteration is a major surgical procedure that involves the *en bloc* removal of some or all of the pelvic organs. **The main indication for the operation is to control isolated central pelvic recurrences of cervical and other gynecologic malignancies, after primary treatment with pelvic radiation therapy.** In geographic regions of the world where modern radiation can be delivered, central control rates have improved, and the need for radical resection of pelvic recurrences has decreased.

While some European centers have advocated pelvic exenteration for patients with advanced primary cervical cancer (1), most centers restrict the operation to patients with a central recurrence following chemoradiation. The only exception would be patients with stage IVA disease and a rectovaginal or vesicovaginal fistula.

Pelvic exenteration provides the only hope for cure in women with recurrent pelvic malignancies after radiation therapy. Most procedures are done for recurrent cervical cancer. Operative morbidity and mortality can be decreased by careful patient selection, attention to intraoperative technique, excellent postoperative care, and early management of complications. The 5-year survival rate is acceptable given the lack of satisfactory alternative treatments. With modern reconstructive and rehabilitative techniques, the patient can maintain a near-normal lifestyle, but sexual functioning will always be significantly impaired.

History of Exenteration

The first series of pelvic exenterations for gynecologic cancer was published in 1946 by Alexander Brunschwig, who summarized the outcome of 22 patients, 5 of whom died of the operation itself (2). The original procedure included sewing both ureters into the colon, which was then brought out as a colostomy. Since these humble beginnings, there have been major improvements in the selection of patients, operative technique, blood product use, antibiotic availability, and intensive postoperative medical management.

The operation gained wider acceptance after Bricker (3) published his technique of isolating a loop of ileum, closing one end, anastomosing the two ureters to this end, and bringing the other out as a stoma. This eliminated the hyperchloremic acidosis and markedly diminished the recurrent pyelonephritis and renal failure that were experienced with the wet colostomy. The popularity of the Bricker ileal loop was aided by the development of watertight stomal appliances.

Failure of the small bowel anastomosis to heal because of radiation fibrosis in some patients led to the use of a segment of nonirradiated transverse colon for the conduit (4). Further reductions in bowel complications occurred with the use of surgical staplers, which decreased the operative time, blood loss, and subsequent medical complications (5). Further refinements in the urinary diversion led to the continent urinary reservoir, which is described in Chapter 20.

As a higher percentage of patients became long-term survivors, the desire to improve quality of life led to reconstructive techniques for the vagina and the colon. Today, the patient undergoing pelvic exenteration may have a colonic J-pouch rectal anastomosis, vaginal reconstruction, and continent urinary diversion, allowing her to enjoy a near-normal quality of life without major alterations in her physical appearance.

The terminology of pelvic exenteration has changed as the operations have been tailored to remove the tumor and only the involved organs. The total exenteration performed by Brunschwig included the bladder, uterus, vagina, anus, rectum, and sigmoid colon (2). It usually included a large perineal phase (Fig. 23.1). This would lead to a permanent colostomy and urinary stoma. Rutledge et al. (6) and Symmonds et al. (7) reported decreased morbidity and acceptable survival when performing anterior exenteration, which removed the uterus, bladder, and various amounts of the vagina (Fig. 23.2). Total pelvic exenteration with rectosigmoid anastomosis (supralevator) became possible with the development of circular staplers. The rectum is excised to within 2 to 3 cm of the anal canal, and the levator support of the anal canal and perineal body is preserved (Fig. 23.3). The *posterior exenteration* removes the uterus, vagina, and portions of the rectosigmoid and anus. It is rarely performed today. Vaginal reconstructive techniques are discussed in Chapter 20.

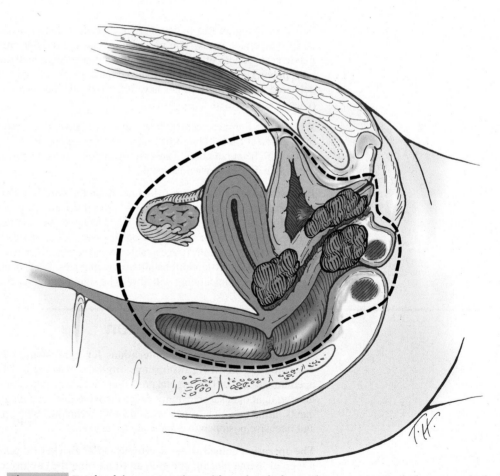

Figure 23.1 Total pelvic exenteration with perineal phase. This operation includes removal of the bladder, uterus, vagina, anus, rectum, and sigmoid colon, as well as performance of a perineal phase.

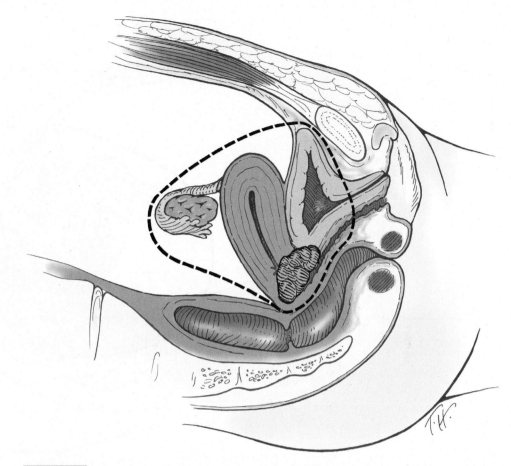

Figure 23.2 **Anterior pelvic exenteration.** This operation includes removal of the bladder, uterus, and varying amounts of the vagina, depending on the extent of disease.

Indications

The most common indication for pelvic exenteration is recurrent or persistent cancer of the cervix after radiation therapy. Some of the early series reported pelvic exenteration as primary therapy for stage IVA cervical cancer, and cancer of the vulva with urethral, vaginal, or rectal invasion. With modern radiation therapy, the use of exenteration as primary therapy is uncommon.

Exenteration has also been used for endometrial carcinoma, vaginal cancer, rhabdomyosarcoma, and other rare miscellaneous tumors, whenever ultraradical central resection of the cancer was feasible and there was no evidence of systemic or lymphatic spread.

Patients with endometrial cancer have a high likelihood of spread beyond the pelvis and are, in general, poor candidates for exenterative surgery. The survival rate for highly selected patients with endometrial cancer undergoing exenteration is less than 20% at 5 years (8). To debulk ovarian cancer optimally, a modified posterior exenteration is often performed, which includes *en bloc* resection of the pelvic peritoneum, uterus, tubes, ovaries, and a segment of rectosigmoid. It usually preserves most of the rectum and allows for a rectal anastomosis. Because there is ovarian cancer left behind, the procedure violates the principle that exenterative surgery is meant to be curative. **In the treatment of ovarian cancer, modified exenteration is performed as part of a cytoreductive procedure and is followed by chemotherapy.**

Patient Selection

The medical evaluation begins with histologic confirmation that cancer is present. The patient should have no other potentially fatal disease, and her general medical condition must be

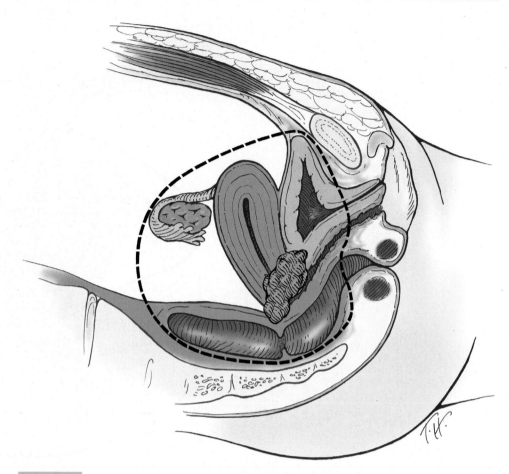

Figure 23.3 **Supralevator total pelvic exenteration.** This operation removes the uterus, vagina, and portions of the rectosigmoid colon above the levator ani muscles, with colonic reanastomosis.

adequate for a prolonged operative procedure (up to 8 hours) with considerable fluid shifts and blood loss.

The search for metastatic disease is imperative. The physical examination should include careful palpation of the peripheral lymph nodes and fine-needle aspiration (FNA) cytologic analysis of anything suspicious. Particular attention should be paid to the groin and supraclavicular nodes. A random biopsy of nonsuspicious supraclavicular lymph nodes has been advocated but is not routinely practiced (9).

Magnetic resonance imaging (MRI) has been evaluated for preoperative assessment of the pelvic disease (10). Popovich et al. evaluated 23 patients before pelvic exenteration for tumor extension to the bladder, rectum, or pelvic sidewall, and presence and location of lymphadenopathy. In four patients (17.4%), the MRI was falsely positive for pelvic sidewall infiltration, and in one patient (4.3%), it was falsely negative.

A more recent MRI study of 50 patients undergoing a pelvic exenteration by Donati et al. from Memorial Sloan-Kettering Cancer Center assessed the accuracy of two readers for bladder, rectal, and pelvic sidewall invasion (11). Of 23 patients with bladder invasion on final pathology, both readers correctly identified 20 patients (86%). There were two false positives for bladder invasion (4%). Rectal invasion occurred in 16 patients and was correctly identified in 13 (81%) and 12 (75%) patients by the two readers, respectively. There was one false positive for rectal invasion (2%). Eight patients had pelvic sidewall invasion; six patients (75%) and seven patients (87.5%) were correctly identified by the two readers, respectively. Similarly, pelvic sidewall invasion was overcalled in 2% and 4% of cases by the two readers.

MRI is a useful modality to evaluate the extent of local recurrence, but overdiagnosis and underdiagnosis of rectal, bladder, and sidewall involvement may occur, particularly in the irradiated pelvis.

A computed tomographic (CT) scan of the chest, pelvis, and abdomen has been considered routine in the past for the detection of lung, liver, and lymph node metastases in particular, but has recently been replaced by positron emission tomography (PET).

Lai et al. from Taipei evaluated the **PET scan for the restaging of cervical carcinoma at the time of first recurrence** (12). Forty patients had a PET scan, together with computed tomography and/ or MRI. Twenty-two patients (55%) had their treatment modified as a result of the PET findings. **PET was significantly superior to CT/MRI (sensitivity = 92% vs. 60%; $p < 0.0001$) in identifying metastatic lesions.** When compared with an earlier cohort of patients who did not undergo restaging with PET, there was a significantly better 2-year overall survival (72% vs. 36%; $p = 0.02$).

Husain et al. used FDG PET to determine metastatic disease prior to pelvic exenteration or radical resection in 27 patients with recurrent cervical or vaginal cancers (13). They found that FDG PET had a high sensitivity (100%), and a specificity of 73% in detecting sites of extrapelvic metastasis.

Chung (14) performed PET/CT scans in 52 patients suspected of having recurrent cervical cancer. Twenty-eight of 32 patients (87.5%) with positive scans were proven to have recurrent disease. Seventeen of 20 patients (85%) with negative PET CT scans had no evidence of disease, giving a sensitivity of 90.2% and a specificity of 81%.

The role of PET/CT in detecting the extent of pelvic recurrence was recently addressed by Burger et al. from Memorial Sloan-Kettering Cancer Center (15). Thirty-one patients had PET/CT within 90 days of a pelvic exenteration. Two readers blindly read the PET/CT to determine invasion of bladder, rectum, vagina, and pelvic sidewall. Bladder invasion was found in 13 patients (42%) and correctly identified in 9 cases (69.2%) by one reader and 10 cases (76.9%) by the second. Rectal invasion was found in nine cases (29%) and correctly identified in six (66.6%) by both readers. Pelvic sidewall invasion is the most important local recurrence to identify for the surgeon. In this paper, pelvic sidewall involvement was found in five patients (16%) at the time of surgery and it was correctly identified in three cases (60%) by one reader and four cases (80%) by the other. Both readers had one (10%) false-positive case for pelvic sidewall involvement. Thus **PET/CT was not effective in detecting pelvic sidewall disease.**

Extension of the tumor to the pelvic sidewall is a contraindication to exenteration; however, this may be difficult for even the most experienced examiner to determine because of radiation fibrosis. If any question of resectability arises, the patient should be given the benefit of exploratory laparotomy and parametrial biopsies.

Laparoscopy has been reported to be useful for the assessment of lymph nodes as well as the resectability of disease in the pelvis. In the hands of a highly skilled laparoscopic surgeon, this may be an option (16).

The clinical triad of unilateral leg edema, sciatic pain, and ureteral obstruction is nearly always indicative of unresectable cancer on the posterolateral pelvic sidewall.

The PET/CT scan is an important addition to the preoperative investigation of a candidate for pelvic exenteration, and should significantly decrease the number of cases that have to be abandoned because of metastatic disease discovered at the time of laparotomy. Miller et al. reported that 111 of 394 patients (28.2%) undergoing exploration at the University of Texas M. D. Anderson Cancer Center before the availability of the PET scan had findings that led to abandonment of the exenterative procedure (17). Reasons included peritoneal disease in 49 patients (44%), nodal metastasis in 45 (40%), parametrial fixation in 15 (13%), and hepatic or bowel involvement in 5 (4.5%). A preoperative PET-CT is presented in Figure 23.4.

Neoadjuvant Chemotherapy

Landoni from Italy has reported the largest series to date using *paclitaxel, ifosfamide,* **and** *cisplatin* **as neoadjuvant chemotherapy) for patients considered to be poor candidates for pelvic exenteration** (18). The criteria for neoadjuvant chemotherapy were large tumor size, diffuse lateral pelvic infiltration, early recurrence within 6 months, or persistence following primary chemoradiotherapy.

Thirty-one patients were identified and compared to 30 patients who had pelvic exenteration without neoadjuvant chemotherapy. There was a 61% response rate for the patients undergoing neoadjuvant chemotherapy, but no complete responders. The neoadjuvant chemotherapy group had a mean tumor size 4.39 cm versus 2.80 cm for the primary surgical group. Lateral infiltration was found in

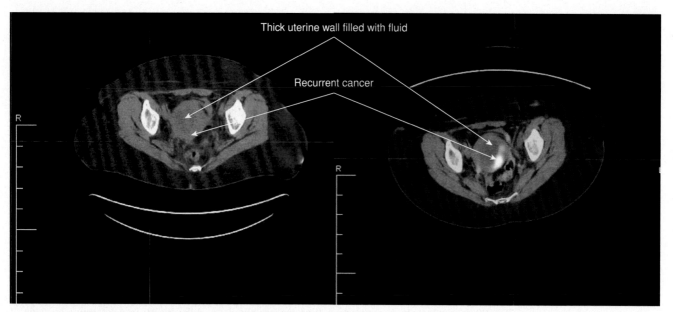

Thick uterine wall filled with fluid

Recurrent cancer

R

R

CT shows fluid filled uterine cavity and thickened wall. PET fusion reveals this to be current cancer of the cervix.

Figure 23.4 **CT and PET scans of a 52-year-old woman who had been treated with primary chemoradiation for Stage IIB squamous cell cancer of the cervix 2 years earlier.** She presented with pelvic pain, and a CT scan showed a fluid-filled mass. The cervix was not visible due to an upper vaginal stricture. A Pap smear was negative, but the PET CT suggested a central recurrence. This was subsequently confirmed histologically, and the patient underwent a total supralevator exenteration.

45% of the neoadjuvant chemotherapy group versus 20% in the primary surgical group. Despite these unfavorable clinical findings, the resection margins were positive in only 26% in the neoadjuvant chemotherapy group versus 20% in the primary surgical group. Intraoperative radiotherapy was given to 4 of 8 patients with positive margins in the neoadjuvant chemotherapy group and 6 of 6 patients in the primary surgical group. After a median follow-up of 31 months, 55% were dead of disease in the neoadjuvant chemotherapy group and none alive with disease. The primary surgical group had 50% dead of disease and 7% alive with disease. There was no significant difference in overall or disease-free survival. The neoadjuvant chemotherapy group did not have any complications related to the chemotherapy.

The results from this paper would indicate that there may be a role for neoadjuvant chemotherapy in patients who have no evidence of metastatic disease on PET/CT but have large tumors with lateral extension.

Preoperative Patient Preparation

The patient must be counseled extensively concerning the seriousness of the operation. She should be prepared to spend several days in the intensive care unit and have a prolonged hospitalization of up to several weeks. She must understand that her sexual functioning will be permanently altered and that she may have one or two stomas. In addition, there can be no guarantee of cure. The most difficult subject to broach is the possibility that she may have unresectable disease and that the procedure will need to be abandoned.

A mechanical bowel preparation is usually given. The patient should have the stoma sites marked by the ostomy team, and management of the ostomies should be discussed. **If the patient is severely malnourished, total parenteral nutrition (TPN) should be started in advance of surgery.** Because these patients may not have significant oral caloric intake for a week or longer, postoperative TPN is commonly given.

Operative Technique

The patient is placed in the low lithotomy position using stirrups that support the hips, knees, and thighs and can be repositioned during the surgery. This position allows the operators to perform the abdominal and perineal phases of the operation simultaneously. **Intermittent pneumatic compression devices are applied to the calves** as prophylaxis against deep venous thrombosis. **Combined epidural and general anesthesia** allow the epidural to be maintained after surgery for better pain control, while keeping the patient alert and able to maintain better respiratory function.

The abdominal incision is made in the midline and should be adequate for exploration of the upper abdomen and for performing the pelvic surgery. The liver and omentum should be palpated carefully. The rest of the abdomen is explored, and the para-aortic nodes are palpated. Both the right and left para-aortic nodes may be sent for frozen-section analysis. If these are negative, the pelvic spaces are opened by dividing the round ligament at the pelvic sidewall. The prevesical, paravesical, pararectal, and presacral spaces are all developed and the ligaments are evaluated for resectability. Enlarged or suspicious pelvic lymph nodes should be removed and sent for frozen-section evaluation. **More than one positive pelvic node, positive para-aortic nodes, peritoneal breakthrough of tumor, or tumor implants in the abdomen or pelvis should lead to abandonment of the operation.**

The procedure begins by ligating the internal iliac artery just after it crosses the internal iliac vein. This sacrifices the uterine artery, vesical artery, and obliterated umbilical artery. The remainder of the hypogastric artery is left intact. It carries the internal pudendal and inferior hemorrhoidal arteries that are important in maintaining the blood supply to the anal canal and lower rectum, where a potential low rectal anastomosis may be performed. The obturator artery should also be preserved because it is the major blood supply to the gracilis muscle, and a gracilis neovagina may be planned. The cardinal ligaments are divided at the sidewall and the broad attachments of the rectum to the sacrum are divided. The vaginal attachments to the tendinous arch are divided. The vaginal arteries and vein are located at the lateral margin of this pedicle. The specimen is completely mobilized and the penetration of the rectum and vagina through the pubococcygeal muscle can be identified. Various sites for ligation of pubococcygeal muscle for total exenteration versus anterior exenteration are identified (Fig. 23.5).

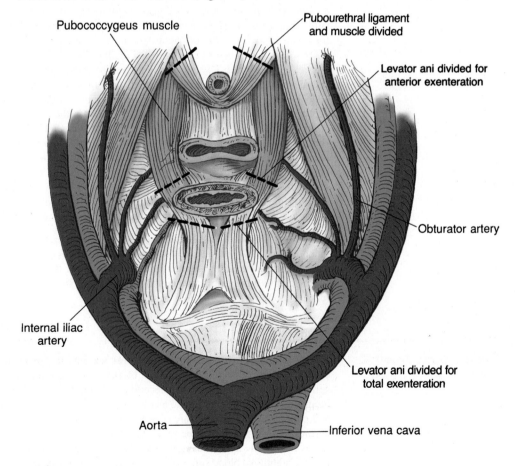

Figure 23.5 Cross-sectional diagram of pelvis showing lines of excision through the pubococcygeus muscle for anterior and total exenterations.

Anterior Exenteration

Anterior exenteration may be planned for lesions confined to the cervix and the anterior upper vagina. The uterus, cervix, bladder, urethra, and anterior vagina are removed, and the posterior vagina and rectum are preserved. Intraoperative bimanual palpation helps select the appropriate patient. The peritoneal reflection of the cul-de-sac can be incised and the rectum dropped away with a finger in the rectum and a finger in the vagina to ensure that the tumor is adequately resected. One surgeon conducts the perineal phase and the other surgeon conducts the abdominal phase.

The perineal incision includes the urethral meatus and the anterior vagina. A long curved clamp is placed beneath the pubis and directed caudad and anterior to the urethra. Another clamp is placed lateral to the pubourethral ligaments and directed out under the symphysis pubis, first at 2 o'clock and then at 10 o'clock. This isolates the right and left pubourethral ligaments, which can be clamped, divided, and ligated. The posterior vaginal incision is made under direct vision from below, insuring a surgical margin of at least 4 cm. The specimen is then ready to be removed. Hemostasis is provided by suture ligatures, and a pelvic pack is placed while the urinary diversion is performed. **The omentum is mobilized and brought down the left paracolic gutter into the pelvis.** It is used to cover the denuded area of the rectum and may provide a receptacle for neovaginal construction by a split-thickness skin graft. The omentum is sewn to the posterior vaginal epithelium, over the rectum and to the pelvic sidewalls. The skin is harvested and placed around a sterile mold, which is then placed into the cylinder formed by the omentum. If there is not enough omentum, the bulbocavernosus flaps may be used (19).

Supralevator Total Exenteration

Supralevator total exenteration with low rectal anastomosis for patients whose disease extends off the cervix on to the posterior vagina should have the segment of rectum removed *en bloc* with the specimen. This usually entails resection of the rectum to within 6 cm of the anal verge (Fig. 23.3). To remove the specimen, it is best to divide the sigmoid with the stapler to allow for easier exposure to the presacral space. The space is developed in the median avascular plane down to where the rectum exits between the levator muscles. The superior rectal and middle rectal arteries are sacrificed. The incision in the vaginal mucosa is 1 to 2 cm inside the hymenal ring. The supralevator attachments of the bladder, urethra, and vagina are divided, leaving the specimen attached only by the rectum. The hand is placed to encircle the rectum and traction is placed cephalad. The thoracoabdominal stapling device is then placed across the lower rectum with a 4-cm margin and the specimen is removed from the field. **Preservation of some of the lower rectum is desirable for the patient to have better continence and stool storage functions.** Hemostasis is provided and a pack is placed while the urinary diversion is performed. The left colon is mobilized, sacrificing the sigmoidal arteries and leaving the inferior mesenteric vessels. **The sigmoid is used for a colonic J-pouch, and a low anastomosis is performed using the stapling device.** The omentum should be mobilized and brought down to reinforce the stapled anastomosis. It also helps to cover the denuded area in the pelvis.

Because there is more of the vagina removed in this operation than in the anterior exenteration, the omentum may not be satisfactory for a split-thickness skin-grafted neovagina. **The patient is more likely to require a myocutaneous graft from the gracilis muscles in the medial thighs or the rectus abdominis muscle.** Because of the smaller opening in the vaginal introitus, the rectus abdominis myocutaneous graft is preferred.

Total Exenteration with Perineal Phase

If the tumor has extended down the lower vagina and involved the levator muscles, it is necessary to remove them for a chance of cure. The specimen is mobilized from above in a way similar to that described in the preceding operations (Fig. 23.6). The perineal incision is made around the anus and as far lateral as necessary to gain clearance from the tumor. The anococcygeal and pubococcygeal muscles are divided as necessary for margins. This leaves a large pelvic and perineal defect, which may be filled with bilateral gracilis myocutaneous flaps. Alternatively, the rectus abdominis muscle can be used. The omentum is harvested and used as a pedicle flap to provide additional blood supply and a barrier to bowel adhesions. A permanent colostomy is placed and urinary diversion is undertaken.

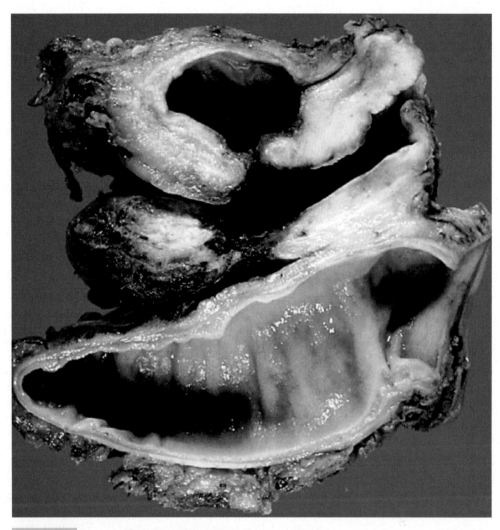

Figure 23.6 **A surgically removed specimen from a total pelvic exenteration.** Note the bladder above with a fistulous tract to the vagina, and the rectum below.

Posterior Exenteration

Posterior exenterations are rarely performed, except occasionally for cancer of the vulva involving the rectum after radiation therapy. When cervical cancer recurs after radiation therapy, even if it is confined to the posterior vagina and rectum, the distal ureters, bladder, and urethra should be removed to avoid the morbidity and mortality of urinary tract fistulae, stenosis, and denervation.

Low Rectal Anastomosis during Pelvic Exenteration

The introduction of the end-to-end circular stapling device greatly facilitated and popularized the performance of low rectal resection and reanastomosis for a variety of general surgical and gynecologic malignancies. **The automatic circular stapling device has many advantages over the traditional hand-sewn anastomosis. It allows use of a shorter anal or rectal stump, causes less tissue inflammation, creates a higher collagen content, and facilitates faster healing** (20). These are most likely the result of a better blood supply at the stapled anastomosis compared with a sutured anastomosis (21,22).

The anastomotic leak rate for low rectal anastomosis is less than 8% in patients without previous radiation (23,24). **The most important variables in the anastomotic leak rate are the distance** from the anus to the anastomosis, the vascularity of the cut ends, the tension on the anastomotic line, and the elimination of the pelvic cavity (25,26). Graffner et al. (26) showed in a randomized series that the anastomotic leak rate in previously unirradiated patients is the same for those patients with diverting colostomies as for those without.

There are a few reports in the gynecologic literature concerning the low rectal anastomosis in women with previous pelvic radiation therapy. Berek et al. (27) reported 11 patients with no anastomotic leaks and 7 of these patients had their bowel continuity reestablished with the end-to-end stapling device. Harris and Wheeless (28) reported 17 patients with a 12.4% anastomotic leak rate and a 12.4% stricture rate. Both groups advised using a diverting colostomy in the previously radiated patient. Hatch et al. (25) reported using a diverting colostomy in 12 of 31 previously irradiated patients. Six patients (50%) later had non–cancer-related rectovaginal fistulae requiring a permanent colostomy. Of the 19 patients without protective colostomies, 6 (31.6%) had non–cancer-related rectovaginal fistulae. In the series of Hatch et al. (25), **the most important factor in fistula prevention was the use of an omental wrap to bring a new blood supply to the irradiated pelvis.** For patients who did not have a diverting colostomy, TPN was used for 14 to 21 days.

Mirhashemi et al. (24) conducted a risk factor analysis of 77 patients at the University of Miami who had low rectal anastomosis after exenterative surgery. The indications for the surgery were recurrent cervical cancer (37); ovarian cancer (31); recurrent vaginal cancer (8); recurrent endometrial cancer (5); colon cancer (4); and endometriosis (4). **Previous radiation was the major factor in anastomotic leak rate, with 35% of the irradiated patients and 7.5% of the nonirradiated patients having a leak or a fistula. Protective colostomy did not make a difference.** Of the 40 patients who had total pelvic exenteration with low rectal anastomosis, 36 had received pelvic radiation therapy. A protective colostomy was used in 12 of these patients and 6 developed fistulae. Of the 24 who did not have protective colostomies, 6 developed an anastomotic leak or fistulae. Only 1 of the 37 patients who had posterior exenteration and low rectal anastomosis had previous radiation therapy, and this patient had an anastomotic leak. Of the remaining 36 patients, 3 had an anastomotic leak. Protective colostomies were not used on any of these patients (24).

Removal of the rectum alters the physiology of stool storage and defecation. The rectum is the reservoir for the collection of feces and transmits impulses to the sensory nerves to initiate the urge to defecate. Inhibitory reflexes from the rectum to the anus are necessary while the rectum is filling to ensure continence. After resection of most of the rectum, reservoir capacity, sensation, and rectoanal reflex are significantly altered (29). **The most important factor in restoring normal bowel function is restoration of the reservoir capacity. Capacity can be increased by preserving as much rectum as possible or by a colonic J-pouch.** The length of rectum necessary for return to acceptable function is 6 cm or more (30,31). When the anastomosis is above 12 cm, there is little alteration of function (32).

The colonic J-pouch was popularized by colorectal surgeons to treat rectal cancer with low rectal resection. It replaced coloanal anastomosis because of its superior results. **Studies comparing colonic J-pouch with coloanal anastomosis have shown (i) a decreased anastomotic leak rate; (ii) a better continence rate; (iii) fewer stools per day; (iv) better control of urgency; and (v) better control of flatus** (33–36). Prospective, randomized trials have confirmed the observational studies (37,38) (Table 23.1).

Table 23.1 Comparison of Colonic J-Pouch versus Coloanal Anastomosis in 100 Patients

Factor	Coloanal (n = 52)	J-Pouch (n = 45)	p Value
Anastomotic leak	8 (15%)	1 (2%)	0.03
Stool frequency	3.5	2	0.001
Incontinence score	5	2	0.001
Use of *loperamide*	19	1	0.001
Medication to induce stooling	10	21	0.07

From **Hallbook O, Pahlman L, Krog M, et al.** Randomized comparison of straight and colonic J pouch anastomosis after low anterior resection. *Ann Surg.* 1996;224:58–65, with permission.

Table 23.2 Randomized Study of 5-cm J-Pouch versus 10-cm J-Pouch			
	5 cm (n = 20)	*10 cm (n = 20)*	*p Value*
Sphincter function			
Resting pressure	97.8	90.6	NS
Squeeze pressure	214	194	NS
Reservoir function			
Threshold volume	40	70	<0.001
Maximum volume	98	129	0.003
Evacuation (mL within 5 min)	430	279	<0.001

NS, not significant.

From **Hida J, Yasutomi M, Fujimoto K, et al.** Functional outcome after low anterior resection with low anastomosis for rectal cancer using the colonic J-pouch: Prospective randomized study for determination of optimum pouch size. *Dis Colon Rectum.* 1996;39:986–991, with permission.

The most significant drawback to the colonic J-pouch is the inability of some patients to empty the pouch. This is most likely because of the length of the staple line used to construct the pouch. Hida et al. (39) prospectively randomized patients to a 5-cm versus a 10-cm pouch and found the 5-cm pouch to be superior for evacuation without compromising the other parameters (Table 23.2). Most authors have reported using a diverting colostomy when creating the colonic J-pouch, which has led to a decrease in the anastomotic leak rate.

Harris et al. have reported the long-term function of J-pouch anal anastomosis in 119 consecutive randomized patients with colorectal cancer from the Cleveland Clinic. Patients who had J-pouch versus coloanal anastomosis had significantly better continence scores at 5 to 9 years after surgery and fewer nocturnal bowel movements (40).

A new procedure called a coloplasty has been developed at the Cleveland Clinic to improve on the poor bowel function after either a coloanal anastomosis or a colonic J-pouch anastomosis (41,42) (see Chapter 20). In a randomized study of the three techniques, the coloplasty and colonic J-pouch patients had significantly more favorable compliance, reservoir volume, and fewer bowel movements per day than the straight anastomotic group. The advantage of the coloplasty was that it could be used in a narrow pelvis. This may apply to the female patient who is having vaginal reconstruction with myocutaneous graphs, where space for anastomosis is diminished (42).

There are some important anatomic considerations for patients undergoing pelvic exenteration with a continent urinary diversion. The continent urinary diversion uses the right colic artery up to its anastomosis with the middle colic artery. A colonic J-pouch uses the sigmoidal and left colic vessels. Adequate mobilization of the descending and left colon requires mobilization of the splenic flexure and rotation of the left colon into the pelvis. If a diverting loop colostomy is performed, it may interrupt the vascular supply from the marginal artery of Drummond. Care must be taken to preserve this vascular supply so that the colonic J-pouch and the resultant colorectal anastomosis have an adequate blood supply.

Husain et al. reported the experience at Memorial Sloan-Kettering in 13 patients who had total pelvic exenteration and low rectal anastomosis with a continent urinary diversion. Of these, seven leaked early and two had fistulae later, for a 30% success rate. They recommend against low rectal anastomosis when a continent diversion is used (43). Because of the vascular problems associated with a loop colostomy, the surgeon should consider a loop ileostomy for diversion of the fecal stream while the bowel anastomoses heal.

The overall survival rate for patients with pelvic exenteration and low rectal anastomosis at the University of Alabama at Birmingham was 68%. This was superior to that of patients with anterior exenteration (53%) (44), although the difference was not statistically significant. For both groups of patients, survival significantly improved if there was no spread of disease beyond the cervix and vagina. **Patients with disease confined to the cervix and vagina who underwent a total pelvic exenteration and a low rectal resection had a corrected survival rate of 94%, versus 70% for patients who underwent an anterior exenteration.** Although this difference is not statistically significant, it suggests that the more extensive procedure may improve survival by virtue of its larger tissue margin around apparently confined tumor. **The survival rate for patients with disease in the bladder, rectum, or parametria was 38%.**

Urinary Diversion

Techniques for urinary diversion are demonstrated in Chapter 20. The selection of the proper urinary diversion technique depends on a number of factors. The majority of women undergoing pelvic exenteration have had high doses of pelvic radiation therapy, which leads to fibrosis and lack of vascularity in the distal ileum. This increases the risk of anastomotic breakdown and bowel and urinary fistulae.

Most centers prefer the transverse colon when a urinary conduit is chosen as the urinary diversion method in a patient who has had full dose radiotherapy. This leads to fewer bowel and ureterocolonic anastomotic leaks (45). The colon absorbs water, sodium, and chlorides. This may lead to hypochloremic acidosis with hyponatremia and hyperkalemia if there is urinary retention caused by stomal stricture, or when a long segment of colon is used. **When a 10 to 15 cm length of colon is used and the stoma remains open, the complications of electrolyte imbalance are rarely encountered.**

Continent urinary diversion is preferred for those patients with motor skills and motivation to maintain the emptying and irrigation that it requires. It gives the advantage of avoiding the external appliance, and helps restore the patient's self-image. **A greater degree of renal function is necessary for the continent reservoirs** versus the conduits. **The glomerular filtration rate (GFT) should be 40 mL/min or greater.** The serum creatinine should be <2 mg/dL and there should be no urinary proteinuria. Because the cecum and ascending colon will absorb electrolytes, it is important that the patient empty the reservoir three times daily and irrigate once daily. The patient may experience diarrhea because the bowel has been shortened and the distal ileum has been taken out of the gastrointestinal stream. This leads to decreased bile acid absorption and steatorrhea. This can be treated with *cholestyramine* and with motility agents such as *lomotil* and *imodium.*

A retrospective analysis by Urh et al. from the M. D. Anderson Cancer Center compared 46 patients who underwent continent urinary division to 87 patients who had incontinent diversion (46). **The rates of pyelonephritis, renal insufficiency, ureteral anastomotic leak, fistula formation, and reoperation were no different between the two groups.** However, urinary stone formation (34.8% vs. 2.3%) and urostomy stricture (13% vs. 1.2%) were more common in continent urinary diversions. Among patients with continent urinary diversion, the incidence of incontinence was 28.3%, and 15.2% had difficulty with self-catheterization.

In a series by Goldberg et al. (47), pyelonephritis and urinary tract infections were more common in patients who had continent diversions. There was no difference in the rate of anastomotic leaks, but 16% of those who had continent operations experienced difficulty with self-catheterization. Others have found no difference in most major complication rates between the two procedures, but the rate of infection was somewhat higher with incontinent operations (48,49). **Preoperative counseling is essential to help both the physician and the patient determine which operation might best suit a particular individual's circumstances** (46).

In the patients who have significant fibrosis in the pelvis after radiation therapy, the ureters should be cut above the pelvic brim so the ureterointestinal anastomosis has a lower fistula and stricture rate. The left ureter will need to be brought across the midline above the inferior mesenteric artery (IMA) to provide the appropriate length and to decrease the risk of stricture caused by the kinking at the level of the IMA. The continent reservoirs and the transverse colon conduit are ideal for patients with short ureters because the anastomosis is in the mid to upper abdomen.

Postoperative Care

Patients are best managed in an intensive care unit with an arterial line and central venous catheter for administration of blood products, colloids, and crystalloids, particularly in those patients whose urine output is not a reliable predictor of fluid status. Patients have a large abdominal and pelvic peritoneal defect that exudes serum, and they may have significant third-space fluid shifts. Inadequate fluid replacement may lead to intravascular compromise and decreased perfusion of the kidneys. The hematocrit should be kept stable above 30% and the prothrombin and partial thromboplastin times should be kept normal with fresh frozen plasma. The central catheter can also be used for TPN.

A first-generation cephalosporin is given immediately before surgery for infectious prophylaxis. It is continued after surgery until the patient has remained afebrile for 48 hours. If febrile episodes persist or become severe, antibiotics are changed based on culture results. If no cultures are available, antibiotic therapy is extended to cover anaerobic and gram-negative organisms. If there is fecal spill during surgery, antibiotic coverage is usually extended to anaerobic and gram-negative organisms.

Complications

Although the present mortality rate is less than 5%, as many as 50% of patients may have a major complication (1,50–70). The most significant intraoperative complication is hemorrhage, with a blood loss of 1,500 to 4,000 mL being typical (71,72). Postoperative hemorrhage is often handled by percutaneous embolization, because re-exploration carries a high morbidity. The length of surgery (4 to 8 hours), large volume of blood loss, and inability to monitor urinary output because of the urinary diversion make the accurate replacement of fluids difficult. The central catheter is invaluable in monitoring the replacement of blood, colloids, and crystalloids, which may reach 1,500 mL/hr during intraoperative management.

Nonsurgical complications, such as myocardial infarction, pulmonary embolism, heart failure, stroke, and multiorgan failure, account for a 2–3% mortality rate, and are slightly more common in the elderly patient.

Gastrointestinal Complications

A small bowel anastomotic leak or fistula is a serious complication, with a mortality rate of 20–50%. **The incidence of small bowel fistulae ranged from 10–32%** (50–53,71–75) **in patients who had an ileo-ileal anastomosis in previously irradiated bowel.** Small bowel fistulae have been virtually eliminated by the use of transverse colon conduits and attention to pelvic floor reconstruction.

The incidence of small bowel obstruction is 4–9%. Initially, conservative management with nasogastric decompression and TPN should be attempted because reoperation is associated with an 8–10% risk of mortality. The obstructions are most common in the distal ileum at the site of the ileal anastomosis. Avoiding the ileal anastomosis and using pelvic floor reconstruction has decreased the morbidity of small bowel obstruction.

Urinary Tract Complications

The standard urinary diversion has been the urinary conduit using a segment of terminal ileum. The high complication rate of the ileo-ileal anastomosis led to development of the transverse colon conduit (76). There have been no bowel anastomotic leaks reported with this technique and ureterocolonic anastomotic leaks are rare.

The continent urinary diversion using the Miami pouch (see Chapter 20) **has a low rate of intestinal fistula formation and urinary leaks.** If urinary leaks or fistulae do occur, conservative management with percutaneous drainage is recommended. The mortality rate from surgical re-exploration for urinary complications may reach 50%.

The most common long-term complication is pyelonephritis, requiring rehospitalization in 14% of patients. The incidence of ureteral stricture has been decreased by the use of ureteral stents and is approximately 8% (77–79).

Results

The 5-year survival rate has improved significantly over time (Table 23.3) (6,7,50,51,54–70,75, 80,81). Patients who have had anterior exenterations have a better survival rate (30–60%) than those with a total exenteration (20–46%), no doubt reflecting the smaller dimensions of the recurrent

Table 23.3 Operative Mortality and 5-Year Survival Rates for Pelvic Exenteration

Author, Year	N	Operative Mortality (%)	5-Year Survival (%)
Brunschwig, 1965 (80)	535	16	20
Symmonds et al., 1975 (7)	198	8.1	33
Rutledge et al., 1977 (6)	296	13.5	42
Shingleton et al., 1989 (81)	143	6.3	50
Lawhead et al., 1989 (75)	65	9.2	23
Soper et al., 1989 (50)	69	7.2	40
Morley et al., 1989 (51)	100	2	61
Stanhope et al., 1990 (54)	133	6.7	41
Berek et al., 2005 (55)	75	4	54
Goldberg et al., 2006 (47)	103	0.97	48
Fleisch et al., 2007 (56)	203	1.8	21
Manggioni et al., 2009 (63)	106	0	52
Fotopoulou et al., 2010 (64)	47	8.5	53
McLean et al., 2011 (65)	44	2	50
Benn et al., 2011 (66)	54	0	34
Forner et al., 2011 (67)	33	0	43
Yoo et al., 2012 (68)	61	0	49
Schmidt et al., 2012 (69)	212	5	64
Baiocchi et al., 2013 (70)	77	6.5	64
Urh et al., 2013 (46)	133	ns	57

disease. **The clinical factors that have been reported to affect survival most significantly are length of time from initial radiation therapy to exenteration** (81), **size of the central mass** (54,56), **and preoperative pelvic sidewall fixation determined by clinical examination** (11,55,68).

The important pathologic factors are positive nodes, positive margins, and spread of tumor to adjacent organs. The occurrence of metastatic cancer in the pelvic lymph nodes after radiation therapy is a poor prognostic finding at the time of exenteration (Table 23.4). Stanhope and Symmonds (58) achieved the highest 5-year survival rate at 23%. In their analysis, they eliminated confounding high-risk factors, such as positive margins and metastasis to other peritoneal surfaces.

Rutledge et al. (6) **in 1977 reported a 6.6% 5-year survival rate in 30 patients with positive nodes.** This publication included patients who had positive pelvic and inguinal nodes and those who died of operative complications. **Ten years later, Rutledge and McGuffee** (59) **reported a 26.3% survival rate in 41 patients with positive nodes.** They noted an increase in the incidence of positive nodes in the later cases, and suggested that the patients were more highly selected to eliminate other risk factors; fewer died of operative complications. There was also a decrease in the number of posterior exenterations performed. These patients had vulvar, urethral, and rectal cancers and were managed more aggressively despite significant risk factors for higher recurrence rates. The 5-year survival rate was 21.9% for recurrent cervical cancer after radiation therapy, after eliminating death from other causes. Given this rate of survival, **patients with positive pelvic nodes and no other poor prognostic factors may be considered candidates for exenteration.**

Morley et al. (51) reported a 73% 5-year survival rate for 57 patients with squamous cell cancer of the cervix versus 22% for 9 patients with cervical adenocarcinoma. Crozier et al. (60) reported a median survival of 38 months for 35 patients with adenocarcinomas and 25 months for 70 control patients with squamous cell carcinomas. They concluded that patients with cervical adenocarcinomas who met the criteria for pelvic exenteration had results similar to those of patients with squamous carcinomas.

Table 23.4 5-Year Survival Based on Lymph Node Status				
	Negative Nodes		*Positive Nodes*	
Author, Year	*N*	5-Year Survival (%)	*N*	5-Year Survival (%)
Barber and Jones, 1971 (57)	299	22	97[a]	5
Symmonds et al., 1975 (7)	68	42	30	15
Rutledge et al., 1977 (6)[b]	NS	NS	30	7
Stanhope and Symmonds, 1985 (58)	NS	NS	26	23
Rutledge and McGuffee, 1987 (59)	NS	NS	41	26
Hatch et al., 1988 (44)	54	52	7	14
Morley et al., 1989 (51)	87	70	13	0
Berek et al., 2003 (55)	59	61	8	0
Fleisch et al., 2007 (56)	NS	35	NS	15
Forner et al., 2011 (67)	9	70	1	35
Schmidt et al., 2012 (69)	91	63	12	26

[a]Thirty-nine patients with gross disease unresected and 10 with metastasis to ovaries.

[b]Includes positive inguinal nodes.

NS, not stated.

Chronologic age is not a contraindication to exenteration. Matthews et al. (72) compared 63 patients aged 65 years or older with 363 patients younger than 65 years who underwent pelvic exenteration. The operative mortality rates were 11% and 8.5%, and the 5-year survival rates were 46% and 45%, respectively.

Intraoperative Radiation Therapy

Intraoperative radiation therapy (IORT) has been utilized in an attempt to improve the poor survival in patients with positive pelvic nodes or positive margins. The technical aspects of IORT can be found in Chapter 4 on radiation therapy.

IORT is delivered at the time of surgery, with a single dose to the area of highest risk for local recurrence. The field can be precisely targeted under direct vision and the bowel moved or shielded out of the field to reduce complications. **The radiation therapy can be delivered with electrons (IOERT), or with high-dose brachytherapy (HDR-IORT).**

The Mayo Clinic experience from 1980 to 2010 with IOERT has been reported by Barney (73). Of the 70 patients with recurrent cervical cancer, 58 had tumor involving the pelvic sidewall. The surgical margins were graded R0 for no residual disease ($n = 35$), R1 for microscopic residual ($n = 30$), and R2 for gross residual ($n = 21$). The dose range was 6.25 to 25 Gy, with a median of 15 Gy, but 71% of patients received additional external beam radiotherapy, the dose being based on the previous dose and field. Mean follow-up of living patients was 2.7 years and median survival was 15 months. The 3-year cumulative incidence of relapse was as follows: central, 23%; locoregional, 39%; and distant, 44%. Cause-specific survival was related to residual disease: R0, 45%; R1, 27%; and R2, 14%. **For the 58 patients who had pelvic sidewall involvement, the cause-specific survival was 25%.**

Gemignani et al. from Memorial Sloan-Kettering Cancer Center published the results of HDR-IORT in 17 patients undergoing radical surgery for recurrent gynecologic malignancies (74). The HDR-IORT was delivered by placing a Harrison–Anderson–Mick applicator and afterloading with Iridium-192. The applicator conformed to the irregular bed of the pelvis, and the bowel was packed out of the way or protected with lead shields. A dose of 12 to 15 Gy was given. **The 3-year local control rate was 83% in patients with complete resection, and 25% in patients with gross residual disease.** The overall survival rate at 3 years was 54%.

Quality of Life

The quality of life after pelvic exenteration is significantly improved by organ reconstruction. Hawigorst-Knapstein et al. (61) reported 28 patients who were periodically assessed in a prospective study by examination, interview, and questionnaires in the postoperative period. The women were divided into groups of two, one, or no ostomies. A separate comparison was made of women with or without vaginal reconstruction. At all points of evaluation, the patients' quality of life was most affected by worries about progression of the tumor. One year after surgery, the patients with two ostomies reported a significantly lower quality of life and poorer body image than patients with no ostomy.

Those women with vaginal reconstruction reported fewer problems in all categories related to quality of life and significantly fewer sexual problems. Ratliff et al. (62) prospectively evaluated 95 patients who underwent pelvic exenteration and gracilis myocutaneous vaginal reconstruction. Forty patients completed the study and 21 (52.5%) reported that they had not resumed sexual activity after surgery. Of the 19 patients who resumed sexual activity, 84% did so within 1 year of surgery. The most common problems were in adjusting to the self-consciousness of the urostomy or colostomy. Vaginal dryness and vaginal discharge were also significant problems. These findings indicate the need for adequate counseling after the exenterative surgery.

References

1. **Hockel M, Dornhofer N.** Pelvic exenteration for gynaecological tumours: Achievements and unanswered questions. *Lancet Oncol.* 2006;7:837–847.
2. **Brunschwig A.** Complete excision of pelvic viscera for advanced carcinoma. *Cancer.* 1948;1:177–183.
3. **Bricker EM.** Bladder substitution after pelvic evisceration. *Surg Clin North Am.* 1950;30:1511–1521.
4. **Orr JW Jr, Shingleton HM, Hatch KD, et al.** Urinary diversion in patients undergoing pelvic exenteration. *Am J Obstet Gynecol.* 1982; 142:883–889.
5. **Orr JW Jr, Shingleton HM, Hatch KD, et al.** Gastrointestinal complications associated with pelvic exenteration. *Am J Obstet Gynecol.* 1983;145:325–332.
6. **Rutledge FN, Smith JP, Wharton JT, et al.** Pelvic exenteration: Analysis of 296 patients. *Am J Obstet Gynecol.* 1977;129:881–892.
7. **Symmonds RE, Pratt JH, Webb MJ.** Exenterative operations: Experience with 198 patients. *Am J Obstet Gynecol.* 1975;121:907–918.
8. **Morris M, Alvarez RD, Kinney WK, et al.** Treatment of recurrent adenocarcinoma of the endometrium with pelvic exenteration. *Gynecol Oncol.* 1996;60:288–291.
9. **Manetta A, Podczaski ES, Larson JE, et al.** Scalene lymph node biopsy in the preoperative evaluation of patients with recurrent cervical cancer. *Gynecol Oncol.* 1989;33:332–334.
10. **Popovich MJ, Hricak H, Sugimura K, et al.** The role of MR imaging in determining surgical eligibility for pelvic exenteration. *Am J Roentgenol.* 1993;160:525–531.
11. **Donati OF, Lakhman Y, Sala E, et al.** Role of preoperative MR imaging in the evaluation of patients with persistent or recurrent gynaecological malignancies before pelvic exenteration. *Eur Radiol.* 2013;23:2906–2915
12. **Lai C-H, Huang K-G, See L-C, et al.** Restaging of recurrent cervical carcinoma with dual phase [18 F] fluoro-2 deoxy-D-glucose positron emission tomography. *Cancer.* 2004;100:544–552.
13. **Husain A, Akhurst T, Larson S, et al.** A prospective study of the accuracy of ^{18}Fluorodeoxyglucose positron emission tomography (^{18}FDG PET) in identifying sites of metastasis prior to pelvic exenteration. *Gynecol Oncol.* 2007;106:177–180.
14. **Burger IA, Vargas HA, Donati OF, et al.** The value of F_Fdg PET/CT in recurrent gynecologic malignancies prior to pelvic exenteration. *Gynecol Oncol.* 2013;129:586–592.
15. **Burger IA, Vargas HA, Donati OF, et al.** The value of 18F-FDG PET/CT in recurrent gynecologic malignancies prior to pelvic exenteration. *Gynecol Oncol.* 2013;129(3):586–592.
16. **Plante M, Roy M.** Operative laparoscopy prior to a pelvic exenteration in patients with recurrent cervical cancer. *Gynecol Oncol.* 1998; 69:94–99.
17. **Miller B, Morris M, Rutledge F, et al.** Aborted exenterative procedures in recurrent cervical cancer. *Gynecol Oncol.* 1993;50: 94–99.
18. **Landoni F, Zanagnolo V, Rosenberg PG, et al.** Neoadjuvant chemotherapy prior to pelvic exenteration in patients with recurrent cervical cancer: Single institution experience. *Gynecol Oncol.* 2013; 130:69–74.
19. **Hatch KD.** Construction of a neovagina after exenteration using the vulvobulbocavernosus myocutaneous graft. *Obstet Gynecol.* 1984;63: 110–114.
20. **Ballantyne GH.** The experimental basis of intestinal suturing. *Dis Colon Rectum.* 1984;27:61–71.
21. **Wheeless CR Jr, Smith JJ.** A comparison of the flow of iodine 125 through three different intestinal anastomoses: Standard, Gambee and stapler. *Obstet Gynecol.* 1983;62:513–518.
22. **McGinn FP, Gartell PC, Clifford PC, et al.** Staples or sutures for low colorectal anastomoses: A prospective randomized trial. *Br J Surg.* 1985;72:603–605.
23. **Hatch KD, Gelder MS, Soong SJ, et al.** Pelvic exenteration with low rectal anastomosis: survival, complications and prognostic factors. *Gynecol Oncol.* 1990;38:462–467.
24. **Mirhashemi R, Averette HE, Estape R, et al.** Low colorectal anastomosis after radical pelvic surgery: A risk factor analysis. *Am J Obstet Gynecol.* 2000;183:1375–1380.
25. **Hatch KD, Shingleton HM, Potter ME, et al.** Low rectal resection and anastomosis at the time of pelvic exenteration. *Gynecol Oncol.* 1988;31:262–267.
26. **Graffner H, Fredlund P, Olsson SA, et al.** Protective colostomy in low anterior resection of the rectum using the EEA stapling instrument: A randomized study. *Dis Colon Rectum.* 1983;26:87–90.
27. **Berek JS, Hacker NF, Lagasse LD.** Rectosigmoid colectomy and reanastomosis to facilitate resection of primary and recurrent gynecologic cancer. *Obstet Gynecol.* 1984;64:715–720.
28. **Harris WJ, Wheeless CR Jr.** Use of the end-to-end anastomosis stapling device in low colorectal anastomosis associated with radical gynecologic surgery. *Gynecol Oncol.* 1986;23:350–357.
29. **Nakahara S, Itoh H, Mibu R, et al.** Clinical and manometric evaluation of anorectal function following low anterior resection with low anastomotic line using an EEA stapler for rectal cancer. *Dis Colon Rectum.* 1988;31:762–766.

30. **Pedersen IK, Christiansen J, Hint K, et al.** Anorectal function after low anterior resection for carcinoma. *Ann Surg.* 1986;204:133–135.

31. **Karanjia ND, Schache DJ, Heald RJ.** Function of the distal rectum after low anterior resection for carcinoma. *Br J Surg.* 1992;79:114–116.

32. **Lewis WG, Holdsworth PJ, Stephenson BM, et al.** Role of the rectum in the physiological and clinical results of coloanal and colorectal anastomosis after anterior resection for rectal carcinoma. *Br J Surg.* 1992;79:1082–1086.

33. **Parc R, Tiret E, Frileux P, et al.** Resection and colo-anal anastomosis with colonic reservoir for rectal carcinoma. *Br J Surg.* 1986;73:139–141.

34. **Mortensen NJ, Ramirez JM, Takeuchi N, et al.** Colonic J-pouch anal anastomosis after rectal excision for carcinoma: Functional outcome. *Br J Surg.* 1995;82:611–613.

35. **Joo JS, Latulippe JF, Alabaz O, et al.** Long-term functional evaluation of straight coloanal anastomosis and colonic J-pouch: Is the functional superiority of colonic J-pouch sustained? *Dis Colon Rectum.* 1998;41:740–746.

36. **Dehni N, Tiret E, Singland JD, et al.** Long-term functional outcome after low anterior resection: Comparison of low colorectal anastomosis and colonic J-pouch anal anastomosis. *Dis Colon Rectum.* 1998;41:817–822.

37. **Seow-Choen F, Goh HS.** Prospective randomized trial comparing J colonic pouch-anal anastomosis and straight coloanal reconstruction. *Br J Surg.* 1995;82:608–610.

38. **Hallbook O, Pahlman L, Krog M, et al.** Randomized comparison of straight and colonic J pouch anastomosis after low anterior resection. *Ann Surg* 1996;224:58–65.

39. **Hida J, Yasutomi M, Fujimoto K, et al.** Functional outcome after low anterior resection with low anastomosis for rectal cancer using the colonic J-pouch: Prospective randomized study for determination of optimum pouch size. *Dis Colon Rectum.* 1996;39:986–991.

40. **Harris GJC, Lavery IC, Fazio VW.** Function of a colonic J pouch continues to improve with time. *Br J Surg.* 2001;88:1623–1627.

41. **Schneider A, Kohler C, Erdemoglu E.** Current developments for pelvic exenteration in gynecologic oncology. *Curr Opin Obstet Gynecol.* 2009;21:4–9.

42. **Mantyh CR, Hull TL, Fazio VW.** Coloplasty in low colorectal anastomosis. *Dis Colon Rectum.* 2001;44:37–42.

43. **Husain A, Curtin J, Brown C, et al.** Continent urinary diversion and low-rectal anastomosis in patients undergoing exenterative procedures for recurrent gynecologic malignancies. *Gynecol Oncol.* 2000;78:208–211.

44. **Hatch KD, Shingleton HM, Soong SJ, et al.** Anterior pelvic exenteration. *Gynecol Oncol.* 1988;31:205–216.

45. **Chiva LM, Lapuente F, González-Cortijo L, et al.** Surgical treatment of recurrent cervical cancer: State of the art and new achievements. *Gynecol Oncol.* 2008;110:S60–S66.

46. **Urh A, Soliman PT, Schmeler KM, et al.** Postoperative outcomes after continent versus incontinent urinary diversion at the time of pelvic exenteration for gynecologic malignancies. *Gynecol Oncol.* 2013;129(3):580–585.

47. **Goldberg GL, Sukumvanich P, Einstein MH, et al.** Total pelvic exenteration: The Albert Einstein College of Medicine/Montefiore Medical Center experience (1987 to 2003). *Gynecol Oncol.* 2006;101:261–268.

48. **Karesenty G, Moutardier V, Lelong B, et al.** Long-term follow-up of continent urinary diversions after pelvic exenteration for gynecologic malignancies. *Gynecol Oncol.* 2005;97:524–528.

49. **Houvenaeghel G, Moutardier V, Karsenty G, et al.** Major complications of urinary diversion after pelvic exenteration for gynecologic malignancies: A 23-year mono-institutional experience in 121 patients. *Gynecol Oncol.* 2004;92:680–683.

50. **Soper JT, Berchuck A, Creasman WT, et al.** Pelvic exenteration: factors associated with major surgical morbidity. *Gynecol Oncol* 1989;35:93–98.

51. **Morley GW, Hopkins MP, Lindenauer SM, et al.** Pelvic exenteration, University of Michigan: 100 patients at 5 years. *Obstet Gynecol.* 1989;74:934–943.

52. **Miller B, Morris M, Gershenson DM, et al.** Intestinal fistulae formation following pelvic exenteration: A review of the University

of Texas M. D. Anderson Cancer Center experience, 1957–1990. *Gynecol Oncol.* 1995;56:207–210.

53. **Fagotti A, Costantini B, Fanfani F, et al.** Risk of postoperative pelvic abscess in major gynecologic oncology surgery: one-year single-institution experience. *Ann Surg Oncol.* 2010;17:2452–2458.

54. **Stanhope CR, Webb MJ, Podratz KC.** Pelvic exenteration for recurrent cervical cancer. *Clin Obstet Gynecol.* 1990;33:897–909.

55. **Berek JS, Howe C, Lagasse LD, et al.** Pelvic exenteration for recurrent gynecologic malignancy: Survival and morbidity analysis of the 45-year experience at UCLA. *Gynecol Oncol.* 2005;99:153–159.

56. **Fleisch MC, Panthe P, Beckman MW, et al.** Predictors of long-term survival after interdisciplinary salvage surgery for advanced or recurrent gynecological cancers. *J Surg Oncol.* 2007;95:476–84.

57. **Barber HR, Jones W.** Lymphadenectomy in pelvic exenteration for recurrent cervix cancer. *JAMA.* 1971;215:1945–1949.

58. **Stanhope CR, Symmonds RE.** Palliative exenteration—what, when, and why? *Am J Obstet Gynecol.* 1985;152:12–16.

59. **Rutledge FN, McGuffee VB.** Pelvic exenteration: Prognostic significance of regional lymph node metastasis. *Gynecol Oncol.* 1987;26:374–380.

60. **Crozier M, Morris M, Levenback C, et al.** Pelvic exenteration for adenocarcinoma of the uterine cervix. *Gynecol Oncol.* 1995;58:74–78.

61. **Hawighorst-Knapstein S, Schonefussrs G, Hoffmann SO, et al.** Pelvic exenteration: effects of surgery on quality of life and body image–a prospective longitudinal study. *Gynecol Oncol.* 1997;66:495–500.

62. **Ratliff CR, Gershenson DM, Morris M, et al.** Sexual adjustment of patients undergoing gracilis myocutaneous flap vaginal reconstruction in conjunction with pelvic exenteration. *Cancer.* 1996;78:2229–2235.

63. **Manggioni A, Roviglione G, Landoni F, et al.** Pelvic exenteration: Ten-year experience at the European Institute of Oncology in Milan. *Gynecol Oncol.* 2009;114:64–68.

64. **Fotopoulou C, Neumann U, Kraetschell R, et al.** Long-term clinical outcome of pelvic exenteration in patients with advanced gynecological malignancies. *Gynecol Oncol.* 2010;101:507–512.

65. **McLean KA, Zhang W, Dunsmoor-Su RF, et al.** Pelvic exenteration in the age of modern chemoradiation. *Gynecol Oncol.* 2011;121:131–134.

66. **Benn T, Brooks RA, Zhang Q, et al.** Pelvic exenteration in gynecologic oncology: a single institution study over 20 years. *Gynecol Oncol* 2011;122:14–1866.

67. **Forner DM, Lampe B.** Exenteration as a primary treatment for locally advanced cervical cancer: Long-term results and prognostic factors. *Am J Obstet Gynecol.* 2011;205:148.e1–e6.

68. **Yoo HJ, Lim MC, Seo SS, et al.** Pelvic exenteration for recurrent cervical cancer: Ten-year experience at National Cancer Center in Korea. *Gynecol Oncol.* 2012;23:242–250.

69. **Schmidt AM, Imesch P, Fink D, et al.** Indications and long-term clinical outcomes in 282 patients with pelvic exenteration for advanced or recurrent cervical cancer. *Gynecol Oncol.* 2012;125:604–609.

70. **Baiocchi G, Guimaraes GC, Faloppa CC, et al.** Does histologic type correlate to outcome after pelvic exenteration for cervical and vaginal cancer? *Ann Surg Oncol.* 2013;20:1694–1700.

71. **Magrina JF, Stanhope CR, Weaver AL.** Pelvic exenterations: Supralevator, infralevator, and with vulvectomy. *Gynecol Oncol.* 1997;64:130–135.

72. **Matthews CM, Morris M, Burke TW, et al.** Pelvic exenteration in the elderly patient. *Obstet Gynecol.* 1992;79:773–777.

73. **Barney BM, Petersen IA, Dowdy SC, et al.** Intraoperative Electron Beam Radiotherapy (IOERT) in the management of locally advanced or recurrent cervical cancer. *Radiat Oncol.* 2013;8:80.

74. **Gemignani ML, Alektiar KM, Leitao M, et al.** Radical surgical resection and high-dose intraoperative radiation therapy (HDR-IORT) in patients with recurrent gynecologic cancers. *Int J Radiat Oncol Biol Phys.* 2001;50:687–694.

75. **Lawhead RA Jr, Clark DG, Smith DH, et al.** Pelvic exenteration for recurrent or persistent gynecologic malignancies: A 10-year review of the Memorial Sloan-Kettering Cancer Center experience (1972–1981). *Gynecol Oncol.* 1989;33:279–282.

76. **Segreti EM, Morris M, Levenback C, et al.** Transverse colon urinary diversion in gynecologic oncology. *Gynecol Oncol.* 1996;63:66–70.

77. **Beddoe AM, Boyce JG, Remy JC, et al.** Stented versus nonstented transverse colon conduits: a comparative report. *Gynecol Oncol.* 1987;27:305–313.

78. **Spahn M, Weiss C, Bader P, et al.** The role of exenterative surgery and urinary diversion in persistent or locally recurrent gynecological malignancy: Complications and survival. *Urol Int.* 2010;85:16–22.

79. **Backes FJ, Tierney BJ, Eisenhauer EL, et al.** Complications after double-barrel wet colostomy compared to separate urinary and fecal diversion during pelvic exenteration: Time to change back? *Gynecol Oncol.* 2013;128:60–64.

80. **Brunschwig A.** What are the indications and results of pelvic exenteration? *JAMA.* 1965;194:274.

81. **Shingleton HM, Soong SJ, Gelder MS, et al.** Clinical and histopathologic factors predicting recurrence and survival after pelvic exenteration for cancer of the cervix. *Obstet Gynecol.* 1989;73:1027–1034.

QUALITY OF LIFE

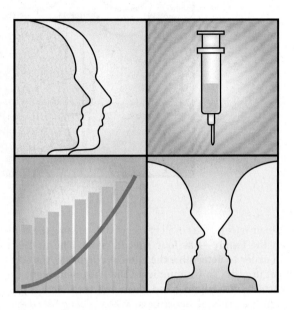

24 Communication Skills

Walter F. Baile

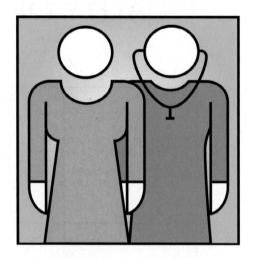

In gynecologic oncology, as in all branches of medicine, **the clinical encounter with the patient—and often the family—has four specific aims. The first is to gather information from the patient in order to determine the clinical diagnosis; the second is to transmit information to the patient in order to communicate the treatment plan; the third is to build a relationship in order to establish rapport and trust; and the fourth is to support the patient and her family through the crisis of her illness.** When accomplished successfully, these aims can achieve the overarching goals of producing objective improvement in the patient's medical condition to the extent medically possible—helping the patient get better—and subjective changes in how she experiences her care—helping the patient to feel better.

The last two aims take on particular significance because the increased survival rates of many cancers can extend the relationship with the oncologist and the clinical team over many years, and encompass a progression of disease crises. The median survival for women with advanced-stage ovarian cancer has increased over the past 20 years, and it is not uncommon for patients to experience remission and recurrence four or five times during the course of their illness (1). **Each disease recurrence can be a crisis in which the patient receives bad news again, and must endure the rigors of a new round of treatment, uncertainty about the outcome, and the threat of death. In these instances, the application of supportive communication skills in the context of a long-standing relationship with the patient can reduce anxiety, facilitate patient coping, and assist in providing the patient with hope** (2–5).

Regardless of whether medical improvement is possible, accomplishment of these goals can produce amelioration of the patient's subjective symptoms. Communication skills are essential for both. This chapter sets out a basic and practical approach for acquiring and improving effective communication skills.

Why Communication Skills Matter

Good communication skills facilitate the clinician's ability to take an accurate clinical history, make a correct diagnosis, and formulate an appropriate plan of management. Communication skills are a central component of every clinician's management techniques. Communication expertise can change the patient's attitude to the entire medical intervention.

Effective communication can change the way a patient feels about the clinical outcome. Communication skills may affect what the patient perceives has happened to her, her assessment

and feelings about her management, her treatment, and her healthcare team (6). **Communication and interpersonal skills matter greatly to patients and are an important determinant of satisfaction with care** (7). The literature suggests that **patients are both likely to choose and to change physicians based on how they perceive their physician communicates and interacts with them** (8).

An important and related issue is that of medical–legal implications. Communication skills have been shown to be a determinant of more objective outcome measures, such as litigation. **Approximately three-fourths of complaints against medical practitioners are caused not by matters of medical management, but by failures or obstacles in communication.** Levinson and Chaumeton (9) have shown that communication skills are a major factor in distinguishing those clinicians who are sued from those who are not.

Patients are very sensitive to communication messages from their oncologists. Using samples of dialogue from interactions between surgeons and their patients, Ambady et al. (10) were reliably able to predict those surgeons most likely to be sued. **Those whose voice communicated lack of empathy and concern toward the patient were more than twice as likely to have had a malpractice claim filed against them.** Many insurance companies in North America reduce their malpractice premiums for physicians who have attended specific programs in communication skills.

Communication skills are particularly essential for ensuring informed consent, enlisting the family in the care of the patient, reducing the uncertainty associated with a new or recurrent illness, and increasing accrual to clinical trials (11–13).

Communication Skills as Learnable Techniques

Why Communication Skills Are So Challenging to Learn

Most oncologists have had little preparation in communicating with patients (11,14,15). Very few have had any formal course work and a fair number learn by observing other clinicians, which is not a guarantee of success. Many clinical encounters are highly emotionally charged, such as breaking bad news and making the transition to palliative care. **The clinician is challenged not only to address the patient's feelings, but also his or her own, which can be characterized by the sense of helplessness and frustration in the face of incurable disease, or self-doubt about having done everything possible for the patient** (12,16). **These feelings may cause the doctor to offer false hope to the patient, avoid discussing issues important to the patient such as disease prognosis and end-of-life issues** (17,18), **or offer treatment when there is little or no chance of success** (19).

Acquiring Communication Skills

Since the late 1970s, clinicians have become increasingly aware of the need for improved communication skills, but defining and testing techniques that can be acquired by practitioners was initially difficult. **In the late 1970s and early 1980s, it was widely believed that communication skills were intuitive, almost inherited talents—*"You've either got the gift or you haven't."*** This was coupled with the belief that somehow the physician would be able to feel or sense what the patient was thinking, to divine what the patient wanted, and be able to respond intuitively in an appropriate way. This belief alienated a large proportion of healthcare professionals, who found the whole topic, as taught at that time, excessively *"touchy-feely,"* intangible, and amorphous, with no guidelines that could lead even a highly motivated practitioner to improve his or her skills.

Since the mid-1980s, researchers and educators have shown that communication skills can be taught and learned and retained over years of practice, and that they are acquired skills, like any other clinical technique, and not inherited or granted as gifts (20–24).

The main part of this chapter describes two practical protocols that can be used by any healthcare professional to improve her or his communication skills. They are (i) **a basic protocol, the CLASS protocol, which may serve for all medical interviews and** (ii) **a variation of that approach, the SPIKES protocol, for breaking bad news.**

Illustrations of Practical Techniques

The CLASS and SPIKES protocols are summarized briefly using simple and practical guidelines or rules. Both protocols have been published in greater detail elsewhere as a textbook (25),

Table 24.1 The CLASS Protocol
C—Physical **context** or setting and **connection**
L—**Listening** skills
A—**Acknowledge** emotions and explore them
S—Management **strategy**
S—**Summary** and closure

a booklet (26), and in illustrated form using videotaped scenarios of interactions between standardized patients (27). Review of this video material can enhance the understanding of these communication techniques.

CLASS: A Protocol for Effective Communication

There are probably an infinite number of ways of summarizing and simplifying medical interviews, but few if any are practical and easy to remember. The five-step basic protocol for medical communication set out in the following sections, which has the acronym *CLASS,* has the virtue of being easy to remember and to use in practice. Furthermore, it offers a relatively straightforward, technique-directed method for dealing with emotions. This is important, because one study showed that most oncologists—more than 85%—believe that dealing with emotions is the most difficult part of any clinical interview (28).

Trust and rapport are especially important to patients at times of medical crisis. Communication skills such as exemplified in the CLASS protocol underpin the establishment of confidence and a working relationship with the patient and her family.

In brief, the CLASS protocol identifies five essential components of the medical interview. They are *Context*—**the physical context or setting, and** *Connection*—**or building rapport,** *Listening skills, Acknowledgment* **of the patient's emotions,** *Strategy* **for clinical management, and** *Summary* **(Table 24.1).**

C—Context—or Setting & Connection—or Building Rapport

The context of the interview means the physical context or setting and connection means the steps that are necessary to begin building rapport or a relationship with the patient. Both these steps are important because they encourage trust on the part of the patient and family, an essential ingredient of any collaborative endeavor. They are especially important in the first encounter, during which the most lasting impressions are often formed. The essential components are listed in Table 24.2. **The first component is to arrange the space optimally. The second is to get your own body language right. It is important to pay attention to eye contact, to whether touch is helpful, and to making introductions.**

A few seconds spent establishing these features of the initial setup of the interview may save many minutes of frustration and misunderstanding later for the professional and the patient. These rules are not complex, but they are easy to forget in the heat of the moment.

Spatial Arrangements

The Setting

Every attempt should be made to ensure privacy. In a hospital setting, if a side room is not available, the curtains should be drawn around the bed. In an office setting, the door should be shut.

Table 24.2 The Elements of Physical Context	
Arrangement	Sitting down, placement of patient, appropriate distance.
Body language	Drop shoulders, sit comfortably, and attentively.
Eye contact	Maintain eye contact except during anger or crying, that is, "not when hot."
Touch (optional)	Touch patient's forearm if you and the patient are comfortable with touch.
Introductions	Tell the patient who you are and what you do. Introduce others.

Any physical objects such as bedside tables, trays, or other impediments **should be moved out of the line between the physician and the patient,** and the television or radio should be turned off. In an office setting, the physician's chair should be moved adjacent to that of the patient. This can create a sense of the physician being more within reach and more connected to the patient (29).

Clutter and papers should be moved away from the area of desk nearest to the patient, and the physician should not talk while reading the chart. If any of these actions seem awkward, an option would be to state *"It may be easier for us to talk if I move the table/if you turn the television off for a moment."*

The most important rule of all is that the physician should sit down. This is an almost inviolable guideline. It is virtually impossible to assure a patient that she has a doctor's undivided attention if he or she remains standing. Anecdotal impressions suggest that when the doctor sits down, the patient perceives the period of time spent at the bedside as longer than if the doctor remains standing. The act of sitting indicates to the patient that she has control at a time when most patients are feeling that it is not they who are "calling the shots." It also indicates that the doctor is there to listen, saves time, and increases efficiency.

Before starting the interview itself, care should be taken to get the patient organized if necessary. After a physical examination, the patient should be allowed time to dress, to restore the sense of personal modesty.

Distance

It is important to be seated at a comfortable distance from the patient. This distance—sometimes called the "body buffer zone"—seems to vary from culture to culture, but a distance of 2 to 3 ft usually serves the purpose for intimate and personal conversation (29). This is another reason why the doctor who remains standing at the end of the bed—"6 ft away and 3 ft up," known colloquially as "the British position"—seems remote and aloof.

The height at which the doctor sits can also be important; normally, his or her eyes should be approximately level with those of the patient. If the patient is already upset or angry, a useful technique is to sit so that the doctor's eyes are below those of the patient. This often decreases the anger. The doctor should try to look relaxed, even if he or she is not feeling that way.

Positioning

The doctor should ensure that he or she is seated closest to the patient whenever possible, and that any friends or relatives are on the other side of the patient. A clear signal should be sent to relatives that the patient has primacy.

Have Tissues Nearby

In almost all oncology settings, it is important to have a box of tissues nearby. If the patient or relative begins to cry, they should be offered tissues. This not only gives overt permission to cry, but also allows the person to feel less vulnerable when crying.

Body Language

It is important to look relaxed and unhurried by sitting down comfortably with both feet flat on the floor, shoulders relaxed and dropped, coat or jacket undone, and hands rested on the knees—often called "the neutral position" in psychotherapy. Attention should be paid to nonverbal behavior, because it may communicate that the doctor is listening and concerned. For example, listening with the arms folded may imply to the patient that the doctor's mind is already made up, and that no further discussion is encouraged.

Eye Contact

Eye contact should be maintained for most of the time while the patient is talking. If the interview becomes intense or emotionally charged—particularly if the patient is crying or is very angry—it is helpful to the patient at that point for the doctor to look away—to break eye contact.

Touching the Patient

Touch may also be helpful during the interview if (i) a nonthreatening area is touched, such as the hand or forearm; (ii) the doctor is comfortable with touch; and (iii) the patient appreciates touch and does not withdraw.

Most clinicians have not been taught specific details of clinical touch at any time in their training (30). They are, therefore, likely to be ill at ease with touching as an interview technique until they have had some practice. Nevertheless, there is considerable evidence, although the data are somewhat soft, that touching the patient, particularly above the patient's waist to avoid misinterpretation, is of benefit during a medical interview (31). It seems likely that **touching is a significant action at times of distress and should be encouraged, with the proviso that the professional should be sensitive to the patient's reaction.** If the patient is comforted by the contact, it should be continued; if the patient is uncomfortable, it should be stopped. Touch can be misinterpreted, for example, as lasciviousness, aggression, or dominance, so the doctor should be aware that touching is an interviewing skill that requires extra self-regulation.

Starting Off

Introductions

The doctor should ensure that the patient knows who he or she is. Many practitioners make a point of getting up and shaking the patient's hand at the outset, although this is a matter of personal preference. Often the handshake may tell something about the family dynamics as well as about the patient. Frequently the patient's spouse will also extend his hand. It is worthwhile making sure that the patient's hand is shaken before that of the spouse, even if the spouse is nearer, to demonstrate that the patient is the most important person in this context. The "white-coat syndrome" is a well-known phenomenon that describes how the medical setting induces anxiety in many patients—often even leading to blood pressure increases—so a friendly greeting may go a long way at putting the patient at ease.

Others in the medical team should also be introduced by the doctor, for example, medical students, nurses, and the patient should introduce her supporters. At times, when there are many relatives present, as is not uncommon when there is a new diagnosis of cancer, it is judicious to ask the patient *"which two people would you like to come with you now?"* In this way except for family meetings, the physician will not be overwhelmed by the number of people that need to be addressed.

L—Listening Skills

As dialogue begins, the professional should show that she or he is in "listening mode." For a general review of interviewing skills, see Lipkin et al. (32). **The four main points to attend are covered in the following sections. They are the use of open questions, facilitation techniques, the use of clarification, and the handling of time and interruptions** (Table 24.3).

Open-Ended Questions

Open questions are simply questions that can be answered in any way or manner of response. In other words, the questions do not direct the respondent or require her to make a choice from a specific range of answers. In taking the medical history, of course, most of the questions are, appropriately, closed questions—*"Do you have swelling of the ankles?" "Have you had any bleeding after your menopause?"* In therapeutic dialogue, when the clinician is trying to be part of the patient's support system, open questions are an essential way of finding out what the patient

---

Table 24.3 Fundamental Listening Skills

Switch on your listening skills and techniques to show that you are an effective listener.

1. **Open Questions**
   Questions that can be answered in any way, for example, *"How are you?" "How did that make you feel?"*

2. **Facilitating**
   Pausing or being silent when patient speaks. Try not to interrupt. Nodding, smiling, saying *"mm hmm," "tell me more about that,"* and the like. Use repetition, that is, repeating one key word from patient's last sentence in your first sentence.

3. **Clarifying**
   Making overt any ambiguous or awkward topic

4. **Handling Time and Interruptions**
   With pagers and phones: Acknowledge the patient who is with you as you answer; tell patient about any time constraints and clarify when discussion will resume

is experiencing as a way of tailoring support for her. Hence, open questions—*"What did you think the diagnosis was?" "How did you feel when you were told that...?" "How did that make you feel?"* are a mandatory part of the "nonhistory" therapeutic dialogue. **A very useful phrase to use when it is unclear what a patient is trying to say is "tell me more," which invites the patient to expand on her thoughts or feelings.**

Facilitation Techniques	### Silence

The first and most important technique in facilitating dialogue between the patient and clinician is silence (33). If the patient is speaking, she should not be talked over. This, the simplest rule of all, is the one most often ignored, and it is most likely to give the patient the impression that the doctor is not listening.

Silences also have other significance: They can be—and often are—revealing about the patient's state of mind. Often, a patient falls silent when she has feelings that are too intense to express in words. A silence, therefore, means that the patient is thinking or feeling something important, not that she has stopped thinking. If the clinician can tolerate a pause or silence, the patient may well express the thought in words a moment later.

If breaking the silence is necessary, the ideal way to do so is to say *"What were you thinking about just then?"* or *"What is it that's making you pause?"* **For the physician, silence is especially important after giving bad news.** The patient's silence should not be addressed with reassurance or other "fix it" statements, which may make the doctor feel better, but which cut off the ability of the patient to process emotion.

Other Simple Facilitation Techniques

Having encouraged the patient to speak, the doctor should prove that he or she is hearing what is being said. This may be demonstrated by the following techniques: Nodding, pausing, smiling, saying *"Yes," "Mmm hmm," "Tell me more,"* or anything similar.

Repetition and Reiteration

Repetition, after sitting down, is probably the second most important technique of all interviewing skills. To show that the doctor is really hearing what the patient is saying, one or two key words from the patient's last sentence should be used in his or her own next sentence: *"I just feel so lousy most of the time"; "Tell me what you mean by feeling lousy."* Reiteration means repeating what the patient has said in the doctor's own words: *"Since I started those new pills, I've been feeling sleepy"; "So you're getting some drowsiness from the new pills."* Both repetition and reiteration confirm to the patient that she has been heard.

Reflection

Reflection is the act of restating the patient's statement in terms of what it means to the clinician. It takes the act of listening one step further and shows that the patient has been heard and interpreted correctly: *"If I understand you correctly, you're telling me that you lose control of your waking and sleeping when you're on these pills."* |
| **Clarification** | Patients often have concerns about treatment or other issues related to their care. When not asked about them directly, they may hint or express them in nuances, protests, or questions that are not clear. Listed below are some examples of how important information may be indirectly communicated.

Statement: *"I don't know how my family can take any more of this."*

Patient means: *"I really feel guilty."*

Statement: *"I just couldn't stand another round of chemo."*

Patient means: *"I felt so awful when my hair fell out."*

Statement: *"Doctor, how long do you think I have to live?"*

Patient means: *"I wonder if I'll see my grandson graduate."*

Statement: *"What will the end be like?"*

Patient means: *"How much will I suffer?"* |

As the patient talks, it is very tempting for the clinician to go along with what the patient is saying, even when the exact meaning or implication is unclear. This may lead very quickly to serious obstacles in the dialogue.

It is important to be honest when the patient's meaning is not understood. Many different phrases can be used—*"I'm sorry—I'm not quite sure what you meant when you said...," "When you say...do you mean that...?"* Clarification gives the patient an opportunity to expand on the previous statement or to amplify some aspect of the statement, now that the clinician has shown interest in the topic. **The key to addressing questions is to use clarifying statements that get at the issue underlying the expressed concern.**

Handling Time and Interruptions

Clinicians have a notorious reputation for being impolite when handling interruptions—by phone, pager, or other people, often appearing to abruptly ignore the patient, and going immediately to the phone, or responding immediately to the pager or to a colleague. This appears as a snub or an insult to the patient.

If calls cannot be ignored or pagers turned off—and most cannot—it is important to express sorrow to the patient about the interruption: *"Sorry, this is another doctor that I must speak to very briefly—I'll be back in a moment." "This is something quite urgent about another patient—I won't be more than a few minutes."* The same is true of time constraints: *"I'm afraid I have to go to the O. R. now, but this is an important conversation. We need to continue this tomorrow morning on the ward round ...").* If it is known that an important phone call is expected, the patient should be informed ahead of time so that she feels respected.

A—Acknowledgment—and Exploration—of Emotions

The Empathic Response

The empathic response is an extremely useful technique in an emotionally charged interview, yet is frequently misunderstood by students and trainees (Table 24.4).

The empathic response has nothing to do with the doctor's personal feelings. Sadness in the patient does not require the doctor to feel sad at that moment. It is simply a technique to acknowledge to the patient that the emotion she is experiencing has been observed. Importantly, **empathic responses are correlated with the degree of support that the patient experiences** (34).

The empathic response consists of three *mental* steps:

1. **Identifying the emotion that the patient is experiencing.**
2. **Identifying the origin and root cause of that emotion.**
3. **Responding in a way that tells the patient that the connection between steps 1 and 2 has been made.**

Often, **the most effective empathic responses follow the format of** *"You seem to be..."* or *"It must be,"* for example, *"It must be very distressing for you to know that all that therapy didn't give*

Table 24.4 Acknowledgment of Emotions: The Empathic Response
Acknowledging the emotional content of the interview is the central skill of being perceived as sensitive and supportive.
The central technique is the empathic response.
1. Identify the emotion
2. Identify the cause or source of the emotion
3. Respond in a way that shows you have made the connection between (1) and (2), for example, *"that must have felt awful," "this information has obviously come as quite a shock"*
The empathic response is a technique or skill—not a feeling. It is not necessary for you to (i) experience the same feelings as the patient or (ii) agree with the patient's view or assessment.

Table 24.5 Management Strategy

A reasonable management plan that the patient understands and will follow is better than an ideal plan that the patient will ignore.

1. **Think what is best medically, then . . .**

2. **Assess the patient's expectations of her condition, treatment, and outcome**—summarize this in your mind, or clarify and summarize aloud, if needed.

3. **Propose a strategy.**

4. **Assess the patient's response,** for example, what stage of action is the patient in: precontemplation, contemplation, implementation, or reinforcement phase?

5. **Agree on a plan** as far as possible.

---

you a long remission" or even *"This must be awful for you."* **The objective of the empathic response is to demonstrate to the patient that the emotion she is experiencing has been identified and acknowledged, thereby giving it legitimacy. It is a way of saying to the patient *"it's ok to feel that way."***

In fact, if the patient is experiencing a strong emotion, for example, anger or crying, and its existence is not acknowledged, all further attempts at communication will fail, and the doctor will be perceived as insensitive. This will render the rest of the interaction useless.

S—Management Strategy

There are several useful techniques to ensure that a management plan is constructed with which the patient concurs and will follow (Table 24.5). The following are useful guidelines:

1. **The optimal medical strategy in the doctor's mind should be determined.**

2. **The patient should be asked about her own expectations of her condition, treatment, and outcome.** When there is a marked mismatch between the patient's view of the situation and the medical facts, it will be more difficult to make the plan appear logical and acceptable.

The conclusions from steps 1 and 2 should be borne in mind when the strategy is proposed to the patient. As it is explained to the patient:

3. **The patient's response should be assessed.** Note should be made of the patient's progress in forming an action plan—the stages are often defined as the precontemplation, contemplation, implementation, and reinforcement phases. The patient's emotions should be acknowledged as they occur, and discussion continued in a contractual fashion until a plan has been determined to which the patient has agreed, and that she will follow. **The patient's understanding should be checked by asking her to repeat what she has been told.**

S—Summary

The summary is the closure of the interview. In gynecologic oncology, the relationship with the patient is likely to be a continuing one and a major component of the patient's treatment. The closure of the interview is an important time to emphasize that point.

It is relatively straightforward to cover three areas in the summary (Table 24.6). They are **(i)** a *précis* or reiteration of the main points covered in the dialogue; **(ii)** an *invitation* for the

---

Table 24.6 Summary and Closure

Ending of the interview has three main components.

1. **A précis or summary of the main topics** you have discussed

2. **Identification of any important issues that need further discussion** even if you do not have time to discuss them in this interview, they can be on the agenda for the next

3. **A clear contract for the next contact**

---

patient to ask questions; and (iii) *a clear arrangement for the next interaction*—"**a clear contract for the contact.**" This part of the interview is not necessarily long, but does require considerable focus and concentration.

SPIKES: a Variation of CLASS for Breaking Bad News

Among the various types of medical interviews, breaking bad news is a special case, and one of exceptional importance for both parties in the clinician–patient relationship (25,35,36).

Bad news can best be defined as any news that seriously adversely affects the patient's view of her future (37). In other words, the "badness" of bad news is the gap between the patient's expectations of the future and the medical reality. This is crucially important because what is good news for one patient, for example, *"I'm really glad they could operate on this tumor,"* may be very bad for another, for example, *"I don't think I can take another operation."* In gynecologic oncology, bad news is common at many stages in a patient's history: (i) Initial diagnosis; (ii) recurrence or disease progression; (iii) clinical deterioration; (iv) development of new complications; and (v) change from therapeutic to palliative intent. It is necessary to have a protocol that will function in all these circumstances.

Both physician communication skills and patient-centered factors are associated with higher patient satisfaction with the gynecologic cancer diagnosis disclosure experience (38). **Patient-centered factors include the perception of physician sensitivity and empathy, having the opportunity to ask questions and express emotion, and setting the pace of conversation. Higher patient satisfaction scores are associated with face-to-face disclosure compared with over the phone disclosure, communication of the information in a private setting compared with an impersonal setting, and an encounter longer than 10 minutes.**

The SPIKES protocol has been designed specifically for these purposes and allows assessment of the patient's expectations before sharing the information (Table 24.7).

S—Setting = Context + Listening Skills

In the SPIKES protocol, for the sake of convenience, two phases of the CLASS protocol have been combined—the *context* (Table 24.2) and *listening skills* (Table 24.3)—into "setting."

P—The Patient's Perception of the Situation

The cardinal rule of breaking bad news is to find out what the patient already knows or suspects before going on to share the information. To condense this into a slogan, it might be said: "Before you tell, ask."

The exact words used to find out how much the patient already understands are a personal choice (Table 24.8)—*"Before I go on to tell you about the results, why don't you tell me what you've been thinking?" "When you first developed that swelling of the abdomen, what did you think was going on?" "Had you been thinking this was something serious?"* or *"What did the referring medical team tell you about your medical condition?"*

As the patient replies, particular attention should be paid to her *vocabulary* and *comprehension* of the subject. When starting to give information, it is very helpful to start at the same level of knowledge as the patient (39).

Table 24.7 The SPIKES Protocol for Breaking Bad News[a]
S—**Setting** = Context, **connection** and **listening skills**
P—**Patient's perception** of her condition and its seriousness
I—**Invitation** from the patient to give information
K—**Knowledge**—giving medical facts
E—**Explore emotions** and empathize as the patient responds
S—**Strategy and summary**

[a]A variant of the basic CLASS approach.

Table 24.8 Patient's Perception of Condition

Ask the patient to say what she knows or suspects about the current medical problem, for example, "What did you think when...?" or "Did you think it might be serious...?"

As the patient replies:

Listen to the level of comprehension and vocabulary.

Note any mismatch between the actual medical information and the patient's perception of it, including denial.

I—Getting a Clear Invitation to Share News

Next, it is important to try to get a clear invitation to share the information (Table 24.9). **Most patients want full disclosure. There has been a steady increase in the desire for honest information since Oken's (40) study in 1961, when 95% of surgeons indicated that they did not disclose a cancer diagnosis to their patients.** Twenty years later, a study by Novack et al. (41) showed a dramatic reversal of this proportion. Regarding the proportion of patients who state they want to be informed, Jones's (42) study in 1981 showed that 50% of British patients wanted to know. Since then, there have been many studies that all put **the proportion of patients who want full disclosure at above 90%** (43–45).

Disguising the information or lying to the patient is highly likely to be unsatisfactory. The phrase used to obtain a clear invitation is again a matter of personal choice and judgment—*"Are you the sort of person who'd like to know exactly what's going on?" "Would you like me to go on and tell you exactly what the situation is and what we recommend?"* or *"How would you like me to handle this information? Would you like to know exactly what's going on?"*

Once this is determined, goals can be set for the interview, for example, *"So now I'm going to explain what the MRI showed."*

It is important to respect cultural norms that may delineate how bad news is discussed. For example, in some Middle Eastern countries, the word "dying" is not used, and in others, bad information is felt to cause the progression of the patient's illness. For example, in some Native American tribes, giving bad news is felt to make the situation worse (46).

K—Knowledge—Explaining the Medical Facts

Having obtained a clear invitation to share information, the medical facts should be given while simultaneously being aware of and sensitive to the patient's reaction to the information—in other words, giving the information and responding to the patient's emotions should proceed simultaneously.

The most important guidelines for giving the medical facts are shown in Table 24.10.

- **The level of comprehension and use the vocabulary that the patient has indicated should be used—this is called aligning.**
- **Plain, intelligible English should be used, avoiding the technical jargon of the medical profession—"medspeak." Information should be given in small amounts.** The assistance of an interpreter is essential when speaking with someone who is not English speaking.
- **The patient's understanding of the information should be checked before going further**—*"Do you follow what I'm saying?" "Is this clear so far?" "Am I making sense so far?"*
- **A narrative approach should be used to make sense of what has occurred; the sequence of events and their implications should be explained**—*"When you became*

Table 24.9 Invitation from Patient to Give Information

Find out from the patient if she wants to know the details of the medical condition or treatment, for example, *"Are you the sort of person who...?"*

Accept patient's right not to know, but offer to answer questions as patient wishes later.

Table 24.10 Knowledge: Giving Medical Facts
Bring the patient toward a comprehension of the medical situation, filling in any gaps.
Use language intelligible to the patient, and start at the level at which he or she finished.
Give information in small pieces.
Check the reception: Confirm that the patient understands what you are saying after each significant piece of information.
Respond to the patient's reactions as they occur.

short of breath, we didn't know whether it was just a chest infection or something more serious. So that's when we did the chest x-ray...."

- **All emotions expressed by the patient should be responded to as they arise,** as discussed below.

E—Emotions—Exploration and Empathic Response

The acknowledgment of emotions is more important in an interview about bad news than it is in most other interviews, for example, see Section "A—Acknowledgment" in the CLASS protocol, previously (Table 24.4).

The doctor can effectively use an empathic response on his or her own feelings if they are becoming intense—*"I'm finding this very upsetting, too."*

The value of all empathic responses lies in the fact that an observation is being made that is almost unemotional in itself about an issue that is heavily charged with emotion—whether the patient's or the doctor's. The fact that this is experienced by the patient as a supportive response is why an empathic response cools the temperature of a fraught moment and facilitates the exploration of the situation without causing escalation.

S—Strategy and Summary

The interview should be closed with a management strategy and closure, as described in the sections "S—Strategy" and "S—Summary" for the CLASS protocol (Table 24.5). It is useful to ask the patient to repeat what she has understood about the plan to ensure appropriate comprehension.

Challenging Conversations

Dealing with Hope and False Hopes

Many clinicians and patients often say *"But you can't take away hope."* **Frequently clinicians use this as an excuse for not telling the patient the truth. Usually, the real rationale behind this attitude is to protect the clinician from discomfort, not the patient.**

Clinicians are more likely to create major problems for themselves if they promise cure when that is not possible or hold out unrealistic hopes. Supporting the patient and reinforcing realistic hopes is part of the foundation of a genuinely therapeutic relationship. Setting realistic goals for treatment early on allows the patient to "hope for the best while preparing for the worst" (47,48).

The important thing is not whether to tell the truth—there is a moral, ethical, and legal obligation to do so if that is what the patient wants—but how to tell the truth. Insensitive and ineffective truth telling may be just as damaging and counterproductive as insensitive lying. In practice, the preceding protocols allow the truth to be told at a pace determined by the patient, and in a way that allows recruitment and reinforcement of the patient's coping strategies.

Clinicians may overlook the fact that patients often have more than one hope. Early on in the disease patients hold on tightly to a hope for cure. As a disease progresses, or when significant and disabling side effects occur, their focus may shift to other goals in life such as time spent with loved ones or anticipated events, such as a daughter's wedding.

Communication in Palliative Care

In palliative care, communication skills can be even more important than in acute care—and may sometimes be the only therapeutic modality available to the clinician (49). **In palliative care, communication may have at least three distinct functions: (i) taking the history; (ii) breaking bad news; and (iii) as therapeutic dialogue, that is, support of the patient.**

Even when the prognosis is acknowledged to be grave, there may be stages in which some hoped-for improvement or stabilization is not achieved. In these circumstances, the SPIKES protocol can be helpful, even when the clinician and the patient already have a long-standing relationship.

At other times, **simply listening to the patient and acknowledging the various emotions and reactions she is experiencing is in itself a therapeutic intervention.** This is particularly true in discussions about dying. **Nonabandonment and acknowledging appreciation of the patient's circumstance may be powerful strategies to pay attention to at the end of life** (50). When a patient realizes and acknowledges that she is dying, there is no "answer" the clinician can give. Instead, listening to the questions, issues, and emotions is a valuable service.

Discussing Prognosis

When patients present with advanced disease, it is often a quandary as to how much to tell the patient about the seriousness of her disease. While many studies have shown that patients want specific information about their prognosis, and estimations of how long they have to live, it is difficult to predict how much information they actually want and its timing. It is important to negotiate the amount of information and modulate its delivery. **Increased question asking and discussion of prognosis have been shown not to increase anxiety, but rather to promote greater patient satisfaction, lower anxiety and depression, and curtail use of alternative therapies** (51,52). **End-of-life discussions about the poor short-term outlook may cut down on use of heroic measures, and encourage more use of supportive care services** (53).

Many patients misunderstand the purpose of treatment, so it is important to be clear about the goals of care. For example, when patients present with advanced disease, the strategy of "hoping for the best but preparing for the worst" may be helpful. The statement that *"your disease is not likely curable, but we will give you the best treatment available"* can serve to maintain hope, while opening the door to further questions from the patient.

Talking to Family Members

Family members are an important component of the psychological context surrounding the patient. Often they may assist the clinician in confirming the medical facts and supporting the patient as she responds to the information. Sometimes, however, **individual family members may be at a different phase of acceptance or understanding of the medical information than the patient. This is called discordance,** and it can be a serious additional problem for the clinician. This is particularly true in a potential conflict, such as when a relative tells a clinician, *"My mother is not to be told the diagnosis."* This is a common and awkward situation. It requires care and effort to emphasize the primacy of the patient's right to knowledge, if that is what she wants; while at the same time underlining the relative's importance and value as part of the patient's support system.

It is often helpful in discordance to ask the family member what they understand about the disease or where the treatment is so that the goals of care can be clarified. In other instances, **it is useful to explore with the family member what they think the patient already knows.** This will often move the discussion to how to best assist the family as they deal with the patient's illness at a time when they may feel helpless.

Another exceptionally difficult situation for the clinician is telling a relative that the patient has died. The central principle is to use a narrative approach to the events, but to be prepared at any instant to respond to the relative if he or she asks whether the patient has died.

Difficult Questions

At times patients or family members may ask questions that are awkward to answer, such as *"how much time do I have?"* or *"how am I going to tell my husband?"* A good rule of thumb is to assume that there is a specific concern behind the question. The patient who asks *"how much time do I have"* often is wondering if they will be able to meet a milestone in their life, such as seeing a grandson graduate from college. It is useful to remember the *"ask before you tell"* strategy, while acknowledging that you heard the patient's question. This might be something such as *"I'd be happy to talk to you about that but first I'd like to understand if there is a specific reason for asking."*

In the second instance, a simple exploratory question such as *"tell me about your concerns regarding your husband"* may reveal important information such as her concern about shocking him, or burdening him with caregiving responsibilities.

Another question that often comes up is *"what would you do doctor?"* A neutral but exploratory response to this question might be *"I can't really answer that because I am not in your situation, but tell me what is troubling you about your decision?"*

Sometimes out of desperation, a patient or family member may ask *"isn't there any more you can do?"* This is best responded to with an empathic statement, for example, *"I can see this is very hard for you,"* followed by a wish statement *"you know I wish there were another therapy that would do more good than harm."*

Communication with Other Healthcare Professionals

Medical professionals are only human, and under great stress, may become short-tempered, rude, aggressive, or impatient, which is difficult to mitigate. With good communication skills, the resulting damage can be minimized.

The two principles that are most useful are (i) clarification and (ii) acknowledgment of the situation using empathic responses. Whenever an emotion is responded to by acknowledging it with a relatively unemotional empathic response, the dispute will deescalate. It is also worth remembering the old adage that *"an ounce of prevention is worth a pound of cure."* Giving information early—a *"preemptive information strike"*—prefaced as a *"for your information"* discussion may prevent major disputes or discontent later—*"Why didn't you tell me...?"*

Motivation and Manners

Like any clinical intervention, effective communication requires motivation to be successful. **If the doctor is motivated to be a good clinical communicator, it is achievable.** Some of it depends on having a basic strategy for the task, and the protocols presented here should be helpful. The rest is largely a matter of being aware of the effect of what is said and done on the patient and her family. There is a great deal of courtesy and common sense mixed in with the specific strategies. It is important to be mindful of the fact that if chosen poorly, words can be scalpels, but if chosen carefully, they can be perceived by the patient and family as a source of comfort and support.

Communication tasks are of enormous importance in the relationship between doctor and patient. As has been said, "Do this part of your job badly and they will never forgive you; do it well and they will never forget you."

Acknowledgement   This chapter is dedicated to its former coauthor **Robert Buckman, MD, PhD**...scholar, wit, and doctor's doctor. Rob left us in 2011...but left behind so much.

References

1. **Armstrong DK.** Relapsed ovarian cancer: Challenges and management strategies for a chronic disease. *Oncologist.* 2002;7(suppl 5): 20–28.
2. **Sardell AN, Trierweiler SJ.** Disclosing the cancer diagnosis: Procedures that influence patient hopefulness. *Cancer.* 1993;72:3355–3365.
3. **Zachariae R, Pedersen CG, Jensen AB, et al.** Association of perceived physician communication style with patient satisfaction, distress, cancer-related self-efficacy, and perceived control over the disease. *Br J Cancer.* 2003;88:658–665.
4. **Kerr J, Engel J, Schlesinger-Raab A, et al.** Doctor-patient communication: Results of a four-year prospective study in rectal cancer patients. *Dis Colon Rectum.* 2003;46:1038–1046.
5. **Dimoska A, Butow PN, Dent E, et al.** An examination of the initial cancer consultation of medical and radiation oncologists using the Cancode interaction analysis system. *Brit J Cancer.* 2008;98:1508–1514.
6. **Kaplan SH, Greenfield S, Ware JE.** Impact of the doctor-patient relationship on the outcomes of chronic disease. In: **Stewart M, Roter D, eds.** *Communicating with Medical Patients.* Newbury Park, CA: Sage Publications; 1989:228–245.
7. **Bredart A, Bouleuc C, Dolbeault S.** Doctor-patient communication and satisfaction with care in oncology. *Curr Opin Oncol.* 2005;17: 351–354.
8. **Gandhi IG, Parle JV, Greenfield SM, et al.** A qualitative investigation into why patients change their GPs. *Fam Pract.* 1997;14:49–57.
9. **Levinson W, Chaumeton N.** Communication between surgeons and patients in routine office visits. *Surgery.* 1999;125:127–134.
10. **Ambady N, Laplante D, Nguyen T, et al.** Surgeons' tone of voice: A clue to malpractice history. *Surgery.* 2002;132:5–9.
11. **Albrecht TL, Ruckdeschel JC, Riddle DL, et al.** Communication and consumer decision making about cancer clinical trials. *Patient Educ Couns.* 2003;50:39–42.
12. **Stewart MA.** Effective physician-patient communication and health outcomes: A review. *CMAJ.* 1995;152:1423–1433.
13. **Epstein AM, Street RL.** *Patient-Centered Communication in Cancer Care: Promoting Healing and Reducing Suffering.* Bethesda, MD: National Cancer Institute; 2007:NIH Publication No. 07–6225.
14. **Hoffman M, Ferri J, Sison C, et al.** Teaching communication skills: An AACE survey of oncology training programs. *J Cancer Educ.* 2004;19:220–224.
15. **Baile WF, Buckman R, Lenzi R, et al.** SPIKES-A six-step protocol for delivering bad news: Application to the patient with cancer. *Oncologist.* 2000;5:302–311.
16. **Wallace J, Hlubocky FJ, Daugherty CK.** Emotional responses of oncologists when disclosing prognostic information to patients with

terminal disease; Results of qualitative data from a mailed survey to ASCO members. *J Clin Oncol.* 2006;24(Suppl 18):8520.

17. **Taylor KM.** "Telling bad news": Physicians and the disclosure of undesirable information. *Sociol Health Illn.* 1988;10:109–132.

18. **Maguire P, Pitceathly C.** Key communication skills and how to acquire them. *BMJ.* 2002;325:697–700.

19. **Harrington SE, Smith TJ.** The role of chemotherapy at the end of life: "When is enough, enough?" *JAMA.* 2008;299:2667–2678.

20. **Garg A, Buckman R, Kason Y.** Teaching medical students how to break bad news. *CMAJ.* 1997;6:1159–1164.

21. **Baile WB, Kudelka AP, Beale EA, et al.** Communication skills training in oncology: Description and preliminary outcomes of workshops on breaking bad news and managing patient reactions to illness. *Cancer.* 1999;86:887–897.

22. **Maguire P, Faulkner A.** Improve the counselling skills of doctors and nurses in cancer care. *BMJ.* 1999;297:847–849.

23. **Simpson M, Buckman R, Stewart M, et al.** Doctor-patient communication: The Toronto consensus statement. *BMJ.* 1991;393: 1985–1987.

24. **Back AL, Arnold RM, Baile WF, et al.** Efficacy of communication skills training for giving bad news and discussing transitions to palliative care. *Arch Intern Med.* 2007;167:453–460.

25. **Buckman R, Kason Y.** *How to Break Bad News: A Guide for Health Care Professionals.* Baltimore, MD: Johns Hopkins University Press; 1992.

26. **Baile W, Buckman R.** *The Pocket Guide to Communication Skills in Clinical Practice.* Toronto, ON: Medical Audio-Visual Communications; 1998.

27. **Buckman R, Baile W, Korsch B.** *A Practical Guide to Communication Skills in Clinical Practice.* CD-ROM or video set. Toronto, ON: Medical Audio-Visual Communications; 1998.

28. **Baile WB, Glober GA, Lenzi R, et al.** Discussing disease progression and end-of-life decisions. *Oncology.* 1999;13:1021–1031.

29. **Hall ET.** *The Hidden Dimension.* New York: Doubleday; 1966.

30. **Older J.** Teaching touch at medical school. *JAMA.* 1984;252:931–933.

31. **Buis C, De Boo T, Hull R.** Touch and breaking bad news. *Earn Pract.* 1991;8:303–304.

32. **Lipkin M, Quill TE, Napodano J.** The medical interview: A core curriculum for residencies in internal medicine. *Ann Intern Med.* 1984;100:277–284.

33. **Frankel RM, Beckman HB.** The pause that refreshes. *Hosp Pract.* 1988;23:62–67.

34. **Pollak KI, Alexander SC, Tulsky JA, et al.** Physician empathy and listening: Associations with patient satisfaction and autonomy. *J Am Board Fam Med.* 2011;24:665–672.

35. **Ptacek JT, Eberhardt L.** The patient-physician relationship: Breaking bad news. A review of the literature. *JAMA.* 1996;276:496–502.

36. **Billings AJ.** *Outpatient Management of Advanced Cancer: Symptom Control, Support, and Hospice-in-the-Home.* Philadelphia, PA: JB Lippincott; 1985:236–259.

37. **Buckman R.** Breaking bad news: Why is it still so difficult? *BMJ.* 1984;288:1597–1599.

38. **Kuoki LM, Zhao Q, Jeffe DB, et al.** Disclosing a cancer diagnosis: Conversations specific to gynecologic oncology patients. *Obstet Gynecol.* 2013;122:1033–1039.

39. **Maynard DW.** On clinicians co-implicating recipients perspective in the delivery of bad news. In: **Drew P, Heritage J, eds.** *Talk at Work: Social Interaction in Institutional Settings.* Cambridge: Cambridge University Press; 1992:331–358.

40. **Oken D.** What to tell cancer patients: A study of medical attitudes. *JAMA.* 1961;175:86–94.

41. **Novack DH, Plumer R, Smith RL, et al.** Changes in physicians' attitudes toward telling the cancer patient. *JAMA.* 1979;241:897–900.

42. **Jones JS.** Telling the right patient. *BMJ.* 1981;283:291–292.

43. **Meredith C, Symonds P, Webster L, et al.** Information needs of cancer patients in west Scotland: Cross-sectional survey of patients' views. *BMJ.* 1996;313:724–726.

44. **Benson J, Britten N.** Respecting the autonomy of cancer patients when talking with their families: Qualitative analysis of semi-structured interviews with patients. *BMJ.* 1996;313:729–731.

45. **Northouse PG, Northouse LL.** Communication and cancer: Issues confronting patients, health professionals and family members. *J Psychosocial Oncol.* 1988;5:17–45.

46. **Baile WF, Lenzi R, Parker PA, et al.** Oncologists' attitudes toward and practices in giving bad news: An exploratory study. *J Clin Oncol.* 2002;20:2189–2196.

47. **Von Roenn JH, von Gunten CF.** Setting goals to maintain hope. *J Clin Oncol.* 2003;21:570–574.

48. **Back AL, Arnold RM, Quill TE.** Hope for the best, and prepare for the worst. *Ann Intern Med.* 2003;138:439–443.

49. **Buckman R.** Communication in palliative care: A practical guide. In: **Doyle D, Hanks GWC, MacDonald N, eds.** *Oxford Textbook of Palliative Care.* Oxford: Oxford University Press; 1998:141–156.

50. **Back AL, Arnold RM, Tulsky J.** *Mastering Difficult End of Life Communications.* New York, NY: Cambridge Press; 2009:121–136.

51. **Chochinov HM, Tataryn DJ, Wilson KG, et al.** Prognostic awareness and the terminally ill. *Psychosomatics.* 2000;41:500–541.

52. **Pruyn JF, Rijckman RM, van Brunschot CJ, et al.** Cancer patients' personality characteristics, physician-patient communication and adoption of the Moerman diet. *Soc Sci Med.* 1989;20: 841–847.

53. **Wright AA, Zhang B, Ray A, et al.** Associations between end-of-life discussions, patient mental health, medical care near death, and caregiver bereavement adjustment. *JAMA.* 2008;300:1665–1673.

25

Symptom Relief and Palliative Care

Rosanne Moses
Jennifer A. M. Philip
J. Norelle Lickiss

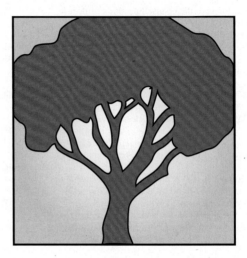

Throughout the course of a woman's illness, anticancer treatment should be coupled with attention to symptom relief, and personal and family support (1). **The development of progressive cancer heralds a point in care where reflection upon the woman's priorities, and clarification of her goals, should be a priority.** Careful exploration of priorities may reveal the importance, for example, of time spent at home, or the need to attend to personal relationships. Ideally, these issues should be raised over time and multiple clinical encounters, rather than suddenly at the time of crisis.

The concept of "parallel care" has been widely advocated (2,3). This concept implies attention to the principles of palliative care (personal and family support, symptom relief, and care planning/death preparation) from the time of diagnosis of a disease with a high likelihood of eventually becoming a fatal illness, for example, advanced ovarian cancer. The alternative approach of introducing palliative care only after anticancer treatments cease has many deficiencies, including potential lack of adequate symptom relief throughout treatment, and perceived abandonment of the patient by the primary physician as care is "handed over" to a new group of healthcare professionals.

The goals of palliative care should be to facilitate comfort, personal rehabilitation, and quality of life in the face of an incurable illness. The patient's quality of life will be determined by many aspects of her life including her values, her relationships, her sense of self-worth, and health-related matters. A woman can achieve much and indeed may report "quality" in a number of areas, even in the face of progressive illness. The challenge for health caregivers is to create a climate in which such achievements may emerge.

The last phase of life is crucial to the completion of a human life. Patients report that important issues at the conclusion of a fulfilled life include relief of pain and other symptoms, clear decision-making, preparation for death, being able to contribute to others, and being affirmed as a whole person (4–6). During this final phase, it is the responsibility of the medical and nursing professions to facilitate maximum autonomy and dignity, through careful symptom relief, good communication and decision-making, and the development or continuation of a supportive relationship.

Practical Aspects of Palliative Care

The palliative care of a woman with advanced gynecologic malignancy involves several components: assessment, clarification and delineation of therapeutic options, implementation of treatment, evaluation of outcome, continuing review and reassessment, and prognostication. Attention to each of these clinical tasks is necessary for a woman to maximize her possibilities in the final part of life.

Assessment

It is essential to make a comprehensive assessment, which includes listening to the patient's experience with her cancer, from the prediagnostic phase to the current time. There should be detailing of responses to treatments, side effects experienced, hopes realized, and, conversely, disappointments encountered. The narrative of the illness experience will give information on the patient's responses and her vulnerabilities and supports. It establishes a shared understanding of what has gone before and is a much more useful therapeutic tool than a checklist approach.

A comprehensive assessment involves at least the following:

1. **Ascertainment of the patient's current symptoms and other problems,** in her order of priorities, because only the woman herself can determine which is affecting her quality of life and requiring attention.

2. **Clarification of the nature and the extent of the neoplastic process,** with careful consideration of any other pathologic process, including comorbidities, that may be contributing to the current problems, or may be likely to contribute in the near future.

3. **Clarification of her understanding of her illness and the treatment goals.**

4. **Delineation of the personal and social context within which the patient is living** and from which she may draw support.

5. **Elucidation of her current goals**—the delineation of such goals and discussion concerning their achievability can do much to enhance a person's sense of self and hence quality of life.

Involvement of family in the consultation, with the woman's permission, is often useful as it provides additional understanding of relationships and supports, and may yield other perspectives that have implications for care. The assessment should be regarded as a continuous process, as both the circumstances of the illness and the woman's priorities are constantly changing.

Clinical Decision-Making

On the basis of a comprehensive assessment, with or without further investigations to elucidate the mechanism of troublesome symptoms, it is normally possible to delineate the reasonable therapeutic possibilities.

The choice between therapeutic options should reflect the patient's priorities. In general, alternatives involving the least dependence on medical facilities and the least use of the patient's time, resources, and personal energy should be recommended, particularly in the setting of advanced disease. For example, it would be inappropriate to resort to intravenous (or spinal) techniques for pain relief if oral, transcutaneous, or subcutaneous techniques had not been adequately explored. **When decision-making is shared and enacted to realize a woman's nominated priorities, quality of life is often improved.** For example, the fulfillment of a goal to return home may be more important to some than a minor extension of life from a further course of antibiotics.

Careful consideration of relevant antitumor measures (surgery, radiation therapy, or chemotherapy) is always mandatory, because control of the neoplastic process usually offers the best chance of alleviating symptoms. **Factors that should be considered when evaluating therapy include the following** (7):

1. **The stage of disease**

2. **The likely natural history of the illness with and without intervention, including the likely symptom patterns**

3. **The burden of investigation and treatment**

4. **The likely success of the intervention**

5. **The potential for rehabilitation (physical, psychological, social, or spiritual)**

6. **The patient's goals and priorities**

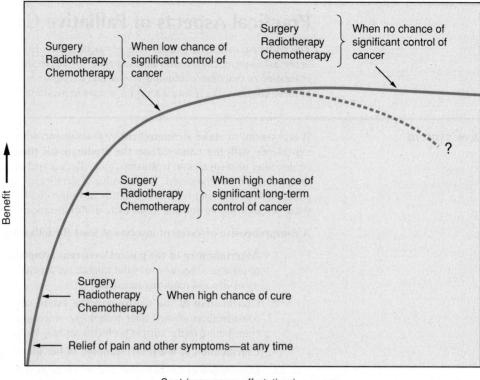

Surgery
Radiotherapy
Chemotherapy } When low chance of
significant control of
cancer

Surgery
Radiotherapy
Chemotherapy } When no chance of
significant control of
cancer

Surgery
Radiotherapy
Chemotherapy } When high chance of
significant long-term
control of cancer

Surgery
Radiotherapy
Chemotherapy } When high chance of cure

Relief of pain and other symptoms—at any time

Benefit

Cost (resources, effort, time)

Figure 25.1 Factors to be taken into account when considering further anticancer therapy: Benefit versus cost.

If cost–benefit issues are considered, **it is essential to avoid "flat of the curve" medicine**. Good symptom relief is almost always high in benefit in relation to cost (broadly considered), whereas anticancer measures may vary in benefit. These matters are represented simply in Figure 25.1.

Clinical decision-making is always undertaken in a context of prevailing values, much influenced by culture, social circumstances, and facts (legal, medical, and resource limitations).

Decisions concerning treatment should usually involve the patient, who should be adequately informed about the advantages and disadvantages of the various options. Such involvement may help the patient to regain control at a potentially chaotic time in her life. **Although the patient should share in decision-making, her attending clinician should indicate the course of action he or she favors** and ultimately take the responsibility for any intervention, so that a distressing outcome does not engender guilt in the patient and her family. This being said, the physician should not compromise his or her better judgment or conscience in the face of patient or family pressure.

The burden of decision-making is considerable and ways of reaching decisions vary according to social, cultural, economic, and medical contexts. When disagreements arise between patients (or their families) and clinicians regarding clinical decisions, it is often useful to consult within the treating team to determine if a range of views exists among clinicians. **A negotiated position between patient and clinician can almost always be reached.** If not, a second opinion or a perceived "independent broker" may be useful (8,9).

There are no circumstances that justify a physician's declaring "there is nothing more that can be done." A decision not to pursue anticancer treatments, but to focus solely on symptomatic measures, does not indicate nihilism or inactivity. It may reflect authentic clinical wisdom with clear goals of comfort and dignity.

**Evaluation of
Outcomes**

Evaluation of palliative interventions is best performed by the informed patient, although the observations of the medical and nursing staff are important. Evaluations should be performed regularly, at intervals consistent with the clinical goal. Pain measurements may, for example, be appropriately performed each time observations such as blood pressure and temperature are undertaken. For patients with advanced disease when the goals of care are centered on comfort and dignity, monitoring only of those parameters that serve these goals is justified. Formal outcome measures based on subjective criteria, of which there are many examples (10–14), should ideally be introduced into routine clinical practice, with outcomes to be measured commensurate with the patient's priorities for comfort and for personal objectives.

Discussing Prognosis	Mention should be made of the art of prognostication, because estimates of survival underlie much of the clinical decision-making. There is a considerable body of literature to guide the clinician when formulating a prognosis (15–17). **Factors to be considered** in such a formulation for patients with advanced cancer **include performance status, symptoms and signs relating to nutritional status such as anorexia, and other key symptoms including dyspnea. Biologic parameters,** including white cell counts, lymphocyte ratios, and serum albumin **also appear to be important** (17). These prognostic factors differ from those for a newly diagnosed cancer, such as tumor size and grade (17).

While it may be possible to determine a probability of survival for a particular patient, the communication of this information to the patient and her family requires thought and care. Such a discussion should occur in the context of a supportive relationship, and when the clinician has sufficient time to devote to the task. If the discussion has been prompted by a question, it is important to clarify what the patient has asked, and what has motivated her to ask it. The patient's understanding of her current situation should be ascertained. It is often helpful to ask the patient what she believes her prognosis to be. **The uncertainty of prognostic elements must be explained, and information should be given slowly, at a pace dictated by the patient** (9).

A reasonable approach for many patients in the face of a question concerning prognosis is to offer some time boundaries within which death is likely to occur. Such boundaries are useful for determining priorities and for planning medical care to best serve those priorities. Time boundaries do not give a patient or her family an agonizing date around which to focus, nor do they suggest that what is still somewhat uncertain can be predicted precisely (9,18,19).

Symptoms and Their Relief

In general, **effective antidisease therapy offers the best chance of good symptom relief if the patient is a "responder,"** but the quality of life of a "nonresponder" to chemotherapy may be worse than that of an untreated patient. Expertise in palliative therapeutics should be made available alongside surgery, chemotherapy, and radiation therapy, and delivered according to clinical needs, not prognosis (1).

Symptoms are subjective and their presence and severity are not necessarily apparent to the observer. A patient in severe pain may show no signs of distress, yet she may admit upon careful questioning that the pain is almost unbearable. Her expressions of pain will be influenced by cultural and environmental factors and by personal and interpersonal relationships. Accurate assessment of symptoms requires skill, patience, and active, supportive listening. **Symptoms vary in their significance for the patient,** and anxiety or distress associated with the development of a particular symptom will inevitably have a psychological impact. **It is important to give the patient a chance to express her fears and to offer some explanation for the symptom,** because this will at least reduce uncertainty.

Symptoms may arise from the tumor itself, from the treatment, and from unrelated causes. Symptoms may precede signs or objective evidence (x-ray or scans) of disease. An example is the development of leg pain from lumbosacral plexus infiltration, which may herald recurrent cervical cancer. Imaging may fail to demonstrate a lesion suspected on the basis of symptoms, but the pain needs treatment even while awaiting a definitive diagnosis. Waiting for objective signs may be disastrous in certain circumstances, such as in the early diagnosis of remediable spinal cord compression.

There is now considerable literature concerning the understanding and therapy of major symptoms in cancer, and attention is given here to those seen more commonly, with emphasis on practical considerations.

Pain Management

Pain is defined by the International Association for the Study of Pain as "an unpleasant sensory and emotional experience associated with actual or potential tissue damage or described in terms of such damage." Thus pain is subjective—all pain is "in the mind." Psychological factors influence the perception of pain. Pain is the experience of a person, not a part of the body, and changing the experience of a person is a major challenge. Effective pain management is dependent upon understanding and delineating the pain mechanisms involved, and prescribing medication based upon these mechanisms. Controversies relevant to gynecologic practice remain, not least being the global inequity in access to pain relief for women with gynecologic cancer (20).

Pain in gynecologic cancer presents in many forms and may occur at any stage in the illness. It may be caused by the disease and its treatment. Pain caused by treatment (e.g., radiation therapy) requires as close attention as that caused by tumor. Many guidelines for the assessment and treatment of cancer pain have been published, including those by the National Comprehensive Cancer Network and the European Society of Medical Oncology (21,22). The following simple steps provide a practical approach in the face of the complexity of recent research and practice (23).

Pain management must begin with a diagnosis of the likely mechanism of the pain at this site and at this time. The mechanism of pain can usually be diagnosed clinically. The history should include the mode of onset, characteristics, distribution, aggravating factors, trends over time, and response to therapeutic endeavors thus far. Therapeutic approaches vary according to the mechanism that is operative. **Following diagnosis of the pain mechanism, management may proceed according to the following four steps** (Fig. 25.2):

1. **Reduce the noxious stimulus at the periphery.**
2. **Raise the pain threshold.**
3. **Consider and use appropriate doses of opioid drugs.**
4. **Recognize residual neuropathic pain and treat it correctly.**

Such steps should be considered in order, but measures relating to all four steps may be instituted simultaneously if the clinical circumstances dictate.

Step One: Reduce the Noxious Stimulus at the Periphery

This step demands an adequate understanding of the mechanism of the pain stimulus in the individual patient. Pain in patients with gynecologic cancer is most commonly due to soft tissue infiltration, bone involvement, neural involvement, muscle spasm (e.g., psoas spasm), infection

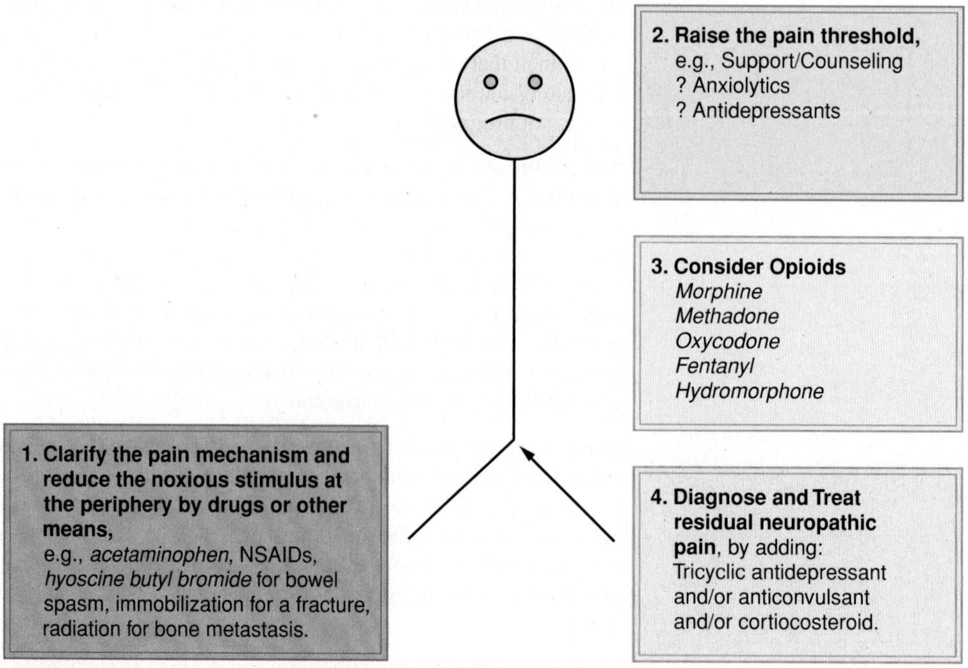

2. Raise the pain threshold,
e.g., Support/Counseling
? Anxiolytics
? Antidepressants

3. Consider Opioids
Morphine
Methadone
Oxycodone
Fentanyl
Hydromorphone

1. Clarify the pain mechanism and reduce the noxious stimulus at the periphery by drugs or other means,
e.g., *acetaminophen*, NSAIDs, *hyoscine butyl bromide* for bowel spasm, immobilization for a fracture, radiation for bone metastasis.

4. Diagnose and Treat residual neuropathic pain, by adding:
Tricyclic antidepressant and/or anticonvulsant and/or cortiocosteroid.

Figure 25.2 Schema for the approach to pain management. NSAIDs, nonsteroidal anti-inflammatory drugs.

within or near tumor masses, or intestinal colic. **Pain felt in the back needs particularly careful consideration, because the causes are many and the treatments are diverse.**

Specific measures to reduce the noxious stimulus may include reducing size of the tumor mass with radiotherapy, treating an unstable fracture by surgical fixation, or performing a peripheral nerve block. Peripherally acting drugs should be used irrespective of these specific therapeutic measures.

Bone metastases frequently cause inflammatory changes with release of inflammatory mediators, including prostaglandins. When the pain is clearly arising from bone metastases, the use of drugs that interfere with prostaglandin synthesis (e.g., nonsteroidal anti-inflammatory drugs [NSAIDs]) is logical. These drugs should be avoided or used with caution in patients who have a history of peptic ulceration, excessive alcohol consumption, bleeding diathesis, renal impairment, or known allergies to aspirin or related drugs. **Where the use of NSAIDs is precluded, *acetaminophen (paracetamol)* is a useful alternative.** While its mechanism of action is yet to be fully elucidated, clinical utility suggests some peripheral action. Evidence for its benefit is yet to be established in large studies (24). *Acetaminophen* is fairly well tolerated and safe, but it should be used in reduced dosage in patients with impaired liver function.

Peripherally acting drugs such as *acetaminophen* and NSAIDs are useful for pain arising in nonosseous sites and for postoperative pain (25). They should rarely be omitted from analgesic regimens, even in bedbound patients. Rectal preparations may prove useful in patients who derive clinical benefit but are unable to take oral drugs.

Muscle spasm requires muscle relaxants and gentle massage. Psoas muscle spasm, usually resulting from direct tumor infiltration, is not infrequent in gynecologic cancer (26). Psoas muscle infiltration should be suspected if there is pain in a lumbosacral plexus distribution associated with difficulty achieving full extension of the hip. While radiation therapy is being considered or applied, relief can usually be achieved by careful adherence to the outlined principles, but will not be adequately managed by opioids alone. ***Acetaminophen* and NSAIDs, an oral opioid (such as *oxycodone*), and a laxative must be supplemented by a drug that is active against spasm in skeletal muscle, such as *diazepam*. Steroids should be considered in the short term (e.g., *dexamethasone* 2 to 4 mg daily). Polypharmacy is justified to relieve pain in the malignant psoas syndrome.** If the pain does not respond to these measures, specialist help must be sought (27).

Regional blockade with a local anesthetic and neurolytic techniques may be a useful measure to reduce the peripheral noxious stimulus if the area of pain is circumscribed and attributable to an accessible peripheral nerve, such as pain in the intercostal region.

Step Two: Raise the Pain Threshold

All persons should be considered to have a threshold above which they will be troubled by pain. It is useful to consider the threshold as "one's sense of mastery of a situation." **Such a threshold is dynamic** and may be influenced by many factors. **The threshold for pain may be raised by explanation, comfort, care, concern, diversion, and various forms of relaxation.** Similarly, **the threshold may be lowered, or a patient's sense of mastery may be affected negatively by sleeplessness, depression, anxiety, uncertainty, loneliness, and isolation.** Threshold issues in general require a nonpharmacologic approach.

A wide range of strategies exist to facilitate coping with pain and simple measures, such as explanation of, for example, the likely cause of pain, should be available to all patients. The diagnosis of a disturbed threshold in an individual patient is difficult, but **the narrative approach to assessment of the patient will give clues.** As the patient tells the story of her diagnosis, treatment, and the pattern of her pain, she imparts information about the cancer and about herself, and **excessive distress can be readily perceived.** Many complementary therapies, such as massage and meditation, assist in the relief of pain and it is likely that their benefits stem from enhancing a patient's sense of mastery.

Occasionally, anxiety and depression are so marked that the patient is impeded in her attempts to relate to her loved ones or to come to terms with her disease, and may manifest as ever increasing pain. In such circumstances, a formal psychiatric consultation may be of assistance and anxiolytics or antidepressants may prove helpful. In general, **threshold issues, including extreme anguish, feelings of futility, loss of sense of meaning, personal guilt, and other forms of spiritual pain, require a nonpharmacologic approach, with help from skilled counselors, pastors, and, above all, those people who are closest to the patient.**

Pain and suffering are related but distinct. Suffering is described as a sense of impending personal disintegration (28). In common parlance, there may be a sense of being about to "go to pieces." Suffering may be triggered by poorly controlled symptoms, perceived loss of dignity, loss of a sense of control or autonomy, fear for the future, and loss of a future. Pain may be the main cause of suffering, or a manifestation (through threshold shifts) of suffering, with the language of suffering expressed through pain.

If suffering is defined as a sense of impending "personal disintegration," then the response to suffering should be "reintegration." Such reintegration may be most assisted by others who have skills in the dimension of care that is focused on existential issues; these may or may not be related to religious matters. But every doctor has the responsibility and privilege to be aware of such dimensions of care, to provide the "space" for patients to consider their existential concerns (notably to ensure that symptoms are well controlled), and to take time to be informed about current reflections on this area (29).

Step Three: Precise and Appropriate Use of Opioid Drugs

There is abundant literature on opioid use to supplement peripherally acting analgesics, with a range of opioids available (30). Despite the initiatives of the World Health Organization, **there are still difficulties obtaining opioids for medical use in some countries** (31). A variety of opioids is available and the principles of choice need to be understood (Table 25.1) (30). In practice, **low-potency opioids such as *codeine* or *dextropropoxyphene*, or high-potency opioids such as *morphine*, are**

Table 25.1 Opioid Analgesics Used for the Treatment of Chronic Pain					
	Dose (mg) Equianalgesic to Morphine 10 mg IM[a]				
Drugs	**PO**	**IM**	**Half-life (hr)**	**Duration (hr)**	**Comment**
Morphine	20–30[b]	10	2–3	2–4	Standard for comparison
Morphine CR	20–30	10	2–3	8–12	Various formulations are not bioequivalent
Morphine SR	20–30	10	2–3	24	
Oxycodone	20	—	2–3	3–4	
Oxycodone CR	20	—	2–3	8–12	
Hydromorphone	7.5	1.5	2–3	2–4	Potency may be greater; for example, IV *hydromorphone*: IV *morphine* = 3:1 rather than 6.7:1 during prolonged use
Methadone	20	10	12–190	4–12	Although 1:1 IV ratio with *morphine* was in single-dose study, there is a change with chronic dosing; large dose reduction (75–90%) is needed when switching to *methadone*
Oxymorphone	10 (rectal)	1	2–3	2–4	Available in rectal and injectable formulations
Levorphanol	4	2	12–15	4–6	
Fentanyl	—	—	7–12	—	Can be administered as a continuous IV or SQ infusion; based on clinical experience, 100 μg/hr is roughly equianalgesic to IV *morphine* 4 mg/hr
Fentanyl TTS	—	—	16–24	48–72	Based on clinical experience, 100 μg/hr is roughly equianalgesic to IV *morphine* 4 mg/hr; a ratio of oral *morphine*: transdermal *fentanyl* of 70:1 may also be used clinically

[a]Studies to determine equianalgesic doses of opioids have used *morphine* by the IM route. The IM and IV routes are considered to be equivalent. (Note: SQ route is generally used for recurrent dosing in most countries.)

[b]Although the PO:IM morphine ratio was 6:1 in a single-dose study, other observations indicate a ratio of 2–3:1 with repeated administration.

IM, intramuscular; PO, oral; CR, controlled release; SR, sustained release; IV, intravenous; SQ, subcutaneous.

From **Derby S, Chin J, Portenoy RK**. Systemic opioid therapy for chronic cancer pain: Practical guidelines for converting drugs and routes of administration. *CNS Drugs.* 1998;9:99–109, with permission.

combined with peripherally acting drugs such as *acetaminophen* or *aspirin*. Low- and high-potency opioids should not be given concurrently, but a change from one opioid to another may be justified (32). While equianalgesic dose calculation tables assist if changing prescription from one opioid to another (Table 25.1), these should be used only as a guide, with clinical surveillance essential to ensure neither toxicity nor too little effect is achieved. When calculating an equivalent dose of an alternative opioid, conservative dosing is recommended. Doses that are 25–50% of the calculated dose may be appropriate, with regular assessment following the change (33). **While for many *morphine* remains the preferred high-potency opioid, consideration is increasingly being given to alternative high-potency opioids such as *oxycodone* and *hydromorphone*,** if available (30,34). Local availability and affordability should inform the choice of opioids.

Regardless of the choice, opioids should be given at regular intervals in accordance with the half-life of the drug concerned, rather than haphazardly in response to a severe pain stimulus. Doses of opioid drugs should be carefully titrated against response and side effects.

A number of oral opioids including morphine, *oxycodone,* and hydromorphone are available in two forms: an immediate-release preparation that reaches a peak within 30 minutes of ingestion, and a sustained release preparation that typically takes several hours to reach peak concentrations (35). As a general rule, for a patient not previously taking opioids, **initial prescribing should involve regular dosing with an immediate-release preparation as a "dose-finding" exercise.** This allows rapid escalation or reduction of dose according to clinical response. When effective doses are reached, the woman may be converted to a convenient, long-acting preparation with the dose prescribed based upon her daily requirements. Any long-acting medication should be given with an immediate-release opioid available, should episodes of "breakthrough" pain occur.

Some types of pain are only partially responsive to opioids (27), **including pain caused by nerve irritation, extreme muscle spasm, incident pain** (i.e., pain exacerbated by a particular activity such as movement), **or pain that is heightened by unaddressed anguish.** Even in these circumstances, for the patient with cancer, opioids remain "partially effective" and should be introduced alongside, for example, neuropathic pain agents, and carefully calibrated to ensure that optimum benefit is achieved while minimizing side effects (36).

Morphine

Immediate-release *morphine* is best given every 4 hours, with a double dose (or 1.5 times the standard dose in the frail) at bedtime, and a break of approximately 8 hours overnight to permit sleep for both patient and caregiver. A reasonable starting dose of oral *morphine* in a patient with severe pain not already on an opioid drug would be 10 mg in an average sized patient, or 3 to 5 mg in a frail or very elderly patient. The original dose should be repeated in 1 to 2 hours if there is inadequate relief of pain. Over the next 24 to 48 hours, dose finding should be undertaken by prescribing regular doses every 4 hours, together with one or two "breakthrough" doses, equal to the standard dose. The correct dose may range from 2 mg to more than 100 mg every 4 hours, but most patients should need less than 50 mg every 4 hours.

When the daily dose requirement has been established, it can be converted to a sustained-release formulation, maintaining supplemental breakthrough doses of the immediate-release preparation. For example, a patient taking 20 mg oral *morphine sulfate* mixture every 4 hours should be converted to 60 mg sustained-release *morphine* each 12 hours, with additional breakthrough doses of 20 mg of *morphine sulfate* mixture if required.

Sustained-release *morphine* (or other sustained-release opioids) should not be used in patients with (i) uncontrolled or unstable pain; (ii) extensive upper abdominal or retroperitoneal disease that is likely to interfere with gastrointestinal motility; or (iii) fecal loading or impaction. Subcutaneous *morphine* is a better choice in such circumstances.

If parenteral *morphine* is essential, the subcutaneous route is appropriate, either with intermittent injections through an indwelling butterfly needle every 4 hours or with a continuous infusion through a battery-driven syringe driver or pump. When a patient is constipated or has a bowel obstruction and pain is not well controlled with simple analgesics such as *acetaminophen (paracetamol),* 4-hourly subcutaneous *morphine* is useful for both pain relief, and calibration of the required dose of *morphine*. After the constipation has been relieved, the subcutaneous 24-hourly dose may be readily converted to oral *morphine*. **The intramuscular route is rarely advantageous.**

In general, a parenteral dose of one-half or one-third of the oral dose appears equianalgesic (37). If oral or subcutaneous *morphine* is efficacious but the side effects are troublesome, the epidural route may be occasionally necessary, but a change to another oral or parenteral opioid should normally be tried first.

Intravenous *morphine* infusions, although sometimes useful (e.g., in a patient with peripheral circulatory failure), do not offer significant advantage over the subcutaneous route for most patients, and generally ensure greater complexity and disruption for the patient. In the setting of rapid dose escalation of intravenous *morphine,* cessation of the infusion and resumption of appropriate subcutaneous doses every 4 hours may be helpful. Simultaneously, it is important to review other aspects of management, such as the possible need for NSAIDs or drugs relevant to neuropathic pain, and to pay appropriate attention to psychological factors.

The efficacy of the regular dosing approach to *morphine* administration may depend on the contribution of an active metabolite (*morphine 6-glucuronide*), which, like *morphine,* is a powerful mu receptor agonist. Hepatic impairment, if severe, interferes with *morphine* metabolism to glucuronides. Renal impairment, even if only moderate, interferes with excretion of the active metabolites. In both these circumstances, dose reduction is essential. In a patient with renal impairment, it may be necessary to extend the dose interval from 4 to 8 or even 12 hours. The use of *morphine* in a patient with marked renal impairment is very complex, and an alternative opioid that does not have active metabolites such as fentanyl may be a better choice (30,38).

Some physicians, nurses, and patients continue to harbor misconceptions about the use of *morphine.* When morphine is to be commenced, counseling should address three issues to counteract widely held fears:

1. The use of *morphine* with careful dose finding and monitoring does not, in the vast majority of patients, lead to addiction (although physical dependence, a separate issue, occurs). Specialist help is needed to use *morphine* appropriately in current or former intravenous *heroin* users.

2. The introduction of *morphine* does not mean that the patient is actually dying, but rather that morphine is the most appropriate opioid at that time. It is the type of pain and its severity, not the prognosis of the patient, that dictates whether an opioid should be introduced. *Morphine,* correctly used, does not hasten death.

3. The introduction of *morphine* does not mean that it will be ineffective at a later stage in the illness, when the situation may be worse. *Morphine* does not lose its effectiveness, but increased doses may be needed later in response to tumor progression.

Use of Alternative Opioids

Other potent opioids should be considered when (i) pain persists despite careful drug calibration; (ii) unacceptable side effects persist (e.g., cognitive impairment, nausea) despite careful drug calibration; or (iii) drowsiness or toxicity occurs at levels of the drug required to control the pain. In these circumstances, after reconsideration of the pain mechanism and the other analgesic steps, an alternative opioid should be considered. Availability varies from country to country, but gynecologic oncologists should become familiar with a narrow range of opioids (Table 25.1). In countries where there is wide availability and affordability of opioids, the choice may depend upon the preferred route of administration (oral versus transdermal). *Oxycodone* (available as immediate-release tablets, suspension, sustained-release preparations, parenteral, and suppositories) is somewhat more potent (20–50%) than *morphine*. *Oxycodone* is most often used in a dose of 5 to 20 mg every 4 to 6 hours. Some patients tolerate *oxycodone* better than *morphine* at the same dose, and vice versa. In general terms, however, the side-effect profile is similar (30).

Methadone is occasionally useful, particularly for those who appear to have pain that is more difficult to control (30,39). Its long half-life is sometimes disadvantageous, particularly in the elderly, and its sedative action may outlast its analgesic activity. It has mechanisms of action that differ slightly from those of *morphine,* being reported to have both opioid receptor activity and activity on the *N*-methyl-D-aspartate (NMDA) receptor pathways (40). Therefore, *methadone* may be occasionally useful when higher doses of other opioids have been reached with only a partial or inadequate response. Conversion from *morphine* to *methadone* may be difficult, with subsequent dose reduction frequently required—specialist assistance is recommended (41). *Methadone* has a similar side-effect profile to *morphine.*

Hydromorphone **is another alternative.** Like *morphine, hydromorphone* is a mu agonist but with far greater solubility. It can be administered orally, intravenously, and subcutaneously with a duration of action and half-life similar to *morphine*. Its high potency allows smaller volume injections (42).

Fentanyl **offers a transdermal route of administration, enabling continuous administration of a short-acting opioid** (43). Dose calibration should usually occur with *morphine, oxycodone,* or subcutaneous or intravenous *fentanyl* before transdermal therapeutic system (TTS) *fentanyl* is applied. **The patch forms a depot of drug in the dermis, resulting in a 12- to 48-hour delay before maximum plasma concentration is reached.** After TTS removal, the terminal half-life is approximately 13 to 25 hours (44). In practice, this means that when the patch is applied, the immediate-release drug should be continued for at least 12 hours. If adverse effects develop, they will continue after TTS *fentanyl* removal and the patient should be monitored closely. When a patient who is using TTS *fentanyl* experiences an increase in pain, a short-acting opioid should be given concurrently and the dose used to calculate the extra opioid requirement, which can then be incorporated into the TTS *fentanyl* dose.

TTS *fentanyl* is an attractive option for many patients because of the convenience of the delivery system and the slightly less troublesome constipation compared with *morphine* (43). Dose escalation is commonly observed, possibly related to the short half-life of the drug. If very rapid dose escalation occurs (without evidence of rapid tumor progression), a change to another opioid may be wise and less expensive.

Buccal and transmucosal *fentanyl citrate* **preparations provide an immediate-release** *fentanyl* **formulation for breakthrough pain that offers rapid onset of analgesia, and similar or improved response compared with immediate release** *morphine* (45). Expense may dictate that traditional preparations are still chosen.

When using TTS *fentanyl,* **it must be remembered that:**

- **It is a delivery system useful only for chronic pain.** It may be hazardous for unstable pain and should not be used after surgery or in rapidly changing pain states.
- **Because of depot formation in the dermis, a delayed response occurs** that is particularly important in toxicity or overdose situations.
- **A short-acting opioid should be available for breakthrough needs** (e.g., immediate-release *morphine,* or transmucosal *fentanyl citrate*).

Meperidine (pethidine) **is of very little value in palliative care.** It is addictive, has poor oral bioavailability, and a short half-life, requiring administration approximately every 2 hours. At high doses (>1 g/d) or when renal failure is present, the metabolites lead to neurotoxicity, including delirium, agitation, and seizures. If a patient is already receiving *meperidine* subcutaneously or intramuscularly, conversion to *morphine* can be achieved with approximately 10% of the *meperidine* dose given as subcutaneous *morphine*, or 30% of the *meperidine* dose given as oral *morphine* every 4 hours.

Side Effects of Opioids

In general, the side effect profile of all opioids is similar, though there may be individual variation in response, particularly around the development of adverse effects. It is likely these individual variations result from cytogenetic differences, though this is an emergent field of knowledge (46). Side effects can be avoided, or at least minimized, in large part by precise prescribing. Although there are some side effects that are almost invariable, such as constipation, individual variation in side-effect profile may be used to advantage by substituting an alternative opioid (30,41).

Constipation occurs in most patients, and prophylactic laxatives should be prescribed. A reasonable laxative prescription would be *senna* and *sodium docusate* tablets twice daily. Fecal impaction, much more likely if opioids are given without a laxative, may cause a variety of distressing symptoms, such as nausea, vomiting, pelvic pain, or confusion. **TTS** *fentanyl* **is slightly less constipating than slow-release** *morphine* (47).

If opioid-induced constipation persists after treatment with the usual laxatives, subcutaneous methylnaltrexone, the opioid antagonist, may be considered, though bowel obstruction should be ruled out prior to administration (30). Compounds have been developed which combine oxycodone with prolonged release naloxone (which displays local, antagonist effects on opioid receptors in the gut wall and has negligible systemic bioavailability) in an attempt to minimize the constipating effects of opioids (48). These offer some benefits in terms of convenience, but have limitations for those patients with higher opioid dose requirements as the fixed ratio between compounds means that the opioid dose cannot be escalated beyond the ceiling dose of methylnaltrexone.

Nausea and vomiting may occur in association with opioid therapy as a result of gastric stasis, stimulation of the chemoreceptor trigger zone, or constipation. Nausea is particularly common when opioids are commenced or when the dose is changing, but tolerance to this side effect develops in many patients within 48 hours. Suitable antinauseants such as *metoclopramide,* 10 mg four times daily or *haloperidol,* 0.5 to 1.5 mg twice daily, both given orally or subcutaneously, should be available if required. Regular prophylactic antiemetics should be prescribed for at least the first 48 hours if the patient is very anxious, or if there is a history of opioid-induced nausea or vomiting. If vomiting persists, an alternative opioid should be substituted. All opioids may cause nausea, but there appears to be individual but unpredictable variability in response between the drugs. The evolving field of pharmacogenetics may provide some ability to predict an individual's response (46).

The prescription of opioids should be individualized. As with a number of other medications (e.g., *digoxin*), if the dose prescribed is inadequate, there will be no clinical response. If the dose is too high, the patient will enter a toxic range and will develop dose-related side effects. **The dose-related side effects of opioids include drowsiness and delirium. At the extreme end of the toxic range is respiratory depression, with reduced respiratory rate.** This is rarely seen in chronic opioid prescribing, and not before the patient has exhibited earlier signs of toxicity such as drowsiness and delirium.

If drowsiness develops and persists for more than 24 hours, the opioid level is probably above the therapeutic range for that patient. Other causes of drowsiness should be excluded, such as sedating drugs or hypercalcemia, and a dose reduction of opioids should be considered.

The development of confusion or hallucinations generally indicates either excessive dosage, or excessive accumulation such as may occur in renal failure, or occasionally, an idiosyncratic reaction. Hydration—orally, subcutaneously, or intravenously—may assist in eliminating troublesome metabolites while dose reduction is undertaken. If the pain is not well controlled in the presence of drowsiness or confusion, another approach is usually required, such as an alternative opioid or an alternative route of administration (e.g., spinal).

Pruritus is troublesome for a small number of patients taking *morphine* because of its histaminogenic properties. It usually settles within 48 hours and **can be managed with judicious use of *promethazine*.** Pruritus is rarely reported for other opioids. Anticholinergic side effects of opioids are usually not troublesome.

Tolerance to opioids may be a significant clinical problem if the drug is not introduced and calibrated correctly. When opioids are used correctly, increased requirements during the course of an illness usually signify an increase in the noxious stimulus because of disease progression, rather than a reduction in the effectiveness of the analgesic. *Ketamine,* a drug used traditionally in anesthesia, has been used occasionally to reverse opioid tolerance for some patients with pain** (49).

Step Four: Recognize Neuropathic Pain and Treat Correctly

Neuropathic pain is a term used to describe those pain syndromes in which the pathophysiology is related to aberrant somatosensory processes that originate with a lesion in the peripheral or central nervous system. Neuropathic pain is a frequent complication in gynecologic cancer, especially in advanced cancer of the cervix. It may be caused by tumor infiltration (notably lumbar plexopathy), or occasionally may result from therapeutic interventions. It may be flashing or burning in nature, but is often an unpleasant ache in an area of altered sensation corresponding to a peripheral dermatome.

When pain is neuropathic in origin, Steps 1 to 3 should usually be supplemented by a tricyclic antidepressant, anticonvulsant, or a corticosteroid (36). An agent should be chosen from a particular class of drug, such as an anticonvulsant (e.g., gabapentin). The choice should be based on tolerability, comorbidities, and any associated symptoms such as anxiety. If ineffective, an alternative agent from that same class should be trialed before moving to another class such as antidepressants (50). In general, medications should be started at low doses and gradually increased as tolerated, but treatment of severe neuropathic pain is a challenge (30,50).

Other Dimensions of Pain

Breakthrough pain is **defined as an episode of worsening pain when the background pain appears to be controlled by the regular analgesia** (45). Breakthrough pain should be distinguished from end of dose failure, where the long-acting opioid dose is insufficient to provide analgesia until the next regular dose is due. In general, a short-acting opioid, either immediate-release oral opioid or buccal or transmucosal fentanyl, should be made available to cover these breakthrough episodes (30). The effective dose required for relief of breakthrough pain is not necessarily related to the baseline scheduled medication (45) so therapy should be initiated using low doses with dose titration thereafter as necessary. For those using an oral opioid, clinical experience has revealed that 1/10th to 1/6th of the 24-hour scheduled medication total dose should be safe.

Ketamine, **when used in subanesthetic doses, has been reported by some to be useful in the management of very complex pain, both somatic and neuropathic in origin** (49). *Ketamine* acts as an antagonist to the NMDA receptor system, a system frequently activated in refractory pain states, when high doses of opioids appear ineffective. Small trials and case series have suggested that low doses of infusional subcutaneous *ketamine* can reduce opioid tolerance and improve analgesia (51). A multisite study investigating ketamine in refractory cancer pain revealed that ketamine was equivalent to placebo in analgesic response, and held substantially greater toxicity (52). Further studies are underway, but it should only be used in consultation with palliative medicine or pain specialists, because of the **significant side effects, such as hallucinations**.

Spinal analgesia may benefit a carefully selected small group of patients. Anesthetic opinion should be considered for patients who continue to have pain despite an adequate trial of analgesia according to Steps 1 to 4, or for those who have very severe incident pain, that is, pain associated with a particular activity, such as weight bearing (53). **The ongoing capacity of the care system to support the spinal analgesic delivery devices** (implantable pumps, intrathecally inserted Port-o-cath devices, or other systems) **must be considered prior to implementation.** For some, the delivery of spinal analgesia requires ongoing hospitalization, because community supports are unavailable. Expense may be very significant.

Pain Prognostic Score

The recognition that patients with cancer-related pain vary considerably in their responses to standard analgesic regimes has led to the development of a classification system for pain. Based on the TNM classification system for cancer, this represents an attempt to group pain such that appropriate comparisons and predictions of outcome can be made (Table 25.2) (54). According to this classification, **the presence of particular pain mechanisms, incident pain** (pain during an activity), **psychological distress, addictive behavior, and disturbed cognitive function are all associated with increasing complexity of pain management.**

Special Considerations in Pain Management

The Patient with Renal Failure

In patients with renal impairment, NSAIDs should be avoided, as they will frequently worsen renal function, while the use of *morphine* will result in the accumulation of active *morphine* metabolites. Therefore, **if prescribing *morphine*, a dose reduction may be necessary** and, more importantly, **the interval between doses should be extended.** Use of **alternative opioids such as *fentanyl* or *methadone*,** which are reported not to have active metabolites, is recommended (38).

Allergy to Opioids

Many patients will report that they are allergic to opioids, or have such an allergy recorded on their medical record. A detailed exploration should be undertaken of the event when an allergy was first cited. Frequently, the original event was the development of nausea and vomiting when opioids were administered. Sometimes it is the report of a confusional state, particularly in the setting of postoperative analgesia. Neither of these constitutes **a true allergic reaction, which is extremely rare**. If it is suspected, palliative care expertise should be sought.

The Patient with Reduced Motility of the Gastrointestinal Tract

The patient who has a hypomotile gastrointestinal tract, most commonly seen in patients with disseminated ovarian cancer, may have impaired peristalsis and impaired absorption of oral medication.

Table 25.2 Edmonton Classification System for Cancer Pain

1. Mechanism of Pain

No—**No** pain syndrome

Nc—Any **noc**iceptive combination of visceral and/or bone or soft tissue pain

Ne—**Ne**uropathic pain syndrome with or without any combination of nociceptive pain

Nx—Insufficient information to classify.

2. Incident Pain

Io—No incident pain

Ii—Incident pain present

Ix—Insufficient information to classify

3. Psychological Distress

Po—No psychological distress

Pp—Psychological distress present

Px—Insufficient information to classify

4. Addictive Behavior

Ao—No addictive behavior

Aa—Addictive behavior present

Ax—Insufficient information to classify

5. Cognitive Function

Co—No impairment. Patient able to provide accurate present and past pain history unimpaired.

Ci—Partial impairment. Sufficient impairment to affect patient's ability to provide accurate present and/or past pain history.

Cu—Total impairment. Patient unresponsive, delirious, or demented to the stage of being unable to provide any present and past pain history.

Cx—Insufficient information to classify

Reproduced with permission from **Fainsinger RL, Nekolaichuk CLA**. A "TNM" classification system for cancer pain: The Edmonton Classification System for Cancer Pain (ECS-CP). *Support Care Cancer.* 2008;16:547–555.

Motility may be further impaired by drugs such as $5HT_3$ blockers (e.g., *ondansetron*), which, although very effective antinauseants for patients undergoing chemotherapy, may induce constipation. **Consideration should be given to delivering analgesics via an alternative route, such as transdermally** (*fentanyl*) **or,** for the very ill, **subcutaneously.** Similarly, alternative routes of analgesic administration should be sought for the patient with established fecal loading.

The Patient with Cognitive Impairment

The cognitively impaired patient may not complain of pain, but if she does, she should be believed. If the location of the cancer is likely to cause pain, then pain should be assumed to be present. **Facial expression may assist in the diagnosis (unless the pain is chronic), as may the presence of any physiologic indicators such as tachycardia (55). Other clues may include restlessness and agitation.** The family should be questioned about any behavioral changes they have observed. Ultimately, diagnosis may require a therapeutic trial of analgesia and observation of the response. Prescribing should be scheduled regularly rather than on an as required basis for those with an expected painful stimulus, such as postoperative patients (55). Regular assessment of response is mandatory.

Particular note should be made of the interaction of the two symptom complexes of pain and delirium, both of which are common in the very ill. Patients with delirium have global cognitive dysfunction, including problems with memory, concentration, and alertness. They frequently have hallucinations and delusions. It is postulated that **usual inhibitory processes are affected with consequent "unmasking" and heightened pain complaints**. When the response to such complaints is to unquestioningly escalate opioid doses, this can further exacerbate the situation, because opioids at high doses (beyond the therapeutic range) may be implicated in causing delirium (55).

When a patient develops this complex set of clinical problems, the following approach is recommended:

1. **Evaluate the likely pain mechanism(s)** and prescribe the analgesic regimes considered most likely to be effective.
2. **Evaluate the likely causes of delirium** and correct where possible.
3. **Consider medication of the symptoms of delirium** with an appropriate antipsychotic such as haloperidol or olanzapine.
4. **Review the opioid dose regularly** and consider opioid substitution if necessary (41).

Difficult-to-Manage Postoperative Pain

Occasionally, the management of pain in the postoperative setting is difficult. Possible reasons could include the following:

1. **Inappropriate use of the patient-controlled analgesic (PCA) device.** Patients who are cognitively impaired (including those developing delirium postoperatively), those who are anxious or depressed, the very frail, and those for whom the language of explanation is not their mother tongue, may all struggle to use a PCA device effectively. In such patients, a careful estimate of probable dosage requirements prescribed regularly may be wiser.
2. **Preoperative use of opioids.** Patients who have a history of previous opioid abuse, especially intravenous drug users, have a level of tolerance that appears to persist even when they have not used opioids for some years, and usually require significantly larger doses of opioids than would be expected (56). There is little literature to guide this complex clinical problem, but experience suggests the following:
   a. **Open discussion** of the concerns with the patient and with other physicians involved in her care. Many former opioid addicts will fear the prescription of opioids for their pain.
   b. **Use of regional anesthetic techniques.**
   c. **Use of opioid-sparing coanalgesics.**
   d. **Possible use of higher doses of opioids.**
   e. **Ensurance of a single point of prescription.**
   f. **Prescription of precise amounts of opioids for relatively short periods of time,** such as 1 week.

   On the other hand, patients who are taking preoperative opioids as part of their current treatment need to continue equivalent opioid doses, with an additional moiety to cover the operative trauma (56).
3. **Extreme patient anxiety.** This significantly disturbs pain threshold levels, and care should be taken not to continue to escalate opioid doses in such cases. Instead, **explanation, support, counseling, and anxiolytics** are likely to be more effective, and to be associated with fewer adverse effects.

Chronic Nonmalignant Pain

While not the focus of this chapter, a word of caution should be made about the management of the patient with chronic nonmalignant pain. In general, the pain management approach for these patients has a rehabilitative focus. In common with cancer pain management is the need for diagnosis, repeated assessment, and use of pharmacologic agents and interventions according to the pain mechanism involved. **The difference between the management of cancer pain and nonmalignant pain lies in the more cautious use of opioids, and the focus on improvement of functional outcomes in the latter.** There is an extensive body of literature examining this particular clinical challenge (57,58).

Gastrointestinal Symptoms

Gastrointestinal symptoms are common in gynecologic cancer, both because of the cancer and because of various aspects of treatment (59).

Anorexia–Cachexia

Anorexia is a common and significant symptom with a multitude of causes and serious nutritional consequences. The best initial approach to management includes careful preparation of small meals, elimination of reversible gastric stasis or constipation, emotional support, and direct nutritional supplements. It is helpful to educate the patient and her family about the importance of these measures. Extensive research has isolated a number of potential therapies, but these remain in trial and developmental phase (60). Until such agents enter clinical practice, the pharmacologic responses available to clinicians include the use of prokinetics, progestational agents, and cautious use of corticosteroids.

Prokinetic agents may be useful when the symptom of early satiety is present, indicating gastric stasis. **Progestational agents** have been demonstrated in randomized, double-blinded, placebo-controlled trials to increase appetite and food intake and to lead to weight gain in a number of patients, without undue side effects (61), but the expense is considerable. **Corticosteroids** have also been shown to improve appetite and daily activity of patients with cancer, but this effect is short lived, usually with a return to baseline responses by 28 days. Because patients must then undergo the problems of corticosteroid withdrawal, patient selection is critical.

Mouth Symptoms

Mouth symptoms, including xerostomia, pain, and altered taste, can be most distressing. A dry mouth can result from many factors in the critically ill patient: oral candidiasis, previous radiation therapy, mouth breathing, nasal oxygen, and drugs, particularly those with anticholinergic effects. Management of xerostomia may include minimization of contributory nonessential medications, frequent small drinks with a small amount of lemon/orange to stimulate saliva production, use of artificial saliva or *glycerin* preparations, and *pilocarpine* drops to stimulate saliva locally with minimal systemic effects.

Frank pain can occur from treatment-related mucositis and infected ulcers, so mouth care is crucial in very ill patients. **Oral candidiasis is often overlooked.** It responds to antifungal agents such as *nystatin* mouthwashes (every 2 to 3 hours), *amphotericin* lozenges and, if necessary, a systemic triazole derivative such as *fluconazole*. Pain from mucositis may be relieved by *sucralfate* suspension and by *acetaminophen* with *morphine* (orally or subcutaneously).

Altered taste, a not uncommon symptom in patients with cancer, is hard to relieve. After all the above causes of mouth pathology are excluded, a dietitian may be able to assist in food choice and encouragement.

Nausea and Vomiting

Nausea and vomiting are common in advanced gynecologic cancer and each symptom requires precise diagnosis so that rational therapy may be applied. Mechanisms of nausea and vomiting are complex (62). Nausea, with or without vomiting, is mediated finally by the vomiting center situated in the reticular formation of the medulla oblongata, an area rich in histaminic and muscarinic receptors. The vomiting center is influenced by several connections, each of which can be the causal pathway for nausea (Fig. 25.3).

Causal pathways include the following:

1. **The cerebral cortex** (e.g., stimulated by anxiety-conditioned responses).
2. **The vestibular center,** which is rich in histaminic (H_1) and muscarinic receptors (e.g., stimulated by cerebral metastases).
3. **The chemoreceptor trigger zone,** which is rich in dopaminergic and serotonergic receptors (e.g., stimulated by hypercalcemia, uremia, and some drugs, including chemotherapeutic agents).
4. **The gastrointestinal tract** (e.g., stimulated by gastric stasis, intestinal obstruction, fecal impaction, abnormalities of gut motility), which has dopaminergic, muscarinic, and serotonergic receptors.

After the likely mechanism has been identified by means of a careful history, physical examination and investigations if indicated, the appropriate antinauseant may be prescribed (Table 25.3). While the evidence base proving the efficacy of this approach remains scant, it continues to be useful in practice and is recommended as an appropriate approach (63).

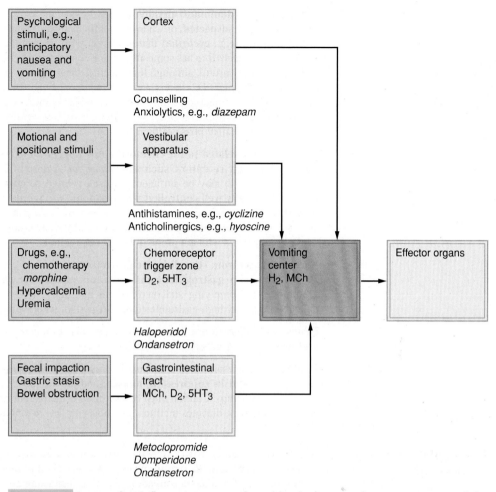

Figure 25.3 Factors that influence nausea and vomiting in the central nervous system and the gastrointestinal tract. Nausea, with or without vomiting, is mediated by the vomiting center. D, dopaminergic; H, histaminic; MCh, muscarinic; 5HT3, hydroxytryptophan.

Table 25.3 Commonly Used Antinauseant Drugs		
Drug	*Dose*	*Comment*
Metoclopramide	10–20 mg q4h (oral or subcutaneous)	Avoid if patient has bowel colic, or high gastrointestinal obstruction
Haloperidol	1–3 mg bid or tid (oral) 0.5–2 mg bid or tid (subcutaneous)	Lower doses required than when used as a sedative
Prochlorperazine	5–10 mg tid or qid (oral) 25 mg bid or tid (rectal)	May be useful if vomiting mechanism is unknown
Cyclizine	25–150 mg/d in divided doses (oral or subcutaneous)	Useful if patient has bowel obstruction
Hyoscine hydrobromide	0.1–0.4 mg q6–8h (subcutaneous)	Central nervous system side effects can occur, particularly drowsiness and confusion
Ondansetron	4–8 mg od or bid oral or IV	Main use is for chemotherapy-related nausea. Constipation can be troublesome

Levomepromazine: start with 6.25 mg bid (orally or subcutaneously, doses greater than 25 mg/d can cause drowsiness, subcutaneous). Progressively increase 12.5 to 25 mg bid q4h, every 4 hrs.

See text and manufacturers' information before prescribing; watch for side effects; review frequently; cease ineffective drugs.

bid, two times a day; tid, three times a day; IV, intravenous.

When anxiety is dominant, anxiolytics may be crucial in reducing the nausea. When vestibular mechanisms are suspected, or when no specific pathway can be identified, relatively less sedating antihistamines (e.g., *cyclizine*) that act directly on the vomiting and vestibular centers may be useful. *Prochlorperazine* has some affinity for dopaminergic, muscarinic, and histaminic receptors and is moderately useful, although less specific. *Levomepromazine (methotrimeprazine)* is a phenothiazine with potent D2- and α1-receptor antagonist and some $5HT_2$-receptor antagonist action. This means it is a broad-spectrum antiemetic, which is most commonly used as a second- or third-line drug when more specific drugs seem ineffective. It is significantly sedating, so is often reserved for patients in the final phase of their life (64).

Nausea clearly related to the chemoreceptor trigger zone requires a drug with high affinity for dopaminergic receptors, such as *haloperidol.* A dose of 1.5 to 3 mg or less at night (orally or subcutaneously) may be sufficient. Nausea related to chemotherapy or abdominal radiotherapy is usually well controlled with serotonin antagonists such as *ondansetron* or *tropisetron.* If delayed emesis resulting from chemotherapy is present, the introduction of haloperidol can be a useful adjunct. Constipation is a potentially distressing side effect of *ondansetron,* particularly in patients who are prone to bowel obstruction.

Nausea arising from stimuli in the gastrointestinal tract associated with slowing of the gut should respond to gastrokinetic antinauseants such as *metoclopramide* or *domperidone,* which promote gastric emptying and increase gut motility. These actions are counterproductive in a patient with a very high gastrointestinal obstruction, when vomiting will be aggravated.

Drugs available by more than one route are advantageous. *Metoclopramide, haloperidol,* and *cyclizine* may be used subcutaneously and orally.

In addition to the established antinauseant drugs, corticosteroids, which act by an unknown mechanism, are useful in suppressing nausea, and are frequently used in premedication programs before chemotherapy. Caution must be exercised if the patient has a history of active peptic ulceration, tuberculosis, diabetes mellitus, psychosis, or severe emotional instability.

Gastrointestinal Hypomotility

A number of women with extensive intra-abdominal disease, usually as a result of ovarian cancer, will present with symptoms of gastrointestinal hypomotility. Typically the initial complaints will be of marked constipation requiring increasing doses of laxatives, followed by early satiety and nausea. Eventually some will progress to develop symptoms of gastrointestinal obstruction. Examination reveals few or absent bowel sounds and plain abdominal radiographs are frequently normal or may show fecal loading without air–fluid levels. The pathophysiology of this syndrome is not well understood, but probably includes tumor infiltration of the myenteric plexus.

Medication is aimed at increasing bowel peristalsis using infusional *metoclopramide,* 60 to 90 mg subcutaneously over 24 hours. Our own experience suggests corticosteroids (*dexamethasone* 4 to 8 mg daily) may be useful to improve symptoms of obstruction in this group (65). Gastrointestinal hypomotility will result in reduced absorption of oral medications, including analgesics.

Hypomotility or dysmotility of the bowel sometimes follows apparently successful surgery for bowel obstruction. The condition may be temporary and related to the surgery, or it may be longer lasting and related to the underlying malignant infiltration. The difficulty facing the clinician is how best to support such patients nutritionally postoperatively. There is little literature to inform such a decision and, as always, it should be based on the patient's disease status, her performance status, the anticancer options still available, and her personal goals.

Constipation

Constipation, a common symptom, may be caused by changing diet, inactivity, opioid use without laxatives, or varying degrees of tumor-induced intestinal obstruction. Constipation can be largely avoided through anticipation and careful prescribing of laxatives. Reviews highlight the diversity both of mechanisms leading to constipation, and of classes of laxatives (Table 25.4) (66). Any prescription of opioids should be accompanied by a laxative, as constipation is an inevitable side effect. In most instances, a combination of a fecal softener and a peristaltic agent such as *sodium docusate* and *senna* will be adequate to prevent opioid-induced constipation. Care should be taken in the use of bulking agents, because those patients with significant frailty may be unable to ingest the volume of water required for their adequate function.

Table 25.4 Classification of Laxatives	
I. Bulking or hydrophilic agents	**B. Diphenylmethane derivatives**
A. Dietary fiber	1. *Phenolphthalein*
B. *Psyllium (plantago)*	2. *Bisacodyl*
C. *Polycarbophil*	3. *Sodium picosulfate*
D. *Methylcellulose, carboxymethylcellulose*	C. Ricinoleic acid (castor oil)
II. Osmotic agents	D. Anthraquinones
A. Poorly absorbed ions	1. *Senna*
1. *Magnesium sulfate (Epsom salt)*	2. *Cascara sagrada*
2. *Magnesium hydroxide (milk of magnesia)*	**IV. Lubricating agent**
3. *Magnesium citrate*	A. Mineral oil
4. *Sodium phosphate*	**V. Neuromuscular agents**
5. *Sodium sulfate (Glauber salt)*	A. Cholinergic agonists
6. *Potassium sodium tartrate (Rochelle salt)*	1. *Bethanechol*
B. Poorly absorbed disaccharides, sugar alcohols	2. *Neostigmine*
1. *Lactulose*	B. 5-HT$_4$ agonists
2. *Sorbitol, mannitol*	1. *Cisapride*
C. *Glycerin*	2. *Prucalopride*
D. Polyethylene glycol	3. *Tegaserod*
III. Stimulant laxatives	C. Prostaglandin agonist
A. Surface-active agents	1. *Misoprostol*
1. *Docusates (dioctyl sulfosuccinate)*	D. *Colchicine*
2. *Bile acids*	E. Opiate antagonists
	1. *Naloxone*
	2. *Naltrexone*

Reproduced with permission from **Schiller LR**. The therapy of constipation (review article). *Aliment Pharmacol Ther.* 2001;15:749–763.

Severe constipation is a common cause of major symptoms, including nausea, vomiting, spurious diarrhea, pain, and even confusion, especially in the elderly. If unrecognized or untreated, it may result in inadequate absorption of oral medications including analgesics, and, rarely, perforation. **Opioid-induced fecal impaction is usually avoidable, but if present, vigorous local treatment is required.** This includes fecal softeners (e.g., *docusate sodium*), large bowel stimulants (e.g., *senna*) and stimulant suppositories, or careful enemas. **Osmotic laxatives (e.g., *lactulose*) may be helpful.** Fecal impaction caused by a holdup at the sigmoid colon (with an empty, dilated rectum) sometimes requires high docusate sodium enemas if oral laxatives fail to provide relief.

Methylnaltrexone is a methylated form of the mu-opioid antagonist *naltrexone,* which blocks the peripheral effects of opioids without affecting the analgesic effect (67). It may be beneficial in the treatment of opioid-induced constipation when first-line aperients are ineffective. It is contraindicated in patients with a bowel obstruction.

Drugs other than opioids may cause constipation. Drugs commonly implicated in this population **would include 5HT$_3$ antagonists (e.g., *ondansetron*) and tricyclic antidepressants.** Constipation caused by mechanical obstruction requires either surgical intervention or acceptance of the problem as an end-stage event.

Medical Management of Intestinal Obstruction

Obstruction may occur at any level of the gastrointestinal tract in patients with gynecologic cancer, and frequently involves several different levels. It is a common late-stage problem, particularly in patients with ovarian cancer. Since the ground-breaking work at St. Christopher's Hospice, London (68), there have been several studies, reviews, and recommendations around the palliative medical management of patients with a bowel obstruction (69,70). The following represents a practical approach for the gynecologist (Table 25.5).

Patients presenting with an acute bowel obstruction should initially be placed on nil by mouth and given intravenous fluids. If there is copious vomiting, nasogastric suction is helpful. **If the obstruction is not relieved within 48 to 72 hours, a choice needs to be made between surgical intervention and medical management.**

In general, surgery provides the best palliative relief of symptoms, if successful. This is particularly true for the few patients who have a nonmalignant cause for the obstruction, such as adhesions from radiation therapy or previous surgery. Similarly, bowel obstruction in a patient for whom chemotherapeutic options have not been exhausted justifies active surgical intervention. **Stents may offer a useful means of bypassing obstruction that is caused by a defined tumor mass,** and are associated with low morbidity and mortality. Stents have little role in the patient with more than one level of obstruction (71). In patients whose life expectancy is limited to less than 2 months, a noninterventional approach is usually preferable.

One option for the conservative management of obstruction at high or low levels is a trial of corticosteroids (e.g., *dexamethasone,* 4 to 8 mg parenterally daily for 3 to 5 days) (65,72). They presumably work by decreasing inflammatory edema, thereby improving luminal diameter. It may be repeated in the future. **There is need for caution when using corticosteroids in patients with a history of diabetes mellitus, peptic ulceration, recent infection, impending bowel perforation, significant psychiatric disorder, or tuberculosis.** Corticosteroids are best used in patients considered unsuitable for surgical intervention.

In a patient with high end-stage obstruction, when the aforementioned measures have failed to relieve the problem, a conservative medical approach may be helpful. In brief, this approach avoids the use of full intravenous fluid replacement. It relies on careful mouth care, with a little food and drink as desired. **The patient remains mildly dehydrated,** but this is beneficial and decreases the amount of vomiting. Centrally acting antinauseants (e.g., *cyclizine*) are used, if necessary, in combination with low doses of opioid analgesics. **Gastrokinetic antinauseants** (e.g., *metoclopramide* or *domperidone*) **are contraindicated.** For many, **gastric drainage via a nasogastric tube or a venting gastrostomy may be required to ensure comfort.**

Hyoscine butyl bromide may serve several purposes in patients with bowel obstruction, reducing gastrointestinal secretions and reducing intestinal tone, **effectively increasing bowel capacity. This alleviates nausea for the patient with complete obstruction and avoids multiple small vomits, although infrequent large-volume vomits continue.**

A subcutaneous butterfly needle, with or without a battery-driven syringe driver, **can be used to deliver appropriate doses of antinauseants, such as** *cyclizine* 25 to 150 mg/d **and** *hyoscine butyl bromide* 10 to 20 mg every 6 hours. With careful calibration of dose, the patient need not be drowsy. *Morphine* may be given in the same syringe as *hyoscine* if pain is present. If colic is not controlled with *morphine,* additional *hyoscine* may be useful. **Rectal** *prochlorperazine,* 50 to 100 mg/d, may be tried instead of *cyclizine. Octreotide,* starting at a dose of 50 µg subcutaneously every 8 hours, can provide additional relief of symptoms by further reducing secretions and colic and has been demonstrated to be superior to *hyoscine hydrobromide,* though it is also more expensive (69). Doses greater than 600 µg/d probably do not afford additional benefit.

Some patients prefer occasional bouts of vomiting to a continuous nasogastric tube. Under all these circumstances, electrolyte imbalance becomes inevitable, but they should neither be monitored nor corrected.

Low-bowel obstruction commences with reduced then absent defecation, followed by severe abdominal distention, pain, and later nausea and vomiting. If colostomy or stenting is not to be undertaken, the focus should be on relief of discomfort with low-dose opioids. **Subcutaneous** *morphine* **or transdermal** *fentanyl* may be the drugs of choice. If nausea occurs, antinauseants may be useful. *Metoclopramide* subcutaneously may help keep the stomach empty, and may be combined with a centrally acting antinauseant such as *cyclizine*. A very light diet may be tolerated if the patient wishes to try to eat.

Diarrhea and Tenesmus

Diarrhea in a patient with advanced gynecologic cancer is probably best considered as a sign of fecal impaction until proven otherwise. True irritative diarrhea can occur by tumor involvement

Table 25.5 Management of Gastrointestinal Obstruction in Patients with Gynecologic Cancer

1. Is it an obstruction?

Clarify by

History

Examination

Investigation

Erect abdominal x-ray

Contrast studies

CT abdomen

Clarify highest level of obstruction and likely mechanism

Treat pain—SQ morphine

Treat nausea—SQ cyclizine

Treat conservatively initially with IV fluids and nasogastric suction

2. Is surgery or stenting an option?

Consider the following in making the decision

Single or multiple levels of obstruction

Likely prognosis—will the patient live at least 8 wks?

Likelihood of a nonmalignant cause of obstruction

Possible anticancer treatments available

Patient performance status

Patient preferences and goals

Likely rehabilitative outcome

3. If surgery or stenting not an option:

Consider trial of corticosteroids
e.g., *dexamethasone* 8 mg/d for 3–5 d

If clearly end stage, ensure goals of care known to patient, family, and treating team

Do not check electrolytes

Continue to relieve discomfort

Continue to relieve nausea with *cyclizine* (SQ)

If "high" obstruction

Decrease fluid intake (negative fluid balance)

Perform exquisite mouth care

Decrease GIT fluid production and relax gastrointestinal tract with *hyoscine hydrobromide* or *octreotide* (SQ)

Will likely require drainage of upper gastrointestinal track using nasogastric tube or venting gastrostomy

If "low" obstruction

Maintain a light diet if tolerated

Consider *metoclopramide* (SQ) to keep upper gastrointestinal tract empty (and reduce vomiting)

SQ, subcutaneously.

of the bowel wall or after radiation therapy. *Loperamide* may be useful in the management of such patients.

When fecal soiling is associated with an enterovaginal or rectovaginal fistula, surgical diversion should be considered if at all possible. If such surgery is not possible, the emphasis should be on nursing procedures calculated to keep the vagina and perineum as clean and comfortable as possible, and to support the patient in her distress. Antibiotics, especially *metronidazole,* locally and systemically, may reduce some of the distressing odor when necrosis occurs. A urinary catheter may assist in restoring urinary continence. Cases have been reported of the successful use of *octreotide* **to reduce small bowel fistula drainage** (73). The use of stool bulking agents (e.g., cellulose) may reduce the amount of fecal ooze if the fistula is colonic.

Tenesmus usually responds to anticholinergic agents, corticosteroids and opioids, often in combination. Anecdotal experience has shown that low-dose *ketamine,* followed by very low dose *methadone,* may be effective for more refractory cases. Occasionally, resection of tumor as a palliative procedure may be justified. In severe cases, spinal local anesthetics or sacral nerve blocks may be necessary.

Many of the gastrointestinal symptoms (which are such a feature of gynecologic cancer) are disturbances of gastrointestinal motility. This subject is a focus of ongoing research and the mechanisms involved are being elucidated (74). The gynecologic oncologist needs to recognize the following:

1. **Gastrointestinal motility disturbances, such as a tendency to constipation and reduced bowel sounds, may be a feature of gynecologic cancer even before any use of opioid drugs.**

2. **Drugs prone to constipate should be used with caution in such patients.** For example, opioid drugs must always be accompanied by laxatives. The use of $5HT_3$ blockers as antinauseants in the postoperative period or as premedication for chemotherapy should be routinely accompanied by appropriate laxatives.

Ascites

Abdominal distention that is due to intractable ascites can be a major cause of distress. Despite being a common complication of advanced cancer, the optimal approach to management is far from clear. **Paracentesis has an important role in diagnosis and in the immediate relief of symptoms.** It should be performed when there is significant abdominal discomfort, and patients should be warned that in the absence of systemic control of the malignancy, ascites will generally reaccumulate. Attempts to reduce the rate of reaccumulation include the institution of diuretics, particularly *spironolactone,* 50 to 150 mg/d, if necessary coupled with a loop diuretic such as *frusemide*. These may prove helpful initially. If ascites is reaccumulating rapidly, the clinician should anticipate the need for recurrent paracenteses and book clinical reviews accordingly. **Shunting procedures are not reliable and have been associated with significant morbidity and mortality. Systemic cytotoxic agents should be considered, although for the heavily pretreated patient with advanced disease, their potential is limited.** Discomfort is usually controlled with a combination of a drug such as *acetaminophen* and a low dose of an opioid.

Respiratory Symptoms

A clinical history, physical examination and chest imaging should differentiate between dyspnea caused by a pleural effusion, bronchial obstruction, diffuse lung involvement, reduced excursion from massive ascites, bronchial asthma, chronic obstructive airway disease, cardiac failure, and respiratory infection. However, **in advanced cancer, dyspnea may be multifactorial, with anemia, advanced cachexia, and resultant muscle asthenia contributing to the situation.** Treatment of contributing comorbidities, such as cardiac failure, should be considered in all patients. **Drainage of a pleural effusion, with early consideration of a pleurodesis, may afford prompt relief of dyspnea, cough, and chest wall discomfort.** Radiation therapy to a bronchial lesion causing hemoptysis, cough, or obstruction may produce prolonged palliation of symptoms.

When the cause of dyspnea is not reversible, the careful use of *morphine* may improve the situation significantly (75). Oral *morphine* should be commenced at doses of 2 to 5 mg every 4 hours and increased until drowsiness develops or until no further benefit is gained. In practice, this usually means doses of approximately 5 to 10 mg every 4 hours. The mechanism by which *morphine* reduces dyspnea is poorly understood, but includes both central and peripheral actions.

If a patient is already receiving *morphine* calibrated correctly for pain relief but becomes dyspneic because of tumor progression, *morphine* may be increased by a further 30–50%.

For the patient with an obstructing bronchial lesion or with carcinomatous lymphangitis, corticosteroids may afford some relief by reducing peritumor edema. This can be achieved with daily doses equivalent to 8- to 16-mg *dexamethasone,* with reduction to the lowest possible dose when an effect has been achieved. For those with bronchial obstruction, there should be an immediate review by a radiation oncologist.

The role of oxygen in dyspneic patients with advanced cancer who are not seriously hypoxic is controversial (76,77). **Some patients find that oxygen masks or even nasal prongs inhibit communication, restrict their movements, and induce claustrophobia.** These patients may find an open window or a fan to be more effective. Other patients appear to benefit from oxygen, and feel unable to manage without it. **The use of oxygen should depend upon the patient's report of improvement of dyspnea** and not on measures of oxygenation. Some patients who have been oxygen dependent because of dyspnea can become less so with careful use of *morphine.*

Anxiolytics may be valuable in modest doses. Benzodiazepines (e.g., 2-mg *diazepam* orally or 0.5-mg *lorazepam* sublingually) may have significant benefit for the anxious patient. For the patient who is in the last few days of life, an infusion of subcutaneous *midazolam* at low doses (e.g., 5 to 15 mg over 24 hours in the patient who is benzodiazepine naive) can afford significant relief of dyspnea.

Urinary Tract Symptoms

Urinary tract symptoms are common in women with advanced gynecologic cancer. Bilateral ureteric obstruction, with subsequent infection, pain, and acute renal failure, may justify mechanical measures such as nephrostomy or ureteric stent insertion if the prognosis on other grounds is for at least several good-quality months of life. Although some patients clearly benefit, fine judgment is required in an individual case, and such patients should be managed in consultation with a gynecologic oncologist. **For patients with no reasonable treatment options and problematic symptoms, it may be prudent to refrain from mechanical intervention.**

Improved patency of ureters may be achieved by short courses of corticosteroids (e.g., oral *dexamethasone,* 4 mg/d for 3 to 5 days), but steroids should only be considered if goals are short term, for example, to prolong life for a few weeks (78).

Bladder symptoms may benefit from the use of NSAIDs to reduce detrusor irritability, or drugs with an anticholinergic action to reduce bladder contractility. Catheterization may be unavoidable in some circumstances. **Urinary incontinence resulting from fistulae to the vagina or rectum is usually best managed by urinary diversion if feasible.** If not, urinary catheterization may assist in keeping the perineum dry.

Edema

Deep venous thrombosis should be excluded, particularly if other signs such as pain, increased temperature of the affected limb, or superficial venous dilatation are present. Anticoagulation in patients who have a deep venous thrombosis may lead to a reduction in symptoms, but the decision to anticoagulate a patient with advanced cancer must be made in the context of the patient's prognosis and goals.

If the swelling is due to lymphatic obstruction, the management must be individualized. Physical therapies, in experienced hands, are most helpful for moderate to severe lymphedema. Massage, bandaging, and fitting of support garments may add much to a patient's comfort (79). Care should be taken when applying compression bandages to grossly edematous legs to ensure venous circulation is not compromised.

Weakness

Weakness or fatigue can be profound when there is a large tumor burden, but there are many reversible causes of this symptom (80). These include nutritional deficiencies, hypotension, hypokalemia, hypoglycemia or hyperglycemia, hypoadrenalism, hypercalcemia, renal failure, infection, and anemia. At least some of these may be readily treated in appropriate circumstances. **Anemia *per se* does not require correction in every patient,** because the benefit may be short lived and not proportionate to the expenditure of resources. A patient who is confined to bed because of advanced disease often tolerates a hemoglobin of 7 g/dL or less. However, **if the hemoglobin is low and weakness is a dominant symptom, transfusion may be justified.**

For a number of patients, fatigue remains a dominant symptom without readily correctible contributory factors. For those women who are maintaining some independence, **evidence suggests that a program which seeks to maintain and increase gentle physical activity improves both fatigue and quality of life** (81).

Hypercalcemia

Hypercalcemia (raised ionized plasma calcium level) **is a recognized complication of malignancy and a potent cause of symptoms, ranging from lethargy, weakness, and constipation to severe nausea, vomiting, confusion, and exacerbation of bone pain.** In general, treatment of hypercalcemia should be coupled with anticancer therapy directed at removing the cause of the hypercalcemia if this is still feasible.

Hypercalcemia usually heralds a poor prognosis and for the relatively asymptomatic or already obtunded patient, aggressive treatment may not be warranted. The presence of troublesome symptoms often makes palliative antihypercalcemic therapy worthwhile (82).

Treatment of hypercalcemia depends on its severity. The following measures are necessary in moderate or severe cases:

1. **Modest rehydration with intravenous normal saline** (2 to 3 L/d or more). The patient should be monitored carefully to avoid fluid overload, especially the elderly, and those with comorbidities such as heart failure.

2. **Infusion of a bisphosphonate** (e.g., *pamidronate* 60 to 90 mg intravenously in 250 mL of crystalloid over 4 to 8 hours, or *zoledronic acid* 4 mg given over 15 minutes) (83). The duration of response varies according to the drug given and the clinical circumstances, but may be in the order of 35 days for *pamidronate*.

Improvement of symptoms with these measures can be expected within a few days, as calcium uptake in bone increases. When the calcium level is extremely high and intravenous bisphosphonate therapy is not causing a rapid reduction, **subcutaneous *calcitonin* administration combined with bisphosphonate therapy may provide a more rapid reduction in calcium levels,** but administration of *calcitonin* always warrants specialist assistance.

Should hypercalcemia recur, the bisphosphonate dose may be repeated. The rate of relapse depends in part on the availability of effective therapy for the underlying tumor, and on the biologic characteristics and tempo of the neoplastic process. Therefore the decision to repeat doses of bisphosphonate must take into account these factors, the likely prognosis, and the symptoms implicated.

Care of the Patient Close to Death

It is important to recognize that a woman is actually dying; this is an important diagnosis with clinical and social implications. What is medically possible at this stage, such as treatment of renal failure, septicemia, or hypercalcemia, may not necessarily be medically wise.

There are many physical indicators that a patient is actually dying and these are well known to clinicians, although not necessarily to family members. **There may be a change in the tempo of the disease, a manifest change in the function of critical organs, or a rapid deterioration in strength or physical performance in the absence of reversible factors.** The patient may become bedbound, semiconscious, only able to take sips of fluid, or no longer able to swallow medications (84).

When it is clear that the patient is dying, the goal is dignity, privacy, peace, and space for the woman to complete those remaining tasks important to "a life well-lived." Care should encompass the following domains:

1. **The rigorous treatment of symptoms.**
2. **The discontinuation of those interventions** and treatments (including medications) **that are not directly involved in maintaining comfort and dignity**.
3. **Sensitive communication** and explanation with the patient and her family.
4. **Attention to social, psychological, and spiritual needs** (84).

Sometimes it is justifiable to offer direct sedation when, in spite of adequate symptom control, distress is extreme and opportunities for verbal communication no longer exist.

There are circumstances in which a patient should be able to sleep peacefully as she dies. **This is particularly the case if an agitated delirium is present** after treating any remediable factors such as fecal impaction, urinary retention, or unrelieved pain. If hallucinations are prominent, an antipsychotic may be most useful, whereas if agitation and distress are present, a benzodiazepine should be used, usually in combination with an antipsychotic (85). **Suitable benzodiazepines include *midazolam*** (2 to 5 mg subcutaneously, intramuscularly, or intravenously stat and 10 to 50 mg over 24 hours by subcutaneous infusion if distress is protracted) **or** sublingual ***lorazepam*** (0.5 to 2.5 mg every 4 to 6 hours). **Antipsychotics used commonly include *haloperidol*,** 0.5 to 5 mg twice daily orally or subcutaneously, ***risperidone*,** 0.5 to 1 mg twice daily orally, or ***olanzapine*,** 2.5 to 10 mg daily orally or buccal wafer. Some of the older sedating antipsychotic agents (such as ***chlorpromazine***) remain useful in this setting.

On rare occasions, distress and agitation may not be relieved with the combination of a benzodiazepine and an antipsychotic. In such circumstances, careful dosing of ***phenobarbital*** (50 to 100 mg given 8 hourly, orally or subcutaneously) may allow calm in the final stages of life. **Large doses of opioids are not appropriate for sedation of the dying.** Ensuring that a patient sleeps most of the time during the last hours or days of her life is not euthanasia.

The development of "rattling" respirations indicating pooling of secretions is common in the patient close to death. Management should include repositioning the patient, and possibly the judicious use of anticholinergic agents (*hyoscine hydrobromide* 0.2 to 0.4 mg subcutaneously up to 4 hourly) to reduce the production of secretions. The latter must be coupled with measures to keep the mouth moist. Reassurance should be given to families that this is usually not distressing to the patient (84).

Complex equipment should be avoided if possible. All measures should be taken to facilitate maximum physical contact with loved ones. Nursing care should particularly emphasize pressure care, mouth care, and "grooming." Teaching family members to assist with the care of their loved one can do much to enhance intimacy, and diminish the sense of helplessness many families feel. In the face of imminent death, respect for individual religious and cultural customs is mandatory.

It is essential that medical and nursing staff accept and understand the personal significance of the final phase of life. It is a crucial period of personal development and a time for clarifying, reconciling, healing, and affirming personal relationships—always a complex task at the close of life.

The issues which patients view as significant in the final part of life are (i) receiving adequate pain and symptom management; (ii) avoiding inappropriate prolongation of dying; (iii) achieving a sense of control; (iv) relieving the burden on caregivers; and (v) strengthening relationships with loved ones (5,6). These issues must inform all care providers.

Good care of patients with incurable, progressive disease is concerned with the enrichment of remaining life, reduction of relievable distress, and support for personal growth and development, even when facing the human task common to all, that of dying. **The inherent dignity of the dying woman can be maintained and enhanced by the care she receives and the respect afforded to her continued relationships with those she loves (86).**

A Final Note

Mention has been made of the suffering of patients, yet nothing has been said of the distress of the health professionals who care for and journey with these patients. Such distress is often not articulated or shared. The sensitive clinician may take comfort from the words of a French oncologist:

Suffering is something like crossing a sea, traversing a mountain or a desert; it is an experience, painful indeed, in which the person will become more oneself and will discover oneself; it is an experience in which a person will experience evil, and yet, at the same time, will be led to discover and express the deepest meaning of one's life. This is true also for the suffering of the doctor (87).

However, the major burden of distress remains with the woman with gynecologic cancer and her family. Competent and compassionate palliative care may salvage dignity and meaning for the individual who is suffering and, in some small way, for the doctor as well. This is the task and the privilege when providing care to those at the end of their life.

References

1. **McDonald N.** The interface between oncology and palliative medicine. In: **Hanks GW, Cherny N, Christakis NA, et al., eds.** *Oxford Textbook of Palliative Medicine.* 4th ed. Oxford: Oxford University Press; 2011:11.
2. **Doyle D, Hanks GW, Cherny N, et al.** Introduction. In: **Doyle D, Hanks GW, Cherny N, et al., eds.** *Oxford Textbook of Palliative Medicine.* Oxford: Oxford University Press; 2009:3.
3. **World Health Organisation.** WHO definition of palliative care. 2013.
4. **Steinhauser K, Clipp E, McNeilly M, et al.** In search of a good death: Observations of patients, families and providers. *Ann Int Med.* 2000;132:825–832.
5. **Steinhauser KE, Christakis NA, Clipp EC, et al.** Preparing for the end of life: Preferences of patients, families, physicians, and other care providers. *J Pain Symptom Manage.* 2001;22(3):727–737.
6. **Zhang B, Nilsson ME, Prigerson HG.** Factors important to patients' quality of life at the end of life. *Arch Intern Med.* 2013;172(15):1133–1142.
7. **Cowcher K, Hanks GW.** Long-term management of respiratory symptoms in advanced cancer. *J Pain Symptom Manage.* 1990;5:705–707.
8. **Philip J, Gold M, Schwarz M, et al.** Anger in palliative care: A clinical approach. *Intern Med J.* 2007;37(1):49–55.
9. **Clayton JM, Hancock KM, Butow PN, et al.** Clinical practice guidelines for communicating prognosis and end-of-life issues with adults in the advanced stages of a life-limiting illness, and their caregivers. *Med J Aust.* 2007;186(12 suppl):S77, S79, S83–S108.
10. **Richardson A, Medina J, Brown V, et al.** Patients' needs assessment in cancer care: A review of assessment tools. *Support Care Cancer.* 2007;15(10):1125–1144.
11. **Kirkova J, Davis MP, Walsh D, et al.** Cancer symptom assessment instruments: A systematic review. *J Clin Oncol.* 2006;24(9):1459–1473.
12. **Vodermaier A, Linden W, Siu C.** Screening for emotional distress in cancer patients: A systematic review of assessment instruments. *J Natl Cancer Inst.* 2009;101(21):1464–1488.
13. **Albers G, Echteld MA, de Vet HC, et al.** Evaluation of quality-of-life measures for use in palliative care: A systematic review. *Palliat Med.* 2010;24(1):17–37.
14. **Holen JC, Hjermstad MJ, Loge JH, et al.** Pain assessment tools: Is the content appropriate for use in palliative care? *J Pain Symptom Manage.* 2006;32(6):567–580.
15. **Lau F, Cloutier-Fisher D, Kuziemsky C, et al.** A systematic review of prognostic tools for estimating survival time in palliative care. *J Palliat Care.* 2007;23(2):93–112.
16. **Maltoni M, Caraceni A, Brunelli C, et al.** Prognostic factors in advanced cancer patients: Evidence-based clinical recommendations-a study by the Steering Committee of the European Association for Palliative Care. *J Clin Oncol.* 2005;23(25):6240–6248.
17. **Glare P, Sinclair CT.** Palliative medicine review: Prognostication. *J Palliat Med.* 2008;11:84–103.
18. **Hancock KM, Clayton JM, Parker SM, et al.** Truth-telling in discussing prognosis in advanced life-limiting illnesses: A systematic review. *Palliat Med.* 2007;21(6):507–517.
19. **Clayton JM, Butow PN, Arnold RM, et al.** Fostering coping and nurturing hope when discussing the future with terminally ill cancer patients and their caregivers. *Cancer.* 2005;103(9):1965–1975.
20. **Lickiss JN.** Pain control in patients with gynecologic cancer. In: **Gershenson DM, Gore M, McGuire WP, et al., eds.** *Gynecologic Cancer: Controversies in Management.* London: Churchill-Livingstone; 2004.
21. **Jost L, Roila F.** Management of cancer pain: ESMO Clinical Practice Guidelines. *Ann Oncol.* 2010;21(suppl 5):v257–v260.
22. **NCCN.** http://www.nccn.org/professionals/physician_gls/f_guidelines.asp-pain. 2013.
23. **Lickiss JN.** Approaching cancer pain relief. *Eur J Pain.* 2001;5(suppl A):5–14.
24. **Tasmacioglu B, Aydinli I, Keskinbora K, et al.** Effect of intravenous administration of paracetamol on morphine consumption in cancer pain control. *Support Care Cancer.* 2009;17(12):1475–1481.
25. **McNicol E, Strassels S, Goudas L, et al.** Nonsteroidal anti-inflammatory drugs, alone or combined with opioids, for cancer pain: A systematic review. *J Clin Oncol.* 2004;15(22):1975–1992.
26. **Stevens MJ, Gonet YM.** Malignant psoas syndrome: Recognition of an oncologic entity. *Australas Radiol.* 1990;34:150–154.
27. **Mercadante S.** Challenging pain problems. In: **Walsh D, ed.** *Palliative Medicine.* Philadelphia, PA: Saunders Elsevier; 2009.
28. **Cassell E.** Suffering. In: **Walsh D, ed.** *Palliative Medicine.* Philadelphia, PA: Saunders Elsevier; 2009.
29. **Lickiss JN.** The human experience of illness. In: **Walsh D, ed.** *Palliative Medicine.* Philadelphia, PA: Saunders Elsevier; 2009.
30. **Caraceni A, Hanks G, Kaasa S, et al.** Use of opioid analgesics in the treatment of cancer pain: Evidence-based recommendations from the EAPC. *Lancet Oncol.* 2012;13(2):e58–e68.
31. **Cherny NI, Baselga J, deConno F, et al.** Formulary availability and regulatory barriers to accessibility of opioids for cancer pain in Europe: A report from the ESMO/EAPC Opioid Policy Initiative. *Ann Oncol.* 2010;21(3):615–626.
32. **Klepstad P, Kaasa S, Brochgrevink PC.** Starting step III opioids for moderate to severe pain in cancer patients: Dose titration: A systematic review. *Palliat Med.* 2011;25(5):424–430.
33. **Fine PG, Portenoy RK.** Establishing "best practices" for opioid rotation: Conclusions of an expert panel. *J Pain Symptom Manage.* 2009;38(3):418–425.
34. **Caraceni A, De Conno F, Kaasa S, et al.** Update on cancer pain guidelines. *J Pain Symptom Manage.* 2009;38(3):e1–e3.
35. **Biancofiore G.** Oxycodone controlled release in cancer pain management. *Ther Clin Risk Manag.* 2006;2:229–234.
36. **Fallon M.** Neuropathic pain in cancer. *Br J Anaesth.* 2013;111(1):105–111.
37. **Berdine HJ, Nesbit SA.** Equianalgesic dosing of opioids. *J Pain Palliat Care Pharmacother.* 2006;20:79–84.
38. **King S, Forbes K, Hanks GW, et al.** A systematic review of the use of opioid medication for those with moderate to severe cancer pain and renal impairment: A European Palliative Care Research Collaborative opioid guidelines project. *Palliat Med.* 2011;25(5):525–552.
39. **Cherny N.** Is oral methadone better than placebo or other oral/transdermal opioids in the management of pain? *Palliat Med.* 2011;25(5):488–493.
40. **Inturrisi CE.** Pharmacology of methadone and its isomers. *Minerva Anestesiol.* 2005;71(7–8):435–437.
41. **Mercadante S, Caraceni A.** Conversion ratios for opioid switching in the treatment of cancer pain: A systematic review. *Palliat Med.* 2011;25(5):504–515.
42. **Pigni A, Brunelli C, Caraceni A.** The role of hydromorphone in cancer pain treatment: A systematic review. *Palliat Med.* 2011;25(5):471–477.
43. **Cachia E, Ahmedzai SH.** Transdermal opioids for cancer pain. *Curr Opin Support Palliat Care.* 2011;5(1):15–19.
44. **Grond S, Radbruch L, Lehmann K.** Clinical pharmacokinetics of transdermal opioids: Focus on transdermal fentanyl. *Clin Pharmacokinet.* 2000;38:59–89.
45. **Zeppetella G.** Opioids for the management of breakthrough cancer pain in adults: A systematic review undertaken as part of an EPCRC opioid guidelines project. *Palliat Med.* 2011;25(5):516–524.
46. **Somogyi AA, Barratt DT, Coller JK.** Pharmacogenetics of opioids. *Clin Pharmacol Ther.* 2007;81(3):429–444.
47. **Tassinari D, Sartori S, Tamburini E, et al.** Adverse effects of transdermal opiates treating moderate-severe cancer pain in comparison to long-acting morphine: A meta-analysis and systematic review of the literature. *J Palliat Med.* 2008;11(3):492–501.
48. **Leppert W.** The role of opioid receptor antagonists in the treatment of opioid-induced constipation: A review. *Adv Ther.* 2010;27(10):714–730.
49. **McQueen AL, Baroletti SA.** Adjuvant ketamine analgesia for the management of cancer pain. *Ann Pharmacother.* 2002;36(10):1614–1619.
50. **Dworkin RH, O'Connor AB, Backonja M, et al.** Pharmacologic management of neuropathic pain: Evidence-based recommendations. *Pain.* 2007;132(3):237–251.
51. **Prommer EE.** Ketamine for pain: An update of uses in palliative care. *J Palliat Med.* 2012;15(4):474–483.
52. **Hardy J, Quinn S, Fazekas B, et al.** Randomized, double-blind, placebo-controlled study to assess the efficacy and toxicity of subcutaneous ketamine in the management of cancer pain. *J Clin Oncol.* 2012;30(29):3611–3617.

53. **Kurita GP, Kaasa S, Sjøgren P.** Spinal opioids in adult patients with cancer pain: A systematic review: A European Palliative Care Research Collaborative (EPCRC) opioid guidelines project. *Palliat Med.* 2011;25(5):560–577.

54. **Fainsinger RL, Nekolaichuk CL.** A "TNM" classification system for cancer pain: The Edmonton Classification System for Cancer Pain (ECS-CP). *Support Care Cancer.* 2008;16(6):547–555.

55. **Buffum MD, Hutt E, Chang VT, et al.** Cognitive impairment and pain management: Review of issues and challenges. *J Rehabil Res Dev.* 2007;44(2):315–330.

56. **Stromer W, Michaeli K, Sandner-Kiesling A.** Perioperative pain therapy in opioid abuse. *Eur J Anaesthesiol.* 2013;30(2):55–64.

57. **Nicolaidis C.** Police officer, deal-maker, or health care provider? Moving to a patient-centered framework for chronic opioid management. *Pain Med.* 2011;12(6):890–897.

58. **Chou R, Fanciullo GJ, Fine PG, et al.** Clinical guidelines for the use of chronic opioid therapy in chronic noncancer pain. *J Pain.* 2009;10(2):113–130.

59. **Marsden DE, Lickiss JN, Hacker NF.** Gastrointestinal problems in patients with advanced gynaecological malignancy. *Best Pract Res Clin Obstet Gynaecol.* 2001;15(2):253–263.

60. **Fearon K, Arends J, Baracos V.** Understanding the mechanisms and treatment options in cancer cachexia. *Nat Rev Clin Oncol.* 2013;10(2):90–99.

61. **Loprinzi CL, Ellison NM, Schaid DJ, et al.** Controlled trial of megestrol acetate for the treatment of cancer anorexia and cachexia. *J Natl Cancer Inst.* 1990;82(13):1127–1132.

62. **Davis MP, Walsh D.** Treatment of nausea and vomiting in advanced cancer. *Support Care Cancer.* 2000;8(6):444–452.

63. **Glare P, Pereira G, Kristjanson LJ, et al.** Systematic review of the efficacy of antiemetics in the treatment of nausea in patients with far-advanced cancer. *Support Care Cancer.* 2004;12(6):432–440.

64. **Twycross RG.** *Palliative Care Formulary.* Oxford: Radcliffe Medical Press; 2002.

65. **Philip J, Lickiss N, Grant PT, et al.** Corticosteroids in the management of bowel obstruction on a gynecological oncology unit. *Gynecol Oncol.* 1999;74(1):68–73.

66. **Schiller LR.** Review article: The therapy of constipation. *Alimen Pharmacol Ther.* 2001;15(6):749–763.

67. **Portenoy RK, Thomas J, Moehl Boatwright ML, et al.** Subcutaneous methylnaltrexone for the treatment of opioid-induced constipation in patients with advanced illness: A double-blind, randomized, parallel group, dose-ranging study. *J Pain Symptom Manage.* 2008;35(5):458–468.

68. **Baines M, Oliver DJ, Carter RL.** Medical management of intestinal obstruction in patients with advanced malignant disease. A clinical and pathological study. *Lancet.* 1985;2(8462):990–993.

69. **Mercadante S, Casuccio A, Mangione S.** Medical treatment for inoperable malignant bowel obstruction: A qualitative systematic review. *J Pain Symptom Manage.* 2007;33(2):217–223.

70. **Ripamonti C, Twycross R, Baines M, et al.** Clinical-practice recommendations for the management of bowel obstruction in patients with end-stage cancer. *Support Care Cancer.* 2001;9(4):223–233.

71. **Dionigi G, Villa F, Rovera F, et al.** Colonic stenting for malignant disease: Review of literature. *Surg Oncol.* 2007;16(suppl 1):S153–S155.

72. **Feuer DJ, Broadley KE.** Corticosteroids for the resolution of malignant bowel obstruction in advanced gynaecological and gastrointestinal cancer. *Cochrane Database Syst Rev.* 2000(2):CD001219.

73. **Curtin JP, Burt LL.** Successful treatment of small intestine fistula with somatostatin analog. *Gynecol Oncol.* 1990;39(2):225–227.

74. **Grundy D, Schemann M.** Enteric nervous system. *Curr Opin Gastroenterol.* 2006;22(2):102–110.

75. **Abernethy AP, Currow DC, Frith P, et al.** Randomised, double blind, placebo controlled crossover trial of sustained release morphine for the management of refractory dyspnoea. *BMJ.* 2003;327(7414):523–528.

76. **Philip J, Gold M, Milner A, et al.** A randomized, double-blind, crossover trial of the effect of oxygen on dyspnea in patients with advanced cancer. *J Pain Symptom Manage.* 2006;32(6):541–550.

77. **Abernethy AP, McDonald CF, Frith PA, et al.** Effect of palliative oxygen versus room air in relief of breathlessness in patients with refractory dyspnoea: A double-blind, randomised controlled trial. *Lancet.* 2010;376(9743):784–793.

78. **Chye R, Lickiss N.** The use of corticosteroids in the management of bilateral malignant ureteric obstruction. *J Pain Symptom Manage.* 1994;9(8):537–540.

79. **Framework L.** *Best Practice for the Management of Lymphoedema: International Consensus.* London: MEP Ltd; 2006.

80. **Barnes EA, Bruera E.** Fatigue in patients with advanced cancer: A review. *Int J Gynecol Cancer.* 2002;12(5):424–428.

81. **Cramp F, Byron-Daniel J.** Exercise for the management of cancer-related fatigue in adults. *Cochrane Database Syst Rev.* 2012;11:CD006145.

82. **Legrand SB.** Modern management of malignant hypercalcemia. *Am J Hosp Palliat Care.* 2011;28(7):515–517.

83. **Clines GA.** Mechanisms and treatment of hypercalcemia of malignancy. *Curr Opin Endocrinol Diabetes Obes.* 2011;18(6):339–346.

84. **Ellershaw J, Ward C.** Care of the dying patient: The last hours or days of life. *BMJ.* 2003;326(7379):30–34.

85. **LeGrand SB.** Delirium in palliative medicine: A review. *J Pain Symptom Manage.* 2012;44(4):583–594.

86. **Chochinov H.** Dignity and the essence of medicine: The ABC and D of dignity-conserving care. *BMJ.* 2007;335:184–187.

87. **Schaerer R.** Suffering of the doctor linked with the death of patients. *Palliat Med.* 1993;7(suppl 2):27–37.

26

Psychological Issues

Kristen C. Williams
Barbara L. Andersen

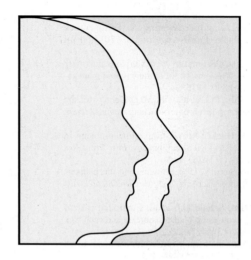

For most women, a diagnosis of gynecologic cancer is a crisis, and it is essential to consider a patient's psychological and behavioral responses when managing her disease. While most patients adapt and recover, cancer becomes a chronic stressor for some, either because the disease has disseminated and can be controlled only with radical treatment, or because a survivor's coping strategies are not adequate. This chapter reviews the data on these issues, and presents practical information that can be used to understand patients' responses and assist patients in coping during diagnosis, treatment, follow-up, and monitoring.

The stress of cancer diagnosis and treatment can have wide-ranging, long-term impacts on patients' mental health at every stage of the cancer experience. Cancer-specific stress triggers significant biologic effects. For example, following surgery and prior to adjuvant treatment, stress among breast cancer patients was associated with immune downregulation, shown across assays for NK cell cytotoxicity (NKCC), the response of NK cells to recombinant interferon gamma (rIFN-g), and T-cell responses, including proliferative responses to concanavalin A (ConA), phytohemagglutinin (PHA), and a T3 monoclonal antibody (MoAb) (1). **Attendance to a patient's psychological distress may have important benefits beyond alleviating the psychological impacts. Evidence suggests that psychological interventions can improve biobehavioral outcomes and potentially the disease course** (2).

Gynecologic Screening and Follow-Up

Research suggests that individuals become distressed during medical screening, long before a cancer diagnosis is suggested (3). **In the case of an abnormal screen, many women will experience significant anxiety, distress, and daily life disruptions.** Ideström et al. described reactions to abnormal Papanicolaou (Pap) test results in a sample of 242 women. More than half of the women surveyed (59%) reported feelings of worry and anxiety after being informed of their abnormal Pap result, and about a third (30%) of women reported that their daily life was disrupted in the time between the initial Pap result and follow-up tests (4). A smaller proportion of women (8%) reported symptoms of sexual dysfunction.

Another large survey of 3,500 women found increased risk for anxiety in response to an abnormal Pap result in women who were younger, had children, were current smokers, or had the highest levels of physical activity (5). Lerman et al. (6) reported that women who received abnormal Pap results worried more about cancer and had significantly more disruptions in mood, daily activities, sexual interest, and sleep patterns when compared to women who received normal results.

With respect to the initial gynecologic oncology consultation, patients have reported significantly elevated psychiatric symptoms, with 42% reporting clinical levels of depressive symptoms and 30% reporting moderate to severe anxiety symptoms, regardless of whether the eventual diagnosis was one of cancer or benign gynecologic disease (7). In a study of women undergoing ovarian cancer screening, most patients who received false-positive results showed little long-term psychological effect other than an increase in worry about cancer, but certain women, including those who underwent a surgical intervention, experienced more significant psychological distress (8).

The relationship between increased psychological distress and nonadherence to screening and treatment recommendations is well documented in cancer patients. **Possible explanations for noncompliance following an abnormal Pap result include fear of the diagnostic procedures, not wanting to know if something is wrong, fear of a cancer diagnosis, belief that the outcomes will be negative (fatalism), and belief that one is too old for treatment** (9).

While screening for ovarian cancer is under continued investigation, the high mortality associated with the disease has led to the adoption of prophylactic oophorectomy as an effective reducer of risk for women with a hereditary risk. This preventative treatment can have many psychological impacts. Although two studies of women receiving a prophylactic oophorectomy have reported that most (86%) participants were satisfied with their decision to undergo the procedure and experienced a reduction in cancer-related anxiety and worry (10,11), another found that such women experienced levels of cancer-related worry similar to those undergoing screening programs (12). All three studies reported that women who underwent the procedure experienced menopausal symptoms and sexual dysfunction (10–12).

Diagnosis

Stress and its negative impact on quality of life begin with diagnosis (13–15). Risk of suicide for women diagnosed with gynecologic cancer is highest during this time, particularly among women with ovarian cancer, and those for whom surgery is not recommended (16). The term existential plight has been used to describe this period, and the emotional turmoil that continues during treatment (17).

Emotions and sources of distress experienced at diagnosis are diverse. They may include the following:

1. **Depression,** from life disruption and doubts concerning the future.
2. **Anxiety,** from anticipating cancer treatment and side effects.
3. **Confusion,** from dealing with a complex medical environment.
4. **Anger,** from the loss of childbearing capacity and the opportunity to choose whether to have children.
5. **Guilt,** from concerns that previous sexual activity may have "caused" the cancer.

An early study conducted in 1989 compared mood disturbance among those recently diagnosed with a gynecologic cancer with two matched groups, one with benign gynecologic disease anticipating surgery, and the other with no disease (i.e., healthy women). All participants completed a self-report inventory on the emotions they experienced during their initial evaluation (18). While both groups with disease reported high anxiety and equivalent levels of fatigue and anger, **only women with cancer reported high levels of confusion and described themselves as having negative moods suggestive of depression.** A similar study conducted in 2011 by Posluszny et al. (15) reported that women with cancer reported higher levels of traumatic stress and perceived threat than matched controls with benign disease.

Data consistently underscore the significant distress experienced by many cancer patients. Mental health disorders among cancer patients are prevalent, largely unrecognized, and usually untreated. It is consistently estimated that 30–50% of cancer patients meet criteria for mood or anxiety disorders, with depressive disorders (major depression, minor depression, adjustment disorder with depressed mood) being the most common (19,20). Specifically, estimates for major depressive disorder (MDD) are 22–29% for patients with early-stage disease (21), 8–40% for patients with advanced disease (22), and higher for patients with recurrence (23). Among breast and gynecologic cancer patients, Zabora et al. (24) found prevalence of MDD to be 33% and 30%, respectively.

Common comorbidities with depression include anxiety (25,26), poorer quality of life (26–28), fatigue (29,30), and more distress from physical symptoms (31). Unfortunately, **cancer patients with depression are often not identified, despite the availability of simple screening measures** (32). For example, among 112 women with major depression undergoing cancer treatment, Ell et al. found that only 12% were receiving antidepressants, and only 5% were receiving psychological therapy (33).

Patients experiencing high levels of distress have many difficulties including (i) **understanding and remembering all that they have been told,** including both simple information (e.g., what time they are to be admitted) and more complex information (e.g., the organs to be surgically removed and the nature of the side effects); (ii) **managing personal affairs** (e.g., contacting their insurance company or arranging for child care during recovery); and (iii) **being a "patient" and allowing others to care for them**.

Even for those with some knowledge of gynecologic surgeries, cancer treatment is qualitatively different. For example, a woman's mother, sister, or a close friend may have related her experiences with hysterectomy. Even if the friend's surgery involved an abdominal rather than a vaginal approach, the preoperative and postoperative experience for the woman with cancer will be notably different (e.g., bowel preparation, length of recovery, vaginal shortening, bladder dysfunction) and more distress will likely result. It is normal for any patient to experience cognitive, emotional, and behavioral difficulties; and **it is the rare patient who does not require supportive assistance as treatment approaches**.

The acute stress associated with a cancer diagnosis may portend later difficulties. When there is an absence of positive coping, patients subsequently report a loss of meaning in their lives (34). Patients with high levels of diagnostic distress have been found to have high depressive symptoms during follow-up and lower quality of life (35).

Cancer Treatments

Despite efforts to allay concerns and provide accurate information about treatment plans, many women have misconceptions about their treatments and anxiety often remains high as patients approach surgery, radiation therapy, or chemotherapy. Many of these concerns are similar across treatment modalities, but others are unique to a particular treatment type. For example, bladder irritation and vaginal stenosis may occur with radiation treatment. Lymphedema, on the other hand, may occur with surgery or radiation. Women experiencing lymphedema report lower quality of life, more cancer worry, more problems with sleep, and more physical and social limitations (36).

Whichever treatment modality is utilized, it is important to consider the cultural implications of treatment effects. In a series of focus groups of women diagnosed with cervical cancer, for example, Latina, African American, Asian, and Caucasian women felt differently regarding their control over their illness, particularly in the assignment of blame (37). **Latinas often blamed themselves for their diagnosis, seeing cancer as a form of punishment for some failure,** while Caucasian, African American, and Asian women often considered their partners as at least partially to blame. **Latina and Asian women also worried about the loss of their purpose as a woman with the loss of their fertility.** These culturally related beliefs might affect a woman's treatment seeking, adherence to treatment, and psychological response following treatment.

Surgery

In 1982, Gottesman and Lewis (38) noted **greater and more lasting feelings of crisis and a stronger sense of helplessness among patients with cancer, compared to patients receiving surgery for benign conditions.** These feelings lasted for as long as 2 months after discharge from hospital. Similar findings have been observed in other studies subsequently. For example, women with advanced cancer have been reported to experience high levels of traumatic stress when compared to those receiving surgery for a benign gynecologic disease (15). Such psychological distress tends to be worse for those with less social support (14).

In addition to stress and anxiety, gynecologic cancer surgery imposes unique burdens. **Women of childbearing age who are nulliparous or have not yet achieved their desired family size may become distraught if they lose their childbearing capability** (39,40). Because the age of childbearing among women in the United States has risen, the likelihood of this situation occurring has increased. Identifying referral sources for information or fertility-preserving resources may prove difficult for those not near cities or major medical centers (39). **Women receiving information about reproductive assistance options experience less distress and depression** (41).

Radical surgery, such as pelvic exenteration, resulting in genital disfigurement or dramatic changes to the pelvis, may produce depression, feelings of isolation, and body image distress (42,43). Other surgeries, such as radical hysterectomy, may produce other effects, such as vaginal shortening and bladder dysfunction. Premature menopause from oophorectomy or ovarian failure may lead to distressing sexual and menopausal symptoms (e.g., atrophic vaginitis, hot flashes). Taken together, bodily changes and the loss of control of bodily functions contribute to decreased quality of life, depression, impaired body image, and anxiety (44). If feasible, less invasive surgeries, such as nerve sparing radical hysterectomy, may mitigate these side effects (44,45).

Radiation Therapy

Most patients report confusion and negative emotions regarding radiation treatments. Misinformation is common, with some patients fearing permanent contamination of themselves or others from treatment, while other patients assume that radiation attacks only "bad" cells, leaving others unaffected. A patient's prior knowledge of radiation therapy may be based on the experiences of a friend or relative, and if their treatment was unsuccessful or difficult, she may enter treatment believing it will be the same for her (46).

External beam therapy brings fears or uneasiness about the size or the safety of treatment machines and, often, distress from being in a radiation therapy department where there are other patients in obvious ill health. For some women, disrobing and exposing the pelvic area is a daily embarrassment, and field-marking tattoos are visible reminders of the cancer. In one study, roughly 80% of patients expressed an unwillingness to discuss these concerns with their physicians (47). This occurs particularly when patients perceive their physicians as disinterested, embarrassed, or too busy. Patients may also feel they cannot ask "intelligent" questions of their physicians.

As the treatment progresses, the daily procedures of radiation therapy become routine, and many patients report less emotional distress. However, side effects of fatigue, diarrhea, and anorexia then begin. Side effects complicate living, requiring activity reductions and dietary modifications. Previously symptom-free patients may begin to feel and think of themselves as "ill" doubting their positive prognosis. Premenopausal women experience hot flashes, a salient and distressing reminder of their loss of fertility.

At the termination of treatment, these patients might be expected to report a drop in anxiety and fear. Instead, gynecologic patients (48) and other patients with cancer (49) report a differing patterns of anxiety responses. **Women with high pretreatment anxiety are less anxious on the last treatment day than on the first, although they remain the most distressed.** Those with moderate levels of pretreatment distress report little diminution in distress by the last treatment, and surprisingly, those with low levels of anxiety at the onset of treatment report significantly greater anxiety on the last treatment day. **Physical symptoms of fatigue, abdominal pain, anorexia, diarrhea, and skin irritation are peaking at this time.** Patients may anticipate that treatment being over will bring a rapid end to symptoms, not knowing that symptoms only diminish with passing months (48).

In contrast to external beam, few patients are familiar with intracavitary radiotherapy. While the replacement of low-dose rate brachytherapy with high-dose rate equipment in most Western countries has reduced isolation times, **intracavitary radiotherapy still presents unique challenges to patients**. During treatment, women have significant physical discomfort, even when there has been liberal analgesic medication (49). Gas pains, burning sensations, and lower backache are typical, and emotional distress can be pervasive. Visitation restrictions limit contact with family and friends, which may be frightening to a patient if it is perceived as isolation from nurses or physicians. It is not surprising that many women are irritable and upset during the treatment.

If a second radiation application is received, physicians may anticipate that this might be an easier experience for patients, but it is not. **Women report feeling more anxious during the treatment,**

and are naturally more debilitated afterward. Even women with lower levels of anxiety before their first intracavitary treatment are reported to experience elevated levels of anxiety after their second application (50).

Without assistance, recovery from the physical and psychological distress of radiation therapy is slow. Nail et al. have documented an incidence of nausea in 5%, anorexia in 15%, diarrhea in 15%, and fatigue in 32% of gynecologic patients as long as 3 months after treatment (51). Complications, such as radiation proctitis or vaginal atrophy emerge across time. While some physical symptoms and quality of life may improve beyond levels seen before treatment by 3 to 4 months, anxiety, depression, and some physical symptoms may persist (52,53).

Sexual dysfunction after radiotherapy is common, severe, and persistent. Decreased lubrication and vaginal tenderness or pain are significant sexual disruptors during recovery, with lack of sexual interest and dyspareunia being major problems for many women. Alterations to the vaginal anatomy, including vaginal shortening and stenosis, begin during radiation treatment (54). Longitudinal data show that **sexual dysfunction persists at least 2 years after radiotherapy treatment** as the vaginal changes continue, with approximately 85% of women reporting low or no sexual interest and 55% experiencing mild to severe dyspareunia (55).

Any patient receiving radiation is at risk for dyspareunia. It is most severe among women receiving both external and intracavitary radiation, although external beam alone also produces dyspareunia (18). The magnitude of pain during intercourse appears to decrease during the months after treatment for women who maintain sexual activity. Atrophic vaginitis is extremely difficult to treat, making a regimen of vaginal care essential for all patients. Ovarian failure worsens these difficulties.

Chemotherapy

Patients' reactions to learning that they need chemotherapy can range from extreme negativity (i.e., feeling nervous, anxious, or depressed) to relief that some kind of treatment is available to them. This mix of emotions reflects distress at having to undergo a difficult treatment, which many believe is only for "hopeless" cancers, and the fear that it will not control the disease. In one study, nearly 60% of women at their first chemotherapy session reported levels of distress high enough to warrant follow-up by an oncologic psychologist (56). To allay patients' concerns, medical personnel usually provide descriptions of, and written materials about, the effects and side effects of treatment. In spite of this, as many as 10% of patients report uncertainty and lack of knowledge when beginning treatment (57). Others may approach chemotherapy optimistically and believe that they will belong to the small subset of people who do not experience any side effects.

Patients experience significant distress throughout chemotherapy that declines slowly with time. As treatment occupies more and more of a patient's life, worries become intrusive, and the intense and noxious side effects generate a clear awareness of illness. Compared to active, positive coping (e.g., seeking information, asking for social support), negative coping (e.g., avoiding information, withdrawal, substance use) is predictive of distress and more frequent reports of physical symptoms (58,59). In addition, women who attempt to control the side effects and fail become more distressed than those who report that they have coped successfully (57).

Anticipatory nausea and vomiting may complicate the course of chemotherapy for approximately 10% of patients (60,61). This refers to nausea and vomiting before the administration of chemotherapy. In most cases this is a conditioned response, resulting from the pairing of the stimuli surrounding the administration of chemotherapy (e.g., needles, smell of alcohol, the clinic) with the occurrence of posttreatment nausea and vomiting. With repeated cycles, the stimuli become conditioned and thus are able to evoke nausea or vomiting before the chemotherapy is administered. Once anticipatory reactions develop, they can become more general (e.g., alcohol-containing substances such as perfume may cause nausea), and they occur progressively earlier (e.g., on entering the hospital, rather than on entering the treatment room).

Factors that place a patient at risk for development of anticipatory nausea and vomiting include (62,63) the following:

- Age less than 50 years
- Lengthy infusion and toxicity of the regimen
- Severe posttreatment nausea or vomiting that is not controlled in the early cycles
- Extreme anxiety and/or depression
- Previous susceptibility to nausea and/or motion sickness

Women with higher levels of state anxiety tend to be more susceptible to both anticipatory and posttreatment nausea and vomiting (64). The likelihood of **anticipatory nausea and vomiting** developing has been reduced with prechemotherapy administration of antiemetics, and the use of second- and third-generation agents with lower gastrointestinal toxicities.

Confusion and cognitive impairment, colloquially referred to as "chemobrain," are prevalent in patients receiving chemotherapy and are distressing symptoms for the patient and her family. In a study of ovarian cancer patients, 69% reported some level of cognitive impairment (65). Pharmacologic effects of chemotherapeutic agents account for some cognitive changes (66), and such changes further emphasize the illness and its consequences to the patient.

Early Posttreatment

Patients often receive little preparation for the unique challenges of concluding active treatment (67). While it is certainly the case that patients are relieved that treatment is over, this is a transition. Daily or weekly contacts with treating physicians and nurses abruptly end, and with it the familiarity of context and support that was a part of being in treatment. Recovery from radiation therapy and chemotherapy is slow. While symptoms may diminish within weeks, residual fatigue will last upward of 12 months.

Reestablishing new routines with family, friends, employment, and so on, begins, and not all the transitions may be smooth. Some individuals may have "powered through" the diagnosis, treatments, and recovery without emotionally processing the cancer experience. This experience is captured in the common sentiment after treatment, "then it hit me…." Taken together, experiences such as these continue up to 2 years following the end of treatment before emotions and general adjustment stabilize. In the general case, physical and psychological symptoms and quality of life improve (15,68–71), but some symptoms may persist. **Sleep disturbances, sexual dysfunction, anxiety, and body image concerns have all been found to persist for even a year or longer** (68,71–77). Younger patients may have a particularly difficult time during this transition (68,70,78).

Survivor Years

The permanent sequelae of gynecologic cancer treatment, while expected, demand new behaviors and coping strategies from survivors. Data indicate that **most patients cope successfully; many report renewed vigor in their approach to life, stronger interpersonal relationships, and a "survivor" adaptation** (79–81). Patients report that **physical sequelae pose the most significant survivorship challenge** (82). Although psychological distress declines for the majority (70%), **approximately 25% of patients experience significant residual anxiety-related or depressive symptoms** (74–76,82,83). In short, physical sequelae and psychological adjustment are not necessarily mitigated by the passage of time (73,83–85). Physical and psychological sequelae covary such that worse psychological outcomes are associated with worse physiologic outcomes and worse quality of life (73,81,83–85), although younger women are at risk for worse psychological and quality-of-life outcomes despite their better physical functioning (81).

Physical side effects of treatment vary by treatment modality, even many years after treatment (73). Survivors' general health-related quality of life is often reported to be comparable with healthy controls, controls with minor medical illness, and standard norms (70,81,85,86). Long-term survivors' disease-specific quality of life, however, has been found to be comparable to scores found shortly after cancer treatment (85). In one study, long-term survivors (average 17 years) reported significantly worse physical health and physical functioning than matched controls without a history of cancer. This suggests that the physical difficulties of survivors may be obscured by more general measures.

Rates of psychiatric disorders—primarily mood or anxiety disorders—are substantial (72,74–76,82,83,85–87). Fear of death or recurrence may contribute for those who have a precancer generalized anxiety disorder. Such fears are common and may persist (81,86). Such reactions are substantial in gynecologic cancer survivors, with traumatic stress symptoms reported in 13–19% (74,88). They may be more common for those undergoing more difficult treatment regimens or those receiving life-altering and/or disfiguring cancer treatments (e.g., pelvic exenteration).

Patients with a prior history of psychiatric treatment and/or traumatic stress have reported greater symptom rates, as have patients who have reported greater rates of unmet supportive care needs (30,74). Although symptom rates were high, only one study has investigated clinically diagnosed posttraumatic stress disorder (PTSD), and it found no clinical cases among 75 women screened for PTSD and followed for 1 month (88). Thus, while it is essential to be attentive to traumatic stress symptoms in gynecologic cancer survivors, depression and anxiety are more prevalent.

Recurrence and Progressive Disease

Compared to earlier phases of gynecologic cancer, information about the psychological impact of recurrent cancer is scarce. In one controlled, prospective study of 227 women followed for 8 years after their diagnosis of breast cancer, 30 were diagnosed with recurrence (89). **Women's reports of cancer-specific stress at recurrence were equivalent to their reports after their initial diagnoses.** Emotional distress, social functioning, and quality of life showed no disruption at recurrence, and were equivalent to that of controls that had not recurred. This suggests that while a recurrent diagnosis is still exceedingly stressful, women may be more resilient at a recurrent diagnosis than they were at their initial diagnosis. Another study reported that such **women may also experience less confusion than women receiving their initial diagnoses** (90).

This is not to suggest, however, that women with recurrent gynecologic cancer do not experience emotional difficulties, particularly when their disease progresses. **In a sample of ovarian cancer patients nearing the end of life, Roberts et al. found that 39% exhibited acute fears, the most common being fear of abandonment (32%) and isolation (17%)** (91). In a study of 217 women with ovarian cancer followed during their last year of life, Price et al. found that quality of life declined sharply in the final 6 months, while symptoms such as nausea, anorexia, and pain increased (92). A cross-sectional study of 60 women with recurrent ovarian cancer suggested that younger age, greater symptom distress, and fewer years in their current relationship were related to worse adjustment to illness (93).

End-of-life care is essential. In a sobering review of the literature, however, Lopez-Acevedo et al. (94) reported that hospice care was underutilized, and used ineffectively when it was utilized, for gynecologic cancer patients. Although palliative care may reduce healthcare utilization while improving physical and psychological symptoms, women are often referred too late to fully benefit (94).

Addressing the Psychological Impacts of Cancer

The psychological and behavioral aspects of gynecologic cancer can be addressed in a number of ways. **Some anxiety and confusion can be mitigated or prevented simply through the provision of information, while depression or generalized anxiety may require more intensive therapy.** Data on the effectiveness of various interventions addressing the psychological needs of gynecologic cancer patients are described below.

Identifying Patients with Symptoms of Anxiety or Depression

Guidelines suggest that all patients should be screened for distress at their initial visit, at appropriate intervals as clinically indicated, with significant changes such as the diagnosis of recurrence, and when the transition to palliative and end-of-life care is made (95). Valid and reliable measures are available such as the Patient Health Questionnaire Nine-Symptom Depression Scale (PHQ-9) (96) for depressive symptoms, or the Generalized Anxiety Disorder (GAD)-7 (97) scale for anxiety symptoms. Measures such as these generate scores with established cut-offs that are clinically meaningful. Whatever strategy is used for screening, it is important that a phased assessment be used that does not rely simply on a symptom count. As a first step for all patients, identification of risk factors for distress is important.

Patients most vulnerable to significant symptoms of anxiety or depression include those with following (95):

- **Prior mood or anxiety disorder,** with or without prior treatment
- **Familial history of depression,** with or without prior treatment
- **Familial history of anxiety disorders,** with or without prior treatment
- **Other psychiatric disorders,** including substance abuse
- **Recurrent, advanced, or progressive disease**
- **Presence of significant chronic illness(es)** in addition to cancer
- **Singleton (single not married, widowed, divorced)** versus partnered
- **Unemployed** or lower socioeconomic status

As a second step, a measure such as the PHQ-9 can be used to assess for the classic depressive symptoms of low mood and anhedonia, and if endorsed, other depressive symptoms can be assessed (98). Many individuals (50–60%) with a diagnosed depressive disorder will have a comorbid anxiety disorder, with generalized anxiety being the most prevalent (99). **It has been recommended that patients be assessed for generalized anxiety disorder, as it is the most prevalent anxiety disorder, and is commonly comorbid with mood disorders or other anxiety disorders** (e.g., social anxiety disorder) (99). If an individual has comorbid anxiety symptoms or disorder(s), the route is usually to treat the depression first.

Informational Needs for all Patients

Effective provision of information is essential, beginning with the initial consultation. For example, Stewart et al. prepared a brief psychoeducational brochure for women who were referred for biopsy after an initial abnormal screen (87). Results demonstrated that women who received the brochure were significantly less distressed. Moreover, 75% of women who received the materials complied with treatment and follow-up 18 to 24 months later compared with 46% of women not receiving the materials. Thus, providing effective information addressed both psychological distress and nonadherence concerns.

It is crucial for a woman to receive information about the treatment plan for her disease. Misconceptions are common and can have important consequences. Detailed descriptions of the procedure, sensations, side effects, and behavioral coping strategies (e.g., relaxation training or distraction exercises for pain management) are useful. **Prepared patients tend to have shorter hospital stays, use fewer medications, and report less severe pain than patients receiving standard hospital care and preoperative nursing information** (100). It is hypothesized that this type of preparation reduces stress by helping to build accurate expectations, and by enhancing feelings of control and predictability for the patient.

In discussions regarding the treatment plan and prognosis, the patient's desire for the quantity and type of information may vary. **Maintenance of hope is important, particularly for patients with advanced disease.** This is compatible with the provision of honest prognostic information. Some patients may prefer quantitative time frames, while others may be more comfortable with vague, qualitative information (101,102).

Information can be provided in a number of ways. Pamphlets and one-on-one conversations are common, but multimedia and internet sources are also useful. In a study of 59 patients with newly diagnosed ovarian cancer, verbal and printed information was provided to all. The patients were then randomized to watch an educational video or a neutral video. The former group recalled more information about their condition than those who viewed a neutral video (103). While such an intervention is unlikely to replace more traditional sources of information, the availability of multiple methods of information provision may help understanding among some patients. A survey of 185 women in a mixed gynecologic oncology clinic suggested that while **pamphlets, one-on-one discussions with providers, and websites were the preferred methods of receiving information,** women were also interested in modalities such as books, group classes, and audio-visual materials (104).

After information about treatment has been delivered, patient understanding needs to be assessed, because many patients become confused or forgetful when too much information is given. One way to ensure understanding is to ask the patient to explain in her own words what she has been told, as if she were telling her husband or a close friend. This strategy provides an opportunity to reinforce her understanding and to correct any misconceptions. **Research on patient preparation suggests that information needs to be simplified and repeated.** Instead of providing all information to patients on one occasion at the start of treatment, an alternative is to repeat portions as particular information becomes more relevant. For example, Israel and Mood provided information about therapeutic procedures early in the treatment, about radiation side effects and their management at the midpoint of treatment, and about emotional issues and the length of recovery toward the end of therapy (105).

Interventions to Reduce Stress, Anxiety, and Depression

Psychological needs go unaddressed for the majority of patients (106)—a fact regularly acknowledged by the Institute of Medicine (IOM) and similar reports (e.g., *Meeting the psychosocial needs of women with breast cancer* [107]; *Cancer care for the whole patient: Meeting psychosocial health needs* [108]; *Living with and beyond cancer in the United Kingdom Cancer Reform Strategy* [109]). This occurs despite the availability of efficacious psychological interventions for reducing cancer stress and enhancing coping, as described below.

While the majority of intervention trials have been conducted with breast cancer patients, the findings are also applicable to gynecologic patients. Many randomized controlled trials (RCTs) have shown efficacy in patients with newly diagnosed cancer (110–112). Regarding psychological support, crisis or brief therapy (8 to 10 sessions), usually conducted in a group context, is effective. **These interventions involve an assessment of the patient's emotional distress and other difficulties, a focus on the immediate problems facing the patient, and focused therapeutic goals.** The therapist is active in making suggestions for coping and problem management. Therapeutic components may include **(i) distress reduction,** such as providing training in relaxation to lower anxiety and bodily tension and to enhance the patient's sense of control; **(ii) the provision of information about the disease and treatment; (iii) the provision of behavioral coping strategies,** for example, role-playing difficult discussions with family or the medical staff; seeking information about the disease or impending treatments; **(iv) the provision of cognitive coping strategies,** such as identifying the patient's troublesome worries and thoughts and providing alternative appraisals; and **(v) the provision of social support and comfort,** which acknowledges the difficulty of the situation, and provides a context for the patient to discuss her fears and anxieties openly.

Fewer RCTs have been conducted with gynecologic cancer patients. Results suggest the efficacy of coping and communication-enhancing interventions, supportive counseling, couple-based coping training, counseling and relaxation training, and acceptance and commitment interventions in reducing distress, anxiety, and depressive symptoms, and in enhancing coping (113–116). Other trials have shown promising outcomes with cognitive behavioral therapy for depression (117,118) and peer support (117,118).

Although patients prefer psychological treatments to pharmacologic treatments (119), **evidence-based practices are underused in the community** (120). For patients coping with depression, multiple trials with noncancer patients have tested the relative and comparative efficacy of the two primary treatments (121): Medication (122) and psychotherapy (123). Among psychotherapies, the most extensively studied and most successful treatment is cognitive behavioral therapy (124,125). **In randomized clinical trials,** cognitive behavioral therapy **has generally been found to be as effective as antidepressant medication** (126), even among the severely depressed. A 2006 report reviewed data on antidepressant medication for patients with cancer and depression (127). The authors found few studies, but concluded that those reported provided some evidence that antidepressants were effective in reducing depressive symptoms in cancer patients. Antidepressants may also enhance adherence to recommended treatment regimens.

In addition to the general psychological effects associated with a gynecologic cancer diagnosis and treatment, psychological interventions may be used to address concerns specific to the effects of various treatment modalities. For example, in a review of 54 studies investigating the efficacy of behavioral intervention methods, the authors concluded that in addition to controlling **anticipatory nausea and vomiting** associated with chemotherapy, interventions integrating several behavioral methods could reduce patients' anxiety and distress concerning other treatments. The review also suggested that although a variety of behavioral methods have been shown to reduce acute treatment-related pain, hypnotic-like methods, involving relaxation, suggestion, and distracting imagery hold the greatest promise for pain management (128).

Sexuality Outcomes and Sexuality Interventions

Commonality of Sexual Morbidity

The long-term impact of gynecologic cancers and cancer treatments on sexual health has been well documented (129–132). While sexual problems may not be a woman's primary concern when she is initially diagnosed, **persistent sexual problems are of concern for most survivors** (133). Often the first symptoms of a gynecologic cancer are related to sexual intercourse, such as dyspareunia or postcoital bleeding (134).

Most healthcare professionals are aware of the likelihood of sexual difficulties for their gynecologic oncology patients, yet assessment, prevention, or referral for treatment is uncommon. Stead et al. interviewed 43 physicians and nurses regularly treating women with ovarian cancer. While 98% reported that they felt sexual issues should be discussed with patients, only 21% reported actually doing so (135). Given that **30–50% of patients experience significant sexual disruption,** women with cancer indicate that sexuality needs to be addressed (42,43,136,137).

Table 26.1 Sexual Dysfunction Diagnoses According to Gynecologic Condition				
	Sexual Dysfunction (% Affected)			
Group	**Desire**	**Excitement**	**Orgasm**	**Dyspareunia**
Cancer	32%	29%	29%	29%
Benign	13%	20%	14%	14%
Healthy	9%	9%	6%	6%

Twelve months posttreatment. From **Andersen BL, Anderson B, deProsse C.** Controlled prospective longitudinal study of women with cancer: I. sexual functioning outcomes. *J Consult Clin Psychol.* 1989; 57:683–691.

Concerns are varied and may be physical, psychological, or interpersonal. Common problems reported by survivors include lack of desire, pain with intercourse (dyspareunia), vaginal atrophy, difficulty achieving orgasm, and negative body image. It is common for problems such as these to be accompanied by concerns about maintaining intimacy, communicating with a partner, and negative changes in a partner's interest in the sexual relationship.

In an early comprehensive study of sexual dysfunction in women with gynecologic cancer from Andersen et al., women with clinical stage I or II cancers ($n = 47$) were compared with two matched comparison groups: Women treated for benign gynecologic disease ($n = 18$) and gynecologically healthy women ($n = 57$) (17,18). All participants were assessed after diagnosis but before treatment, and then reassessed 4, 8, and 12 months later. **The frequency of intercourse declined for women treated for disease, whether malignant or benign. Women with disease experienced significant declines in sexual excitement;** the difficulty was more severe and distressing for women with cancer, possibly because of significant coital and postcoital pain, premature menopause, and/or treatment-related side effects. Changes in the desire, orgasm, and resolution phases of the sexual response cycle were also substantial. **Sexual dysfunction was diagnosed in approximately 30% of women treated for cancer.** Table 26.1 provides a summary of the rates of sexual dysfunction 12 months after treatment. In all cases, the rates of dysfunction were 2–3 times those found among healthy women.

Sexual morbidity persists long into gynecologic cancer survivorship. In a recent study, Carpenter et al. (138) examined sexuality in a sample of 175 gynecologic cancer survivors 2 to 10 years after initial treatment. Despite prevalent sexual difficulties, most resumed intercourse at rates comparable to available norms for similarly aged women (139), but sexual satisfaction and responsiveness were significantly impaired. Taken together, **these data suggest that resumption of sexual intercourse is not necessarily an adequate marker for improved sexual health, and that assessment of impaired sexual responses and sexual difficulties requires a comprehensive approach.**

The Role of the Gynecologic Oncology Team

Physicians and nurses need to be familiar with the adverse sexual outcomes for patients treated for gynecologic cancer. In the study by Stead et al., reasons clinicians listed for not discussing sexual sequelae included lack of knowledge and experience with such information, embarrassment, and lack of resources to provide support if needed (135). The acquisition of such knowledge is crucial for the gynecologic oncology service provider, and it is best if this information is part of a broad understanding of normal female sexual function and response. **Patients make few inquiries, despite their concerns, so providers need to initiate discussion of sexuality and provide information to all patients.** When questions do arise, an informed and understanding response encourages future discussion.

A brief sexual history should be obtained from all patients before treatment. Obtaining a sexual assessment can achieve three goals:

1. **It identifies sexuality as an area of well-being that the medical team considers important.**

2. **It provides the baseline data** necessary to evaluate any future changes in sexual functioning without the biases associated with retrospective reports.

3. **It provides an informed context for future discussions** about sexuality between the patient and the medical team.

A pretreatment sexual history is best obtained by questioning the patient directly. Questionnaires can be used to assess such topics as sexual behavior (136,140) or sexual arousal (17). Even for the older woman or the woman who is not currently sexually active, such information is desirable. The most important determinant of the frequency of sexual activity for a woman is not age, but the presence of a healthy and interested sexual partner (141). Further, women who are not currently sexually active may wish to be so in the future, and need to know how their functioning may be changed.

The following areas are important in considering risk for sexual difficulties:

- **Marital status** and availability of a current sexual partner(s)
- **Body image concerns**
- **Frequency of sexual activity** (intercourse or an equivalent intimate activity)
- **Presence of current sexual dysfunction** (e.g., lack of desire, orgasmic difficulties)
- **Presence of current sexual dysfunction in the partner** (e.g., premature ejaculation, erectile difficulties, sexual difficulties secondary to medication usage)

Sexual dysfunction is generally categorized based on the general model of sexual response put forward by Masters and Johnson (142). Thus, problems following treatment for gynecologic cancer may occur in the phases of desire (e.g., lack of desire for sex, negative body image), excitement/arousal (e.g., vaginal dryness, pain with penetration), orgasm (e.g., lack of orgasm), or resolution (e.g., residual pain). Consideration of both the phase and the cause are important.

The Importance of Information Provision

If the sexual problems resulting from gynecologic cancer and its treatments are to be minimized, investment of time, energy, and resources is necessary. **Departments caring for patients with gynecologic cancer need a plan for providing psychosexual assistance.** For the individual patient, **preventive rather than rehabilitative efforts are desirable.** There are at least three components that are essential in a sexual functioning intervention: (i) **information about sexuality** (e.g., male and female sexual anatomy, the sexual response cycle, sexual dysfunctions, and potential sources of difficulty after cancer treatment); (ii) **surgical or medical interventions** (e.g., hormonal therapy, reconstructive surgery); and (iii) **specific sexual therapeutic suggestions.**

Information *per se* is an important component of sexual therapeutic interventions (109). Longitudinal data indicate that if sexual difficulties develop, most are evidenced in the early months of recovery (143); therefore, **information should be provided before and immediately after treatment, as patients resume sexual activity.** At the time of diagnosis and treatment, patients should be well informed of the potential direct effects that the treatments might have on sexuality, such as changed general health (e.g., chronic fatigue), structural changes to the genitalia, hormonal changes, and interference with the physiologic components of the sexual response cycle (144). During recovery, healthcare professionals should discuss the sexual complications, such as atrophic vaginitis, and strategies for overcoming them. Such information aids in preventing problems resulting from ignorance or misconception, and potentially decreasing the severity of problems that arise from other factors.

The Importance of Treating Atrophic Vaginitis

Specific medical interventions may enhance sexual functioning for selected patients (145,146). Although **vaginal dilator therapy** has long been suggested, particularly for patients recovering from radiation therapy, a meta-analysis has shown insufficient evidence to support this practice (147). **Hormonal medication** may be used for menopausal symptoms; a **Fenton's operation** may be necessary to treat introital stenosis after vulvectomy. Patients with vaginal dryness should be instructed to use **lubricants** during vaginal intercourse and **vaginal moisturizers** daily. Despite these efforts, certain sexual activities may remain difficult. If vaginal stenosis is severe, patients and partners may need to reorient themselves to a sexual lifestyle focused on alternatives to vaginal intercourse.

The Importance of Referral to Sexual Health Professionals

Patients with significant sexual difficulties should be referred to a professional who is trained broadly in sexual therapy, and familiar with the specific difficulties of the patient with gynecologic cancer. There have been few clinical (148,149) or empirical (116,144,150,151) reports of sexual therapies for cancer patients. Some interventions have provided brief counseling to patients with gynecologic cancer on a variety of topics, and these often have included a sexuality module

(150,151). A handful of interventions specifically addressing sexuality have applied strategies from established psychotherapies, such as cognitive behavioral therapy, mindfulness training (152,153), sex therapy (148), and couples therapy (116,154). Results of these studies have suggested the effectiveness of psychotherapies in ameliorating sexual functioning after gynecologic cancer. **For many patients, behaviorally oriented sex therapy offers the most promise for change as the individual's specific sexual problems** (e.g., loss of desire) **are targeted.**

References

1. **Andersen BL, Farrar WB, Golden-Kreutz D, et al.** Stress and immune responses after surgical treatment for regional breast cancer. *J Natl Cancer Inst.* 1998;90(1):30–36.
2. **Antoni MH.** Psychosocial intervention effects on adaptation, disease course and biobehavioral processes in cancer. *Brain Behav Immun.* 2013;30 (suppl):S88–S98.
3. **Wardle J, Pope R.** The psychological costs of screening for cancer. *J Psychosom Res.* 1992;36(7):609–624.
4. **Idestrom M, Milsom I, Andersson-Ellstrom A.** Women's experience of coping with a positive Pap smear: A register-based study of women with two consecutive Pap smears reported as CIN 1. *Acta Obstet Gynecol Scand.* 2003;82(8):756–761.
5. **Gray NM, Sharp L, Cotton SC, et al.** Psychological effects of a low-grade abnormal cervical smear test result: Anxiety and associated factors. *Br J Cancer.* 2006;94(9):1253–1262.
6. **Lerman C, Miller SM, Scarborough R, et al.** Adverse psychologic consequences of positive cytologic cervical screening. *Am J Obstet Gynecol.* 1991;165(3):658–662.
7. **Fowler JM, Carpenter KM, Gupta P, et al.** The gynecologic oncology consult: Symptom presentation and concurrent symptoms of depression and anxiety. *Obstet Gynecol.* 2004;103(6):1211–1217.
8. **Wardle J, Pernet A, Collins W, et al.** False positive results in ovarian cancer screening: One year follow-up of psychological status. *Psychol Health.* 1994;10(1):33–40.
9. **Yabroff KR, Kerner JF, Mandelblatt JS.** Effectiveness of interventions to improve follow-up after abnormal cervical cancer screening. *Prev Med.* 2000;31(4):429–439.
10. **Madalinska JB, Hollenstein J, Bleiker E, et al.** Quality-of-life effects of prophylactic salpingo-oophorectomy versus gynecologic screening among women at increased risk of hereditary ovarian cancer. *J Clin Oncol.* 2005;23(28):6890–6898.
11. **Tiller K, Meiser B, Butow P, et al.** Psychological impact of prophylactic oophorectomy in women at increased risk of developing ovarian cancer: A prospective study. *Gynecol Oncol.* 2002;86(2):212–219.
12. **Fry A, Busby-Earle C, Rush R, et al.** Prophylactic oophorectomy versus screening: Psychosocial outcomes in women at increased risk of ovarian cancer. *Psychooncology.* 2001;10(3):231–241.
13. **Pearman T.** Quality of life and psychosocial adjustment in gynecologic cancer survivors. *Health Qual Life Outcomes.* 2003;1:33.
14. **Petersen RW, Graham G, Quinlivan JA.** Psychologic changes after a gynecologic cancer. *J Obstet Gynaecol Res.* 2005;31(2):152–157.
15. **Posluszny DM, Edwards RP, Dew MA, et al.** Perceived threat and PTSD symptoms in women undergoing surgery for gynecologic cancer or benign conditions. *Psycho-Oncology.* 2011;20(7):783–787.
16. **Mahdi H, Swensen RE, Munkarah AR, et al.** Suicide in women with gynecologic cancer. *Gynecol Oncol.* 2011;122(2):344–349.
17. **Andersen BL, Anderson B, deProsse C.** Controlled prospective longitudinal study of women with cancer: I. Sexual functioning outcomes. *J Consult Clin Psychol.* 1989;57(6):683–691.
18. **Andersen BL, Anderson B, deProsse C.** Controlled prospective longitudinal study of women with cancer: II. Psychological outcomes. *J Consult Clin Psychol.* 1989;57(6):692–697.
19. **Massie MJ.** Prevalence of depression in patients with cancer. *J Natl Cancer Inst Monogr.* 2004;(32):57–71.
20. **van't Spijker A, Trijsburg RW, Duivenvoorden HJ.** Psychological sequelae of cancer diagnosis: A meta-analytical review of 58 studies after 1980. *Psychosom Med.* 1997;59(3):280–293.
21. **Raison CL, Miller AH.** Depression in cancer: New developments regarding diagnosis and treatment. *Biol Psychiatry,* 2003;54(3):283–294.
22. **Hotopf M, Chidgey J, Addington-Hall J, et al.** Depression in advanced disease: A systematic review Part 1. Prevalence and case finding. *Palliat Med.* 2002;16(2):81–97.
23. **Burgess C, Cornelius V, Love S, et al.** Depression and anxiety in women with early breast cancer: Five year observational cohort study. *BMJ.* 2005;330(7493):702.
24. **Zabora J, BrintzenhofeSzoc K, Curbow B, et al.** The prevalence of psychological distress by cancer site. *Psychooncology.* 2001;10(1):19–28.
25. **Dausch B, Compas BE, Beckjord E, et al.** Rates and Correlates of DSM-IV diagnoses in women newly diagnosed with breast cancer. *J Clin Psychol Med Settings.* 2004;11(3):159–169.
26. **Schwartz L, Drotar D.** Posttraumatic stress and related impairment in survivors of childhood cancer in early adulthood compared to healthy peers. *J Pediatr Psychol.* 2006;31(4):356–366.
27. **Deshields T, Tibbs T, Fan MY, et al.** Differences in patterns of depression after treatment for breast cancer. *Psychooncology.* 2006;15(5):398–406.
28. **Peters L, Sellick K.** Quality of life of cancer patients receiving inpatient and home-based palliative care. *J Adv Nurs.* 2006;53(5):524–533.
29. **Sadler IJ, Jacobsen PB, Booth-Jones M, et al.** Preliminary evaluation of a clinical syndrome approach to assessing cancer-related fatigue. *J Pain Symptom Manage.* 2002;23(5):406–416.
30. **Smith EM, Gomm SA, Dickens CM.** Assessing the independent contribution to quality of life from anxiety and depression in patients with advanced cancer. *Palliat Med.* 2003;17(6):509–513.
31. **Mystakidou K, Tsilika E, Parpa E, et al.** Assessment of anxiety and depression in advanced cancer patients and their relationship with quality of life. *Qual Life Res.* 2005;14(8):1825–1833.
32. **Thekkumpurath P, Walker J, Butcher I, et al.** Screening for major depression in cancer outpatients. *Cancer.* 2011;117(1):218–227.
33. **Ell K, Sanchez K, Vourlekis B, et al.** Depression, correlates of depression, and receipt of depression care among low-income women with breast or gynecologic cancer. *J Clin Oncol.* 2005;23(13):3052–3060.
34. **Jim HS, Richardson SA, Golden-Kreutz DM, et al.** Strategies used in coping with a cancer diagnosis predict meaning in life for survivors. *Health Psychol.* 2006;25(6):753–761.
35. **Golden-Kreutz DM, Andersen BL.** Depressive symptoms after breast cancer surgery: Relationships with global, cancer-related, and life event stress. *Psychooncology.* 2004;13(3):211–220.
36. **Dunberger G, Lindquist H, Waldenström AC, et al.** Lower limb lymphedema in gynecological cancer survivors-effect on daily life functioning. *Support Care Cancer.* 2013;21(11):3063–3070
37. **Ashing-Giwa KT, Kagawa-Singer M, Padilla GV, et al.** The impact of cervical cancer and dysplasia: A qualitative, multiethnic study. *Psychooncology.* 2004;13(10):709–728.
38. **Gottesman D, Lewis MS.** Differences in crisis reactions among cancer and surgery patients. *J Consult Clin Psychol.* 1982;50(3):381–388.
39. **Trivers KF, Patterson JR, Roland KB, et al.** Issues of ovarian cancer survivors in the USA: A literature review. *Support Care Cancer.* 2013;21(10):2889–2898.
40. **Carter J, Chi DS, Brown CL, et al.** Cancer-related infertility in survivorship. *Int J Gynecol Cancer.* 2010;20(1):2–8.
41. **Carter J, Raviv L, Applegarth L, et al.** A cross-sectional study of the psychosexual impact of cancer-related infertility in women: Third-party reproductive assistance. *J Cancer Surviv.* 2010;4(3):236–246.
42. **Andersen BL, Hacker NF.** Treatment for gynecologic cancer: A review of the effects on female sexuality. *Health Psychol.* 1983;2(2):203–211.

43. **Andersen BL, Hacker NF.** Psychosexual adjustment after vulvar surgery. *Obstet Gynecol.* 1983;62(4):457–462.
44. **Carter J, Stabile C, Gunn A, et al.** The physical consequences of gynecologic cancer surgery and their impact on sexual, emotional, and quality of life issues. *J Sex Med.,* 2013;10:21–34.
45. **Pieterse QD, Kenter GG, Maas CP, et al.** Self-reported sexual, bowel and bladder function in cervical cancer patients following different treatment modalities: Longitudinal prospective cohort study. *Int J Gynecol Cancer.* 2013;23(9):1717–1725.
46. **Peck A, Boland J.** Emotional reactions to radiation treatment. *Cancer.* 1977;40(1):180–184.
47. **Mitchell GW, Glicksman AS.** Cancer patients: Knowledge and attitudes. *Cancer.* 1977;40(1):61–66.
48. **Andersen BL, Tewfic H.** Psychological aspects of gynaecological cancer. In: **Broome AK, Wallace L, eds.** *Psychology and Gynaecological Problems.* London: Tavistock/Routledge; 1985:117–141.
49. **Andersen BL, Tewfik HH.** Psychological reactions to radiation therapy: Reconsideration of the adaptive aspects of anxiety. *J Pers Soc Psychol.* 1985;48(4):1024–1032.
50. **Mages NL, Mendelsohn GA.** Effect of cancer on patients' lives: A personological approach. In: **Stone GC, Cohen F, Adler NE, eds.** *Health Psychology.* San Francisco, CA: Jossey-Bass; 1979:255–284.
51. **Nail LN, King KB, Johnson JE.** Coping with radiation treatment for gynecologic cancer: Mood and disruption in usual function. *Psychosom Obstet Gynaecol.* 1986;5(4):271–281.
52. **Vaz AF, Conde DM, Costa-Paiva L, et al.** Quality of life and adverse events after radiotherapy in gynecologic cancer survivors: A cohort study. *Arch Gynecol Obstet.* 2011;284(6):1523–1531.
53. **Yavas G, Dogan NU, Yavas C, et al.** Prospective assessment of quality of life and psychological distress in patients with gynecologic malignancy: A 1-year prospective study. *Int J Gynecol Cancer.* 2012;22(6):1096–1101.
54. **Katz RC, Flasher L, Cacciapaglia H, et al.** The psychosocial impact of cancer and lupus: A cross validation study that extends the generality of "benefit-finding" in patients with chronic disease. *J Behav Med.* 2001;24(6):561–571.
55. **Jensen PT, Groenvold M, Klee MC, et al.** Longitudinal study of sexual function and vaginal changes after radiotherapy for cervical cancer. *Int J Radiat Oncol Biol Phys.* 2003;56(4):937–949.
56. **Johnson RL, Gold MA, Wyche KF.** Distress in women with gynecologic cancer. *Psychooncology.* 2010;19(6):665–668.
57. **Leventhal H, Easterling D, Coons H, et al.** Adaptation to chemotherapy treatments. In: **Andersen BL, ed.** *Women with Cancer: Psychological Perspectives.* New York, NY: Springer-Verlag; 1986:192–193.
58. **Lutgendorf S, Anderson B, Sorosky JI, et al.** Interleukin-6 and use of social support in gynecologic cancer patients. *Int J Behav Med.* 2000;7(2):127–142.
59. **Yang HC, Brothers BM, Andersen BL.** Stress and quality of life in breast cancer recurrence: Moderation or mediation of coping? *Ann Behav Med.* 2008;35(2):188–197.
60. **Akechi T, Okuyama T, Endo C, et al.** Anticipatory nausea among ambulatory cancer patients undergoing chemotherapy: Prevalence, associated factors, and impact on quality of life. *Cancer Science.* 2010;101(12):2596–2600.
61. **Roila F, Herrstedt J, Aapro M, et al.** Guideline update for MASCC and ESMO in the prevention of chemotherapy- and radiotherapy-induced nausea and vomiting: Results of the Perugia consensus conference. *Ann Oncol.* 2010;21(suppl 5):v232–v243.
62. **Andrykowski MA.** Defining anticipatory nausea and vomiting: Differences among cancer chemotherapy patients who report pretreatment nausea. *J Behav Med.* 1988;11(1):59–69.
63. **Carey MP, Burish TG.** Etiology and treatment of the psychological side effects associated with cancer chemotherapy: A critical review and discussion. *Psychol Bull.* 1988;104(3):307–325.
64. **Andrykowski MA.** The role of anxiety in the development of anticipatory nausea in cancer chemotherapy: A review and synthesis. *Psychosom Med.* 1990;52(4):458–475.
65. **Stavraka C, Ford A, Ghaem-Maghami S, et al.** A study of symptoms described by ovarian cancer survivors. *Gynecol Oncol.* 2012;125(1):59–64.
66. **Silberfarb PM, Maurer LH, Crouthamel CS.** Psychosocial aspects of neoplastic disease: I. Functional status of breast cancer

patients during different treatment regimens. *Am J Psychiatry.* 1980;137(4):450–455.
67. **Stanton AL.** What happens now? Psychosocial care for cancer survivors after medical treatment completion. *J Clin Oncol.* 2012;30(11):1215–1220.
68. **Chan YM, Ngan HY, Li BY, et al.** A longitudinal study on quality of life after gynecologic cancer treatment. *Gynecol Oncol.* 2001;83(1):10–19.
69. **Clevenger L, Schrepf A, Degeest K, et al.** Sleep disturbance, distress, and quality of life in ovarian cancer patients during the first year after diagnosis. *Cancer.* 2013;119(17):3234–3241.
70. **Dahl L, Wittrup I, Væggemose U, et al.** Life after gynecologic cancer–a review of patients quality of life, needs, and preferences in regard to follow-up. *Int J Gynecol Cancer.* 2013;23(2):227–234.
71. **Ferrandina G, Mantegna G, Petrillo M, et al.** Quality of life and emotional distress in early stage and locally advanced cervical cancer patients: A prospective, longitudinal study. *Gynecol Oncol.* 2012;124(3):389–394.
72. **Harrington CB, Hansen JA, Moskowitz M, et al.** It's not over when it's over: Long-term symptoms in cancer survivors–a systematic review. *Int J Psychiatry Med.* 2010;40(2):163–181.
73. **Carlsson M, Strang P, Bjurstrom C.** Treatment modality affects long-term quality of life in gynaecological cancer. *Anticancer Res.* 2000;20(1B):563–568.
74. **Hodgkinson K, Butow P, Hunt GE, et al.** Life after cancer: Couples' and partners' psychological adjustment and supportive care needs. *Support Care Cancer.* 2007;15(4):405–415.
75. **Li C, Samsioe G, Iosif C.** Quality of life in long-term survivors of cervical cancer. *Maturitas.* 1999;32(2):95–102.
76. **Li C, Samsioe G, Iosif C.** Quality of life in endometrial cancer survivors. *Maturitas.* 1999;31(3):227–236.
77. **Matthews AK, Aikens JE, Helmrick S, et al.** Sexual functioning and mood among long-term survivors of clear-cell adenocarcinoma of the vagina or cervix. *J Psychosoc Oncol.* 2000;17(3–4):27–45.
78. **Juraskova I, Butow P, Robertson R, et al.** Post-treatment sexual adjustment following cervical and endometrial cancer: A qualitative insight. *Psycho-oncology.* 2003;12(3):267–279.
79. **Andersen BL, Anderson B.** Psychosomatic aspects of gynecologic oncology: Present status and future directions. *J Psychosom Obstet Gynaecol.* 1986;5(4):233–244.
80. **Taylor SE.** Adjustment to threatening events: A theory of cognitive adaptation. *Am Psychol.* 1983;38(11):1161–1173.
81. **Roland KB, Rodriguez JL, Patterson JR, et al.** A literature review of the social and psychological needs of ovarian cancer survivors. *Psychooncology.* 2013;22(11):2408–2418.
82. **Wenzel L, Huang HQ, Monk BJ, et al.** Quality-of-life comparisons in a randomized trial of interval secondary cytoreduction in advanced ovarian carcinoma: A Gynecologic Oncology Group study. *J Clin Oncol.* 2005;23(24):5605–5612.
83. **Wenzel LB, Donnelly JP, Fowler JM, et al.** Resilience, reflection, and residual stress in ovarian cancer survivorship: A gynecologic oncology group study. *Psychooncology.* 2002;11(2):142–153.
84. **Miller BE, Pittman B, Case D, et al.** Quality of life after treatment for gynecologic malignancies: A pilot study in an outpatient clinic. *Gynecol Oncol.* 2002;87(2):178–184.
85. **Carpenter KM, Fowler JM, Maxwell GL, et al.** Direct and buffering effects of social support among gynecologic cancer survivors. *Ann Behav Med.* 2010;39(1):79–90.
86. **Hodgkinson K, Butow P, Fuchs A, et al.** Long-term survival from gynecologic cancer: Psychosocial outcomes, supportive care needs and positive outcomes. *Gynecol Oncol.* 2007;104(2):381–389.
87. **Stewart DE, Lickrish GM, Sierra S, et al.** The effect of educational brochures on knowledge and emotional distress in women with abnormal Papanicolaou smears. *Obstet Gynecol.* 1993;81(2):280–282.
88. **Guglietti CL, Rosen B, Murphy KJ, et al.** Prevalence and predictors of posttraumatic stress in women undergoing an ovarian cancer investigation. *Psychol Serv.* 2010;7(4):266–274.
89. **Andersen BL, Shapiro CL, Farrar WB, et al.** Psychological responses to cancer recurrence. *Cancer.* 2005;104(7):1540–1547.
90. **Yang HC, Thornton LM, Shapiro CL, et al.** Surviving recurrence: Psychological and quality-of-life recovery. *Cancer.* 2008;112(5):1178–1187.

91. **Roberts JA, Brown D, Elkins T, et al.** Factors influencing views of patients with gynecologic cancer about end-of-life decisions. *Am J Obstet Gynecol.* 1997;176(1 Pt 1):166–172.

92. **Price MA, Bell ML, Sommeijer DW, et al.** Physical symptoms, coping styles and quality of life in recurrent ovarian cancer: A prospective population-based study over the last year of life. *Gynecol Oncol.* 2013;130(1):162–168.

93. **Ponto JA, Ellington L, Mellon S, et al.** Predictors of adjustment and growth in women with recurrent ovarian cancer. *Oncol Nurs Forum.* 2010;37(3):357–364.

94. **Lopez-Acevedo M, Lowery WJ, Lowery AW, et al.** Palliative and hospice care in gynecologic cancer: A review. *Gynecol Oncol.* 2013; 131(1):215–221..

95. **Andersen BL, DeRubeis RJ, Berman BS, et al.** Screening, assessment, and care of anxiety and depressive symptoms in adults with cancer: An American Society of Clinical Oncology guideline adaptation. *J Clin Oncol.* 2014;32(15):1605–1619.

96. **Kroenke K, Spitzer RL, Williams JB.** The PHQ-9: validity of a brief depression severity measure. *J Gen Intern Med.* 2001;16: 606–613.

97. **Spitzer RL, Kroenke K, Williams JB, et al.** A brief measure for assessing generalized anxiety disorder: The GAD-7. *Arch Intern Med.* 2006;166(10):1092–1097.

98. **Arroll B, Goodyear-Smith F, Crengle S, et al.** Validation of PHQ-2 and the PHQ-9 to screen for major depression in the primary care population. *Ann Fam Med.* 2010;8:348–353.

99. **Kessler RC, Chiu WT, Demler O, et al.** Prevalence, severity, and comorbidity of 12-month DSM-IV disorders in the National Comorbidity Survey Replication. *Arch Gen Psychiatry.* 2005;62(6): 617–627.

100. **Hayward J.** *Information: A Prescription Against Pain.* London: Royal College of Nursing; 1975.

101. **Innes S, Payne S.** Advanced cancer patients' prognostic information preferences: A review. *Palliat Med.* 2009;23(1):29–39.

102. **Smith TJ, Dow LA, Virago E, et al.** Giving honest information to patients with advanced cancer maintains hope. *Oncology (Williston Park).* 2010;24(6):521–525.

103. **Geller MA, Downs LS, Judson PL, et al.** Learning about ovarian cancer at the time of diagnosis: Video versus usual care. *Gynecol Oncol.* 2010;119(2):370–375.

104. **Papadakos J, Bussière-Côté S, Abdelmutti N, et al.** Informational needs of gynecologic cancer survivors. *Gynecol Oncol.* 2012;124(3): 452–457.

105. **Israel MJ, Mood DW.** Three media presentations for patients receiving radiation therapy. *Cancer Nurs.* 1982;5(1):57–63.

106. **Forsythe LP, Kent EE, Weaver KE, et al.** Receipt of psychosocial care among cancer survivors in the United States. *J Clin Oncol.* 2013; 31(16):1961–1969.

107. **Hewitt ME, Herdman R, Holland JC, et al.** *Meeting Psychosocial Needs of Women with Breast Cancer.* Washington, DC: National Academies Press; 2004:278.

108. **Adler NE, Page A, National Institue of Medicine (U.S.).** Committee on Psychosocial Services to Cancer Patients/Families in a Community Setting. *Cancer Care for the Whole Patient: Meeting Psychosocial Health Needs.* Washington, DC: National Academies Press; 2008:xxii, 429.

109. **National Health Service.** *Living with and Beyond Cancer: The Improvement Story so Far.* Leicester: National Health Service, NHS Improvement; 2007.

110. **Andersen BL.** Psychological interventions for cancer patients to enhance the quality of life. *J Consult Clin Psychol.* 1992;60(4): 552–568.

111. **Blake-Mortimer J, Gore-Felton C, Kimerling R, et al.** Improving the quality and quantity of life among patients with cancer: A review of the effectiveness of group psychotherapy. *Eur J Cancer.* 1999; 35(11):1581–1586.

112. **Fawzy FI.** Psychosocial interventions for patients with cancer: What works and what doesn't. *Eur J Cancer.* 1999;35(11): 1559–1564.

113. **Manne SL, Rubin S, Edelson M, et al.** Coping and communication-enhancing intervention versus supportive counseling for women diagnosed with gynecological cancers. *J Consult Clin Psychol.* 2007; 75(4):615–628.

114. **Petersen RW, Quinlivan JA.** Preventing anxiety and depression in gynaecological cancer: A randomised controlled trial. *BJOG.* 2002; 109(4):386–394.

115. **Rost AD, Wilson KG, Buchanan E, et al.** Improving psychological adjustment among late-stage ovarian cancer patients: Examining the role of avoidance in treatment. *Cogn Behav Pract.* 2012;19(4): 508–517.

116. **Scott JL, Halford WK, Ward BG.** United we stand? The effects of a couple-coping intervention on adjustment to early stage breast or gynecological cancer. *J Consult Clin Psychol.* 2004;72(6):1122–1135.

117. **Brothers BM, Yang HC, Strunk DR, et al.** Cancer patients with major depressive disorder: Testing a Biobehavioral/Cognitive Behavioral intervention. *J Consult Clin Psychol.* 2011;79(2):253–260.

118. **Pistrang N, Jay Z, Gessler S, et al.** Telephone peer support for women with gynaecological cancer: Recipients' perspectives. *Psychooncology.* 2012;21(10):1082–1090.

119. **McHugh RK, Whitton SW, Peckham AD, et al.** Patient preference for psychological vs pharmacologic treatment of psychiatric disorders: A meta-analytic review. *J Clin Psychiatry.* 2013;74(6): 595–602.

120. **Herschell AD, Kolko DJ, Baumann BL, et al.** The role of therapist training in the implementation of psychosocial treatments: A review and critique with recommendations. *Clin Psychol Rev.* 2010;30(4): 448–466.

121. **Marangell LB.** Augmentation of standard depression therapy. *Clin Ther.* 2000;22(suppl A):A25–A38; discussion A39–A41.

122. **Rapaport MH, Gharabawi GM, Canuso CM, et al.** Effects of risperidone augmentation in patients with treatment-resistant depression: Results of open-label treatment followed by double-blind continuation. *Neuropsychopharmacology* 2006;31(11):2505–2513.

123. **Delgado PL, Zarkowski P.** Treatment of mood disorders. In: Panksepp J, ed. *Textbook of Biological Psychiatry.* Hoboken, NJ: Wiley-Liss; 2004:231–266.

124. **Butler AC, Chapman JE, Forman EM, et al.** The empirical status of cognitive-behavioral therapy: A review of meta-analyses. *Clin Psychol Rev.* 2006;26(1):17–31.

125. **Hollon SD, Stewart MO, Strunk D.** Enduring effects for cognitive behavior therapy in the treatment of depression and anxiety. *Annu Rev Psychol.* 2006;57:285–315.

126. **Strunk DR, DeRubeis RJ.** Cognitive therapy for depression: A review of its efficacy. *J Cogn Psychother.* 2001;15(4):289–297.

127. **Williams S, Dale J.** The effectiveness of treatment for depression/depressive symptoms in adults with cancer: A systematic review. *Br J Cancer.* 2006;94(3):372–390.

128. **Redd WH, Montgomery GH, DuHamel KN.** Behavioral intervention for cancer treatment side effects. *J Natl Cancer Inst.* 2001; 93(11):810–823.

129. **Bodurka DC, Sun CC.** Sexual function after gynecologic cancer. *Obstet Gynecol Clin North Am.* 2006;33(4):621–30, ix.

130. **Stead ML, Fallowfield L, Selby P, et al.** Psychosexual function and impact of gynaecological cancer. *Best Pract Res Clin Obstet Gynaecol.* 2007;21(2):309–320.

131. **Abbott-Anderson K, Kwekkeboom KL.** A systematic review of sexual concerns reported by gynecological cancer survivors. *Gynecol Oncol.* 2012;124(3):477–489.

132. **Gilbert E, Ussher JM, Perz J.** Sexuality after gynaecological cancer: A review of the material, intrapsychic, and discursive aspects of treatment on women's sexual-wellbeing. *Maturitas.* 2011;70(1): 42–57.

133. **Brotto LA, Heiman JR.** Mindfulness in sex therapy: Applications for women with sexual difficulties following gynecologic cancer. *Sex Relation Ther.* 2007;22(1):3–11.

134. **Andersen BL, Lachenbruch PA, Anderson B, et al.** Sexual dysfunction and signs of gynecologic cancer. *Cancer.* 1986;57(9): 1880–1186.

135. **Stead ML.** Sexual dysfunction after treatment for gynaecologic and breast malignancies. *Curr Opin Obstet Gynecol.* 2003;15(1):57–61.

136. **Andersen BL, Broffitt B.** Is there a reliable and valid self-report measure of sexual behavior? *Arch Sex Behav.* 1988;17(6):509–525.

137. **Wright EP, Kiely MA, Lynch P, et al.** Social problems in oncology. *Br J Cancer.* 2002;87(10):1099–1104.

138. **Carpenter KM, Andersen BL, Fowler JM, et al.** Sexual self schema as a moderator of sexual and psychological outcomes for gynecologic cancer survivors. *Arch Sex Behav.* 2009;38(5):828–841.

139. **Laumann EO, Gagnon JH, Michael RT, et al.** *The Social Organization of Sexuality: Sexual Practices in the United States.* Chicago, IL: University of Chicago Press; 1994.

140. **Derogatis LR, Melisaratos N.** The DSFI: A multidimensional measure of sexual functioning. *J Sex Marital Ther.* 1979;5(3):244–281.

141. **Bachmann GA, Leiblum SR, Kemmann E, et al.** Sexual expression and its determinants in the post-menopausal woman. *Maturitas.* 1984;6(1):19–29.

142. **Masters WH, Johnson VE.** *Human Sexual Response.* New York: Bantam Books; 1966.

143. **Andersen BL.** Predicting sexual and psychologic morbidity and improving the quality of life for women with gynecologic cancer. *Cancer.* 1993;71(4 suppl):1678–1690.

144. **Gamel C, Hengeveld M, Davis B.** Informational needs about the effects of gynaecological cancer on sexuality: A review of the literature. *J Clin Nurs.* 2000;9(5):678–688.

145. **Berek JS, Andersen BL.** In: **Hoskins WJ, Perez CA, Young RC, eds.** *Sexual Rehabilitation: Surgical and Psychological Approaches, in Gynecologic Oncology: Principles and Practice.* Philadelphia, PA: JB Lippincott; 1992:401–416.

146. **Denton AS, Maher EJ.** Interventions for the physical aspects of sexual dysfunction in women following pelvic radiotherapy. *Cochrane Database Syst Rev.* 2003;(1):CD003750.

147. **Miles T, Johnson N.** Vaginal dilator therapy for women receiving pelvic radiotherapy. *Cochrane Database Syst Rev.* 2010;(9): CD007291.

148. **Caldwell R, Classen C, Lagana L, et al.** Changes in sexual functioning and mood among women treated for gynecological cancer who receive group therapy: A pilot study. *J Clin Psychol Med Settings.* 2003;10(3):149–156.

149. **Witkin M.** Helping husbands adjust to their wives' mastectomies. *Med Aspects Hum Sex.* 1978;12:93–94.

150. **Capone MA, Good RS, Westie KS, et al.** Psychosocial rehabilitation of gynecologic oncology patients. *Arch Phys Med Rehabil.* 1980;61(3):128–132.

151. **Christensen DN.** Postmastectomy couple counseling: An outcome study of a structured treatment protocol. *J Sex Marital Ther.* 1983; 9(4):266–275.

152. **Brotto LA, Heiman JR, Goff B, et al.** A psychoeducational intervention for sexual dysfunction in women with gynecologic cancer. *Arch Sex Behav.* 2008;37(2):317–329.

153. **Brotto LA, Erskine Y, Carey M, et al.** A brief mindfulness-based cognitive behavioral intervention improves sexual functioning versus wait-list control in women treated for gynecologic cancer. *Gynecol Oncol.* 2012;125(2):320–325.

154. **Scott JL, Kayser K.** A review of couple-based interventions for enhancing women's sexual adjustment and body image after cancer. *Cancer J.* 2009;15(1):48–56.

Index

Note: Page numbers followed by *f* and *t* indicate figures and tables respectively.

laparoscopic, in cervical cancer, 830
lymphedema with, 352
modified, in cervical cancer, 341
postextirpation, 347
recurrence, 375–376
sexual dysfunction, 351
stage IB2 cancer, 352–357, 353*f*, 355*f*
**Radiation Therapy Oncology Group
(RTOG),** 363
Radioresistance, in hypoxic cells, 92
Randomized controlled trials (RCT),
ovarian cancer, 443
Rapamycin, 45
ras family of G proteins, 11
cervical cancer, 31
endometrial cancer, 23
ras proteins, 11
Receptor tyrosine kinases receptors, 9
**RECIST (Response Evaluation Criteria in
Solid Tumors) criteria,** combination
chemotherapy, 69–70
Reconstructive operations
grafts, 812–813
pelvic floor, 819–820
vaginal, 813–816
vulvar and perineal, 817–819
Rectovaginal fistula, 365
Rectum, radiation therapy, 96
Recurrent cancer
breast cancer, 135, 136*f*
cervical cancer, 375–380
radiation therapy, 114
endometrial, 421–425
hormonal therapy, 422–423
isolated vaginal recurrence, 421–422
prognosis, 425, 425*t*
systematic recurrence, 422
of ovary
chemotherapy for, 509–517
hormonal therapy for, 514
Redistribution, radiation therapy, 91
Regulatory T (Treg) cells, 47
Reid Colposcopic Index, 275, 276*t*
Reinke crystals, 201
Relative biological effectiveness, radiation
therapy, 92–93
Relative risk (RR), 225
Relative survival, 224
Remission, combination chemotherapy and,
68–69, 69*t*
Renal disease, grade 3 surgery with, 728*t*
Renal insufficiency, fluids, and electrolytes,
744
acid–base disorders, 738–741
acute kidney injury, 735–738, 736*t*
hypercalcemia, 744
hyperkalemia, 742–744
hypernatremia, 741–742
hypokalemia, 742–744
hyponatremia, 741–742, 743*f*
maintenance fluids, 741
metabolic acidosis, 740*t*
serum creatinine, algorithm for
management of, 739*f*
urinary diagnostic indices, 737*t*
Renewing tissue growth, 60
Reoxygenation, radiation therapy, 91, 91*f*
Repair mechanisms, fractionated radiation,
88
Repopulation, radiation therapy, 90
Reproductive function, ovarian cancer risk
and, 24
Resection, upper abdominal cytoreduction,
802

Respiratory failure, 731–735
adult respiratory distress syndrome, 734
algorithm for management of, 732*f*
chronic, 734
hypoxic, 733
mechanical ventilation, 734–735
ventilatory failure, 733–734
Retinoblastoma, 7*t*, 13
Retinoblastoma gene, 13, 14*f*
human papilloma virus, 259
Retrograde pyelography, 806
Retrospective cohort study, 226
Revised Cardiac Risk Index, 706, 706*t*
Rhabdomyosarcoma, 600–601
cervical mesenchyma tumors, 145
embryonal, vagina, 146, 149*f*
Rhomboid flap, 817, 820
Rhomboid pedicle graft, 817
Risk of malignancy index (RMI), 450, 475
Risk of Ovarian Cancer (ROC), 443, 447
**Risk of Ovarian Malignancy Algorithm
(ROMA),** 447–448
Rituximab, 51
Robotic surgery, 847–865
adoption of, 848*f*
complications, 862–863, 862*t*
docking techniques, 853–855, 855*f*
gynecologic oncology, applications in,
855–860
cervical cancer, 858–860, 859*t*
endometrial cancer, 856*t*, 857–858,
857*t*
ovarian cancer, 860
instrumentation, 853–855, 853*f*
MIS technology, 848–852
overview, 847–848
patient positioning, 853–855
pelvic exenteration, 860
robotic system, 849–852
components, 850–852
computer interface, 849*f*, 851
operating room with, 850*f*
patient-side cart, 850–851, 850*f*
Surgeon Console, 851–852, 851*f*–852*f*
sentinel lymph nodes, 861, 861*t*
trocar placement sites for, 854*f*
utilization, 863–865
cost-effectivene, 863, 864*t*
technological advances, 865
training and education, 863–865
Rome pouch, 812
Roticulator 55, 797
Rucaparib, 40*t*

S
Salpingo-oophorectomy, 472
hereditary nonpolyposis colon cancer
syndrome and, 22
Sanctuary sites, chemotherapy
pharmacology, 67
Sarcoma botryoides, 372
vagina, 146, 149*f*
Sarcomas, 551
cervical cancer, 371–372
uterine sarcomas, 425–434
chemotherapy, 428
classification, 425–426
radiation therapy, 428
smooth muscle tumors, 426–427
staging, 427–429
surgical treatment, 427–428
of vulva, 600–601
dermatofibrosarcoma protuberans, 601
leiomyosarcoma, 600

malignant schwannoma, 601
proximal-type epithelioid, 600
rhabdomyosarcoma, 600–601
synovial cell sarcoma, 601
Scalene triangle, 780–781
Schauta–Stoeckel technique, 830
Schiller's test, cervical colposcopy, 274
Screening procedures
automated screening, 137
cancer prevention, 235*t*, 236
cervical intraepithelial neoplasia,
265–268
for cervical cancer, 443
ovarian cancer, 233–234, 443–444, 468–469
Secondary cytoreduction, 509
Secondary malignancies
chemotherapy and, 75
Secondary skin closure, 789
Secondary therapy, ovarian cancer
chemotherapy, 509–517
intestinal obstruction, 517
secondary cytoreduction, 509
Second-look operation, 509
SEER. *See* **Surveillance Epidemiology and
End Results program (SEER)**
SEER database, 464
cervical cancer diagnosis and staging,
340
Selection bias, 228
Selumetinib, 44
Semipermanent lines, surgical technique,
782–785, 783*f*
Senescence, cellular, 5–6
Sentinel lymph nodes, 835, 836*t*, 861, 861*f*
Sentinel node biopsy (SNB), in endometrial
cancer, 409–410
Serous borderline tumors, of ovary,
183–185, 184*f*
extraovarian disease, 185
lymph node involvement in, 187*f*
with micropapillary pattern, 183, 184*f*
noninvasive implant of, 185*f*
stromal microinvasion in, 183–185, 185*f*
Serous carcinoma
cervical cancer, 371
endometrium, 164–166, 165*f*
**Serous tubal intraepithelial carcinoma
(STIC) lesions,** 445
Serous tumors, of ovary, 183–188
benign, 183
high grade, 188, 188*f*
low grade, 185–188, 187*f*
serous psammocarcinoma, 186–188
Sertoli–Leydig tumors, 550*f*
prognosis, 551
treatment, 550–551
Serum biomarkers, 359
Groningen multicenter observational
study, 359
Sex-cord-stromal tumors
classification of, 547*t*
granulosa–stromal-cell tumors,
546–550
of ovary, 196–201
adult granulosa cell tumor, 197, 197*f*
with annular tubules, 199, 200*f*
fibroma–thecoma, 199–201
gynandroblastoma, 199
juvenile granulosa cell tumor, 198, 198*f*
Leydig cell tumors, 201
sclerosing stromal cell tumors, 201
Sertoli–Leydig cell tumors, 198–199,
199*f*
steroid cell tumors, 201

CCS1014